PEDIATRIC PARAMETERS AND EQUIPMENT

	Premie	Newborn	6 mo	1 yr	2-3 yr	4-6 yr	7-10 yr	11-15 yr	>16 yr
WT (kg)	1-3	2-4	6-8						>50
BAG VALVE MASK	Infant	Infant	Small chi						Adult
NASAL AIRWAY (Fr)	12	12	14-16						22-36
ORAL AIRWAY	Infant 50 mm	Small 60 mm	Small 60 m						Med 90 mm
BLADE	MIL 0	MIL 0	MIL 1						MIL 2, MAC 3
ETT	2.5-3.0	3.0-3.5	3.5					6.0-6.5	7.0-8.0
LMA	1	1	1.5	2	2	2.5	2.5-3	3	4
GLIDESCOPE	1	1 or 2	2	2	3	3	3	3 or 4	3 or 4
IV CATH (ga)	22-24	22-24	20-24	20-24	18-22	18-22	18-22	18-20	18-20
CVL (Fr)	3	3-4	4	4-5	4-5	5	5	7	7
NGT/OGT (Fr)	5	5-8	8	10	10-12	12-14	12-14	14-18	14-18
CHEST TUBE (Fr)	10-12	10-12	12-18	16-20	16-24	20-28	20-32	28-38	28-42
FOLEY (Fr)	6	8	8	8	8	8	8	10	12

ESTIMATED BLOOD PRESSURE BY AGE

Measurement	50th %	5th %
Systolic BP [Diastolic BP is usually 2/3 systolic BP]	90 + (age × 2)	60 (neonate); 70 (1 mo-1 yr) 70 + (age × 2) (for 2-10 yr) 90 (>10 yr)
MAP	55 + (age × 1.5)	40 + (age × 1.5)

NORMAL VITAL SIGNS BY AGE

Age	Heart Rate (beats/min)	Blood Pressure (mmHg)	Respiratory Rate (breaths/min)
Premie	120-170	55-75/35-45 (gestational age approximates normal MAP)	40-70
0-3 mo	100-150	65-85/45-55	35-55
3-6 mo	90-120	70-90/50-65	30-45
6-12 mo	80-120	80-100/55-65	25-40
1-3 yr	70-110	90-105/55-70	20-30
3-6 yr	65-110	95-110/60-75	20-25
6-12 yr	60-95	100-120/60-75	14-22
>12 yr	55-85	110-135/65-85	12-18

ENDOTRACHEAL TUBE FORMULAS

Uncuffed ETT size: age (years)/4 + 4; Cuffed ETT size: age (years)/4 + 3
ETT depth (from lip to mid-trachea): ETT internal diameter (size) × 3

GLASGOW COMA SCALE

Activity	Score	Child/Adult	Score	Infant
Eye opening	4	Spontaneous	4	Spontaneous
	3	To speech	3	To speech/sound
	2	To pain	2	To painful stimuli
	1	None	1	None
Verbal	5	Oriented	5	Coos/babbles
	4	Confused	4	Irritable cry
	3	Inappropriate	3	Cries to pain
	2	Incomprehensible	2	Moans to pain
	1	None	1	None
Motor	6	Obeys commands	6	Normal spontaneous movement
	5	Localizes to pain	5	Withdraws to touch
	4	Withdraws to pain	4	Withdraws to pain
	3	Abnormal flexion	3	Abnormal flexion (decorticate)
	2	Abnormal extension	2	Abnormal extension (decerebrate)
	1	None (flaccid)	1	None (flaccid)

Adapted from Hunt EA, Nelson-McMillan K, Levin A, O'Brien C, McNamara L, Hutchins L. The Johns Hopkins Children's Center Kids Kard, 2021.

RESUSCITATION MEDICATIONS

Adenosine Supraventricular tachycardia	**0.1 mg/kg IV/IO RAPID BOLUS (over 1-2 sec), Flush with 10 mL normal saline** May repeat at 0.2 mg/kg IV/IO, then 0.3 mg/kg IV/IO after 2 min Max first dose 6 mg, max subsequent dose 12 mg Administer using a 3-way stopcock attached to a 10 mL NS flush Prolonged asystole may occur following administration
Amiodarone Ventricular tachycardia Ventricular fibrillation	**5 mg/kg IV/IO** No Pulse: Push Undiluted Pulse: Dilute and give over 20-60 minutes Max first dose 300 mg, max subsequent dose 150 mg Max total dose 15 mg/kg/24 hours OR 2200 mg/24 hours Strongly consider pretreating with IV calcium in patients with a pulse to prevent hypotension. Monitor for hypotension after administration
Atropine Bradycardia (increased vagal tone) Primary AV block	**0.02 mg/kg IV/IO/IM, 0.04–0.06 mg/kg ETT** Max single dose 0.5 mg Repeat once in 5 minutes if needed to max total dose 1 mg. Max total dose 3 mg used in adults. 1 mg/mL concentration recommended for IM or ETT use
Calcium chloride (10% elemental calcium) Hypocalcemia Hyperkalemia Hypermagnesemia Calcium channel blocker overdose	**20 mg/kg IV/IO** Max dose 1 gram May administer peripherally during an arrest
Calcium gluconate (10% elemental calcium) Hypocalcemia Hyperkalemia Hypermagnesemia Calcium channel blocker overdose	**60 mg/kg IV/IO** Max dose 3 grams
Dextrose Hypoglycemia	**Weight-Based Dosing: 0.5–1 gram/kg** **Volume-Based Dosing ("Rule of 50"):** **<5 kg: 10% dextrose 5-10 mL/kg IV/IO** **5-44 kg: 25% dextrose 2-4 mL/kg IV/IO** **≥45 kg: 50% dextrose 1-2 mL/kg IV/IO** **Max single dose 25 grams = 50 mL**
Epinephrine Pulseless arrest Bradycardia (symptomatic) Anaphylaxis	**0.01 mg/kg IV/IO (0.1 mg/mL) every 3–5 min (max single dose 1 mg)** **0.1 mg/kg ETT (1 mg/mL) every 3–5 min (max single dose 2.5 mg)** **Anaphylaxis:** **0.01 mg/kg IM (1 mg/mL) in thigh every 5-15 min PRN; max single dose 0.5 mg** **Standardized/Autoinjector:** **<7.5 kg: no autoinjector, see above** **7.5 to <15 kg: 0.1 mg IM** **15 to <30 kg: 0.15 mg IM** **≥30 kg: 0.3 mg IM**
Hydrocortisone Adrenal Crisis/Insufficiency	**2 mg/kg IV/IM/IO** Max dose 100 mg
Insulin (Regular or Aspart) Hyperkalemia	**0.1 units/kg IV/IO with 0.5 gram/kg of dextrose** Max dose 5 units Doses less than 5 units require dilution. Consider using a 1 unit/mL dilution.
Lidocaine Antiarrhythmic	**1 mg/kg IV/IO, 2-3 mg/kg ETT** Max single dose 100 mg May repeat every 5 min to max total dose 3 mg/kg
Magnesium sulfate Torsades de pointes Hypomagnesemia	**50 mg/kg IV/IO** No Pulse: Dilution recommended; infusion rate dependent on indication Pulse: Dilute and give over 20-60 minutes Max single dose 2 grams Monitor for hypotension/bradycardia

Naloxone Opioid overdose Coma	**Respiratory Depression: 0.001-0.005 mg/kg/dose IV/IO/IM/SUBQ (max 0.1 mg first dose, may titrate to effect)** **Full Reversal/Arrest Dose: 0.1 mg/kg IV/IO/IM/SUBQ (max dose 2 mg)** ETT dose 2–3 times IV dose, IN dose up to 8 mg. May give every 2 min PRN
Sodium Bicarbonate **(8.4% = 1 mEq/mL)** Administer only with clear indication: Metabolic acidosis Hyperkalemia Tricyclic antidepressant overdose	**1 mEq/kg IV/IO** ≥10kg: Administer undiluted 1 mEq/mL product <10kg: Dilute 8.4% sodium bicarbonate 1:1 with sterile water to a final concentration of 4.2% = 0.5 mEq/mL Hyperkalemia: Max single dose 50 mEq

ETT Meds (NAVEL: naloxone, atropine, vasopressin, epinephrine, lidocaine)—dilute meds to 5 mL with NS, follow with positive-pressure ventilation.

Adapted from Hunt EA, Nelson-McMillan K, Levin A, O'Brien C, McNamara L, Hutchins L. The Johns Hopkins Children's Center Kids Kard, 2021; and the American Heart Association. PALS Pocket Card, 2020.

IV Infusions*

Medication	Dose (mCg/kg/min)	Dilution in 100 mL in a Compatible IV Fluid	IV Infusion Rate
Alprostadil (prostaglandin E₁)	0.05–0.1	0.3 mg/kg	1 mL/hr = 0.05 mCg/kg/min
Amiodarone	5–15	6 mg/kg	1 mL/hr = 1 mCg/kg/min
DOBUTamine	2–20	6 mg/kg	1 mL/hr = 1 mCg/kg/min
DOPamine	5–20	6 mg/kg	1 mL/hr = 1 mCg/kg/min
EPINEPHrine	0.05-2	0.6 mg/kg	1 mL/hr = 0.1 mCg/kg/min
Lidocaine, post resuscitation	20–50	6 mg/kg	1 mL/hr = 1 mCg/kg/min
Phenylephrine	0.1–2, up to 5 in severe circumstances	0.3 mg/kg	1 mL/hr = 0.05 mCg/kg/min
Terbutaline	0.1–4 (up to 10 has been used)	0.6 mg/kg	1 mL/hr = 0.1 mCg/kg/min
Vasopressin (pressor)	0.17–8 milliunits/kg/min	6 units/kg	1 mL/hr = 1 milliunit/kg/min

*Standardized concentrations and use of smart infusion pumps are recommended when available. For additional information, see Larsen GY, Park HB et. al. Standard drug concentrations and smart-pump technology reduce continuous-medication-infusion errors in pediatric patients. *Pediatrics.* 2005;116(1):e21-e25.

Special thanks to LeAnn McNamara, PharmD for her expert guidance with IV infusion and resuscitation medication guidelines.

A MANUAL FOR PEDIATRIC HOUSE OFFICERS

TWENTY-THIRD
EDITION

THE
HARRIET
LANE
HANDBOOK

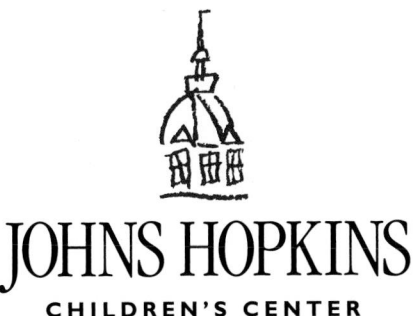

JOHNS HOPKINS
CHILDREN'S CENTER

A MANUAL FOR PEDIATRIC HOUSE OFFICERS

TWENTY-THIRD
EDITION

THE
HARRIET
LANE
HANDBOOK

THE HARRIET LANE HOUSE STAFF AT
THE CHARLOTTE R. BLOOMBERG CHILDREN'S CENTER OF
THE JOHNS HOPKINS HOSPITAL

EDITORS
CAMILLE C. ANDERSON, MD
SUNAINA KAPOOR, MD, MPH
TIFFANY E. MARK, MD

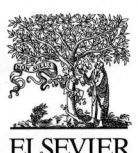

ELSEVIER

Elsevier
1600 John F. Kennedy Blvd.
Ste 1800
Philadelphia, PA 19103-2899

THE HARRIET LANE HANDBOOK,
TWENTY-THIRD EDITION ISBN: 978-0-323-87698-8
INTERNATIONAL EDITION ISBN: 978-0-323-87880-7
Copyright © 2024 by Elsevier Inc. All rights reserved.

Notice

Previous editions copyrighted 2021, 2018, 2015, 2012, 2009, 2005, 2002, 2000,
1996, 1993, 1991, 1987, 1984, 1981, 1978, 1975, 1972, and 1969.

Senior Content Strategist: Marybeth Thiel
Senior Content Development Manager: Meghan Andress
Publishing Services Manager: Julie Eddy
Senior Project Manager: Cindy Thoms
Design Direction: Patrick Ferguson

Printed in China

Last digit is the print number: 9 8 7 6 5 4 3 2

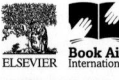

Working together
to grow libraries in
developing countries

www.elsevier.com • www.bookaid.org

To our families

Bill and Robin Anderson, thank you for encouraging me to dream big and pursue a life that brings me meaning and joy. You have helped me every step of the way and I love you more than I can say. Tess Anderson, you inspire me every day with your unending well of kindness and generosity – thank you for being a wonderful sister. Jordan Perry, you make all hard things seem possible; I couldn't have done this without you. To the friends who have supported me like family, thank you for being on this journey with me.

Atul and Nupur Kapoor, thank you for the endless sacrifices, constant support, and unconditional love that allowed me to live out my dreams – I owe it all to you. Anirudh Arun, thank you for being the most caring and supportive husband – I cherish our journey of becoming physicians, life partners, and parents together. Ankit Kapoor, thank you for always challenging me to be the best sister, daughter, and doctor I can be. Sheela Kapoor, thank you for being my biggest cheerleader, my fund of virtue, and my rock – I miss you dearly. Mowgli and Meeko, you bring us endless joy. And finally, to my son Ishaan, this is all for you – you are the bright star in our future.

Charlie and Elizabeth Mark, thank you for being my greatest source of encouragement in pursuing my dreams of becoming a medical doctor. I would not be where I am today without your unwavering support all these years. To my brother, Patrick Mark, thank you for being the greatest and most caring older brother, always showing me the importance of family and love. To my extended family and friends, thank you for all the encouragement, kind words, laughter, and joy throughout my life – you all have made this journey possible.

To our patients and their families

Thank you for teaching us and for trusting in us. You have made us pediatricians.

To our residents

Your tireless advocacy and care for our patients inspires us constantly. Thank you for all of the sacrifices you have made.

To the wonderful pediatricians who trained us, especially
Nicole Shilkofski

To the Children's Center leaders we have learned from
Margaret Moon, Tina Cheng, and George Dover

To the frontline providers of the COVID-19 pandemic
Thank you for your bravery in a time of uncertainty.

Preface

"Why this child? Why this disease? Why now?"

—**Barton Childs, MD**

The Harriet Lane Handbook was first developed in 1953 after Harrison Spencer (chief resident in 1950–1951) suggested that residents should write a pocket-sized "pearl book." As recounted by Henry Seidel, the first editor of *The Harriet Lane Handbook,* "Six of us began without funds and without [the] supervision of our elders, meeting sporadically around a table in the library of the Harriet Lane Home." The product of their efforts was a concise yet comprehensive handbook that became an indispensable tool for the residents of the Harriet Lane Home. Ultimately, Robert Cooke (department chief, 1956–1974) realized the potential of the Handbook and the fifth edition was published for widespread distribution by Year Book. Since that time, the handbook has been regularly updated and rigorously revised to reflect the most up-to-date information and available clinical guidelines. It has grown from a humble Hopkins resident "pearl book" to become a nationally and internationally respected clinical resource. Now translated into many languages, the handbook is still intended as an easy-to-use manual to help pediatricians provide current and comprehensive pediatric care.

Today, *The Harriet Lane Handbook* continues to be updated and revised *by* house officers *for* house officers. Recognizing the limit to what can be included in a pocket guide, additional information has been placed online and for use via mobile applications. The online-only content includes references, expanded text, and additional tables, figures, and images.

In addition to including the most up-to-date guidelines, practice parameters, and references, we will highlight some of the most important improvements in the twenty-third edition of *The Harriet Lane Handbook:*

The **Traumatic Injuries** chapter now contains a detailed description of considerations for the primary survey, as well as emergent labs.

The **Neurology** chapter has been reorganized into emergent and chronic or progressive diagnoses and includes a new section on functional neurologic disorders.

The **Analgesia and Procedural Sedation** chapter has a new section detailing the evaluation of pain in children with significant neurological impairment.

The **Infectious Disease** chapter now includes a summary of parasitic and fungal infections.

The **Cardiology and Rheumatology** chapters now include information on diagnosis and management of multisystem inflammatory syndrome in children (MIS-C).

The **Biostatistics** chapter has been restructured to reflect principles of practicing evidence based medicine (EBM).

The **Development, Behavior, and Developmental Disability** chapter now includes information about adverse childhood experiences.

Also new to *The Harriet Lane Handbook* this year are supplemental Harriet Lane Audio Companion Case Files. These audio files adopt a case-based interview format with content experts in order to take a more conversational and discussion-based approach into important topics within pediatrics (see Audio P.1).

The Harriet Lane Handbook, designed for pediatric house staff, was made possible by the extraordinary efforts of this year's Johns Hopkins Harriet Lane Pediatric Residency Program senior resident class. It has been an honor to watch these fine doctors mature and refine their skills since internship. They have balanced their busy work schedules and personal lives while authoring the chapters that follow. We are grateful to each of them, along with their faculty advisors, who selflessly dedicated their time to improve the quality and content of this publication. The high quality of this handbook is representative of our residents, who are the heart and soul of our department.

	Chapter	Author	Faculty Advisor
1	Emergency and Critical Care Management	Tai Kyung S. Hairston, MD LeAnn McNamara, PharmD	Justin M. Jeffers, MD, MEHP Nicole Shilkofski, MD, MEd
2	Traumatic Injuries	Radhika Ghodasara, MD	Jennifer F. Anders, MD Paul D. Sponseller, MD, MBA
3	Toxicology	Sophie Crinion, MD	Elizabeth Hines, MD
4	Procedures	Maite E. Del Valle Rolón, MD	Thuy Ngo, DO, MEd
5	Adolescent Medicine	Amitte Rosenfeld, MD Yasamin Ege Sanii, MD	Rachel H. Alinsky, MD, MPH Renata Arrington Sanders, MD, MPH, ScM
6	Analgesia and Procedural Sedation	Alexander Jaksic, MD Divya Madhusudhan, MD	Rajeev Wadia, MD
7	Cardiology	Alexander Tang, MD James Ting, MD	Caridad M. de la Uz, MD William Ravekes, MD W. Reid Thompson III, MD
8	Dermatology	Katherine Cummings, MD Allison Haley, MD	Bernard Cohen, MD
9	Development, Behavior, and Developmental Disability	Brenna M. Beck, MD, MEd Christle Nwora, MD	Harolyn Belcher, MD
10	Endocrinology	Rashmi Pashankar, MD	Kristin Arcara, MD
11	Fluids and Electrolytes	Joniqua Ceasar, MD	Leonard S. Feldman, MD
12	Gastroenterology	Elshaddai Ephrem, MD	Darla Shores, MD, PhD
13	Genetics: Metabolism and Conditions with Distinctive Appearance	Jacqueline Wood, MD, MA	Joann Bodurtha, MD, MPH Ada Hamosh, MD, MPH
14	Hematology	Joan Park, MD	James F. Casella, MD Courtney Elizabeth Lawrence, MD, MS Emily S. Rao, MD, MA, MS
15	Immunology and Allergy	Samantha Leong, MD, PhD	Robert Wood, MD
16	Immunoprophylaxis	Lindsay Sheets, MD, MPH	Pranita D. Tamma, MD, MHS
17	Microbiology and Infectious Disease	Amali Gunawardana, MD Ashley Wallace Wu, MD	Alice Jenh Hsu, PharmD Sanjay K. Jain, MD John McAteer, DO, MPH Nadine Peart, MD Erica Prochaska, MD
18	Neonatology	Elizabeth Lee, MD	Maureen M. Gilmore, MD

19	Nephrology	Ryan Handoko, MD	Jeffrey Fadrowski, MD, MHS Cozumel Pruette, MD, MHS, MS
20	Neurology	Hannah E. Edelman MD, PhD Maera J. Stratton, MD	Matthew J. Elrick, MD, PhD Eric H. Kossoff, MD Christopher Oakley, MD Lisa R Sun, MD
21	Nutrition and Growth	Audrey Companiony Hopkins, MD	Darla Shores, MD, PhD Jennifer Thompson, MS, RD, CSP, LDN
22	Oncology	Lawrence Gersz MD, MBA Rebecca Xi, MD	Nicole Arwood, PharmD Stacy Cooper, MD
23	Palliative Care	Sapna Desai, MD	Melanie L. Brown, MD, MSE Matt Norvell, MDiv, BCC
24	Psychiatry	Jelina Marie V. Castillo, MD, MPH	Nadia Zaim, MD
25	Pulmonology and Sleep Medicine	Saskia Groenewald, MD	Laura M. Sterni, MD
26	Radiology	Urveel Mukesh Shah, MD	Emily A. Dunn, MD
27	Rheumatology	Emma Vaimberg, MD	Ekemini Akan Ogbu, MD, MSc
28	Blood Chemistry and Body Fluids	Camille C. Anderson, MD	Nadia Ayala-Lopez, PhD Lori Sokoll, PhD
29	Biostatistics and Evidence-Based Medicine	Michael R. Rose, MD, MPH	Leonard S. Feldman, MD
30	Drug Dosages	Carlton K.K. Lee, PharmD, MPH	
31	Drugs in Kidney Failure	Elizabeth A.S. Goswami, PharmD Katherine Hapgood, PharmD	Carlton K.K. Lee, PharmD, MPH

HARRIET LANE AUDIO COMPANION CASE FILE AUTHORS

Audio Case File	Associated Chapter	Author(s)	Content Expert
P.1 Introduction to Audio Case Files		Camille C. Anderson, MD, Sunaina Kapoor, MD, MPH, and Tiffany E. Mark, MD	
1.1 Advocacy, gun violence, and healthcare utilization	Emergency and Critical Care Management	Rachel Darko, MD	Katherine E. Hoops, MD, MPH
3.1 Pediatric ingestions, workup, and management	Toxicology	Zainab Khan, MD	Roselyn Appenteng, MD
5.1 An interactive walk through the HEADSS assessment, and next steps	Adolescent Medicine	Andrea Silvas, MD	Errol Fields, MD, PhD, MPH
6.1 Medications for analgesia and sedation	Analgesia and Procedural Sedation	Matthew Kosasih, MD	Sapna Kudchadkar, MD, PhD
7.1 Auscultation and heart sounds	Cardiology	Kyla Cordrey, MD Rebecca Dryer, MD	W. Reid Thompson III, MD
7.2 Tetralogy of Fallot: Review of the congenital heart disease and accompanying cardiac surgeries	Cardiology	Fred Lam, MD	W. Reid Thompson III, MD
12.1 A framework for gastrointestinal bleeding by age	Gastroenterology	Kaysha Henry, MD, MPH	Steven Miller, MD
13.1 Newborn screening	Genetics: Metabolism and Conditions With Distinctive Appearance	Nadav Weinstock, MD, PhD	Shira G. Ziegler, MD, PhD

14.1 Hemophilia & Emicizumab	Hematology	Anna Bitners, MD	Courtney Lawrence, MD
17.1 Resistance mechanisms in Gramnegative rods	Microbiology and Infectious Disease	Ashley Wallace Wu, MD and Amali Gunawardana, MD	John McAteer, DO, MPH
18.1 Ventilation strategies in the neonatal ICU	Neonatology	Megan Gates, MD	Kartikeya Makker, MBBS
20.1 Seizure mimics: an age-based approach	Neurology	Maria Molinaro, MD Molly Himmelrich, MD Alexander Testino, MD	Eric H. Kossoff, MD
21.1 Pediatric food insecurity	Nutrition and Growth	Edward Corty, MD	Melissa Lutz, MD
22.1 Initial presentation and workup of acute lymphoblastic leukemia	Oncology	Katelyn Williams, MD Nathaniel J. Silvestri, MD	Michelle Hudspeth, MD
23.1 End of life decision making in the adolescent palliative care patient	Palliative Care	Juliet Joseph, MD	Emily Johnson, CRNP
27.1 A systematic approach to differentiating the various childhood arthritic conditions	Rheumatology	Tolulope Fatola, MD	Julia F. Shalen, MD
29.1 Evidence based medicine: A discussion on race-based clinical practice guidelines	Biostatistics and Evidence-Based Medicine	Rafi Faria, MD Cecilia Di Caprio, MD	Marquita Genies, MD, MPH

The Formulary is complete, concise, and up-to-date thanks to the tireless efforts of Carlton K.K. Lee, PharmD, MPH. With each edition, he carefully updates, revises, and improves the section. His herculean efforts make the Formulary one of the most useful and cited pediatric drug reference texts available.

We are grateful and humbled to have the opportunity to build on the great work of the preceding editors: Drs. Henry Seidel, Harrison Spencer, William Friedman, Robert Haslam, Jerry Winkelstein, Herbert Swick, Dennis Headings, Kenneth Schuberth, Basil Zitelli, Jeffery Biller, Andrew Yeager, Cynthia Cole, Peter Rowe, Mary Greene, Kevin Johnson, Michael Barone, George Siberry, Robert Iannone, Veronica Gunn, Christian Nechyba, Jason Robertson, Nicole Shilkofski, Jason Custer, Rachel Rau, Megan Tschudy, Kristin Arcara, Jamie Flerlage, Branden Engorn, Helen Hughes, Lauren Kahl, Keith Kleinman, Lauren McDaniel, and Matthew Molloy. Many of these previous editors continue to make important contributions to the education of the Harriet Lane house staff, none more than Dr. Nicole Shilkofski, our residency program director. Her dedication to the residents and to educating future pediatricians impresses us constantly. As recent editors, Drs. Keith Kleinman, Lauren McDaniel, and Matthew Molloy also have been instrumental in helping us to navigate this process. We are honored to follow in their footsteps.

An undertaking of this magnitude could not have been accomplished without the support and dedication of some extraordinary people. First, we would like to thank Dr. Nicole Shilkofski, our residency program director, and our associate residency program directors: Drs. Jeffrey Fadrowski, Marquita Genies, Cozumel Pruette, and Nakiya Showell. Thank you for entrusting us with the opportunity to serve as chief residents and *The Harriet Lane*

Handbook editors. We would also like to offer special thanks to our program coordinators: Kathy Mainhart and Yinka Omosule, invaluable assets to our program. We are so appreciative of your support and without you, we would be lost. And finally, thank you to our Department Director, Dr. Margaret Moon, for your tireless leadership of the Children's Center.

Residents	Interns
Saher Ali	Ricci Allen
Halei Benefield	Danielle Amundsen
Anna Bitners	Sarah Benett
Kyla Cordrey	Alec Berman
Edward Corty	David Berman
Rachel Darko	Rikiara Brown
Ian Drummond	
Rebecca Dryer	Carolei Bryan
Tolulope Fatola	Amber Bulna
Devki Gami	Cecilia Di Caprio
Megan Gates	Chizorbam Diribe
Ross Gilbert	Sarah Ehrenberg
Jillian Heckman	Rafi Faria
Laura Henderson	Whitney Fidelis
Kaysha Henry	Jeanette Freeman
Molly Himmelrich	Elena Georges
Zainab Khan	Rachel Gilbert
Andrew Kleist	Dana Goplerud
Matthew Kosasih	Adrienne Johnson
Jacqueline Kruglyakova	Juliet Joseph
Fred Lam	Adam Ketchum
Vianca Masucci	Andrew Koltun
Maria Molinaro	Chiara Pandolfi de Rinaldis
Teresa Oszkinis	Zaw Phyo
Roshni Patel	Megan Rescigno
Kristen Penberthy	
Mallika Rajamani	Claire Rhee
Maneesha Sakhuja	Harper Robinson
Nisha Shah	Sarika Sachdeva
Andrea Silvas	Raquel Sofia Sandoval
Nathaniel Silvestri	Vincent Shieh
William Squiers	Rohan Soman
Alexander Testino	Anthony Spellman
Nadav Weinstock	Melissa Trofa
Katelyn Williams	Sarah Vogel
	Priscilla Yong

Camille C. Anderson
Sunaina Kapoor
Tiffany E. Mark

Contents

PART I

PEDIATRIC ACUTE CARE

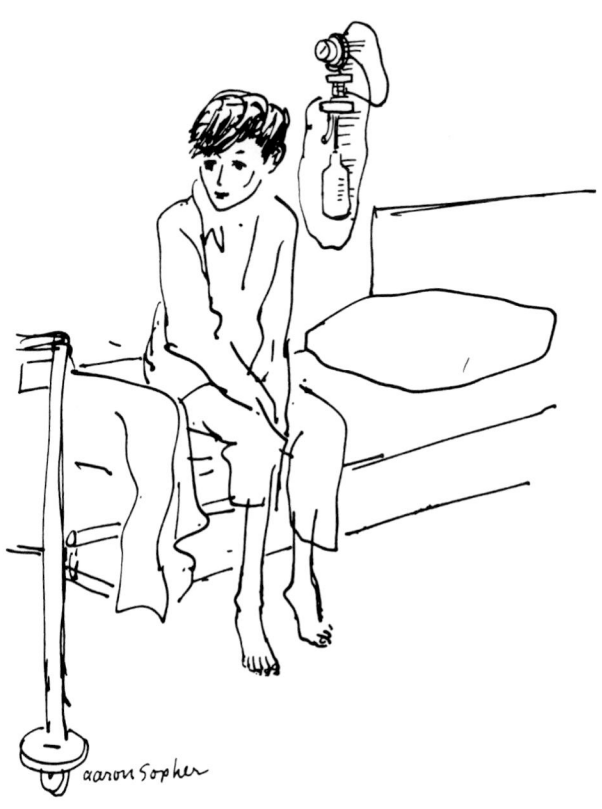

PART 1

PEDIATRIC ACUTE CARE

Chapter 1

Emergency and Critical Care Management

Tai Kyung Hairston, MD and LeAnn McNamara, PharmD

🜛 See additional content online.

🔊 **Audio Case File 1.1** Advocacy, gun violence, and healthcare utilization

This chapter is presented in accordance with the universal acronym **C-A-B** (compressions/circulation, airway, breathing) to emphasize the reduction of "no blood flow" time.[1-3] However, given the high prevalence of asphyxial cardiac arrest in the pediatric population, ventilation remains fundamental to the resuscitation of the critically ill child.[4] This chapter functions as a guide to caring for "sick" children, spanning the principles of resuscitation and stabilization, as well as management of the most common pediatric medical emergencies.

I. APPROACH TO THE UNRESPONSIVE CHILD

A. Circulation[1-3,5-11]

1. Assessment
   a. **Pulse:** Spend no more than **10 seconds** assessing pulse. Assess brachial pulse in infants, carotid or femoral pulse in children.
   b. **Perfusion:** Check for pallor, mottling, or cyanosis. Capillary refill time >2 seconds is delayed and <1 to 2 seconds or "flash" may indicate warm shock.
   c. **Rate:** Bradycardia **<60 beats/min** with **poor perfusion** requires immediate cardiopulmonary resuscitation (CPR). Tachycardia **>220 beats/min** suggests pathologic tachyarrhythmia.
   d. **Rhythm:** Attach patient to defibrillator or continuous electrocardiography. In arrest, check rhythm every 2 minutes with minimal interruptions in chest compressions (e.g., during compressor change).
   e. **Blood pressure (BP):** Hypotension in a pediatric patient is a **late** manifestation of circulatory compromise.
   f. **Urine output:** Normal output is 1.5 to 2 mL/kg/hr in infants and young children and 1 mL/kg/hr in older children.
2. Management: Initiate CPR immediately if patient is pulseless or bradycardic (<60 beats/min) with poor perfusion.
   a. **Chest compressions:** See Box 1.1 for an outline of the five components of **high-quality CPR.**

BOX 1.1

FIVE COMPONENTS OF HIGH-QUALITY CARDIOPULMONARY RESUSCITATION

- "Push fast": Target rate of **100–120 compressions/min.**
- "Push hard": Target depth of **at least $\frac{1}{3}$ anteroposterior diameter of chest.**
  - Place step stool at side of bed to assist compressor.
  - Slide backboard under patient or place on hard surface.
  - Use the compression technique that achieves the best results.
    - Consider two-handed, one-handed, two-finger, or two-thumb-encircling hands techniques.
  - Aim for 1 fingerbreadth below intermammary line in infants, 2 fingerbreadths in prepubertal children, and the lower half of the sternum in adolescents.
- Allow **full chest recoil** between compressions.
- **Minimize interruptions** in chest compressions.
  - Rotate compressor every 2 min or sooner if fatigued.
  - Check cardiac rhythm at time of compressor change.
- Avoid excessive ventilation.
  - If no advanced airway (endotracheal tube, laryngeal mask airway, tracheostomy) secured, perform **30:2 compression-ventilation ratio** (with single rescuer or for any adolescent/adult) or **15:2 ratio** (in an infant/child only if 2 rescuers present).
  - If advanced airway secured, give **one breath every 2–3 sec (20–30/min)** with continuous compressions.
  - Ventilation volume should produce no more than minimal, visible chest rise.

---

b. **Monitoring:** Continuous capnography and invasive hemodynamic monitoring may guide effectiveness of chest compressions.
   (1) Target **end-tidal CO_2** ($EtCO_2$) **>20 mmHg.** If consistently less than 20 mmHg, improve compressions and assess for excessive ventilation.
   (2) Abrupt and sustained rise in $EtCO_2$ is often observed just prior to clinical return of spontaneous circulation (ROSC).
   (3) If a patient has an indwelling arterial catheter, assess waveform for feedback to evaluate chest compressions. Target **diastolic BP >25 mmHg** in infants and **>30 mmHg** in children.
c. **Defibrillation:** Shockable arrest rhythms include **ventricular fibrillation** and **pulseless ventricular tachycardia.** Nonshockable arrest rhythms include asystole, pulseless electrical activity, and bradycardia with poor perfusion.
   (1) Use age- and size-appropriate pads as recommended per manufacturer.
   (2) Initial shock dose is **2 J/kg**, second dose is **4 J/kg**, subsequent doses are ≥**4 J/kg (maximum 10 J/kg or adult maximum dose).**
d. **Cardioversion:** A synchronized electrical shock delivered for hemodynamically **unstable** patients with **tachyarrhythmias** (i.e., supraventricular tachycardia, atrial flutter, ventricular tachycardia) and **palpable pulses.**
   (1) Initial dose is **0.5 to 1 J/kg.** Increase to **2 J/kg** if ineffective, repeating doses if necessary. Reevaluate diagnosis if rhythm does not convert to sinus.

     (2) Consultation with a pediatric cardiologist is recommended for elective cardioversion for stable patients with tachyarrhythmias.

e. Resuscitation

   (1) **Access:** Place intraosseous access immediately if in arrest or if intravenous (IV) access difficult.

     (a) If previously established, central access is preferred for drug administration.

     (b) Endotracheal tube (ETT) drug administration is acceptable if required. Naloxone, atropine, vasopressin, epinephrine, and lidocaine (NAVEL) can be administered via endotracheal route.

   (2) **Pharmacotherapy:** See Table 1.1 detailing medications for pediatric resuscitation. If actual body weight is unavailable, use length-based habitus-modified (e.g., Mercy method, PAWPER tape) estimation methods, parental estimates, or length-based (e.g., Broselow tape) estimation methods, in order of accuracy.

     (a) For nonshockable rhythms, early epinephrine administration after CPR initiation (within 5 minutes) is recommended.

   (3) **Fluids:** Administer isotonic crystalloid for treatment of shock even if BP is normal.

     (a) Administer up to 60 mL/kg of isotonic crystalloid in 20 mL/kg increments in nonneonates during the first 20 minutes until perfusion improves. Frequently reassess for hepatomegaly, pulmonary crackles, and respiratory distress.

     (b) Special consideration for **cardiogenic shock:**

       (i) Administer an initial fluid bolus of 5 to 10 mL/kg over 10 to 20 minutes if cardiac insufficiency suspected or unknown (consider in neonate).

       (ii) Be prepared to support oxygenation and ventilation in case of pulmonary edema.

     (c) Special consideration for **septic shock:** Specific goals of therapy include $ScvO_2$ (central venous saturation) $\geq 70\%$, adequate BP, normalized heart rate (HR), and appropriate end-organ perfusion.

       (i) Administer balanced fluid in 10 mL/kg or 20 mL/kg aliquots with frequent reassessment. Lactated Ringer's solution (LR) preferred.

f. **Extracorporeal-CPR (E-CPR):** Rapid deployment of venoarterial (VA) or venovenous (VV) extracorporeal membrane oxygenation (ECMO) to artificially provide oxygenation, ventilation, and circulation as a means of CPR for in-hospital arrest refractory to conventional interventions. Contraindications are limited but may include extremes of prematurity or low birth weight, lethal chromosomal abnormalities, uncontrollable

TABLE 1.1

PEDIATRIC RESUSCITATION MEDICATIONS[5,7,13,19]

Medication	Indication	Dosing	Mechanism	Side Effects
Adenosine	SVT secondary to AV node reentry or accessory pathways	Initial: 0.1 mg/kg IV (max 6 mg) Sec: 0.2 mg/kg IV (max 12 mg) Third: 0.3 mg/kg IV (max 12 mg) Wait 2 min between doses Administer with three-way stopcock rapid push/flush technique	Purine nucleoside blocks AV node conduction	Brief period of asystole (10–15 sec)
Amiodarone	Shock-refractory VF or pVT, refractory SVT	5 mg/kg (max 300 mg) IV/IO No pulse: Push undiluted dose Pulse: Dilute and run over 20–60 min Repeat dosing: 5 mg/kg (max 150 mg) up to 15 mg/kg total Infusion: 5–15 mcG/kg/min (max 15 mg/kg/day or 2200 mg/day)	Potassium-channel blockade suppresses AV node, prolongs QT and QRS	Risk of polymorphic VT, hypotension, decreased cardiac contractility
Atropine	Bradycardia from increased vagal tone, cholinergic drug toxicity, second- and third-degree AV block	0.02 mg/kg IV/IO/IM (min 0.1 mg/dose, max 0.5 mg/dose; larger doses may be needed for organophosphate poisoning) or 0.04–0.06 mg/kg ET Repeat dosing: May repeat once after 5 min; max total dose 1 mg (child). Max total dose 3 mg used in adults.	Cholinergic blockade accelerates atrial pacemakers, enhances AV conduction	Tachycardia, risk of myocardial ischemia, paradoxical bradycardia with lower than minimal dosing
Calcium chloride	Hypocalcemia, hyperkalemia, hypermagnesemia, calcium channel blocker overdose	20 mg/kg (max 1 g) IV/IO Administer over 5 min Consider calcium gluconate in nonarrest if access is peripheral only	Binds myocardial troponin to increase cardiac contractility	Risk of myocardial necrosis, severe tissue injury with peripheral infiltration
Dextrose	Documented hypoglycemia	0.5–1 g/kg IV/IO Newborn: 5–10 mL/kg D$_{10}$W Infants, children: 2–4 mL/kg D$_{25}$W Adolescents: 1–2 mL/kg D$_{50}$W	Restores energy metabolite	Risk of poor neurologic outcomes in setting of hyperglycemia

Epinephrine	Asystole, PEA, VF, pVT, diastolic hypotension, bradycardia	Bolus: 0.01 mg/kg IV/IO (0.1 mg/mL; max 1 mg) or 0.1 mg/kg ET (1 mg/mL; max 2.5 mg) Repeat dosing: Bolus every 3–5 min as needed Infusion: 0.05–2 mcg/kg/min	α-agonism increases aortic diastolic pressure and coronary perfusion	Tachycardia, ectopy, tachyarrhythmias, hypertension
Lidocaine	Shock-refractory VF or pVT (second-line after amiodarone)	Bolus: 1 mg/kg (max 100 mg) IV/IO, 2–3 mg/kg ET Repeat dosing: 1 mg/kg (max 100 mg) every 5 min up to 3 mg/kg in first hr Infusion: 20–50 mcg/kg/min	Sodium-channel blockade decreases automaticity	Myocardial depression, altered mental status, seizures, muscle twitching
Magnesium sulfate	Torsades de pointes, hypomagnesemia	50 mg/kg (max 2 g) IV/IO No pulse: Dilution recommended; infusion rate dependent on indication Pulse: Dilute and administer over 20–60 min	Calcium antagonist depresses abnormal secondary depolarizations and AV node conduction	Hypotension, bradycardia
Naloxone	Opioid overdose	Full reversal: 0.1 mg/kg/dose (max 2 mg/dose) IV/IO/IM/SUBQ, 0.2 mg/kg to 1 mg/kg/dose ET, or 2–8 mg IN (use full applicator available) Repeat dosing: every 2 min as needed	Opioid antagonist reverses opioid-induced respiratory depression, sedation, analgesia, and hypotension	Rapid withdrawal, agitation, pain, pulmonary edema
Procainamide	Refractory SVT, atrial flutter, atrial fibrillation, VT	Load: 15 mg/kg IV/IO, infuse over 30–60 min Infusion: 20–80 mcg/kg/min (max 2 g/24 hr)	Sodium-channel blockade prolongs effective refractory period, depresses conduction velocity	Proarrhythmic, polymorphic VT, hypotension
Sodium bicarbonate	Routine use in arrest is **not** recommended; hyperkalemia, arrhythmias in tricyclic overdose	1 mEq/kg IV/IO Hyperkalemia: Max single dose 50 mEq	Buffers acidosis by binding hydrogen ions to improve myocardial function, reduce SVR and inhibit defibrillation	May impair tissue oxygen delivery, hypokalemia, hypocalcemia, hypernatremia, impaired cardiac function

AV, Atrioventricular; $D_{10}W$, dextrose 10% in water; *ET*, endotracheal; *HR*, heart rate; *ICP*, intracranial pressure; *IM*, intramuscular; *IO*, intraosseous; *IV*, intravenous; *IN*, intranasal; *mcg*, microgram; *PEA*, pulseless electrical activity; *pVT*, pulseless ventricular tachycardia; *SUBQ*, subcutaneous; *SVR*, systemic vascular resistance; *SVT*, supraventricular tachycardia; *VF*, ventricular fibrillation; *VT*, ventricular tachycardia.

hemorrhage, or irreversible brain damage. Should not be offered if likely to be futile.

g. **Post—cardiac arrest care:** Postresuscitation care optimizes oxygenation and perfusion, preserves organ function, and maintains blood glucose levels.

    (1) Obtain chest x-ray to verify ET tube placement, arterial blood gas to correct acid/base disturbances, hemoglobin and hematocrit to assess need for transfusion.

    (2) Maintain oxygen saturation between 94% and 99% and $PaCO_2$ between 35 and 45 mmHg or appropriate to the patient's underlying condition.

    (3) Monitor core temperature continuously and prevent/treat fever to reduce metabolic demand.

        (a) For comatose patients after out-of-hospital cardiac arrest, either maintenance of normothermia or controlled therapeutic hypothermia may be reasonable.

    (4) Maintain systolic blood pressure >5th percentile for age.

    (5) Continuous electroencephalography (EEG) is recommended for the detection of seizures following cardiac arrest in patients with persistent encephalopathy.

    (6) It is recommended that pediatric cardiac arrest survivors be evaluated for rehabilitation services.

B. Airway and Breathing[1,7,8,13-19]

1. Assessment

  a. **Airway patency:** Perform head tilt and chin lift or jaw thrust to open airway. Avoid overextension in infants.

  b. **Spontaneous respirations:** Assess spontaneous patient effort.

    (1) If the patient is breathing regularly, place the patient in **recovery position** (turn onto side).

    (2) If the patient has a palpable pulse but inadequate breathing, give 1 rescue breath every 2 to 3 seconds (20—30 breaths/min).

    (3) When performing CPR in infants and children with an advanced airway, target a respiratory rate range of 1 breath every 2 to 3 seconds (20—30 breaths/min), accounting for age and clinical condition. Rates exceeding this may compromise hemodynamics.

  c. **Adequacy of respiration:** Evaluate for symmetric chest rise. Auscultate for equal breath sounds with good aeration.

  d. **Distress:** Recognize tachypnea, grunting, flaring, retractions, stridor, or wheeze. Infants may exhibit head bobbing.

2. Securing airway

  a. **Bag-Valve-Mask ventilation** (BVM): May be used indefinitely if ventilating effectively.

    (1) Avoid pushing mask down, which can obstruct airway. Bring face into mask.

(2) Consider **oropharyngeal** airway in the **unconscious** patient with obstruction. Correct size will extend from corner of mouth to mandibular angle.

(3) Consider **nasopharyngeal** airway in the **conscious** (gag reflex intact) or unconscious patient with obstruction. Correct size will extend from tip of nose to tragus of ear.

(4) Cricoid pressure (Sellick maneuver) may be used to minimize gastric inflation and aspiration. Avoid excess pressure leading to tracheal obstruction.

b. **Laryngeal mask airway** (LMA)**:** Supraglottic airway placed blindly. Useful to emergently secure access to a difficult airway.

(1) Use manufacturer-specific weight-based mask size estimation systems or the combined width of the patient's index, middle, and ring fingers to estimate mask size.

(2) Continuous chest compressions can be performed once LMA is placed.

c. **Endotracheal intubation:** Rapid sequence intubation is indicated in patients presenting with (presumed) full stomach. Immediately sequential sedation and neuromuscular blockade help to avert the need for positive pressure ventilation, minimizing aspiration risk.

(1) **Preparation:** Always have a secondary plan to manage the airway if intubation is unsuccessful.

(a) **Preoxygenation:** Deliver 100% oxygen via a nonrebreather mask for at least 3 minutes. Children have higher oxygen consumption than adults and can rapidly become hypoxemic.

(b) **Equipment:** Collect monitoring, suctioning, and oxygen delivery equipment.

(i) If available, quantitative **EtCO$_2$** is recommended as primary method to confirm ventilation.

(ii) Place suction catheter at head of bed. Set suction device from **−80 mmHg to −120 mmHg.**

(iii) Consider nasogastric tube for stomach decompression. See Chapter 4 for placement.

(c) **Airway supplies:** Use cuffed ETTs over uncuffed ETTs for intubating infants and children. When a cuffed ETT is used, attention should be paid to ETT size, position, and cuff inflation pressure (<20−25 cm H$_2$O).

(i) If available, use a length-based estimator (e.g., Broselow tape) of ETT size and laryngoscope blade size.

(ii) To estimate age-based ETT size (internal diameter) for patients 2 to 10 years:

Cuffed ETT(mm) = (age in years/4) + 3.5

Uncuffed ETT(mm) = (age in years/4) + 4.0

(iii) To approximate depth of insertion:

Depth(cm) = ETT size × 3

(iv) Choose laryngoscope blade type and size based on patient age and airway.

(v) Straight (i.e., Miller) blades are typically reserved for children <2 years age or difficult airways.

   (a) Miller #00-1 for premature to 2 months age

   (b) Miller #1 for 3 months to 3 years age

   (c) Miller #2 for >3 years age

(vi) Curved (i.e., Mac) laryngoscope blades are often more effective for children >2 years age.

   (a) Mac #2 for >2 years age

   (b) Mac #3 for >8 years age

(d) **Pharmacology:** See Table 1.2 for rapid sequence intubation medications.

(e) **Positioning:** Place patient in "sniffing" position with neck slightly extended to align the airway.

   (i) Infants and toddlers may require towel roll beneath **shoulders** due to large occiput.

   (ii) Children and adolescents may require towel roll beneath **neck.**

(2) **Procedure:** Advanced airways should be placed by experienced healthcare providers with appropriate training.

   (a) Routine use of cricoid pressure is not recommended during endotracheal intubation of pediatric patients.

   (b) Confirm placement by detecting $EtCO_2$, observing chest wall movement, auscultating for symmetric breath sounds, and monitoring oxygen saturation. Evaluate placement via chest radiograph.

(3) **Failure:** Acute respiratory failure in an intubated patient may signify **D**isplacement of the ETT, **O**bstruction, **P**neumothorax, or **E**quipment failure **(DOPE).**

d. **Surgical airway:** Consider needle or surgical cricothyrotomy if BVM, endotracheal intubation, and LMA fail. If available, consult emergently with difficult airway specialists (pediatric anesthesiologist, intensivist, and/or otolaryngologist).

3. Oxygenation and ventilation

   a. Oxygen delivery systems:

   (1) Low-flow systems (e.g., nasal cannula, simple face mask) **do not meet** the inspiratory flow demand of the patient. Delivery of set fraction of inspired oxygen (FiO_2) is difficult due to room air mixing.

TABLE 1.2

RAPID SEQUENCE INTUBATION MEDICATIONS[13,17-19,22]

Medication	Benefit	Indication	Dosing	Side Effects
1. ADJUNCTS				
Atropine	Prevent bradycardia associated with laryngoscope insertion, decrease oral secretions	Bradycardia in any patient, infants <1 year, children 1–5 years receiving succinylcholine, children >5 years receiving a second dose of succinylcholine	0.02 mg/kg IV/IO/IM (max 0.5 mg)	Tachycardia, pupil dilation
Glycopyrrolate	Decrease oral secretions, prevent bradycardia; may cause less tachycardia than atropine, preserves pupillary exam in trauma	Hypersalivation	0.004–0.01 mg/kg IV/IM/IO (max 0.1 mg)	Tachycardia
Lidocaine	Blunts rise in ICP associated with laryngoscopy	Elevated ICP, shock, arrhythmia, and status asthmaticus	1 mg/kg IV/IO (max 100 mg)	Myocardial depression, altered mental status, seizures, muscle twitching
2. INDUCTION AGENTS				
Etomidate (sedative)	Minimal cardiovascular side effects, minimally decreases ICP	Multitrauma patient at risk for increased ICP and hypotension. Caution in patients with adrenal suppression; avoid in septic shock	0.3 mg/kg IV/IO (max 20 mg)	Suppresses adrenal corticosteroid synthesis, vomiting, myoclonus, lowers seizure threshold
Fentanyl (analgesic, sedative)	Minimal cardiovascular effect	Shock	1–5 mcg/kg slow IV/IM push (max 100 mcg)	Chest wall rigidity, bradycardia, respiratory depression
Ketamine (sedative, analgesic)	Catecholamine release causes bronchodilation, abates bradycardia associated with laryngoscope insertion, increases HR and SVR, produces a "dissociative amnesia"	Status asthmaticus, shock and hypotensive patients. Caution in patients at risk for elevated ICP or glaucoma history	1–2 mg/kg IV/IO (max 150 mg) 4–6 mg/kg IM	Vomiting, laryngospasm, hypersalivation, emergence reactions (hallucinations)

Continued

TABLE 1.2

RAPID SEQUENCE INTUBATION MEDICATIONS[13,17-19,22]**—CONT'D**

Medication	Benefit	Indication	Dosing	Side Effects
Midazolam (sedative, amnestic, anxiolytic)	Minimal cardiovascular effect	Mild shock	0.05–0.1 mg/kg IV/IM/IO (max single dose 6–10 mg depending on age (see Formulary)	Dose-dependent respiratory depression, hypotension
Propofol (sedative)	Ultra-short acting	Avoid in shock or patients who require maintenance of CPP	2 mg/kg IV	Hypotension, myocardial depression, metabolic acidosis; may cause paradoxical hypertension in children
3. NEUROMUSCULAR BLOCKADE				
Succinylcholine (depolarizing)	Rapid-onset, short-acting neuromuscular blockade agent, reversible with acetylcholinesterase inhibitor	Role limited due to adverse events Contraindicated in neuromuscular disease, myopathies, spinal cord injury, crush injury, burns, renal insufficiency	IV: ≤2 years: 2 mg/kg >2 years: 1 mg/kg (30–60 sec onset, 4–6 min duration) IM: 3–4 mg/kg (3–4 min onset, 10–30 min duration) Max dose: 150 mg/dose IM	Hyperkalemia, trigger of malignant hyperthermia, masseter spasm, bradycardia, muscle fasciculations, increased intracranial, intraocular, and intragastric pressure
Rocuronium (nondepolarizing)	Minimal cardiovascular effect, reversible with sugammadex	Caution in patients with difficult airway	1.2 mg/kg IV/IM/IO (30–90 sec onset, 30–45 min duration) Max dose: 100 mg	Prolonged duration in hepatic failure
Vecuronium (nondepolarizing)	Minimal cardiovascular effect, reversible with sugammadex	Caution in patients with difficult airway	0.15–0.2 mg/kg IV/IO (1–3 min onset, 30–40 min duration) Max dose: 10 mg	Prolonged duration in hepatic failure, longer time to paralysis than rocuronium

CPP, Cerebral perfusion pressure; *HR*, heart rate; *ICP*, intracranial pressure; *IM*, intramuscular; *IV*, intravenous; *IO*, intraosseous; *mCg*, microgram; *RSI*, rapid sequence intubation; *SVR*, systemic vascular resistance.

(2) High-flow systems (e.g., nonrebreather, oxygen hood) **do meet** the inspiratory flow demand of the patient. Measurable FiO_2 is delivered.

(3) High-flow nasal cannula **(HFNC):**

    (a) High-flow, noninvasive respiratory support provides a heated and humidified air-oxygen mixture that may improve gas exchange by providing airway-distending pressure.

    (b) Optimal and maximal flow rates are unknown. Consensus supports a maximum flow rate of up to **2 L/kg/min** or 12 L/min for infants and toddlers, 30 L/min for children, and up to 50 L/min for adolescents and adults.

b. Noninvasive positive pressure ventilation **(NIPPV):**

  (1) **CPAP:** Delivery of a continuous, distending positive airway pressure independent of patient inspiratory effort.

  (2) **BiPAP:** Pressure-limited ventilatory mode in which the clinician sets an inspiratory positive airway pressure (IPAP) and expiratory positive airway pressure (EPAP).

    (a) EPAP is started at 4 to 5 cmH_2O and increased to a maximum of 8 to 12 cmH_2O.

    (b) Set 4 to 6 cmH_2O of pressure support, or the difference between IPAP and EPAP.

    (c) Consider setting a "backup rate," or respiratory rate just shy of the spontaneous respiratory rate to be delivered in case of apnea.

c. Mechanical ventilation:

  (1) **Parameters:**

    (a) Rate: Number of mechanical breaths delivered per minute

    (b) FiO_2: Fraction of oxygen in inspired gas

    (c) PIP: Peak inspiratory pressure attained during respiratory cycle

    (d) Positive end-expiratory pressure (PEEP): Distending pressure that increases functional residual capacity (FRC), or volume of gas at the end of exhalation

    (e) Mean airway pressure (P_{aw}): Average airway pressure over entire respiratory cycle, which correlates to mean alveolar volume

    (f) Tidal volume (V_T): Volume of gas delivered during inspiration

    (g) Time: May indicate a function of time spent in inspiration (T_i), in high pressure (T_{high}), or in low pressure (T_{low})

  (2) Modes of ventilation:

    (a) **Controlled ventilation:** Ventilation is completely mechanical with no spontaneous ventilation efforts expected from the patient.

      (i) Pressure-controlled ventilation **(PCV):** A preset respiratory rate and T_i deliver a pressure-limited breath (the set pressure is maintained during inspiration). V_T is determined by the preset pressure as well as lung compliance and resistance.

      (ii) Volume-controlled ventilation **(VCV):** A preset respiratory rate and T_i deliver a preset V_T.

   (b) Intermittent mandatory ventilation **(IMV):** Allows the patient to breathe spontaneously between a preset number of (mandatory) mechanical breaths

      (i) Synchronized IMV **(SIMV):** If patient initiates spontaneous breath, mandatory breath is synchronized with patient effort rather than spaced evenly over each minute.

      (ii) If spontaneous breathing rate is less than mandatory rate, some mandatory breaths will be delivered in the absence of patient effort.

      (iii) Delivered breaths may be volume regulated or pressure limited.

   (c) Airway-pressure-release ventilation **(APRV):** Most of the respiratory cycle is spent at a high distending pressure (a functionally high CPAP phase) with intermittent, short release to a low pressure for a brief ventilation phase. Spontaneous breathing can be superimposed at any point in the cycle.

   (d) **Support ventilation:** Mechanical breaths support patient-initiated breaths, but no mandatory breaths are provided.

      (i) Pressure support **(PS):** Delivers a preset amount of pressure to assist spontaneous respiratory effort

      (ii) Often used in combination with other modes of ventilation to support spontaneous breaths greater than preset respiratory rates

   (e) High-frequency oscillatory ventilation **(HFOV):** Gas flow pressurizes the system to the preset P_{aw} while a piston moves backward and forward to force and withdraw a small V_T (that approximates anatomic dead space) into the lungs at rates exceeding normal respiratory rates.

(3) **Management:** The three subdivisions of mechanical ventilatory support are the acute (lung recruitment), maintenance (lung recovery), and weaning phases.

   (a) **Acute:** See Table 1.3 for ventilation parameter initial settings and titration effects.

   (b) **Maintenance:** To avoid volutrauma, barotrauma, or oxygen toxicity, maintain V_T at 4–6 mL/kg, PIP <35 cmH$_2$O, and FiO$_2$ ≤60%.

TABLE 1.3

MECHANICAL VENTILATION PARAMETER SETTINGS AND EFFECTS[13,16,19]

Parameter	Initial Setting	Effect of ↑ on PaCO₂	Effect of ↑ on PaO₂
PIP	≤28 cmH₂O or ≤29–32 cmH₂O for reduced chest wall compliance	↓↓	↑
PEEP	3–5 cmH₂O	↑	↑↑
V$_T$	5–8 mL/kg or 3–6 mL/kg for poorly compliant lungs	↓↓	↑
Rate	Normal rate for age	↓↓	Minimal ↑
I:E ratio	(33%) 1:2 (67%)	No change	↑
FiO₂	<50% and/or to maintain PaO₂ between 80 and 100 mmHg and SpO₂ ≥95%	No change	↑↑
HIGH-FREQUENCY VENTILATION PARAMETERS			
Amplitude (ΔP)	Set to produce a visible wiggling motion to the level of the lower abdomen	↓	No change
Frequency (Hz)	Range from 3–20 Hz (180–1200 breaths per min)	↑↑	↓
P$_{aw}$	5 cmH₂O > P$_{aw}$ of previous conventional ventilation	Minimal ↓	↑

FiO₂, Fraction of inspired oxygen; *I:E*, inspiratory to expiratory; *Hz*, hertz; *P$_{aw}$*, mean airway pressure; *PaCO₂*, partial pressure of carbon dioxide (arterial); *PaO₂*, partial pressure of oxygen (arterial); *PEEP*, positive end-expiratory pressure; *PIP*, peak inspiratory pressure; *V$_T$*, tidal volume.

- (c) **Weaning:**
  - (i) Assess daily for clinical signs of readiness, such as spontaneous breathing efforts.
  - (ii) Standard indices indicating readiness include FiO₂ <50%, PEEP of 5 cmH₂O, PIP <20 cmH₂O, normalized rate for age, and absence of hypercapnia or acidosis.
  - (iii) The general approach combines gradual weaning of parameters and reliance on pressure-support modes.
- (d) Extubation:
  - (i) Provide humidified inspired oxygen after extubation.
  - (ii) In case of uncuffed tube or the absence of an air leak at delivered pressure <30 cmH₂O, consider 24 hours of dexamethasone (airway edema dosing) to prevent postextubation stridor.

II. MANAGEMENT OF SHOCK[3,5,7,12,13]

A. Definition: Physiologic state characterized by inadequate oxygen and nutrient delivery to meet tissue demands

1. **Compensated:** Perfusion to vital organs is maintained by compensatory mechanisms.
   a. Tachycardia is often the first and most sensitive vital sign change.

    b. Blood flow is redirected from nonvital organs and tissues to vital organs by a selective increase in systemic vascular resistance (SVR), resulting in reduced peripheral perfusion and decreased urine volume.

    c. Cardiac contractility increases to maintain cardiac output.

    d. Increased venous smooth muscle tone improves preload and stroke volume.

2. **Decompensated:** Perfusion to vital organs is compromised. Denoted by **hypotension,** poor perfusion, oliguria/anuria, and altered mental status.

B. Etiology: Categorized into four basic types:

1. **Hypovolemic:** Inadequate fluid intake, increased fluid losses (hemorrhage, gastroenteritis, burns). Assess for tachycardia, narrow pulse pressure, delayed capillary refill, cool extremities.

2. **Cardiogenic:** Congenital heart disease, myocarditis, cardiomyopathy, arrhythmia. Assess for increased respiratory effort from pulmonary edema, hepatomegaly, jugular venous distention, and cyanosis.

3. **Distributive:** Sepsis, anaphylaxis, neurogenic (e.g., high cervical spine injury)

    a. Assess for tachycardia, fever, and petechial, purpuric, or urticarial rash.

    b. Warm septic shock is characterized by bounding peripheral pulses, flash capillary refill, and wide pulse pressure.

    c. Cold septic shock is characterized by decreased peripheral pulses, delayed capillary refill, and narrow pulse pressure.

    d. Neurogenic shock is characterized by hypotension with a wide pulse pressure, normal HR or bradycardia, and hypothermia.

4. **Obstructive:** Tension pneumothorax, cardiac tamponade, pulmonary embolism, ductal-dependent congenital cardiac abnormalities

    a. Early clinical presentation is indistinguishable from hypovolemic shock. Progression of shock leads to signs and symptoms similar to cardiogenic shock.

    b. Cardiac tamponade is characterized by muffled heart sounds and pulsus paradoxus.

    c. Ductal-dependent lesions may be characterized by higher preductal versus postductal BP or arterial oxygen saturation.

C. Management

1. Administer 100% supplemental oxygen initially regardless of oxygen saturation to optimize oxygen delivery. Once perfusion restored, titrate as able to avoid adverse effects from hyperoxia.

2. See Table 1.4 for type- and etiology-specific pathophysiology and management of shock.

3. See Table 1.5 for vasoactive agents to support cardiac output. Vasoactive agents affect SVR (vasodilators and vasoconstrictors), cardiac contractility (inotropes), or HR (chronotropes). Some agents increase blood flow via contractility and vasodilation (inodilators) or increase perfusion pressure via contractility and vasoconstriction (inoconstrictors).

TABLE 1.4

PATHOPHYSIOLOGY AND MANAGEMENT OF SHOCK[3,5]

Type	HR	Preload	Contractility	SVR	Management
Hypovolemic	↑	↓↓	Normal or ↑	↑	Rapid administration of isotonic crystalloids Replace blood loss with 10 mL/kg PRBC boluses Consider colloids if response is poor to crystalloids and loss of protein-containing fluids is suspected
Distributive	↑ or ↓	Normal or ↓	Normal or ↓	↓ (may progress to ↑)	Administer isotonic crystalloids to expand intravascular volume Support with vasopressors if fluid-refractory
Septic	↑	↓↓	Normal or ↓	↓	**Within 1st hour:** Administer fluid boluses (balanced/buffered crystalloid preferred) and broad-spectrum antibiotics, and consider stress-dose hydrocortisone **Warm:** Support with norepinephrine **Cold:** Support with epinephrine
Neurogenic	Normal or ↓	↓↓	Normal	↓↓	Position patient flat or head-down Administer a trial of isotonic crystalloid therapy If fluid-refractory, support with norepinephrine or epinephrine Maintain normothermia
Cardiogenic	↑	↑	↓↓	↑	Consider cautious administration (10–20 min) of isotonic crystalloid (5–10 mL/kg); stop if fluid overload develops Support with inodilator milrinone Decrease metabolic demand with oxygen therapy, ventilatory support, and antipyretics
Obstructive	↑	±	Normal	↑	Correct underlying cause Start prostaglandin E_1 if ductal-dependent lesion suspected Consider cautious administration (10–20 min) of isotonic crystalloid (5–10 mL/kg); stop if fluid overload develops

HR, Heart rate; *PRBC*, packed red blood cell; *SVR*, systemic vascular resistance.

TABLE 1.5

MEDICATIONS TO SUPPORT CARDIAC OUTPUT[5,7,13]

Medication	Dose	Mechanism	Comments
Dobutamine	2—20 mCg/kg/min	Selective β_1 agonist	Inotrope May predispose to arrhythmia Indicated for normotensive, poorly perfused shock
Dopamine	5—20 mCg/kg/min	Direct dopamine receptor agonist, indirect β and α agonist (stimulates norepinephrine release), direct α agonist at high dose (>15 mCg/kg/min)	Low to moderate dose: inotrope, chronotrope, splanchnic vasodilator High dose: vasopressor Indicated for shock with poor contractility and/or low SVR and cold septic shock if epinephrine unavailable
Epinephrine	0.05—2 mCg/kg/min	β_1 and β_2 agonist at low dose (<0.3 mCg/kg/min), α_1 agonist at high dose (>0.3 mCg/kg/min)	Low dose: inotrope, chronotrope, vasodilator High dose: vasopressor Indicated for hypotensive shock with marked circulatory instability and cold septic shock
Milrinone	Loading: 50 mCg/kg over 15 min, then 0.25—0.75 mCg/kg/min	Type III phosphodiesterase-inhibitor	Inodilator Improves cardiac output with little effect on heart rate Indicated for normotensive shock with myocardial dysfunction and cold septic shock refractory to epinephrine
Norepinephrine	0.05—2.5 mCg/kg/min	α_1 and β_1 agonist	Vasoconstrictor, mild inotrope Indicated for shock with low SVR (warm septic, anaphylactic, spinal) and cold shock refractory to epinephrine if diastolic BP low
Phenylephrine	Loading: 5—20 mCg/kg/dose (max 500 mCg), then 0.1—2 mCg/kg/min	Pure α_1 agonist	Vasoconstrictor Rapid increase in BP may cause reflex bradycardia
Vasopressin (ADH)	0.17—8 milliUnits/kg/min	Vasopressin receptor agonist	Vasoconstrictor Consider for cardiac arrest, refractory hypotension in septic shock and GI hemorrhage

ADH, Antidiuretic hormone; *BP*, blood pressure; *GI*, gastrointestinal; *mCg*, microgram; *NO*, nitric oxide; *SVR*, systemic vascular resistance.

a. Use epinephrine or norepinephrine for fluid-refractory septic shock as initial vasoactive infusion (or dopamine if these are unavailable) and consider the addition of stress-dose steroids.
b. For hemorrhagic shock following trauma, administer blood products when available instead of crystalloid.

III. MANAGEMENT OF COMMON EMERGENCIES

A. Anaphylaxis[20]

1. **Definition:** Severe, systemic hypersensitivity reaction. Usually rapid in onset and characterized by compromise in airway, breathing, and/or circulation. May involve multiple organ systems, including the following:
   a. **Cutaneous/mucosal** (80% to 90%): Flushing, urticaria, pruritis, angioedema
   b. **Respiratory** (70%): Laryngeal edema, bronchospasm, dyspnea, wheezing, stridor, hypoxemia
   c. **Gastrointestinal** (45%): Vomiting, diarrhea, nausea, crampy abdominal pain
   d. **Circulatory** (45%): Tachycardia, hypotension, syncope
2. **Management:**
   a. **Stop exposure** to precipitating antigen.
   b. While performing A-B-Cs, immediately give intramuscular **(IM) epinephrine** into midanterolateral thigh.
      (1) For child, administer **0.01 mg/kg of 1 mg/mL solution** up to a max dose of 0.3 mg/dose. For adult-sized patients, first administer **0.2 to 0.5 mg of 1 mg/mL solution,** increasing as necessary up to max single dose of 0.5 mg.
      (2) Autoinjector dosing: 7.5 to <15 kg use **0.1 mg,** 15 to <30 kg use **0.15 mg,** ≥30 kg use **0.3 mg.**
      (3) Repeat dosing every 5 to 15 minutes as needed.
   c. Provide oxygen and ventilatory assistance. Consider early endotracheal intubation.
   d. Obtain IV access. For management of shock, resuscitate with 20 mL/kg isotonic crystalloid fluid boluses and vasoactive agents as needed.
   e. Place patient in Trendelenburg position (head 30 degrees below feet).
   f. Consider adjuvant pharmacologic agents:
      (1) **Histamine receptor antagonist:** Diphenhydramine (H1-antagonism) and famotidine (H2-antagonism)
      (2) **Corticosteroid:** Methylprednisolone or dexamethasone
      (3) **Inhaled β_2 agonist:** Albuterol
   g. Symptoms may recur ("biphasic anaphylaxis") up to 72 hours after initial recovery.
      (1) Observe for a minimum of 4 to 10 hours for late-phase symptoms.

    (2) Discharge with an epinephrine autoinjector and an anaphylaxis action plan.

B. Upper Airway Obstruction

1. **Epiglottitis**[21-22]
   a. **Definition:** Life-threatening, rapidly progressive inflammation (usually infectious) of the supraglottic region
      (1) Most often affects children between 1 and 8 years but may occur at any age
      (2) May be caused by infection, thermal injury, caustic ingestion, or foreign body
      (3) Most common infectious organisms include *Haemophilus influenzae* (unvaccinated), *Streptococcus pneumoniae*, group A streptococci, and *Staphylococcus aureus.*
      (4) Patients often present febrile, toxic-appearing, and tripoding in respiratory distress. Drooling, dysphagia, and inspiratory stridor are common. Barky cough is absent.
   b. **Management:** Avoid *any agitation* of the child prior to securing airway to prevent impending complete obstruction.
      (1) Allow child to assume a position of comfort. Unobtrusively provide blow-by oxygen. Monitor with pulse oximetry.
      (2) To secure airway, emergently consult difficult airway personnel (pediatric anesthesiologist, intensivist, and/or otolaryngologist).
         (a) If unstable (unresponsive, cyanotic, bradycardic), emergently intubate.
         (b) If stable with high suspicion, escort patient to OR for laryngoscopy and intubation under general anesthesia. Equipment for tracheotomy should be readily available.
         (c) If stable with moderate or low suspicion, obtain lateral neck radiograph to assess for "thumb sign" of an inflamed epiglottis.
      (3) Initiate broad-spectrum antibiotic therapy (e.g., vancomycin and ceftriaxone).

2. **Croup**[23-24]
   a. **Definition:** Common respiratory illness of the larynx, trachea, and bronchi.
      (1) Most common in infants aged 6 to 36 months
      (2) 75% of infections are caused by parainfluenza virus.
      (3) Patients present with fever, barking cough, inspiratory stridor, and increased work of breathing, often worse at night.
   b. **Management:**
      (1) Administer oxygen to children with hypoxemia or severe respiratory distress. Consider humidified air, although current consensus suggests it is ineffective for mild to moderate disease.

(2) If **no stridor at rest,** give dexamethasone. Consider nebulized budesonide in patients vomiting or who lack IV access.

(3) If **stridor at rest,** give dexamethasone and nebulized racemic epinephrine. Observe for 2 to 4 hours given short duration of action of nebulized epinephrine.

(4) Indications for hospitalization include >1 racemic epinephrine nebulization required, atypical age (<6 months), severe respiratory distress, or dehydration.

(5) Consider heliox (helium and oxygen mixture) to improve turbulent airflow in moderate to severe croup, although benefit is controversial.

3. Foreign body aspiration[1,22,25]

   a. **Definition:** Acute airway obstruction from aspiration of an organic (e.g., nuts, seeds, grapes, hot dogs) or inorganic (e.g., coins, pins, beads, balloons, small toy parts) foreign body

      (1) Male children younger than 3 years of age are most susceptible.

      (2) Patients (<40%) present with classic triad of paroxysmal cough, wheezing, and decreased air entry. Other manifestations include cyanosis, fever, stridor, and persistent pneumonia or notably may be asymptomatic.

      (3) The most common location is the right main bronchus (45% to 57%), then left main bronchus (18% to 40%), and trachea (10% to 17%).

   b. **Management:** Care is taken to avoid converting a partial airway obstruction into complete obstruction.

      (1) If **not** breathing (no cough or sound):

         (a) Infant: Deliver repeated cycles of 5 back blows followed by 5 chest compressions until object is expelled or victim becomes unresponsive.

         (b) Child: Perform subdiaphragmatic abdominal thrusts (Heimlich maneuver) until object is expelled or victim becomes unresponsive.

         (c) Patients should be taken to the OR for emergent removal under direct laryngoscopy and bronchoscopy.

      (2) If **breathing** (forcefully coughing, phonating):

         (a) Obtain posteroanterior chest (including neck) radiograph to screen for radiopaque body or mediastinal shift. Consider inspiratory and expiratory films (or bilateral lateral decubitus in young patients) to assess for air trapping. A normal chest radiograph does not rule out foreign body.

         (b) If clinical concern is high, consider urgent bronchoscopy or laryngoscopy.

      (3) If patient becomes **unresponsive:** initiate CPR immediately.

         (a) After 30 chest compressions, open airway and remove foreign body if visible. Do **not** perform blind sweep.

(b) Attempt to give two breaths and continue with cycles of chest compressions and ventilations until object expelled.

C. Status Asthmaticus[26-31]

1. **Definition:** Inflammatory airflow obstruction secondary to triad of airway edema, bronchoconstriction, and hyperresponsiveness

2. **Examination:** Assess breathlessness, speech, alertness, respiratory rate, accessory muscle use, wheezing, HR, pulsus paradoxus, peak expiratory flow, SpO_2, and pCO_2.

3. **Management:**
   a. Provide oxygen to achieve SpO_2 ≥90%. If hypoxemia not readily corrected with supplemental oxygen, consider pneumothorax, pneumonia, methemoglobinemia, or other process.
   b. See Table 1.6 for pharmacologic agents used in acute asthma exacerbations. Consider using Pediatric Asthma Score to recognize exacerbation severity and guide treatment (Table 1.7).

TABLE 1.6

STATUS ASTHMATICUS MEDICATIONS[26-30]

Medication	Dose	Comments
SHORT-ACTING β_2 AGONIST		
Albuterol	**Mild to moderate:** Administer up to 3 doses in the first hour MDI: 4–8 puffs (90 mCg/puff) Q20 min–4 hr Nebulizer: 0.15 mg/kg (min 2.5 mg, max 5 mg) Q20 min–4 hr **Severe:** Continuous nebulization: 0.5 mg/kg/hr (max 30 mg/hr)	Inhaler (with spacer) is preferred delivery method given equal or greater efficacy, fewer side effects, and shorter length of stay
ANTICHOLINERGICS		
Ipratropium bromide	Administer Q20 min for 3 doses with albuterol MDI: 4–8 puffs (17 mCg/puff) Nebulizer: 0.25–0.5 mg	No additional benefit shown in inpatient setting
SYSTEMIC CORTICOSTEROIDS		
Dexamethasone	**Mild to moderate:** 0.6 mg/kg/day PO/IV/IM for 1–2 days (max 16 mg/day)	Equally as efficacious as prednisone or prednisolone with fewer side effects, better compliance and palatability
Prednisone, prednisolone Methylprednisolone	**Mild to severe:** 2 mg/kg/day PO for 5–7 days (max 60 mg/day) **Severe:** Loading: 2 mg/kg IV (max 80 mg) Maintenance: 2 mg/kg/day IV divided Q6–12 hr (max <12 years 60 mg/day, ≥12 years 80 mg/day)	Taper if course ≥7 days or bounce back from recent exacerbation No known advantage in severe exacerbations for higher dosing or IV administration over oral therapy, provided normal GI transit and absorption

INJECTED β$_2$ AGONIST		
Epinephrine	0.01 mg/kg of 1 mg/mL IM (max 0.5 mg) Q15—20 min for up to 3 doses	Consider for severe exacerbation with minimal air entry Consider quickly accessed autoinjector
Terbutaline	SUBQ: 0.01 mg/kg (max 0.25 mg/dose) Q20 min for up to 3 doses, then as needed Q2—6 hr IV load: 4—10 mCg/kg IV IV continuous: 0.2—5 mCg/kg/min (doses as high as 10 mCg/kg/min have been used)	Consider for severe exacerbation with minimal air entry IV administration may decrease the need for mechanical ventilation

ADJUNCT THERAPIES		
Magnesium sulfate	25—75 mg/kg/dose IV (max 2 g), infuse over 20 min	Smooth muscle relaxant May cause hypotension; consider simultaneous fluid bolus Reduces hospitalization rates in severe exacerbations
Ketamine	1—2 mg/kg IV load followed by 1 mg/kg/hr infusion, titrated to effect	Used as a sympathomimetic adjuvant in effort to avoid endotracheal intubation Preferred induction-sedative agent for endotracheal intubation in asthma
Aminophylline	6 mg/kg IV load over 20 min followed by 0.5—1.2 mg/kg/hr infusion (age-dependent, see formulary)	Use limited to severe exacerbations refractory to traditional interventions May improve lung function and oxygen saturation but is associated with greater length of stay and time to symptom improvement
Heliox	Optimal helium-oxygen ratio unknown, most commonly 70:30 or 80:20 mixture	Low density gas that promotes laminar airflow and improves β$_2$ agonist delivery to distal airways Useful in severe or very severe exacerbations
Inhaled anesthetics (e.g., halothane, isoflurane, sevoflurane)	Consultation with pediatric anesthetist recommended	Rescue therapy for intubated patients with life-threatening exacerbation Associated with prolonged length of stay and increased cost Isoflurane may cause hypotension Sevoflurane may cause renal tubular injury, hepatotoxicity, neuropathy

GI, Gastrointestinal; *IM*, intramuscular; *IV*, intravenous; *mCg*, microgram; *MDI*, metered-dose inhaler; *PO*, by mouth; *SUBQ*, subcutaneous.

TABLE 1.7

PEDIATRIC ASTHMA SCORE

Examination Component	1	2	3
Respiratory rate			
1–4 yr	≤34	35–39	≥40
4–6 yr	≤30	31–35	≥36
6–10 yr	≤26	27–30	≥31
>12 yr	≤23	24–27	≥28
O_2 requirement	>95% on room air	90%–95% on room air	<90% on room air or any oxygen
Retractions	None or intercostal	Intercostal and substernal	Intercostal, substernal, and supraclavicular
Work of breathing (count to 10)	Speaks in sentences, coos and babbles	Speaks in partial sentences, short cry	Speaks in single words/short phrases, grunting
Auscultation	Normal breath sounds to end-expiratory wheezes only	Expiratory wheezing	Inspiratory and expiratory wheezing to diminished breath sounds

Data from Nievas IF, Anand KJ. Severe acute asthma exacerbation in children: a stepwise approach for escalating therapy in a pediatric intensive care unit. *J Pediatr Pharmacol Ther.* 2013;18(2):88–104. https://doi.org/10.5863/1551-6776-18.2.88

   c. Ventilation interventions:
     (1) Normalizing pCO_2 can be a sign of impending respiratory failure.
     (2) NIPPV (e.g., BiPAP) may be used in patients with impending respiratory failure to avoid intubation but requires a cooperative patient with spontaneous respirations.
     (3) Intubation should be approached cautiously given the risk of worsening air-trapping and difficulty in managing the transition from extremely negative to positive pressure ventilation.
       (a) Indications include severe airway obstruction, markedly increased work of breathing, refractory hypoxemia, and impending respiratory arrest.
       (b) Ventilation strategies include slower rates with prolonged expiratory phase, minimal end-expiratory pressures, and short inspiratory times to minimize hyperinflation and air trapping.
     (4) Consider inhaled anesthetics or ECMO as rescue therapies.

D. Pulmonary Hypertensive Crisis[13,32]

1. **Definition:**
   a. Pulmonary hypertension (PH) is defined as resting elevated mean pulmonary artery pressure (PAP) ≥**25 mmHg** in children >3 months of age.

b. A **pulmonary hypertensive crisis** is a sudden increase in PAP and pulmonary vascular resistance (PVR) that causes acute right-sided heart failure.
   (1) May be triggered by pain, anxiety, tracheal suctioning, hypoxia, acidosis, or respiratory illness. Most commonly described after cardiac surgery or in the setting of rapid withdrawal of PH-specific therapies.
   (2) Patients present with systemic hypotension, oxygen desaturation (if atrial or ventricular communication present), and decreased $EtCO_2$ on capnography (reduced pulmonary blood flow).
   (3) Assess for increased intensity of systolic murmur (worsening tricuspid regurgitation) and increased hepatomegaly.

2. **Management:** Timely consultation with providers with expertise in managing PH is recommended.
   a. Implement efforts to keep patient calm. Consider opiates, sedatives, and neuromuscular blockade to reduce stress response, especially postoperatively. Avoid agents that decrease SVR.
   b. Oxygen is a pulmonary vasodilator and should be administered to treat hypoxemia. Avoid acute hypercarbia and acidosis, which abruptly increase PVR. Consider brief hyperventilation or sodium bicarbonate infusions.
   c. Diuretics treat congestive symptoms. Avoid excessive reduction in intravascular volume leading to decreased cardiac output.
   d. NIPPV may improve oxygenation, treat hypoventilation, and reduce work of breathing. Weigh benefits against increasing patient anxiety and delaying mechanical ventilation.
   e. PH-specific pharmacologic therapies aim to induce pulmonary vasodilation, support the right ventricle, and maintain cardiac output.
      (1) **Inhaled pulmonary vasodilators:** Nitric oxide
         (a) Indicated to reduce need for ECMO in patients with an oxygen index >25
         (b) Rapid withdrawal of low doses may cause rebound PH. Gradually decrease dose when weaning.
         (c) Monitor for methemoglobinemia.
      (2) **Synthetic prostacyclin analogs** (epoprostenol [Flolan], treprostinil, iloprost):
         (a) Administered by continuous IV or subcutaneous route. Iloprost is inhaled.
      (3) **Phosphodiesterase type-5 inhibitors:** Sildenafil, tadalafil
         (a) Often used to prevent rebound PH associated with cessation of nitric oxide
         (b) Monitor for acute hypotension or hypoxemia secondary to increased alveolar-arterial gradient.

    (4) **Endothelin receptor antagonist:** Bosentan

  f. Consider ECMO or emergent atrial septostomy in case of failed medical management.

E. Hypertensive Crisis[13,33]

1. **Definition:**
   a. For normal BP values based on age and height, see Chapter 19.
   b. **Hypertensive emergency:** Acutely elevated BP (usually significantly >99th percentile for age and gender) with evidence of end-organ damage
      (1) Most commonly secondary to renal disease, catecholamine-producing tumors, endocrine syndromes, toxidromes, medication withdrawal, or elevated intracranial pressure (ICP)
      (2) Presents with encephalopathy (e.g., headaches, vomiting, seizures, altered mental status), vision disturbance, congestive heart failure (e.g., dyspnea, peripheral edema, gallop rhythm), and acute kidney injury
   c. **Hypertensive urgency:** Acutely elevated BP (usually >5 mmHg greater than the 99th percentile for age and gender) without evidence of end-organ damage
      (1) Most commonly primary hypertension in children >7 years age, followed by renal disease
      (2) Present with minor complaints (e.g., headaches, nausea)

2. **Management:**
   a. Rule out increased ICP before instituting antihypertensive treatment given critical need to maintain cerebral perfusion.
   b. Goal is to reduce BP by ≤**25%** in the **first 8 hours,** then gradual normalization over the next **24 to 48 hours.**
   c. See Table 1.8 for hypertensive emergency and urgency medications.

F. Pulmonary Embolism[34]

1. **Definition:** Acute obstruction of the pulmonary artery or one of its branches by material that originated downstream.
   a. Risk factors include central venous catheters, OCPs, cancer, immobility, infection, nephrotic syndrome, inflammatory conditions (lupus, IBD), recent surgery, preexisting DVT, and inherited thrombophilia syndromes.
   b. The classic triad of symptoms (pleuritic chest pain, shortness of breath, and hemoptysis) may not always be seen in children, who may only present with persistent tachypnea.
   c. Massive PE, defined as an embolus that completely obstructs pulmonary blood flow, can present with hemodynamic instability and sudden death.
   d. Assess for signs of respiratory distress.
   e. Diagnosis with CT-PA has high sensitivity and specificity. Evaluation may also include EKG, echocardiogram, CXR, or V/Q scan.

TABLE 1.8
HYPERTENSIVE CRISIS MEDICATIONS[13,33]

Drug	Dose	Pharmacokinetics	Mechanism	Side Effects
PARENTERAL THERAPY				
Esmolol	Bolus: 100–500 mCg/kg Infusion: 25–250 mCg/kg/min (max 1000 mCg/kg/min)	Onset: Immediate Duration: 10–30 min	β1 blocker	Bradycardia, bronchospasm (at high doses)
Hydralazine	0.1–0.2 mg/kg/dose IV/IM (max 2 mg/kg/dose or 20 mg) Q4–6 hr PRN	Onset: 5–30 min Duration: 1–4 hr	Direct arteriole vasodilator	Reflex tachycardia, flushing, lupus-like syndrome
Labetalol	Bolus: 0.2–1 mg/kg (max 40 mg) Infusion: 0.25–1 mg/kg/hr (max 3 mg/kg/hr)	Onset: 2–5 min Duration: 2–12 hr	β1, β2, and α1 blocker	Hyperkalemia, bronchospasm; caution in liver failure due to prolonged duration of action
Nicardipine	Start at 0.5–1 mCg/kg/min (max 5 mCg/kg/min or 15 mg/hr)	Onset: 5–15 min Duration: 4–6 hr	Calcium channel blocker	Reflex tachycardia
Nitroprusside	0.3–4 mCg/kg/min (max 10 mCg/kg/min)	Onset: 30 sec to 2 min Duration: 1–10 min	Arterial and venous vasodilation via NO	Cyanide toxicity
ENTERAL THERAPY				
Captopril	0.3–0.5 mg/kg (max 6 mg/kg/day or 450 mg/24 hr)	Onset: 15–30 min Duration: 2–6 hr	ACE inhibitor; lowers blood pressure without causing tachycardia	Hyperkalemia, neutropenia, angioedema, cough; contraindicated in bilateral renal artery stenosis or solitary kidney
Clonidine	1–10 mCg/kg/dose Q6–8 hr (max 25 mCg/kg/24 hr up to 0.8 mg/24 hr)	Onset: 30–60 min Duration: 6–10 hr	Central α agonist	Bradycardia, rebound hypertension, sedation
Nifedipine	0.1–0.25 mg/kg/dose Q4–6 hr PO/SL (max 10 mg/dose, 1–2 mg/kg/24 hr)	Onset: 15–30 min Duration: 4–6 hr	Calcium channel blocker	Precipitous hypotension, reflex tachycardia

ACE, Angiotensin-converting enzyme; *IM,* intramuscular; *IV,* intravenous; *mCg,* microgram; *NO,* nitric oxide; *PO,* oral; *PRN,* as needed; *SL,* sublingual.

(1) Normal D-dimer does not rule out PE.

(2) EKG can show right heart strain and/or atrial enlargement, sinus tachycardia, right axis deviation, RBBB, and ST-T segment changes as well as the classic S1-Q3-T3 pattern. Normal EKG does not rule out PE.

2. **Management:**
   a. Initiate anticoagulation with unfractionated heparin or low-molecular-weight heparin (see Formulary for dosing and monitoring).
   b. Medical thrombolysis using tissue plasminogen activator (alteplase) is indicated in PE with any hemodynamic instability.
   c. Surgical interventions such as thrombolysis, thrombectomy, or embolectomy are indicated in massive PE when medical thrombolysis is contraindicated.

G. Hypercyanotic Crisis ("Tet Spell")[22,35]

1. **Definition:** Cyanotic emergency secondary to an acute worsening of a preexisting right ventricular outflow tract obstruction (e.g., in a patient with tetralogy of Fallot) that prevents pulmonary blood flow and induces a right-to-left intracardiac shunt.
   a. Peak incidence occurs between 2 and 4 months of age.
   b. Usually occurs in the morning after crying, feeding, or defecation.
   c. Patients present with extreme cyanosis, hyperpnea, tachypnea, and agitation.
2. **Management:** Follow stepwise approach, escalating if spell is not broken.
   a. Make every effort to calm the child. Allow parent to comfort. Consider oral sucrose analgesia (e.g., Sweet-Ease).
   b. Bring knees to chest in infants or encourage squatting in older children to increase SVR and decrease shunting.
   c. Administer 100% oxygen **if patient tolerates**, although effect is limited given absence of effective pulmonary blood flow.
   d. For stepwise pharmacologic abortive management, see Table 1.9.
   e. Consider isotonic crystalloid resuscitation (5 to 10 mL/kg boluses) to ensure adequate preload if patient is dehydrated.
   f. Treat acidosis with sodium bicarbonate.
   g. For refractory spells, consider general anesthesia and emergent surgery for palliation with a systemic to pulmonary shunt or full repair.

H. Altered Level of Consciousness[22,36]

1. **Definition:** A spectrum of impaired consciousness spanning confusion, disorientation, agitation, stupor, lethargy, and coma.
   a. Fluctuations in level of consciousness are common and progression may occur rapidly.
   b. **Coma:** Refers to an unarousable state
   c. **Lethargy:** Refers to a depressed consciousness resembling sleep from which a patient can be aroused but immediately returns to depressed state

TABLE 1.9

HYPERCYANOTIC CRISIS ABORTIVE MEDICATIONS[22,35]

Medication	Dose	Comment
Ketamine	1—2 mg/kg IM or IV, administer IV dose over 60 sec	Sedating, increases SVR
Morphine	0.05—0.2 mg/kg IM, SUBQ or IV; do *not* wait for IV access	Calms agitation, suppresses hyperpnea Monitor for respiratory depression
Phenylephrine	5—20 mCg/kg IV bolus Max single dose 200 mCg	α Agonist, increases SVR
Propranolol	0.15—0.25 mg/kg, via slow IV push Max initial dose 1 mg	β Blockade decreases heart rate, promoting ventricular filling Monitor for hypotension

IM, Intramuscular; *IV,* intravenous; *SUBQ,* subcutaneous; *SVR,* systemic vascular resistance.

  d. **Stupor:** Refers to a state of depressed response to external stimuli but not totally asleep

  e. Standard descriptors of level of responsiveness include:

    (1) The **Glasgow Coma Scale** (and modified scale for infants): See Table 1.10 to score level of responsiveness.

    (2) **AVPU** mnemonic: Graded as **A** if alert, **V** if responsive to verbal stimulation, **P** if responsive to painful stimulation, or **U** if unresponsive

TABLE 1.10

COMA SCALES[20]

Grading	Glasgow Coma Scale	Modified Coma Scale for Infants
EYE OPENING		
4	Spontaneous	Spontaneous
3	To speech	To speech
2	To pain	To pain
1	None	None
VERBAL		
5	Oriented	Coos or babbles
4	Confused	Irritable
3	Inappropriate words	Cries to pain
2	Nonspecific sounds	Moans to pain
1	None	None
MOTOR		
6	Follows commands	Normal, spontaneous movements
5	Localizes pain	Withdraws to touch
4	Withdraws to pain	Withdraws to pain
3	Abnormal flexion	Abnormal flexion
2	Abnormal extension	Abnormal extension
1	None	None

Data from Shaw KN, Bachur RG. *Fleisher & Ludwig's Textbook of Pediatric Emergency Medicine.* 7th ed. Lippincott Williams & Wilkins; 2016.

   f. Broad differential considerations include **D**rugs, **I**nfection, **M**etabolic, and **S**tructural causes (DIMS).

   g. See Table 1.11 for common etiologies and targeted workup recommendations.

2. **Management:** Stabilize initially. Further management is aimed at correcting underlying etiology.

   a. **Airway, Breathing, Circulation:**

     (1) Administer supplemental oxygen to patients presenting with seizure or with signs of shock, regardless of pulse oximetry reading.

TABLE 1.11

ETIOLOGIES AND TARGETED EVALUATION OF ALTERED LEVEL OF CONSCIOUSNESS

Category	Etiologies	Workup
Drugs	Opiates (e.g., oxycodone, fentanyl, heroin) Sympathomimetics (e.g., cocaine, MDMA) Anticholinergics (e.g., diphenhydramine, TCAs) Cholinergics (e.g., organophosphates) Serotonin syndrome (e.g., SSRIs, dextromethorphan)	Urine toxicology screen Acetaminophen level ASA level Ethanol level ECG Blood gas Serum chemistry
Infection	Systemic sepsis Meningitis Encephalitis Abscess	Blood culture Complete blood count Urine analysis and culture CSF analysis and culture (if indicated)
Metabolic	Hypoglycemia Electrolyte abnormalities (e.g., hypernatremia/ hyponatremia) Uremic encephalopathy Hyperammonemic encephalopathy Diabetic ketoacidosis Inborn error of metabolism Hepatic failure Renal failure	Blood gas Lactate Glucose Electrolytes Liver enzymes Renal function Ammonia Serum amino acids Urine organic acids Acylcarnitine profile Coagulation studies Serum/urine osmolarity
Structural	Space-occupying lesions (e.g., tumor, blood, abscess, cyst, cerebral edema secondary to trauma) Obstructions to cerebral blood flow (e.g., thrombus, vasculitis)	Head CT or MRI
Other	Anoxia Hypothermia/hyperthermia Seizure/postictal state Psychiatric/psychogenic	EEG

ASA, Acetylsalicylic acid (aspirin); *CSF*, cerebral spinal fluid; *CT*, computed tomography; *ECG*, electrocardiogram; *EEG*, electroencephalogram; *MDMA*, 3,4-Methylenedioxymethamphetamine (ecstasy); *MRI*, magnetic resonance imaging; *SSRI*, selective serotonin reuptake inhibitor; *TCAs*, tricyclic antidepressants.

Data from Krmpotic K. A clinical approach to altered level of consciousness in the pediatric patient. *Austin Pediatr.* 2016;3(5):1046.

    (2) Intubation is indicated in patients unable to protect their airway.

    (3) Consider delaying administration of atropine unless necessary secondary to the loss of pupillary light reflex.

    (4) Avoid hypercarbia, maintaining $PaCO_2$ in normal range. Prophylactic hyperventilation is not recommended.

b. **Dextrose:** Correct hypoglycemia immediately with a 5 to 10 mL/kg bolus of 10% dextrose or 2 to 4 mL/kg of 25% dextrose. After bolus, start a continuous infusion of dextrose-containing fluids to avoid recurrent hypoglycemia.

c. **Imaging:** Request emergency head computed tomography (CT) if patient stable for transport. Consult with neurosurgical team if indicated.

d. **Hyponatremia:** Often asymptomatic unless sodium decreases rapidly or becomes severe (i.e., <125 mmol/L)

    (1) Treat **symptomatic** hyponatremia immediately with a 3 to 5 mL/kg bolus of 3% hypertonic saline over 15 to 30 minutes until seizure activity ceases or serum sodium level is >125 mmol/L.

    (2) See Chapter 11 for subsequent, slow correction of asymptomatic hyponatremia.

e. **Infection:** If presentation concerning for severe sepsis, treat empirically with broad-spectrum antibiotics (e.g., ceftriaxone and vancomycin) within the first hour. Include antiviral therapy (e.g., acyclovir) if viral encephalitis is suspected. Lumbar puncture should be performed only if there is no clinical suspicion of increased ICP and the patient is stable.

f. **Ingestion:** General management includes decreasing absorption, altering metabolism, and enhancing elimination.

    (1) Contact the regional poison control center for specific treatment recommendations.

    (2) See Chapter 3 for toxicology management.

g. **Naloxone:** If patients have a definite pulse but abnormal breathing or only gasping, administer opioid antagonist (full reversal: 0.1 mg/kg/dose IV/IM/subcutaneous [SUBQ], max 2 mg/dose) if opioid ingestion is suspected. Repeat dosing every 2 to 3 minutes. Short duration of action may necessitate multiple doses.

    (1) For patients in respiratory arrest, rescue breathing or bag-mask ventilation should be initiated.

    (2) For patients in cardiac arrest, in the absence of proven benefit from the use of naloxone, standard resuscitative measures should take priority over naloxone administration, with a focus on high-quality CPR.

h. **Thiamine:** Consider administration prior to glucose for patients with eating disorders, chronic disease, or alcoholism to prevent Wernicke encephalopathy.

i. If patient is an infant or toddler, consider evaluation for inborn error of metabolism, hepatic failure, renal failure, or nonaccidental trauma.

I. Status Epilepticus[37-38]

1. **Definition:** Prolonged seizure (clinical or electrographic) or recurrent seizure activity without return to baseline lasting **5 minutes** or more
   a. Common acute etiologies: Febrile seizures, metabolic disturbances, sepsis, head trauma, stroke/hemorrhage, drug toxicity, inadequate antiepileptic therapy, hypoxia, hypertensive encephalopathy, autoimmune encephalitis
   b. Common chronic etiologies: Preexisting epilepsy, tumor, stroke, inborn error of metabolism, ethanol abuse
2. **Management:** Timely administration of anticonvulsant therapy is associated with a greater likelihood of seizure termination and better neurologic outcomes. See Table 1.12 for timed evaluation and treatment outline.

J. Increased Intracranial Pressure[39-41]

1. **Definition:** An increase in the volume of an intracranial component (brain, blood, or cerebrospinal fluid) within the fixed volume of the skull that exceeds the limits of compensation, generally accepted as a sustained increase **≥20 mmHg**
   a. Intricately related to cerebral perfusion via the following equation:

Cerebral perfusion pressure (CPP) = Mean arterial pressure (MAP) − ICP

TABLE 1.12

STATUS EPILEPTICUS TREATMENT GUIDELINE[37-38]

IMMEDIATE APPROACH (0–5 MIN)

Management:

Protect airway, intubate if needed

Assess vitals

Bedside fingerstick blood glucose

Establish peripheral IV access: Administer emergent AED, fluid resuscitation, nutrient resuscitation (thiamine, dextrose)

Labs: laboratory blood glucose, CBC, BMP, calcium, magnesium, antiseizure medication drug levels

Medication	Dose	Comment
Diazepam	0.15–0.2 mg/kg IV (max 10 mg/dose)	Monitor for hypotension, respiratory depression
	2–5 years: 0.5 mg/kg PR (max 20 mg/dose)	
	6–11 years: 0.3 mg/kg PR (max 20 mg/dose)	
	≥12 years: 0.2 mg/kg PR (max 20 mg/dose)	
	May repeat dose once in 5 min	
Lorazepam	0.1 mg/kg IV (max 4 mg/dose)	Monitor for hypotension, respiratory depression
	May repeat dose once in 5–10 min	
Midazolam	0.2 mg/kg IV/IM/IN	Monitor for hypotension, respiratory depression
	0.5 mg/kg buccal	
	Max: 10 mg all forms	
	Single dose recommended	

URGENT APPROACH (5–15 MIN)

Management:

Secondary AED control therapy

Initiate vasopressor support if indicated

Neurological examination

CT if indicated

Labs: Liver function tests, coagulation studies, toxicology screen, inborn error of metabolism screening

Neurologic consultation

Medication	Dose	Comment
Fosphenytoin	20 mg PE/kg IV/IM (max 1500 mg PE/dose) May give additional 10 mg PE/kg repeat dose	Monitor for arrhythmia, hypotension Max administration rate 150 mg PE/min or 2 mg PE/kg/min
Levetiracetam	60 mg/kg IV (max 4500 mg/dose)	Minimal drug interactions Not hepatically metabolized
Phenobarbital	15–20 mg/kg IV (max 1000 mg/dose) May give additional 5–10 mg/kg repeat dose	Monitor for hypotension, respiratory depression
Phenytoin	20 mg/kg IV (max 1500 mg/dose) May give additional 10 mg/kg repeat dose	Monitor for arrhythmia, hypotension, purple glove syndrome
Valproic acid	20–40 mg/kg IV May give additional 20 mg/kg repeat dose (max 3000 mg/dose)	Use with caution in TBI Rarely used in children <2 years due to risk of fatal hepatotoxicity (see Formulary) Monitor for hyperammonemia, pancreatitis, hepatotoxicity, thrombocytopenia

REFRACTORY APPROACH (15–60 MIN)

Management:

Refractory AED control therapy

Continuous EEG monitoring if indicated

MRI if indicated

Lumbar puncture if indicated

Consider broad-spectrum antibiotics and antivirals if indicated

Intracranial pressure monitoring if indicated

Urinary catheter

Medication	Dose	Comment
Midazolam (continuous infusion)	Load: 0.2 mg/kg Infusion: 0.05–2 mg/kg/hr Breakthrough: 0.1–0.2 mg/kg bolus	Tachyphylaxis with prolonged use Monitor for respiratory depression, hypotension
Pentobarbital	Load: 5–15 mg/kg Infusion: 0.5–5 mg/kg/hr Breakthrough: 5 mg/kg bolus	Monitor for hypotension, respiratory depression, cardiac depression, paralytic ileus
Propofol	Load: 1–2 mg/kg Infusion: 20–65 mCg/kg/min Breakthrough: 1 mg/kg bolus	Monitor for hypotension, respiratory depression, cardiac failure, rhabdomyolysis, metabolic acidosis, renal failure, hypertriglyceridemia, pancreatitis (propofol-related infusion syndrome)

AED, Antiepileptic drug; *BMP,* basic metabolic panel; *CBC,* complete blood count; *CT,* computed tomography; *EEG,* electroencephalogram; *IM,* intramuscular; *IN,* intranasal; *IV,* intravenous; *mCg,* microgram; *PE,* phenytoin equivalent; *PR,* per rectum; *TBI,* traumatic brain injury.

b. Most commonly caused by brain trauma, tumors, or intracranial infections

c. Patients present with headache, diplopia, nausea, vomiting, or decreased level of consciousness.

d. Assess for signs of trauma, ataxia, pupillary asymmetry, papilledema, cranial nerve dysfunction, bulging fontanelle, or abnormal posturing.
   (1) Foramen magnum herniation: Hypertension, bradycardia, irregular respirations (Cushing triad)
   (2) Transtentorial herniation: Ipsilateral pupillary dilation, contralateral hemiparesis

e. Evaluation may include infectious studies, electrolytes, toxicology screen, and stat CT head. Lumbar puncture is contraindicated due to herniation risk if cause is obstructive.

2. **Management:** Adequate CPP **(>40 mmHg)** is critical to overcome the resistance of increased ICP.

a. Stabilize initially as per resuscitation guidelines.
   (1) Maintain normal oxygenation and ventilation to treat increased metabolic demand and avoid hypercarbia-related cerebral vasodilation.
   (2) Consider hyperventilation (EtCO$_2$ target between 25 and 30) for patients with **active** evidence of herniation. Prophylactic hyperventilation is otherwise not recommended.
   (3) Support MAP with adequate isotonic fluid resuscitation and vasoactive agents.

b. Consultation with neurosurgical team is recommended and required immediately if evidence of herniation is present.

c. Administer **mannitol** (0.5 to 1 g/kg) and/or **hypertonic saline** (5 to 10 mL/kg of 3% hypertonic saline) in case of acute neurologic deterioration or cerebral herniation.
   (1) Continuous infusions of 3% hypertonic saline (0.1 to 1.0 mL/kg/hr) may be titrated as necessary to maintain ICP less than 20 mmHg.
   (2) Rapid osmotic diuresis from mannitol may cause hypovolemia and hypotension, especially in polytrauma patients.

d. Request **noncontrast head CT** to evaluate for emergent surgical pathology.

e. Treat acute seizure activity given the associated increased cerebral metabolic rate and subsequent increased cerebral blood flow. Consider prophylactic antiseizure therapy (e.g., phenytoin, levetiracetam) if transport or delayed definitive care is anticipated.

f. Sedation and analgesia prevent increases in ICP related to pain and agitation, although benefit is balanced with risk of hypotension and alteration of neurologic exam.

g. Avoid secondary brain injury by maintaining neuroprotective parameters: Maintain head midline and elevated at 30 degrees, normoglycemia, normonatremia, normothermia, and correct acidosis.

   h. If elevated ICP is refractory to medical management, consider draining an existing ventriculoperitoneal shunt or acute neurosurgical intervention (external ventricular drain or decompressive craniectomy).

   i. For elevated ICP refractory to medical and surgical management, consider barbiturate coma.

IV. CRITICAL CARE REFERENCE DATA

1. Minute ventilation (V_E):

$$V_E = \text{Respiratory rate} \times \text{Tidal volume} (V_T)$$

2. Alveolar gas equation:

$$P_AO_2 = [FiO_2(P_{atm} - PH_2O)] - (P_aCO_2 / R)$$

   a. P_AO_2 = Alveolar partial pressure of oxygen
   b. FiO_2 = Inspired fraction of oxygen (0.21 at room air)
   c. P_{atm} = Atmospheric pressure (760 mmHg at sea level; adjust for high altitude)
   d. PH_2O = Water vapor pressure (47 mmHg)
   e. P_aCO_2 = Arteriolar partial pressure of carbon dioxide (measured via arterial blood gas)
   f. R = Respiratory quotient (0.8; CO_2 produced/O_2 consumed)

3. Alveolar-arterial oxygen gradient (A-a gradient):

$$A - a \text{ gradient} = P_AO_2 - P_aO_2$$

   a. P_AO_2 = Alveolar partial pressure of oxygen (estimated from alveolar gas equation)
   b. P_aO_2 = Arteriolar partial pressure of oxygen (measured via arterial blood gas)
   c. Normal gradient is 20 to 65 mmHg on 100% oxygen or 5 to 20 mmHg on room air.
   d. The A-a gradient is increased in hypoventilation, diffusion limitations, pulmonary blood-flow shunts, and ventilation/blood flow (V/Q) mismatch.

4. Oxygenation index (OI):

$$OI = P_{aw} \times FiO_2 \times 100/P_aO_2$$

   a. P_{aw} (mmHg) = Mean airway pressure
   b. OI >40 in hypoxemic respiratory failure is historically considered an indication for extracorporeal life support.

REFERENCES

A complete list of references can be found online.

Chapter 2

Traumatic Injuries

Radhika Ghodasara, MD

⊗ See additional content online.

I. COMPONENTS OF THE TRAUMA ASSESSMENT

A. Primary Survey

1. The primary survey involves assessment of ABCDE: Airway, Breathing, Circulation, Disability, Exposure.[1]
   a. **Airway:**
      (1) Can the patient maintain their own airway? Consider their neurologic status.
      (2) Is the airway patent? Is there an upper airway obstruction or stridor?
      (3) Do they have a head/neck injury that would make endotracheal intubation difficult? Will they need a surgical airway?
      (4) Ensure C-spine stability when assessing and managing a patient's airway.
      (5) Have backup—call anesthesia or an intensivist for difficult airways.
   b. **Breathing:**
      (1) Does the patient have an intervenable process (e.g., hemorrhagic, obstructive, compressive) affecting oxygenation/ventilation that can be addressed with rapid procedural intervention (such as a medical airway, needle decompression, or a chest tube)?
      (2) If the patient is not breathing on their own, is the bag-valve-mask ventilation technique being optimized until a more secure airway is placed? Confirm a good mask seal, appropriate patient positioning, appropriate respiratory rate and volume for age/size, equal chest rise, and end-tidal CO_2 monitoring.
   c. **Circulation:**
      (1) Is the patient actively hemorrhaging? Identify and control external bleeding quickly.
      (2) Does the patient show signs of pericardial tamponade (e.g. distended neck veins, distant heart sounds, and decreased pulse pressure)?
      (3) Assess for shock: hypotension, tachycardia, altered mental status, and decreased urine output. Does the patient have

access? Place two large-bore IVs. If intravenous access is difficult or limited, promptly consider intraosseous (IO) access.

(4) Are pulses strong or thready? Check centrally (carotid, femoral, brachial) and distally (radial, pedal). Is their skin warm or cool? Assess capillary refill.

(5) What are the vital signs? Tachycardia may be the only abnormal vital sign in early shock.

(6) Consider the need for fluid resuscitation and/or blood product administration. Cases of severe hemorrhage may benefit from early activation of massive transfusion protocols.

(7) Large-volume resuscitation is not a substitute for prompt control of external hemorrhage in the injured patient.

d. **Disability:**
   (1) What is the patient's neurologic status? Assess pupil size, symmetry, reactivity.
   (2) Calculate Glasgow Coma Score (see Chapter 1): "intubate when less than 8"; motor score may identify spinal cord injury.
   (3) What was the mechanism of the traumatic injury? (e.g., high-speed motor vehicle collision with traumatic brain injury or house fire with significant burns)
   (4) Does the patient need fast-acting pain control and/or sedation? Consider risk of respiratory depression with opioids. Confirm medical history and drug allergies when possible.

e. **Exposure:**
   (1) Expose skin completely for thorough evaluation. Remove injurious debris and clothing.
   (2) Could there have been a medication overdose or drug intoxication associated with the trauma?

2. Note: The Advanced Trauma Life Support algorithm developed by the American College of Surgeons continues to support prioritizing the rapid assessment and treatment of life-threatening airway and breathing problems ahead of circulation problems (ABC). For nontraumatic cardiorespiratory arrest, the circulation, airway, and breathing (CAB) sequence is currently in use by the American Heart Association as part of the Pediatric Advanced Life Support algorithm (see Chapter 1).

B. Secondary Survey (Fig. 2.1)

C. Labs/Workup to Consider in the Emergent Setting

1. Critical care labs: Hemoglobin, blood gas, lactate, glucose, electrolytes
2. Coagulation studies (PT, aPTT, INR, fibrinogen): especially for operative planning
3. Type and screen/cross: Preparing crossmatched blood is important for anticipated surgical intervention. Emergency blood release may be needed in cases of severe hemorrhage.

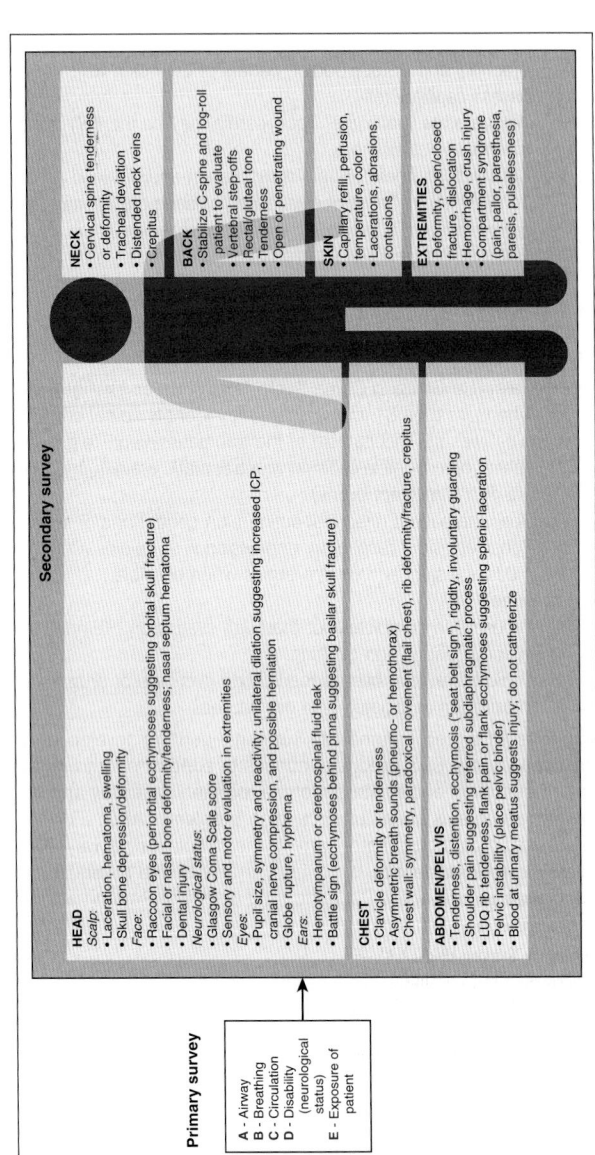

Primary survey

A - Airway
B - Breathing
C - Circulation
D - Disability (neurological status)
E - Exposure of patient

Secondary survey

HEAD
Scalp:
• Laceration, hematoma, swelling
• Skull bone depression/deformity
Face:
• Raccoon eyes (periorbital ecchymoses suggesting orbital skull fracture)
• Facial or nasal bone deformity/tenderness; nasal septum hematoma
• Dental injury
Neurological status:
• Glasgow Coma Scale score
• Sensory and motor evaluation in extremities
Eyes:
• Pupil size, symmetry and reactivity; unilateral dilation suggesting increased ICP, cranial nerve compression, and possible herniation
• Globe rupture, hyphema
Ears:
• Hemotympanum or cerebrospinal fluid leak
• Battle sign (ecchymoses behind pinna suggesting basilar skull fracture)

CHEST
• Clavicle deformity or tenderness
• Asymmetric breath sounds (pneumo- or hemothorax)
• Chest wall: symmetry, paradoxical movement (flail chest), rib deformity/fracture, crepitus

ABDOMEN/PELVIS
• Tenderness, distention, ecchymosis ("seat belt sign"), rigidity, involuntary guarding
• Shoulder pain suggesting referred subdiaphragmatic process
• LUQ rib tenderness, flank pain or flank ecchymoses suggesting splenic laceration
• Pelvic instability (place pelvic binder)
• Blood at urinary meatus suggests injury; do not catheterize

NECK
• Cervical spine tenderness or deformity
• Tracheal deviation
• Distended neck veins
• Crepitus

BACK
• Stabilize C-spine and log-roll patient to evaluate
• Vertebral step-offs
• Rectal/gluteal tone
• Tenderness
• Open or penetrating wound

SKIN
• Capillary refill, perfusion, temperature, color
• Lacerations, abrasions, contusions

EXTREMITIES
• Deformity, open/closed fracture, dislocation
• Hemorrhage, crush injury
• Compartment syndrome (pain, pallor, paresthesia, paresis, pulselessness)

FIGURE 2.1
Trauma secondary survey.

4. Lactate: If level is elevated, consider poor tissue perfusion, organ/vascular injury, internal hemorrhage.
5. Urinalysis: Hematuria may indicate kidney, urinary tract, or pelvic injury.
6. Creatinine and BUN (acute kidney injury); liver transaminases (direct liver trauma or shock liver); lipase (traumatic pancreatitis)
7. CBC: Initial hemoglobin can be normal in acute hemorrhage.
8. Pregnancy test: Obtain for all females of child-bearing age.

II. HEAD AND NECK TRAUMA

A. Head Imaging

1. PECARN algorithm developed by the Pediatric Emergency Care Applied Research Network (Fig. 2.2)[2]
   a. A well-validated, pediatric clinical decision aid that predicts need for computed tomography (CT) head imaging after pediatric head injury by assessing risk factors
   b. Allows providers to identify pediatric patients at very low risk of clinically important traumatic brain injuries (ciTBI)
   c. CT imaging carries known risks of lethal radiation-induced malignancy, which is higher in children than adults (the risk decreases with age).
   d. Only applies to children with GCS scores ≥14.
2. If signs of traumatic brain injury on CT, consider consultation with pediatric intensivists, neurosurgery, and/or trauma surgery.
   a. For management of increased intracranial pressure, see Chapter 1.

B. Cervical Spine and Neck Imaging

1. There are currently no unified protocols or clinical guidelines for pediatric cervical spine clearance after blunt trauma.[3]
2. Based on Pediatric Emergency Care Applied Research Network (PECARN) C-spine criteria,[3] consider obtaining imaging if any of the following are present in a pediatric patient:
   a. Altered mental status
   b. Focal neurologic deficits
   c. Complaint of neck pain
   d. Torticollis
   e. Substantial injury to the torso
   f. Predisposing condition
   g. High-risk motor vehicle crash
   h. Diving accident
3. Of note, many institutions alternatively or adjunctly use NEXUS criteria for clinical C-spine clearance, though it is not validated in children ≤8 years.[3]

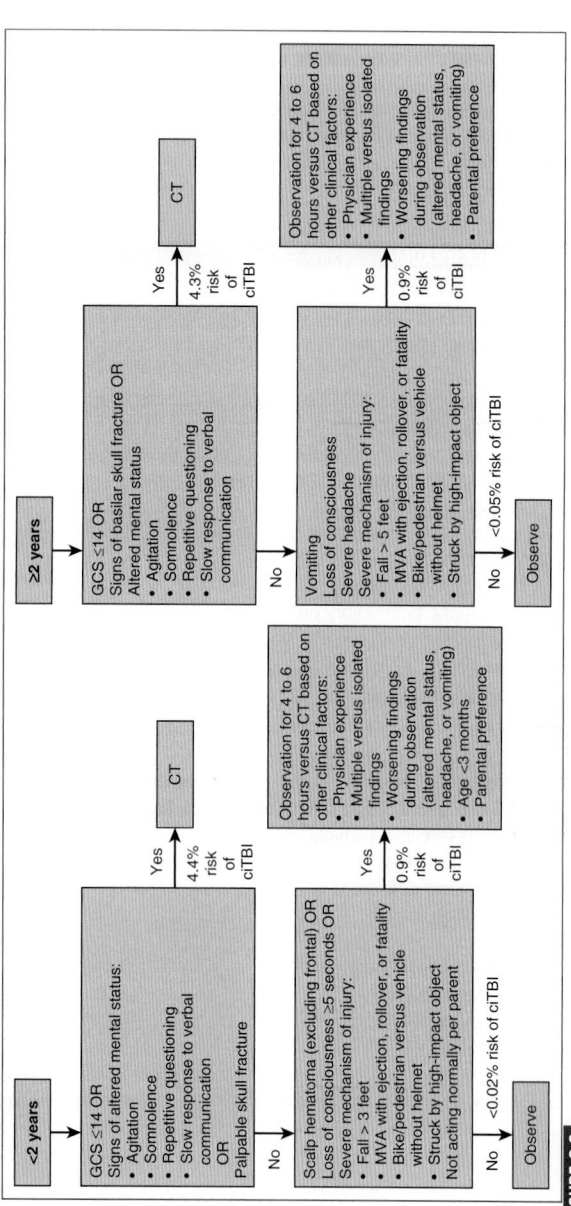

FIGURE 2.2

PECARN algorithm for identifying children at very low risk of clinically important traumatic brain injury (ciTBI).[2]

The criteria state that if any of the below are present, imaging is indicated[4,5]:

   a. Midline cervical tenderness

   b. Altered level of alertness

   c. Evidence of intoxication

   d. Neurologic deficit

   e. Presence of a painful distracting injury

4. Unlike the NEXUS criteria, the PECARN criteria include consideration of mechanism of injury and suggest that cervical spine imaging should be considered even in those who cooperate and are pain free if a high-risk mechanism of injury exists.

5. Recent guidelines by the Pediatric Cervical Spine Clearance Working Group Algorithm[6] additionally highlight the following factors:

   a. When clinical C-spine clearance is not possible, the preferred imaging modality for children who are ≤3 years old is radiography (see Chapter 26).

   b. Clinical clearance can be done regardless of mechanism of injury in a child who is ≥3 years old if they are asymptomatic with normal mental status and normal physical examination.

   c. Clinical clearance cannot be performed if the child or their parent reports persistent neck pain, abnormal head posture, or difficulty in neck movement.

6. Other clinical considerations[7]:

   a. Evaluate carefully children who display marking from seatbelt restraints in a motor vehicle collision, as this may indicate that extreme flexion of the cervical spine has occurred.

   b. It should be stressed that the subsequent development of neck tenderness is an important diagnostic sign. Parents should always be encouraged to return to care if pain develops later or the child develops reluctance to move their neck.

C. Specific Imaging Studies

1. A C-spine x-ray with minimum of two views (lateral, anteroposterior, and/ or odontoid views) has 90% sensitivity in identifying bony cervical spine injury.[8]

2. Consider CT scan if there is high level of concern for a cervical vertebrae fracture and plain radiographs are inconclusive.[9]

3. Consider magnetic resonance imaging (MRI) scan for further evaluation of ligamentous and cervical spinal cord injury.[9,10]

4. 30%–40% of children with traumatic myelopathy have SCIWORA (spinal cord injury without radiographic abnormality)—clinical symptoms of traumatic myelopathy with no radiographic or CT features of spinal fracture or instability. MRI should be considered in these cases.[11]

   a. SCIWORA is most common in children 8 years of age and under.

5. If signs of spinal column or vascular injury on imaging, consider consultation by trauma, vascular, spine, and/or head and neck surgeon.

III. CONCUSSION

A. Concussion Evaluation

1. Concussions can encompass a constellation of symptoms following traumatic head injury, thought to result from neurometabolic dysfunction rather than structural injury. They are typically associated with normal structural neuroimaging findings. Most concussion symptoms clinically resolve in 1 to 3 weeks.[12]
2. Concussion symptoms can be physical, cognitive, emotional, or related to sleep:[13]
    a. Headache
    b. Feeling foggy, fatigued
    c. Confusion, difficulty focusing
    d. Photophobia, phonophobia
    e. Forgetfulness
    f. Nausea ± vomiting
3. Patients with symptoms lasting more than 3 weeks, worsening symptoms, or history of multiple concussions may benefit from a more detailed, longitudinal assessment by a medical provider (pediatrician, neurologist, sports medicine specialist, concussion specialist).[13]
4. The Centers for Disease Control and Prevention (CDC) HEADS UP website is a valuable resource center grounded in an education campaign focused on increasing awareness of concussion among children to prevent and reduce adverse outcomes.[14]
5. The CDC's Acute Concussion Evaluation (ACE) is a tool that can be used in multiple settings, including the clinic and emergency department. The form provides a thorough definition of what a concussion is and signs/symptoms for which to assess. There is also an ACE care plan for patients to help guide their recovery.[14]
6. CDC's HEADS UP resource links for patients and providers:
    a. General website: https://www.cdc.gov/headsup
    b. ACE Forms and Work/School Care Plans: https://www.cdc.gov/headsup/providers/tools.html

B. Return-to-School and Return-to-Play Guidelines (Table 2.1)

1. The overarching goal is to allow healing from injury and prevent cumulative brain trauma.

IV. INTRATHORACIC, ABDOMINAL, AND PELVIC TRAUMA[16]

A. Assessment and Management Pearls

1. See Fig. 2.1 for physical exam findings during the secondary survey.
2. Tension pneumothorax or massive hemothorax

TABLE 2.1

RETURN-TO-PLAY AND RETURN-TO-SCHOOL FOR CONCUSSION

Return-to-School Guidelines[13]	Return-to-Play Guidelines[15]
• If symptoms affect concentration or if unable to tolerate stimulation for more than 30 minutes without symptoms, encourage rest with light mental activities, so long as symptoms are not provoked or worsened. Minimize computer use, texting/phone use, television, and video games.	6 gradual steps to help safely return an athlete to play:
	• Steps should not be completed in one day but instead over days, weeks, or months as tolerated by the individual.
	• Move to the next level of activity only if no new/worsening symptoms are experienced.
	• If symptoms return/worsen, patients should stop activities and notify a medical provider for clinical reevaluation.
• If able to tolerate stimulation for minimum of 30—45 min without symptoms, consider returning to learning with modifications—see below.	• After rest and resolution of symptoms, patients should resume play at the previous tolerated step of the return to play guidelines.
• Students should be performing at their academic baseline before returning to sports, full physical activity, or other extracurricular activities.	**Step 1:** Back to regular activities (such as school)
	Step 2: Light aerobic activity
• Most students with a concussion will recover within 3 weeks.	• 5—10 minutes of walking, light jogging, light stationary biking
	• No weightlifting
• For students with symptoms lasting longer than 3 weeks, consider further medical management and accommodations	**Step 3:** Moderate activity
Suggested school modifications:	• Incorporating more head or body movement
• Shortened school days	• Moderate jogging, brief running, moderate-intensity stationary biking, moderate-intensity weightlifting (reduced time and/or reduced weight from typical routine)
• Frequent breaks during classes	
• Extra time to complete assignments	**Step 4:** Heavy noncontact activity
• Decreased homework load	• Sprinting/running, high-intensity stationary biking, regular weightlifting routine, noncontact sport-specific drills
• No significant examinations or standardized testing at this time	**Step 5:** Full contact in controlled practice
• Consider 504 Plan and/or Individualized Education Plan (IEP)	**Step 6:** Full contact in competition/game play

    a. Symptoms: Respiratory distress, unequal/abnormal breath sounds, hypotension, tachycardia, altered mental status

    b. Iatrogenic causes: Positive-pressure-related barotrauma, procedures (subclavian or internal jugular central line placement), following CPR

    c. Traumatic causes: Penetrating or blunt trauma, rib fractures

    d. Emergent treatment: Immediate needle decompression (tension pneumothorax), chest tube placement (pneumothorax, hemothorax), volume resuscitation/blood transfusion (hemothorax)

3. Cardiac tamponade

    a. Symptoms: Chest pain, difficulty breathing, muffled/distant heart sounds, tachycardia, hypotension, altered mental status, electrical alternans on ECG/cardiac telemetry

    b. Emergent treatment: Pericardiocentesis, volume resuscitation

4. Aortic dissection
   a. Symptoms: Severe chest/abdominal pain, shortness of breath, loss of consciousness, stroke symptoms, pulse differential between arms or between arms and legs, poor distal perfusion, leg pain, difficulty walking
   b. More stable patients can be considered for inotropy-reducing treatment (β-blockers) and endovascular repair.
   c. Transfer should be initiated to the nearest trauma center if indicated and possible.
   d. Hemodynamically unstable patients with concern for dissection should be taken to the operating room for laparotomy/thoracotomy.
5. Rib fractures and flail chest
   a. Patients with multiple acute rib fractures typically warrant admission to a pediatric trauma center for:
      (1) Pain control to improve respiratory function
      (2) Age-appropriate pulmonary physiotherapy to prevent atelectasis
   b. Splinting rib fractures with external devices can worsen ventilatory compromise and should be avoided.
   c. Patients with rib fractures who require tube thoracostomy to relieve pneumo- or hemothorax should have tubes placed at sites separate from the areas of fracture.
   d. Children younger than 3 years of age with rib fractures and without a history of high-force trauma warrant evaluation for possible child abuse.
   e. Children with flail chest (which occurs when the chest wall loses stability as the result of multiple rib fractures) should receive respiratory support. Those with respiratory distress or failure should be intubated and receive positive-pressure ventilation for adequate oxygenation and ventilation as well as to optimally expand and internally splint the injured segments.
   f. Due to more compliant chest walls, more kinetic energy can be transmitted to the intrathoracic structures without thoracic bony injury in children. For this reason, pulmonary contusion without rib fracture occurs more often in children than adults. Significant force is required to produce thoracic bony injury in children.
6. Abdominal injury (vascular, bowel or other organ) requiring surgery
   a. PECARN rule for blunt abdominal trauma
      (1) A pediatric patient with all of the below patient history and physical examination findings (without laboratory or ultrasonographic information) has a very low risk for intra-abdominal injury (IAI) requiring acute intervention (99% sensitivity in internal and external retrospective validation studies).[17,18]
         (a) No evidence of abdominal wall trauma or seatbelt sign
         (b) Glasgow Coma Scale score greater than 13
         (c) No abdominal tenderness
         (d) No evidence of thoracic wall trauma

(e) No complaints of abdominal pain
(f) No decreased breath sounds
(g) No vomiting

b. Peritonitis (severe pain, abdominal wall guarding/rigidity, avoidance of motion, flexed hips to relieve abdominal wall tension, hypoactive-to-absent bowel sounds, distention) can indicate intra-abdominal vascular or organ/bowel injury.

(1) Peritonitis due to intra-abdominal hemorrhage may take several hours to develop.

c. "Seatbelt sign" (bruising/visible injury in the distribution of a seatbelt restraint) is a significant predictive factor for surgical abdominal injury after blunt trauma (sensitivity 70.6%, specificity 82.4%).[19]

d. Emergency laparotomy is the accepted standard of care in patients with a penetrating torso injury who are hemodynamically unstable and have a clinical indication for exploratory laparotomy, such as evisceration or gastrointestinal bleeding.

7. Unstable pelvic fracture
   a. Place a pelvic stabilization device.
   b. Can be associated with pelvic organ injury, internal bleeding, and/or urinary tract injury

B. Imaging Studies to Consider

1. Ultrasound—FAST (focused assessment with sonography in trauma) exam
   a. May identify free fluid early and guide need for further imaging, observation, or surgery
   b. In a 2017 randomized trial of 925 hemodynamically stable children comparing standard trauma workup or standard workup plus FAST, there was no difference in the proportion obtaining CT, missed intra-abdominal injury (IAI), length of stay, or cost.[20]
   c. In a 2021 systematic review and meta-analysis of hemodynamically stable pediatric patients presenting with blunt abdominal trauma, the FAST exam had a pooled sensitivity of 35% and specificity of 96% for IAI.[21]
      (1) A positive FAST examination result means that IAI is likely and could warrant CT imaging.
      (2) A negative examination result alone cannot preclude further diagnostic workup (e.g., CT scan, serial FAST exams).
      (3) See Fig. 2.3 for an algorithm that incorporates the FAST exam and other findings to identify patients at very low risk for IAI.[22]

2. Radiographs
   a. Chest x-ray: Evaluate for rib fracture, pneumothorax/hemothorax, pulmonary contusion, pneumomediastinum.
   b. Abdominal and pelvic x-rays: Evaluate for free air, fluid, pelvic fracture.

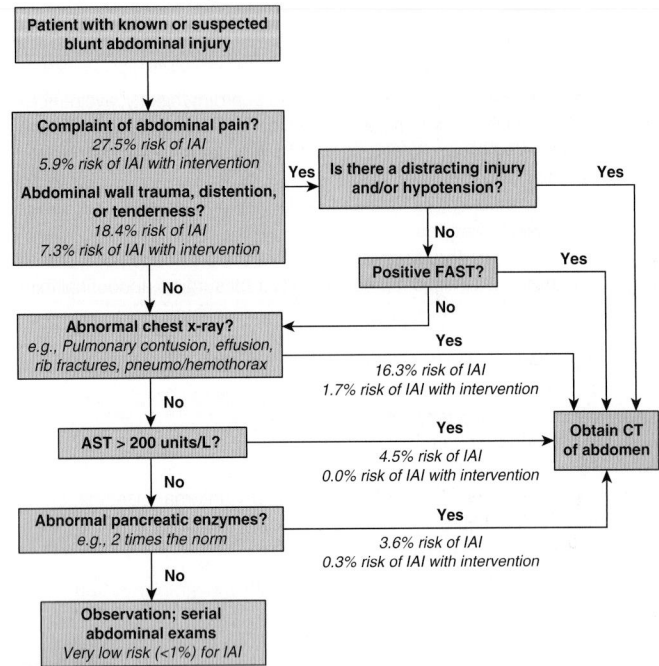

FIGURE 2.3

Workup of intra-abdominal injury (IAI) in pediatric blunt abdominal trauma.[22]

3. Abdominal/pelvic CT with IV contrast:
   a. CT is the gold standard for diagnosis of IAI; however, radiographs should be obtained first if there is concern for additional injuries that would compromise clinical stability.
   b. CT is commonly used to rule out IAI in children, despite associated cost and radiation exposure. The Pediatric Surgery Research Collaborative developed a clinical prediction rule to identify children at very low risk for IAI after blunt abdominal trauma, for whom a CT scan of the abdomen could be avoided. (Fig. 2.3).[22]
      (1) The algorithm includes 5 clinical factors associated with IAI in the order of availability: reported abdominal pain, abnormal abdominal exam, abnormal chest x-ray, AST >200 U/L, and abnormal pancreatic enzymes.
   c. In stable patients with blunt abdominal trauma, CT with routine oral contrast is not necessarily indicated, whereas IV contrast should be used to help to identify visceral, vascular, or bowel injury.
   d. For penetrating abdominal trauma (gunshot wounds, impalement, stab wounds), triple contrast (oral, rectal, IV) CT can be used to

identify peritoneal penetration or intra-abdominal organ injury in stable patients.

e. If gross hematuria or urinalysis with microscopic hematuria ≥50 RBCs per high-powered field, the patient may have genitourinary tract trauma. Consider CT pelvis with/without IV contrast or serial urinalyses/physical exams in consultation with surgery or urology.

4. If any workup is positive for thoracic or abdominal trauma, immediate consultation with nearest pediatric trauma center/surgeon is indicated if not available on site.

V. LIMB AND LONG BONE TRAUMA[16]

A. Assessment and Management Pearls

1. See Fig. 2.1 for physical exam findings during the secondary assessment.
2. Children are difficult to examine, especially when they are in pain. A painful orthopedic injury can distract from other internal injury.
3. Neurovascular assessment:
   a. Choose motor/sensory tests that are easy to perform quickly.
   b. Use Doppler to aid in identifying pulses and monitoring for compartment syndrome.
4. Bleeding
   a. Consider arterial bleed if absent pulses and cool extremity with bleeding.
   b. Consider venous bleed if persistent pulse with bleeding.
   c. Obtain time of tourniquet placement if done in prehospital setting.
5. Compartment syndrome:
   a. Circumferential, constrictive swelling leads to vascular and nerve compromise.
   b. Can develop soon after significant trauma—especially in crush injuries, burns, animal bites/stings, vascular injuries of limbs, long bone fractures, limb gunshot wounds
   c. Symptoms include pain (especially out of proportion to apparent injury or with passive extension), paresthesias, pallor, pulselessness (if unable to palpate pulse, use Doppler), paresis
6. If signs/symptoms of compartment syndrome or fracture, immediate consultation with an orthopedic surgeon is recommended.
7. Consider need for tetanus prophylaxis. Refer to Chapter 16 for details.

B. Imaging

1. Children's bones are less densely calcified, have thickened periosteum, and have growth plates, all of which increase their vulnerability to fractures.
2. Consider obtaining radiographs if bony point tenderness or deformity, decreased sensation, decreased range of motion, or overlying skin discoloration.
3. Radiographs with anterior-posterior (AP) and lateral views ± oblique and including areas above and below the suspected area of injury are recommended.

C. Traumatic Fractures in Children

1. Physeal or Salter-Harris fractures: Fractures involving growth plates (see Chapter 26)
2. Plastic fractures: Pliability of bones in response to compressive and transverse forces
   a. Torus or buckle fracture: Compression injury with buckled cortex
   b. Greenstick fracture: Fracture on one side of the diaphysis with cortex intact on other side of diaphysis
   c. Bowing or bending fractures
3. Avulsion fractures: Tendon or ligament dislodging a bone fragment-these are more common among adolescents participating in sports.
4. Dislocations in children are relatively unusual, generally related to major trauma, and associated with fractures. This is due to stronger ligaments with comparatively less bony strength.
   a. Subluxation of the radial head or "nursemaid elbow" reduction can often be done by an emergency provider. Most other dislocations should be referred to orthopedic surgery.
5. See Chapter 4 for basic splinting and musculoskeletal procedures.

D. Fractures Requiring Urgent Orthopedic Surgeon Consultation

1. Open fractures
2. Unacceptably displaced fractures
3. Fractures with associated neurovascular compromise (consider emergent reduction to improve neurovascular status if orthopedic surgery is not available on site)
4. Significant growth plate or joint injuries
5. Complete or displaced fractures of the long bones of the extremities
6. Pelvic fractures (other than minor avulsions)
7. Spinal fractures
8. Dislocations of major joints other than the shoulder

E. Fractures That Are Appropriate to Manage Acutely With Outpatient Referral to Orthopedics (Table 2.2)

VI. DENTAL TRAUMA

A. Components of a Tooth (Fig. 2.4)
B. Differences Between Primary and Permanent Teeth (Fig. 2.5)

1. Primary teeth appear 6 months to 3 years of age, are relatively smaller, thinner, and whiter; the roots are shorter and the front teeth have a smooth biting surface.
2. Permanent teeth appear 6 years to 21 years of age, relatively larger with a longer root; front teeth have a ridged biting surface.

C. Dental Injuries

1. Avulsion[23]
   a. Complete displacement of the tooth and its root from the bony alveolar socket

TABLE 2.2

COMMON PEDIATRIC ORTHOPEDIC INJURIES AND MANAGEMENT

Injury	ED Management	Follow-Up
Clavicle fracture without tenting or displacement (if present, orthopedic surgery consultation required)	Sling	Primary care provider in 2 weeks
Acromioclavicular joint separation	Sling	Orthopedics within 1 week
Proximal humerus fracture without deformity, displacement, or neurovascular injury	Sling	Orthopedics within 1 week
Distal radius or ulna fracture without deformity, displacement, or neurovascular injury	Volar splint	Orthopedics within 1 week
Salter-Harris Type 1—Distal radius	Volar splint	Orthopedics within 1 week
Salter-Harris Type 1—Distal fibula	Posterior splint, crutches	Orthopedics within 1 week
Distal radius buckle fracture without deformity, displacement, or neurovascular injury	Volar splint	Orthopedics within 1 week
Phalanx fractures without displacement or open deformity	Splint/buddy tape	Primary care provider in 2 weeks

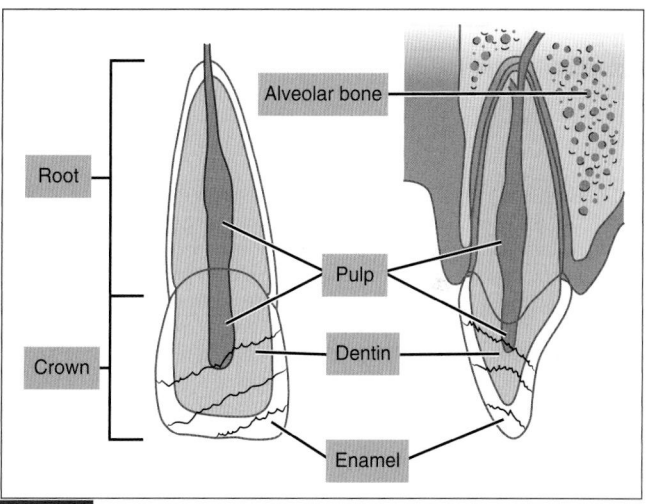

FIGURE 2.4

Normal anatomy of a tooth.[16]

b. If a primary tooth, reimplantation should not be attempted and outpatient dental follow-up is appropriate.
c. If a permanent tooth, this is a dental emergency. If possible and safe, immediate reimplantation should occur within 60 minutes to maximize tooth and periodontal ligament viability.

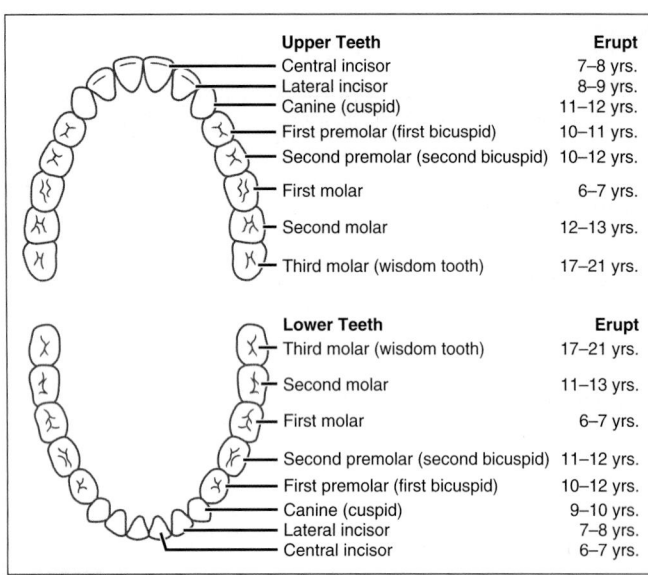

FIGURE 2.5

Development from primary to permanent teeth by location. (Modified from American Dental Association. https://www.mouthhealthy.org)

 (1) Good prognosis is very much dependent on early actions and reimplantation at the place of accident or during emergency care management.

 d. For a permanent tooth, reimplantation should always be attempted. If reimplantation is not possible, place the tooth in a suitable storage medium (in descending order of preference: milk, Hank's balanced salt solution, expectorated saliva, saline) and refer to a dentist emergently for reimplantation and splinting.

  (1) Situations when reimplantation is not indicated: primary tooth avulsion, severe caries or periodontal disease, an uncooperative patient, risk of choking, severe cognitive impairment, sedation, immunosuppression, severe cardiac conditions, unstable patient

 e. Reimplantation steps:

  (1) Pick up the avulsed tooth by the crown and avoid touching the root.

  (2) Wash the tooth and alveolar socket with sterile saline, removing clotted blood if necessary.

(3) Administer local anesthesia (without a vasoconstrictor) into the gum if necessary.

(4) Insert the root into the alveolar socket with concave part facing the tongue, and apply slight manual pressure.

(5) Ask the patient to bite on gauze or cloth to hold it in position.

(6) The patient should be seen by a dentist or dental professional emergently for splinting and follow-up care.

2. Luxation[24]

  a. Luxation injuries result from physical displacement of tooth within the alveolar socket itself. Luxation can be associated with tearing of the periodontal ligament or injury to the alveolar bone.

    (1) Luxation injuries are the most common traumatic dental injuries in the primary dentition.

  b. Primary tooth:

    (1) If tooth is loose and there is an increased risk of aspiration, the tooth may be extracted by using firm pressure with gauze.

    (2) If tooth is not loose, it may need repositioning and splinting.

    (3) In both situations, refer to a dentist for evaluation within 48 hours.

  c. Permanent tooth:

    (1) Immediate dental evaluation required if significant tooth mobility; otherwise, outpatient evaluation within 48 hours is appropriate

3. Subluxation[24]

  a. Subluxation is characterized by tooth injury with minor mobility but without displacement.

  b. Regardless of whether permanent or primary tooth, outpatient dental follow-up, ideally within 48 hours, is needed to rule out root fracture.

4. Tooth fracture[24]

  a. Classify the fracture per involvement of enamel, dentin, and pulp.

  b. For management guidelines, see Table 2.3.

D. Anticipatory Guidance Following Dental Trauma

1. Avoid contact sports until cleared by a dentist

TABLE 2.3

TOOTH FRACTURE TYPES AND FOLLOW-UP RECOMMENDATIONS[26]

Fracture Type	Follow-Up Recommendations
Enamel fracture	Dental evaluation outpatient for possible binding of tooth fragment, if available
Enamel-dentin fracture	Dental evaluation 48–72 hr to place a dressing of calcium hydroxide to prevent injury to the pulp
Enamel-dentin-pulp fracture	Immediate dental evaluation within 48 hr
Alveolar ridge fracture	Emergent dental evaluation

2. Analgesics as needed for pain control (e.g., acetaminophen, ibuprofen, cold compresses)
3. Soft diet
4. Use a soft toothbrush, if able to brush teeth.
5. Regular follow-up with a dentist

VII. OPHTHALMOLOGIC TRAUMA[16]

A. Chemical Injury to the Eye

1. Immediate and continued irrigation of eyes with water, isotonic saline, or lactated Ringer's solution is necessary.
2. Consult with Poison Control.
    a. Call (800) 222-1222—will route to local center.
    b. Available 24 hours a day
3. Determine if substance is an acid or alkali. Alkali solutions tend to be more damaging because they penetrate more deeply.
    a. Obtain a baseline pH by touching Litmus paper to the conjunctiva. This is a crude but practical way to determine the type of substance if otherwise unknown.
        (1) Consider acidic substance if pH <7, and alkali if >7.4.
        (2) Continue irrigation for a minimum of 20 minutes or until 2 liters of fluid have been used to irrigate the eye(s).
        (3) Evert the eyelid and continue lavage.
        (4) Remeasure pH every 15 to 30 minutes until pH becomes neutral (7.0 to 7.4). Normalization of pH for most eye exposures typically takes 30 to 60 minutes.
4. Measure and trend visual acuity if possible.
5. Urgent ophthalmologic evaluation should be considered in cases with severe vision changes or vision loss, uncontrolled pain, significant mucosal injury, or persistent pH abnormality despite diligent irrigation.
6. In the United States, injury from chemical ocular burns occurs most often in residential settings, with preschool-aged children being the most common victims.[16]

B. Ruptured Globe

1. A ruptured globe is caused by laceration or puncture of the cornea and/or sclera following projectile or blunt trauma.
2. Warrants emergent ophthalmology consultation.
3. Key physical exam findings include teardrop-shaped pupil pointing toward perforation, hyphema (hemorrhage in the anterior chamber), subconjunctival hemorrhage, severe pain, decreased visual acuity, edema.
    a. When hyphema is present, sickle cell trait is a significant risk factor for complications including secondary hemorrhage, increased intraocular pressure, and permanent visual impairment in children.[25]

4. Stop the exam and place a rigid eye shield. Do not instill eye drops.
5. Elevate the head of the bed.
6. Keep patient as calm as possible and control symptoms (e.g., antiemetics and pain control) to avoid increased globe pressure and further extrusion of vitreous/aqueous humor.
7. Administer appropriate antibiotics.

C. Corneal Abrasion

1. Symptoms: Red eye with tearing, intense pain, resistance to eye opening, photophobia, foreign body sensation
2. Consider application of topical anesthetic before examination, which can support diagnosis if providing immediate relief.
   a. Although topical anesthetic eye drops may be used during the initial examination, they should not be regularly used or prescribed for the treatment of corneal abrasion pain due to risk of patient misuse or complications. Repeat application of an ocular anesthetic can delay or compromise healing and increase infection risk.
3. Evert eyelids to look for retained foreign body; irrigate eye if necessary.
4. Apply fluorescein staining and examine with Wood's lamp. Focal uptake indicates abrasion.
   a. Staining should be deferred until the eye examination is complete and an open globe is excluded.
5. Treatment: Artificial tears and/or ophthalmic ointment for lubrication, topical ophthalmic antibiotic ointment, oral analgesics or ophthalmic NSAIDs, ophthalmologic follow-up as indicated, ± patching depending on severity or patient cooperation.
6. Consider ophthalmologic consultation in the ED if concern for larger corneal abrasions associated with vision changes, corneal laceration, ulceration, embedded foreign body, or prolonged healing (i.e., symptoms not improving after several days).

D. Eyelid Glued Shut due to Cyanoacrylate (Superglue)

1. Can consider trimming eyelashes as needed with blunt-tip scissors. Do not try to force eyes open.
2. Consider ophthalmology consultation, especially in the case of glue bonding to the eye.
3. The use of around-the-clock eye/mucosa-safe oil-based ointments can help accelerate dissolution of the glue bonds. Can cover eye with gauze or a patch to prevent the patient from touching it.
4. Consider consultation with ophthalmology if a few days of ointment is unsuccessful.
5. A 2017 report by physicians at the University of Alabama at Birmingham Hospital discusses the Jameson muscle hook technique, which has been successfully used there without complications to safely relieve eyelid adhesions due to cyanoacrylate glue without the use of general anesthesia in pediatric and adult patients.[26]

a. With this method, topical anesthetic is applied through an explored opening in the eye. Then, a Jameson muscle hook is inserted into an opening between the eyelids and pulled parallel to the lid margins through the site of adhesion, while counter pressure is applied against the direction of the hook.

E. Eyelid Laceration

1. Do not initiate closure of an eyelid laceration prior to excluding injury to the globe or foreign body.
   a. Ocular injury (i.e., open globe, traumatic hyphema, corneal abrasion) may accompany eyelid laceration in up to two-thirds of cases.
2. Consult with ophthalmology if full-thickness lacerations (exposed adipose tissue), laceration through the lid margin, lacerations involving lacrimal canaliculi (medial third of the upper/lower lids), ptosis (unequal lifting of lids with upward gaze would suggest this), or other concerning symptoms.
3. Lacerations to the eyelid should be repaired within 24 hours of injury to prevent scarring and promote appropriate alignment of the eyelid tissues.
4. Superficial, simple lacerations that are horizontal, follow the skin lines, and involve less than 25% of the lid will usually heal well without suturing. Providers can use antibiotic ointment or adhesive surgical tape (i.e., Steri-strips) to approximate wound edges.

F. Orbital Floor Fractures

1. This injury is usually caused by blunt trauma. The weakest area of the orbital bones is the orbital floor/maxillary roof.
2. For children, the most common mechanisms of orbital fracture injury are falls, being struck by a ball, and physical assaults.
3. Key physical exam findings include eyelid swelling, ecchymosis, exophthalmos, ptosis, diplopia, anesthesia of the cheek (involvement of infraorbital nerve), and restricted extraocular eye movements (intraocular muscle entrapment).
4. Often associated with significant traumatic injury. Evaluate for other globe injuries (including retinal trauma, ruptured globe, hyphema) and intracranial injuries/bleeds.
   a. Injury to the globe is commonly associated with an orbital fracture (29% to 50% of patients, depending upon the setting).
5. In addition to ophthalmology, consider consultation with plastic surgery and/or head and neck surgery.
6. CT imaging should be performed for a patient with periorbital trauma and any of the following findings:
   a. Evidence of a fracture on physical examination
   b. Limitation of extraocular movement
   c. Decreased visual acuity

d. Severe pain
e. Inadequate examination (usually because of soft tissue swelling)
f. Altered mental status

G. Other Instances Requiring Ophthalmologic Consultation

1. Traumatic iritis is associated with blunt trauma and may present as painful red eye, pupillary constriction, and photophobia, often with delayed presentation of symptoms (24 to 72 hours) after trauma.
2. Sudden loss of vision could suggest retrobulbar hemorrhage or retinal detachment.

VIII. ANIMAL BITES[16]

A. Risk of Infection and Antibiotic Prophylaxis

1. Risk factors include:
   a. Underlying immunosuppression (including diabetes) or asplenia
   b. Bite involving the hand, foot, genitalia, or joint surface
   c. Bite in an extremity with underlying venous and/or lymphatic compromise
   d. Bite near or in a prosthetic joint or vascular graft
   e. Crush injury or puncture wound
   f. Cat bite (given propensity for deep puncture wounds)
   g. Human bite
   h. Delayed presentation ($\geq$12 hours after a bite on the extremities and $\geq$24 hours after a bite on the face)
2. Antibiotic prophylaxis is suggested for:
   a. Patients with risk factors above
   b. Lacerations undergoing primary closure
   c. Wounds requiring surgical repair
3. Empiric antibiotic treatment (Table 2.4)
   a. Consider IV antibiotics if patient is critically ill or unable to tolerate PO intake.
   b. Tetanus postexposure prophylaxis: See Chapter 16.
   c. Rabies postexposure prophylaxis: See Chapter 16.

TABLE 2.4

ANTIBIOTIC MANAGEMENT OF ANIMAL AND HUMAN BITES

Type of Bite	Organisms	Treatment
Animal bite	*Staphylococcus aureus, Streptococci*, oral anaerobes, *Pasteurella, Capnocytophaga canimorsus*	• Amoxicillin/clavulanate for 5 days • TMP/SMX and clindamycin, if allergy to penicillin
Human bite	*Streptococcus viridans, S. aureus*, oral anaerobes, *Eikenella corrodens*	• Amoxicillin/clavulanate for 5 days • Clindamycin and ciprofloxacin, if allergy to penicillin

B. Physical Exam Assessment

1. Evaluate wounds carefully for foreign material.
2. Neurovascular assessment should be routinely performed in areas distal to the wounds.
3. The median time to showing symptoms of infection following a dog bite is approximately 24 hours; the median time following a cat bite is typically shorter—approximately 12 hours.

C. Imaging

1. Imaging is not necessary for most clinically uninfected, superficial bites.
2. Deep bite wounds, including those near joints, warrant radiographs to evaluate for evidence of foreign bodies (such as embedded teeth), fracture, or joint disruption.

D. Decision to Suture and Infection Risk

1. Avoidance of primary closure is generally preferred unless wound is present on the face (cosmetic importance and has a lower rate of infection relative to other areas).
2. Wounds left open to heal by secondary intention should be debrided, irrigated copiously, dressed, and evaluated daily for signs of infection.
3. Lacerations closed primarily should be clinically uninfected and ideally <24 hours old (facial lacerations) or <12 hours old (sites other than the face). Meticulous debridement and irrigation should be performed prior to closure.
4. Bite wounds should not be closed with tissue adhesive glue (e.g., Dermabond) due to increased infection risk.
5. Surgical consultation (i.e. plastic, orthopedic, otolaryngology, ophthalmology) warranted in:
   a. Large/complex wounds
   b. Wounds that involve tendons, joints, deep fascia, major vasculature, or bones
   c. Deep infection (abscess, necrotizing soft tissue infection, septic arthritis, osteomyelitis)
   d. Infection associated with neurovascular compromise
   e. Presence of crepitus
   f. Rapidly progressive infection

IX. BURNS[27,28]

A. First Aid and Emergency Management

1. See Fig. 2.6 for an algorithmic approach to burn evaluation in the emergency setting.
2. Triaging burn severity
   a. Estimate of the total body surface area (TBSA) of burns (see Fig. 2.7 for modified Lund-Browder chart)
      (1) Only include partial- and full-thickness burns in this calculation (exclude superficial burns).

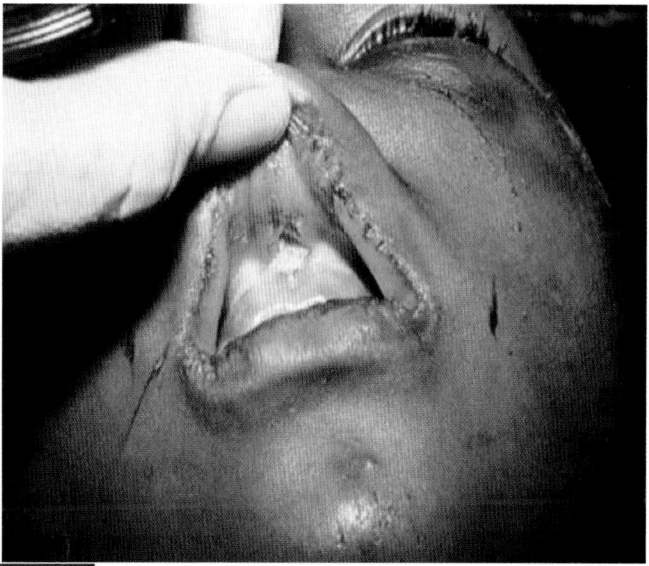

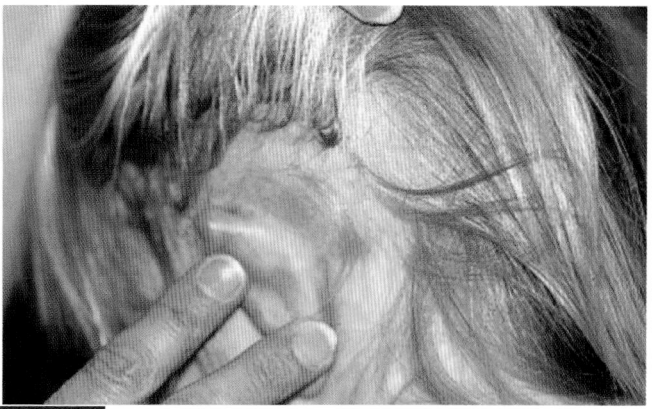

FIGURE 2.9

Frenulum tear due to direct blow to the face. (Modified from Zitelli BJ, McIntire SC, Nowalk, AJ. *Atlas of Pediatric Physical Diagnosis.* 7th ed. Elsevier; 2018.)

FIGURE 2.10

Postauricular bruising. (Modified from Zitelli BJ, McIntire SC, Nowalk, AJ. *Atlas of Pediatric Physical Diagnosis.* 7th ed. Elsevier; 2018.)

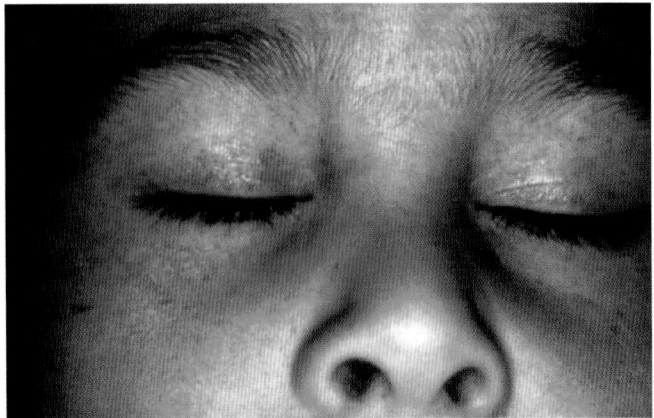

FIGURE 2.11

Petechial lesions due to choking. (Modified from Zitelli BJ, McIntire SC, Nowalk, AJ. *Atlas of Pediatric Physical Diagnosis.* 7th ed. Elsevier; 2018.)

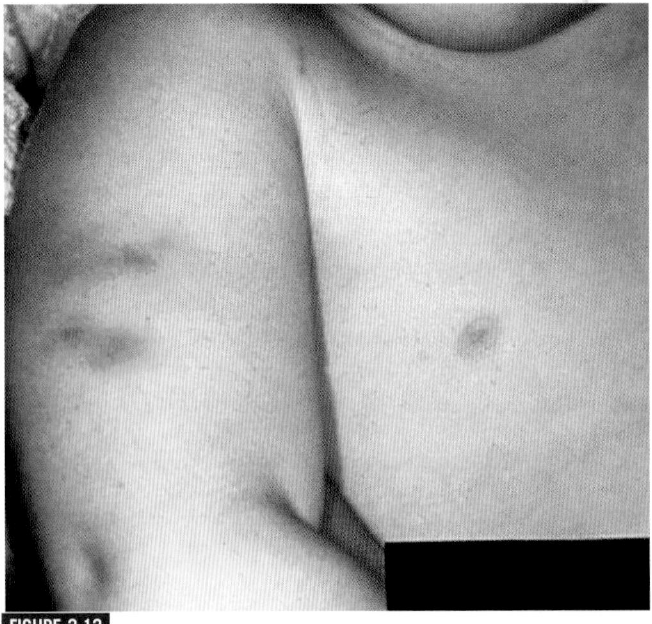

FIGURE 2.12

Pinch marks signified by two small bruises separated by clear space. (Modified from Zitelli BJ, McIntire SC, Nowalk, AJ. *Atlas of Pediatric Physical Diagnosis.* 7th ed. Elsevier; 2018.)

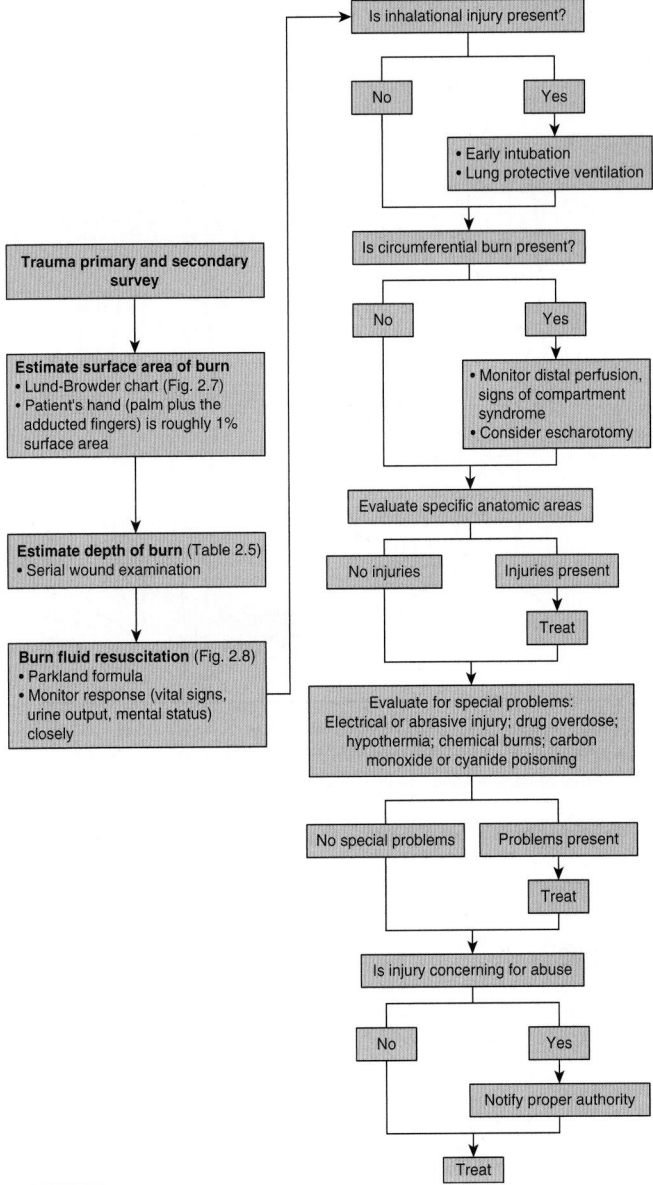

FIGURE 2.6

Initial burn management.[28]

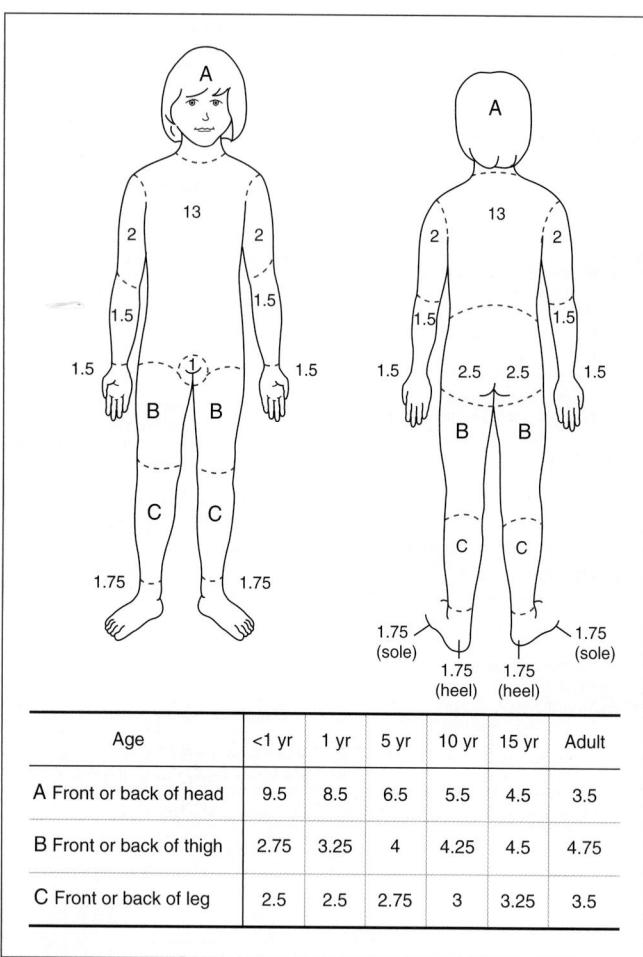

Age	<1 yr	1 yr	5 yr	10 yr	15 yr	Adult
A Front or back of head	9.5	8.5	6.5	5.5	4.5	3.5
B Front or back of thigh	2.75	3.25	4	4.25	4.5	4.75
C Front or back of leg	2.5	2.5	2.75	3	3.25	3.5

FIGURE 2.7

Burn assessment (modified Lund-Browder chart). All numbers are percentages. Only include partial and full thickness burns in calculation. (Modified from Barkin RM, Rosen P. *Emergency Pediatrics: A Guide to Ambulatory Care.* 6th ed. Mosby; 2003.)

      (2) The hand of the person who is burned (palm and adducted 5 fingers) is approximately 1% of the TBSA; this can be an easier way to measure TBSA of burns in the emergent setting

  b. Determine the depth of the burn (see Table 2.5).

3. Burns that should prompt consideration of elective/early intubation

TABLE 2.5

BURN CLASSIFICATION

Wound Depth	Layer Involved	Clinical Findings
Superficial	Epidermis	• Dry, painful, erythematous (like a sunburn)
Partial thickness	Dermis	• Moist, painful, erythematous • Blistering, blanching • Disruption of nails, hair, sebaceous glands
Full thickness	Subcutaneous, fascia, muscle, bone	• Pale, charred, waxy, leathery • Insensate (nerve endings burned) • No bleeding or blanching (capillary bed burned)

   a. Signs of smoke inhalational injury (e.g., singed nasal hairs, soot at the nares, oropharyngeal erythema)

   b. Early onset stridor

   c. Severe burns of face and/or mouth

   d. Signs of worsening oxygenation/ventilation

4. Fluids

   a. See Fig. 2.8 for fluid resuscitation guide in patients with burns.

     (1) Fluid resuscitation should be considered a dynamic process guided by frequent reassessments as opposed to an absolute volume, to prevent over- or under-resuscitation.

   b. Consider central venous access for burns greater than 25% TBSA.

   c. Withhold potassium from IV fluids for the first 48 hours (release of potassium from damaged tissues).

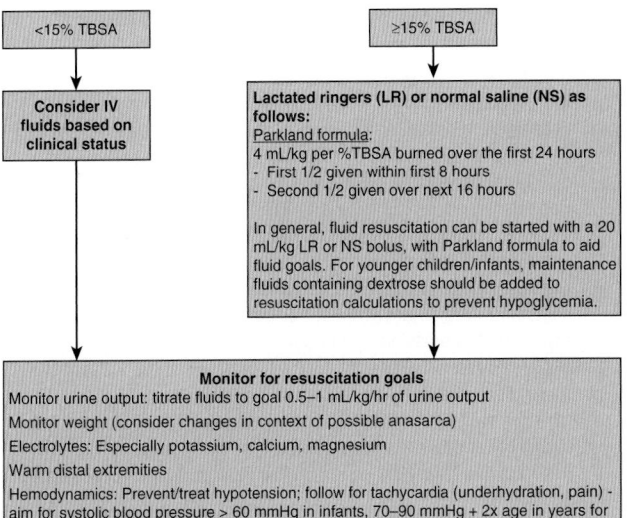

FIGURE 2.8

Formulaic fluid resuscitation for pediatric burn patients.[16,28]

    d. Foley catheter placement is recommended to monitor urine output during fluid resuscitation phase.

5. Analgesia
   a. Consider conscious/procedural sedation versus general anesthesia for cases requiring significant debridement.
   b. Children with major burns typically require opioid analgesics for pain relief.
   c. Most burn centers use morphine for wound care pain. Fentanyl may be a safer choice for initial pain management for patients whose cardiovascular status is unstable.
   d. Acetaminophen and NSAIDs alone or in combination with opioids for less severe burns.

6. Indications for transfer to a burn center
   a. Partial-thickness (second-degree) burns ≥10% TBSA burn
   b. Any significant burn to the face, hands, feet, genitalia, perineum, or major joints
   c. Full-thickness (third-degree) burns
   d. Electrical burns, including lightning injury
   e. Chemical burns
   f. Inhalation injury
   g. Any child with burns and traumatic injury (i.e., fractures) in whom the burn injury poses the greatest risk of morbidity or mortality
   h. Burns in children with preexisting conditions that could complicate management, prolong recovery, or affect mortality.
      (1) Children requiring social, emotional, or rehabilitative factors
      (2) Burned children in hospitals without qualified personnel and equipment for the care of children

7. Risk of shock
   a. Immediately following the burn injury, vasoactive mediators (cytokines, prostaglandins, oxygen radicals) are released from damaged tissue, causing increased capillary permeability and risk of distributive shock.
   b. Patients with large burns (≥15% TBSA for young children and ≥20% for older children and adolescents) often develop systemic inflammatory responses.
   c. Tissue damage and release of cell contents can cause electrolyte shifts and cardiac arrhythmia. For patients with 40% TBSA or more, myocardial depression can occur.

8. Criteria for admission to a local hospital for observation, intravenous fluid administration, and pain management include:
   a. Children with 5%–10% TBSA burn (depending upon parental capability and social circumstances)
   b. Full thickness burn 2%–5% TBSA, if local pediatric surgical expertise is available
   c. Circumferential burn
   d. Medical problem predisposing to infection
   e. Concern for nonaccidental trauma or unsafe home environment

9. Wound evaluation and care
   a. Debridement
      (1) Debridement of devitalized tissue (including ruptured blisters) decreases the risk of infection.
      (2) The depth of burn wounds can be determined with better accuracy when the wound bed is inspected directly.
      (3) Initial debridement can usually be accomplished with sterile saline-soaked gauze.
      (4) Experts generally recommend that large blisters and those that are painful (regardless of size) be removed.
   b. Wound dressing
      (1) For patients who are being rapidly transferred to a burn unit, burns should be covered with dry, sterile dressings. Moist dressings, ointments, or creams should not be applied because they can hinder initial wound assessment and care at the burn center.
      (2) Superficial burns (epidermal and superficial partial-thickness burns) are generally managed with topical antimicrobial agents with an overlying dressing.
         (a) A moist wound environment should be maintained for optimal healing.
         (b) For optimum effect and pain relief, the dressing should maintain maximum contact with the wound without adhering to it. It should be easy to apply and remove.
   c. Management of less severe burns (superficial and partial thickness)
      (1) Clean with warm saline or mild soap and water.
      (2) For superficial burns (including sunburns), application of nonperfumed moisturizing cream or ointment is typically all that is required, without need for a topical antibiotic or dressing.
      (3) Sloughed or necrotic skin, including ruptured blisters, should be debrided before applying a dressing.
      (4) For partial-thickness burns, apply topical antibacterial agent such as bacitracin (requires daily dressing changes) or silver-impregnated dressings (dressing can be left in place until follow-up) and cover with nonadherent dressing.
      (5) Follow-up inspections of burn wounds should occur the day after injury (to adjust pain medications and to assess the patient's/family's competence performing dressing changes). Subsequent follow-up can then be done on a weekly basis until wound epithelialization occurs.

B. Other Special Considerations With Burns

1. Circumferential burns rapidly begin to contract and can lead to compartment syndrome.
2. Children involved in a house/building fire or fire in an enclosed space are at risk for carbon monoxide and cyanide poisoning; consider empiric use of appropriate therapy (e.g. hyperoxygenation or hydroxocobalamin).

3. For patients with electrical burns from exposure to high voltage (>1000 V) or lightning:
    a. May have associated conditions such as cardiac arrhythmias—consider cardiac monitoring for 48 hours
    b. Risk of fractures, compartment syndromes, and rhabdomyolysis/myoglobinuria (with related renal injury)
    c. Increased risk of compression spine fractures or spinal cord injury due to tetany
4. Household outlets are 120 to 240 V, and household electrical burns rarely cause serious injuries or cardiac arrhythmias.[27]
    a. Mobile babies, toddlers, and young children can chew on or bite electrical cords that are plugged into an outlet. Electrical burn from this can lead to significant mouth/facial injury.
5. Tetanus prophylaxis is warranted with burns. Refer to Chapter 16 for details.
6. See Section X for signs of nonaccidental traumatic burns.

X. NONACCIDENTAL TRAUMA[16]

A. Physical Abuse

1. Red flags in history
    a. History is inconsistent with age, pattern, or severity of the injury.
    b. History is inconsistent with child's physical or developmental capabilities.
    c. Inconsistent/incomplete/vague/changing explanations for significant injury
    d. Delay in presentation
    e. Different witnesses provide different explanations.
2. Red flags in physical exam
    a. Bruises
        (1) In protected areas—chest, abdomen, back, buttocks
        (2) Multiple
        (3) In various stages of healing
        (4) Do not fit history or developmental stage of child
        (5) In unusual places (e.g., postauricular, neck, inner aspect of arms)
        (6) Consistent with slap of hand or pinch
    b. Burns
        (1) Scald burns that have a sharply demarcated edge
        (2) Burns in the distinct shape of an object
        (3) Small circular burns matching a cigarette or cigar tip
        (4) Burns on the perineal area with sparing of inguinal/flexural creases, matching a "dip-in" pattern (child dipped into scalding water)
        (5) Multiple burns in various places
        (6) Stocking/glove distribution burns

(7) Symmetrically burned palms/soles, buttocks, and/or lower legs; mirror image burns of extremities

c. Frenulum tears

d. Loop marks from cord or cable

e. Welts

f. Bites

g. See Figs. 2.9 through 2.12 (color plates) and eFigs. 2.1 through 2.4 for examples.

3. Imaging guidelines[29-31]

a. Skeletal survey

(1) In children less than 2 years of age, use a skeletal survey to evaluate for bony injury. This includes frontal and lateral views of the skull, lateral views of the cervical spine and thoracolumbosacral spine, and single frontal views of the long bones, hands, feet, chest, and abdomen.

(2) In children greater than 5 years of age, targeted imaging to the area(s) of suspected injury is usually appropriate. The utility of screening with skeletal survey diminishes after 5 years of age.

(3) In children 2 to 5 years of age, decisions about type of imaging are open to clinical judgement.

(4) Do not use "babygrams" (i.e., whole-body x-rays) because of the high rate of false negatives.

(5) Follow-up skeletal survey approximately 2 weeks after the initial examination should be performed when abnormal or equivocal findings are found on initial study or to identify fractures missed on initial survey.

(6) Fractures associated with child abuse include posterior rib fractures, bucket handle and metaphyseal corner fractures, spine and scapula fractures, and skull fractures.

b. Head CT without contrast if:

(1) Less than 6 months of age with suspected abuse

(2) Neurological changes, altered mental status

(3) Significant facial injuries concerning for abuse

c. Additional imaging/consultation

(1) Ophthalmologic evaluation for retinal hemorrhages

(2) MRI may identify lesions/injury not detected by CT.

4. What to do if child abuse is suspected:

a. Medical stabilization is the immediate goal; prevention of further injuries is the long-term goal.

b. All healthcare providers are mandated by law to report suspected child maltreatment to the local police and/or child welfare agency.

c. The professional who makes a report is immune from any civil or criminal liability.

d. Consider consultation of local child injury/abuse specialist.

    e. It is important to obtain a workup to rule out medical causes of injurie (bleeding disorder, osteogenesis imperfecta).

5. Carefully and legibly document the following:
    a. Reported and suspected history and mechanisms of injury
    b. Any history given by the victim in their own words (use quotation marks)
    c. Information provided by other providers or services
    d. Physical examination findings, including photos or drawings of injuries and details of dimensions, color, shape, and texture. Conside early use of police crime laboratory photography to document injuries If taking photos, start with full patient, then part of patient, then zoomed into wound, and then take a separate photo of wrist identification band.

B. Sexual Abuse[32]

1. What to do if sexual abuse is suspected:
    a. Sexual abuse evaluations are best performed in a nonemergency setting, such as a child abuse advocacy center.
    b. Urgent evaluation is necessary under the following circumstances and typically occurs in an emergency setting:
        (1) The alleged abuse occurred within 72 to 96 hours, depending upon jurisdiction.
        (2) There are genital or anal injuries that require treatment.
        (3) There is obvious forensic evidence on the patient's clothes or body that must be collected.
        (4) There is danger of continued abuse or reprisal by the alleged perpetrator.
        (5) The victim has reported homicidal or suicidal ideation.
    c. Avoid re-traumatizing the patient with invasive exams unless medically necessary. Keep in mind that most genital examinations are normal in cases of sexual abuse.

2. The medical evaluation of childhood sexual abuse has several immediate goals:
    a. Identify injuries or other conditions that require treatment.
    b. Screen for, empirically treat, and/or diagnose sexually transmitted infections (STIs).
    c. Evaluate for and, if possible/desired, reduce the risk of pregnancy.
    d. Document findings of potential forensic value.

3. STI testing
    a. In adolescents, recommended for all patients presenting with concern for sexual abuse
    b. In prepubertal children presenting with concern for sexual abuse, consider testing if any of the below factors are met:
        (1) Penetration of the vagina or anus
        (2) Abuse by a stranger

      (3) Abuse by a perpetrator known to be infected with an STI or at high risk of being infected (IV drug use, sex trafficking concerns, multiple sexual partners)

      (4) Child with sibling or another household member with STI

      (5) Child living in an area with high rate of STI in the community

      (6) Signs/symptoms of an STI

      (7) Has already been diagnosed with one STI

  c. Tests include:

      (1) Serum: HIV, syphilis

      (2) Specimen cultures for gonorrhea/chlamydia/trichomonas, which can be collected from the penis, vagina, anus, and pharynx

  d. Consider the need for postexposure HIV prophylaxis (see Chapter 17).

REFERENCES

A complete list of references can be found online.

Chapter 3

Toxicology

Sophie Crinion, MD

⊗ See additional content online.

◀) **Audio Case File 3.1** Pediatric ingestions, workup, and management

Whenever ingestion is suspected, contact local poison control at 1-800-222-1222.

Each year the American Association of Poison Control Centers records about 1.2 million childhood poisoning exposures. Of these exposures, 75% occur in children younger than the age of 6 years. Exposures in young children are often unintentional, whereas adolescents are more likely to have intentional ingestions.[1]

I. INITIAL EVALUATION

When to suspect ingestion: always, but especially with altered mental status or seizure. Begin the evaluation with an assessment of circulation, airway and breathing, and manage accordingly.[2]

A. History

Keep in mind that history may be inaccurate and provide supportive care and treatment in accordance with clinical condition and toxidrome.[2]

1. **Exposure history**

Obtain history from witnesses and/or close contacts: Route, timing, and number of exposures (acute, chronic, or repeated ingestion), prior treatments or decontamination efforts.

2. **Substance identification and quantity ingested**

Attempt to identify exact name of substance(s) ingested, including product name, active ingredients, possible contaminants, expiration date, concentration, and dose. Attempt to estimate the missing volume of liquid or the number of missing pills from a container. Poison control can assist with pill identification.[2,3]

3. **Environmental information**

Accessible items in the house or garage, open containers, spilled tablets, household members taking medications, other caregivers, herbs, or other complementary medicines[2,3]

B. Workup and Laboratory Investigation

1. **Electrocardiogram (ECG):** Several medications will cause ECG changes, including QTc and QRS prolongation.
2. **Blood tests**
   a. Venous blood gas, blood glucose, and serum electrolytes

b. Individual drug levels such as acetaminophen, aspirin, and ethanol are helpful general screenings in an acute, unknown ingestion.

c. Acetaminophen levels are especially important to test in suicidal ingestions. Many medications for pain or upper respiratory symptoms contain acetaminophen.

3. **Urine toxicology screens**

a. Basic screens include amphetamines, cocaine, opiates, phencyclidine (PCP), and tetrahydrocannabinol (THC).

b. Positive results are presumptive only; must be confirmed by gas chromatography/mass spectrometry[4]

C. Clinical Diagnostic Aids: Table With Clinical Signs and Possible Intoxicants (eTable 3.1)

II. TOXIDROMES

See Table 3.1.

III. INGESTIONS AND ANTIDOTES

See Table 3.2.

A. Decontamination

1. **Activated charcoal**[5]

a. Most effective when used within first hour after ingestion but can be given after first hour, especially for sustained-release preparations

b. Should be given PO to an awake and alert patient. Nasogastric (NG) tube should be used only if a patient is intubated due to risk of aspiration.

c. Substances not absorbed by charcoal: Iron, alcohols, lithium

d. Contraindications: Unprotected airway, caustic ingestion, disrupted gastrointestinal tract, concern for aspiration

2. **Whole bowel irrigation**

a. Indicated for evacuation of substances not bound to activated charcoal, such as iron, lead-containing foreign bodies, fatal sustained-release products, drug packing

b. Use a polyethylene glycol electrolyte solution preparation to irrigate the bowel. Recommended rates: 9 months to 6 years (500 mL/hr), 6 to 12 years (1000 mL/hr), more than 12 years (1500 to 2000 mL/hr). Often will need two NG tubes and pumps to maintain these rates.[6]

B. Enhanced Removal

1. Hemodialysis or exchange transfusions may be indicated to remove a drug/toxin.

2. Ingestions that may require enhanced removal therapies: Salicylate, lithium, methanol, ethylene glycol, metformin-associated lactic acidosis, valproate, theophylline

TABLE 3.1

TOXIDROMES

Drug Class	Temp	HR	RR	BP	Pupils	Skin	Mental Status	Other Signs	Causative Agents
Anticholinergic "Mad as a hatter, red as a beet, blind as a bat, hot as a hare, dry as a bone"[a]	↑	↑	↑/nl	↑/nl	Dilated	Dry, flushed	Delirium, psychosis, paranoia	Urinary retention, decreased bowel sounds, thirst, garbled speech	Antihistamines, atropine, antipsychotics, phenothiazines, scopolamine, TCAs
Cholinergic "SLUDGE, Killer Bs"[a]	nl	↓	↑ (bronchospasm)	↓/nl	Constricted	Sweaty	Depressed, confused	Salivation, lacrimation, urination, defecation, emesis. Liquid nicotine can cause fasciculations and paralysis.	Organophosphates, pesticides, nerve agents, tobacco, liquid nicotine
Opioids	↓/nl	↓ /nl	↓ (hypoventilation)	↓/nl	Constricted	No change	Sedated	At risk for seizures, coronary vasospasm	Morphine, fentanyl, oxycodone, methadone
Sympathomimetics	↑/nl	↑	↓/nl	↑	Dilated	Sweaty	Agitated	At risk for seizures, coronary vasospasm	Amphetamines, cocaine
Sedative/hypnotics "Coma with normal vitals"	nl	nl	↓/nl	↓/nl	Normal	No change	Depressed		Benzodiazepines, barbiturates, ethanol
Serotonergic	↑	↑	↑	↑/nl	Dilated	Flushed	Confusion	Shivering, muscle rigidity, at risk for seizures, hyperreflexia and clonus of lower extremities	SSRIs, SNRIs, MAOIs, trazodone, dextromethorphan, LSD, TCAs, MDMA (ecstasy)

[a]The "mad as a hatter" mnemonic references delirium, flushed skin, mydriasis, hyperpyrexia, and dry skin/urinary retention seen in the anticholinergic toxidrome. The "SLUDGE" mnemonic references salivation, lacrimation, urination, diaphoresis, gastrointestinal distress (including diarrhea), and emesis seen in the cholinergic toxidrome. The "Killer Bs" mnemonic references bronchospasm, bronchorrhea, and bradycardia seen in the cholinergic toxidrome.
↑ refers to increased or elevated vital sign, ↓ refers to decreased or depressed vital sign, *nl* refers to vital sign within normal limits.
BP, Blood pressure; *HR,* heart rate; *LSD,* lysergic acid diethylamide; *MAOIs,* monoamine oxidase inhibitors; *MDMA,* 3,4-methylenedioxymethamphetamine; *RR,* respiratory rate; *SNRIs,* serotonin and norepinephrine reuptake

TABLE 3.2

COMMONLY INGESTED AGENTS

Ingested Agent	Signs and Symptoms	Antidote[a]
Acetaminophen	See Section IV.	
Amphetamines	See sympathomimetics toxidrome in Table 3.1.	Supportive care Benzodiazepines for agitation
Anticholinergics	See anticholinergic toxidrome in Table 3.1.	Physostigmine
Anticholinesterase inhibitors (carbamates, donepezil)	See cholinergic toxidrome in Table 3.1.	Atropine
Antihistamines	See anticholinergic toxidrome in Table 3.1; paradoxical CNS stimulation, dizziness, seizures, prolonged QT	Supportive care
Button batteries	Electrical injury and necrosis in esophagus and surrounding tissues	Location: Esophagus: EMERGENT ENDOSCOPIC/SURGICAL REMOVAL Stomach/beyond stomach: Consult GI
Benzodiazepines	See sedative/hypnotic toxidrome in Table 3.1.	Flumazenil
β-Blockers	Bradycardia, hypotension, AV conduction block, bronchospasm, hypoglycemia	Glucagon See insulin/dextrose treatment in calcium channel blockers below. High-dose pressors
Household bleach (small volume)	Oral irritation	Supportive care
Calcium channel blockers	Bradycardia, hypotension, AV conduction block, pulmonary edema, hyperglycemia	Calcium chloride (10%) Calcium gluconate (10%) Glucagon High-dose insulin/dextrose[12]: 1 unit/kg bolus → infuse at 1–10 unit/kg/hr; give with $D_{25}W$ at 0.5 g/kg/hr. Monitor BG frequently. High-dose pressors
Clonidine	Symptoms resemble an opioid toxidrome. CNS depression, coma, lethargy, hypothermia, miosis, bradycardia, profound hypotension, respiratory depression	Naloxone Supportive care
Cocaine	See sympathomimetics toxidrome in Table 3.1.	Supportive care
Detergent pods	Vomiting, sedation, aspiration, respiratory distress	Supportive care
Ecstasy	Hallucinations, teeth grinding, hyperthermia, hyponatremia, seizures	Supportive care
Ethanol	See sedative/hypnotic toxidrome in Table 3.1. Hypoglycemia in young children	Supportive care

Continued

Ingested Agent	Signs and Symptoms	Antidote[a]
Ethylene glycol/ methanol	Similar to ethanol; additionally, blurry or double vision (methanol), renal failure/hypocalcemia (ethylene glycol), osmol gap with severe anion gap metabolic acidosis	Fomepizole Ethanol (only to be used as second-line agent when fomepizole unavailable; risk of inappropriate dosing, CNS depression, aspiration, and hypoglycemia) Consider dialysis.
Iron	Vomiting, diarrhea, hypotension, lethargy, anion gap metabolic acidosis, cardiogenic shock, renal failure	Deferoxamine
Lead	See Section V.	
Nicotine	Vomiting and see cholinergic toxidrome in Table 3.1	Supportive care
NSAIDs	Nausea, vomiting, epigastric pain, headache, gastrointestinal hemorrhage, renal failure	Supportive care
Opioids	See opioid toxidrome in Table 3.1.	Naloxone
Organophosphates	See cholinergic toxidrome in Table 3.1.	Atropine Pralidoxime
Salicylates	Gastrointestinal upset, tinnitus, tachypnea, hyperpyrexia, dizziness, lethargy, dysarthria, seizure, coma, cerebral edema	Sodium bicarbonate: $1-2$ mEq/kg IV push, followed by $D_5W + 140$ mEq/L $NaHCO_3$ and 20 mEq/L KCl at $1.5\times$ maintenance fluid rate with goal serum pH $7.45-7.55$ Consider dialysis.
Serotonergic agents	See serotonergic toxidrome in Table 3.1.	Benzodiazepines (first-line) Cyproheptadine
Sulfonylureas	Hypoglycemia, dizziness, agitation, confusion, tachycardia, diaphoresis	Food (if able) Dextrose: $0.5-1$ g/kg ($2-4$ mL/kg of $D_{25}W$) *After euglycemia achieved:* Octreotide: $1-1.25$ mCg/kg SQ Q6–12 hr (max. dose 50 mCg) if rebound hypoglycemia
Synthetic cannabinoids	Agitation, altered sensorium, tachycardia, hypertension, vomiting, mydriasis, hypokalemia	Supportive care
TCAs	Tachycardia, seizures, delirium, widened QRS possibly leading to ventricular arrhythmias, hypotension	*For wide QRS complex:* Sodium bicarbonate: $1-2$ mEq/kg IV push, followed by $D_5W + 140$ mEq/L $NaHCO_3$ and 20 mEq/L KCl at $1.5\times$ maintenance fluid rate with goal serum pH $7.45-7.55$
Warfarin	Bleeding	Phytonadione/vitamin K_1

[a]See Formulary for dosing recommendations.

BG, Blood glucose; *CNS*, central nervous system; *KCl*, potassium chloride; *NaHCO₃*, sodium bicarbonate; *NSAIDs*, nonsteroidal antiinflammatory drugs; *TCA*, tricyclic antidepressant.

Data from Gummin DD, Mowry JB, Beuhler MC, et al. 2020 Annual Report of the American Association of Poison Control Centers' National Poison Data System (NPDS): 38th Annual Report. *Clin Toxicol.* 2021;59(12):1282–1501.

C. Other Considerations

1. Many ingestions are managed primarily with supportive care of any associated toxic effects, such as hypotension or hyperpyrexia.
2. Seizures: First-line agents are benzodiazepines. Barbiturates or propofol should be considered as second-line agents. Phenytoin has no role in the treatment of toxin-induced seizures.[7]
3. Patients with severe poisoning and refractory cardiorespiratory failure after ingestion are potential extracorporeal membrane oxygenation (ECMO) candidates because the toxic effects are transient.

IV. ACETAMINOPHEN OVERDOSE[8]

NAPQI metabolite is hepatotoxic.

A. Four Phases of Intoxication

1. **Phase 1 (first 24 hours):** Nonspecific symptoms such as nausea, malaise, vomiting
2. **Phase 2 (24 to 72 hours):** Above symptoms resolve; right upper quadrant pain, hepatomegaly, and increasing transaminases develop
3. **Phase 3 (72 to 96 hours):** Return of nonspecific symptoms as well as evidence of liver failure (increased prothrombin time, lactate, phosphate), renal failure, and encephalopathy
4. **Phase 4 (4 days to 2 weeks):** Recovery or death

B. Treatment Criteria

1. **Serum acetaminophen** concentration above the possible toxicity line on the Rumack-Matthew nomogram after single acute ingestion (Fig. 3.1)
2. **History of ingesting more than 200 mg/kg or 10 g** (whichever is less) and serum concentration not available or time of ingestion not known
3. **If time of ingestion is unknown or multiple/chronic ingestion,** check acetaminophen level and AST. Treat if either is elevated.

C. Antidote: N-Acetylcysteine (See Formulary in Chapter 30)

1. **PO:** 140 mg/kg loading dose (max 15 g/dose) followed by 70 mg/kg/dose (max 7.5 g/dose) Q4 hours continue treatment until transaminases and INR have peaked and are decreasing substantially towards normal. Repeat dose if vomiting occurs within 1 hour of administration.
2. **Intravenous (IV):** 150 mg/kg N-acetylcysteine IV loading dose (max 15 g/dose) over 60 minutes, followed by 50 mg/kg/dose (max 5 g/dose) over 4 hours, followed by 100 mg/kg/dose (max 10 g/dose) over 16 hours for a total infusion time of 21 hours. Some patients may require more than 21 hours of N-acetylcysteine administration. See Formulary for weight-based drug dilution volumes.
3. **Liver failure:** Continue the 100 mg/kg over 16 hours infusion until resolution of encephalopathy, AST less than 1000 units/L, and INR less than 2.

D. Consider Referral to Liver Transplant Center if Patient Meets King's College Criteria

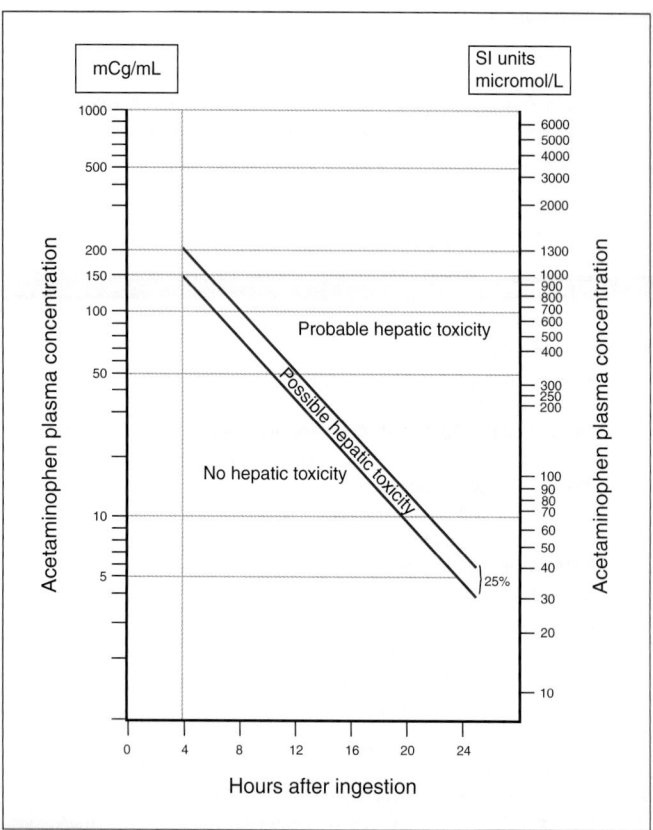

FIGURE 3.1

Rumack-Matthew nomogram. Semilogarithmic plot of plasma acetaminophen levels versus time. This nomogram is valid for use after single acute ingestions of acetaminophen. The need for treatment cannot be extrapolated based on a level before 4 hr. (Data from *Pediatrics* 1975;55:871, and Micromedex.)

V. LEAD POISONING[9]

A. Definition
Centers for Disease Control and Prevention (CDC) defines a reference level of 3.5 µg/dL to identify children with elevated blood lead levels (BLLs).[10]

B. Sources of Exposure
Paint, dust, soil, drinking water, cosmetics, cookware, toys, caregivers with occupations and/or hobbies using lead-containing materials or substances, and bullets if in joint spaces or pleura

C. Overview of Symptoms by Blood Lead Level

1. **BLL ≥40 μg/dL:** Irritability, vomiting, abdominal pain, constipation, anorexia
2. **BLL ≥70 μg/dL:** Lethargy, seizure, and coma. **Note:** Children may be asymptomatic with lead levels greater than 100 μg/dL.

D. Management

1. See Tables 3.3 and 3.4 for general management and repeat testing guidelines.
2. Chelation therapy[2]
   a. Asymptomatic children with BLL 45 to 69 mCg/dL
      Succimer: 1050 mg/m^2/day PO divided Q8 hours × 5 days, then 700 mg/m^2/day divided Q12 hours × 14 days. See Formulary for more details.
   b. Asymptomatic children with BLL ≥70 mCg/dL
      (1) **Succimer:** Per above dosing
      (2) **Edetate (EDTA) calcium disodium:** 1000 mg/m^2 (max dose 2 to 3 g) as 24-hour IV infusion × 5 days. Begin 2 hours after first dose of succimer. Monitor renal function closely.
      Warning: Do not mistake edetate disodium for edetate calcium disodium. Edetate *calcium* disodium is the correct medicine used for the treatment of lead poisoning.
   c. Symptomatic children unable to take PO (e.g., lead encephalopathy, seizure)

TABLE 3.3

MANAGEMENT OF LEAD POISONING[11]

Blood Lead Level (BLL)	Recommended Guidelines (*See Table 3.4 for Repeat Testing Guidelines.*)
3.5—19 μg/dL	1. Obtain detailed environmental exposure history to assess for possible sources. 2. Provide education about reducing environmental lead. 3. Consider CBC, iron studies, and multivitamin with iron supplementation. 4. Environmental investigation may be available based on local resources.
10—19 μg/dL	1. As above for BLL 5—9 μg/dL 2. Environmental investigation may be available based on local resources.
20—44 μg/dL	1. As above for BLL 5—9 μg/dL 2. Environmental investigation 3. Iron level, complete blood cell count (CBC), abdominal radiography with bowel decontamination if indicated 4. Complete exam, including neurodevelopmental assessment
45—69 μg/dL	1. As above for BLL 20—44 μg/dL 2. Administer oral chelation therapy, consider hospitalization.
≥70 μg/dL	1. Hospitalize and commence chelation therapy. 2. Contact local poison control.

TABLE 3.4

REPEAT BLOOD LEAD TESTING GUIDELINES[11]

If Screening BLL Is: (μg/dL)	Time Frame of Confirmation of Screening BLL	Follow-Up Testing (After Confirmatory Testing)	Later Follow-Up Testing After BLL Declining
>3.5–9	3 months	3 months	6–9 months
10–19	1 month[a]	1–3 months	3–6 months
20–44	2 weeks[a]	2 weeks–1 month	1–3 months
>45	48 hours	As soon as possible	As soon as possible

[a]Per provider discretion.

BLL, Blood lead level.

(1) **Dimercaprol (BAL):** 450 mg/m^2/day IM divided Q4 hours × 3 to 5 days (number of days based on clinical course). Do not give to patients with peanut allergy. Do not use concomitantly with iron, as BAL-iron complex is a potent emetic. Use with caution in patients with G6PD deficiency, as it may cause hemolysis.

(2) **Edetate (EDTA) calcium disodium:** 1500 mg/m^2 (maximum dose 2 to 3 g) as 24-hour IV continuous infusion × 5 days. Begin 4 hours after first dose of BAL.

VI. WEB RESOURCES

- American Association of Poison Control Centers: http://www.aapcc.org/
- American Academy of Clinical Toxicology: http://www.clintox.org/index.cfm
- Centers for Disease Control and Prevention, Section on Environmental Health: http://www.cdc.gov/nceh

REFERENCES

A complete list of references can be found online.

Chapter 4

Procedures

Maite E. Del Valle Rolón, MD

See additional content online.

I. GENERAL GUIDELINES

A. Consent
Before any procedure is performed, it is crucial to obtain informed consent from the parent or guardian by explaining the procedure, the indications, and any risks involved; answer questions; and discuss possible alternatives. Obtaining consent should not impede lifesaving, emergent procedures.

B. Documentation
It is important that the physician performing the procedure document the informed consent process. Include the date, time, additional providers present (if applicable), brief summary of the consent conversation, the diagnosis, recommended procedure, specific risks and benefits, and alternative treatments. It is equally important to document if a patient refuses a procedure and that the risks associated with refusal were discussed.

C. Risks
1. All invasive procedures involve pain, risk for infection and bleeding, and potential injury to neighboring structures.
2. Sedation and analgesia should be planned, and the risks of such explained to the parent and/or patient as appropriate. (See Chapter 6 and the AAP Guidelines for Monitoring and Management of Pediatric Patients Before, During, and After Sedation for Diagnostic and Therapeutic Procedures.[1])
3. Universal precautions and proper sterile technique should be followed for all patient contact that exposes the healthcare provider to bodily fluids.

D. Attending to the Needs of a Fearful Child[2]
Children represent a vulnerable population in that they often lack the capacity to understand why a potentially uncomfortable procedure is being performed. All efforts should be made to provide information about the procedure to the child at an age-appropriate level. Utilize child life specialists as able.

1. **Observe:** Monitor how child reacts when you enter the room. If they are visibly fearful, you should take some time for them to get used to your presence.
2. **Engage:** Talk about an unrelated subject to get their attention. When possible, allow the child to touch medical equipment. Mimic parts of the exam on toys or others so that the child can see the exam before experiencing it.

3. **Monitor:** If your initial interaction was not successful, step back and try a different approach.

II. ULTRASOUND FOR PROCEDURES[2a]

A. Introduction to Ultrasound

Ultrasound has become an increasingly important bedside diagnostic and procedural aid, and it can improve visualization of subcutaneous structures during procedures.

B. Ultrasound Basics

1. **Probe selection**
    a. Linear transducers use higher frequencies than curvilinear or phased-array transducers to produce higher-resolution images near the body's surface and are primarily used for procedures in pediatrics. A wide area of contact at the skin surface facilitates needle placement in procedures. Linear transducers have poor resolution of deep structures in the body.
    b. Curvilinear transducers use low to midrange frequencies and permit deep structure visualization. Though they provide a wide area of skin contact to facilitate procedures near concave and convex surfaces, larger curvilinear probes are difficult to use in small children.
    c. There are a variety of other probes (i.e., phased-array, microconvex, intracavitary) that generate sector-shaped images but are predominantly used for diagnostic purposes.

2. **Image optimization**
    a. Ensure adequate contact by using enough ultrasound gel and applying comfortable pressure on the skin.
    b. Gain: Measure of image brightness, which is used for optimizing images and reducing artifact
    c. Frequency: Increase to improve image resolution of shallow structures. Decrease to improve imaging of deep structures.
    d. Depth: Adjust to visualize structure of interest and at least a centimeter of tissue below that structure.

III. NEUROLOGIC PROCEDURES: LUMBAR PUNCTURE[3-5]

A. Indications

Examination of spinal fluid for suspected infection, inflammatory disorder, malignancy, instillation of intrathecal chemotherapy, diagnosis of subarachnoid hemorrhage, or measurement of opening pressure

B. Complications

Local pain, apnea due to positioning, headache, bleeding, infection, subarachnoid epidermal cyst, ocular muscle palsy, epidural CSF leak, spinal hematoma, and/or brainstem herniation

C. Cautions and Contraindications

1. Increased intracranial pressure (ICP): Before lumbar puncture (LP), perform a funduscopic examination. Presence of papilledema, retinal hemorrhage, or clinical suspicion of increased ICP should prompt further evaluation and may be a contraindication to the procedure. A sudden

drop in spinal canal fluid pressure by rapid release of cerebrospinal fluid (CSF) may cause fatal herniation. Computed tomography (CT) may be indicated before LP if there is suspected intracranial bleeding, focal mass lesion, or increased ICP. A normal CT scan does not rule out increased ICP but usually excludes conditions that may put the patient at risk for herniation. Decision to obtain CT should not delay appropriate antibiotic therapy, if indicated.

2. Bleeding diathesis: Platelet count greater than 50,000/mm^3 is desirable before LP, and correction of any clotting factor deficiencies can minimize the risk for bleeding and subsequent cord or nerve root compression.
3. Overlying skin infection may result in inoculation of CSF with organisms.
4. A mass or evidence of trauma to lumbar vertebrae
5. LP should be deferred in unstable patients, and appropriate therapy should be initiated, including antibiotics, if indicated.

D. Procedure

1. Apply local anesthetic cream if sufficient time is available.
2. Position child (Fig. 4.1) in either the sitting position or lateral recumbent position, with hips, knees, and neck flexed. Keep shoulders and hips aligned to avoid rotating the spine. *Do not* compromise a small infant's cardiorespiratory status with positioning.
3. Locate the desired intervertebral space (either L3 to L4 or L4 to L5) by drawing an imaginary line between the top of the iliac crests. Alternatively, ultrasound can be used to mark the intervertebral space (see Section XI [online content]).
4. Prepare the skin in a sterile fashion. Drape conservatively to make monitoring the infant possible. Use a 20- to 22-gauge spinal needle with stylet (1.5, 2.5, or 3.5 inch, depending on the size of the child). A smaller-gauge needle will decrease the incidence of spinal headache and CSF leak.
5. Overlying skin and interspinous tissue can be anesthetized with 1% lidocaine using a 25-gauge needle.
6. Puncture the skin in the midline just caudad to the palpated spinous process, angling slightly cephalad toward the umbilicus. Advance several millimeters at a time, and withdraw stylet frequently to check for CSF flow. **Needle may be advanced without the stylet once it is completely through the skin.** In small infants, one may *not* feel a change in resistance or "pop" as the dura is penetrated.
7. If resistance is met initially and the needle cannot be advanced, withdraw needle to just under the skin surface and redirect the angle of the needle slightly.
8. Send CSF for appropriate studies. In general, send the first tube for culture and Gram stain, the second tube for measurement of glucose and protein levels, and the last tube for cell count and differential. Additional tubes can be collected for viral cultures, polymerase chain reaction (PCR), or CSF metabolic studies, if indicated. If subarachnoid hemorrhage or traumatic tap is suspected, send the first and fourth tubes

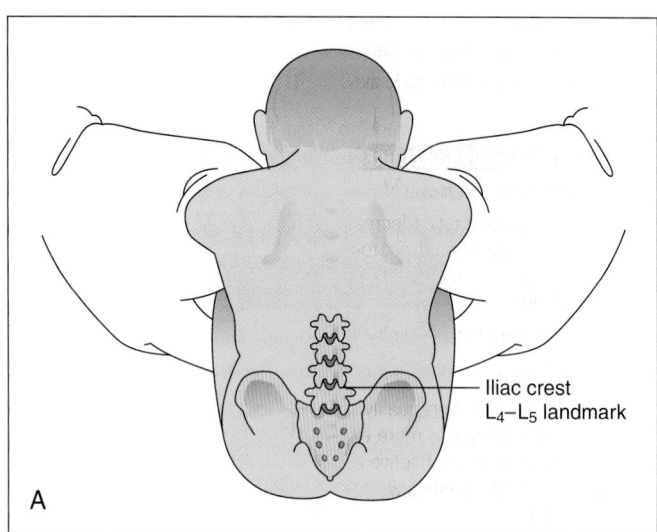

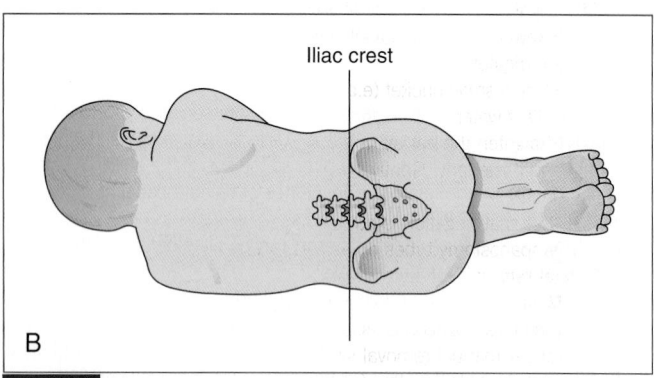

FIGURE 4.1

Lumbar puncture site. (A) Infant placed in sitting position. (B) Infant placed in lateral (recumbent) position. (From Dieckmann R, Fiser D, Selbst S. *Pediatric Emergency and Critical Care Procedures.* Mosby; 1997.)

for cell count, and ask the laboratory to examine the CSF for xanthochromia.
9. Accurate measurement of CSF pressure can be made only with the patient lying quietly on their side in an unflexed position. It is not a reliable measurement in the sitting position. Once the free flow of spinal fluid is

obtained, attach the manometer and measure CSF pressure. Opening pressure is recorded when the CSF level is steady.

E. A video on lumbar punctures is available on the *New England Journal of Medicine*'s website

IV. OTOLARYNGOLOGIC PROCEDURES

A. Cerumen Impaction Removal[6,7]

1. **Indications:** Symptomatic (decreased hearing, pain) and/or assessment of the ear. Clinicians should *not* routinely disimpact asymptomatic patients whose ears can be adequately assessed.
2. **Complications:** Allergic reaction to cerumenolytics, trauma, earache, dizziness, nystagmus, retention of water, tympanic membrane perforation
3. **Procedures**
   a. **Cerumenolytics**
      (1) There is no high-quality evidence suggesting that one cerumenolytic is more effective than another. Water and saline are equally as effective as cerumenolytics. Hydrogen peroxide has reduced efficacy.
   b. **Irrigation**
      (1) Direct visualization is not necessary.
      (2) Irrigation of the ear canal with a large syringe containing lukewarm water is equally effective as a commercial mechanical jet irrigator.
      (3) Place a small bucket (e.g., emesis bin) under the patient's ear to collect water.
      (4) Straighten the ear as much as possible by lifting the auricle up and posteriorly. Gently apply a continuous stream upward in the canal.
      (5) Note that irrigation is contraindicated in patients with tympanostomy tubes or perforated tympanic membranes
   c. **Manual removal/instrumentation**
      (1) Most useful for cerumen removal in the outer one-third of the ear
      (2) Direct visualization is essential and an uncooperative patient may render manual removal impossible.
      (3) Tools include curettes (plastic or metal), spoons, alligator forceps. Do not attempt to break through the cerumen. Advance the loop of the curette behind the cerumen and retrieve.
   d. **A video on** cerumen removal **is available on the *New England Journal of Medicine*'s website.**

B. Foreign Body Removal From Ear[3,8]

1. **Indications:** Retained foreign body in the external auditory canal
2. **Contraindications:** Urgent referral to an otolaryngologist **prior** to attempted removal is indicated if object is a button battery or penetrating the ear canal (e.g., pencil, cotton-tipped swab).
3. **Complications:** External auditory canal trauma (most common), perforation of the tympanic membrane, retained foreign object, ossicular disruption

4. **Procedure:**
   a. Insects should be killed with mineral oil, ethanol, or lidocaine prior to attempted removal.
   b. Irrigation is useful for hard objects resistant to grasping that are nonocclusive. It is contraindicated for removal of vegetables/legumes (increases swelling) and button batteries (enhances current flow)
   c. Instrumentation is most successful for irregularly shaped objects that are graspable.
   d. Studies suggest that referral to ENT should be made after a single provider fails to remove the foreign body.
5. **A video on** removal of foreign bodies from the ear and nose **is available on the *New England Journal of Medicine*'s website.**

C. Foreign Body Removal From Nose[9,10,3]

1. **Indications:** Retained foreign body in the nasal cavity. Button batteries and magnets attached to the nasal septum require emergent removal.
2. **Contraindications:** Most nasal foreign bodies do not require subspecialty referral. Consider otolaryngology referral for posterior objects, button batteries, penetrating injuries, and unsuccessful initial attempts.
3. **Complications:** Epistaxis, perforation of cribriform plate, aspiration, mucosal injury, rhinosinusitis, retained foreign object (which may lead to necrosis of septum and mucosa).
4. **Procedure:** Topical lidocaine, a vasoconstrictor (e.g., crushed ice or spray), may be used to minimize bleeding and edema.
   a. **Self-removal:** The easiest and least invasive method. Typically, only effective for patients older than 3 years. Instruct the patient to occlude the unobstructed nostril and blow their nose.
   b. **Parent kiss:** Provides up to a 60% successful removal rate.
      (1) Instruct the caregiver to place their lips around the patient's lips (similar to a "mouth-to-mouth" resuscitation breath) and occlude the uninvolved nostril with one finger.
      (2) Quickly and forcefully exhale one puff into the child's mouth. This maneuver often expels the foreign body.
   c. **High-flow oxygen:** Best for foreign bodies that *completely* occlude the anterior nasal cavity. Place suction tubing into the unobstructed nostril while the child's mouth is closed. Deliver 10 to 15 L/min of oxygen flow through the tubing.
   d. **Instrumentation:** Best for foreign bodies that are *nonocclusive*.
      (1) Equipment: alligator forceps, right-angle hook, Foley catheter (5 to 8 Fr) or Katz extractor, irrigating devices
      (2) Use alligator forceps to extract compressible objects that have rough surfaces.
      (3) Use a right-angle hook for smooth objects that cannot be easily grasped.
      (4) Use a Foley catheter for small, round objects (e.g., marble). Lubricate the catheter, advance the uninflated catheter past the object, inflate the catheter balloon, and withdraw the catheter and the object.

D. Management of Epistaxis[9,11]

1. **Indications:** Simple nosebleed. Most cases of epistaxis in children have a benign etiology. Referral to an otolaryngologist is indicated for uncontrollable bleeding, posterior epistaxis, hemodynamic instability, or anatomic abnormalities (e.g., tumors, polyps). See Chapter 14 for management of epistaxis in patients with hemophilia, von Willebrand disease, immune thrombocytopenia, or other bleeding disorders.

2. **Complications:** Persistent bleeding, swallowing blood, toxic shock syndrome (from packing material), septal hematomas/abscesses from traumatic packing, sinusitis

3. **Procedure:** The child should sit upright and bent forward at the waist to minimize swallowing blood. Remove blood clots, which promote fibrinolysis.

   a. **Direct compression:** Instruct the child or parent to compress the nasal alae against the septum with two fingers for 5—15 minutes. Most simple bleeds will clot after 5 to 10 minutes.

   b. **Topical vasoconstriction:** Use oxymetazoline-soaked cotton pledgets or gauze. Phenylephrine is associated with morbidity when used topically and should be avoided in patients younger than 6 years of age. However, if bleeding is refractory to other interventions, the minimum dose of phenylephrine needed to cease bleeding should be used. Use a squirt bottle or apply the vasoconstrictor on a piece of cotton, applying direct pressure on the nose for 5 to 10 minutes.

   c. **Nasal packing**

      (1) Apply topical anesthetic on a cotton pledget and insert into the nasal cavity. Remove after 5—10 minutes.

      (2) Rub antibiotic ointment into a quarter-inch × 72-inch gauze ribbon. Using a nasal speculum or forceps, pack the nasal cavity by grasping the gauze ribbon approximately 6 inches from its end and placing the packing as far back as possible. Ensure that the free end protrudes from the nose and secure with tape.

      (3) Maintain packing for 72 hours. If bleeding persists after 72 hours, packing should be replaced and the child referred to an otolaryngologist.

V. CARDIOVASCULAR PROCEDURES

A. Vagal Maneuvers for Supraventricular Tachycardia (SVT)[12-14]

1. **Indications:** Supraventricular tachycardia, 2:1 atrioventricular (AV) block, evaluation of cardiac murmurs

2. **Contraindications:** Carotid sinus massage is to be avoided in patients with prior stroke within the past 3 months, significant carotid stenosis or bruit, or any history of ventricular arrhythmia.

3. **Complications:** Typically transient (resolve within seconds to minutes) and include prolonged sinus pause, hypertension (increased intrathoracic pressure), hypotension (decreased venous return/decrease in intrathoracic pressure on exhalation)

4. **Procedure:**
   a. **Cold stimulus to the face:** Briefly place an icepack or washcloth soaked in ice water on the forehead or bridge of the nose. The ice should not be applied for longer than 30 seconds to avoid frostbite.
   b. **Valsalva maneuver:** Place the patient in supine position and instruct to exhale forcefully against a closed glottis. The strain should be maintained for 10 to 15 seconds before resuming normal breathing.
   c. **Modified Valsalva maneuver:** Place the patient in a semirecumbent position (45-degree angle) and apply standard Valsalva strain. Immediately reposition supine with 15 seconds of passive leg raise at a 45-degree angle. (This has greater success rate at restoring sinus rhythm than standard Valsalva.)
   d. **Carotid sinus massage:** Place the patient in a supine position with neck extension. Apply steady pressure for 5 to 10 seconds to **one** carotid sinus (inferior to the angle of the mandible where pulsation is detected). If unsuccessful, wait 1 to 2 minutes and repeat on the contralateral side.
   e. **See Chapter 1 for further management of SVT.**

B. **Heelstick and Fingerstick[15]**

1. **Indications:** Blood sampling in infants, obtaining point-of-care whole blood samples such as serum glucose
2. **Complications:** Infection, bleeding, osteomyelitis
3. **Procedure:**
   a. Warm heel or finger.
   b. Clean with alcohol.
   c. Using a lancet, puncture heel on the lateral aspect (avoiding the posterior area) or finger on the distal palmar lateral pad.
   d. Wipe away the first drop of blood, and then collect the sample using a capillary tube or container.
   e. Alternate between squeezing blood from the leg toward the heel (or from the hand toward the finger) and then releasing the pressure for several seconds.

C. **Peripheral Intravenous Access[15]**

1. **Indications:** Blood sampling and access to peripheral venous circulation to deliver fluid, medications, or blood products
2. **Complications:** Thrombosis, infection
3. **Procedure:**
   a. Apply tourniquet around the extremity proximal to chosen site.
   b. Prepare site with alcohol or chlorhexidine.
   c. Insert IV catheter, bevel up, at an angle almost parallel to the skin, advancing until a *flash* of blood is seen in the catheter hub. Advance the plastic catheter only, remove the needle, and secure the catheter.
   d. After removing tourniquet, attach a syringe and apply gentle negative pressure to withdraw blood for serum sampling. Then, attach T connector filled with saline to the catheter, flush with normal saline (NS) to ensure patency of the IV line.

4. **Ultrasound-guided procedure:**
   a. With linear ultrasound probe, identify a vein that does not appear to be prohibitively tortuous or stenotic. Perform this by sliding the probe along the course of the vessel and identifying its direction and branching. The saphenous veins in the calves, veins in the forearms, antecubital areas, inside of the upper arms, and external jugular veins are areas where ultrasound guidance can help. An ideal vessel appears less than 1 cm below the skin surface. Deeper vessels are prone to through-and-through perforation of the vessel. Infiltration around deeper vessels is also a risk, as a shorter length of catheter resides in the vessel after insertion.
   b. Prepare the site, and in the case of limb vessels, place a tourniquet proximal to the insertion site.
   c. Under ultrasound visualization, insert the needle into the skin at a shallow (usually <30 degrees) angle to the skin at the midline of the probe near where it contacts the skin. With the probe visualizing the vessel transversely, slowly advance the needle and follow the tip of the needle by sliding the probe away from you. Advance the ultrasound probe until the needle punctures the vessel wall.
   d. Proceed with cannulation of the vessel and secure the intravenous catheter per standard procedure.
5. **Infiltration and extravasation**[16]**:** This is a common injury secondary to fluid infusion into subcutaneous tissues around the venipuncture site and typically occurs due to puncture of the vein or if the catheter slips out of the vein. The difference between infiltration and extravasation is the type of fluid that has leaked (nonvesicant vs. vesicant). Infiltrations are generally benign, although they can still inflict damage via exertion of mechanical forces on surrounding structures. Extravasation due to a vesicant can cause blistering and burns, leading to necrosis of the tissue. To determine if infiltration/extravasation has occurred, firmly occlude the vein 1 to 2 inches proximal to the insertion site. Continued infusion without resistance indicates infiltration. Immediately stop the infusion. Refer to institutional policy for guidelines regarding application of medication (e.g., hyaluronidase, phentolamine, nitroglycerin ointment). Elevate the affected limb to reduce swelling; apply a warm compress for 10 to 15 minutes; encourage movement of the affected arm. Reevaluate the site every 8 hours.
6. **A video on** peripheral IV placement **is available on the *New England Journal of Medicine*'s website.**
7. **A video on** ultrasound-guided peripheral IV placement **is available on the *New England Journal of Medicine*'s website.**

D. External Jugular Puncture and Catheterization (See Section XI [Online Content])
E. Radial Artery Puncture and Catheterization[3,4,15]

1. **Indications:** Arterial blood sampling or frequent blood gas and continuous blood pressure monitoring in an intensive care setting

2. **Complications:** Infection, bleeding, occlusion of artery by hematoma or thrombosis, ischemia if ulnar circulation is inadequate
3. **Procedure:**
   a. Before the procedure, test adequacy of ulnar blood flow with the Allen test: Clench the hand while simultaneously compressing ulnar and radial arteries. The hand will blanch. Release pressure from the ulnar artery and observe the flushing response. Procedure is safe to perform if the entire hand flushes.
   b. Locate the radial pulse. It is optional to infiltrate the area over the point of maximal impulse with lidocaine. Avoid infusion into the vessel by aspirating before infusing. Prepare the site in a sterile fashion.
   c. Puncture: Insert a butterfly needle attached to a syringe at a 30- to 60-degree angle over the point of maximal impulse. Blood should flow freely into the syringe in a pulsatile fashion. Suction may be required for plastic tubes. Once the sample is obtained, apply firm, constant pressure for 5 minutes and then place a pressure dressing on the puncture site.
   d. Catheter placement: Secure the patient's hand to an arm board. Leave the fingers exposed to observe any color changes. Prepare the wrist with sterile technique and infiltrate over the point of maximal impulse with 1% lidocaine. Insert an IV catheter with its needle at a 30-degree angle to the horizontal until a flash of blood is seen in the catheter hub. Advance the plastic catheter and remove the needle. Alternatively, pass the needle and catheter through the artery to transfix it, and then withdraw the needle. Very slowly, withdraw the catheter until free flow of blood is noted, then advance the catheter and secure in place using sutures or tape. Seldinger technique (Fig. 4.2) using a guidewire can also be used. Apply a sterile dressing and infuse heparinized isotonic fluid (per institutional protocol) at a minimum of 1 mL/hr. A pressure transducer may be attached to monitor blood pressure.
   e. Suggested size of arterial catheters based on weight:
      (1) Infant (<10 kg): 24 Gauge
      (2) Child (10 to 40 kg): 22 Gauge
      (3) Adolescent (>40 kg): 20 Gauge
4. **Ultrasound-guided procedure:**
   a. Use the linear probe. After the sterile field has been prepped, apply gel to the probe and place within a sterile cover. Place the ultrasound probe transverse to the artery on the radial, posterior tibial, or dorsalis pedis pulse. Identify the artery, which will appear pulsatile with some compression. Once the artery has been identified, center the probe over the vessel (Fig. 4.3). Insert the needle into the skin at a 45-degree angle at the midline of the probe near where it contacts the skin. With the probe visualizing the vessel transversely, slowly advance the needle and follow the tip of the needle by sliding the probe away. Advance the ultrasound probe until the needle punctures

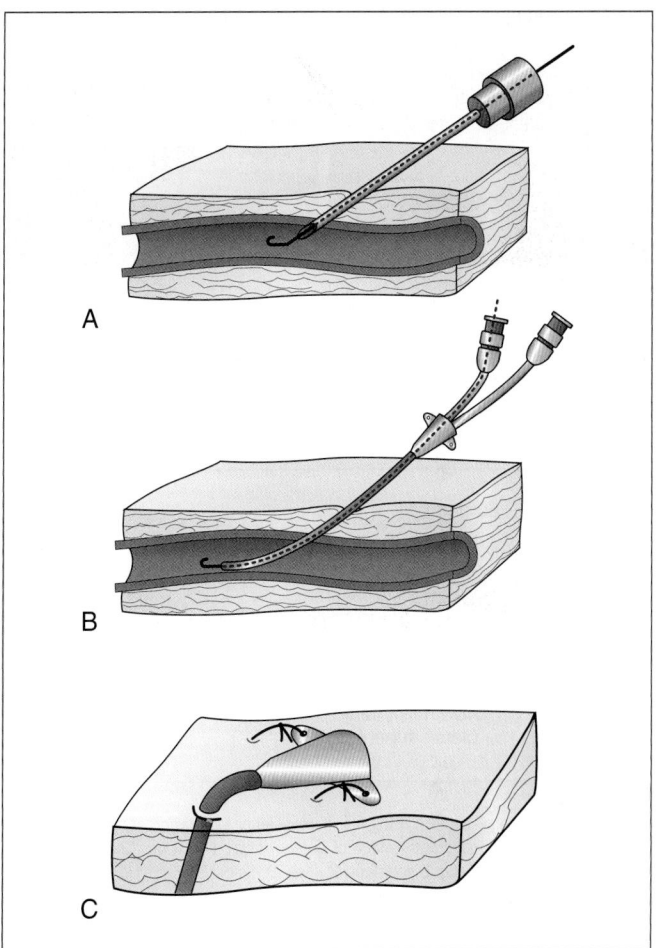

FIGURE 4.2

Seldinger technique. (A) Guidewire is placed through introducer needle into lumen of vessel. (B) Catheter is advanced into vessel lumen along guidewire. (C) Hub of catheter is secured to skin with suture. (Modified from Fuhrman B, Zimmerman J. *Pediatric Critical Care.* 4th ed. Mosby; 2011.)

the vessel wall. Proceed with the rest of the procedure after vessel puncture, as described previously.
5. **Videos on** arterial puncture **and** radial artery catheterization **are available on the *New England Journal of Medicine*'s website.**

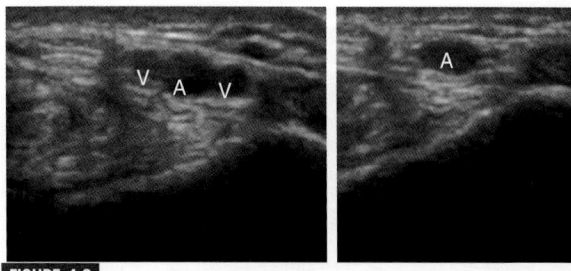

FIGURE 4.3

Ultrasound transverse view of radial artery. In the left image, the radial artery is seen in cross section with veins on either side. On the right image, pressure has been applied and the veins are collapsed while the artery remains patent. *A,* Artery; *V,* vein. (From Weiner MM, Geldard P, Mittnacht AJC. Ultrasound guided vascular access: a comprehensive review. *J Cardiothorac Vasc Anesth.* 2013;27[2]:345–360.)

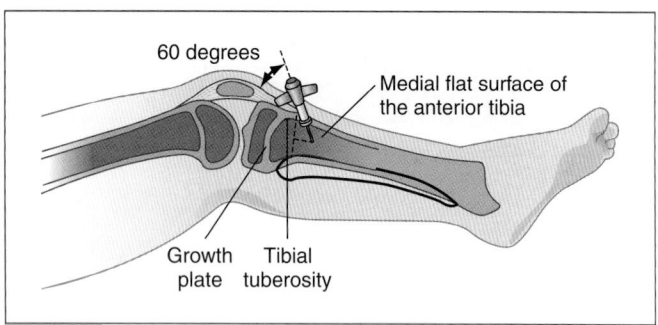

FIGURE 4.4

Intraosseous needle placement using standard anterior tibial approach. Insertion point is in the midline on medial flat surface of anterior tibia, 1 to 3 cm (2 fingerbreadths) below tibial tuberosity. (From Dieckmann R, Fiser D, Selbst S. *Pediatric Emergency and Critical Care Procedures.* Mosby; 1997.)

6. **A video on** ultrasound-guided radial artery catheterization **is available on the *New England Journal of Medicine*'s website.**

F. Intraosseous (IO) Access[3,4,17] (Fig. 4.4)

1. **Indications:** Obtain emergency access in children during life-threatening situations. This is very useful during cardiopulmonary arrest, shock, burns, and life-threatening status epilepticus. Any crystalloid, blood product, or drug that may be infused into a peripheral vein may also be infused into the IO space. The IO needle should be removed once adequate vascular access has been established. Insertion of IO needle into fractured bones should be avoided.

2. **Complications:**
   a. Extravasation of fluid from incomplete or through-and-through cortex penetration, infection, bleeding, osteomyelitis, compartment syndrome, fat embolism, fracture, epiphyseal injury.
   b. Frequency of complications increases with prolonged infusions.
3. **Sites of entry (in order of preference):**
   a. Anteromedial surface of the proximal tibia, 1 to 2 cm below and slightly medial to the tibial tuberosity on the flat part of the bone
   b. Distal femur 3 cm above the lateral condyle in the midline
   c. Medial surface of the distal tibia 1 to 2 cm above the medial malleolus (may be a more effective site in older children than the distal femur)
   d. Proximal humerus, 2 cm below the acromion process into the greater tubercle with the arm held in adduction and internal rotation
   e. Anterosuperior iliac spine at a 90-degree angle to the long axis of the body
4. **Procedure:**
   a. Prepare the selected site in a sterile fashion.
   b. If the child is conscious, anesthetize the puncture site down to the periosteum with 1% lidocaine (optional in emergent situations).
   c. Choose between a manual IO or drill-powered IO insertion device:
      (1) For manual IO needle: Insert a 15-gauge (for all children) or 18-gauge (for infants and neonates) IO needle perpendicular to the skin at an angle away from the epiphyseal plate, and advance to the periosteum. With a boring rotary motion, penetrate through the cortex until there is a decrease in resistance, indicating that you have reached the marrow. The needle should stand firmly without support. Secure the needle carefully.
      (2) For drill-powered IO needle: Enter skin with the needle perpendicular to the skin, as with the manual needle, and press the needle until you meet the periosteum. Then apply easy pressure while gently depressing the drill trigger until you feel a decrease in resistance. Remove the drill while holding the needle steady to ensure stability prior to securing the needle. Use an EZ-IO AD 15-mm needle (pink hub) for patients 3 to 39 kg and a 25-mm needle (blue hub) for patients 40 kg and greater.
   d. Remove the stylet and attempt to aspirate marrow. (Note that it is not necessary to aspirate marrow.) Flush with crystalloid solution. Observe for fluid extravasation. Marrow can be sent to determine glucose levels, chemistries, blood types and crossmatches, hemoglobin levels, blood gas analyses, and cultures. Note that sending serum laboratory tests from IO aspirates is institution-dependent.
   e. Secure the IO needle. Attach standard IV tubing. Increased pressure (through pressure bag or push) may be necessary for infusion. There is a high risk for obstruction if continuous high-pressure fluids are not flushed through the IO needle.

5. **A video on** IO catheter placement **is available on the *New England Journal of Medicine*'s website.**

G. Umbilical Artery and Umbilical Vein Catheterization[3,18]

1. **Indications:** Vascular access (via umbilical vein [UV]), blood pressure monitoring (via umbilical artery [UA]), or blood gas monitoring (via UA) in critically ill neonates

2. **Complications:** Infection; bleeding; perforation of vessel; thrombosis with distal embolization, ischemia or infarction of lower extremities, bowel, or kidney; arrhythmia if catheter is in the heart; air embolus

3. **Contraindications:** Omphalitis, peritonitis, possible/confirmed necrotizing enterocolitis, intestinal hypoperfusion

4. **Line placement:**
   a. Umbilical arterial catheter (UAC) line: Low line vs. high line
      (1) Low line: Tip of catheter should lie just above the aortic bifurcation between L3 and L4.
      (2) High line: Tip of catheter should be above the diaphragm between T6 and T9. A high line has fewer complications and lesser need for replacement than a low line.
   b. Umbilical venous catheter (UVC) lines should be placed in the inferior vena cava above the level of the ductus venosus and the hepatic veins and below the level of the right atrium.
   c. Catheter length: Determine the length of catheter required using either a standardized graph based on shoulder-umbilical length or the following birth weight (BW) regression formula:
      (1) UAC high line (cm) = $(3 \times \text{BW [kg]}) + 9$
      (2) UVC length (cm) = $0.5 \times \text{UAC high line (cm)} + 1$

5. **Procedure for UAC line (Fig. 4.5):**
   a. Determine the length of the catheter to be inserted for either high (T6 to T9) or low (L3 to L4) position.
   b. Restrain infant. Maintain the infant's temperature during the procedure. Prepare and drape the umbilical cord and adjacent skin using sterile technique.
   c. Flush the catheter with sterile saline solution before insertion. Ensure that there are no air bubbles in the catheter or attached syringe.
   d. Tie sterile umbilical tape around the base of the cord, tight enough to prevent bleeding. Cut through the cord horizontally about 1.5 to 2 cm from the skin.
   e. Identify the one large, thin-walled UV and two smaller, thick-walled arteries. Use one tip of open, curved forceps to gently probe and dilate one artery. Then use both points of closed forceps and dilate artery by allowing forceps to open gently.
   f. Grasp the catheter 1 cm from its tip with toothless forceps and insert the catheter into the lumen of the artery. Aim the tip toward the feet and gently advance the catheter to the desired distance. *Do not force.*

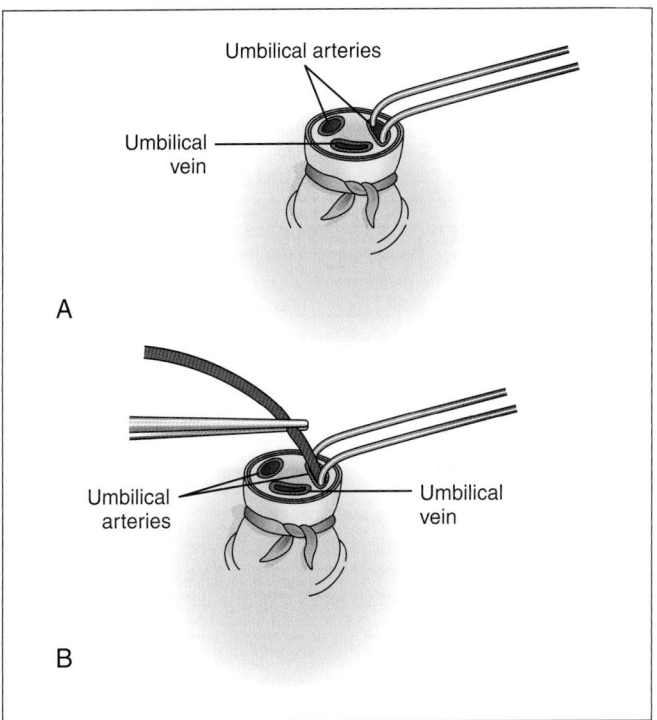

FIGURE 4.5

Placement of umbilical arterial catheter. (A) Dilating lumen of umbilical artery. (B) Insertion of umbilical artery catheter. (From Dieckmann R, Fiser D, Selbst S. *Pediatric Emergency and Critical Care Procedures.* Mosby; 1997.)

If resistance is encountered, try loosening umbilical tape, applying steady and gentle pressure, or manipulating the angle of the umbilical cord to the skin. Often the catheter cannot be advanced because of the creation of a "false luminal tract." There should be good blood return when the catheter enters the iliac artery.

g. Confirm catheter tip position with x-ray or ultrasound. Secure catheter with a suture through the cord, a marker tape, and a tape bridge. The catheter may be pulled back but *not* advanced once the sterile field is broken.

h. Observe for complications: Blanching or cyanosis of lower extremities, perforation, thrombosis, embolism, or infection. If any complications occur, the catheter should be removed.

i. Use isotonic fluids containing heparin per institutional policy. Never use hypoosmolar fluids in the UA.

6. **Procedure for UVC line (see** Fig. 4.5**):**
   a. Determine the desired length and follow steps "5a" through "5d" for UA catheter placement.
   b. Isolate the thin-walled UV, clear thrombi with forceps, and insert catheter, aiming the tip toward the right shoulder. Gently advance the catheter to the desired distance. *Do not force.* If resistance is encountered, try loosening the umbilical tape, applying steady and gentle pressure, or manipulating the angle of the umbilical cord to the skin. Resistance is commonly met at the abdominal wall and again at the portal system. *Do not* infuse anything into the liver.
   c. Confirm catheter tip position with x-ray or ultrasound. Secure catheter with a suture through the cord, a marker tape, and a tape bridge. The catheter may be pulled back but *not* advanced once the sterile field is broken.
7. **A video on** UVC/UAC line placement **is available on the *New England Journal of Medicine*'s website.**

VI. PULMONARY PROCEDURES

A. Use of Metered-Dose Inhalers and Spacers[9]

1. **Indications:** Delivery of medication to distal airways in the lungs
2. **Complications:** Failure of medication delivery. **Note** that there are risks associated with the medication rather than the delivery method.
3. **Procedure:**
   a. Shake the inhaler, remove the cap, and attach it to the spacer device.
   b. Instruct the child to exhale completely.
   c. Place the mouthpiece of the spacer into the patient's mouth and instruct the child to make a complete seal with the lips. Alternatively, a spacer with a mask can be placed over the child's mouth if they are unable to make a seal with their lips.
   d. Spray 1 puff from the inhaler into the spacer and instruct the patient to breathe slowly and deeply. Older children should hold a single large breath for 10 seconds; younger children can take 4 to 5 breaths.
   e. Wait 1 minute and repeat as indicated.

B. Needle Cricothyrotomy[9,19]

1. **Indications:** When an emergency airway is required and the clinician is unable to use bag-valve-mask (BVM) ventilation or secure an orotracheal or nasotracheal airway. Common indications include facial fractures, blood or vomitus in the airway, airway obstruction (e.g., foreign body, tumor, edema from trauma).
2. **Contraindications:** Relative contraindications include inability to locate landmarks, laryngotracheal damage, coagulopathy, bleeding dyscrasia, laryngeal fracture or tracheal transection.
3. **Complications:** Bleeding, hypoxia, pneumothorax, esophageal laceration, vocal cord injury, posterior tracheal wall perforation, infection

4. **Procedure:**
   a. Immobilize the larynx with the nondominant hand and identify the cricothyroid membrane. This is located by palpating the laryngeal prominence at midline of the thyroid cartilage and then moving distally 1 to 2 cm to a small depression. This depression overlies the cricothyroid membrane.
   b. Insert a 12- to 14-gauge angio-catheter caudally at a 30- to 45-degree angle through the cricothyroid membrane. Attach a 3-mL syringe with saline, aspirating as the needle is inserted. Advance until air is aspirated into the syringe.
   c. Advance the catheter over the needle and remove the needle. Attach a 3.0 endotracheal tube (ETT) adapter to the angio-catheter and then attach an oxygen source that can deliver roughly 30 psi. Alternatively, a bag-valve device can be connected using a 7.0 ETT adapter and a 3-mL syringe with plunger removed.
   d. Intermittent ventilation can be achieved by cutting a small hole in the oxygen tubing and covering the hole in the tubing. Allow for expiration by uncovering the hole for 2 to 9 seconds.

C. Needle Thoracostomy[3,20]

1. **Indications:** Evacuation of a tension pneumothorax
2. **Complications:** Infection; bleeding; pneumothorax; hemothorax; pulmonary contusion or laceration; puncture of diaphragm, spleen, or liver; or bronchopleural fistula
3. **Procedure:**
   a. Prepare and drape the skin as clean as possible, with goal of sterility.
   b. Insert a large-bore angio-catheter (14- to 22-gauge, based on patient size and likely depth of the chest wall) into the anterior second intercostal space in the midclavicular line. Insert needle over superior aspect of rib margin to avoid neurovascular structures. If the angio-catheter permits, a 3- to 10-mL syringe with 1 to 2 mL of saline can be connected to it. Aspirating the syringe while inserting the IV will pull air bubbles through the saline if an air collection exists. A rush of bubbles signifies successful access.
   c. When pleural space is entered, withdraw needle and attach a three-way stopcock and syringe to the catheter, and aspirate air. The stopcock is used to stop air flow through the catheter when sufficient evacuation has been performed.
   d. Subsequent insertion of a chest tube is necessary for ongoing release of air. It is advised not to completely evacuate chest prior to placement of chest tube to avoid pleural injury.
4. **A video on** needle decompression of spontaneous pneumothorax **is available on the *New England Journal of Medicine*'s website.**

D. Bag-Valve-Mask Ventilation[21,22]

1. **Indication:** Respiratory failure, apnea
2. **Contraindication:** Complete upper airway obstruction
3. **Complications:** Gastric distention

4. **Procedure:**
   a. Child's head should be positioned so that nose and mouth are pointing toward the ceiling. A shoulder roll may be needed to improve position. If cervical spine injury is suspected, do not move the neck.
   b. Place mask on patient's face. For effective BVM ventilation, the mask must fit properly (covering the patient's mouth and nose).
   c. Use the E-C clamp technique. For the "E" use the little, ring, and middle fingers to lift the jaw. The thumb and index finger form the "C" to hold the mask to the face, forming a seal between the mask and the face.
   d. Two-person BVM ventilation is more effective. One rescuer will do the E-C clamp technique with both hands while the other person compresses the ventilation bag.

E. Endotracheal intubation: Please refer to Chapter 1

VII. GASTROINTESTINAL PROCEDURES

A. Nasogastric Tube Placement[3,9,23]

1. **Indications:** Enteral nutrition, administration of medications, treatment of ileus or obstruction, gastric decompression, gastric lavage
2. **Contraindications:** Esophageal stricture, esophageal varices, severe midface trauma (cribriform plate disruption), bleeding diatheses, alkaline ingestion
3. **Complications:** Malposition, coiling of tube, esophageal perforation, pneumothorax, aspiration
4. **Procedure:**
   a. Approximate the length of 5- to 18-Fr tube insertion by positioning the tube from the nares or mouth to the ear, then to the mid-xyphoid-umbilicus. Mark this length on the tube with marker.
   b. The patient should be sitting as upright as possible. The head should be tilted toward the chest.
   c. Lubricate the tube and insert the tube through the nose. Advance the tube to the length mark, asking the patient to swallow while the tube is inserted. It may be helpful to provide a cup of water with a straw.
   d. Confirm placement of the tube with a radiograph of the lower chest/upper abdomen. Ensure that the tube is located distal to the carina, crosses the diaphragm, and rests in a central position in the gastric region. The tube should not cross the midline. Additional confirmation can be obtained by testing the pH of aspirated contents. A pH <4 confirms proper positioning. Alternatively, insert a small amount of air (20 to 30 mL) through the tube while listening to the gastric area with a stethoscope.
   e. Secure the tube.

B. Gastrostomy Tube Replacement[3,9,24]

1. **Indications:** Dislodged, blocked, or replacement of gastrostomy tube (G-tube) or gastrostomy button.

2. **Complications:** Perforation, bleeding, pneumoperitoneum, creation of "false tract" particularly if tube is newly placed. **Note** that misplacement and associated complications are rare for children with a mature G-tube tract undergoing tube replacement in a pediatric emergency room.
3. **Relative contraindications:** Tube has been displaced for 24 hours or more, tube was placed less than one month ago, suspicion of peritonitis
4. **Procedure:**
   a. Deflate balloon completely with a syringe and pull the tube out steadily.
   b. Insert new tube in the stoma and inflate balloon fully with water. Gently tug on the tube to assess whether the balloon is inflated. Secure the tube.
   c. Confirm intragastric placement by aspirating gastric contents.
   d. If replacement tube is not immediately available, a Foley catheter of similar size may be placed using the method above to maintain tract patency.
   e. If the G-tube tract is too constricted for placement of G-tube, consider upsizing with Foley catheter serial dilation.
5. **A video on** gastrostomy tube exchange **is available on the *New England Journal of Medicine*'s website.**

VIII. GENITOURINARY PROCEDURES

A. Urinary Bladder Catheterization[9,25]

1. **Indications:** To obtain urine for urinalysis and sterile culture, to accurately monitor hydration status, and bladder decompression
2. **Complications:** Hematuria, infection, trauma to urethra or bladder, intravesical knot of catheter (rarely occurs)
3. **Contraindications:** Pelvic fractures, known trauma to the urethra, or blood at the meatus
4. **Catheter selection:** 6 Fr for newborns, 6 to 8 Fr for infants, 8 to 10 Fr for prepubertal females, and up to 12 Fr for adolescents
5. **Procedure:**
   a. For collection of urinalysis and/or urine culture, the infant/child should not have voided within 1 hour of procedure.
   b. Prepare the urethral opening using sterile technique.
   c. In males, apply gentle traction to the penis to straighten the urethra. In uncircumcised male infants, expose the meatus with gentle retraction of the foreskin. The foreskin must be retracted only far enough to visualize the meatus.
   d. In females, the urethral orifice may be difficult to visualize but is usually immediately superoanterior to the vaginal orifice.
   e. Gently insert a lubricated catheter into the urethra. Slowly advance catheter until resistance is met at the external sphincter. Continued pressure will overcome this resistance, and the catheter will enter the bladder. Only a few centimeters of advancement are required to reach

the bladder in females. In males, insert a few centimeters longer than the shaft of the penis.

    f. Carefully remove the catheter once specimen is obtained, and cleanse skin of iodine.

    g. If indwelling Foley catheter is inserted, inflate balloon with sterile water or saline as indicated on bulb, then connect catheter to drainage tubing attached to urine drainage bag. Secure catheter tubing to inner thigh.

6. **Videos on** catheterization of the male urethra **and** catheterization of the female urethra **are available on the *New England Journal of Medicine*'s website.**

B. Suprapubic Bladder Aspiration[3,4]

1. **Indications:** To obtain urine in a sterile manner for urinalysis and culture in children younger than 2 years (avoid in children with genitourinary tract anomalies, coagulopathy, or intestinal obstruction), bladder decompression. This bypasses distal urethra, thereby minimizing risk for contamination.

2. **Complications:** Infection (cellulitis), hematuria (usually microscopic), intestinal perforation

3. **Procedure** (Fig. 4.6):

    a. Anterior rectal pressure in females or gentle penile pressure in males may be used to prevent urination during the procedure. Child should not have voided within 1 hour of procedure.

    b. Restrain child in the supine, frog leg position. Prepare suprapubic area in a sterile fashion.

    c. The site for puncture is 1 to 2 cm above the symphysis pubis in the midline. Use a syringe with a 22-gauge, 1.5-inch needle, and puncture at a 10- to 20-degree angle to the perpendicular, aiming slightly caudad.

    d. Ultrasound guidance:

        (1) Ultrasound can be used to visualize the urinary bladder for this procedure as follows: Use the curvilinear or linear probe depending on the size of the child. Apply the probe in transverse position in the midline of the lower abdomen, positioning it to locate the bladder. The bladder is a midline structure with a dark center and bright margins. The shape of the bladder is usually rounded; however, it can appear spherical, pyramidal, or even cuboidal (Fig. 4.7).

        (2) The bladder may be empty as well with no dark cavity. If no clear structure, give fluids and reassess in 30 minutes. This technique can also be used in the evaluation of anuric patients, to differentiate between decreased urine production and urinary retention. This is also useful in the case of patients with a urinary catheter as the catheter is usually visible. If it is visualized and the bladder also has urine around it, the catheter is likely malfunctioning.

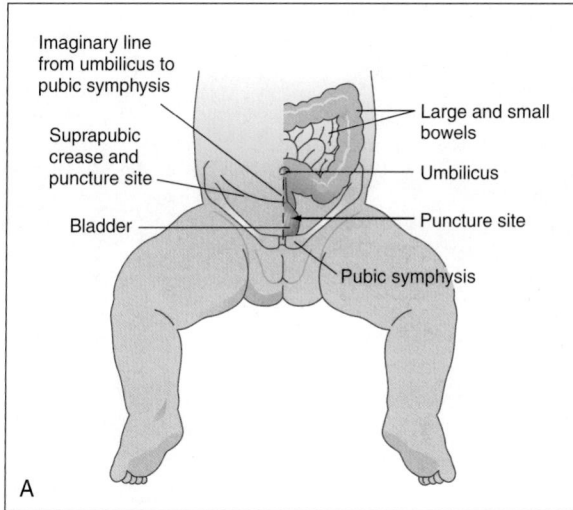

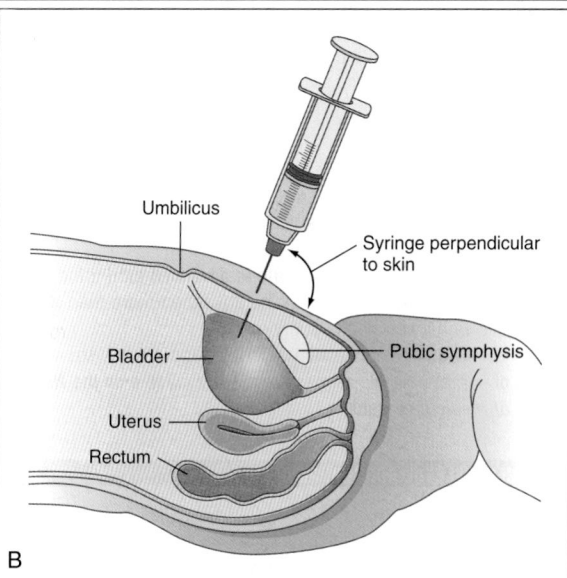

FIGURE 4.6

Landmarks for suprapubic bladder aspiration. (Modified from Dieckmann R, Fiser D, Selbst S. *Pediatric Emergency and Critical Care Procedures.* Mosby; 1997.)

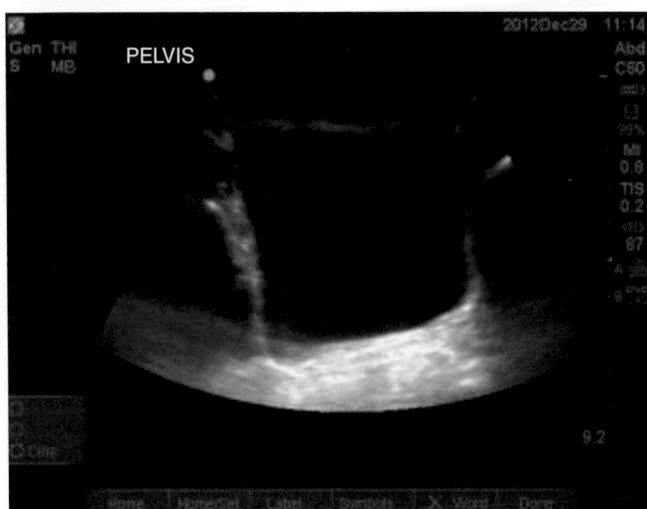

FIGURE 4.7

Ultrasound of bladder. In this transverse midline view of the pelvis the bladder appears black (anechoic) and cuboid in the midline. This is the typical appearance of a full bladder on ultrasound, although the shape may vary. (From Leeson K, Leeson B. Pediatric ultrasound: applications in the emergency department. *Emerg Med Clin North Am.* 2013;31[3]:809–829.)

      (3) Aspiration can be performed after marking the site with ultrasound, proceeding with preparing and draping the patient, and proceeding to puncture.

    e. **Gently exert suction as the needle is advanced until urine enters syringe.** The needle should not be advanced more than 3 cm. Aspirate urine with gentle suction.

    f. Remove needle, cleanse skin of iodine, and apply a sterile bandage.

4. **A video of** suprapubic bladder aspiration **is available on the *New England Journal of Medicine*'s website.**

IX. MUSCULOSKELETAL PROCEDURES

A. Basic Splinting[3]

1. **Indications:** To provide short-term stabilization of limb injuries while accommodating swelling associated with acute injuries

2. **Complications:** Pressure sores, dermatitis, neurovascular impairment

3. **Procedure:**

    a. Determine style of splint needed (see Section IX.B).

    b. Measure and cut fiberglass or plaster to appropriate length. If using plaster, upper-extremity splints require 8 to 10 layers and lower-extremity splints require 12 to 14 layers.

   c. Pad extremity with copious cotton roll padding, taking care to overlap each turn by 50%. In prepackaged fiberglass splints, additional padding is not generally required. Bony prominences may require additional padding. Place cotton between digits if they are in a splint.

   d. Immerse plaster slabs into room temperature water until bubbling stops. Smooth out wet plaster slab, avoiding any wrinkles. Fiberglass splints will harden when exposed to air.

   e. Position splint over extremity and mold to desired contour. Wrap with an elastic bandage to hold molded splint onto extremity in position of function, overlapping each turn by 50%. Continue to hold desired form of splint upon extremity until fully hardened.

   f. **NOTE:** Plaster and fiberglass become warm while drying. Using warm water will decrease drying time. This may result in inadequate time to mold splint. Turn edge of the splint back on itself to produce a smooth surface. Take care to cover the sharp edges of fiberglass.

   g. Use crutches or slings as indicated.

   h. The need for orthopedic referral should be individually assessed.

   i. Emergent orthopedic referral may be required, including when there is concern for neurovascular compromise or compartment syndrome of the affected extremity.

4. **Postsplint care:**
   a. Standard rest, ice, and elevation of affected extremity should be performed.
   b. Avoid weight bearing on splinted extremity.
   c. Do not get splint wet. Splints can be wrapped in water-resistant items such as a plastic bag or a specially designed splint bag to allow for showering. Use a hair dryer in instances where the splint has accidentally gotten wet.
   d. Do not stick items such as a pen or clothes hanger to scratch inside the splint.
   e. If areas in or distal to the splint develop numbness, tingling, or increased pain; turn blue or pale; or become swollen, patient should loosen the elastic bandage of the splint. Instruct to seek immediate medical care if this does not quickly (<30 minutes) resolve these symptoms.

5. **A video on** basic splinting techniques **is available on the *New England Journal of Medicine*'s website.**

B. Selected Splints and Indications (Fig. 4.8)

1. **Long arm posterior splint**
   a. **Indications:** Immobilization of elbow and forearm injuries
   b. **Procedure:** Elbow flexed at 90 degrees, forearm in neutral position, slight dorsiflexion of the wrist. Splint extends from palmar crease of the hand to mid upper arm along the ulnar side of the forearm and the posterior aspect of the humerus. Width should be semicircumferential.

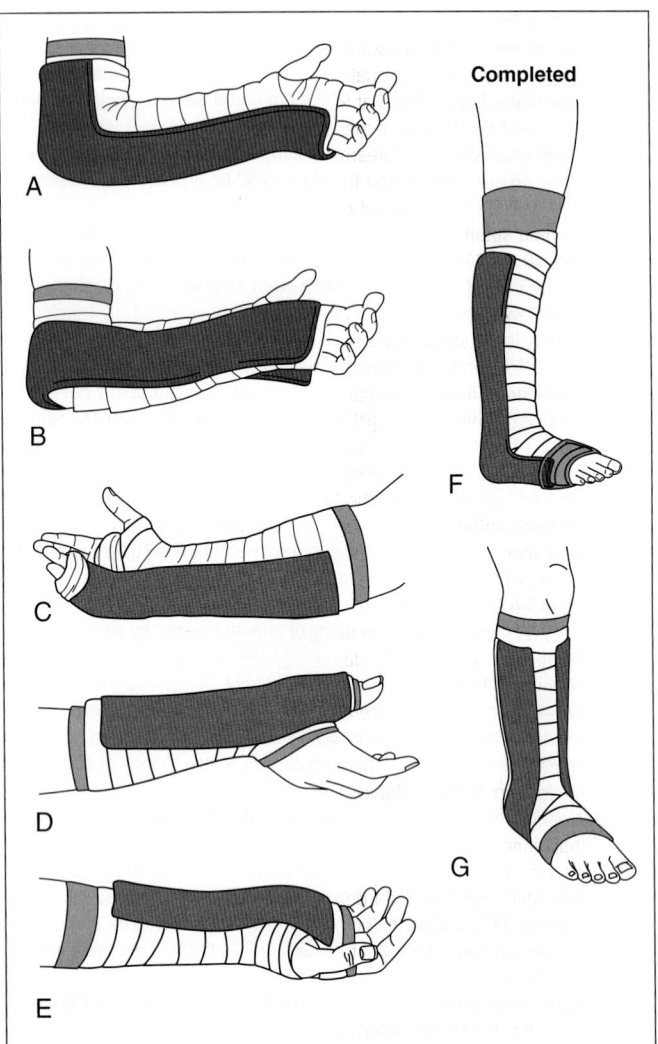

FIGURE 4.8

Selected splint types. Light purple layer is stockinette, white layer is cotton roll, dark purple layer is the splint. (A) Long arm posterior splint. (B) Sugar tong forearm splint. (C) Ulnar gutter splint. (D) Thumb spica splint. (E) Volar splint. (F) Posterior ankle splint. (G) Ankle stirrup splint.

2. **Sugar tong forearm splint**
   a. **Indications:** For distal radius and wrist fractures; to immobilize the elbow and minimize pronation and supination
   b. **Procedure:** Elbow flexed at 90 degrees, forearm in neutral position, and slight dorsiflexion of the wrist. Splint extends from palmar crease along volar aspect of forearm, around elbow, and dorsally to the metacarpals. Fingers and thumb remain free. Width should support arm on both sides but not overlap.
3. **Ulnar gutter splint**
   a. **Indications:** Nonrotated fourth or fifth (boxer) metacarpal metaphyseal fracture with less than 20 degrees of angulation, uncomplicated fourth and fifth phalangeal fracture.
   b. Assess for rotation, displacement (especially Salter I type fracture), angulation, and joint stability before splinting.
   c. **Procedure:** Elbow in neutral position, wrist in slight dorsiflexion, metacarpophalangeal (MP) joint at 60 to 90 degrees, interphalangeal (IP) joint at 20 degrees. Apply splint in U shape from the tip of the fifth digit to 3 cm distal to the volar crease of the elbow. Splint should be wide enough to enclose the fourth and fifth digits.
4. **Thumb spica splint**
   a. **Indications:** Nonrotated, nonangulated, nonarticular fractures of the thumb metacarpal or phalanx, ulnar collateral ligament injury (gamekeeper's or skier's thumb), scaphoid fracture, or suspected scaphoid fracture (pain in anatomic snuff box)
   b. **Procedure:** Wrist in slight dorsiflexion, thumb in some flexion and abduction, IP joint in slight flexion. Apply splint in U shape along radial side of forearm extending from tip of thumb to mid-forearm. Mold the splint along the long axis of the thumb so that thumb position is maintained. This will result in a spiral configuration along the forearm with maintained apposition of the index finger and thumb.
5. **Volar splint**
   a. **Indications:** Wrist immobilization for wrist sprains, strains, or certain uncomplicated fractures
   b. **Procedure:** Wrist in slight dorsiflexion. Apply splint on palmar surface from the MP joint to 2 to 3 cm distal to the volar crease of the elbow. It is useful to curve the splint to allow the MP joint to rest at an 80- to 90-degree angle.
6. **Posterior ankle splint**
   a. **Indications:** Immobilization of ankle sprains and fractures of the foot, ankle, and distal tibia and/or fibula
   b. **Procedure:** Place patient in prone position with ipsilateral knee flexed at 90 degrees and affected ankle held in flexion at 90 degrees. Splint should extend from base of toes to upper portion of the calf. Width should match that of the foot. An ankle stirrup (sugar tong) splint can be added to increase stability for ankle fractures.
7. **Ankle stirrup splint**
   a. **Indications:** Immobilization of the ankle

b. **Procedure:** Ankle held in flexion at 90 degrees. Splint extends in U-shaped fashion from fibular head underneath the ankle to just below the knee. Width should be one-half of the narrowest circumference of the lower leg and not overlapping. May be used alone or in combination with (placed after) posterior ankle splint.

C. Radial Head Subluxation (Nursemaid's Elbow) Reduction[26,27]

1. **Presentation:** Commonly occurs in children aged 1 to 4 years with a history of inability to use an arm after it was pulled. Child presents with affected arm held at the side in pronation, with elbow slightly flexed.
2. **Caution:** Rule out a fracture clinically before doing procedure. Consider radiograph if mechanism of injury or history is atypical or if exam is concerning for fracture (e.g., swelling, bruising, tenderness).
3. **Procedure:**
   a. Two most common techniques include hyperpronation (HP) and traditional supination-flexion (SF) maneuvers. Meta-analyses of randomized trials evaluating the two techniques favor HP for both efficacy and pain tolerance.
   b. Support the elbow with one hand and place your thumb laterally over the radial head at the elbow applying pressure medially. With your other hand, grasp the child's hand in a handshake position or at the wrist.
   c. HP method: Forcefully pronate the wrist. You may feel a click as reduction occurs.
   d. SF method: Quickly and deliberately supinate and externally rotate the forearm, and simultaneously flex the elbow.
   e. Most children will begin to use the arm within 15 minutes, some immediately after reduction. If reduction occurs after a prolonged period of subluxation, it may take the child longer to recover use of the arm. In this case, the arm should be immobilized with a posterior splint.
   f. If procedure is unsuccessful, consider obtaining a radiograph. Maneuver may be repeated if needed.
4. **A video on** reduction of nursemaid's elbow **is available on the *New England Journal of Medicine*'s website.**

D. Finger/Toe Dislocation Reduction[3]

1. **Indications:** IP and MP/metatarsophalangeal dislocations
2. **Complications:** Fracture of phalanges, entrapment of neurovascular structures
3. **Cautions:** Volar dislocations and dorsal dislocations with interposition of the volar plate or entrapment of the metacarpal/metatarsal head often cannot be performed using closed reduction.
4. **Procedure:**
   a. Assess for neurovascular compromise in the affected digit. Perform radiographs to evaluate for possible fracture.
   b. Consider procedural sedation or a digital block prior to procedure.
   c. Grasp the digit proximal to the fracture to allow for stabilization.

    d. Grasp the tip of the distal digit and apply longitudinal traction, with the joint typically slipping into place.

    e. Alternatively, grasp the distal phalanx and mildly hyperextend to accentuate the deformity while applying longitudinal traction.

    f. After reduction, again evaluate neurovascular status and obtain radiographs to ensure proper position and to further evaluate for fracture.

    g. Immobilize the joint using a padded splint using full extension for distal IP joints and 20 to 30 degrees of flexion for proximal IP joints.

E. Knee Arthrocentesis[3]

1. **Indications:** Evaluation of fluid for the diagnosis of disease, including infectious, inflammatory, and crystalline disease, and removal of fluid for relief of pain and/or functional limitation

2. **Contraindications:** Bleeding diathesis, local fracture, overlying skin infection

3. **Complications:** Pain, bleeding, infection

4. **Procedure:**

    a. Place child supine on exam table with knee in slight flexion, with use of a padded roll underneath the knee for support, if unable to slightly flex.

    b. The lateral or medial approach can be made, with the lateral approach preferred to avoid the vastus medialis muscle.

    c. The puncture point should be at the posterior margin of the patella in both cases.

    d. Prepare the overlying skin in a sterile fashion, and once cleaned, numb the area using 1% lidocaine with a small-gauge needle. Then, using an 18-gauge needle attached to a syringe, puncture the skin at a 10- to 20-degree downward angle, and advance under continuous syringe suction until fluid is withdrawn, indicating entry into the joint space.

    e. In large effusions, several syringes may be needed for complete fluid removal if so desired, and the needle may have to be redirected to access pockets of fluid.

    f. Upon completion, withdraw the needle and cover the wound with a sterile gauze dressing.

    g. Synovial fluid can then be sent for studies as indicated.

5. **A video on** knee arthrocentesis **is available on the *New England Journal of Medicine*'s website.**

F. Hematoma Blocks[28]

1. **Indications:** Analgesia for closed fracture of the extremity that requires manipulation or closed reduction. It can be an adjunct or an alternative when procedural sedation is not possible or is impractical.

2. **Contraindications:** Allergic reactions to local anesthetic agents, open fracture, cellulitis overlying fracture site, presence of a neurologic or vascular deficit

3. **Complications:** Rare, but include compartment syndrome, local anesthetic toxicity (circumoral and tongue numbness, dizziness, tinnitus, and visual disturbances), and osteomyelitis

4. **Procedure:**
   a. Perform using aseptic technique.
   b. Draw up the local anesthetic solution into a syringe with a 22- or 23-gauge, 2-inch-long needle. Bupivacaine is desired and can be used alone or mixed with lidocaine in a 50:50 ratio. (See Chapter 6 for dosage maximum.)
   c. Apply a wheal of 1% lidocaine subcutaneously over the fracture site. Wait 1 to 2 minutes for the anesthetic to take effect.
   d. Slowly insert and advance the needle attached to the local anesthetic solution through the skin wheal and aimed at the fracture site. C-arm fluoroscopy can aid fracture/hematoma localization. Slowly advance the needle.
      (1) Aspirate with the syringe to **ensure there is no free flow of blood,** which indicates that the needle is within a blood vessel. If there is free blood flow, do not inject the local anesthetic solution.
      (2) A flash, without flow, of blood indicates entry of the tip of the needle into the hematoma.
      (3) Redirect needle if you strike bone or if no flash of blood is returned.
   e. Once flash, without flow, is obtained, slowly inject the local anesthetic solution into the hematoma.
   f. Reposition the needle to different areas within the hematoma and inject small amounts of the local anesthetic into each area. This distributes the local anesthetic solution to increase the efficacy of the hematoma block and minimizes the risk of intravascular injection of the entire dose of local anesthetic.
   g. Withdraw the needle, apply a bandage to the skin puncture site, and await analgesia.

X. SKIN/DERMATOLOGIC PROCEDURES

A. Immunization and Medication Administration[9,29]

NOTE: Please see Chapters 16 and 30 for relevant vaccines and medications and their appropriate administration routes.

1. **Subcutaneous injections**
   a. **Indications:** Immunizations and medications
   b. **Complications:** Bleeding, infection, allergic reaction, lipohypertrophy, or lipoatrophy after repeated injections
   c. **Procedure:**
      (1) Locate injection site: Upper outer arm or outer aspect of upper thigh.
      (2) Cleanse skin with alcohol.

(3) Insert $\frac{5}{8}$-inch, 23- or 25-gauge needle into subcutaneous layer at a 45-degree angle to the skin. Aspirate for blood; if none present, inject medication/immunization.

2. **Intramuscular (IM) injections**
    a. **Indications:** Immunizations and medications
    b. **Complications:** Bleeding, infection, allergic reaction, nerve injury
    c. **Cautions:**
        (1) Avoid IM injections in a child with a bleeding disorder or thrombocytopenia.
        (2) Maximum volume to be injected is 0.5 mL in a small infant, 1 mL in an older infant, 2 mL in a school-aged child, and 3 mL in an adolescent.
    d. **Procedure:**
        (1) Locate injection site: Anterolateral upper thigh in smaller child or outer aspect of upper arm (deltoid) in older one. The dorsal gluteal region is less commonly used because of risk for nerve or vascular injury. To find the ventral gluteal site, form a triangle by placing your index finger on the anterior iliac spine and your middle finger on the most superior aspect of the iliac crest. The injection should occur in the middle of the triangle formed by the two fingers and the iliac crest.
        (2) Cleanse skin with alcohol.
        (3) Isolate the muscle by spreading the skin tight. Insert a 1-inch, 22- or 25-gauge needle until hub is flush with skin surface. The needle should be perpendicular to the skin. Aspirate for blood; if none present, inject medication.

B. Basic Laceration Repair[3,9]

1. **Wound irrigation**[30,31]**:** Numerous studies, including a large Cochrane review, conclude that there is no difference in the infection rates of wounds irrigated with either tap water or sterile NS. The volume of irrigation depends on the location and size of the wound; 100 mL per 1 cm of laceration is a good approximation for relatively uncontaminated wounds.

2. **Suturing:**
    a. Basic suturing technique (Fig. 4.9):
        (1) Simple interrupted: Basic closure of most uncomplicated wounds
        (2) Horizontal mattress: Provides eversion of wound edges
        (3) Vertical mattress: For added strength in areas of thick skin or areas of skin movement; provides eversion of wound edges
        (4) Running intradermal: For cosmetic closures
        (5) Deep dermal: For bringing together deeper portions of wounds with dissolving sutures to allow improved approximation and closure of superficial surfaces
    b. **Procedure:**
        (1) See Tables 4.1 to 4.3 for sutures material, size, and time for removal.[32]

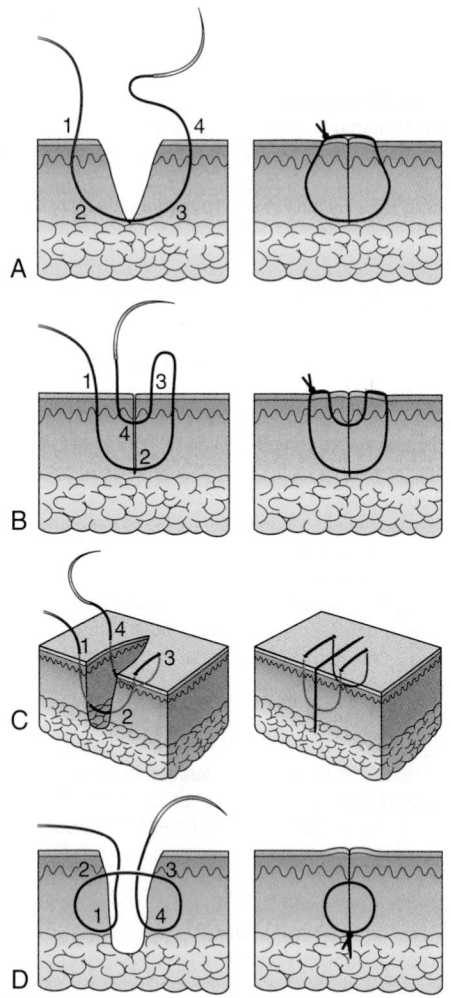

FIGURE 4.9

Suture techniques. (A) Simple interrupted. (B) Vertical mattress. (C) Horizontal mattress. (D) Deep dermal. (Modified from Srivastava D, Taylor RS. Suturing technique and other closure materials. In: Robinson JK, Hanke CW, Siegel DM, et al., eds. *Surgery of the Skin.* 3rd ed. Elsevier; 2015:193–213.)

(2) **NOTE:** Lacerations of the face, lips, hands, genitalia, mouth, or periorbital area may require consultation with a specialist. Ideally, lacerations at increased risk for infection (areas with

TABLE 4.1

GUIDELINES FOR SUTURE MATERIAL, SIZE, AND REMOVAL[32]

Body Region	Nonabsorbable	Absorbable	Duration (Days)
Scalp	5—0 or 4—0	4—0	5—7
Face	6—0	5—0	3—5
Eyelid	7—0 or 6—0	—	3—5
Eyebrow	6—0 or 5—0	5—0	3—5
Trunk	5—0 or 4—0	3—0	5—7
Extremities	5—0 or 4—0	4—0	7—10
Joint surface	4—0	—	10—14
Hand	5—0	5—0	7
Foot sole	4—0 or 3—0	4—0	7—10

TABLE 4.2

CHARACTERISTICS OF COMMON ABSORBABLE SUTURES[32]

Material	Type	Tensile Strength	Absorption Time (Weeks)	Uses
Vicryl	Braided	75% at 14 days 50% at 21 days 5% at 30 days	8—10	Subcutaneous closure, vessel ligature
Vicryl rapide	Braided	50% at 5 days 0 at 14 days	6	Mucosa, dermis
Surgical gut plain	Twisted	Poor at 7—10 days	6—8	Subcutaneous closure
Surgical gut chromic	Twisted	Poor at 21—23 days	8—10	Subcutaneous closure
Monocryl	Monofilament	60%—70% at 7 days 30%—40% at 14 days	13—17	Subcuticular

TABLE 4.3

CHARACTERISTICS OF COMMON NONABSORBABLE SUTURES[32]

Material	Type	Tensile Strength
NYLON (USED FOR SKIN CLOSURE)		
Ethilon	Monofilament	20% per year
Dermalon	Monofilament	20% per year
Surgilon	Braided	Good
Nurolon	Braided	Good
POLYPROLENE (USED FOR SCALP, EYEBROWS)		
Prolene	Monofilament	Permanent
Surgilene	Monofilament	Permanent

poor blood supply, contamination, or crush injury) should be sutured within 6 hours of injury. Clean wounds in cosmetically important areas may be closed up to 24 hours after injury in the absence of significant contamination or devitalization. In general, bite wounds should not be sutured except in areas of high cosmetic importance (face) or if significant gaping is present. These wounds can be closed loosely to aid in healing by secondary intention. The longer sutures are left in place, the greater potential for scarring and infection. Sutures in cosmetically sensitive areas should be removed as soon as possible. Sutures in high tension areas (e.g., extensor surfaces) should stay in longer.

(3) Prepare child for procedure with appropriate sedation, analgesia, and restraint. Utilize Child Life Specialist or age-appropriate distraction.

(4) Anesthetize the wound with topical anesthetic or with lidocaine mixed with bicarbonate (with or without epinephrine) by injecting the anesthetic into the subcutaneous tissues (see Chapter 6).

(5) Copiously irrigate the wound as per above. This is the most important step in preventing infection.

(6) Prepare and drape the patient for a sterile procedure.

(7) Debride the wound when indicated. Probe for foreign bodies as indicated. Consider obtaining a radiograph if a radiopaque foreign body is suspected.

(8) Select suture type for indicated wound closure (see Tables 4.1 to 4.3).

(9) Match layers of injured tissues. Carefully match the depth of the bite taken on each side of the wound when suturing. Take equal bites from both wound edges. Apply slight thumb pressure on the wound edge as the needle is entering the opposite side. Pull the sutures to approximate wound edges but not too tightly, to avoid tissue necrosis. In delicate areas, sutures should be approximately 2 mm apart and 2 mm from the wound edge. Larger bites are acceptable where cosmesis is less important.[3]

(10) When suturing is complete, apply topical antibiotic and sterile dressing. If laceration is in proximity of a joint, splinting of the affected area to limit mobility often speeds healing and prevents wound dehiscence.

(11) For active children, keep the wound covered until sutures are removed.

(12) Check wounds at 48 to 72 hours in cases where tissue is of questionable viability, if wound was packed, or for patients prescribed prophylactic antibiotics. Change dressing at checkup.

(13) For hand lacerations, close skin only; do not use subcutaneous stitches. Elevate and immobilize the hand. Consider consulting a hand or plastics specialist.

(14) Consider the need for tetanus prophylaxis (see Chapter 16).

   c. **Wound care at home:**
      (1) Keep the wound dry and clean for the initial 24 hours. The child may shower and dry the wound after.
      (2) Avoid swimming or bathing until sutures are removed.
      (3) Wear sunscreen to minimize pigment changes.
      (4) Counsel on signs of wound infection and dehiscence.
      (5) Return for suture removal as indicated.
   d. **A video on** basic laceration repair **is available on the *New England Journal of Medicine*'s website.**

3. **Skin staples**[33]
   a. **Indications:**
      (1) Best for scalp, trunk, extremity lacerations
      (2) More rapid application than sutures, but can be more painful to remove
      (3) Lower rates of wound infection
   b. **Contraindications:**
      (1) Not for areas that require meticulous cosmesis
      (2) Avoid in patients who require magnetic resonance imaging (MRI) or CT.
   c. **Procedure:**
      (1) Apply topical anesthetic, as above. Injection of lidocaine is not routinely used when using staples.
      (2) Clean and irrigate wound, as with suturing.
      (3) Appose wound edges, press stapler firmly against skin at center of apposed edges, and staple.
      (4) Apply antibiotic ointment and sterile bandage.
      (5) Leave in place for the same length of time as sutures (see Table 4.1)
      (6) To remove, use dedicated staple remover.

4. **Tissue adhesives**[3,34]
   a. **Indications:**
      (1) For use with superficial lacerations with clean edges
      (2) Excellent cosmetic results, ease of application, and reduced patient anxiety
      (3) Lower rates of wound infection
   b. **Contraindications:**
      (1) Not for use in areas under large amounts of tension (e.g., hands, joints)
      (2) Use caution with areas near the eye or over areas with hair such as the eyebrow.
   c. **Procedure:**
      (1) Use pressure to achieve hemostasis and clean the wound as explained previously.
      (2) Hold together wound edges.
      (3) Apply adhesive dropwise along the wound surface. Avoid applying adhesive to the inside of the wound. Hold in place for 20 to 30 seconds.

(4) If the wound is misaligned, remove the adhesive with forceps and reapply. Petroleum jelly or similar substance can aid in removal of skin adhesive.

(5) Adhesive will slough off after 5 to 10 days.

(6) Antibiotic ointments or other creams/lotions should not be applied to the adhesive, as this can cause premature loosening of the glue and subsequent wound dehiscence.

(7) No need to return for removal.

5. **Hair apposition technique**[35,36]
   a. **Indication:** Linear lacerations of the scalp
   b. **Contraindications:** It does not provide hemostasis, so it is not recommended for bleeding wounds.
   c. **Procedure:**
      (1) Separate a few strands of hair on each side of the wound (parallel).
      (2) Cross the strands once and add tissue adessive where the strands cross.
      (3) No need to return for removal

C. Incision and Drainage (I&D) of Abscess[3]

1. **Indications:** Diagnostic and therapeutic drainage of soft tissue abscess
2. **Complications:** Inadequate abscess drainage, local tissue injury, pain, scar formation, and, in rare cases, fistula formation. Consider specialized surgical evaluation for abscesses in cosmetically or anatomically sensitive areas (the face, neck, breast, or anogenital region) or for recurrent and multiple interconnected abscesses.
3. **Ultrasound identification:** Ultrasound imaging can be used to differentiate cellulitis from abscess.
   a. Use a linear probe; place the probe over the area of interest, and scan it systematically such that the entire area of interest is examined.
   b. Cellulitis characteristics on ultrasound:
      (1) Increased edema; tissue may appear slightly darker and will have distorted, indistinct margins
      (2) Areas may have a "cobblestone" appearance caused by edema (Fig. 4.10).
   c. Abscess characteristics on ultrasound:
      (1) Dark fluid collection distinct from surrounding tissue (see Fig. 4.10)
      (2) Often round or oval
      (3) Doppler can help to distinguish between lymph nodes and fluid collections.
4. **Procedure:**
   a. Consider procedural sedation based upon the child's expected tolerance of the procedure and the location/size/complexity of the abscess.

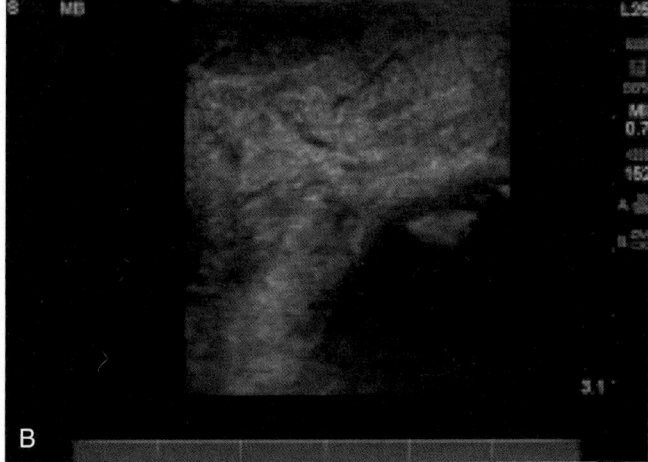

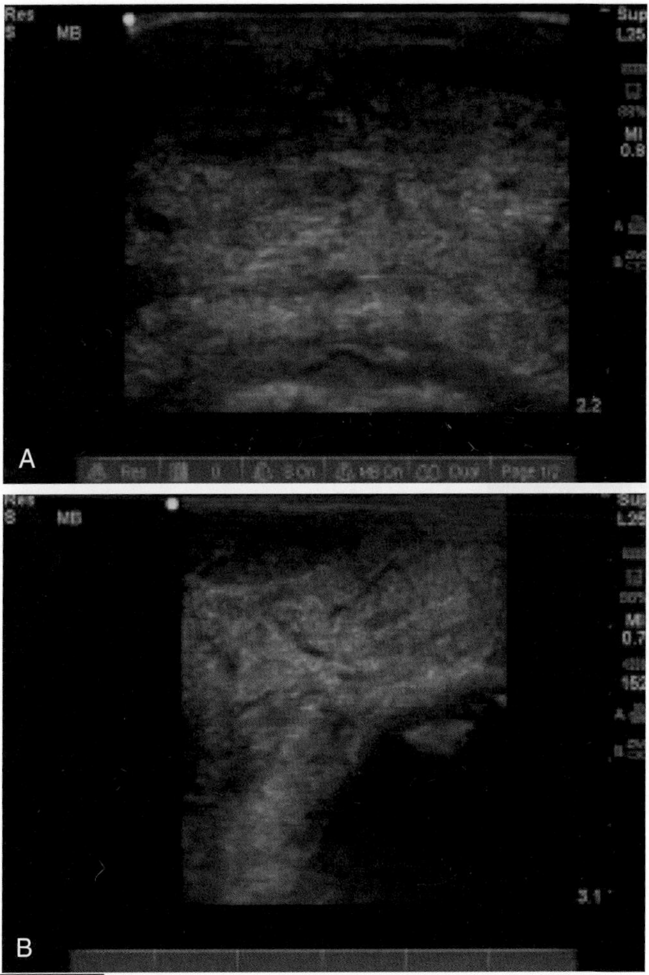

FIGURE 4.10

Ultrasound characteristics of soft tissue cellulitis and *abscess*. (A) Cellulitis characterized by bright (hyperechoic) tissue due to edema and inflammation in the tissue. (B) This image demonstrates the classic "cobblestone" appearance which is a later ultrasound finding in cellulitis.

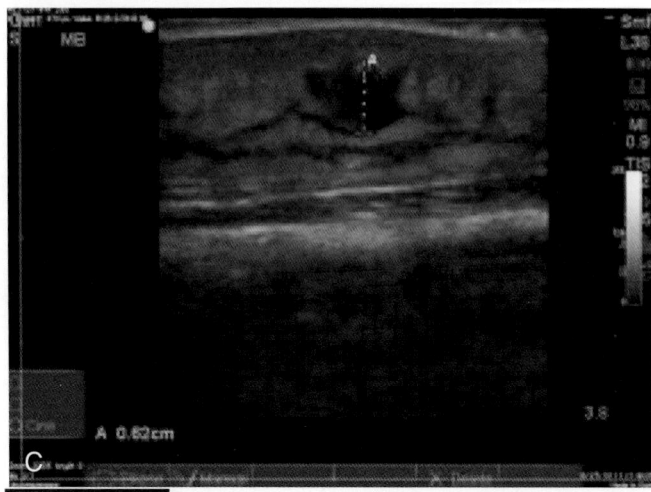

FIGURE 4.10, cont'd

(C) A black (anechoic) rounded structure is noted in the soft tissue, which is charac-teristic of a soft tissue abscess. Some abscesses may appear dark gray depending on the characteristics of the fluid within the abscess. (From Leeson K, Leeson B. Pediatric ultrasound: applications in the emergency department. *Emerg Med Clin North Am.* 2013;31[3]:809–829.)

b. Apply topical anesthetic cream to the abscess to numb the superficial epidermis (see Chapter 6).

c. Prepare the overlying skin in a sterile fashion and, once cleaned, numb the area using 1% lidocaine and a small-gauge needle, performing first a circumferential field block of the abscess area followed by direct injection to the planned incision site.

d. Make a simple linear incision over the total length of the abscess down to the superficial fascia using a scalpel blade, cutting parallel to the natural crease of the skin.

e. Using a hemostat, bluntly widen and undermine the incision to break up any septations or loculated fluid collections. Vigorously irrigate the wound using sterile saline to improve removal of purulent material.

f. If desired, introduce a sterile packing strip into the wound using a hemostat, making sure to fill in an outside-to-inside pattern without overfilling. Leave a 2- to 3-cm tail outside the wound to facilitate removal and cover the wound with an absorbent dressing. Packing material should be removed in 1 to 2 days with a minimum of daily dressing changes until healed.

g. Consider starting antibiotics that cover staphylococcus and streptococcal species per local guidelines and resistance patterns.

Consider obtaining Gram stain, culture, and susceptibility testing of purulent fluid.

5. **A video on** I&D of Abscesses **is available on the** *New England Journal of Medicine*'s **website.**

D. Tuberculin Skin Test Placement[37]

1. **Indications:** Concern for exposure to tuberculosis
2. **Contraindications:** History of severe reactions to prior placements (e.g., necrosis, anaphylactic shock, ulcerations). **Note** that there is no contraindication for any other individuals including infants, children, pregnant women, or persons who have been vaccinated with Bacillus Calmette-Guérin (BCG). Vaccination with live viruses may interfere with the tuberculin skin test (TST), so the test should be done either the same day as the vaccination or at least 1 month after administration of the vaccine.
3. **Complications:** Pain, necrosis
4. **Procedure:** Inject 0.1 mL of tuberculin purified protein derivative (PPD) with a tuberculin syringe (bevel up) into the forearm at a 5- to 15-degree angle. It is an intradermal injection. The injection should produce a pale elevation of the skin 6 to 10 mm in diameter.
5. **Follow-up:** A TST should be read between 48 and 72 hours after administration. The reaction is measured across the forearm (perpendicular to the long axis) in millimeters of induration (palpable, raised, hardened area or swelling). Do not measure erythema.
6. **Interpretation:** See Chapter 17.

E. Tick Removal[38,39]

1. **Indications:** Visualization of tick. Urgent removal is essential, as the risk of Lyme disease transmission significantly increases after 24 hours of attachment.
2. **Complications:** Retention of tick fragments (particularly mouthparts), infection, granuloma formation
3. **Procedure:**
   a. Use clean, fine-tipped tweezers to grasp the tick at the skin surface. Lift up firmly, applying steady pressure and without a twisting motion. Do not squeeze the body of the tick, because its fluid may leak infectious material.
   b. Clean the bite area with rubbing alcohol or soap and water.

REFERENCES

A complete list of references can be found online.

PART II

DIAGNOSTIC AND THERAPEUTIC INFORMATION

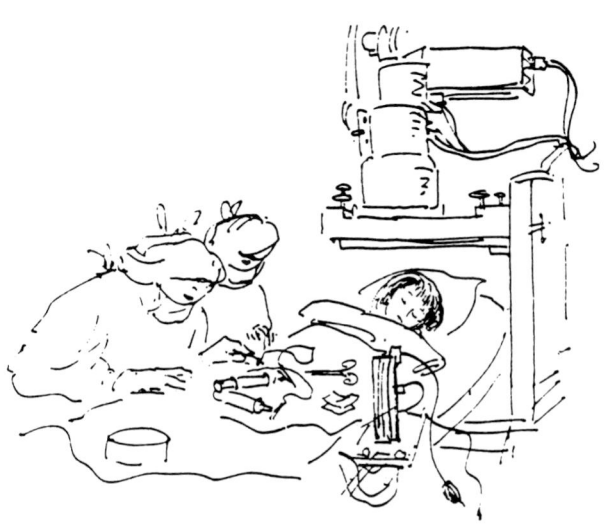

Chapter 5

Adolescent Medicine

Yasamin Ege Sanii, MD and Amitte Rosenfeld, MD

🌐 See additional content online.

🔊 **Audio Case File 5.1** An interactive walk through the HEADSSS assessment, and next steps

I. THEORY OF ADOLESCENCE/INTRODUCTION

Adolescence is defined by both an age range, typically encompassing ages 10 to 25, as well as a life stage consisting of rapid physical, psychological, and social growth and development.[1] Adolescence is a foundational time that lays groundwork for future identity, health, and well-being. Progression through adolescence is characterized by cognitive, psychosocial, and emotional development, which help adolescents to establish their identity and autonomy.[2] See eTable 5.1 for detailed psychosocial development by age. The goal of adolescence is to gain independence and develop a secure identity, spanning a period of legal and medical dependency and independency.[2] The health habits and behaviors formed during this time can have long-lasting impact on future health status and well-being.[3] Helping adolescents effectively navigate these changes and junctures enables safe and supported growth and development.

II. STRUCTURAL FACTORS IMPACTING ADOLESCENTS AND THEIR HEALTH

Structural factors have significant impact on the health and well-being of adolescents. Adverse childhood experiences have been associated with chronic health problems, mental illness, and substance use issues in adulthood[4] (see Chapter 9 for further discussion). Consideration and integration of these issues into care for adolescence is essential to providing effective care.

A. Examples

This is not meant to be an exhaustive list, but rather a starting point for discussion of selected factors. For further information please see References.

1. **Racism**[5]
   a. Institutional: Education, environmental/location, legal (police-instigated violence, juvenile justice system)
   b. Personally mediated: Explicit/implicit bias, interpersonal relationships
   c. Internalized: Stereotypes, stereotype threat

2. **Environmental/neighborhood disparities:** Lack of outdoor spaces, clean air and water, exposure to environmental toxins, exposure to trauma and violence

3. **Documentation status and immigration:** Limited access to services and higher education, concerns for family separation

4. **Reproductive justice:** Restriction of services based on geography, insurance status

B. Role Clinicians Can Play[5]

1. **Individual patient interactions/relationships:** Clinicians can work to create a culturally safe space for patients and their families by examining their own biases and employing a patient- and family-centered and evidence-based approach to care for all patients. Additionally, strategies can be used such as "Raising Resistors"[6] to provide anticipatory guidance to support patients and families in resisting internalized messages of racism and instead promote positive and value-based identity formation.

2. **Community engagement and advocacy:** Clinicians can work with their local communities, governments, and community-based organizations to advocate for systems and policies that reduce inequity and improve access, thereby reducing exposure to adverse childhood experiences and optimizing outcomes for youth.

III. CONFIDENTIALITY

Confidentiality is a crucial component of adolescent healthcare because adolescents report that they may be delayed in seeking care, preferentially seek care at sites offering confidential care and information shared on sensitive topics may be limited.[7,8] Begin integrating one-on-one time between the provider and patient into adolescent visits as early as age 11 to provide teens with regular opportunities to discuss concerns and sensitive topics in an open manner.[9] This time also provides the foundation for their transition to adulthood, helping them learn how to talk to their doctor on their own and take responsibility for their health. Providers should be aware of barriers to confidentiality related to consent laws and billing/explanation of benefits by insurance companies.[10]

A. Consent Laws

All states within the United States, including the District of Columbia, allow minors to consent to sexually transmitted infection (STI) services (diagnosis and treatment), although some states have a minimum age to consent. No states explicitly prohibit minors' consent to pre-exposure prophylaxis (PrEP), although it is often not explicitly addressed.[11] Laws surrounding consent to HIV testing and treatment, contraception, abortion, mental health/substance use disorder treatment, and other healthcare services vary by state. Current information on consent laws by state can be found at the Guttmacher Institute's website (https://www.guttmacher.org/state-policy/explore/overview-minors-consent-law).[12]

B. Breach of Confidentiality

Confidentiality must be breached if the adolescent is at risk of harming themselves or others (e.g., suicidal or homicidal ideation). Parents/guardians should be informed if there is concern for self-harm and for safety concerns, patients should be taken to an emergency room, and/or police should be called. Providers should familiarize themselves with the "duty to warn" (harm to others) laws in their jurisdiction—the responsibility of a provider to warn an identifiable third party of a potential threat of harm to their health.[13] Cases of child abuse or neglect must be reported to child protective services. The definition of statutory rape and reporting laws vary by state, with minimum age to consent to sexual activity ranging from 16 to 18 years old. Current information on reporting laws by state can be found at the Rape, Abuse & Incest National Network's website (https://rainn.org/public-policy-action).[14] See Chapter 2 for more information on evaluation and management of suspected sexual abuse. When confidentiality must be breached, special care must be taken to maintain the physician-patient relationship with the adolescent to the extent possible. This can be done by involving the adolescent in the conversation by offering choices about what exactly is shared and how it is shared (e.g., with whom, by whom) so that they are part of the decision-making process. It is also helpful to share with adolescents at the beginning of the confidential component of their visits the reasons that would necessitate breaking confidentiality so that it does not come as a surprise if concerns do arise.

C. Documentation and Billing

Confidentiality can be inadvertently breached if providers are not careful about documentation and do not have sufficient understanding of who has access. In the United States, the 21st Century Cures Act necessitates open notes, but providers can choose to keep notes on sensitive topics confidential. Providers in the United States should explore with their own hospital and/or legal counsel how to do this. Other providers should explore local laws and regulations to be able to share with patients what can and cannot be kept confidential. In some places insurance disclosures such as "Explanations of Benefits" may also inadvertently breach confidentiality.[10] Providers should be aware of the local regulations around what will be sent to the primary insurance holder. Government-funded and other programs outside of insurance such as US Title X services and local health departments can be possible solutions to overcome this barrier.

IV. HEALTH MAINTENANCE ELEMENTS UNIQUE TO THE ADOLESCENT PATIENT

A. History (HEEADSSS Assessment) and Screenings[15]

Medical history should include all areas typically covered; however, there are some areas that require specific focus during adolescence. Most of the well visit is often spent exploring the psychosocial aspects of an adolescent's health. HEEADSSS is a useful mnemonic to remember these essential components.

1. **H—Home:** Household composition, family dynamics and relationships, recent changes, housing stability

2. **E—Education/employment:** School performance and attendance, goals for the future, after-school job or other work history, vocational training programs
   a. See Chapter 9 for more information on learning disabilities

3. **E—Eating**
   a. Body image and dieting
   b. Eating disorders (see Chapter 24 for more information)
   c. Obesity and weight management in adolescence (see Chapter 21 for more information)
      (1) Developing lifelong habits and new independence in decision making around lifestyle. Overweight in adolescence is a predictor of lifelong morbidity and mortality.[16]
      (2) Family practices around food: who does the shopping/cooking, what (if any) responsibility the adolescent holds, how often do they eat out, do they eat all together or separately, where do people eat in the home (e.g., at a table vs. in front of the TV)
      (3) Lipid and diabetes mellitus (DM) screening recommendations (Table 5.1)
   d. Food security: Can use validated two-item survey ("often true" or "sometimes true" is a positive screen vs. "never true")[17]:
      (1) Within the past 12 months we worried whether our food would run out before we got money to buy more.
      (2) Within the past 12 months the food we bought just didn't last and we didn't have money to get more.

4. **A—Activities:**
   a. Social media[18]: Explore how social media is used and for what quantity of time.
      (1) Benefits: Communication and engagement
      (2) Risks of excessive/inappropriate use: Impaired sleep, attention, and learning; obesity; depression; viewing of unsuitable content; decrease in caregiver-child interactions; compromised privacy; meeting high-risk sexual partners or sexual predators, sexting, and cyberbullying
      (3) Guidance for teens and families: https://downloads.aap.org/AAP/PDF/Bright%20Futures/BF4_HealthySocialMedia.pdf
      (4) American Academy of Pediatrics (AAP) Family Media Use Plan: https://www.healthychildren.org/MediaUsePlan
   b. Screen time: Provide guidance on limiting use.
   c. Physical activity: Goal of at least 60 minutes of moderate to vigorous physical activity daily.[19] Work with adolescents and their families to identify safe and creative ways they can achieve this while acknowledging limitations and inequities in access to safe outdoor space.
   d. Hobbies and interests
   e. Sleep

5. **D—Drugs** (Substance use: tobacco, EtOH, illicit substances, prescription drugs not prescribed to the individual)

TABLE 5.1	

PREVENTATIVE HEALTH LABS AND PROCEDURES

Preventative Health Topic	Recommendations and Further References
Immunizations	See Chapter 16
Cholesterol[98,9]	Once between ages 9 and 11 and again between 17 and 21
Diabetes[99]	Screen with A1c, fasting plasma glucose, or oral glucose tolerance test for adolescents with: 1. BMI ≥85% for age and sex AND 2. One or more risk factors, such as family history, acanthosis nigricans, HTN, HLD, PCOS, or other signs of or conditions associated with insulin resistance If normal, repeat at minimum every 3 years or sooner based on changes in risk profile.
Blood pressure[100]	See Chapter 19. BP should be checked annually in all adolescents and at every healthcare encounter if they have obesity or are taking medications known to increase BP, have renal disease, a history of aortic arch obstruction or coarctation, or DM.[103]
Sexual health	See Section V.
Cervical cancer[101,102]	1. <21 years old: no screening 2. Aged 21–29 years: Cytology alone every 3 years 3. Immunocompromised (living with or without HIV): screening within 1 year of first insertional sexual activity. Annually for 3 years, then every 3 years (cytology only) Recommended screening intervals and follow-up depend on patient's risk of CIN3+ based on combination of pap smear results, and past history. Web-based decision tool can be found at https://app.asccp.org/
Infectious diseases[9]	1. HIV: Universal screening beginning at age 15: See Section V for details based on risk. 2. *N. gonorrhoeae* and *C. trachomatis*: See Section V for recommendations and discussion. 3. Hepatitis C Virus (HCV)[104]: • Universal screening for age 18+ • Screening for all adolescents (regardless of age) who have ever injected or used intranasal drugs, have a history of incarceration, with HIV infection and/or prior to starting PrEP

A lack of evidence has led to variability in guidelines for topics such as screening for dyslipidemia, iron-deficiency anemia, diabetes, and tuberculosis. The recommendations in this table are largely based on the AAP,[9] CDC, U.S. Preventive Services Task Force (USPSTF),[98] and the American College of Obstetricians and Gynecologists (ACOG).

a. **Epidemiology**
   (1) In 2021 almost half of 12th graders in the United States reported using alcohol in the last year, and a similar number reported using illicit drugs in their lifetime, with cannabis being by far the most frequent.[20]
   (2) Roughly a third of 12th graders in the United States reported vaping nicotine in the past year, down from a peak of 40% in 2019.[20]

(3) Substance use during adolescence increases likelihood of developing a substance use disorder (SUD) later, with greater risk conferred with earlier use.[22]

b. **Screening, brief intervention, and referral to treatment (SBIRT):** The AAP and SAMHSA recommend universal screening as part of routine healthcare. This can be done wherever and whenever adolescents receive medical care.[23]

(1) **S**creening: Must be done with a validated tool. Start by asking how many days adolescent has used any alcohol, marijuana, or anything else to get high in the past 12 months, followed by risk stratification/brief assessment using a validated tool specifically designed for adolescents. May require comprehensive assessment if problem suggested (see below).[22]

(a) Validated self-report tools are generally considered to be a credible method for screening and found to corroborate with other sources of information, making other methods such as urine drug testing unnecessary.

(b) Tools *(a few examples, many others available):* Screening to Brief Intervention (S2BI)[24] and Brief Screener for Tobacco, Alcohol and other Drugs (BSTAD)[25] are available online through the National Institute on Drug Abuse (NIDA)[26] (https://nida.nih.gov/nidamed-medical-health-professionals/ screening-tools-resources/screening-tools-adolescent-substance-use). CRAFFT[27] (Box 5.1) can be used after positive initial screen to "any use" question and identifies potentially problematic behavior associated with the substance use, as well as calculates the probability that the patient has a substance use disorder.

(c) Important to also screen for co-occurring mental health disorders (see Chapter 24)

(2) **B**rief **I**ntervention: Counseling based on risk stratification; motivational interviewing as appropriate

---

BOX 5.1

CRAFFT QUESTIONNAIRE

C—Have you ever ridden in a **C**AR driven by someone (or yourself) who was "high" or had been using alcohol or drugs?

R—Do you ever use alcohol or drugs to **R**ELAX, feel better about yourself, or fit in?

A—Do you ever use alcohol/drugs while you are **A**LONE?

F—Do your family or **F**RIENDS ever tell you that you should cut down on your drinking or drug use?

F—Do you ever **F**ORGET things you did while using alcohol or drugs?

T—Have you gotten into **T**ROUBLE while you were using alcohol or drugs?

NOTE: Answering yes to two or more questions is a positive screen.

From Gephart H: Rating scales, questionnaires, and behavior checklists. In ADHD Complex: Practicing Mental Health in Primary Care. Philadelphia, Elsevier, 2019, pp 1–7.

(a) Low risk (abstinent): Reinforce decisions with praise and provide anticipatory guidance regarding riding in a car with a driver under the influence.

(b) Yes to "Car" question: Counsel and encourage safety plan.

(c) Substance use without an SUD: Advise cessation of substance use, educate regarding health risks of continued use, and praise personal attributes.

(d) Mild to moderate SUD: Conduct in-depth assessment using motivational interviewing (MI) (see eTable 5.2). MI is a counseling technique aimed at helping a patient identify their goals and values and use these to strengthen their motivation for change.

(e) Severe SUD: In-depth assessment and MI as above plus referral to treatment (see IV.A.5.d.(3))

(3) **R**eferral to **T**reatment (see IV.A.5.d.(3))

c. Peer and family use/exposure

d. Substance use disorders

(1) **Epidemiology:** In the United States, in 2020 an estimated 6.3% of adolescents aged 12 to 17 and 24.4% aged 18 to 25 met criteria for an SUD in the past year based on DSM-5 criteria.[28]

(2) **Diagnosis:** DSM-5 defines substance use disorders with the same criteria for all substances: A pattern of continued use and clinically/functionally significant impairment with ≥2 of the symptoms in Table 5.2

(3) **Treatment and referral**[22]

(a) Spectrum of service levels: Outpatient services to intensive outpatient/partial hospital to residential/inpatient services and medically managed intensive inpatient services

(b) Utilize multidimensional assessment for a holistic, biopsychosocial approach to service planning and treatment[29,22]

(c) Medication for addiction treatment[30]: For opioid use disorder, buprenorphine is FDA approved for ages 16+ but is often used off-label for younger ages; naltrexone is FDA approved for ages 18+, and methadone is approved for 18 and up, with limited accessibility in certain circumstances for <18 years old. Medications for other SUDs such as with alcohol and tobacco/nicotine are largely approved for 18+, though may be used off-label.

(4) HCV screening (see Table 5.1)

6. S—Sexuality and gender

a. Terminology and definitions (Table 5.3): While gender and sexuality are often conflated, they are independent components of identity, each with multiple subcomponents. Gender identity is a person's intrinsic sense of self, as male, female, or other gender.[31] Sexuality is how one relates to others sexually. There are three components of sexual orientation: identity, behavior, and attraction.

TABLE 5.2

DSM-5 CRITERIA FOR SUBSTANCE USE DISORDERS (SUD)[a]

Category	Criteria
Impaired control	• Using more or longer than intended • Persistent desire or unsuccessful attempts to cut down or quit • Excessive time spent obtaining, using, or recovering from substances • Intense desire to use or cravings
Social impairment	• Failure to fulfill academic, work, or home responsibilities • Use causing or exacerbating interpersonal problems • Giving up or reducing important social, occupational, or recreational activities because of use
Risky use	• Recurrent substance use in physically hazardous situations • Continued use despite physical or psychological problems due to use
Pharmacologic criteria[b]	• Tolerance (diminished effect of same dose, needing higher dose to achieve effect) • Withdrawal symptoms with cessation of substance use

[a]No longer separated into substance dependence and abuse (DSM-IV); all categorized as substance use disorder.
[b]If medication is being taken only as prescribed, then tolerance and withdrawal do not count toward SUD diagnosis.
≥ 2 = positive for SUD; 2-3 = mild SUD; 4-5 = moderate SUD; 6+ = severe SUD.
Data from American Psychiatric Association. *Diagnostic and Statistical Manual of Mental Disorders* (DSM-5). American Psychiatric Publishing; 2013.

TABLE 5.3

GENDER AND SEXUALITY TERMINOLOGY AND DEFINITIONS

Term	Definition
Gender identity	A person's internal sense of self and how they fit into the world, from the perspective of gender
Gender expression	The outward manner in which an individual expresses or displays their gender. This may include choices in clothing and hairstyle, or speech and mannerisms. This may differ from gender identity.
Sex assigned at birth	Based on assessment of external genitalia, as well as chromosomes and gonads
Sexual orientation	There are three components: identity, behavior, and attraction; not directly related to gender identity. The sexual orientation of transgender people should be defined by the individual.
Transgender	An individual whose gender identity differs from the sex assigned at birth
Cisgender	An individual whose gender identity is the same as the sex assigned at birth
Gender diverse	Includes individuals whose gender identity and/or role does not conform to a binary understanding of gender as limited to the categories of man or woman, male or female. May be more complex, fluid, multifaceted, or otherwise less clearly defined than a transgender person
Gender dysphoria	Discomfort or distress caused by discrepancy between a person's gender identity and sex assigned at birth. DSM-5 criteria recommend a diagnosis occur after 6 months of continuous incongruence. For prepubescent children, defined by DSM-5 as a marked incongruence between one's experienced/expressed gender and assigned gender.[95]

Adapted from World Professional Association for Transgender Health[34] and UCSF Transgender Care.[96] Others as referenced in table.

(1) One teaching tool to assist with this concept can be found at https://genderbread.org and https://thegenderbook.com.

b. Taking a sexual history: Should be done as part of routine healthcare. Employ a patient-centered, nonjudgmental approach, keeping in mind potential histories of trauma or abuse. The "Five Ps" approach is outlined below.[32] See https://www.cdc.gov/std/treatment/sexualhistory.htm for full list of questions and example script.

(1) **P**artners: Number of lifetime and current partners

(2) **P**ractices: Type of sexual contact, parts of body involved, history of exchanging sex for needs

(3) **P**rotection from STIs: Knowledge of contraception and STI prevention

(4) **P**ast History of STIs: Prior testing for STIs/HIV

(5) **P**regnancy Intention: Reproductive life plan and prior pregnancies and/or abortions

(6) Additionally inquire about history of nonconsensual intimate physical contact or sex and performance or function concerns

c. Development of identity and behaviors during adolescence

(1) The AAP recommends routinely asking about sexual orientation and gender identity during adolescent visits as sexual identity emerges during adolescence.[33] It is important to provide a safe environment for adolescents to discuss questions about their sexual identity and behavior and to ask questions about sexual activities regardless of sexual orientation, and keep information that they are not ready to share confidential.

(2) Mirror language used by adolescents for body parts and for their identified gender and sexual orientation or behaviors. This is particularly important for lesbian, gay, bisexual, transgender (LGBT), and other gender diverse youth. Terms used by adolescents may not match what the provider expects based on reported activity or sexual orientation.

d. Considerations for transgender and gender-diverse adolescents

(1) Several societies put out standards of care, which can be used to guide management:

(a) The World Professional Association for Transgender Health (WPATH) standards of care[34]: https://www.wpath.org/publications/soc

(b) UCSF Health Considerations for Gender Non-Conforming Children and Transgender Adolescents[35]: https://transcare.ucsf.edu/guidelines/youth

(c) Endocrine Society Clinical Practice Guideline[36]

(2) Gender affirmation: Table 5.4

(3) Timing: Timing of treatment interventions is based on clinical evaluation, including age and pubertal status, input from the patient and their family, and shared decision making. Interventions range from fully reversible to partially irreversible to fully irreversible. It is recommended that these be carried out in a

TABLE 5.4

GENDER AFFIRMATION FOR TRANSGENDER AND GENDER-DIVERSE YOUTH

Type	Components	Reversibility and Timeline
Social	• Changes to name, pronoun, clothing, or appearance (e.g., binders, stand-to-pee devices, silicone breasts) • Parental support and education to create a safe environment for the child	Reversible; all ages; familial support of social transition for transgender children has been associated with better mental health outcomes.[97]
Legal	Legally changing name and gender identifier	Reversible; all ages
Medical	Pubertal suppression: GnRH analogue (e.g., leuprolide and histrelin)	Reversible; starting at Tanner stage II (recommended that adolescent experience the onset of puberty in order to make informed decision about pubertal delay); can relieve distress of pubertal development and can provide time to explore gender identity further
	Hormone therapy: for example, estradiol, progesterone, testosterone, spironolactone	Partially irreversible; sufficient mental capacity to give informed consent (generally by the age of 16 years). Treatment can be considered as early as age 13.5 to 14 years.
Surgical	For example, gonadectomy, hysterectomy, mastectomy, and genital surgery	Irreversible; typically not recommended until age of majority

Adapted from Rafferty et al,[37] World Professional Association for Transgender Health,[34] and Olson-Kennedy et al.[35]

staged approach, prioritizing reversible interventions earlier.[34,37] See Table 5.4 for more details.

(4) Fertility and family planning: It is important to discuss with adolescents and their families who are considering gender affirmation interventions how these may impact future sexual function, fertility, and family planning. Fertility preservation options should be offered early in the process.[37]

(5) Family acceptance is an important protective factor for the mental health and well-being of transgender and gender-diverse youth.[38] Clinicians can support and facilitate these relationships through open conversations and providing resources such as[37]:

(a) The Family Acceptance Project: https://familyproject.sfsu.edu

(b) Parents, Families & Friends of Lesbians and Gays (PFLAG): https://community.pflag.org

(c) The Parents Project: https://www.theparentsproject.com

7. **S—Suicide/depression (see Chapter 24 for further details)**

a. History of depression or other mental health problems

b. Current or prior suicidal thoughts or attempts or other self-harming or injurious behavior

c. Screening: PHQ-A[39] is a validated depression screening tool for adolescents. Screening tools also exist for other mental health disorders such as anxiety (GAD7),[40] although they are not specific to adolescents: https://www.aacap.org/AACAP/Families_and_Youth/ Resource_Centers/Depression_Resource_Center/Resources_for_ Clinicians_Depression.aspx

    d. National disasters, such as pandemics, can impact mental health. Isolation has been associated with negative health outcomes,[41] and the COVID-19 pandemic specifically has resulted in higher rates of a range of mental health concerns including anxiety, depression, eating disorders, and substance use.[42]

    e. Sociocontextual factors: Social determinants of health, racism (see Section II for more in-depth discussion)

8. **S—Safety**

    a. Screening for history of ACEs/trauma (see Chapter 9 for more details)

    b. Feeling unsafe at home, school, or in the community

    c. Bullying

    d. Guns or other weapons at home or access to them

    e. Interactions with police/police-instigated violence and police brutality[43]

        (1) Significant racial disparities: Black youth experience nearly ninefold-more encounters with police compared with White counterparts and are more likely to experience use of force and injury.

        (2) Police exposures are associated with adverse health outcomes for Black youth, including increased rates of adverse mental health, sexual risk behaviors, and substance use.

    f. Fighting, arrests, gang membership

9. **Other aspects of medical history with relevance during adolescence:**

    a. Review of symptoms: STI symptoms, obstructive sleep apnea symptoms (see Chapter 25), sleep (how much, sleep hygiene habits)

    b. Menstrual history

        (1) Age of menarche, last menstrual period (LMP), frequency/ regularity, quality, duration, associated symptoms and severity (missing school/work, requiring medication, etc.)

        (2) Menarche for majority will occur between ages 11 and 15; lack of menarche by age 16 is defined as primary amenorrhea and warrants further workup.[45] Clinical consideration of overall course of growth and development also important

        (3) See Chapter 10 for more regarding expected pubertal development timing and concern for polycystic ovary syndrome (PCOS).

    c. Medications: Any over-the-counter supplements, protein powders, weight loss meds, etc.

B. Physical Examination Elements Unique to the Adolescent[46,47]

1. Conducting a trauma-informed examination[48]

    a. Definition: Incorporating awareness of known or potential history of trauma into the physical exam: intentional use of clinical language, modesty draping and professional touch, and prioritizing patient autonomy whenever possible

b. Screen all patients for history of trauma prior to any sensitive exam.

c. Language: Use clinical rather than colloquial language. Verbally walk patient through entire exam prior to starting.

d. Optimize patient autonomy during the exam whenever possible. This can include strategies (based on patient comfort and desire) such as self-swabbing for STI screening (see Section V.A for more details), self-insertion of the speculum, keeping the head of the table up during a pelvic exam, or others determined through shared decision making.[49]

2. **Dentition and gums:** Caries, enamel defects from tobacco use, and enamel erosion from induced vomiting

3. **Skin:** Acne (see Chapter 8 for treatment guidelines), hirsutism, atypical nevi, acanthosis nigricans, rashes, evidence of cutting, piercings, and tattoos

4. **Thyroid:** Size, nodules. Hypo-/hyperthyroidism can affect puberty.

5. **Breasts:**
   a. Female normal breast development: Tanner staging, also known as Sexual Maturity Rating (Fig. 5.1A), masses (most commonly fibrocystic changes and fibroadenomas in females, or gynecomastia in males), breast asymmetry (common occurrence in adolescence; more pronounced between Tanner pubertal stages 2 and 4)
   b. Physiologic gynecomastia in males:
      (1) Epidemiology: Generally, occurs in middle to late stages of puberty (usually peaks in Tanner pubertal stage 3); occurs in 50% of boys (50% unilateral, 50% bilateral)
      (2) Etiology: Breast growth stimulated by estradiol
      (3) Clinical course: Regression usually occurs over a 2-year period.
      (4) Physical examination: Firm glandular tissue in a concentric mass beneath the areola/nipple is consistent with physiologic gynecomastia. A testicular examination should also be performed.
      (5) Differential diagnosis: Nonphysiologic gynecomastia. Common causes include medication or substance use (particularly cannabis), primary or secondary hypogonadism, cirrhosis, hyperthyroidism, tumors, and pseudogynecomastia (excess adipose tissue on exam).
      (6) Red flags: Symptom duration over 2 years, nipple discharge, skin changes, breast masses, and coincident testicular abnormalities
      (7) Treatment: Often no treatment is necessary. Severe or nonregressing cases may warrant referral to pediatric surgeon, endocrinologist, or oncologist, depending on suspected etiology.

6. **Genitalia:** For both male and female genital examinations, in addition to trauma-informed guidance discussed previously, a chaperone should be present (parent, guardian, or family member not included), an explanation should occur before the examination, and findings should be

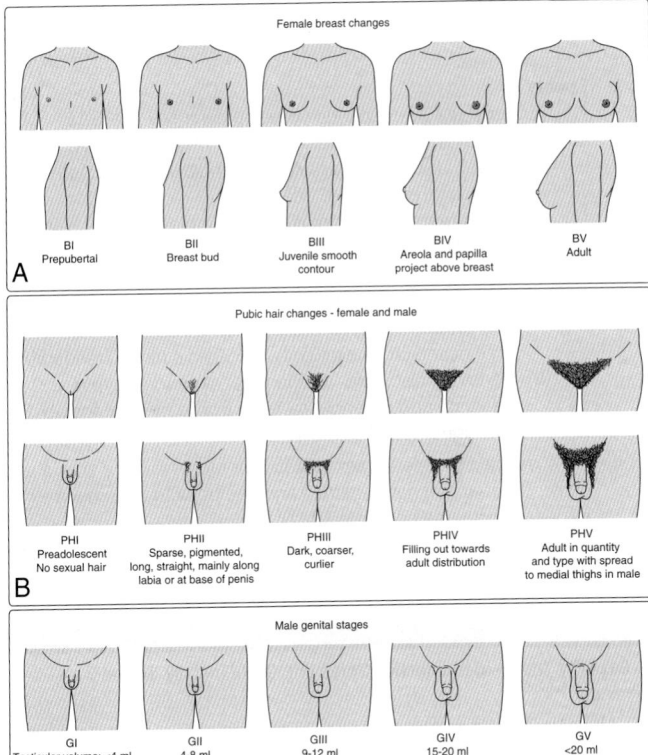

FIGURE 5.1

Tanner stages of puberty. (A) Breast development in females. (B) Pubic hair development in males and females. (C) Male genital development. (Modified from Rodgers A, Salkind J. *Crash Course: Paediatrics*. 5th ed. Elsevier; 2019. Figure 7.3 with data from Emmanuel M, Bokor BR. Tanner Stages. [Updated December 15, 2021]. In: *StatPearls*. StatPearls Publishing; 2022. https://www.ncbi.nlm.nih.gov/books/NBK470280/)

discussed. Tanner staging should be done separately for genitalia and pubic hair to identify issues with the hypothalamic-pituitary-gonadal (HPG) vs. hypothalamic-pituitary-adrenal (HPA) axis.

a. **Male**[50]

(1) Tanner staging of genital development: Fig. 5.1C

(2) Tanner staging of pubic hair development: Fig. 5.1B

(3) Assess for signs of STIs (rashes, warts, ulcers, erosions, discharge), inguinal hernias, masses, hydroceles, varicoceles, and evidence of trauma. If there are symptoms of proctitis with

history of receptive anal intercourse (e.g., rectal pain, rectal bleeding, or tenesmus), a digital rectal examination should be performed.

b. **Female**[51,52]
   (1) Tanner staging of pubic hair development: see Fig. 5.1B
   (2) Assess for signs of STIs (rashes, warts, ulcers, erosions, discharge), discharge suggestive of candidiasis or bacterial vaginosis, and evidence of trauma.
   (3) Speculum exams are not routinely recommended for healthy asymptomatic women.[53] Indications for bimanual exam or speculum exam include:
      (a) Vaginal discharge with or without lower abdominal or pelvic pain (assess cervix for mucopurulent discharge, friability, large ectropion, foreign body, or cervical motion tenderness)
      (b) Menstrual disorders (amenorrhea, abnormal vaginal bleeding, or dysmenorrhea refractory to medical therapy)
      (c) Pap smear (see Table 5.1)

c. For suspected or reported sexual abuse or rape, refer to a specialized center if not appropriately trained and equipped to document evidence of trauma and collect forensic specimens.
   NOTE: See Chapter 10 for information about precocious and delayed puberty.

V. SEXUAL HEALTH

A. Sexually Transmitted Infection Screening Guidelines by Sexual Behaviors[15,52-55]

1. **All adolescents over age 13:** The CDC recommends universal screening for HIV (via HIV 1/2 antigen/antibody test) at least once using an opt-out approach, or more frequently based on risk factors.

2. **Receptive vaginal intercourse:**
   a. **With one lifetime partner:** Screen once with HIV 1/2 antigen/antibody test; self- or provider-collected vaginal NAAT for gonorrhea and chlamydia (routine screening recommended annually in sexually active women under age 25), can add trichomonas in high-prevalence settings.
      (1) *Vaginal swab* is the preferred method to screen for gonorrhea and chlamydia; self-collected specimens may have higher patient acceptability. Vaginal swabs are as sensitive and specific as cervical swabs, and both are more accurate than urine samples.[56-58]
   b. **With risk factors (new partner, multiple partners, partner with STI, incarceration, transactional sex):** Screen for syphilis and trichomonas in high-prevalence settings, HIV testing when being evaluated for other STIs, continued gonorrhea and chlamydia testing annually in women >25 years old. Repeat testing 3 months after treatment of

gonorrhea or chlamydia due to high risk for re-infection. Repeat as indicated by sexual risk.

3. **Penetrative penile intercourse:**
   a. **With one lifetime partner:** Screen once with HIV 1/2 antigen/antibody test. Insufficient evidence on gonorrhea and chlamydia urine NAAT screening benefits; consider in high-risk clinical settings (adolescent clinics, sexual health clinic).
   b. **With risk factors (new partner, multiple partners, partner with STI, incarceration, transactional sex):** HIV testing whenever being evaluated for STIs, rapid plasma reagin (RPR), and NAAT for gonorrhea and chlamydia in high-risk clinical settings. Repeat as indicated by sexual risk.

4. **Receptive anal intercourse:** HIV testing indicated if unknown status or previously negative and patient or their partner has had more than one sex partner since last test; RPR annually, and gonorrhea and chlamydia NAAT (test swab of rectum) are recommended if receptive intercourse in the last year.
   a. Consider 3- to 6-month interval STI testing for those at increased risk (e.g., new sexual partner without a condom).

5. **Oral intercourse:** Gonorrhea NAAT (test swab of pharynx) if receptive oral intercourse in the last year, pharyngeal chlamydia screening not recommended. If positive for pharyngeal gonorrhea, should return in 7 to 10 days for test of cure. If still positive, should complete culture before re-treating.

6. **Pregnant women:** Screenings at first prenatal visit include HIV, hepatitis B (HBsAg), hepatitis C, syphilis (RPR), HIV, gonorrhea, and chlamydia.
   a. If positive gonorrhea or chlamydia, recommend test of cure 4 weeks after treatment with repeat screening 3 months after and during the third trimester.
   b. Repeat testing with patients at high risk for infection, including cisgender women with current or recent injection-drug use, STI during pregnancy, multiple sex partners during pregnancy, or new sexual partner during pregnancy.
      (1) Repeat syphilis screen (RPR) at 28 weeks' gestation.
      (2) Repeat HIV screen in third trimester (preferably before 36 weeks' gestation).
      (3) Repeat hepatitis B testing should be completed at time of admission to the hospital for delivery.

7. **Transgender/gender diverse:** Given the diversity of transgender persons regarding patterns of sexual behavior, hormone use, and surgery, clinicians should assess STI risk based on the patient's sexual behaviors and current anatomy (the latter of which should guide method of NAAT testing, if indicated).

8. **Correctional facilities recommended screenings via opt-out approach:**
   a. Women less than or equal to 35 years old: gonorrhea, chlamydia, and trichomonas

    b. Men less than or equal to 30 years old: gonorrhea and chlamydia

    c. Syphilis testing in high-prevalence locations

    d. All people should receive HIV and hepatitis A, B, and C screening.

9. **Concern for recent exposure to STI:**

    a. Fourth-generation HIV 1/2 antigen/antibody tests detect acute infection within 10 to 14 days. If there is concern for acute or early HIV exposure, consider an HIV RNA nucleic acid test.[59]

    b. Screen with RPR, gonorrhea, and chlamydia NAT (method of testing as described earlier by sexual behavior), and vaginal trichomonas NAT as indicated.

    c. Consider HSV PCR testing in individuals presenting for STI evaluation with genital lesion(s). There is no role for HSV antibody testing.

10. **Persons living with HIV:** Screen at initial visit and at least annually with RPR, gonorrhea and chlamydia NAAT (screening at anatomic site of exposure), and vaginal trichomonas NAAT as indicated. Hepatitis B screening at initial diagnosis, hepatitis C screening at initial diagnosis, and annually thereafter. Screen more frequently if indicated by sexual risk behaviors.

B. Sexually Transmitted Infection Evaluation and Management (Tables 5.5 to 5.7)[52]

1. **HIV:** See Chapter 17 for information on diagnosis and treatment of HIV, Pre-exposure prophylaxis (PrEP), and postexposure prophylaxis (PEP). PrEP should be initiated in the primary care setting, when possible.

2. **Syphilis[52]**

    a. Etiology: *Treponema pallidum*

    b. Early syphilis (within 1 year of initial infection)

       (1) Primary syphilis (chancre): Firm, usually painless sore(s) or ulcer(s) develop at the site of initial infection (genital, rectal, or oral). Chancres typically develop within 3 weeks of infection and heal 3 to 6 weeks after development in the absence of treatment.

       (2) Secondary syphilis: Within weeks to months after a chancre appears, patients may develop body rash involving palms and soles, mucocutaneous lesions, lymphadenopathy, constitutional symptoms, and/or early neurosyphilis (e.g., meningitis or ocular syphilis).

       (3) Early latent syphilis: Asymptomatic stage

       (4) Late syphilis (over 1 year after initial infection)

          (a) Late latent syphilis: Asymptomatic stage

          (b) Tertiary syphilis: Organ involvement may progress to cardiovascular syphilis (e.g., aortitis), late neurosyphilis (e.g., tabes dorsalis or paresis), or gummatous syphilis.

    c. Diagnosis: Testing algorithm varies by laboratory and typically includes a nontreponemal test (RPR or Venereal Disease Research Laboratory [VDRL] test) and a treponemal test (e.g., fluorescent

TABLE 5.5

SEXUALLY TRANSMITTED AND GENITOURINARY INFECTIONS: GUIDELINES FOR MANAGEMENT[a,52]

Infection	Clinical Diagnosis	Empiric Therapy[a]	Comments
Chlamydia infections	Uncomplicated infection of the cervix, urethra, or rectum	Doxycycline 100 mg PO 2×/day for 7 days *Alt regimen:* Azithromycin OR levofloxacin	• Consider empiric treatment for gonococcal infection in patient at high risk for gonorrhea. • Repeat test in 3 months due to high rates of reinfection.
	Lymphogranuloma venereum (LGV)	Doxycycline 100 mg PO 2×/day for 21 days *Alt regimen:* Azithromycin OR erythromycin	
Gonorrhea infections	Uncomplicated infection of the cervix, urethra, or rectum of adolescents <150 kg	Ceftriaxone 500 mg IM once *Alt for cephalosporin allergy:* Gentamicin PLUS azithromycin *If ceftriaxone administration not available:* Cefixime	• Empiric treatment for chlamydia should be provided if chlamydia cannot be excluded with doxycycline 100 mg orally 2×/day for 7 days. • Repeat test in 3 months due to high rates of reinfection.
	Infection of the pharynx in adolescents <150 kg	Ceftriaxone 500 mg IM once	• Test of cure at 7–14 days
	Infection of cervix, urethra, rectum, or pharynx of adolescents >150 kg	Ceftriaxone 1 gm IM once	
	Disseminated gonococcal infections	Ceftriaxone 1 gm IV/IM daily *Alt regimen:* Cefotaxime OR ceftizoxime	• Can switch to oral therapy 24–48 hr after clinical improvement. Total course: 7 days
Epididymitis	Acute epididymitis most likely caused by gonorrhea and chlamydia	Ceftriaxone 500 mg IM once PLUS doxycycline 100 mg PO 2×/day for 10 days	
	Acute epididymitis most likely caused by gonorrhea, chlamydia, or enteric organisms (men who practice insertive anal sex)	Ceftriaxone 500 mg IM once PLUS levofloxacin 500 mg PO 1×/day for 10 days	

Continued

TABLE 5.5

SEXUALLY TRANSMITTED AND GENITOURINARY INFECTIONS: GUIDELINES FOR MANAGEMENT[a,52]—CONT'D

Infection	Clinical Diagnosis	Empiric Therapy[a]	Comments
Pelvic inflammatory disease (PID)	Acute epididymitis caused by enteric organisms only	Levofloxacin 500 mg PO 1×/day for 10 days	
	Parenteral treatment	Ceftriaxone 1 gm IV Q24 hr *PLUS* doxycycline 100 mg PO or IV Q12 hr *PLUS* metronidazole 500 mg PO or IV Q12 hr *Alt regimen:* Cefotetan *PLUS* doxycycline *OR* Cefoxitin *PLUS* doxycycline	• Can transition to oral therapy 24–48 hr after clinical improvement. • If tubo-ovarian abscess present, should be observed >24 hr.
	IM or oral treatment	Ceftriaxone 500 mg IM once *PLUS* doxycycline 100 mg PO 2×/day for 14 days *PLUS* metronidazole 500 mg PO 2×/day for 14 days *OR* Cefoxitin *PLUS* probenecid *PLUS* doxycycline *PLUS* metronidazole	
Nongonococcal urethritis (NGU)	Initial	Doxycycline 100 mg PO 2×/day for 7 days *Alt regimen:* Azithromycin	
	Persistent NGU test for *Mycoplasma genitalium* (NAAT) and resistance	*Refer to treatment for Mycoplasma genitalium below.*	

Mycoplasma genitalium	Persistent urethritis, cervicitis, or PID despite appropriate treatment	*Macrolide sensitive:* Doxycycline 100 mg PO 2×/day for 7 days, *FOLLOWED BY:* Azithromycin 1 gm PO once, *FOLLOWED BY:* Azithromycin 500 mg PO 1×/day for 3 days (2.5 gm total) *Macrolide resistant OR unable to complete resistance testing:* Doxycycline 100 mg PO 2×/day for 7 days, FOLLOWED BY: Moxifloxacin 400 mg PO 1×/day for 7 days
Syphilis	Primary, secondary, or early latent syphilis	Benzathine penicillin G 2.4 million units IM once (single dose)	Dosing applies to pregnant patients and patients with HIV.
	Late latent syphilis	Benzathine penicillin G 7.2 million units total, 3 doses of 2.4 million units IM each at 1-week intervals	Dosing applies to pregnant patients and patients with HIV.
Trichomonas vaginalis	Men with nongonococcal urethritis, test for trichomonas in men who have penile-vaginal intercourse in high-prevalence areas	Metronidazole 2 gm PO once *Alt regimen:* Tinidazole	Molecular diagnostic options more sensitive than wet mount. Repeat test in 3 months due to high rates of reinfection.
	Women, see Table 5.6	Metronidazole 500 mg PO 2×/day for 7 days *Alt regimen:* Tinidazole	
Herpes (genital, nonneonatal)	First clinical episode genital herpes	Acyclovir 400 mg PO 3×/day for 7–10 days OR famciclovir 250 mg PO 3×/day for 7–10 days OR valacyclovir 1 gm PO 2×/day for 7–10 days	
	Suppressive therapy for recurrent genital herpes	Acyclovir 400 mg PO 2×/day OR valacyclovir 500 mg PO 1×/day OR valacyclovir 1 gm PO 1×/day OR famciclovir 250 mg PO 2×/day	Suppressive therapy can be offered in patients with severe recurrent HSV-2 infections; suppression also effective for less frequent recurrences and decreases transmission of HSV-2 to partner.

Continued

TABLE 5.5

SEXUALLY TRANSMITTED AND GENITOURINARY INFECTIONS: GUIDELINES FOR MANAGEMENT[a,52]—CONT'D

Infection	Clinical Diagnosis	Empiric Therapy[a]	Comments
	Episode therapy for recurrent genital herpes	Acyclovir 800 mg PO 2×/day for 5 days *Alt regimen:* Alternative dosing of acyclovir, famciclovir, or valacyclovir	• HSV-1 genital herpes is much less likely to result in recurrence, rapid decrease in shedding during first year of infection. Minimal data on suppressive therapy, should be reserved for those with frequent recurrences. • Low concern for adverse events or antiviral resistance.

[a]For dosing for children aged ≤8 years or weighing less than 45 kg, for dosing of alternative regimens, or for details on treatment in pregnancy or patients who are HIV positive, please refer to the CDC Treatment Guidelines, 2021: https://www.cdc.gov/std/treatment-guidelines/wall-chart.pdf. Partner notification and treatment are recommended for most sexually transmitted infections. Patients treated for a sexually transmitted infection should refrain from all sexual activity for 7 days posttreatment.

Alt, Alternative; *IM,* intramuscular; *IV,* intravenous; *PO,* per os.

TABLE 5.6

DIAGNOSTIC FEATURES AND MANAGEMENT OF VAGINAL INFECTIONS[52]

	No Infection/Physiologic Leukorrhea	Vulvovaginal Candidiasis	Trichomoniasis	Bacterial Vaginosis[a]
Etiology	—	Candida albicans and other candida species	Trichomonas vaginalis	High concentration of anaerobic bacteria: Gardnerella vaginalis, Prevotella, Mobiluncus, etc.
Typical symptoms	None	Pruritus, vaginal soreness, dyspareunia, external dysuria, ↑ discharge	Malodorous frothy discharge, vulvar irritation	Malodorous, ↑ discharge
Discharge amount	Variable; usually scant	Scant to moderate	Profuse	Moderate
Discharge color	Clear or white	White	Yellow-green	Usually white or gray
Discharge consistency	Heterogenous	Clumped; adherent plaques	Homogenous	Homogenous, low viscosity (milk consistency)
Vulvar/vaginal inflammation	No	Yes	Yes, may see strawberry-appearance cervix on pelvic exam	No
pH of vaginal fluid[b]	Usually <4.5	Usually <4.5	Usually >5.0	Usually >4.5
Amine ("fishy") odor with 10% potassium hydroxide (KOH)	None	None, but KOH helps with visualization of yeast	May be present	Present, positive "whiff-amine" test
Microscopy[c]	Normal epithelial cells; Lactobacillus predominates	Leukocytes, epithelial cells, yeast, mycelia, or pseudomycelia in 40%–80% of cases	Leukocytes; motile trichomonads wet mount with low sensitivity of 44%–68%, sensitivity decreases 21$ within 1 hour after collection	Clue cells, few leukocytes; Lactobacillus outnumbered by profuse mixed flora (nearly always including G. vaginalis plus anaerobes)

Continued

TABLE 5.6

DIAGNOSTIC FEATURES AND MANAGEMENT OF VAGINAL INFECTIONS[52]—CONT'D

	No Infection/Physiologic Leukorrhea	Vulvovaginal Candidiasis	Trichomoniasis	Bacterial Vaginosis[a]
Usual treatment	None	Fluconazole 150 mg PO once *OR* intravaginal azole cream	Metronidazole 500 mg PO 2×/ day for 7 days *OR* tinidazole 2 gm PO once	Metronidazole 500 mg PO 2×/day for 7 days *OR* metronidazole gel 0.75% 5 gm intravaginally daily for 5 days *OR* clindamycin cream 2% 5 gm intravaginally daily for 7 days

[a]Despite more sensitive and specific laboratory tests, cost and practicality make the Amsel criteria the best in-office method to diagnose bacterial vaginosis (BV). To diagnose BV, at least three criteria must be present: (1) homogenous, thin, gray/white discharge; (2) vaginal pH >4.5; (3) positive whiff-amine test; (4) clue cells on wet mount.

[b]pH determination is not useful if blood is present.

[c]To detect fungal elements, vaginal fluid is mixed with 10% KOH before microscopic examination; to examine for other features, fluid is mixed with saline.

DIAGNOSTIC FEATURES AND MANAGEMENT OF GENITAL ULCERS AND WARTS[52]

Infection	Clinical Presentation	Presumptive Diagnosis	Definitive Diagnosis	Treatment/Management of Sex Partners
Genital herpes	Grouped vesicles, painful shallow ulcers to mild clinical manifestation (redness, pain, excoriations); HSV-2 more common cause of genital lesions	HSV virologic testing by NAAT or culture from active lesion. HSV NAAT 90%–100% sensitive and very specific. Previously used cytologic detection of cellular changes in HSV is less sensitive and specific (Tzanck preparation)	HSV NAAT or culture HSV PCR should be used in systemic or CNS HSV infections.	No known cure. Prompt initiation of therapy shortens duration of first episode. For severe recurrent disease, initiate therapy at start of prodrome or within 1 day. Transmission can occur during asymptomatic periods. See Table 5.5.
Chancroid	Etiology: *Haemophilus ducreyi* Painful and deep genital ulcer(s); tender, suppurative inguinal adenopathy	Clinical presentation of genital ulcer and, if present, regional lymphadenopathy No evidence of *Treponema pallidum* (syphilis) on dark-field microscopy or NAAT of ulcer exudate/fluid, serologic syphilis testing negative 7–14 days after symptom onset; negative HSV NAAT or culture of ulcer exudate/fluid	Use of special media (not widely available in United States); no FDA-cleared NAAT for *H. ducreyi* in the United States	Azithromycin 1 gm PO once *OR* ceftriaxone 250 mg IM once *OR* ciprofloxacin 500 mg PO 2×/day for 3 days *OR* erythromycin base 500 mg PO 3×/day for 7 days Partners should be examined and treated, regardless of whether symptoms are present, or if they have had sex within 10 days preceding onset of patient's symptoms. Reexamine in 3–7 days, symptoms should improve within 3 days of treatment, objective improvement of ulcer within 7 days. Larger ulcers may take longer to heal, may take longer to heal if concomitant with HIV or if lesion is under foreskin in uncircumcised patient.
Primary syphilis (chancre)	Indurated, well-defined, usually single painless ulcer or chancre; nontender inguinal adenopathy	Nontreponemal serologic test: VDRL, RPR, or STS	Treponemal serologic test: FTA-ABS, dark-field microscopy or direct fluorescent antibody tests of lesion exudates or tissue	Parenteral penicillin G (see Table 5.5 for preparation[s], dosage, and length of treatment)

Continued

TABLE 5.7

DIAGNOSTIC FEATURES AND MANAGEMENT OF GENITAL ULCERS AND WARTS[52]—CONT'D

Infection	Clinical Presentation	Presumptive Diagnosis	Definitive Diagnosis	Treatment/Management of Sex Partners
HPV infection (anogenital warts)	Soft, fleshy, flat, papular, or pedunculated, painless growths, painless most often around vaginal introitus, under foreskin in uncircumcised men, shaft of the penis or intra-anal area; no inguinal adenopathy	Typical clinical presentation and visual inspection	Can complete biopsy for atypical lesions, immunocompromised patients, or those who do not respond to therapy	Treatment does not eradicate infection. 1. **Patient-administered therapies include:** Podofilox gel *OR* imiquimod cream *OR* sinecatechins ointment 2. **Clinician-applied therapies include:** Cryotherapy with liquid nitrogen or cryoprobe *OR* surgical removal *OR* trichloroacetic acid (TCA) or bichloroacetic acid (BCA) • HPV that causes genital warts (most often strains 6 and 11) typically not the same as HPV that causes cancer. • Due to period of communicability being unknown, current and future partners should be informed. • Previous partners can be evaluated for STIs; however, typically no HPV testing necessary, should be made aware that they may have contracted HPV even if asymptomatic.

NOTE: Chancroid, lymphogranuloma venereum (LGV), and granuloma inguinale should be considered in the differential diagnosis of genital ulcers if the clinical presentation is atypical and tests for herpes and syphilis are negative. *EIA*, Enzyme immunoassay; *FTA-ABS*, fluorescent treponemal antibody absorbed; *HPV*, human papillomavirus; *HSV*, herpes simplex virus; *IM*, intramuscular; *RPR*, rapid plasma reagin; *STS*, serologic test for syphilis; *TP-PA*, *T. pallidum* passive particle agglutination assay; *VDRL*, Venereal Disease Research Laboratory.

treponemal antibody absorbed [FTA-ABS] test, enzyme immunoassay) for confirmation.

d. Treatment: See Table 5.5. Clinical and serologic evaluation should be performed 6 and 12 months after treatment to ensure a fourfold reduction in nontreponemal titers or seroreversion. Monitor for Jarisch-Herxheimer reaction (fever, headache, and myalgias) within 24 hours of treatment.

e. Partner treatment: Partners with sexual contact within 90 days of a patient's diagnosis should be treated presumptively for early syphilis, even if serologic testing is negative. Partners with sexual contact over 90 days prior to diagnosis should be treated presumptively for early syphilis if serologic results are not immediately available or opportunity for follow-up is uncertain. If serologic test results are available and negative, treatment is not necessary. If serologic tests are positive, treatment should be based on clinical and serologic evaluation and syphilis stage.

f. See Chapter 17 for information on neonatal syphilis and interpretation of maternal and neonatal syphilis testing.

3. **Chlamydia and gonorrhea**[52]

a. Etiology: *Chlamydia trachomatis* and *Neisseria gonorrhoeae*

b. Clinical manifestations: Urethritis, cervicitis, pharyngitis, proctitis, epididymitis, prostatitis, pelvic inflammatory disease. Other manifestations include:

(1) Lymphogranuloma venereum (LGV): Lymphoproliferative reaction caused by *C. trachomatis* serovars L1 to L3 that most frequently presents as proctitis and lymphadenopathy in patients who have receptive anal intercourse or are HIV positive

(2) Disseminated gonococcal infection: Bacteremic spread of *N. gonorrhoeae* results in septic arthritis or arthritis-dermatitis syndrome (polyarthralgia, tenosynovitis, and dermatitis). May also involve CNS or cardiovascular system manifestations. In addition to urogenital, rectal, and pharyngeal NAAT, workup should include blood, synovial, or CSF cultures, as applicable.

c. Diagnosis: Site-specific NAAT, including urogenital (urine NAAT in males, urine or vaginal NAAT in females [see Section II.A.2.b]), pharyngeal, and rectal

d. Treatment: See Table 5.5. In order to prevent re-infection, patients should be advised to abstain from sexual intercourse for 7 days after a single-dose therapy (standard gonorrhea treatment) or until completion of a 7-day regimen (standard chlamydia treatment), until resolution of symptoms and until all sexual partners have been treated.

e. Partner treatment: Partners should be treated if they had sexual contact with the patient 60 days preceding onset of symptoms or are the last sexual contact of the patient. For partners for whom providers are concerned about access to prompt clinical evaluation and treatment, expedited partner therapy may be an option depending on local and state laws.

4. **Pelvic inflammatory disease (PID):** Acute infection of the female upper genital tract, may include tubo-ovarian abscess (TOA)[52]

   a. Etiology: Often polymicrobial in nature; however, *N. gonorrhoeae* and *C. trachomatis* are the most identified pathogens, followed by *Mycoplasma genitalium*

   b. Differential diagnosis: Endometriosis, ovarian cyst, ovarian torsion, ectopic pregnancy, acute appendicitis, inflammatory bowel disease (IBD), pyelonephritis, dysmenorrhea, septic/threatened abortion

   c. Workup: Pelvic and bimanual examination, gonorrhea/chlamydia and HIV testing, human chorionic gonadotropin (hCG), wet preparation, erythrocyte sedimentation rate (ESR), C-reactive protein (CRP), and urinalysis/urine culture if clinically indicated. Consider testing for *M. genitalium* in persistent PID despite appropriate treatment. Consider a complete blood cell count (CBC) with differential and pelvic ultrasound if the patient is ill appearing, has an adnexal mass on bimanual examination, or is not improving after antibiotics.

   d. Minimum diagnostic criteria: Uterine, adnexal, or cervical motion tenderness without other identifiable causes. One or more of the following additional criteria enhances specificity: fever (>38.3°C), mucopurulent vaginal or cervical discharge, cervical friability, leukocytes on saline microscopy, increased ESR or CRP, laboratory documentation of chlamydial or gonorrhea infection.

   e. Treatment: See Table 5.5.

   f. Hospital admission criteria: Cannot exclude acute surgical abdomen, presence of TOA, pregnancy, immunodeficiency, severe illness, inability to tolerate or follow outpatient oral regimen, failure to respond to appropriate outpatient therapy, or follow-up cannot be ensured

5. **Trichomoniasis**[52]

   a. Etiology: *Trichomonas vaginalis*

   b. Clinical manifestations: See Table 5.6.

   c. Diagnosis and treatment: See Table 5.6. Patients should be advised to abstain from sexual intercourse until they and their partners have completed therapy and symptoms have resolved.

   d. Follow-up: Women treated for trichomoniasis should be retested 3 months after treatment due to high rates of reinfection.

   e. Partner treatment: Partners should be treated to prevent reinfection.

6. *Mycoplasma genitalium*[52]

   a. Etiology: *M. genitalium*

   b. Clinical manifestations: Persistent urethritis, cervicitis, or PID despite appropriate treatment

   c. Diagnosis: FDA-cleared NAAT of *M. genitalium* for urine and urethral, penal meatal, endocervical, and vaginal swab samples. Due to high rates of macrolide resistance, if resistance testing is available, it should be completed to guide therapy.

    d. Treatment: See Table 5.5.

7. **Vaginal infections, genital ulcers, and warts**
   a. Diagnostic features of vaginal infections (see Table 5.6) can assist in differentiating normal vaginal discharge from bacterial vaginosis, trichomoniasis, and yeast vaginitis.
   b. Diagnostic features of genital lesions, as well as management of warts and ulcers, are presented in Table 5.7.

C. Contraception[60,61]

1. **Special considerations in adolescents:**
   a. Approximately 40% to 50% of adolescents in the United States have had penile-vaginal sexual intercourse, and nearly half of adolescent pregnancies are unplanned.[62-64]
   b. Barriers to contraception may include confidentiality concerns (e.g., fear of parental disclosure), fear of pelvic examination, and fear of medication side effects.
   c. **Long-acting reversible contraception (LARC)** methods have well-established safety and efficacy and are first-line contraceptive methods according to the ACOG and the AAP. Adherence and continuation rates of LARC methods in adolescents are superior to short-acting contraceptives. To avoid a delay in initiation, quick-start methods should be considered for most adolescents.[65]
   d. Providers should pay special attention to informed consent, confidentiality, parental involvement, insurance coverage, and cost. If an adolescent does not have or does not want to use their insurance coverage, refer to a clinic with Title X or other public funding (https://www.hhs.gov/opa/).
   e. Counseling should include discussion of the need for barrier method to prevent STIs.

2. **Method comparison (Fig. 5.2)[66]**

3. **Contraception selection and initiation:**
   a. **Selecting a contraceptive method:** Refer to the CDC Medical Eligibility Criteria (https://www.cdc.gov/reproductivehealth/contraception/pdf/summary-chart-us-medical-eligibility-criteria_508tagged.pdf) for relative and absolute contraindications for each hormonal contraceptive method and the CDC's Selected Practice Recommendations (https://www.cdc.gov/reproductivehealth/contraception/mmwr/spr/summary.html) for minimum requirements to start each method.
      (1) To start a hormonal method, the basic medical history should include assessment of clotting risk, blood pressure, pregnancy status, migraines with aura, family history, and any other pertinent medical comorbidities.
      (2) Combined hormonal contraception (contraception that includes estrogen) is associated with a small increase in risk for thrombosis, including deep venous thrombosis, myocardial infarction, and stroke.[67] The risk is higher in women who smoke

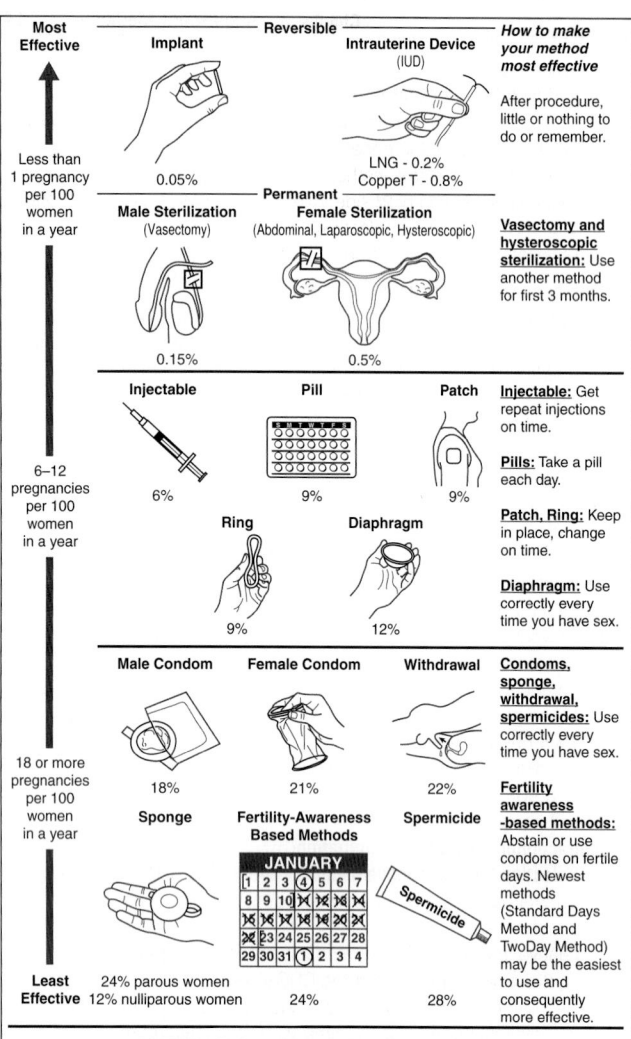

**CONDOMS SHOULD ALWAYS BE USED TO REDUCE
THE RISK OF SEXUALLY TRANSMITTED INFECTIONS**

Other Methods of Contraception

Lactational Amenorrhea Method: LAM is a highly effective, *temporary* method of contraception.

Emergency Contraception: Emergency contraceptive pills or a copper IUD after unprotected intercourse substantially reduces risk of pregnancy.

FIGURE 5.2

Comparing effectiveness and side effects of family planning methods. (From Centers for Disease Control and Prevention. U.S. selected practice recommendations for contraceptive use, 2016. *MMWR Recomm Rep.* 2016;65[4];1–66. Patient-friendly chart per U.S. Food & Drug Administration available at: https://www.fda.gov/consumers/free-publications-women/birth-control-chart)

more than 15 cigarettes a day, women over 35 years old, women with history of migraine with aura, and women with other risk factors for cardiovascular disease.

(3) To support adherence and continuation, use a patient-centered approach, review method effectiveness, and provide anticipatory guidance regarding side effects of each method when assisting an adolescent in selecting a new contraceptive method.

b. **Quick start** (Fig. 5.3): Starting a method of contraception on the day of the visit (not waiting until a new menstrual cycle begins) should be considered for most adolescents. Can be used for all methods, including LARC, if there is reasonable certainty that the patient is not pregnant (Box 5.2). A urine pregnancy test should be performed when using this approach, and patients should be advised to use a second form of birth control for 7 days.[68]

4. **Specific contraceptive methods:**

NOTE: Contraceptive methods are described in order of effectiveness.

a. **Subdermal implant:** Progestin-only LARC, 4-cm rod inserted into the upper arm. Newer model (Nexplanon) is radio-opaque. FDA approved for 3 years; studies show efficacy for up to 5 years.[69] Minimal or no effect on bone density; can cause irregular bleeding, mood swings, depressed mood, headache, or acne.[70] Return to fertility is rapid after removal. May be less effective for women who are overweight or obese. The most effective form of birth control

(1) Efficacy: Number of expected pregnancies per 100 women is less than 1.[71]

(2) Persistent irregular bleeding is the most common complaint resulting in implant removal, but continuation rates among adolescents remain high.[72] As opposed to levonorgestrel IUD, bleeding changes persist throughout duration of use. The bleeding pattern in the first 3 months of use is predictive of future bleeding. Important to provide pre-insertion anticipatory guidance. Consider postinsertion management of bleeding with NSAIDs or combined OCPs.[66,73]

b. **Intrauterine device (IUD)[65]:** LARC inserted into the uterus through the cervix. Safe to use among adolescents, may be inserted without difficulty in most adolescents and nulliparous women. Rate of expulsion is between 0.05% and 8%, typically occurs within the first 3 months. Does not increase risk of infertility; baseline fertility returns rapidly after removal. Previously thought that risk of pelvic infection was increased with placement; however, recent reviews do not support this and demonstrate similar risks of PID in women with asymptomatic gonorrhea or chlamydia regardless of IUD insertion.[74] Women should be tested for STIs on day of insertion depending on their risk factors. Insertion should not be delayed for test results; treatment can occur without IUD removal.[75]

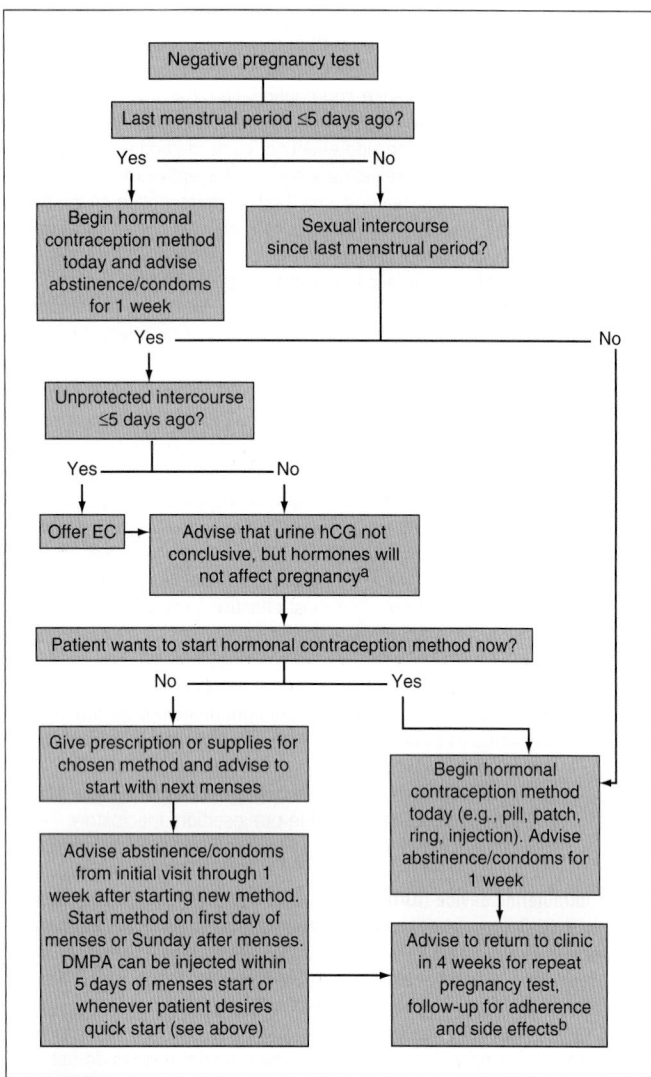

FIGURE 5.3

Algorithm for quick start initiation of contraception (https://www.aafp.org/afp/2006/0701/p105.html).

[a]Pregnancy tests may take 2 to 3 weeks after sex to be accurate.

[b]Consider pregnancy test at second depot medroxyprogesterone acetate (*DMPA* [Depo-Provera]) injection if quick start regimen was used and patient failed 4-week follow-up visit. (Lesnewski R, Prine L. Initiating hormonal contraception. *Am Fam Physician.* 2006;74[1]:105–112. PMID: 16848384.)

BOX 5.2

HOW TO BE REASONABLY CERTAIN THAT A WOMAN IS NOT PREGNANT

If the patient has no symptoms or signs of pregnancy and meets any of the following criteria:
1. Is ≤7 days after the start of normal menses
2. Has not had sexual intercourse since the start of last normal menses
3. Has been correctly and consistently using a reliable method of contraception
4. Is ≤7 days after spontaneous or induced abortion
5. Is within 4 weeks postpartum
6. Is fully or nearly fully breastfeeding, amenorrheic, and <6 months postpartum

Adapted from Curtis KM, Jatlaoui TC, Tepper NK, et al. U.S. selected practice recommendations for contraceptive use, 2016. *MMWR Recomm Rep.* 2016;65(4):1–66.

---

(1) Efficacy: Among the most effective forms of birth control. Number of expected pregnancies per 100 women is less than 1.[71]
(2) Types of IUDs
  (a) Copper (Paragard): Hormone-free, FDA approved for 10 years of use, although data support potential efficacy for an additional 1 to 2 years[65,76]
  (b) Progestin-containing (levonorgestrel): There are four types with differing amounts of progestin. Mirena is FDA approved for 5 years; data support an additional 2 years.[65,69] Kyleena is FDA approved for 5 years. Liletta is FDA approved for 4 years; data support an additional year.[65,77] Skyla is FDA approved for 3 years.
(3) Side Effects: Changes in bleeding patterns are common in the first months of use. Copper IUD may cause heavier menses and cramping. Many women using the levonorgestrel IUD will have a decrease in bleeding over time or amenorrhea.[70] First-line treatment for bleeding and spotting is NSAIDs.[78] Bleeding concerns that are not associated with device insertion should be evaluated for other etiologies.

c. **Depot medroxyprogesterone acetate (DMPA [Depo-Provera]) injection**[67,74]: Progestin-only, IM injection every 13 weeks or subcutaneous injection every 12 to 14 weeks. Delayed return to fertility (9 to 18 months).[79] Menstrual irregularity is common but often resolves after several cycles. Other side effects include headaches, abdominal pain, and weight gain.[86] Average weight gain within 1 year is <2 kg, increase of weight by 5% within 6 months is associated with continued excessive weight gain and patients should be counseled appropriately.[80,81]
  (1) Efficacy: Number of expected pregnancies per 100 women is 6.
  (2) Patient should be encouraged to receive adequate calcium and vitamin D due to association with decrease in bone mineral density.

(3) In 2004 an FDA black box warning was issued on DMPA, stating it should not be used for longer than 2 consecutive years, unless other forms of birth control are inadequate due to bone mineral density concerns. However, further studies have shown that bone density substantially, if not completely returns after discontinuation. Therefore, risk of potential loss of bone mineral density should be weighed against the need for effective contraception in the context of each adolescent.[68]

d. **Combined hormonal methods:** Combined estrogen-progestin–containing methods of contraception have similar efficacy with 9% failure rate if used correctly. They may result in side effects of breast tenderness, nausea, and headache, symptoms that usually improve with time.[70] These estrogen-containing methods are medically contraindicated in patients 35 years or older who smoke 15 or more cigarettes per day or have a history of stroke, thrombosis, cardiovascular disease, hypertension, migraine with aura, breast cancer, valvular heart disease, or certain forms of liver disease.[75]

(1) **Combined hormonal oral contraceptive pills (OCPs):** Combination of estrogen and progestin taken daily. "Low-dose" (35 mCg or less of ethinyl estradiol) pills are the recommended dosing for adolescents. First-line treatment for dysmenorrhea and endometriosis as combined hormonal OCPs make menstruation lighter, shorter, and more regular and decrease pain.[79] Newer formulations exist, known as extended-cycle regimens, which reduce the number of menstrual cycles per year.

(a) The first pill should be taken either on the day of the visit (quick start) or between the first and seventh day after the start of the menstrual period (most commonly Sunday).

(b) Some pill packs have 28 pills; others have 21 pills. When the 28-day pack is empty, immediately start taking pills from a new pack. When the 21-day pack is empty, wait 1 week (7 days), then begin taking pills from a new pack.

(c) If a pill is missed, it should be taken as soon as remembered, even if it means taking two pills in 1 day. If two or more pills are missed, two pills should be taken daily until back on schedule and a backup method should be used for 7 days.

(2) **Transdermal (patch) contraceptive:** Apply one patch for 3 weeks, then remove for 1 week for withdrawal bleed. Place on abdomen, upper torso, upper outer arm, or buttocks. Greater exposure to estrogen than with other methods; may have more estrogen-related side effects. There may be a greater risk for thromboembolism compared to OCPs, though the data are not clear.[82] May be less effective in obese women

(3) **Vaginal ring:** Flexible latex-free ring. Placed in vagina for 3 weeks, removed for 1 week for withdrawal bleeding. May be used continuously (avoiding week of menses) by replacing with a new ring every 4 weeks (or the same day every month) to help reduce

pelvic pain and dysmenorrhea. May be removed for up to 3 hours (not recommended in adolescents). Requires user comfort with insertion and removal[70]

e. **Progestin-only pills:** Can be used for those with contraindications to estrogen-containing formulations. Require daily use and are more sensitive to timing (should be taken at same time each day); have no pill-free interval. Considered less effective than combined hormonal methods. Irregular bleeding is a common adverse effect. Norethindrone is a commonly used progestin-only pill; however, a new formulation, Drospirenone, has also been approved. Drospirenone has a higher dose of hormone and, though there are limited data at this time, is thought to be more effective than norethindrone. Drospirenone has anti-mineralocorticoid effects similar to spironolactone and therefore a theoretical possibility of causing hyperkalemia, though data are still limited.[79,80]

f. **Barrier methods:** Require placement prior to sexual intercourse. Include cervical sponge, cervical cap, cervical shield, diaphragm (these methods are used in conjunction with spermicide), as well as female and male condoms. Male condom is the most used birth control among adolescents with a failure rate of 18% with typical use.[66,70] Use latex condoms only with water-based lubricants; oil-based lubricants are not recommended due to increased breakage.[81] While barrier methods are less effective than other methods of contraception, their use should still be emphasized for prevention of STIs. For patient education materials on how to properly use a condom, please visit https://www.cdc.gov/condomeffectiveness/external-condom-use.html.

g. **Fertility awareness-based methods of pregnancy prevention:** Involves following a woman's menstrual cycle to help prevent pregnancy. Many smartphone apps are available for use.

h. **Other forms of nonhormonal birth control:** Spermicide is a gel, foam, cream, or suppository applied to vagina prior to sexual intercourse. Most spermicides contain nonoxynol-9, a detergent that works by damaging a sperm's body and flagella, making it immobile and inactive. Spermicide has a failure rate of 28%. Side effects include allergic reaction, irritation, and UTI.[70] A pH-regulating gel, Phexxi, was approved in 2020. This gel of lactic acid must be applied prior to intercourse and maintains a lower vaginal pH even when alkaline sperm is present, immobilizing sperm. Initial studies demonstrate 86.3% effectiveness with side effects of vulvovaginal burning, pruritus, UTI, BV, and mycotic infection. However, rates of UTI, BV, and yeast infections were reduced from baseline data, demonstrating it may protect for vulvovaginal infections.[83]

5. **Emergency contraception (EC)[84]:** Used to prevent pregnancy following unprotected sex (including sexual assault) or a recent possible failure of another method of contraception. A patient-friendly handout on forms of emergency contraception, efficacy, and how to obtain EC is available

at https://beyondthepill.ucsf.edu/sites/beyondthepill.ucsf.edu/files/EC-English-043019.pdf

a. Mechanism: Hormonal methods work by delaying ovulation. Copper IUD inhibits fertilization by affecting sperm viability and function. Recent studies demonstrate that hormonal IUDs may also be used for emergency contraception.[85] All methods are only effective before implantation takes place and will not disrupt an implanted pregnancy.

b. Efficacy[86]: Copper or hormonal IUDs are the most effective method, with failure rates less than 0.1% if inserted within 5 days, but require a clinic visit for insertion.[87] Ulipristal is the next most effective but requires a prescription and is less effective in women over 195 pounds. Levonorgestrel is the next most effective and is available over the counter. The Yuzpe regimen is the least effective with at least 75% efficacy and has the most side effects.[88]

c. Timing: Hormonal methods are most effective when given as soon as possible. Efficacy declines linearly with time, but there is efficacy up to 120 hours after intercourse. Ulipristal and an IUD maintain high efficacy when taken up to 120 hours after intercourse.

d. Pregnancy should be excluded based on history, physical exam, or pregnancy testing before prescribing ulipristal or placing an IUD, as they may adversely affect an established pregnancy.

e. Methods:
   (1) Progestin only: Levonorgestrel. Take 1.5 mg orally once within 72 hours of coitus. Only method offered over the counter without prescription
   (2) Antiprogestins: Ulipristal. Take 30 mg orally once as soon as possible, but at least within 120 hr. Mifepristone is an alternative agent used in some countries as EC but is not available in the United States. Provider prescription required
   (3) Ethinyl estradiol plus levonorgestrel (Yuzpe regimen): Patients take multiple OCPs from packets designed for 28-day use. Take equivalent of 100 mCg of ethinyl estradiol plus 500 mCg of levonorgestrel. Twelve hours later, take the same dose.
   (4) Copper or hormonal IUD may be inserted within 120 hours of coitus to prevent pregnancy from occurring.

f. General recommendations[89-91]:
   (1) Counseling about EC should be a routine part of anticipatory guidance for all female and male adolescents. Advance prescriptions should be considered for all adolescents.
   (2) Antiemetics can be used to prevent nausea and should be used prophylactically in the Yuzpe regimen.
   (3) May be combined with other ongoing methods of birth control
   (4) OCPs may be started immediately after progestin-only or combined hormonal EC dosing has been completed. DMPA may be given the same day.

   (5) Patient should abstain from sexual intercourse or use barrier contraception for 7 days (14 if using ulipristal) or until next menses, whichever comes first.
   (6) Scheduled follow-up is not required after use of EC. However, women whose menses are delayed by a week or more, or have any signs of pregnancy (e.g., irregular menses, abdominal cramping), should be evaluated clinically or have a pregnancy test.

6. **Follow-up recommendations for contraception:** Two or three visits per year to monitor compliance, blood pressure, side effects, and satisfaction with chosen birth control option

D. Pregnancy[92,93]

If pregnancy is suspected in an adolescent patient, take a sexual history and explore how the patient feels about a possible pregnancy in order to guide the rest of the visit.

1. Diagnosis:
   a. Perform urine hCG testing to diagnose the pregnancy. False-positives and false-negatives are possible; repeat urine testing or quantitative serum hCG testing may be indicated.
   b. If pregnancy is diagnosed, estimate the gestational age using the LMP. Confirm with a brief exam of uterine size. When in doubt, arrange an ultrasound and obstetric consultation promptly, as gestational age will affect counseling options.
   c. Share the diagnosis with the patient privately. Encourage them to involve a parent or legal guardian and facilitate the discussion, if necessary. Be familiar with local confidentiality laws, which vary by state. State-specific information can be found at https://www.plannedparenthoodaction.org/abortion-access-tool/US
   d. Review the patient's medications to ensure they are safe for pregnancy. Start patient on prenatal vitamin if not taking and review general pregnancy recommendations for diet, exercise, and abstinence from substance use.

2. **Prenatal testing:** All pregnant adolescents should be tested for HIV, syphilis, hepatitis B, hepatitis C, chlamydia, and gonorrhea at the first prenatal visit. If an infection is suspected or if there may be a delay in obstetric care, the pediatrician should perform the testing.[52]

3. **Options counseling:** Counsel the adolescent on the importance of making a timely decision. The options depend on gestational age but may include continuing the pregnancy and raising the infant, continuing the pregnancy and making an adoption plan, or terminating the pregnancy. If a pediatrician has personal limitations in offering a discussion of all three options, they should make a prompt referral to a colleague or consultant. Medical and surgical abortion may be available depending on the gestational age of the pregnancy, coexisting medical conditions, and state laws. Medical abortion is generally available under 9 weeks of gestation; surgical abortion is generally available under 20 to 24 weeks of gestation.

4. **Complications:** First-trimester complications include ectopic pregnancy and spontaneous abortion; immediate obstetric referral may be indicated for abdominal pain and/or vaginal bleeding in the pregnant patient.

VI. TRANSITIONING ADOLESCENTS INTO ADULT CARE[94]

All adolescents, particularly those with special healthcare needs or chronic conditions, benefit from careful attention to the process of transitioning to an adult model of care. Transition planning should routinely occur during well visits and should start at age 12. Resources for how to approach and organize the transition process, including guidance on transition readiness and planning, are available at https://www.gottransition.org/. See Chapter 9 for discussion of transition to adult care for youth with developmental disorders and disabilities.

VII. WEB RESOURCES

A. Websites for Clinicians
- Centers for Disease Control and Prevention (CDC) on contraception: http://www.cdc.gov/reproductivehealth/unintendedpregnancy/contraception.htm
- CDC on sexually transmitted infections (STI): https://www.cdc.gov/std/life-stages-populations/adolescents-youngadults.htm
- CDC Wall Chart, Quick Reference for STI Treatment: https://www.cdc.gov/std/treatment-guidelines/wall-chart.pdf
- Society for Adolescent Health and Medicine: http://www.adolescenthealth.org

B. Websites for Patients
- Drug abuse: http://www.teens.drugabuse.gov
- Sexual health: http://www.plannedparenthood.org/, http://www.bedsider.org
- CDC resources for Lesbian, Gay, Bisexual, & Transgender (LGBT) youth: https://www.cdc.gov/lgbthealth/youth-resources.htm

REFERENCES

A complete list of references can be found online.

Chapter 6

Analgesia and Procedural Sedation

Alexander James Jaksic, MD and
Divya Madhusudhan, MD

🌐 See additional content online.

🔊 **Audio Case File 6.1** Medications for analgesia and sedation

I. TYPES OF PAIN

A. Definition

1. Pain can be defined as "An unpleasant sensory and emotional experience associated with, or resembling that associated with, actual or potential tissue damage."[1]
2. Pain can be classified as nociceptive or neuropathic.

B. Types of Pain: Table 6.1

II. PAIN ASSESSMENT

A. Infant[5]

1. **Physiologic response**
   a. Characterized by oxygen desaturation, crying, diaphoresis, flushing or pallor, and increases in blood pressure, heart rate, and respiratory rate
   b. Seen primarily in acute pain; can subside with continuing/chronic pain
2. **Behavioral response**
   a. Observe characteristics and duration of cry, facial expressions, visual tracking, body movements, and response to stimuli.
   b. Neonatal Infant Pain Scale (NIPS): Behavioral assessment tool for the preterm neonate and full-term neonate up to 6 weeks after birth.
   c. FLACC scale (Table 6.2): Measures and evaluates pain interventions by quantifying pain behaviors, including **F**acial expression, **L**eg movement, **A**ctivity, **C**ry, and **C**onsolability, with scores ranging from 0 to 10.[6] The Revised FLACC scale (r-FLACC) is reliable in children with cognitive impairment.[7]

B. Preschooler

1. In addition to physiologic and behavioral responses, the **FACES** pain scale revised (FPS-R) can be used to assess pain intensity in children as young as 3 years of age by having the patient point to the image on the scale that best characterizes their pain (Fig. 6.1).

TABLE 6.1

TYPES OF PAIN

Category[2-4]	Mechanism/Role	Common Clinical Features
Nociceptive	An adaptive (protective) pain. Sensed by functional pain receptors (nociceptors) that respond to thermal, mechanical, or chemical stimuli (inflammation/tissue injury). Associated with physiologic processes and behaviors intended to benefit the affected individual. • Somatic pain: Injury to bones, joints, muscles, skin • Visceral pain: Pain from organs (bladder, bowel, ovaries/testes)	• Somatic: More easily localized. Stabbing, sharp, aching, throbbing, squeezing, "pressure-like" • Visceral: Poorly localized. Deep, diffuse. Dull, "gnawing," crampy, achy
Neuropathic/dysfunctional	A maladaptive pain that provides no clear protective benefit. It is thought to be caused by damage to, or dysfunction of, sensory nerves. Can result from uncontrolled chronic nociceptive pain. • Neuropathic pain—Pain due to nerve injury. Commonly caused by compression, surgical transection, ischemia, or infiltration of nerve (i.e., neuropathy, neuromas, trigeminal and postherpetic neuralgia) or uncontrolled chronic pain. • Dysfunctional pain—Pain without known neurologic etiology. Related to abnormal processing of signals (i.e., fibromyalgia, irritable bowel syndrome, interstitial cystitis).	• Burning, shooting, shock-like, pins/needles, tingling • Frequently difficult to describe for patients

C. School-Age and Adolescent

1. Evaluate physiologic and behavioral responses; ask about description, location, and character of pain. Starting at the age of 7 years, children can use the standard subjective pain rating scale, in which 0 is no pain and 10 is the worst pain ever experienced.

D. Children With Significant Neurological Impairment (SNI)[4]

1. Pain is often underrecognized and undertreated in children with SNI.
2. The behavioral responses to pain in children with SNI can be quite similar or disparate from pain responses in children without SNI. Having meaningful input from a consistent care provider who is familiar with the child's baseline behaviors and responses to painful and nonpainful (such as hunger) stimuli is crucial.
3. Identifying observable pain behaviors in children with SNI: Table 6.3

TABLE 6.2

FLACC PAIN ASSESSMENT TOOL

FACE

0—No particular expression or smile
1—Occasional grimace or frown, withdrawn, disinterested
2—Frequent to constant frown, quivering chin, clenched jaw

LEGS

0—Normal position or relaxed
1—Uneasy, restless, tense
2—Kicking or legs drawn up

ACTIVITY

0—Lying quietly, normal position, moves easily
1—Squirming, shifting back and forth, tense
2—Arched, rigid, or jerking

CRY

0—No cry (awake or asleep)
1—Moans or whimpers, occasional complaint
2—Crying steadily, screams or sobs, frequent complaints

CONSOLABILITY

0—Content, relaxed
1—Reassured by occasional touching, hugging, or being talked to; distractible
2—Difficult to console or comfort

Modified from Manworren R, Hynan L. Clinical validation of FLACC: preverbal patient pain scale. *Pediatr Nurs.* 2003;29:140–146.

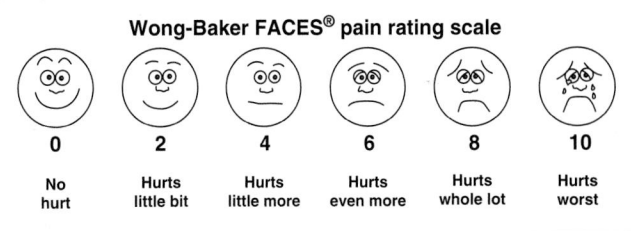

Wong-Baker FACES® pain rating scale

0	2	4	6	8	10
No hurt	Hurts little bit	Hurts little more	Hurts even more	Hurts whole lot	Hurts worst

FIGURE 6.1

Wong-Baker FACES pain rating scale. (From Wong-Baker FACES Foundation. Wong-Baker FACES pain rating scale. 2016. Retrieved with permission from http://www. WongBakerFACES.org. Originally published in *Whaley & Wong's Nursing Care of Infants and Children*. Elsevier.)

4. Pain assessment tools that incorporate the input of a parent or longitudinal caregiver such as the r-FLACC scale can be of great benefit to better identify and quantify pain and determine response to interventions provided.

TABLE 6.3

OBSERVABLE PAIN BEHAVIORS IN CHILDREN WITH SNI

Category	Examples
Vocalization	Crying, moaning, gasping, sharp intake of breaths
Facial Reaction	Grimacing, squinting, frowning, teeth grinding/clenched
Interaction	Inconsolable, withdrawn, seeking comfort
Sleep	Disturbed sleep, increased or decreased sleep
Activity/Tone	Increased baseline movement/tone, restless/fidgety, startles easily, pulls away when touched, twists or turns, posturing [arching/stiffening], resists motion
Physiologic	Tachycardia, shivering, color change/pallor, tears
Atypical Features	Breath holding, withdrawn/lack of facial expression, laughter, self-injurious behavior

From Hauer J, Houtrow AJ. Pain assessment and treatment in children with significant impairment of the central nervous system. Section on Hospice & Palliative Medicine Council on Children with Disabilities. *Pediatrics.* 2017 Jun.

    a. Like the FLACC, the r-FLACC scale is a 5-item pain assessment tool with a score ranging from 0 to 10. Constructed to allow parents to individualize by adding behaviors specific to their child, which can be particularly beneficial for children with atypical pain behaviors

    b. Sample r-FLACC scale[8] (Table 6.4)

      (1) The descriptors in italics are validated in children with SNI.[8]

      (2) Review descriptors in each category with family; assess if there are better indicators of pain in their child and incorporate them into the appropriate category.

      (3) Observe child for 1–2 minutes (longer if asleep) with their legs/body uncovered. Observe activity or reposition child, if possible, to assess for tenseness and tone. Initiate consoling interventions if needed.

III. ANALGESICS[5]

A. Medications to Avoid in Children

1. Combined analgesics

    a. Danger of acetaminophen toxicity when using combined opioid-acetaminophen products (oxycodone or hydrocodone with acetaminophen)

    b. **Preferable to prescribe opioids and acetaminophen separately**

2. Codeine

    a. **Not recommended for use in children**

    b. Five percent of the population show ultra-rapid metabolism of codeine to morphine (the active metabolite), which can lead to dangerously high levels. This is especially unsafe after tonsillectomy and adenoidectomy (T&A) performed for sleep apnea.[9]

    c. Little to no analgesic effect in newborns and approximately 10% of the US population.[10]

TABLE 6.4

R-FLACC SCALE[a]

Category	0	1	2
Face	• No particular expression or smile	• Occasional grimace/frown; withdrawn or disinterested	• Consistent grimace or frown; frequent/constant quivering chin, clenched jaw • *Distressed-looking face; expression of fright or panic* Individual Behavior:
Legs	• Normal position or relaxed • *Usual tone and motion to limbs*	• Uneasy, restless, tense • *Occasional tremors*	• Kicking, or legs drawn up • *Marked increase in spasticity, constant tremors or jerking* Individual Behavior:
Activity	• Lying quietly, normal position, moves easily • *Regular, rhythmic respirations*	• Squirming, shifting back and forth • *Tense or guarded movements; mildly agitated (head back and forth, aggression); shallow, splinting respirations, intermittent sighs*	• Arched, rigid or jerking • *Severe agitation; head banging; shivering (not rigors); breath holding, gasping or sharp intake of breaths, severe splinting* Individual Behavior:
Cry	• No cry/verbalization	• Moans or whimpers; occasional complaint • *Occasional verbal outburst or grunt*	• Crying steadily, screams or sobs, frequent complaints • *Repeated outbursts, constant grunting* Individual Behavior:
Consolability	• Content and relaxed	• Reassured by occasional touching, hugging or being talked to. Distractible	• Difficult to console or comfort • *Pushing away caregiver, resisting care/comfort measures* Individual Behavior:

[a]Italicized text in above table indicates the additional or revised aspects of the r-FLACC scale compared to the FLACC scale.

3. Meperidine
   a. Not recommended for use in children due to risk of neurotoxicity (agitation, tremors, myoclonus, and seizures), especially when renal dysfunction is present.[11]
   b. Contraindicated in patients receiving monoamine oxidase (MAO) inhibitors.
4. Tramadol
   a. Opioid pain reliever, with additional effects on nonopioid receptors.
   b. May be overmetabolized to an active opiate metabolite, resulting in potentially fatal respiratory depression.
   c. In 2017 the FDA issued its strongest warning against use in children; therefore, administration is considered off label.[12]

B. Nonopioid Analgesics

Weak analgesics with antipyretic activity are commonly used to manage mild to moderate pain of nonvisceral origin. Can be administered alone or in combination with opioids.

1. **Acetaminophen (by mouth [PO]/per rectum [PR]/intravenous [IV]):** Weak analgesic with no antiinflammatory activity, platelet inhibition, or gastrointestinal (GI) irritation. Hepatotoxicity can occur with high doses.
2. **Aspirin (PO/PR):** Associated with platelet inhibition and GI irritation. Avoid use as analgesia in children due to risk of Reye syndrome.
3. **Nonsteroidal antiinflammatory drugs (NSAIDs):** Ibuprofen (PO/IV), ketorolac (IV/intramuscular [IM]/PO/intranasal [IN]), naproxen (PO), diclofenac (PO/IV), and celecoxib (PO)
   a. Use with extreme caution in children less than 6 months of age due to concern for adverse GI effects and risk of renal failure.
   b. Especially useful for sickle cell disease and pain of bony, rheumatic, or inflammatory etiology.
   c. Concurrent histamine-2-receptor blocker or proton pump inhibitor is recommended with prolonged use given GI side effects.
   d. Other adverse effects include interference with platelet aggregation, hepatitis, bronchoconstriction, hypersensitivity reactions, and azotemia. Avoid in patients with severe renal disease, dehydration, or heart failure.

NOTE: Ketorolac is a potent analgesic. Limit duration of therapy to less than 5 days to minimize renal toxicity.

C. Opioids (Table 6.5)

Produce analgesia by binding to μ receptors in the brain and spinal cord.

1. **Side effects:** Pruritus, nausea, vomiting, constipation, urine retention, sedation, respiratory depression and hypotension. Prescribe a bowel regimen when prescribing opioids.
2. **Patients with renal failure**
   a. **Morphine:** Avoid use. Decreased excretion of the active metabolite may result in respiratory depression.
   b. **Preferred choices:** Fentanyl, remifentanil, methadone, hydromorphone, oxycodone

TABLE 6.5

COMMONLY USED OPIOIDS

Drug	Morphine Equivalence Ratio	Onset (min)	Duration (hr)	Side Effects	Comments
Fentanyl	80–100	IV: 1–2	0.5–1	Pruritus Bradycardia **Chest wall rigidity with doses >5 mCg/kg** (but can occur at all doses); treat with naloxone or neuromuscular blockade.	Risk of cardiovascular instability is lower than other opioids, making it relatively safer in hypovolemia, congenital heart disease, or head trauma. Respiratory depressant effect much longer (4 hr) than analgesic effect Most commonly used opioid for short, painful procedures, but transdermal route is more effective in chronic pain[a]
Hydromorphone	4–7	IV/SQ: 5–10 PO: 30–60	3–4		Less sedation, nausea, and pruritus than morphine
Methadone	0.25–1[b]	IV: 5–10 PO: 30–60	4–24		Initial dose may produce analgesia for 3–4 hr, duration of action is increased with repeated dosing. Useful for neuropathic pain and opioid weaning due to unique mechanism of NMDA blockade
Morphine	1	IV: 5–10 IM/SQ: 10–30 PO: 30–60	IV: 3–4 IM/SQ/PO: 4–5	Seizures in neonates Can cause significant histamine release	Available in sustained-release form for chronic pain
Oxycodone	1.5		30–60	3–4		Available in sustained-release form for chronic pain

[a]Removing a transdermal fentanyl patch does not stop opioid uptake from the skin; fentanyl will continue to be absorbed for 12–24 hours after patch removal (fentanyl 25 mCg patch administers 25 mCg/hr of fentanyl).

[b]Morphine-to-methadone conversion in the tolerant/dependent patient is variable. Consider starting at the lowest conversion ratio: 0.25.

IM, Intramuscular; *IV*, intravenous; *mCg*, microgram; *PO*, by mouth; *SQ*, subcutaneous.

Data from Yaster M, Cote C, Krane E, et al. *Pediatric Pain Management and Sedation Handbook.* Mosby; 1997:29–50.

6

3. Long-acting opioids, such as extended-release tablets, transdermal patches, and PO methadone, are not recommended for acute pain management.

4. Although opioids are essential for the treatment of moderate to severe pain, a thoughtful approach is recommended with the quantity that is dispensed, as studies have shown that over 50% of opioid doses dispensed are not consumed.[13] There is need for further research to develop evidence-based opioid prescribing guidelines for treating acute pain in children.

D. Local Anesthetics[14–17]

Administered topically or subcutaneously to surround peripheral nerves (peripheral block) or centrally (epidural/spinal block). Temporarily block nerve conduction at the sodium channel.

1. **For all local anesthetics, 1% solution = 1 g/100 mL = 10 mg/mL**
2. **Topical local anesthetics (**Table 6.6)[17]
3. **Injectable local anesthetics (**Table 6.7):
   a. Subcutaneous infiltration of the skin at the site: Used for painful procedures such as wound closure or lumbar puncture
   b. Use of a 27- to 30-gauge needle, alkalization, warming the solution to 37°C to 42°C, and a slow injection can reduce stinging from injection. Alkalinize by adding 1 mL (1 mEq [milliequivalent]) sodium bicarbonate to 9 mL lidocaine (or 29 mL bupivacaine).
   c. To enhance efficacy and duration, add epinephrine (5 to 10 mCg of epinephrine to 1 mL of local anesthetic) to decrease vascular uptake. **Never use local anesthetics with epinephrine in areas supplied by end arteries (e.g., pinna, fingers, toes, nasal tip, penis).**
   d. **Maximum volume (mL) = (maximum mg/kg dose × weight in kg)/(% solution × 10).** See Table 6.7 for maximum doses.
   e. **Toxicity:** Central nervous system (CNS) and cardiac toxicity are of greatest concern. CNS symptoms are seen before cardiovascular collapse. Calculate the maximum volume of the local anesthetic and always draw up less than that. Bupivacaine is associated with more severe cardiac toxicity than lidocaine.
      (1) Progression of symptoms: Perioral numbness → dizziness → auditory disturbances → muscular twitching → loss of consciousness → seizures → coma → respiratory arrest → cardiovascular collapse
      (2) Summary of American Society of Regional Anesthesia and Pain Medicine (ASRA) Checklist for Treatment of Local Anesthetic Systemic Toxicity (LAST) (Fig. 6.2)[18]
      (3) If concerned for systemic toxicity, contact an anesthesiologist and call Poison Control (1-800-222-1222).

E. Nonpharmacologic Measures of Pain Relief[19,20]

1. **Sucrose for neonates (Sweet-Ease):**
   a. Indications: Painful minor procedures (heel lance, venipuncture, and intramuscular injection) in neonates and infants. Has not been shown to be effective for relief of circumcision pain. Strongest evidence for

TABLE 6.6

COMMONLY USED TOPICAL LOCAL ANESTHETICS

	Components	Indications	Peak Effect	Duration[a]	Cautions
EMLA	Lidocaine 2.5% Prilocaine 2.5%	Intact skin only Venipuncture, circumcision, LP, abscess drainage, BMA	60 min	90 min	Methemoglobinemia: Not for use in patients predisposed to methemoglobinemia (e.g. G6PD deficiency) Infants <3 months of age: Use sparingly (up to 1 g is safe)
LMX	Lidocaine 4%	Same as EMLA	30 min	60 min	Same as EMLA
LET	Lidocaine 4% Epinephrine 0.1% Tetracaine 0.5% Can be mixed with cellulose to create a gel	Safe for nonintact skin/lacerations Can be used to attain hemostasis with simple lacerations	30 min	45 min	Vasoconstriction: Contraindicated in areas supplied by end arteries (e.g., pinna, nose, penis, digits) Avoid contact with mucous membranes Not for use in contaminated wounds
Viscous lidocaine	Lidocaine 2% (May be mixed with aluminum/ magnesium hydroxide/simethicone [Maalox] and diphenhydramine in a 1:1:1 ratio for palatability when administered orally)	Safe for nonintact skin Mucous membranes (e.g., urethral catheter placement, mucositis)	10 min	30 min	Overuse can lead to life-threatening toxicity Not to be used for teething

[a]Approximate.

BMA, Bone marrow aspiration; *EMLA,* eutectic mixture of local anesthetics; *G6PD,* glucose-6-phosphate dehydrogenase; *LP,* lumbar puncture; *min,* minutes.

Data from Krauss B, Green SM. Sedation and analgesia for procedures in children. *N Engl J Med* 2000;342:938–945; Zempsky W, Cravero J. Relief of pain and anxiety in pediatric patients in emergency medical systems. *Pediatrics.* 2004;114:1348–1356.

6

TABLE 6.7

COMMONLY USED INJECTABLE LOCAL ANESTHETICS

Agent	Concentration (%)[a]	Max Dose (mg/kg)	Onset (min)	Duration (hr)
Lidocaine	0.5—2	5	3	0.5—2
Lidocaine with epinephrine	0.5—2	7	3	1—3
Bupivacaine	0.25—0.75	2.5	15	2—4
Bupivacaine with epinephrine	0.25—0.75	3	15	4—8
Bupivacaine with lidocaine mixture	Variable	[b]	3—15	0.5—4

[a]1% solution = 10 mg/mL.

[b][(mg/kg used of bupivacaine)/2.5 mg/kg × 100] + [(mg/kg used of lidocaine)/5 mg/kg × 100]. **Toxicity occurs when the sum is >100%.**

Data from St Germain BA. The management of pain in the emergency department. *Pediatr Clin North Am.* 2000;47:651—679; Yaster M, Cote C, Krane E, et al. *Pediatric Pain Management and Sedation Handbook.* Mosby; 1997:51—72.

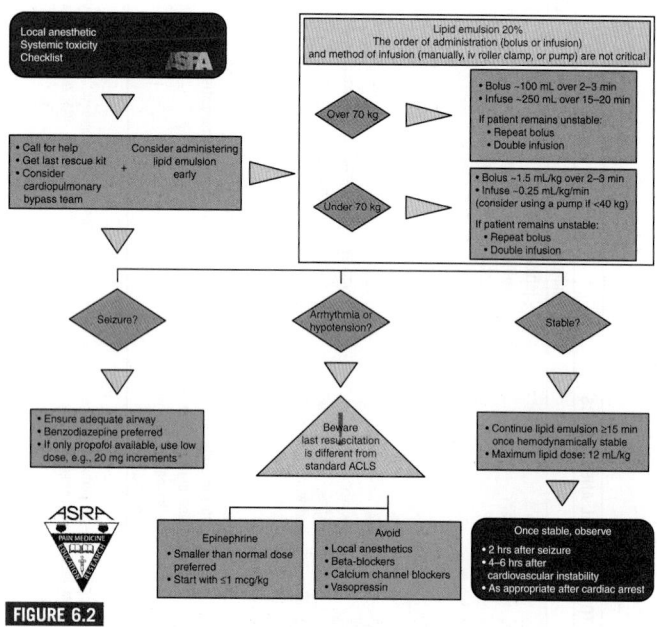

FIGURE 6.2

Checklist for Treatment of Local Anesthetic Systemic Toxicity (LAST). (From American Society of Regional Anesthesia and Pain Medicine. Local Anesthetic Systemic Toxicity Checklist. 2020. https://www.asra.com/images/default-source/asra-products/local-anesthetic-systemic-toxicity-rgb.jpg?sfvrsn=61e2f4b3_3) infants less than 1 month old,[19] but additional evidence suggests efficacy up to 12 months.[20]

b. Procedure: Administer up to 2 mL of 24% sucrose into the infant's mouth by syringe or from a nipple/pacifier ~2 minutes before the procedure. Effective doses in very low-birth-weight infants may be as low as 0.05 to 0.1 mL.

c. An additional dose may be administered within a relatively short period of time for multiple procedures, but it should not be administered more than twice in 1 hour.

d. Use with other age-appropriate nonpharmacologic measures.

e. Avoid if patient is unable to appropriately feed by mouth or cannot safely handle oral secretions.

2. **Other:** Parental presence/holding, distraction with toys, child life specialists, guided meditation/coping skills, virtual reality simulations, hot or cold packs.

IV. PATIENT-CONTROLLED ANALGESIA (PCA)

A. Definition

1. PCA enables a patient to receive a limited number of small bolus doses of an analgesic with or without a continuous (basal) infusion on an as-needed basis. In children younger than 6 years old or with physical/mental disability, a family member, caregiver, or nurse may administer bolus doses.

2. Practitioner specifies: Dose, minimum time period between doses (lockouts), basal infusion rate, maximum dose per hour.

B. Indications

1. Moderate to severe pain of acute or chronic nature. Commonly used in sickle cell disease, postsurgery, posttrauma, burns, and cancer

2. Useful for preemptive pain management (e.g., dressing changes)

C. Routes of Administration

1. IV

2. Epidural: This route should be prescribed and managed by an anesthesiologist.

D. Agents (Table 6.8)

TABLE 6.8

ORDERS FOR PATIENT-CONTROLLED ANALGESIA

Drug	Basal Rate (mCg/kg/hr)	Bolus Dose (mCg/kg)	Lockout Period (min)	Boluses (hr)	Max Dose (mCg/kg/hr)
Morphine	10–30	10–30	6–10	4–6	100–150
Hydromorphone	3–5	3–5	6–10	4–6	15–20
Fentanyl	0.5–1	0.5–1	6–10	2–3	2–4

mCg, Microgram.
Data from Yaster M, Cote C, Krane E, et al. *Pediatric Pain Management and Sedation Handbook*. Mosby; 1997:100.

E. Adjuvants

1. Low-dose **naloxone** (Narcan) infusion reduces incidence of pruritus and nausea associated with narcotic administration.
2. Low-dose **ketamine** infusion is an analgesic with a narcotic sparing effect. It is especially helpful in chemotherapy-induced mucositis, visceral pain, and neuropathic pain. Its mechanism of action is by N-methyl-D-aspartate (NMDA) blockade. May be used with, or as an alternative to, methadone.

F. Side Effects of Opioid Patient-Controlled Analgesia

1. Please refer to III. Analgesics; C. Opioids; 2. Side Effects

V. OPIOID TAPERING

A. Indications

1. Because of the development of dependence and potential for withdrawal, a tapering schedule is required if the patient has received frequent opioid analgesics for >5 days.

B. Withdrawal

1. See Box 18.1 for symptoms of opioid withdrawal.
2. Onset of signs and symptoms: 6 to 12 hours after the last dose of morphine and 36 to 48 hours after the last dose of methadone
3. Duration: 7 to 14 days, with a peak intensity reached within 2 to 4 days

C. Recommendations for Tapering

1. **Conversion:** All drugs should be converted to a single equianalgesic member of that group (see Table 6.5).
2. **PCA wean:** Drug dosing should be changed from continuous/intermittent IV infusion to PO basal/bolus therapy. If the patient is on PCA, once the first PO dose is administered, the PCA basal infusion should be stopped 30 to 60 minutes later. PCA bolus doses should be continued but reduced by 25% to 50%. If no further bolus doses are administered in the next 6 hours, the PCA should be discontinued. If the patient continues to experience pain, consider increasing scheduled PO dose, administering a rescue one-time PO bolus dose, or adding an adjuvant analgesic (e.g., NSAID).
3. **Slow dose decrease:** During an intermittent IV/PO wean, the total daily dose should be decreased by 10% to 20% of the original dose every 1 to 2 days (e.g., to taper a morphine dose of 40 mg/day, decrease the daily dose by 4 to 8 mg every 1 to 2 days).
4. **Oral regimen:** If not done previously, IV dosing should be converted to equivalent PO administration 1 to 2 days before discharge, and titration should be continued as outlined previously.
5. **Adjunctive therapy:**
   a. **Clonidine** in combination with an opioid decreases the length of time needed for opioid weaning in neonatal abstinence syndrome, with few short-term side effects. Long-term safety has yet to be thoroughly

investigated, but follow-up after 1 year on motor, cognitive, and language scores showed no difference in those treated with clonidine.[21,22]

b. PO and transdermal clonidine have a potential role for sedation, analgesia, and iatrogenic drug withdrawal in critically ill children, but current reports are retrospective or small clinical trials with significant heterogeneity in dosing, so further research is necessary. Transdermal dosing should not be used in children aged <1 year due to altered skin absorption.[23]

c. Studies have shown efficacy of α_2-adrenergic agonists in treating opioid withdrawal and reducing doses of methadone, but the duration of treatment was longer with α_2-adrenergic agonists, and there were fewer adverse effects with methadone.[24]

d. **Dexmedetomidine** is an α_2-adrenoreceptor agonist, which produces sedation and mild analgesia, with minimal to no respiratory depression. Administered as a continuous infusion, it has been shown to reduce opioid requirements and facilitate opioid weaning.

6. **Examples**
   a. See eBox 6.1 for example of opioid wean.

VI. PROCEDURAL SEDATION[5,14−17,25−27]

A. Definitions

1. **Mild sedation (anxiolysis):** Intent is anxiolysis with maintenance of consciousness.

2. **Moderate sedation:** Formerly known as *conscious sedation*. A controlled state of depressed consciousness during which airway reflexes and patency are maintained. Patient responds appropriately to age-appropriate commands (e.g., "Open your eyes") and light touch. This level of sedation often obtained with a combination of a low-dose sedative-hypnotic and an analgesic.

3. **Deep sedation:** A controlled state of depressed consciousness during which *airway reflexes and patency may **not** be maintained*, though cardiovascular function is usually maintained. The child will have purposeful response to repeated or painful stimulation. In practice, deep sedation is required for most painful procedures in children. This level of sedation may be achieved with propofol or a combination of a sedative-hypnotic and an analgesic agent.

4. **Dissociative sedation:** Unique state of sedation achieved with ketamine characterized by a deep level of depressed consciousness and analgesia. Airway reflexes and patency are generally maintained; however, excessive oral secretions may become problematic, occasionally resulting in micro-aspiration or laryngospasm.

B. Preparation

1. The patient should be **NPO** (nothing by mouth) for solids and liquids (Table 6.9).[25] Per American Society of Anesthesiologists (ASA) and American Academy of Pediatrics (AAP) guidelines, children receiving

TABLE 6.9

FASTING RECOMMENDATIONS FOR ANESTHESIA

Food Type	Minimum Fasting Period (hr)
Clear liquids	2
Breast milk	4
Nonhuman milk, formula	6
Solids	8

Data from *Practice Guidelines for Preoperative Fasting and the Use of Pharmacologic Agents to Reduce the Risk of Pulmonary Aspiration: Application to Healthy Patients Undergoing Elective Procedures.* A report by the American Society of Anesthesiologists Task Force on Preoperative Fasting and Use of Pharmacological Agents to Reduce the Risk of Pulmonary Aspiration. https://anesthesiology.pubs.asahq.org/article.aspx?articleid=1933410

moderate sedation for elective procedures should follow the same fasting guidelines as those for general anesthesia.[26,28] For urgent/emergent sedation when children are not NPO, the risks of sedation and possible aspiration must be balanced against the benefits of performing the procedure promptly. Recent studies suggest that NPO status for liquids and solids may not be statistically associated with aspiration, although studies are limited because aspiration is a relatively uncommon complication.[29]

2. **Focused patient history:**
   a. Allergies, medications, and any history of a previous reaction to anesthesia or sedation
   b. Assess for the possibility of an adverse airway event occurring with sedation (e.g., hypoxemia, hypercarbia, inability to mask ventilate). This can occur from: (1) mechanical airway obstruction (micrognathia, tonsillar and/or adenoid hypertrophy, large tongue, history of snoring, presence of noisy breathing, diagnosis of obstructive sleep apnea, obesity, presence of a craniofacial syndrome), (2) lung disease (history of prematurity, chronic lung disease, asthma), or (3) presence of a recent upper respiratory infection (URI). A history of a URI increases the risk of laryngospasm and/or bronchospasm; therefore, one must weigh the risks/benefits of providing sedation after a recent URI versus need for immediate interventional procedure. For elective procedures requiring sedation, it is best to wait 2 to 4 weeks after resolution of illness to reduce the risk of an adverse event.[30]
      (1) There is currently insufficient data regarding how long to wait after symptomatic COVID-19 infection before undergoing an elective procedure.
   c. Assess aspiration risk (neuromuscular disease, esophageal disease, altered mental status, obesity, pregnancy).
   d. Presence of kidney/liver disease (may prolong sedative effect) and cardiac disease (potential for hemodynamic instability with sedative administration)

3. **Physical examination:** Specific attention to mouth opening and neck extension. Use the Mallampati classification system to assess the airway for likelihood of difficult direct laryngoscopy and intubation (Fig. 6.3).
4. **Determine ASA Physical Status Classification** (Table 6.10)**:** Class I and II patients are generally good candidates for mild, moderate, or deep sedation outside of the operating room.[26]
5. **Always have an emergency plan ready:**
   a. Make sure qualified backup personnel and equipment are close by.

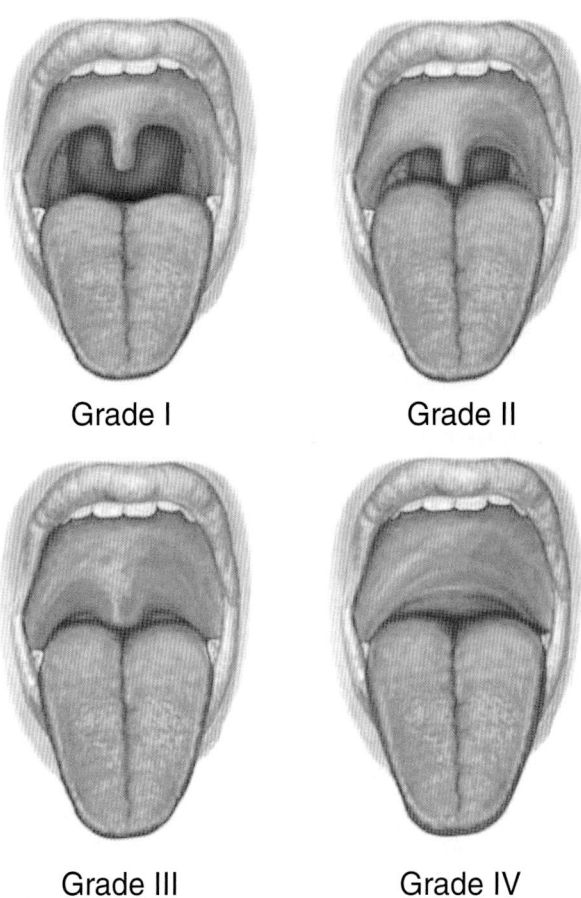

Grade I   Grade II

Grade III   Grade IV

FIGURE 6.3

Mallampati classification system.

TABLE 6.10	
ASA PHYSICAL STATUS CLASSIFICATION	
Class I	A normally healthy patient
Class II	A patient with mild systemic disease (e.g., controlled reactive airway disease)
Class III	A patient with severe systemic disease (e.g., a child who is actively wheezing)
Class IV	A patient with severe systemic disease that is a constant threat to life (e.g., a child with status asthmaticus)
Class V	A moribund patient who is not expected to survive without the operation (e.g., a patient with severe cardiomyopathy requiring heart transplantation)
Class VI	A declared brain-dead patient whose organs are being removed for donor purposes

    b. Complications most often occur 5 to 10 minutes after administration of IV medication and immediately after a procedure is completed (when the stimuli associated with the procedure are removed).[16]

6. **Personnel:** Two providers are required. One provider should perform the procedure, and a separate provider should monitor the patient during sedation and recovery.

7. **Ensure IV access** prior to induction by flushing with saline. Subcutaneous infiltration of a sedative can cause unpredictable or prolonged sedation.

8. **Have airway/intubation equipment immediately available** (see Chapter 1).

9. **Emergency medications:** Always have emergency medications for rapid sequence intubation and CPR immediately available.

10. **Reversal agents** should be readily available (naloxone, flumazenil).

C. Monitoring[31]

1. **Vital signs:** Baseline vital signs should be obtained. The following should be monitored throughout sedation:

    a. Oxygenation: Continuous pulse oximetry with variable pitch pulse tone and audible low threshold alarm

    b. Circulation: Continuous EKG, with arterial blood pressure and heart rate evaluated at least every 5 minutes

    c. Ventilation: Frequent evaluation of respiratory rate and airway patency (via direct visualization and auscultation) during any sedation, and continuous capnography (end-tidal carbon dioxide [CO_2]) during moderate or deep sedation

        (1) Unrecognized apnea is often followed by desaturation within 1 to 2 minutes when not receiving supplemental oxygenation. Administration of supplemental oxygen can further delay recognition of apnea because the onset of desaturation may occur more than 2 minutes after apnea.

D. Pharmacologic Agents

1. **Goal of procedural sedation:** The administration of medications to provide appropriate levels of analgesia, sedation, and anxiolysis so that the procedure can occur without the need to secure the airway.

2. **CNS, cardiovascular, and respiratory depression** may always occur; occurs more commonly when combining sedative drugs and/or opioids, or with rapid drug administration. It is always best to titrate medications to the desired level of sedation.

3. **Common sedative/hypnotic agents (Box 6.1).** Also see Table 6.5 and Table 6.11 for more information on opioids, barbiturates, and benzodiazepines.

BOX 6.1

PROPERTIES OF COMMON SEDATIVE/HYPNOTIC AGENTS

Sedating Antihistamines (Diphenhydramine, Hydroxyzine)

- Mild sedative-hypnotics with antiemetic and antipruritic properties; used for sedation and treatment of opioid side effects
- No anxiolytic or analgesic effects

Barbiturates

- Contraindicated in patients with porphyria
- Suitable only for nonpainful procedures
- Not reversible with flumazenil
- Narrower margin of safety than benzodiazepines
- No anxiolytic or analgesic effects

Benzodiazepines

- Reversible with flumazenil
- Anxiolytic effects; no analgesic effects

Opioids

- Reversible with naloxone
- Analgesic effects; no anxiolytic effects

Ketamine[5,15–19]

- Causes potent dissociative amnesia and analgesia
- Nystagmus indicates likely therapeutic effect
- Vocalizations/movement may occur even with adequate sedation
- Onset: IV, 0.5–2 min; IM, 5–10 min; PO/PR, 20–45 min
- Duration: IV, 20–60 min; IM, 30–90 min; PO/PR, 60–120+ min
- **CNS effects:** Emergence delirium with auditory, visual, and tactile hallucinations
- **Cardiovascular effects:** Inhibits catecholamine reuptake, thereby causing increased HR, BP, SVR, and PVR. Rarely causes hemodynamic instability; however, in catecholamine-deplete patients (e.g., shock) it can cause direct myocardial depression and hypotension.
- **Respiratory effects:** Bronchodilation (useful in patients with asthma), increased secretions (can result in laryngospasm), maintenance of ventilatory response to hypoxia, relative maintenance of airway reflexes

---

Continued

BOX 6.1—CONT'D

- **Other effects:** Increased muscle tone, myoclonic jerks, nausea, emesis
- **Contraindications:** Hypertension and preexisting psychotic disorders
  - Controversy exists on its safety in patients with elevated ICP or IOP. Evidence suggesting ketamine elevates intracranial pressure or causes harm in these patients is limited.

Propofol

- For deep sedation or general anesthesia
- Administered as single or multiple IV boluses ± infusion
- Rapid onset and brief recovery (5–15 min) with bolus administration
- Can have antiemetic and euphoric effects
- **Caution:** Respiratory depression, apnea, hypotension
- No analgesic effects

Dexmedetomidine[32-36]

- α_2 agonist
- Sedative, anxiolytic, and analgesic effects
- Administration
  - IV: load over 10 min followed by infusion
  - Intranasal: administered via drops or atomizer, no IV access required, plasma levels theoretically equal to IV dose
- Slower onset of action compared to other IV sedative-hypnotics
- Favorable due to low risk of respiratory depression, decreased irritability/agitation during recovery
- Can cause hypotension (with initial bolus), hypertension (with high doses, multiple boluses), and bradycardia (avoid in patients on atrioventricular nodal blocking medications)

Data from Yaster M, Cote C, Krane E, et al. *Pediatric Pain Management and Sedation Handbook.* Mosby; 1997:376–382; St Germain BA. The management of pain in the emergency department. *Pediatr Clin North Am.* 2000;47:651–679; Cote CJ, Lerman J, Todres ID, et al. *A Practice of Anesthesia for Infants and Children.* WB Saunders; 2001.

---

4. Reversal agents:
   a. Naloxone: Opioid antagonist. See Box 6.2 for naloxone administration protocol.
   b. Flumazenil: Benzodiazepine antagonist.

E. Discharge Criteria[26]

1. The patient can maintain a patent airway without requiring supplemental oxygen. There should also be no compromise in cardiovascular function.
2. The patient should be easily arousable with intact protective airway reflexes (swallow, cough, and gag).
3. The patient should have the ability to talk and sit up unaided (if age appropriate). Alternatively, for very young or intellectually disabled children, the goal is to return to their presedation level of responsiveness.
4. Ensure ability to maintain adequate hydration (i.e., the patient can tolerate enteral fluids).

TABLE 6.11

COMMONLY USED BENZODIAZEPINES[a] AND BARBITURATES

Drug Class	Duration of Action	Drug	Route	Onset (min)	Duration (hr)	Comments
Benzodiazepines	Short	Midazolam (Versed)	IV	1–3	1–2	Has rapid and predictable onset of action, short recovery time
			IM/IN	5–10		Causes amnesia
			PO/PR	10–30		Results in mild depression of hypoxic ventilatory drive
	Intermediate	Diazepam (Valium)	IV (painful)	1–6	0.25–1	Poor choice for procedural sedation
			PR	7–15	2–6	Excellent for muscle relaxation or prolonged sedation
			PO	30–60	2–6	Pain on IV injection
	Long	Lorazepam (Ativan)	IV	1–5	3–4	Poor choice for procedural sedation
			IM	10–20	3–6	Ideal for prolonged anxiolysis, seizure treatment
			PO	30–60	3–6	
Barbiturates	Short	Methohexital	PR[b]	5–10	0.5–1.5	PR form used as sedative for nonpainful procedure
	Intermediate	Pentobarbital	IV	1–10	1–4	Predictable sedation and immobility for nonpainful procedures
			IM	5–15	2–4	Minimal respiratory depression when used alone
			PO/PR	15–60	2–4	Associated with slow wake up and agitation

[a]Use IV solution for PO, PR, and IN administration. Rectal diazepam gel (Diastat) is also available.

[b]IV administration produces general anesthesia; only PR should be used for sedation.

IM, Intramuscular; *IN,* intranasal; *IV,* intravenous; *min,* minute; *PO,* by mouth; *PR,* per rectum.

Data from Yaster M, Cote C, Krane E, et al. *Pediatric Pain Management and Sedation Handbook.* Mosby; 1997:345–374; St Germain BA. The management of pain in the emergency department. *Pediatr Clin North Am.* 2000;47:651–679; Cote CJ, Lerman J, Todres ID, et al. *A Practice of Anesthesia for Infants and Children.* WB Saunders; 2001.

6

BOX 6.2

NALOXONE (NARCAN) ADMINISTRATION[a]

Indications: Patients Requiring Naloxone (Narcan) Usually Meet All the Following Criteria

- Shallow respirations or respiratory rate <8 breaths/min[b]
- Pinpoint pupils
- Unresponsive to physical stimulation

Procedure

1. **Stop opioid administration** (as well as other sedative drugs), assess **ABCs** (**A**irway, **B**reathing, **C**irculation), and **call for help.**
2. **Dilute naloxone:**
   a. If child >40 kg: Mix 0.4 mg (1 ampule) of naloxone with 9 mL of normal saline (final concentration 0.04 mg/mL = 40 mCg/mL).
   b. If child <40 kg: Mix 0.4 mg (1 ampule) of naloxone with 9 mL of normal saline to make a concentration of 40 mCg/mL (as above). **Then, repeat dilution** by mixing 1 mL of the 40 mCg/mL solution with 9 mL of normal saline for final concentration of 4 mCg/mL.
3. **Administer and observe response:** Administer dilute naloxone *slowly* (1–2 mCg/kg/dose IV over 2 minutes). Observe patient response.
4. **Titrate to effect:** Within 1–2 minutes, patient should open eyes and respond. If not, continue until a total dose of 10 mCg/kg is given. If no response is obtained, evaluate for other cause of sedation/respiratory depression.
5. **Discontinue naloxone administration:** Discontinue naloxone as soon as patient responds (e.g., takes deep breaths when directed).
6. **Caution:** Another dose of naloxone may be required within 30 min of first dose (duration of action of naloxone is shorter than that of most opioids).
7. **Monitor patient:** Assign a staff member to monitor sedation/respiratory status and remind patient to take deep breaths as necessary.
8. **Alternative analgesia:** Provide nonopioids for pain relief. Resume opioid administration at half the original dose when the patient is easily aroused, and respiratory rate is >9 breaths/min.

---

[a]Naloxone administration for patients being treated for pain. Higher doses may be necessary for patients found in the community or those with signs of cardiopulmonary failure. Please see Formulary for additional dosing.
[b]Respiratory rates that require naloxone vary according to infant's/child's usual rate.
Modified from McCaffery M, Pasero C. *Pain: Clinical Manual.* Mosby; 1999:269–270.

F. Examples of Sedation Protocols (Table 6.12 and eTable 6.1)

TABLE 6.12

EXAMPLES OF SEDATION PROTOCOLS

Protocol/Doses	Comments
Ketamine × 1–3 doses	Lowest rates of adverse events when ketamine used alone[a]
Ketamine + midazolam + atropine ("ketazolam") Ketamine × 1–3 doses Midazolam × 1 dose Atropine × 1 dose	Atropine = antisialagogue Midazolam = counters emergence delirium Can be given IM or IV. If giving IM, combine all 3 agents in 1 syringe (using the smallest volume possible, preferably <3 mL total).
Midazolam + fentanyl Midazolam × 3 doses PRN Fentanyl × 3 doses PRN	High likelihood of respiratory depression Give fentanyl no more frequently than every 3 min Risk of rigid chest—give no faster than 1 mCg/kg/min
Dexmedetomidine	Can be given IN or IV Risk of hypotension, hypertension, and bradycardia with bolus

[a]Green SM, Roback MG, Krauss B, et al. Predictors of emesis and recovery agitation with emergency department ketamine sedation: an individual-patient data meta-analysis of 8,282 children. *Ann Emerg Med.* 2009;54:171–180.

IM, Intramuscular; *IN,* intranasal; *IV,* intravenous; *mCg,* microgram; *PRN,* as needed.

Modified from Yaster M, Cote C, Krane E, et al. *Pediatric Pain Management and Sedation Handbook.* Mosby; 1997.

VII. WEB RESOURCES

- International Association for the Study of Pain: http://childpain.org/
- American Pain Society: https://painmed.org/
- American Society of Anesthesiologists: http://www.asahq.org/

REFERENCES

A complete list of references can be found online.

Chapter 7

Cardiology

Alexander Tang, MD and James Ting, MD

🌐 See additional content online.

🔊 **Audio Case File 7.1** Auscultation and heart sounds

🔊 **Audio Case File 7.2** Tetralogy of Fallot: Review of the congenital heart disease and accompanying cardiac surgeries

I. PHYSICAL EXAMINATION

A. Heart Rate

Refer to the first page of this book for normal heart rate (HR) by age.

B. Blood Pressure

1. Blood pressure (BP):

   See Chapter 19 for normal BP values by age.

2. **Mean arterial pressure (MAP)**

   a. MAP = diastolic pressure + 1/3 pulse pressure OR MAP = 1/3 systolic pressure + 2/3 diastolic pressure

   b. Preterm infants and newborns: Normal MAP = gestational age in weeks

3. Abnormalities in BP

   a. Four-limb BP measurements can be used to assess for coarctation of the aorta.

   b. Pulsus paradoxus: Exaggeration of the normal drop in systolic blood pressure (SBP) with inspiration. Determine SBP at the end of exhalation and during inhalation; difference >10 mmHg, consider pericardial effusion, tamponade, pericarditis, severe asthma, or restrictive cardiomyopathies.

4. Hypertension (HTN)

   a. See Chapter 1 for management of acute HTN.

   b. See Chapter 19 for screening, workup, and management of chronic HTN.

C. Heart Sounds

1. **S_1:** Associated with closure of mitral and tricuspid valves; heard best at the apex or left lower sternal border (LLSB)

2. **S_2:** Associated with closure of pulmonary and aortic valves; heard best at the left upper sternal border (LUSB) and has normal physiologic splitting that increases with inspiration

3. **S_3:** Heard best at the apex or LLSB

4. **S_4:** Heard at the apex

D. Systolic and Diastolic Sounds

See Box 7.1 for abnormal heart sounds.[1]

E. Murmurs

Clinical characteristics are summarized in Table 7.1.[1]

1. **Grading of heart murmurs:** Intensified by states of higher cardiac output (e.g., anemia, anxiety, fever, exercise)[1]
   a. Grade I: Barely audible
   b. Grade II: Murmur softer than heart sounds, but audible
   c. Grade III: Murmur moderately loud, equally loud as heart sounds, not accompanied by a thrill
   d. Grade IV: Murmur louder than heart sounds, associated with a thrill
   e. Grade V: Audible with a stethoscope barely on the chest
   f. Grade VI: Audible with a stethoscope off the chest
2. Benign heart murmurs[2]:
   a. Caused by a disturbance of the laminar flow of blood; frequently produced as the diameter of the blood's pathway decreases and velocity increases
   b. Present in >80% of children sometime during childhood, most commonly beginning at age 3 to 4 years
   c. Accentuated in high-output states, especially with fever and anemia
   d. Normal electrocardiogram (ECG) and radiographic findings

   NOTE: ECG and chest radiograph are not routinely used, nor are they cost-effective screening tools for distinguishing benign from pathologic murmurs.

BOX 7.1

SUMMARY OF ABNORMAL HEART SOUNDS

- **Widely split S_1:** Ebstein anomaly, RBBB
- **Widely split and fixed S_2:** Right ventricular volume overload (e.g., ASD, PAPVR), pressure overload (e.g., PS), electrical delay in RV contraction (e.g., RBBB), early aortic closure (e.g., MR), occasionally heard in normal child
- **Narrowly split S_2:** Pulmonary hypertension, AS, delay in LV contraction (e.g., LBBB), occasionally heard in normal child
- **Single S_2:** Pulmonary hypertension, one semilunar valve (e.g., pulmonary atresia, aortic atresia, truncus arteriosus), P_2 not audible (e.g., TGA, TOF, severe PS), severe AS, occasionally heard in normal child
- **Paradoxically split S_2:** Severe AS, LBBB, Wolff-Parkinson-White syndrome (type B)
- **Abnormal intensity of P_2:** Increased P_2 (e.g., pulmonary hypertension), decreased P_2 (e.g., severe PS, TOF, TS)
- **S_3:** Occasionally heard in healthy children or adults or may indicate dilated ventricles (e.g., large VSD, CHF)
- **S_4:** Always pathologic, indicative of decreased ventricular compliance
- **Ejection click:** Heard with stenosis of the semilunar valves, dilated great arteries in the setting of pulmonary or systemic HTN, idiopathic dilation of the PA, TOF, persistent truncus arteriosus
- **Midsystolic click:** Heard at the apex in mitral valve prolapse
- **Diastolic opening snap:** Rare in children; associated with TS/MS

AS, Aortic stenosis; *ASD,* atrial septal defect; *CHF,* congestive heart failure; *LBBB,* left bundle-branch block; *LV,* left ventricle; *MR,* mitral regurgitation; *MS,* mitral stenosis; *PA,* pulmonary artery; *PAPVR,* partial anomalous pulmonary venous return; *PS,* pulmonic stenosis; *RBBB,* right bundle-branch block; *RV,* right ventricular; *TGA,* transposition of the great arteries; *TOF,* tetralogy of fallot; *TS,* tricuspid stenosis; *VSD,* ventricular septal defect.
Modified from Park MK. *Pediatric Cardiology for Practitioners.* 5th ed. Elsevier; 2008:25.

TABLE 7.1

COMMON INNOCENT HEART MURMURS

Type (Timing)	Description of Murmur	Age Group
Classic vibratory murmur (Still murmur; systolic)	Maximal at LMSB or between LLSB and apex Grade 2–3/6 in intensity Low-frequency vibratory, twanging string, groaning, squeaking, or musical	3–6 years; occasionally in infancy
Pulmonary ejection murmur (systolic)	Maximal at LUSB Early to midsystolic Grade 1–3/6 in intensity Blowing in quality	8–14 years
Pulmonary flow murmur of newborn (systolic)	Maximal at LUSB Transmits well to left and right chest, axilla, and back Grade 1–2/6 in intensity	Premature and full-term newborns Usually disappears by 3–6 months
Venous hum (continuous)	Maximal at right (or left) supraclavicular and infraclavicular areas Grade 1–3/6 in intensity Inaudible in supine position Intensity changes with rotation of head and disappears with compression of jugular vein	3–6 years
Carotid bruit (systolic)	Right supraclavicular area over carotids Grade 2–3/6 in intensity Occasional thrill over carotid	Any age

LLSB, Left lower sternal border; *LMSB*, left middle sternal border; *LUSB*, left upper sternal border.
From Park MK. *Pediatric Cardiology for Practitioners*. 5th ed. Elsevier; 2008:36.

3. **A murmur is more likely to be pathologic when one or more of the following are present:** Symptoms (e.g., chest pain, dyspnea with exertion, syncope with exertion); cyanosis; a systolic murmur that is loud (grade ≥3/6), harsh, pansystolic, or long in duration; diastolic murmur; abnormal heart sounds; presence of a click; abnormally strong or weak pulses[1,2]
4. Systolic and diastolic heart murmurs (Box 7.2)

II. ELECTROCARDIOGRAPHY

A. Basic Electrocardiography Principles

1. Lead placement (Fig. 7.1)
2. ECG complexes
   a. P wave: Represents atrial depolarization
   b. QRS complex: Represents ventricular depolarization
   c. T wave: Represents ventricular repolarization
   d. U wave: May follow the T wave and represents late phases of ventricular repolarization

---

BOX 7.2

SYSTOLIC AND DIASTOLIC HEART MURMURS

RUSB

Aortic valve stenosis (supravalvular, subvalvular)
Aortic regurgitation

LUSB

Pulmonary valve stenosis
Atrial septal defect
Pulmonary ejection murmur, innocent
Pulmonary flow murmur of newborn
Pulmonary artery stenosis
Aortic stenosis
Coarctation of the aorta
Patent ductus arteriosus
Partial anomalous pulmonary venous return (PAPVR)
Total anomalous pulmonary venous return (TAPVR)
Pulmonary regurgitation

LLSB

Ventricular septal defect, including atrioventricular septal defect
Vibratory innocent murmur (Still murmur)
HOCM (IHSS)
Tricuspid regurgitation
Tetralogy of Fallot
Tricuspid stenosis

Apex

Mitral regurgitation
Vibratory innocent murmur (Still murmur)
Mitral valve prolapse
Aortic stenosis
HOCM (IHSS)
Mitral stenosis

Murmurs listed by the location at which they are best heard. *Diastolic murmurs are in italics.*
HOCM, Hypertrophic obstructive cardiomyopathy; *IHSS,* idiopathic hypertrophic subaortic stenosis; *LLSB,* left lower sternal border; *LUSB,* left upper sternal border; *RUSB,* right upper sternal border.
From Park MK. *Pediatric Cardiology for Practitioners.* 5th ed. Elsevier; 2008:30.

3. **Systematic approach for evaluating ECGs** (Table 7.2 shows normal ECG parameters)[1,3]:
    a. **Rate**
        (1) Standardization: Paper speed is 25 mm/sec. One small square = 1 mm = 0.04 second. One large square = 5 mm = 0.2 second. Amplitude standard: 10 mm = 1 mV
        (2) Calculation: HR (beats/min) = 60 divided by the average R-R interval in seconds, or 300 divided by the number of large boxes between 2 R waves (1 large box = 300 bpm, 2 large boxes = 150 bpm) (Fig. 7.2)

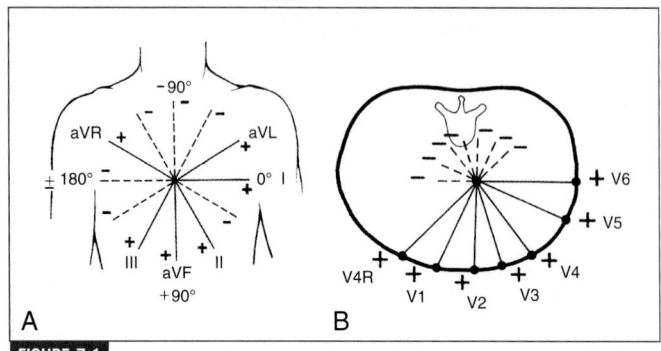

(A) Hexaxial reference system. (B) Horizontal reference system. (Modified from Park MK, Guntheroth WG. *How to Read Pediatric ECGs*. 4th ed. Elsevier; 2006:3.)

b. **Rhythm**
  (1) Sinus rhythm: Every QRS complex is preceded by a P wave and normal P-wave axis (upright P in leads I and aVF).
  (2) There is normal respiratory variation of the R-R interval without morphologic changes of the P wave or QRS complex.
c. **Axis:** The direction of the QRS in leads I and aVF should be observed, the quadrant determined, and comparison made with age-matched normal values (Fig. 7.3 and Table 7.2).
d. **Intervals** (PR, QRS, QTc)
  (1) See Table 7.2 for normal PR and QRS intervals.
  (2) The QTc is calculated using the Bazett formula:
    QTc = QT (sec) measured/$\sqrt{\text{R-R}}$ (use the shortest R-R interval on the ECG measured in lead II or V_5).
  (3) The QT interval (in seconds) is measured from the beginning of the QRS complex to the end of the T wave. Divide this value by the square root of the preceding R-R interval (also measured in seconds) to obtain the QTc.
  (4) **Normal values for QTc are:**
    (a) 0.44 second is the 97th percentile for infants 3 to 4 days old.[4]
    (b) ≤0.45 second in all males aged >1 week and in prepubescent females
    (c) ≤0.46 second for postpubescent females
e. **P-wave size and shape:** A normal P wave duration should be <0.09 second (2.5 small boxes) in children and <0.07 second (2 small boxes) in infants. Normal P wave amplitude (height) is <0.3 mV (3 mm or 3 small boxes in height, with normal standardization).
f. **R-wave progression:** In general, there is a normal increase in R-wave size and a decrease in S-wave size from leads V_1 to V_6 (with dominant S waves in the right precordial leads V_1,V_2 and dominant R waves in the left precordial leads V_4,V_5, representing dominance of left

TABLE 7.2
NORMAL PEDIATRIC ELECTROCARDIOGRAM PARAMETERS

Age	Heart Rate (bpm)	QRS Axis[a]	PR Interval (sec)[b]	QRS Duration (sec)[b]	Lead V$_1$ R-Wave Amplitude (mm)[b]	Lead V$_1$ S-Wave Amplitude (mm)[b]	Lead V$_1$ R/S Ratio	Lead V$_6$ R-Wave Amplitude (mm)[b]	Lead V$_6$ S-Wave Amplitude (mm)[b]	R/S Ratio
0–7 days	95–160 (125)	+30 to +180 (+110)	0.10 (0.12)	0.05 (0.07)	13 (24)	7 (18)	1.5	5 (15)	3 (10)	2
1–3 weeks	105–180 (145)	+30 to +180 (+110)	0.10 (0.12)	0.05 (0.07)	13 (24)	7 (18)	1.5	5 (15)	3 (10)	2
1–6 months	110–180 (145)	+10 to +125 (+70)	0.10 (0.14)	0.055 (0.075)	10 (19)	5 (15)	1.5	13 (22)	3 (9)	4
6–12 months	110–170 (135)	+10 to +125 (+60)	0.10 (0.14)	0.055 (0.075)	10 (20)	7 (18)	1.2	13 (23)	2 (7)	6
1–3 years	90–150 (120)	+10 to +125 (+60)	0.11 (0.14)	0.055 (0.075)	9 (18)	8 (21)	0.8	13 (23)	2 (7)	20
4–5 years	72–135 (108)	+20 to +120 (+60)	0.13 (0.17)	0.06 (0.075)	8 (16)	11 (23)	0.65	15 (26)	2 (5)	20
6–8 years	65–135 (100)	+20 to +120 (+60)	0.13 (0.17)	0.06 (0.075)	8 (16)	11 (23)	0.65	15 (26)	2 (5)	20
9–11 years	65–130 (90)	+20 to +120 (+60)	0.15 (0.18)	0.06 (0.085)	5 (12)	12 (25)	0.5	17 (26)	1 (4)	20
12–16 years	60–120 (85)	+20 to +120 (+60)	0.15 (0.19)	0.07 (0.085)	4 (10)	11 (22)	0.3	14 (23)	1 (4)	10
>16 years	60–100 (80)	+30 to +105 (+50)	0.15 (0.21)	0.08 (0.10)	3 (14)	10 (23)	0.3	10 (21)	1 (13)	9

[a]Normal range and (mean).
[b]Mean and (98th percentile).
Data from Park MK, Salamat M. *Pediatric Cardiology for Practitioners.* 7th ed. St Louis: Elsevier; 2021; and Davignon A, et al. Normal ECG standards for infants and children. *Pediatr Cardiol.* 1979;1:123–131.

7

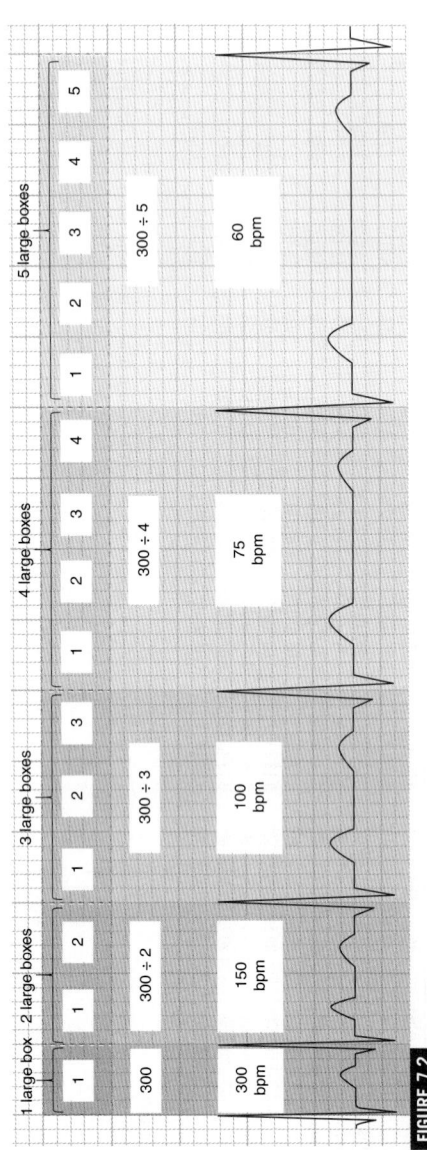

FIGURE 7.2

Calculation of approximate rate.

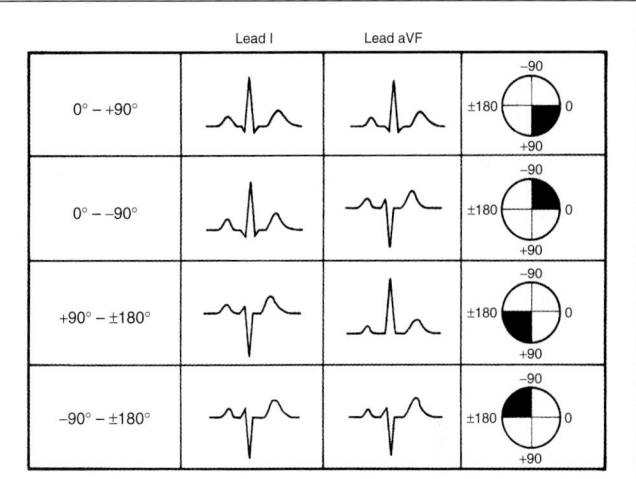

	Lead I	Lead aVF	
0° – +90°			
0° – –90°			
+90° – ±180°			
–90° – ±180°			

FIGURE 7.3

Location of quadrants of the mean QRS axis from leads I and aVF. (From Park MK, Guntheroth WG. *How to Read Pediatric ECGs*. 4th ed. Elsevier; 2006:17.)

ventricular forces. However, newborns and infants have a normal dominance of the right ventricle and therefore larger R waves in V_1, V_2, and smaller R waves in V_5, V_6.

g. **Q waves:** Normal Q waves are usually <0.04 second in duration and <25% of the total QRS amplitude. Normal Q waves are ≤5.5 mm deep in the left precordial leads V_4, V_5 and aVF in children >3 years of age, and ≤6 mm deep in lead III for children age <3 years. Q waves of >0.04 second duration are likely pathologic. Excessively deep Q waves in III, V_5, and V_6 may indicate left ventricular hypertrophy.

h. **ST-segment** (Fig. 7.4): ST-segment elevation or depression of >1 mm in two contiguous limb leads and >2 mm in two contiguous precordial leads (V_1-V_6) is consistent with myocardial ischemia or injury. Diffuse ST elevation of <1 mm in the limb leads and <2 mm in the precordial leads may indicate early repolarization, which is a normal variant.

i. **T wave:**
   (1) Inverted T waves in V_1 and V_2 can be normal in children up to adolescence (Table 7.3).
   (2) Tall, peaked T waves may be seen in hyperkalemia. A normal T wave is less than one-half the amplitude of its corresponding R wave.[1,3]
   (3) Flat or low T waves may be seen in hypokalemia, hypothyroidism, normal newborns, myocardial/pericardial ischemia, and inflammation.

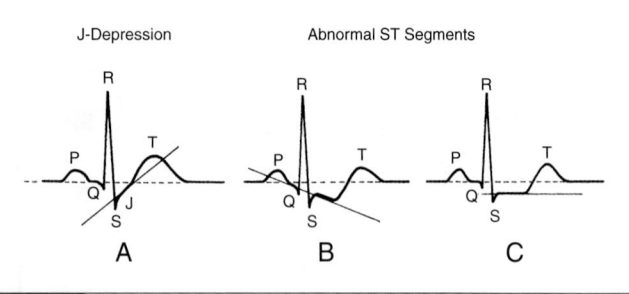

FIGURE 7.4

Nonpathologic (nonischemic) and pathologic (ischemic) *ST* and *T* changes. (A) Characteristic nonischemic ST-segment alteration called J-depression (note that ST slope is upward), B to C. Ischemic or pathologic ST-segment alterations: (B) downward slope of ST segment; (C) horizontal segment is sustained. (From Park MK, Guntheroth WG. *How to Read Pediatric ECGs.* 4th ed. Elsevier; 2006:107.)

TABLE 7.3

NORMAL T-WAVE AXIS

Age	V_1, V_2	AVF	I, V_5, V_6
Birth to 1 day	±	+	±
1–4 days	±	+	+
4 days to adolescent	−	+	+
Adolescent to adult	+	+	+

+, T wave positive; −, T wave negative; ±, T wave normally either positive or negative.

    j. **Hypertrophy/enlargement**
      (1) Atrial enlargement: P wave duration exceeding these norms may indicate left atrial enlargement. P wave amplitude greater than 3 mm may indicate right atrial enlargement (Fig. 7.5).
      (2) Ventricular hypertrophy: Diagnosed by QRS axis, voltage, and R/S ratio (Box 7.3; see also Table 7.4).

B. ECG Abnormalities

1. **Nonventricular arrhythmias** (Table 7.4; Fig. 7.6)[5]
2. **Ventricular arrhythmias** (Table 7.5; Fig. 7.7)
3. **Nonventricular conduction disturbances** (Table 7.6; Fig. 7.8)[6]
4. **Ventricular conduction disturbances** (Table 7.7)

C. ECG Findings Secondary to Electrolyte Disturbances, Medications, and Systemic Illnesses (Table 7.8)[5,7]

D. Long QT

1. **Diagnosis:**
    a. In general, normal QTc is similar in males and females from 6 months until late adolescence (0.37 to 0.44). In newborns and small infants, the upper limit is 0.47 in the first week and 0.45 in the first 6 months.
    b. In adults, prolonged QTc is generally >0.45 second in males and >0.46 second in females after adolescence.
    c. In ~10% of cases, patients may have a normal baseline QTc. Patients may also have a family history of long QT associated with

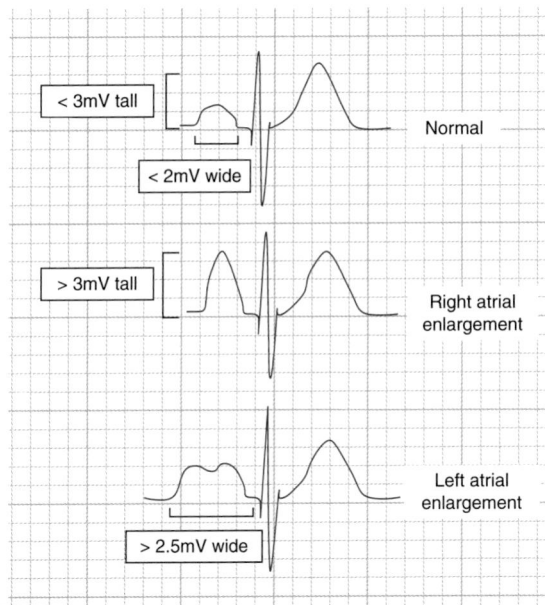

FIGURE 7.5

Criteria for atrial enlargement (From Park MK, Guntheroth WG: *How to Read Pediatric ECGs,* 4th ed. Philadelphia, Mosby, 2006.)

BOX 7.3

VENTRICULAR HYPERTROPHY CRITERIA

Right Ventricular Hypertrophy (RVH) Criteria

Must have at least one of the following:
- Upright T wave in lead V_1 after 3 days of age to adolescence
- Presence of Q wave in V_1 (QR or QRS pattern)
- Increased right and anterior QRS voltage (with normal QRS duration):
  - R in lead V_1, V_2, or aVR >98th percentile for age
  - S in lead V_6, >98th percentile for age
- Right ventricular strain (associated with inverted T wave in V_1 with tall R wave)

Left Ventricular Hypertrophy (LVH) Criteria

- Left ventricular strain (associated with inverted T wave in leads V_6, I, and/or aVF)
- Left axis deviation (LAD) for patient's age
- Volume overload (associated with Q wave >5 mm and tall T waves in V_5 or V_6)
- Increased QRS voltage in left leads (with normal QRS duration):
  - R in lead V_6 (and I, aVL, V_5), >98th percentile for age
  - S in lead V_1, >98th percentile for age

TABLE 7.4

NONVENTRICULAR ARRHYTHMIAS

Name/Description	Cause	Treatment
SINUS		
Tachycardia		
Normal sinus rhythm with HR >95th percentile for age (usually infants: <220 beats/min and children: <180 beats/min)	Hypovolemia, shock, anemia, sepsis, fever, anxiety, CHF, PE, myocardial disease, drugs (e.g., β-agonists, albuterol, caffeine, atropine)	Address underlying cause.
Bradycardia		
Normal sinus rhythm with HR <5th percentile for age	Normal (especially in athletic individuals), increased ICP, hypoxia, hyperkalemia, hypercalcemia, vagal stimulation, hypothyroidism, hypothermia, drugs (e.g. opioids, digoxin, β-blockers), long QT	Address underlying cause; if symptomatic, refer to inside back cover for bradycardia algorithm.
SUPRAVENTRICULAR[a]		
Premature Atrial Contraction (PAC)		
Narrow QRS complex; ectopic focus in atria with abnormal P-wave morphology	Digitalis toxicity, medications (e.g., caffeine, theophylline, sympathomimetics), normal variant	Treat digitalis toxicity; otherwise no treatment needed
Atrial Flutter		
Atrial rate 240–360 beats/min; characteristic saw-tooth or flutter pattern with variable ventricular response rate and normal QRS complex	Dilated atria, previous intra-atrial surgery, valvular or ischemic heart disease, idiopathic in newborns	Synchronized cardioversion or overdrive pacing; treat underlying cause
Atrial Fibrillation		
Irregular; atrial rate 350–600 beats/min, yielding characteristic fibrillatory pattern (no discrete P waves) and irregular ventricular response rate of about 110–150 beats/min with normal QRS complex	Those listed previously for atrial flutter (except idiopathic), alcohol exposure, familial	Synchronized cardioversion; then may need anticoagulation based on stroke risk

SVT

Sudden run of three or more consecutive premature supraventricular beats at >220 beats/min (infant) or >180 beats/min (child), with narrow QRS complex and absent/abnormal P wave; either sustained (>30 sec) or non-sustained

Wolff-Parkinson-White syndrome, idiopathic, may be seen in congenital heart disease (e.g., Ebstein anomaly, single ventricle)

Vagal maneuvers, adenosine; if unstable, need immediate synchronized cardioversion (0.5 J/kg up to 1 J/kg); consult cardiologist; refer to the back of the book for tachycardia with poor perfusion and tachycardia with adequate perfusion algorithms

I. *AV Reentrant:* Presence of accessory bypass pathway, in conjunction with AV node, establishes cyclic pattern of reentry independent of SA node; most common cause of nonsinus tachycardia in children (see Wolff-Parkinson-White syndrome, Table 7.7)

II. *Junctional:* Automatic focus; simultaneous depolarization of atria and ventricles yields invisible P wave or retrograde P wave

Cardiac surgery, idiopathic

Adjust for clinical situation; consult Cardiology

III. *Ectopic atrial tachycardia:* Rapid firing of ectopic focus in atrium

Idiopathic

AV nodal blockade, ablation

NODAL ESCAPE/JUNCTIONAL RHYTHM

Abnormal rhythm driven by AV node impulse, giving normal QRS complex and invisible P wave (buried in preceding QRS or T wave) or retrograde P wave (negative in lead II, positive in aVR); seen in sinus bradycardia

Common after surgery of atria

Often requires no treatment; if rate is slow enough, may require pacemaker

7

aAbnormal rhythm resulting from ectopic focus in atria or AV node, or from accessory conduction pathways. Characterized by different P-wave shape and abnormal P-wave axis. QRS morphology usually normal. See Fig. 7.6.[6]
AV, Atrioventricular; *CHF,* congestive heart failure; *HR,* heart rate; *ICP,* intracranial pressure; *PE,* pulmonary embolism; *SA,* sinoatrial; *SVT,* supraventricular tachycardia.

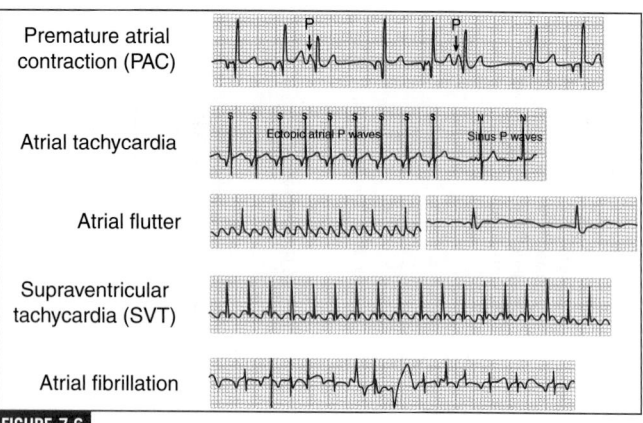

Premature atrial contraction (PAC)	
Atrial tachycardia	
Atrial flutter	
Supraventricular tachycardia (SVT)	
Atrial fibrillation	

FIGURE 7.6

Supraventricular arrhythmias. *P*, Premature atrial contraction. (From Park MK, Guntheroth WG. *How to Read Pediatric ECGs.* 4th ed. Elsevier; 2006:129.)

TABLE 7.5

VENTRICULAR ARRHYTHMIAS

Name/Description	Cause	Treatment
PREMATURE VENTRICULAR CONTRACTION (PVC)		
Ectopic ventricular focus causing early depolarization. Abnormally wide QRS complex appears prematurely, usually with full compensatory pause. May be unifocal or multifocal **Bigeminy:** Alternating normal and abnormal QRS complexes **Trigeminy:** Two normal QRS complexes followed by an abnormal one **Couplet:** Two consecutive PVCs	Myocarditis, myocardial injury, cardiomyopathy, long QT, congenital and acquired heart disease, drugs (catecholamines, theophylline, caffeine, anesthetics), MVP, anxiety, hypokalemia, hypoxia, hypomagnesemia; can be normal variant	None; more worrisome if associated with underlying heart disease or syncope, if worse with activity, or if they are multiform (especially couplets); address underlying cause; rule out structural heart disease
VENTRICULAR TACHYCARDIA		
Series of three or more PVCs at rapid rate (120–250 beats/min), with wide QRS complex and dissociated, retrograde, or no P wave	See causes of PVCs (70% have underlying cause)	Refer to front of book for tachycardia with poor perfusion and tachycardia with adequate perfusion algorithms
VENTRICULAR FIBRILLATION		
Depolarization of ventricles in uncoordinated asynchronous pattern, yielding abnormal QRS complexes of varying size and morphology with irregular, rapid rate; rare in children	Myocarditis, MI, postoperative state, digitalis or quinidine toxicity, catecholamines, severe hypoxia, electrolyte disturbances, long QT	Requires immediate defibrillation; refer to back of book for asystole and pulseless arrest algorithm

MI, Myocardial infarction; *MVP,* mitral valve prolapse.

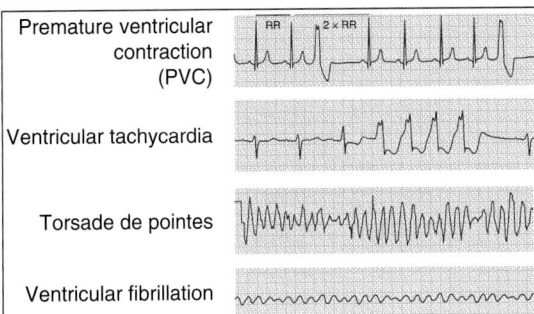

Premature ventricular contraction (PVC)	
Ventricular tachycardia	
Torsade de pointes	
Ventricular fibrillation	

FIGURE 7.7

Ventricular arrhythmias. *RR*, R-R interval. (From Park MK, Guntheroth WG. *How to Read Pediatric ECGs*. 4th ed. Elsevier; 2006:138.)

TABLE 7.6

NONVENTRICULAR CONDUCTION DISTURBANCES

Name/Description[a]	Cause	Treatment
FIRST-DEGREE HEART BLOCK		
Abnormal but asymptomatic delay in conduction through AV node, yielding prolongation of PR interval	Acute rheumatic fever, tickborne (e.g., Lyme) disease, connective tissue disease, congenital heart disease, cardiomyopathy, digitalis toxicity, postoperative state, normal children	No specific treatment except to address the underlying cause
SECOND-DEGREE HEART BLOCK: MOBITZ TYPE I (WENCKEBACH)		
Progressive lengthening of PR interval until a QRS complex is not conducted; common finding in asymptomatic teenagers	Myocarditis, cardiomyopathy, congenital heart disease, postoperative state, MI, toxicity (digitalis, β-blocker), normal children, Lyme disease, lupus	Address underlying cause, or none needed
SECOND-DEGREE HEART BLOCK: MOBITZ TYPE II		
Loss of conduction to ventricle without lengthening of the PR interval; may progress to complete heart block	Same as for Mobitz type I	Address underlying cause; may need pacemaker
THIRD-DEGREE (COMPLETE) HEART BLOCK		
Complete dissociation of atrial and ventricular conduction, with atrial rate faster than ventricular rate; P wave and PP interval regular; RR interval regular and much slower	Congenital due to maternal lupus or other connective tissue disease. Acquired due to same causes as Mobitz type I.	If bradycardic and symptomatic, consider pacing; refer to back of the book for bradycardia algorithm

[a]High-degree AV block: Conduction of atrial impulse at regular intervals, yielding 2:1 block (two atrial impulses for each ventricular response), 3:1 block, etc.

AV, Atrioventricular; *MI,* myocardial infarction.

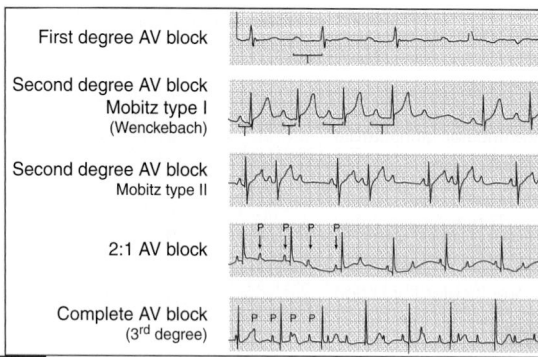

First degree AV block	
Second degree AV block Mobitz type I (Wenckebach)	
Second degree AV block Mobitz type II	
2:1 AV block	
Complete AV block (3rd degree)	

FIGURE 7.8

Conduction blocks. *P*, P wave. (From Park MK, Guntheroth WG. *How to Read Pediatric ECGs.* 4th ed. Elsevier; 2006:141.)

TABLE 7.7

VENTRICULAR CONDUCTION DISTURBANCES

Name/Description	Criteria	Causes/Treatment
RIGHT BUNDLE-BRANCH BLOCK (RBBB)		
Delayed right bundle conduction prolongs RV depolarization time, leading to wide QRS	1. Prolonged or wide QRS with terminal slurred R′ (M-shaped RSR′ or RR′) in V_1, V_2, aVR 2. Wide and slurred S wave in leads I and V_6	ASD, surgery with right ventriculotomy, occasionally seen in normal children
LEFT BUNDLE-BRANCH BLOCK (LBBB)		
Delayed left bundle conduction prolongs septal and LV depolarization time, leading to wide QRS with loss of usual septal signal; there is still a predominance of left ventricle forces; rare in children	1. Wide negative QRS complex in lead V_1 with loss of septal R wave 2. Wide R or RR′ complex in lead V_6 with loss of septal Q wave	Hypertension, ischemic or valvular heart disease, cardiomyopathy
WOLFF-PARKINSON-WHITE (WPW)		
Atrial impulse transmitted via anomalous conduction pathway to ventricles, bypassing AV node and normal ventricular conduction system; leads to early and prolonged depolarization of ventricles; bypass pathway is a predisposing condition for SVT	1. Shortened PR interval 2. Delta wave 3. Wide QRS	Acute management of SVT if necessary, as previously described; consider ablation of accessory pathway if recurrent SVT; all patients need Cardiology referral

ASD, Atrial septal defect; *LV*, left ventricle; *RV*, right ventricle; *SVT*, supraventricular tachycardia.

TABLE 7.8

SYSTEMIC EFFECTS ON ELECTROCARDIOGRAM

	Short QT	Long QT-U	Prolonged QRS	ST-T Changes	Sinus Tachycardia	Sinus Bradycardia	AV Block	Ventricular Tachycardia	Miscellaneous
CHEMISTRY									
Hyperkalemia			X	X			X	X	Low-voltage P waves; peaked T waves
Hypokalemia		X		X					
Hypercalcemia	X					X	X	X	
Hypocalcemia		X			X		X		
Hypermagnesemia							X		
Hypomagnesemia		X							
DRUGS									
Digitalis	X			X		T	X	T	
Phenothiazines		T						T	
Phenytoin	X								
Propranolol	X					X	X		
Tricyclic antidepressants		T	T	T	T		T	T	
Verapamil						X	X		

Continued

TABLE 7.8

SYSTEMIC EFFECTS ON ELECTROCARDIOGRAM—CONT'D

	Short QT	Long QT-U	Prolonged QRS	ST-T Changes	Sinus Tachycardia	Sinus Bradycardia	AV Block	Ventricular Tachycardia	Miscellaneous
MISCELLANEOUS									
CNS injury		X		X	X	X	X		
Friedreich ataxia				X	X			X	Atrial flutter, SVT
Duchenne muscular dystrophy				X	X			X	Atrial flutter, SVT
Myotonic dystrophy			X	X		X	X		SVT
Collagen vascular disease				X			X	X	
Hypothyroidism						X	X		Low voltage
Hyperthyroidism			X	X	X		X		SVT
Lyme disease							X		
Maternal lupus							X		

CNS, Central nervous system; T, present only with drug toxicity; X, present.

Data from Garson A Jr. *The Electrocardiogram in Infants and Children: A Systematic Approach.* Lea & Febiger; 1983:172; and Walsh EP, Alexander ME, Cecchin F. Electrocardiography and introduction to electrophysiologic techniques. In: Keane JF, Lock JE, Fyler DC, eds. *Nadas' Pediatric Cardiology.* Elsevier; 2006:168.

unexplained syncope, seizure, SIDS, or cardiac arrest, with or without prolongation of QTc on ECG at baseline.
d. Treadmill exercise testing and QT prolonging medications may prolong the QTc and may induce arrhythmias.

2. **Complications:** Associated with ventricular arrhythmias (torsades de pointes), syncope, and sudden death

3. **Management:**
   a. Congenital long QT: β-blockers and/or defibrillators and avoidance of QT-prolonging medications; rarely requires cardiac sympathetic denervation or cardiac pacemakers
   b. Acquired long QT: Treatment of arrhythmias, discontinuation of precipitating drugs, and correction of metabolic abnormalities

E. Hyperkalemia

ECG changes dependent on the serum potassium (K^+) level; however, the ECG may be normal with serum K^+ levels between 2.5 and 6 mEq/L

1. **Serum K^+ <2.5 mEq/L:** Depressed ST segment, biphasic T wave, prominent U wave
2. **Serum K^+ >6 mEq/L:** Tall T wave
3. **Serum K^+ >7.5 mEq/L:** Long PR interval, wide QRS, tall T wave
4. **Serum K^+ >9 mEq/L:** Absent P wave, sinusoidal

III. CONGENITAL HEART DISEASE

A. Pulse Oximetry Screening for Critical Congenital Heart Disease

1. **To be done as late as possible but before discharge from nursery, preferably >24 hours of life, due to decreased false-positive rate.** Recommended to use the right hand and one foot, either in parallel or direct sequence
2. **The screening result would be considered positive if:**
   a. Any oxygen saturation measures <90%
   b. Oxygen saturation <95% in both extremities on three measures, each separated by 1 hour
   c. There is a >3% absolute difference in oxygen saturation between the right hand and foot on three measures, each separated by 1 hour

B. Common Syndromes Associated With Cardiac Lesions (Table 7.9)
C. Acyanotic Lesions (Table 7.10)
D. Cyanotic Lesions (Table 7.11)

A hyperoxia test is used to evaluate the etiology of cyanosis in neonates. A baseline arterial blood gas (ABG) with saturation at $FiO_2 = 0.21$ is obtained. Then the infant is placed in an oxygen hood at $FiO_2 = 1$ for a minimum of 10 minutes, and the ABG is repeated. In cardiac disease, there will not be a significant change in PaO_2 following the oxygen challenge test. A PaO_2 of >200 after exposure to FiO_2 of 1.0 is considered normal, and >150 indicates pulmonary rather than cardiac disease. **NOTE:** Pulse oximetry is not useful for following changes in oxygenation once saturation has reached 100% (approximately a PaO_2 of >90 mmHg).[8-17] See eTable 7.1 for interpretation of oxygen challenge test (hyperoxia test). Hyperoxia test is not commonly performed anymore to known adverse effects of hyperoxemia and alkalosis.

TABLE 7.9	
MAJOR SYNDROMES ASSOCIATED WITH CARDIAC DEFECTS	
Syndrome	**Dominant Cardiac Defect**
CHARGE	TOF, truncus arteriosus, aortic arch abnormalities
DiGeorge	Aortic arch anomalies, TOF, truncus arteriosus, VSD, PDA
Trisomy 21	Atrioventricular septal defect, VSD
Marfan	Aortic root dilation, mitral valve prolapse
Loeys-Dietz	Aortic root dilation with higher risk of rupture at smaller dimensions
Noonan	Supravalvular pulmonic stenosis, LVH
Turner	COA, bicuspid aortic valve, aortic root dilation as a teenager
Williams	Supravalvular aortic stenosis, pulmonary artery stenosis
FAS	Occasional: VSD, PDA, ASD, TOF
IDM	TGA, VSD, COA, cardiomyopathy
VATER/VACTERL	VSD
VCFS	Truncus arteriosus, TOF, pulmonary atresia with VSD, TGA, interrupted aortic arch

ASD, Atrial septal defect; *CHARGE*, a syndrome of associated defects including **C**oloboma of the eye, **H**eart anomaly, choanal **A**tresia, **R**estriction of growth and development, and **G**enital and **E**ar anomalies; *COA*, coarctation of aorta; *FAS*, fetal alcohol syndrome; *IDM*, infant of diabetic mother; *LVH*, left ventricular hypertrophy; *PDA*, patent ductus arteriosus; *TGA*, transposition of the great arteries; *TOF*, tetralogy of Fallot; *VATER/VACTERL*, association of **V**ertebral anomalies, **A**nal atresia, **C**ardiac anomalies, **T**racheo**e**sophageal fistula, **R**enal/radial anomalies, **L**imb defects; *VCFS*, velocardiofacial syndrome; *VSD*, ventricular septal defect.

From Park MK. *Pediatric Cardiology for Practitioners*. 5th ed. Elsevier; 2008:10–12.

IV. ACQUIRED HEART DISEASE

A. Myocardial Infarction (MI) in Children (Box 7.4; Fig. 7.9)

B. Endocarditis

1. **Common causative organisms noted in Nationwide Inpatient Sample Database (2000–2010):**

   a. In children with underlying heart disease, viridans streptococci are the most common organisms (33%), with other streptococci making up 17%. *Staphylococcus aureus* is the second most common (28%), with other staphylococcus species making up 7%. Gram-negative bacilli (5%) and polymicrobial infections (11%) make up the remaining cases.

   b. In children without underlying heart disease, *S. aureus* is the most common organism (47%), with other staphylococcus species making up 6%. Viridans streptococci are the second most common (18%), with other streptococci making up 10%. Gram-negative bacilli (8%) and polymicrobial infections (12%) make up the remaining cases.[14]

   c. In neonates and immunocompromised children, fungi and HACEK organisms (*Haemophilus*, *Actinobacillus*, *Cardiobacterium*, *Eikenella*, and *Kingella*) are more common, accounting for 17% to 30% of cases.[15]

TABLE 7.10

ACYANOTIC CONGENITAL HEART DISEASE

Lesion Type	Examination Findings	ECG Findings	Chest Radiograph Findings
Ventricular septal defect (VSD)	2–5/6 holosystolic or early systolic murmur, loudest at the LLSB, ± systolic thrill ± apical diastolic rumble with large shunt With large VSD and pulmonary hypertension, S₂ may be narrow	Small VSD: Normal Medium VSD: LVH ± LAE Large VSD: BVH ± LAE, pure RVH	May show cardiomegaly and increased PVMs, depending on amount of left-to-right shunting
Atrial septal defect (ASD)	Wide, fixed split S₂ with grade 2–3/6 SEM at the LUSB May have mid-diastolic rumble at LLSB	Small ASD: Normal Large ASD: RAD and mild RVH or RBBB with RSR′ in V₁	May show cardiomegaly with increased PVMs if hemodynamically significant ASD
Patent ductus arteriosus (PDA)	40%–60% in VLBW infants 1–4/6 continuous "machinery" murmur loudest at LUSB Wide pulse pressure	Small–moderate PDA: Normal or LVH Large PDA: BVH	May have cardiomegaly and increased PVMs, depending on size of shunt
Atrioventricular septal defects	Most occur in Down syndrome Hyperactive precordium with systolic thrill at LLSB and loud S₁ ± grade 3–4/6 holosystolic regurgitant murmur along LLSB ± systolic murmur of MR at apex ± mid-diastolic rumble at LLSB or at apex ± gallop rhythm	Superior QRS axis RVH and LVH may be present	Cardiomegaly with increased PVMs
Pulmonary stenosis (PS)	Ejection click at LUSB with valvular PS; click intensity varies with respiration, decreasing with inspiration and increasing with expiration S₂ may split widely with P₂ diminished in intensity SEM (2–5/6) ± thrill at LUSB with radiation to back and sides	Mild PS: Normal Moderate PS: RAD and RVH Severe PS: RAE and RVH with strain	Normal heart size with normal to decreased PVMs

Continued

TABLE 7.10

ACYANOTIC CONGENITAL HEART DISEASE—CONT'D

Lesion Type	Examination Findings	ECG Findings	Chest Radiograph Findings
Aortic stenosis (AS)	Systolic thrill at RUSB, suprasternal notch, or over carotids Ejection click that does not vary with respiration if valvular AS. Harsh SEM (2–4/6) at second RICS or third LICS, with radiation to neck and apex ± early diastolic decrescendo murmur due to AR Narrow pulse pressure, if severe stenosis	Mild AS: Normal Moderate–severe AS: LVH ± strain	Usually normal
Coarctation of aorta may present as: 1. Infant in CHF 2. Child with HTN 3. Child with murmur	Male/female ratio of 2:1 2–3/6 SEM at LUSB, radiating to left interscapular area Bicuspid valve is often associated, so may have systolic ejection click at apex and RUSB BP in lower extremities will be lower than in upper extremities Pulse oximetry discrepancy of >5% between upper and lower extremities is also suggestive of coarctation	*In infancy:* RVH or RBBB *In older children:* LVH	Marked cardiomegaly and pulmonary venous congestion Rib notching from collateral circulation usually not seen in children younger than 5 years because collaterals not yet established

AR, Aortic regurgitation; *ASD,* atrial septal defect; *BP,* blood pressure; *BVH,* biventricular hypertrophy; *CDG,* congenital disorders of glycosylation; *CHD,* congenital heart disease; *CHF,* congestive heart failure; *HTN,* hypertension; *LAE,* left atrial enlargement; *LICS,* left intercostal space; *LLSB,* left lower sternal border; *LUSB,* left upper sternal border; *LVH,* left ventricular hypertrophy; *MR,* mitral regurgitation; *PVM,* pulmonary vascular markings; *RAD,* right axis deviation; *RAE,* right atrial enlargement; *RBBB,* right bundle-branch block; *RICS,* right intercostal space; *RUSB,* right upper sternal border; *RVH,* right ventricular hypertrophy; *SEM,* systolic ejection murmur; *VLBW,* very low birth weight (i.e., <1500 g); *VSD,* ventricular septal defect.

TABLE 7.11

CYANOTIC CONGENITAL HEART DISEASE

Lesion	Examination Findings	ECG Findings	Chest Radiograph Findings
Tetralogy of Fallot: 1. Large VSD 2. RVOT obstruction 3. RVH 4. Overriding aorta Degree of RVOT obstruction will determine whether there is clinical cyanosis; if PS is mild, there will be a left-to-right shunt, and child will be acyanotic; increased obstruction leads to increased right-to-left shunting across VSD, and child will be cyanotic	Loud SEM at LMSB and LUSB and a loud, single S_2; ± thrill at LMSB and LLSB *Tet spells*: Occur in young infants; as RVOT obstruction increases or systemic resistance decreases, right-to-left shunting across VSD occurs; may present with tachypnea, increasing cyanosis, and decreasing murmur	RAD and RVH	Boot-shaped heart with normal heart size ± decreased PVMs
Transposition of great arteries	Nonspecific; extreme cyanosis; loud, single S_2; no murmur unless there is associated VSD or PS	RAD and RVH (due to RV acting as systemic ventricle); after 3 days of age, upright T wave in V_1 may be only abnormality	Classic finding: "egg on a string" with cardiomegaly; possible increased PVMs
Tricuspid atresia (absent tricuspid valve and hypoplastic RV and PA; must have ASD, PDA, or VSD to survive)	Single S_2 + grade 2–3/6 systolic regurgitation murmur at LLSB if VSD is present. Occasional PDA murmur	Superior QRS axis; RAE or CAE and LVH	Normal or slightly enlarged heart size; may have boot-shaped heart

Continued

TABLE 7.11

CYANOTIC CONGENITAL HEART DISEASE—CONT'D

Lesion	Examination Findings	ECG Findings	Chest Radiograph Findings
Total anomalous pulmonary venous return: Instead of draining into LA, pulmonary veins drain into the following locations (must have ASD or PFO for survival): *Supracardiac (most common):* SVC *Cardiac:* Coronary sinus or RA *Subdiaphragmatic:* IVC, portal vein, ductus venosus, or hepatic vein *Mixed type*	Hyperactive RV impulse, quadruple rhythm, S_2 fixed and widely split, 2–3/6 SEM at LUSB, and mid-diastolic rumble at LLSB	RAD, RVH (RSR′ in V_1); may see RAE	Cardiomegaly and increased PVMs; classic finding is "snowman in a snowstorm," but this is rarely seen until after age 4 months
OTHER			
Cyanotic CHDs that each occur at a frequency of <1% include pulmonary atresia, Ebstein anomaly, truncus arteriosus, single ventricle, and double outlet right ventricle			

ASD, Atrial septal defect; *CAE,* common atrial enlargement; *CHDs,* congenital heart diseases; *ECG,* electrocardiogram; *IVC,* inferior vena cava; *LA,* left atrium; *LLSB,* left lower sternal border; *LMSB,* left midsternal border; *LUSB,* left upper sternal border; *LVH,* left ventricular hypertrophy; *PA,* pulmonary artery; *PDA,* patent ductus arteriosus; *PFO,* patent foramen ovale; *PVM,* pulmonary vascular markings; *PS,* pulmonary stenosis; *RA,* right atrium; *RAD,* right-axis deviation; *RAE,* right atrial enlargement; *RV,* right ventricle; *RVH,* right ventricular hypertrophy; *RVOT,* right ventricular outflow tract; *SEM,* systolic ejection murmur; *SVC,* superior vena cava; *VSD,* ventricular septal defect.

BOX 7.4

MYOCARDIAL INFARCTION IN CHILDREN[18,19]

Etiologies	Diagnosis
Anomalous origin of coronary artery	**ECG findings[20,21]:** See Fig. 7.9.
Kawasaki disease	**History and Exam:** See Fig. 7.13.
Congenital heart disease	**Biomarkers**
Dilated cardiomyopathy	Troponin I, CK-MB nonspecific for ischemic injury in children
Severe hypertension	
SLE	
Myocarditis	
Drug ingestion (cocaine, adrenergic drugs)	

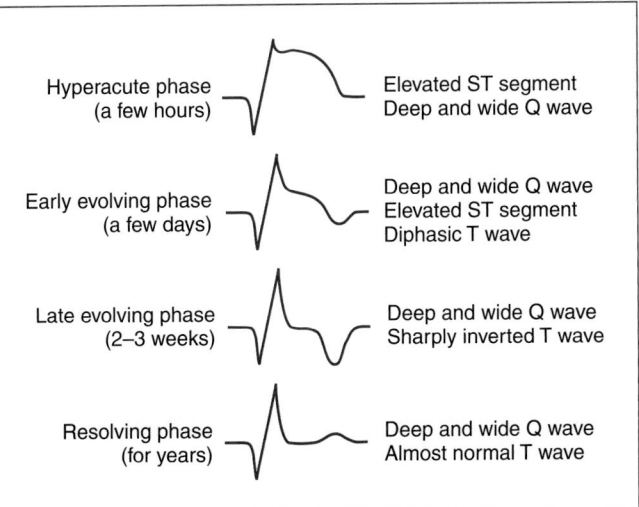

Hyperacute phase (a few hours)	Elevated ST segment Deep and wide Q wave
Early evolving phase (a few days)	Deep and wide Q wave Elevated ST segment Diphasic T wave
Late evolving phase (2–3 weeks)	Deep and wide Q wave Sharply inverted T wave
Resolving phase (for years)	Deep and wide Q wave Almost normal T wave

FIGURE 7.9

Sequential changes during myocardial infarction. (From Park MK, Guntheroth WG. *How to Read Pediatric ECGs.* 4th ed. Elsevier; 2006:115.)

2. **Presentation:** Heart murmur, recurrent fever, splenomegaly, petechiae, fatigue, Osler nodes (tender nodules at the fingertips), Janeway lesions (painless hemorrhagic areas on the palms or soles), splinter hemorrhages, Roth spots (retinal hemorrhages)

3. **Diagnosis**—Duke criteria:
   a. Pathologic criteria:
      (1) Direct evidence of endocarditis based upon histologic findings
      (2) Gram stain positive or cultures of specimens
   b. Clinical criteria: 1 major criterion and 1 minor OR 3 minor criteria:
      (1) Major: Persistently positive blood cultures (2 sets 12 hours apart), positive echocardiogram for vegetations, new regurgitant murmur, single positive blood culture for *Coxiella burnetii*
      (2) Minor: Fever, predisposing valvular condition (prosthetic heart valve, valve lesion OR intravenous drug user [IVDU]), vascular phenomenon (e.g., emboli), immunologic phenomenon (e.g., Roth spots, Osler nodes), positive blood cultures that do not meet major criteria
4. Management: Daily blood cultures while febrile; support heart failure symptoms with diuretics, digoxin, etc.

C. Bacterial Endocarditis Prophylaxis

See Box 7.5 for cardiac conditions that meet criteria for prophylaxis.[16]

1. **All dental procedures** that involve treatment of gingival tissue, the periapical region of the teeth, or oral mucosal perforation
2. **Invasive procedures** that involve incision or biopsy of respiratory mucosa, such as tonsillectomy and adenoidectomy
3. **Not recommended** for genitourinary or gastrointestinal tract procedures; solely for bacterial endocarditis prevention
4. **Treatment:** Amoxicillin is preferred PO; ampicillin if unable to take PO; cephalexin if allergic to penicillins[16]

D. Myocardial Disease

1. **Dilated cardiomyopathy:** End result of myocardial damage leading to atrial and ventricular dilation with decreased systolic contractile function of the ventricles
   a. Treatment: Management of congestive heart failure (CHF) (digoxin, diuretics, vasodilation, angiotensin-converting enzyme [ACE] inhibitors)
   b. Anticoagulants should be considered to decrease the risk of thrombus formation. Cardiac transplant may eventually be required.

BOX 7.5

CARDIAC CONDITIONS FOR WHICH ANTIBIOTIC PROPHYLAXIS IS RECOMMENDED

- Prosthetic cardiac valve
- Previous bacterial endocarditis
- Congenital heart disease (CHD)—Limited to the following conditions:
  - Unrepaired cyanotic defect, including palliative shunts and conduits
  - Completely repaired CHD with prosthetic material/device (placed by surgery or catheterization), during first 6 months after procedure
  - Repaired CHD with residual defects at or adjacent to the site of prosthetic patch or device (which inhibits endothelialization)
  - Cardiac transplantation patients who develop cardiac valvulopathy

---

Data from Wilson W, Taubert KA, Gewitz M, et al. Prevention of infective endocarditis: Guidelines from the American Heart Association: A guideline from the American Heart Association Rheumatic Fever, Endocarditis, and Kawasaki Disease Committee, Council on Cardiovascular Disease in the Young, and the Council on Clinical Cardiology, Council on Cardiovascular Surgery and Anesthesia, and the Quality of Care and Outcomes Research Interdisciplinary Working Group. *Circulation.* 2007;116(15):1736–1754.

2. **Hypertrophic obstructive cardiomyopathy (HOCM):** Abnormality of myocardial cells leading to significant ventricular hypertrophy (usually left ventricle) with small to normal ventricular dimensions. Increased contractile function, impaired filling secondary to stiff ventricles. Most common type is asymmetrical septal hypertrophy with (HOCM) or without left ventricular outflow obstruction. There is a 4% to 6% incidence of sudden death in children and adolescents.

   a. Treatment: Moderate restriction of physical activity, negative inotropes (β-blocker, calcium channel blocker) to help improve filling, and maintenance of adequate hydration. If at increased risk for sudden death, may consider implantable defibrillator. If symptomatic with subaortic obstruction, may benefit from myectomy

   b. Additional management: HOCM is a preload-dependent lesion; therefore patient may benefit from higher rates of fluid administration. Avoid inotropes, tachycardia, and afterload reduction.

3. **Restrictive cardiomyopathy:** Myocardial or endocardial disease (usually infiltrative or fibrotic) resulting in stiff ventricular walls with restriction of diastolic filling but normal contractile function. Results in atrial enlargement. Associated with a high mortality rate. Very rare in children. Treatment is supportive with diuretics, anticoagulants, calcium channel blockers, a pacemaker for heart block, and cardiac transplantation, if severe.

4. **Myocarditis:** Inflammation of myocardial tissue
   a. Etiology:
      (1) Infectious: Viral (coxsackie virus, echovirus, adenovirus), bacterial, rickettsial, fungal, parasitic
      (2) Other: Immune-mediated disease (Kawasaki disease, acute rheumatic fever), collagen vascular disease, toxin-induced
   b. Presentation: Symptoms can be nonspecific, including fatigue, shortness of breath, emesis. Exam includes signs of CHF, soft systolic murmur, arrhythmia.
   c. Testing:
      (1) Imaging: ECG: Low QRS voltages throughout (<5 mm), ST-segment and T-wave changes (e.g., decreased T-wave amplitude), prolongation of QT interval, arrhythmias (especially premature contractions, first- or second-degree AV block); echo shows enlarged chambers and impaired LV function
      (2) Labs: CK, troponin
   d. Treatment: Bed rest, diuretics, inotropes (dopamine, dobutamine, milrinone), digoxin, gamma globulin, ACE inhibitors, possibly steroids
   e. May require ventricular assist device and/or heart transplantation (~20% to 25% of cases)

E. Pericardial Disease

1. **Pericarditis:** Inflammation of visceral and parietal layers of pericardium. It is often self-limited.
   a. Presentation: Chest pain (often pleuritic in nature), fever, tachycardia, distant heart sounds, friction rub
   b. EKG: Diffuse ST-segment elevation in almost all leads (representing inflammation of adjacent myocardium); PR-segment depression

    c. Treatment: Address underlying condition and provide symptomatic treatment with rest, analgesia, and antiinflammatory drugs

2. **Pericardial effusion:** Accumulation of excess fluid in pericardial sac
   a. Etiology: Acute pericarditis, serous effusion from increased hydrostatic pressure (CHF), decreased plasma oncotic pressure, increased capillary permeability
   b. Presentation: Can be asymptomatic, chest or abdominal pain, muffled heart sounds, dullness to percussion, vital sign instability from cardiac compression (e.g., hypotension)
   c. EKG: Decreased QRS voltage, electrical alternans
   d. Treatment: Address underlying condition. Observe if asymptomatic; use pericardiocentesis if there is sudden increase in volume or hemodynamic compromise. Nonsteroidal antiinflammatory drugs (NSAIDs) or steroids may be of benefit, depending on etiology.

3. **Cardiac tamponade:** Accumulation of pericardial fluid under high pressure causing compression of cardiac chambers, limiting filling, and decreasing stroke volume and cardiac output
   a. Etiology: Same as pericardial effusion
   b. Presentation: Dyspnea, fatigue, signs of CHF (jugular venous distension, hepatomegaly, edema, tachypnea/rales), pulsus paradoxus
   c. EKG: Same as pericardial effusion
   d. Echocardiogram: RV collapse in early diastole, RA/LA collapse in end diastole and early systole
   e. Treatment is pericardiocentesis with temporary catheter left in place if necessary; pericardial window or stripping, if it is a recurrent condition

F. Kawasaki Disease[17]

Acute febrile vasculitis of unknown etiology, which is common in children aged <8 years and is the leading cause of acquired childhood heart disease (in the form of coronary artery dilation/aneurysm) in developed countries

1. **Etiology:** Unknown; thought to be immune regulated in response to infectious agents or environmental toxins

2. **Diagnosis:**
   a. Complete/typical Kawasaki disease (KD): Based on clinical criteria. These include high fever lasting 5 days or more, plus at least four of the following five criteria below. If at least four of the below criteria are present, the diagnosis of KD can be made with 4 days of fever.
      (1) Bilateral, painless, bulbar, limbic-sparing conjunctival injection without exudate
      (2) Erythematous mouth and pharynx, strawberry tongue, or red, cracked lips
      (3) Polymorphous exanthem (may be morbilliform, maculopapular, or scarlatiniform)
      (4) Swelling of hands and feet with erythema of palms and soles
      (5) Cervical lymphadenopathy (>1.5 cm in diameter), usually single and unilateral
   b. Incomplete/atypical Kawasaki disease: A suspicion of KD with fewer than four of the diagnostic criteria present. Laboratory criteria and echocardiogram are assessed to support the diagnosis. There is no

difference in the risk of developing coronary artery lesions between complete KD and incomplete KD.[22]

(1) More often seen in infants. Incomplete KD should be considered in any infant <6 months with fever of 7 days or greater duration with or without clinical criteria, and in patients of any age with unexplained fever of 5 or more days with two or three clinical criteria of KD. Baseline echocardiogram should be strongly considered for any infant <6 months with fever of 7 days or greater duration, even in the absence of clinical or laboratory criteria.

(2) See Fig. 7.10 for evaluation of incomplete Kawasaki disease.

(3) Supplemental laboratory criteria: Albumin ≤3.0 g/dL, anemia for age, elevation of alanine aminotransferase, platelets after 7 days ≥450,000/mm^3, white blood cell count ≥15,000/mm^3, and urine white blood cells/hpf ≥10 (non-catheterized specimen)

3. **Other clinical findings:** Often associated with extreme irritability, abdominal pain, diarrhea, vomiting. Also seen are arthritis and arthralgia, hepatic enlargement, jaundice, acute acalculous distention of the gallbladder, carditis

4. **Laboratory findings:** Leukocytosis with left shift, neutrophils with vacuoles or toxic granules, elevated C-reactive protein (CRP) or erythrocyte sedimentation rate (ESR) (seen acutely), thrombocytosis, normocytic and normochromic anemia, sterile pyuria (33%), increased transaminases (40%), hyperbilirubinemia (10%)

5. **Subacute phase (11 to 25 days after onset of illness):** Resolution of fever, rash, and lymphadenopathy. Often, desquamation of the fingertips or toes and thrombocytosis occur. Cardiovascular complications: If untreated, 20% to 25% develop coronary artery aneurysms and dilation in subacute phase (peak prevalence occurs about 2 to 4 weeks after onset of disease; rarely appears after 6 weeks) and are at risk for coronary thrombosis acutely and coronary stenosis chronically. Carditis; aortic, mitral, and tricuspid regurgitation; pericardial effusion; CHF; MI; left ventricular dysfunction; and ECG changes may also occur.

6. **Convalescent phase:** ESR, CRP, and platelet count return to normal. Those with coronary artery abnormalities are at increased risk for MI, arrhythmias, and sudden death.

7. **Management** (see also eTable 7.2)[17]

a. Intravenous immunoglobulin (IVIG)

(1) Shown to reduce incidence of coronary artery dilation to <3% and decrease duration of fever, if given in the first 10 days of illness. Current recommended regimen is a single dose of IVIG, 2 g/kg over 10 to 12 hours.[17]

(2) Can be given to children after 10th day of fever if ESR or CRP elevated with persistent fever

(3) Approximately 10% of patients treated with IVIG fail to respond (persistent or recurrent fever ≥36 hours after IVIG completion). Re-treat with second dose.[17]

b. Aspirin is recommended for both its antiinflammatory and antiplatelet effects. In the United States, high-dose aspirin (80 to 100 mg/kg/day divided in four doses) is recommended until 48 to 72 hours after

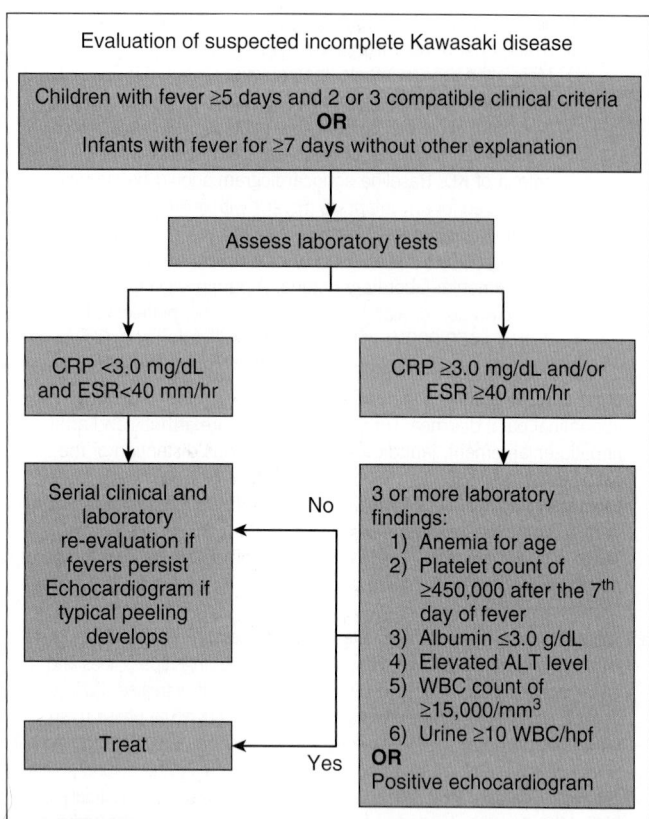

FIGURE 7.10

Evaluation of incomplete Kawasaki disease. (From Diagnosis, treatment, and long-term management of Kawasaki disease: a scientific statement for health professionals from the American Heart Association. *Circulation* 2017; Mar 29.)

defervescence. Some centers use moderate-dose aspirin (30 to 50 mg/kg/day), as there is no evidence to suggest either dosing is superior, and because of the increased potential for adverse effects with the higher dosing. This is given in addition to IVIG. Low-dose aspirin (3 to 5 mg/kg/day as a single daily dose) is continued for 6 to 8 weeks or until platelet count and ESR are normal (if there are no coronary artery abnormalities). Aspirin may be continued indefinitely, if coronary artery abnormalities persist. Concomitant use of ibuprofen antagonizes the antiplatelet effect of aspirin and, as such, should be avoided in patients with coronary artery aneurysms taking aspirin for its platelet-inhibiting effects.[17]

c. High-dose pulse glucocorticoids (usually intravenous methylprednisolone) or infliximab are sometimes used for IVIG-resistant patients.[17]

   d. Follow-up: Serial echocardiography is recommended to assess coronary arteries and left ventricular function (at time of diagnosis, at 2 weeks, at 6 to 8 weeks, and at 12 months [optional]). More frequent intervals and long-term follow-up are recommended if abnormalities are seen on echocardiography. A higher baseline z-score of the coronary arteries on echocardiogram is strongly associated with worse cardiac outcomes.[17] Cardiac catheterization may be necessary.

   e. Follow up with a pediatric cardiologist depending on presence of coronary aneurysms and z-score of aneurysm (see eTable 7.2).

G. Multisystem Inflammatory Syndrome in Children

Please see Chapter 27 for a full discussion of multisystem inflammatory syndrome in children (MIS-C). The cardiac monitoring for MIS-C is discussed here. Cardiac dysfunction is a principal concern in the management of MIS-C. In various case series, the reported incidence of cardiac dysfunction in patients with MIS-C has ranged from 35% to 100%.[23] As there are still relatively few data for MIS-C and practice varies from center to center, these are general principles surrounding the cardiac monitoring for patients with suspected MIS-C.

1. **Lab monitoring:** B-type natriuretic peptide and troponin levels should be obtained at baseline, and if elevated, should be monitored serially and as clinically indicated.

2. **ECG:** At minimum, a baseline 12-lead ECG is indicated in patients with suspected MIS-C, and serial ECGs every 1–2 days is suggested. Should there be concern for significant abnormality, namely AV block (in two studies, first-degree AV block occurred in approximately 20% of hospitalized patients with MIS-C[24,25]), telemetry should be considered. Similarly, if there is any concern for hemodynamic instability, continuous cardiac monitoring should be strongly considered.

3. **Echocardiography:** All patients with suspected MIS-C should have a baseline echocardiogram to assess for ventricular function, valvar function, coronary artery dimensions, presence of effusion, or other abnormalities. Timing of repeat echocardiogram will depend on the presence and degree of abnormality noted on baseline echocardiogram. Typically, if the baseline echocardiogram is abnormal, echocardiogram will be repeated while inpatient as clinically indicated. Namely, if there are coronary artery changes, current recommendations are to repeat an echocardiogram every 2 to 3 days until the size is stable, then determine frequency based upon the Kawasaki disease guidelines. If the baseline echocardiogram is within normal limits, a repeat can be done in 1 to 2 weeks and can be done outpatient.

4. **Outpatient follow-up:** Current expert opinion frameworks based on initial data and Kawasaki disease guidelines recommend outpatient follow-up for at least one year after the acute episode of illness with an echocardiogram and ECG at all appointments. Cardiac enzymes should be repeated if not normalized at discharge. If arrhythmia or AV block is noted at any point, a Holter monitor should be considered. Recommendations also depend upon the presence or absence of ventricular dysfunction of coronary artery change, as these factors may warrant more frequent follow-up. Proposed timing of these follow-up evaluations are as follows:

BOX 7.6

GUIDELINES FOR DIAGNOSIS OF INITIAL ATTACK OF RHEUMATIC FEVER (JONES CRITERIA)

Major Manifestations	Minor Manifestations
Carditis	Clinical findings:
Polyarthritis	Arthralgia
Chorea	Fever
Erythema marginatum	Laboratory findings:
Subcutaneous nodules	Elevated acute-phase reactants (erythrocyte
	sedimentation rate, C-reactive protein)
	Prolonged PR interval

Plus Supporting Evidence of Antecedent Group A Streptococcal Infection

- Positive throat culture or rapid streptococcal antigen test
- Elevated or rising streptococcal antibody titer

NOTE: If supported by evidence of preceding group A streptococcal infection, the presence of two major manifestations or of one major and two minor manifestations indicates a high probability of acute rheumatic fever.

---

    a. 1–2 weeks

    b. 4–6 weeks

    c. A cardiac MRI can be considered at the 3-month follow-up if there is a history of ventricular dysfunction or significantly elevated cardiac enzymes.

    d. 9–12 months[23,24]

5. **Activity restriction:** Current practice for activity restriction following MIS-C is based upon guidelines for return to sport participation following acute myocarditis. In those guidelines, restriction for 3 to 6 months following diagnosis is recommended due to myocardial involvement. Additionally, subsequent preparticipation screening may be prudent to ensure the safety of return to athletic activity.[23]

H. Rheumatic Heart Disease

1. **Etiology:** Believed to be an immunologically mediated, delayed sequela of group A streptococcal pharyngitis

2. **Clinical findings:** History of streptococcal pharyngitis 1 to 5 weeks before onset of symptoms. Often with pallor, malaise, easy fatigability

3. **Diagnosis:** Jones criteria (Box 7.6)

4. **Management:** Penicillin, bed rest, salicylates, supportive management of CHF (if present) with diuretics, digoxin, morphine

V. IMAGING

A. Chest Radiograph (Fig. 7.11)

B. Echocardiography (eTable 7.3)

VI. PROCEDURES

A. Cardiac Surgery (Fig. 7.12, Table 7.12)

B. Cardiac Catheterization[9,10] (Table 7.13)

1. Relatively common complications to be aware of: Arrhythmias (SVT, AV block, bradycardia, etc.), vascular complications (thrombosis, decreased/absent pulses), intervention-related (balloon rupture, etc.), bleeding

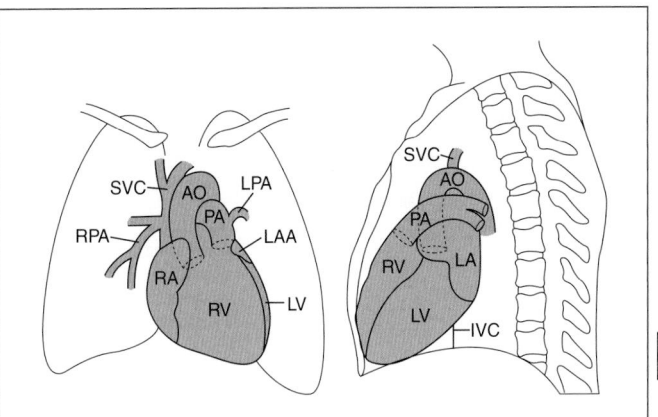

FIGURE 7.11

Radiological contours of the heart. *AO*, Aorta; *IVC*, inferior vena cava; *LA*, left atrium; *LAA*, left atrial appendage; *LPA*, left pulmonary artery; *LV*, left ventricle; *PA*, pulmonary artery; *RA*, right atrium; *RPA*, right pulmonary artery; *RV*, right ventricle; *SVC*, superior vena cava.

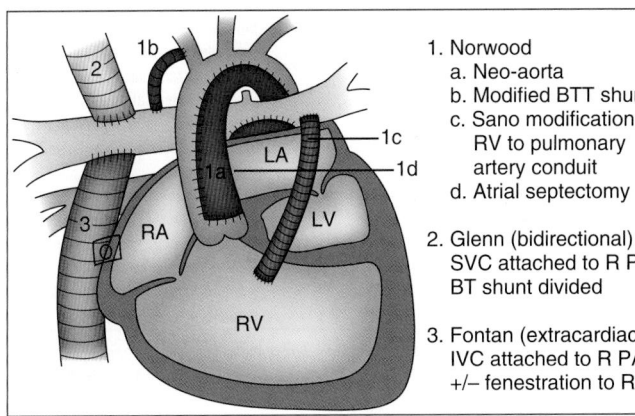

1. Norwood
   a. Neo-aorta
   b. Modified BTT shunt
   c. Sano modification – RV to pulmonary artery conduit
   d. Atrial septectomy

2. Glenn (bidirectional) SVC attached to R PA BT shunt divided

3. Fontan (extracardiac) IVC attached to R PA +/− fenestration to RA

FIGURE 7.12

Schematic diagram of cardiac shunts, including the modified Blalock-Taussig-Thomas *(BTT)*, Sano modification, bidirectional Glenn, and Fontan shunts.

2. Other less common complications: Myocardial/vessel staining, cardiac perforation, cardiac tamponade, air embolus, infection, allergic reaction, cardiac arrest, and death

TABLE 7.12

CARDIAC SURGERIES[30]

Intervention	Indication	Procedure
Palliative systemic-to-pulmonary artery shunts (e.g., Blalock-Taussig-Thomas shunt)	Lesions with impaired pulmonary perfusion (TOF, HLHS, tricuspid atresia, pulmonary atresia)	Shunt created to increase pulmonary blood flow
Norwood procedure, stage 1 (neonatal period)	HLHS	MPA anastomosis to aorta with arch reconstruction Modified BTTS or Sano performed to provide pulmonary blood flow ASD created for decompression of left atrium Expected oxygen saturation 75%–85%
Bidirectional Glenn shunt or hemi-Fontan (3–6 months)	HLHS Intermediate step between Norwood 1 and Fontan	Bidirectional Glenn shunt or hemi-Fontan to reduce volume overload of single right ventricle Expected oxygen saturation 80%–85%
Fontan procedure	Functionally single ventricle (tricuspid atresia, HLHS)	Anastomosis of right atria and/or IVC to pulmonary arteries, separates systemic and pulmonary circulations Expected oxygen saturation >92%
Modified Fontan	Single ventricle	Completely separates systemic and pulmonary circulations Expected oxygen saturations >92%
Arterial switch	TGA	Connects aorta to LV and PA to RV, reconnects coronary arteries to aorta Normal oxygen saturations
Ross procedure ("switch procedure")	Aortic stenosis	Pulmonary valve used to replace diseased aortic valve, pulmonary valve replaced by homograft, avoids long-term anticoagulation Normal oxygen saturations

ASD, Atrial septal defect; *BTTS*, Blalock-Taussig-Thomas shunt; *HLHS*, hypoplastic left heart syndrome; *LV*, left ventricle; *MPA*, main pulmonary artery; *PA*, pulmonary artery; *RV*, right ventricle; *TAPVR*, total anomalous pulmonary venous return; *TGA*, transposition of great arteries; *TOF*, tetralogy of Fallot.

VII. COMMON CARDIAC COMPLAINTS

A. Nontraumatic Chest Pain[18]

1. **Etiologies**
   a. Life-threatening causes
      (1) Cardiac: Congenital heart disease (CHD) with left ventricular outflow tract obstruction, coronary artery abnormality, pericarditis, myocarditis, dilated cardiomyopathy, aortic root dissection; cardiac etiologies are rare in children (prevalence <6%)[26]

TABLE 7.13

CARDIAC CATHETERIZATION

Intervention	Indication	Procedure
Diagnostic catheter	Pre- or postcardiac procedure, monitoring progression of disease severity	Measurement of flow and pressures within different parts of the heart and large vessels
Patent ductus arteriosus (PDA) stent	Duct-dependent cyanotic lesions	Stent placed within PDA to allow mixing of blood between aorta and pulmonary artery
Balloon atrial septostomy	Common: TGA, HLHS with restrictive atrial septum Less common: tricuspid/mitral/aortic/pulmonary atresia, TAPVR	Opening between left and right atria created to allow mixing of blood between systemic and pulmonary systems
Device closure of ASD	ASD	Placement of device within atrial septal defect to close connection between right and left atria
Balloon valvuloplasty	Common: aortic or pulmonary valve stenosis	Inflation of balloon within valve to enlarge opening to reduce narrowing
Transcatheter valve replacement	Aortic/pulmonary/mitral/tricuspid valve stenosis or regurgitation	Placement of new valve within old valve to replace functionality to either improve stenosis or regurgitation
Catheter ablation	Certain arrhythmias, including pre-excitation, atrial ectopic tachycardia	Utilization of energy to scar tissue to limit production of ectopic beats or aberrant pathways

ASD, Atrial septal defect; *BTTS*, Blalock-Taussig-Thomas shunt; *HLHS*, hypoplastic left heart syndrome; *LV*, left ventricle; *MPA*, main pulmonary artery; *PA*, pulmonary artery; *RV*, right ventricle; *TAPVR*, total anomalous pulmonary venous return; *TGA*, transposition of great arteries; *TOF*, tetralogy of Fallot.

    (2) Noncardiac: Pneumothorax, pulmonary embolism, pulmonary HTN, acute chest syndrome
  b. Common, noncardiac causes (94% to 99% patients): Musculoskeletal (costochondritis), respiratory (asthma, pneumonia, pleuritic), gastrointestinal (gastroesophageal reflux disease [GERD]), psychiatric (panic attack, hyperventilation syndrome)
2. **When to consider referral to cardiologist:** Symptoms that suggest cardiac etiology (palpitations, syncope with exertion, and decreased exercise tolerance), ECG changes, new murmur

B. Syncope[19]

1. **Etiologies**
  a. Cardiac etiologies:
    (1) Electrical disturbances: Long QT syndrome, Brugada syndrome, congenital short QT syndrome, catecholaminergic polymorphic ventricular tachycardia
    (2) Structural heart disease: Hypertrophic cardiomyopathy, coronary artery anomalies, valvular aortic stenosis, dilated cardiomyopathy, acute myocarditis, pulmonary HTN
  b. Noncardiac etiologies[19]:

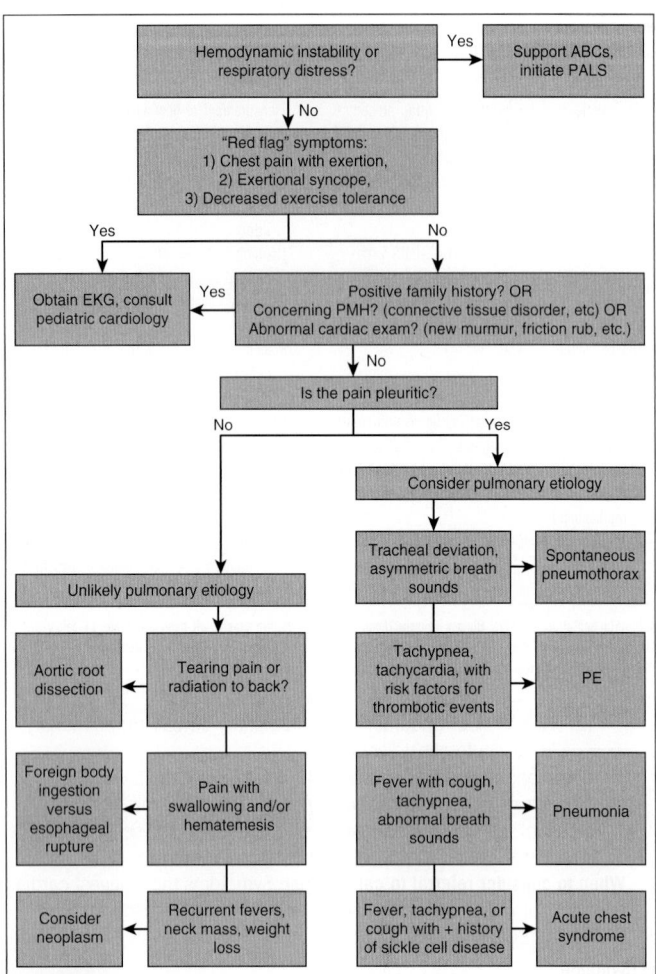

FIGURE 7.13

Algorithm for the evaluation of nontraumatic chest pain. *ABCs,* Airway, breathing, and circulation; *EKG,* electrocardiogram; *PALS,* pediatric advanced life support; *PE,* pulmonary embolism; *PMH,* past medical history.

(1) Common: Vasovagal syncope (50% pediatric syncope), breath-holding spells, orthostatic hypotension
(2) Life-threatening: Heat illness/stroke, anaphylaxis, toxic ingestion, hypoglycemia

2. **When to consider referral to cardiologist:**
   a. History: Congenital/acquired heart disease, syncope with exertion, associated chest pain or palpitations
   b. Family history: Early sudden cardiac death, arrhythmia, cardiomyopathy
   c. Evaluation: Abnormal cardiac exam or abnormal ECG

VIII. EXERCISE RECOMMENDATIONS FOR PATIENTS WITH CONGENITAL HEART DISEASE

See eTable 7.4 for exercise recommendations for patients with CHD.[27]

IX. LIPID MONITORING RECOMMENDATIONS

A. Screening of Children and Adolescents[28]

1. **Universal screening:** Children 9 to 11 years old (prior to onset of puberty) and at 17 to 21 years
2. **Targeted screening:** 2 to 8 years old and 12 to 16 years old with risk factors:
   a. Moderate or high-risk medical condition: History of prematurity, very low birth weight, CHD (repaired or unrepaired), recurrent urinary tract infections, renal or urologic malformations, family history of congenital renal disease, solid organ transplant, malignancy or bone marrow transplant, treatment with drugs known to raise BP, other systemic illness associated with HTN (e.g., neurofibromatosis, tuberous sclerosis), evidence of elevated intracranial pressure
   b. Other cardiovascular risk factors, including diabetes, HTN, body mass index ≥95th percentile, cigarette use
   c. Family history of early cardiovascular disease (CVD) or severe hypercholesterolemia:
      (1) Parent or grandparent who at <55 years old (males) or <65 years old (females) suffered an MI or sudden death, underwent a coronary artery procedure, or who had evidence of coronary atherosclerosis, peripheral vascular disease, or cerebrovascular disease.
      (2) Parent with total cholesterol ≥240 mg/dL or known dyslipidemia

B. Goals for Lipid Levels in Childhood[28]

1. **Total cholesterol**
   a. Acceptable (<170 mg/dL): No additional testing.
   b. Borderline (170 to 199 mg/dL): Dietary or other lifestyle modifications. Could repeat testing in 1 year.
   c. High (≥200 mg/dL): Repeat and average values. If persistently ≥200, obtain lipoprotein analysis. Could consider pharmacotherapy.
2. **Low-density lipoprotein (LDL) cholesterol**
   a. Acceptable (<110 mg/dL)
   b. Borderline (110 to 129 mg/dL)
   c. High (≥130 mg/dL)

X. CARDIOVASCULAR SCREENING

A. Sports[29,30]

There is no established or mandated preparticipation sports screening. There is a recommended history and physical examination screening from the AHA.[29] Routine ECGs are not required unless there is suspicion of underlying cardiac disease (see eBox 7.1).

B. Attention–Deficit/Hyperactivity Disorder (ADHD)[31]

1. Obtain a good patient and family history as well as physical examination.
2. There is no increased risk of sudden cardiac death in children without cardiac disease taking ADHD medications. There is no consensus on universal ECG screening. ECGs should be obtained in those who screen with positive answers on history, in cases of polypharmacy, in those with tachycardia while on medications, and in those with a history of significant cardiac disease. If a patient has significant heart disease or concern for cardiac disease, have patient evaluated by a pediatric cardiologist.

XI. WEB RESOURCES

- Cove Point Foundation: Congenital Heart Disease: http://www.pted.org
- MurmurQuiz: https://murmurquiz.org

REFERENCES

A complete list of references can be found online.

Chapter 8

Dermatology

Allison Haley, MD and Katherine Cummings, MD

⊗ See additional content online.

I. EVALUATION AND CLINICAL DESCRIPTIONS OF SKIN FINDINGS

A. Primary Skin Lesions

1. **Macule:** Small, flat, well-circumscribed discolored lesion (<1 cm)
2. **Patch:** Large macule (≥1 cm)
3. **Papule:** Small, elevated, firm, well-circumscribed superficial lesion (<1 cm)
4. **Plaque:** Large papule (≥1 cm)
5. **Pustule:** Small, well-circumscribed elevation of skin containing purulent material (<1 cm)
6. **Vesicle:** Small, well-circumscribed elevation of skin containing serous fluid (<1 cm)
7. **Bulla:** Large vesicle (≥1 cm)
8. **Wheal:** Transient, raised, well-circumscribed lesion with erythematous periphery and central pallor
9. **Nodule:** Soft or firm lesion in dermis or subcutaneous fat (≥1 cm)
10. **Tumor/mass:** Solid, firm lesion (typically ≥2 cm)

B. Secondary Skin Lesions

1. **Scale:** Small, thin plates (scales) shedding from the surface of the skin
2. **Crust:** Solidified exudative material from erosions or ruptured vesicles/pustules
3. **Erosion:** Loss of the most superficial layers of the epidermis from friction, pressure, or inflammation that heals without scarring
4. **Ulcer:** Full-thickness loss of the epidermis and at least a part of the dermis, with clearly defined edges, that heals with scarring
5. **Fissure:** Linear or wedge-shaped epidermal tear that reaches into the dermis and may be associated with inflammation and pain
6. **Excoriation:** Any loss of substance of the skin secondary to scratching
7. **Lichenification:** Thickening of the epidermis with accentuated skin lines, secondary to chronic inflammation and/or scratching
8. **Scar:** Formation of new connective tissue after full-thickness injury to skin, leaving permanent change in skin

C. Shapes and Arrangements

1. **Linear:** Distributed along a line
2. **Dermatomal:** Following a dermatome
3. **Filiform:** Thread-like

4. **Serpiginous:** Wavy, coiled, serpentine pattern
5. **Annular:** Ring-like configuration
6. **Nummular/discoid:** Disk-like, coin-shaped lesion
7. **Targetoid:** Resembling a bull's-eye target with central erythema surrounded by pale edema with a peripheral border of erythema
8. **Clustered:** Lesions in a group
9. **Herpetiform:** Clustered vesicular lesions on erythematous bases (herpes simplex pattern)
10. **Reticulated:** Net or lacey distribution
11. **Geographic:** Resembling outlines on a map such as a continent
12. **Morbilliform:** Eruption of erythematous to dusky coalescing macules with interspersed healthy skin

II. VASCULAR ANOMALIES[1]

A. Vascular Tumors

1. Infantile hemangiomas (Fig. 8.1, Color Plates)[2,3]
    a. **Pathogenesis:** Benign vascular tumor with rapid proliferation followed by spontaneous involution. Most present before 4 weeks of age. Undergo rapid growth between 1 and 2 months of age, with 80% of size reached by 3 months. Most begin to regress between 6 and 12 months of age, with the majority of tumor regression occurring by 4 years of age. 50% to 70% resolve completely.
    b. **Clinical presentation:** Newborns may demonstrate pale macules with overlying or surrounding, thread-like telangiectasias that later develop into hemangiomas. May be superficial, deep, or mixed. Pattern may be focal (neat round lesions) or segmental (following embryologic segments). After involution, can have residual skin changes including scarring and atrophy
    c. Indicators that should prompt consideration for early treatment:
        (1) Potential for life-threatening complications: Airway hemangiomas, liver hemangiomas (associated with high-output heart failure and severe hypothyroidism), and profuse bleeding from an ulcerated hemangioma
        (2) Risk of functional impairment: Interference with the development of vision (if near eye) and interference with feeding (if near mouth)
        (3) Ulceration: Most common complication (5% to 21%). Can be extremely painful and usually scars; risk greatest in large hemangiomas and those located in skin creases, particularly the diaper area
        (4) Associated structural anomalies: PHACES syndrome (**P**osterior cranial fossa malformations, large segmental facial **H**emangiomas, **A**rterial lesions, **C**ardiovascular anomalies [aortic anomalies], **E**ye anomalies, **S**ternal cleft anomalies/ supraumbilical raphes[4]) and LUMBAR syndrome (**L**ower body hemangioma, **U**rogenital anomalies, **U**lceration, **M**yelopathy,

Bony deformities, **A**norectal malformations, **A**rterial anomalies, **R**enal anomalies)

(5) Potential for disfigurement: Risk of permanent scarring or distortion of anatomic landmarks

d. **Diagnosis:** Usually diagnosed clinically. Atypical clinical findings, growth pattern, and equivocal imaging should prompt tissue biopsy to exclude other neoplasms or unusual vascular malformations. See Table 8.1 for indications to order imaging.

(1) Consult the free International Society Study of Vascular Anomalies (ISSVA) classification online for characterization and differentiation between benign and aggressive vascular tumors

e. **Treatment:**

(1) Most are uncomplicated and can be observed with watchful waiting. Photo documentation is used to follow the growth and regression process.

(2) If an infantile hemangioma is identified as high risk, the child should be evaluated by a hemangioma specialist promptly, as there is a narrow window of opportunity in which to intervene and prevent poor outcomes.

(3) β-adrenergic blockers such as propranolol are considered first-line therapy for complicated infantile hemangiomas and should be initiated under supervision of a pediatric dermatologist or experienced practitioner.[5] While patients should be clinically screened for cardiac disease, EKG and/or echocardiogram are not required unless there is clinical concern. Contraindications include: reactive airways, sinus bradycardia, decompensated heart failure, greater than first-degree heart block, hypotension, hypoglycemia, hypersensitivity to propranolol. Off-label use of selective β-blockers may be considered in certain patients. Duration should be at least 6 months and up to 12 months of age.[6]

TABLE 8.1

INDICATIONS TO OBTAIN IMAGING OF INFANTILE HEMANGIOMAS

Indication	Imaging Modality
1. Diagnosis of infantile hemangiomas (IH) is uncertain (e.g., atypical appearance or behavior)	Ultrasound with Doppler
2. Five or more cutaneous IH	Abdominal ultrasound with Doppler (screen for hepatic IH)
3. Associated structural abnormalities (e.g., PHACE syndrome or LUMBAR syndrome) are suspected	1. If PHACE syndrome is suspected, MRI/MRA head/neck with and without contrast; echocardiography 2. If LUMBAR syndrome is suspected, spinal ultrasound and abdominal ultrasound with Doppler are initial screen, with MRI likely to follow 3. May wish to consult with hemangioma specialist on exact imaging to be ordered

From Krowchuk D, Frieden IJ, Mancini AJ, et al. Clinical practice guideline for the management of infantile hemangiomas. *Pediatrics.* 2019;143(1):1–28.

    (4) Corticosteroids are considered second line. Similar efficacy to propranolol in a prospective, randomized, investigator-blinded trial, but propranolol is better tolerated and with fewer severe side effects.[7]

    (5) Topical timolol is effective in superficial, uncomplicated hemangiomas (recommend 0.5% gel forming solution).

    (6) Ulcerated hemangiomas may respond to pulsed dye laser therapy or topical or systemic steroids.

2. Pyogenic granuloma (lobular capillary hemangioma) (Fig. 8.2, Color Plates)

    a. **Clinical presentation:** Benign vascular tumor, appears as small (usually 3 to 10 mm but occasionally much larger), bright red papule that grows over several weeks to months into sessile or pedunculated papule with a "collarette," scale, or crust. Can bleed profusely with minor trauma and can ulcerate. Rarely spontaneously regresses. Seen in all ages; average age of diagnosis 6 months to 10 years. Located on head and neck, sometimes in oral mucosa but can be at any skin site and often misdiagnosed as hemangiomas

    b. **Treatment:** Usually required, given frequent bleeding and ulceration. Options include shave excision or curettage with cautery of base, surgical excision, carbon dioxide laser excision, or pulsed dye laser therapy. For most cases, shave and cautery are quick, safe, low risk, and can be performed quickly with local anesthesia. Small, intact lesions may respond to topical timolol therapy.

B. Vascular Malformations

Include capillary (port-wine stains and salmon patch/stork bite/angel kiss), lymphatic, venous, and arteriovenous malformations

    NOTE: For a comparison of vascular malformations to vascular tumors, please see eTable 8.1.[8]

III. INFECTIONS

A. Viral

1. Warts

    a. **Pathogenesis:** Human papillomaviruses (HPVs) of the epithelium or mucus membrane

    b. **Clinical presentation:**

        (1) Common warts: Skin-colored, rough, minimally scaly papules and nodules found most commonly on the hands, although can occur anywhere. Can be solitary or multiple, range from a few millimeters to several centimeters, may form large plaques or a confluent linear pattern secondary to autoinoculation. Sometimes persistent in immunocompromised patients and persistence may be a marker for underlying immunodeficiency.

        (2) Flat warts: Flesh to brown/yellow-colored, smooth, flat-topped papules commonly found over the hands, arms, and face. Usually <2 mm in diameter and often present in clusters

        (3) Plantar warts: Occur on soles of feet as inward-growing, hyperkeratotic plaques and papules. Trauma on weight-bearing surfaces results in small black dots (petechiae from thrombosed vessels on the surface of the wart). Can be painful

  c. **Diagnosis:** Clinical diagnosis; using a magnifier may help confirm clinical diagnosis

  d. **Treatment**[9]:

      (1) Spontaneous resolution occurs in greater than 75% of warts in otherwise healthy individuals within 3 years. No specific treatment clearly better than placebo, except possibly topical salicylic acid. Cryotherapy is sometimes combined with salicylic acid, but the efficacy of this combination has not been proven.

      (2) Keratolytics (topical salicylates): Particularly effective in combination with adhesive tape occlusion. Response may take 4 to 6 months.

      (3) Intralesional bleomycin, topical or intralesional fluorouracil, laser therapy, topical sensitizers, and imiquimod have been used for refractory warts, but the efficacy has not been proven. Destructive techniques, *Candida* antigen, cantharidin, or "beetle juice" are not clearly more effective than placebo. Additionally, destructive techniques can be painful and cause scarring, particularly on the digits. These options are not routinely recommended in children.

2. Molluscum contagiosum (Fig. 8.3, Color Plates)

  a. **Pathogenesis:** Large DNA poxvirus. Spread by skin-to-skin contact

  b. **Clinical presentation:** Dome-shaped, often umbilicated, translucent to white papules that range from 1 mm to 1 cm. Occur anywhere but only rarely on palms and soles, most commonly on the trunk and intertriginous areas. Can occur in the genital area and lower abdomen when obtained as a sexually transmitted infection in sexually active adolescents and autoinoculation in younger children. May be pruritic and can be surrounded by erythema, resembling eczema. The surrounding red, scaly reaction is referred to as "the beginning of the end" (see Treatment).

  c. **Diagnosis:** Clinical diagnosis; magnifier can be used to distinguish from warts and other papular lesions

  d. **Treatment:** Most spontaneously resolve within 6 to 18 months and do not require intervention other than monitoring for secondary bacterial infection. Surrounding eczematous changes may indicate an immunologic reaction and serve as a harbinger of regression. Treatment may cause scarring and may not be more effective than placebo. For symptomatic lesions curettage, topical irritants and sensitizers, and cantharidin may be an option. Recurrences are common.

3. Herpes simplex virus

  a. **Pathogenesis:** Either HSV-1 or HSV-2 may be implicated, regardless of lesion location. During the initial outbreak, oral lesions last 2 to

3 weeks, whereas genital lesions may last 2 to 6 weeks. Recurrent episodes are usually much shorter.

b. **Clinical presentation (Fig. 8.5, Color Plates):** Symptoms include prodrome of tingling, itching, or burning followed by painful vesicles on erythematous base that may last 7 to 10 days, break open, and crust prior to healing; flu-like symptoms; dehydration (gingivostomatitis); dysuria (genital); ophthalmologic symptoms (keratitis). May be triggered by stress, illness, sun exposure, and menstruation. The first outbreak is typically the worst.

c. **Intrauterine HSV skin findings:** Recent case series show that cutaneous manifestation of HSV acquired in utero includes erosions, ulcerations, crusted papules or plaques, calcinosis cutis, excoriations, macules (erythematous, scaring with hypopigmented or hyperpigmented lesions), cutaneous atrophy, contractures, and bruising in addition to vesicles with erythematous base.

d. **Diagnosis:** Diagnosed clinically and, in many centers, with viral DNA PCR (more sensitive than culture). To culture a lesion, clean with alcohol, un-roof lesion with sterile needle or wooden side of cotton swab, collect vesicular fluid on sterile swab, and send in viral transport medium.

e. **Treatment:** Acyclovir or valacyclovir for 7 to 14 days (see Formulary for dosing). For children with herpetic gingivostomatitis, antiviral therapy should be initiated within 72 to 96 hours of onset if they are unable to drink or have significant pain. Valacyclovir is generally preferred as it is more bioavailable than acyclovir and, as a result, is dosed less frequently. See infectious disease chapter for more details on neonatal HSV.

4. Erythema infectiosum ("fifth disease")

a. **Pathogenesis:** Parvovirus B19

b. **Clinical presentation:** Pediatric presentation of nonspecific febrile illness with headache, coryza, and gastrointestinal complaints. Two to five days after onset of symptoms, the classic malar rash with "slapped cheek" appearance erupts, followed by a reticular rash to the trunk several days later. Associated signs and symptoms include arthralgias (more common in adults) and a transient aplastic crisis, which may be more of a problem in patients with hemoglobinopathies and pregnant women.

c. **Diagnosis:** Clinical diagnosis, serum IgM, or serum DNA PCR

d. **Treatment:** Supportive care. Avoid people who are pregnant as virus can cause hydrops fetalis.

5. Pityriasis rosea (PR, Figs. 8.9 and 8.10, Color Plates)

a. **Pathogenesis:** Possible viral etiology (HHV-6, -7) as some cases are preceded by a prodrome of headache and malaise. No association with bacterial or fungal organisms has been found.

b. **Clinical presentation:** Classically presents with a "herald" patch, a single salmon-colored oval patch 2 to 5 cm in diameter, with central clearing. In the following days, similar but smaller oval patches appear, usually on the trunk and proximal extremities. On the back, the confluence of patches may appear in a "Christmas tree" pattern. The rash usually spreads from top down or centrifugally. In young children, lesions more often involve the scalp, face, and groin and can spare the trunk. Symptoms resolve in 4 weeks to several months.

   c. **Diagnosis:** Clinical diagnosis, but KOH scrapings to differentiate from tinea may be necessary. In sexually active patients, testing is recommended to rule out secondary syphilis, which may mimic the rash of PR.

   d. **Treatment:** Will self-resolve without treatment. Symptomatic therapy with topical medium-potency steroids may reduce pruritis.

6. Roseola infantum (Fig. 8.11, Color Plates)

   a. **Pathogenesis:** Human herpesvirus 6 (HHV-6, less commonly HHV-7)

   b. **Clinical presentation:** Typically diagnosed in children <2 years old with peak 7 to 13 months. Febrile phase of 3 to 5 days of high fever (often >40°C), viremia, and irritability. As febrile phase resolves, patients develop a morbilliform rash on neck and trunk that spreads centripetally to face and extremities for 1 to 2 days.

   c. **Diagnosis:** Clinical diagnosis

   d. **Treatment:** Self-resolving

7. Hand, foot, and mouth disease

   a. **Pathogenesis:** Most commonly coxsackievirus A serotypes

   b. **Clinical presentation:** Oral lesions on the tongue, buccal mucosa, and palate that initially are 1- to 5-mm erythematous macules and evolve to vesicles and ulcers with a thin erythematous halo. Erythematous, nonpruritic 1- to 10-mm macules, papules, and/or vesicles on the palms and soles. Typically resolve in 3 to 4 days. Usually nontender, unless caused by coxsackie A6 (may be associated with high fevers, widespread lesions, longer duration [12 days], palmar and plantar desquamation, and nail dystrophy)

   c. **Diagnosis:** Clinical diagnosis. Most infections are now caused by coxsackie A6, and the rash tends to be worse in areas with normal skin trauma (face, extremities, diaper area). Moreover, lesions may be dramatic in areas with irritated skin such as in patches of eczema.

   d. **Treatment:** Supportive care

8. Reactive erythema (Fig. 8.4; Figs. 8.5 to 8.11, Color Plates)

   a. **Pathogenesis:** Represent cutaneous reaction patterns triggered by endogenous and environmental factors (e.g., viral infections, drug reactions, immunizations)

   b. **Clinical presentation:** Group of disorders characterized by erythematous patches, plaques, and nodules that vary in size, shape, and distribution and may develop purpura, urticarial plaques, and erythema multiforme-like lesions

B. Parasitic

1. Scabies (Figs. 8.12 to 8.14, Color Plates)

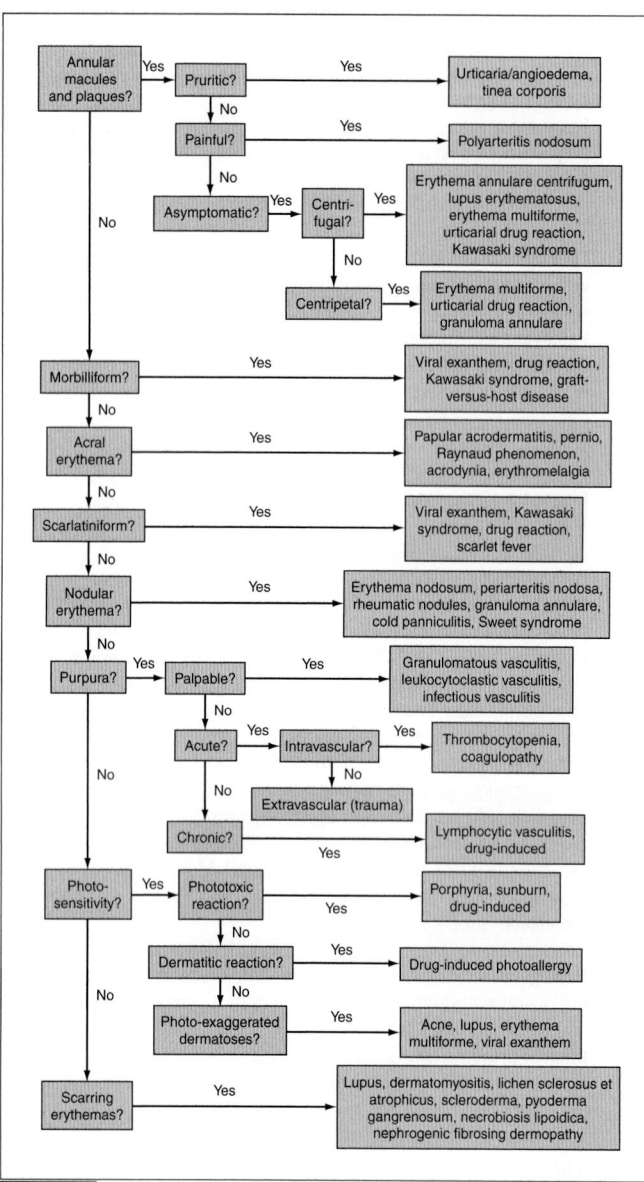

FIGURE 8.4

Reactive erythema. (Modified from Cohen BA. *Atlas of Pediatric Dermatology.* 4th ed. Elsevier Limited; 2013:206.)

a. **Pathogenesis:** Caused by the mite *Sarcoptes scabiei*. Spread by skin-to-skin contact and through fomites. Can live for 2 days away from a human host. Female mites burrow and lay eggs under the skin.

b. **Clinical presentation:** Initial lesion is a small, erythematous papule that is easy to overlook. Can have burrows (elongated, edematous papulovesicles, often with a pustule at the advancing border) that are pathognomonic. Most commonly located in interdigital webs, wrist folds, elbows, axilla, genitals, buttocks, and belt line but can become widely disseminated. In temperate climates, the face and scalp are usually spared. In young infants, the palms and soles are also commonly involved. Burrows are most dramatic in patients who are unable to scratch (e.g., infants). An immunologically mediated disseminated eczematous (Id) eruption results in generalized severe pruritus, especially at night. Can become nodular, particularly in intertriginous areas, or be susceptible to superinfection due to frequent excoriations. Immunosuppressed patients may develop diffuse, scaly, crusted eruption and lack pruritus and may progress to "crusted scabies" or infection with very high numbers of mites, requiring more intensive topical and oral therapy.

c. **Treatment**[10]:

   (1) Permethrin cream: 5% cream applied to skin from neck down in normal hosts, including under fingernails and toenails. Rinse off after 8 to 14 hours. Can repeat in 7 to 10 days

   (2) Ivermectin (off-label use): Single 200 mCg/kg dose; can repeat in 2 weeks. Efficacy comparable to permethrin cream. May be the best choice for immunodeficient patients for whom total body application may be difficult but is not considered first line for pregnant patients or children weighing less than 15 kg

   (3) Spinosad: 0.9% topical suspension, approved for treatment of scabies in adults and children 4 years of age and older. This treatment was approved in 2021, and its efficacy compared to prior treatments has not been well established.

   (4) Environment: Mites cannot live away from human skin for more than 2 to 3 days. Launder clothing and sheets. Bag and seal stuffed animals and pillows for 2 to 3 days. Consider treatment of close contacts.

2. Head lice: Pediculosis capitis

a. **Pathogenesis:** Caused by *Pediculus humanus capitis*. Female louse lays eggs (nits) on the base of the hair shaft, which hatch into nymphs that mature to adult lice in 1 week. Transmission occurs through direct contact with the head of a person with lice, and transmission through towels, brushes, or hats is controversial. Lice do not fly or jump.

b. **Clinical diagnosis:** Should be suspected in child with scalp pruritus or persistent pyoderma around hairline. Diagnosis is confirmed by visualization of live lice, best done by using a fine-toothed nit comb through wet hair.

c. **Treatment:** First-line treatment is topical pediculicides (permethrin, topical ivermectin, malathion, benzyl alcohol, topical dimethicone). Wet combing with a fine-toothed nit comb is an alternative for infants or patients who prefer to avoid medication. There is concern that lice are becoming resistant to topical permethrin and malathion; however, the most common cause of persistent head lice is poor adherence to treatment and continued exposure to other infected individuals. If resistance, independent from reinfection, is suspected, then oral ivermectin can be used.

C. Fungal (Figs. 8.15 to 8.19, Color Plates)

1. Tinea capitis (Fig. 8.15, Color Plates)
   a. **Pathogenesis:** Mostly caused by fungi of the genus *Trichophyton* in North America (95%), less commonly *Microsporum* (5% or less), and spread through direct contact and fomites
   b. **Epidemiology:** Usually occurs in young children, with higher incidence in type 4 hair follicles
   c. **Clinical presentation:**
      (1) Black dot: Most common. Slowly growing, minimally scaly patches, sometimes erythematous but often with little or no inflammation until later in the course. These areas develop alopecia, and black dots are visible on scalp where hair has broken.
      (2) Gray patch ("seborrheic dermatitis type"): Erythematous, scaling, well-demarcated patches that grow centrifugally. Hair breaks off a few millimeters above the scalp and takes on a gray/frosted appearance.
      (3) Kerion (Fig. 8.16, Color Plates): Complication of tinea capitis or tinea corporis. Type IV hypersensitivity to fungus. Raised, boggy/spongy lesions, often tender and covered with purulent exudate. Most commonly occurs months after primary infection
      (4) All can be associated with posterior cervical lymphadenopathy.
      (5) Secondary infection usually from *Staphylococcus aureus* may be associated with tender pustules requiring treatment with oral antibiotic.
   c. **Diagnosis:** Can be made clinically, but since oral antifungal therapy is indicated, tinea capitis should be confirmed by direct microscopic exam of a potassium hydroxide (KOH) preparation of the proximal ends of hairs, gently and painlessly scraped from the affected area. Cultures should be obtained on all patients by using a sterile toothbrush or cotton swab. The scale can be scraped directly into a sterile plastic cup and/or the cotton swab tips can be broken off and placed into the sterile plastic cups.
   d. **Treatment[11]: (Intent for Clinical Review submitted by Section of Dermatology (SOD) of American Academy of Pediatrics (AAP))** Always requires systemic therapy. First-line therapy includes oral griseofulvin for 10 to 12 weeks (which should be taken with fatty foods for improved absorption) or terbinafine for 6 weeks (see

Formulary for dosing). Most experts consider terbinafine superior to griseofulvin for *T. tonsurans* because of its shorter duration of therapy and superior effectiveness. The FDA recommends baseline and follow-up hepatic function testing in children taking terbinafine, though most clinicians forego laboratory testing in healthy children without history of liver disease if treatment is 6 weeks or less. Though not FDA approved for tinea capitis, fluconazole at 6 mg/kg/day (max 400 mg/day) for 6 weeks is recommended by the AAP Red Book as an alternative treatment of tinea capitis in children younger than 2 years old.[12] All family members, particularly other children, should be examined carefully for subtle infection. Selenium sulfide 2.5% shampoo may shorten the period of shedding of fungal organisms and reduce risk of infection of unaffected family members. Off-label treatment with itraconazole 5 to 6 mg/kg/day for 6 weeks (comes in liquid formulation as well, which makes it easier to use in infants and toddlers). For kerion, can use high-potency topical steroid for 1 to 2 weeks at same time that start oral therapy but if severe maybe 1 to 2 weeks of oral steroid; treat secondary bacterial infection with 1 to 2 weeks of oral antibiotic.

2. Tinea corporis and pedis[11] (Figs. 8.17 and 8.18, Color Plates)
   a. **Pathogenesis:** Spread through direct contact and fomites, especially in sports with close contact (e.g., tinea gladiatorum)
   b. **Clinical presentation:** Pruritic, erythematous, annular patch or plaque with central clearing and a scaly raised border. Typically affects hair-free skin, but any skin can be affected
   c. **Diagnosis:** Usually diagnosed clinically, but a KOH preparation or fungal culture can be used to help guide diagnosis and treatment. If widespread and considering oral therapy, send fungal culture to confirm diagnosis.
   d. **Treatment:** Topical antifungals (terbinafine, miconazole, clotrimazole, ketoconazole) through 1 to 2 weeks past lesion resolution. Widespread eruption may require oral antifungals.

3. Tinea (pityriasis) versicolor (Fig. 8.19, Color Plates)
   a. **Pathogenesis:** Caused by *Malassezia*. Exacerbated by hot/humid weather, hyperhidrosis, topical skin oil use. Most people are colonized with *Malassezia*, but only a small number are prone to develop clinical lesions. Not associated with poor hygiene. Not contagious
   b. **Clinical presentation:** Well-demarcated, minimally scaly, hypopigmented macules or patches. Hypopigmented areas tend to be more prominent in the summer because affected areas do not tan. Lesions often have a fine scale that may be noted following gentle rubbing and can be mildly pruritic but are usually asymptomatic.
   c. **Diagnosis:** KOH microscopy reveals pseudohyphae and yeast cells that appear like "spaghetti and meatballs."
   d. **Treatment:** Topical antifungal shampoos and/or creams (miconazole, oxiconazole, ketoconazole) or selenium sulfide are effective. Given the risk of hepatotoxicity, oral azole antifungals are reserved for

resistant or widespread disease. Oral terbinafine is not effective. Pigmentation changes may take months to resolve despite successful treatment.

4. Id reaction
   a. **Pathogenesis:** Possible delayed-type hypersensitivity response to fungal antigens, also referred to as "autoeczematization" or "dermatophytid reaction"
   b. **Clinical presentation:** A new onset pruritic, papular, vesicular rash in a patient with tinea pedis, tinea manuum, tinea cruris, tinea corporis, or tinea capitis. Typically occurs after treatment of the dermatophyte has been initiated. Often presents as patient or caregiver concern for allergy to the antifungal treatment
   c. **Diagnosis:** Clinical
   d. **Treatment:** Continue treatment for underlying dermatophyte. Topical corticosteroids or other antipruritic treatment may be used.

D. Bacterial

1. Impetigo
   a. **Pathogenesis:** Contagious bacterial infection of the skin, most commonly caused by *Staphylococcus aureus* (99% MSSA), with a minority of cases caused by Group A *Streptococcus*
   b. **Clinical presentation:**
      (1) Nonbullous impetigo: Papules that evolve into erythematous pustules or vesicles that break and form thick, honey-colored crusts and plaques. Commonly overlying any break to skin barrier. Primarily face and extremities
      (2) Bullous impetigo: Painless vesicles that evolve into flaccid bullae and crusted patches with undermined border. Seen more in infants and young children. Caused by *Staphylococcus aureus* exfoliative toxin A
   c. **Diagnosis:** Clinical diagnosis
   d. **Treatment:** When impetigo is contained to a small area, topical mupirocin may be used for 5 days. When the infection is widespread, an oral antibiotic such as cephalexin should be used for 7 days. Consider broader coverage if MRSA is suspected, although MSSA accounts for most infections.

2. Staph scalded skin syndrome
   a. **Pathogenesis:** *Staphylococcus aureus* infections of the skin with hematogenous dissemination of exfoliative toxin A or B to the epidermis
   b. **Clinical presentation:** Typical presentation is Ritter disease (generalized exfoliation) in a 3- to 7-day-old infant who initially is febrile and irritable with conjunctivitis and perioral erythema. In addition to newborns, this presentation is seen in young children who do not have antibodies to the toxin and often do not clear the toxin-antibody complex quickly due to decreased renal excretion. It many also occur in older children and adults with renal failure who cannot

clear the toxin/antibody complex. One to two days after the prodromal onset, patient develops diffuse erythema, fragile, flaccid bullae, and erosions that are Nikolsky positive (mild rubbing of skin causes skin to slough off) in areas of mechanical stress such as intertriginous areas. Lesions are not scarring as they are intraepidermal. Older children tend to have a localized bullous impetigo with tender scarlatiniform eruption. Infants and toddlers usually have a combination of the presentations seen in neonates and older children followed 7 to 10 days later by white to brown thick flaking and desquamation of the entire body, especially hands, feet, face, and neck.

   c. **Diagnosis:** Typically clinically. However, cultures should be obtained from any potential source site of infection, if there is a primary site of infection. If there is no primary site of infection, look for sites of colonization such as the medial canthi, nares, or umbilical stump in newborns.

   d. **Treatment:** Nearly all cases are MSSA, with an increasing number being clindamycin resistant. First-line treatment may include oral penicillinase-resistant beta-lactams such as first- or second-generation cephalosporins. Vancomycin should be considered in patients who fail to respond to treatment and/or in areas with a high prevalence of MRSA. Management should also include supportive care with topical emollients and close monitoring of fluid and electrolyte status.

3. Scarlet fever (Fig. 8.20, Color Plates)

   a. **Pathogenesis:** Exotoxin-mediated response to a *Streptococcus pyogenes* infection, typically pharyngitis

   b. **Clinical presentation:** Sandpaper-like, coarse, erythematous, blanching rash that originates in the groin and axilla, then spreads to the trunk, then extremities but spares the palms and soles. May have Pastia lines (pink/red lines in skin creases). Associated with pharyngitis, circumoral pallor, and a strawberry tongue

   c. **Diagnosis:** Clinical diagnosis. May benefit from rapid strep test and throat culture

   d. **Treatment:** No additional treatment aside from treating the patient's *Strep* pharyngitis. Failing to correctly diagnose and treat increases risk of patient developing rheumatic fever.

4. Cellulitis: See Chapter 17.

IV. HAIR LOSS (FIG. 8.22, COLOR PLATES)

A. Telogen Effluvium

1. **Pathogenesis:** Most common cause of diffuse hair loss. Telogen is the resting phase of hair growth that typically lasts 3 months, followed by hair shedding. Normally, 10% of hairs are in resting phase. Acute events (such as infection, fever, anesthesia, certain medications) can trigger premature telogen that results in a larger number of hairs shed 3 months later.

2. **Clinical presentation:** Diffuse hair thinning 3 months after a stressful event (major illnesses or surgery, pregnancy, severe weight loss)
3. **Treatment:** Self-limited. Regrowth usually occurs over several months.

B. Alopecia Areata

1. **Clinical presentation:** Chronic inflammatory (probably autoimmune) disease that starts with well-circumscribed small bald patches and normal-appearing underlying skin. New lesions may demonstrate subtle erythema and be pruritic. Bald patches may enlarge to involve large areas of the scalp or other hair-bearing areas. Many experience good hair regrowth within 1 to 2 years, although most will relapse. A minority progress to total loss of all scalp (alopecia totalis) and/or body hair (alopecia universalis).
2. **Diagnosis:** Usually clinical diagnosis, but examination with magnification will show yellow dots, black dots, and exclamation point hairs. If diagnosis is unclear, a skin biopsy can also be obtained to confirm diagnosis.
3. **Treatment[13]:** First-line therapy is topical steroids. Referral to dermatology is warranted for consideration of other treatments. No evidence-based data that any therapy is better than placebo. Older children, adolescents, and young adults with long-standing localized areas of hair loss have the best prognosis. New agents including JAK inhibitors show promise for treatment of resistant and/or persistent alopecia areata.

C. Traction Alopecia (Fig. 8.22, Color Plates)

1. **Pathogenesis:** Hairstyles that apply tension for long periods of time
2. **Clinical presentation:** Noninflammatory linear areas of hair loss at margins of hairline, part line, or scattered regions, depending on hairstyling procedures used
3. **Treatment:** Avoidance of styling products or styles that result in traction. If traction remains for long periods, condition may progress to permanent scarring hair loss.

D. Trichotillomania and Hair Pulling

1. **Pathogenesis:** Alopecia due to compulsive urge to pull out one's own hair, resulting in irregular areas of incomplete hair loss. Mainly on the scalp; can involve eyebrows and eyelashes. Onset is usually after age 10 and should be distinguished from hair twirling/pulling in younger children that resolves without treatment in most cases.
2. **Clinical presentation:** Characterized by hair of differing lengths; area of hair loss can be unusual in shape
3. **Treatment:** Behavioral modification and consider psychiatric evaluation (can be associated with anxiety, depression, and obsessive-compulsive disorder)

V. ACNE VULGARIS

A. Pathogenetic Factors

Follicular hyperkeratinization, increased sebum production, *Cutibacterium acnes* (formerly *Propionibacterium acnes*) proliferation, and inflammation

B. Risk Factors

Androgens, family history, stress, and medications such as topical and oral steroids, antidepressants, antiepileptics, cyclosporin, B vitamins. No strong evidence that dietary habits affect acne

C. Clinical Presentation

1. **Noninflammatory lesions**
   a. Closed comedone (whitehead): Accumulation of sebum and keratinous material, resulting in white/skin-colored papules without surrounding erythema
   b. Open comedone (blackhead): Dilated follicles filled with keratinocytes, oils, and melanin
2. **Inflammatory lesions:** Papules, pustules, nodules, and cysts with evidence of surrounding inflammation. Typically appear later in the course of acne. Nodulocystic presentations are more likely to lead to hyperpigmentation and/or permanent scarring.

D. Treatment[14-16] (Table 8.2)

Topical minocycline foam, topical clascoterone (anti-androgen for males and females), encapsulated benzoyl peroxide and tretinoin, topical trifarotene (a fourth-generation retinoid approved for face and trunk)

1. **Skin care:** Gentle nonabrasive cleaning. Avoid picking or popping lesions. Vigorous scrubbing and abrasive cleaners can worsen acne.
2. **Topical first-line therapies:** Recommended for mild to moderate acne

TABLE 8.2

PEDIATRIC TREATMENT RECOMMENDATION FOR MILD, MODERATE, AND SEVERE ACNE

Acne Classification	Initial Treatment	Inadequate Response
Mild	Benzoyl peroxide (BPO) or topical retinoid **OR** *Topical combination therapy:* BPO + Antibiotic or retinoid + BPO or retinoid + Antibiotic + BPO	Add BPO or retinoid if not already prescribed OR change topical retinoid concentration, type, and/or formulation OR change topical combination therapy.
Moderate	*Topical combination therapy:* Retinoid + BPO or retinoid + BPO + Antibiotic **OR** Oral antibiotic + Topical retinoid + BPO or Topical retinoid + Topical antibiotic + BPO	Change topical retinoid concentration, type, and/or formulation and/or change topical combination therapy OR add or change oral antibiotic. Consider oral isotretinoin (dermatology referral). Females: Consider hormonal therapy.
Severe	*Combination therapy:* Oral antibiotic + Topical retinoid + BPO ± Topical antibiotic	Consider changing oral antibiotic AND consider oral isotretinoin. Females: Consider hormonal therapy. Strongly consider referral to dermatology.

Topical fixed-combination prescriptions available.

Data from Eichenfield LF, Krakowski AC, Piggott C, et al. Evidence-based recommendations for the diagnosis and treatment of pediatric acne. *Pediatrics.* 2013;131:S163–S186.

   a. Retinoids (eTable 8.2)

     (1) Normalize follicular keratinization and decrease inflammation

     (2) A pea-sized amount should be applied to cover the entire face (not spot treatment). Avoid eyes, creases of nose. Start two to three times weekly, titrate to nightly as tolerated. Can take 2 months to see effect

     (3) Risks: Cause irritation and dryness of skin. Retinoids should be used at night because they can cause photosensitivity and decreased effectiveness when exposed to sunlight. Use daily SPF sunscreen. This class should not be used during pregnancy.

     (4) Three topical retinoids (tretinoin, adapalene, and tazarotene) are available by prescription in the United States. Adapalene 0.1% gel has been approved for over-the-counter (OTC) use with significant efficacy.[17]

   b. Benzoyl peroxide (BPO)

     (1) Oxidizing agent with antibacterial and mild anticomedolytic properties

     (2) Washes may be most convenient formulation, as they can be used in the shower.

     (3) Recommend daily use, typically in the morning.

     (4) Risks: Can bleach hair, clothing, towels, and sheets

   c. Salicylic acid: Topical comedolytic agent that may be found in OTC face washes and serves as an alternative to a topical retinoid

3. **Topical antimicrobials:**

   a. Azelaic acid: Antimicrobial, comedolytic, and antiinflammatory. Recommended by the American Academy of Dermatology (AAD) for the treatment of postinflammatory dyspigmentation Available in a 15% gel and a 20% cream (more efficacious)[18]

   b. Erythromycin and clindamycin: Avoid topical antibiotics as monotherapy. Topical BPO should be concurrently used to optimize efficacy and avoid bacterial resistance.

   c. New topicals undergoing review are clascoterone and minocycline foam.

4. **Oral antibiotics** (eTable 8.3): Recommended for moderate to severe inflammatory acne that is resistant to topical treatment. These medications should be used with BPO or topical retinoid. Do not use as monotherapy. Limit to 3 months to minimize bacterial resistance.

   a. ≥8 years old: Doxycycline or minocycline

   b. <8 years old, pregnancy, or tetracycline allergy: Azithromycin, erythromycin, or trimethoprim/sulfamethoxazole

   c. Erythromycin should be used with care due to increased risk of resistance. The AAD recommends reserving trimethoprim/sulfamethoxazole for patients who have failed other treatments or are unable to tolerate tetracyclines and macrolides.

5. **Hormonal therapy:** Reduces sebum production and androgen levels. Good option for pubertal females who have sudden onset of moderate to

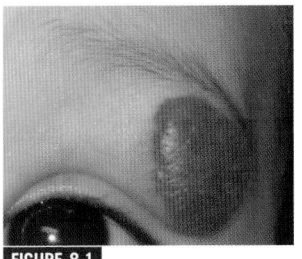

FIGURE 8.1

Infantile hemangioma. (From Cohen BA. *Atlas of Pediatric Dermatology*. 3rd ed. Mosby; 2005:126.)

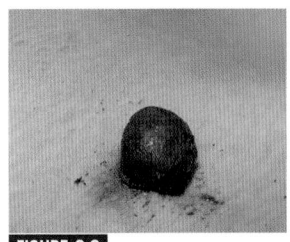

FIGURE 8.2

Pyogenic granuloma. (From Cohen BA. *Dermatology Image Atlas*; 2001. http://www.dermatlas.org/)

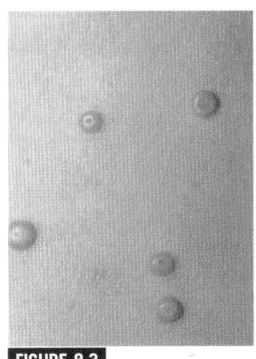

FIGURE 8.3

Molluscum contagiosum. (From Cohen BA. *Atlas of Pediatric Dermatology*. 4th ed. Elsevier Limited; 2013:131.)

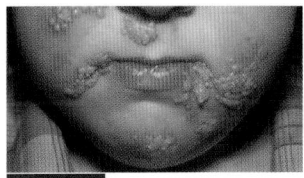

FIGURE 8.5

Herpetic gingivostomatitis. (Modified from Cohen BA. *Atlas of Pediatric Dermatology*. 4th ed. Elsevier Limited; 2013:106.)

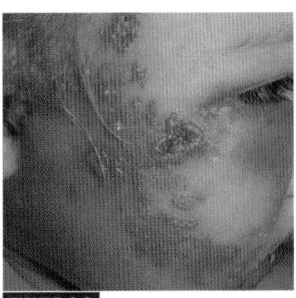

FIGURE 8.6

Herpes zoster. (From Cohen BA. *Atlas of Pediatric Dermatology*. 4th ed. Elsevier Limited; 2013:110.)

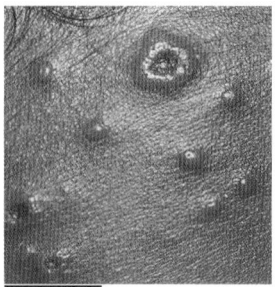

FIGURE 8.7

Varicella. (From Cohen BA. *Atlas of Pediatric Dermatology*. 4th ed. Elsevier Limited; 2013:108.)

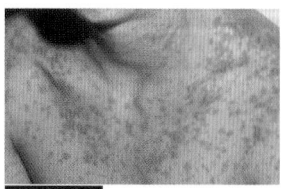

FIGURE 8.8

Measles. (From Cohen BA. *Atlas of Pediatric Dermatology*. 4th ed. Elsevier Limited; 2013:175.)

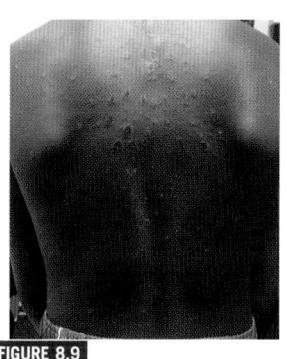

FIGURE 8.9

Pityriasis rosea. (From Cohen BA. *Atlas of Pediatric Dermatology*. 5th ed. Elsevier Limited; 2021.)

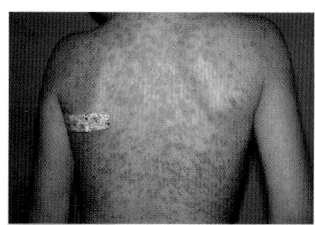

FIGURE 8.10

Pityriasis rosea. (From Cohen BA. *Atlas of Pediatric Dermatology*. 5th ed. Elsevier Limited; 2021.)

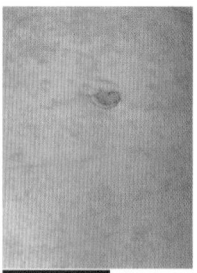

FIGURE 8.11

Roseola. (From Cohen BA. *Atlas of Pediatric Dermatology*. 4th ed. Elsevier Limited; 2013:177.)

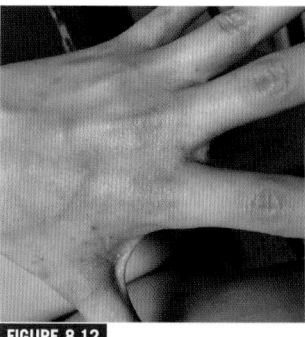

FIGURE 8.12

Scabies; finger webbing. (From Cohen BA. *Atlas of Pediatric Dermatology*. 3rd ed. Mosby; 2005:126.)

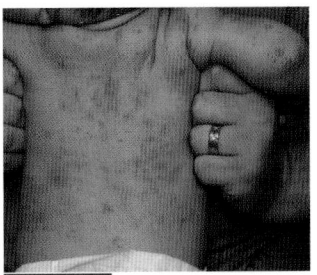

FIGURE 8.13

Scabies. (From Cohen BA. *Atlas of Pediatric Dermatology.* 5th ed. Elsevier Limited; 2021.)

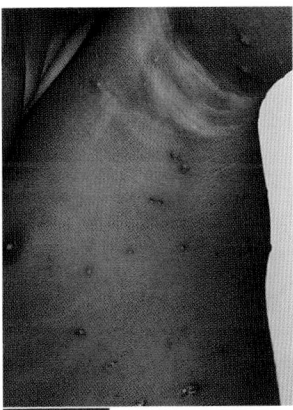

FIGURE 8.14

Scabies. (From Cohen BA. *Atlas of Pediatric Dermatology.* 5th ed. Elsevier Limited; 2021.)

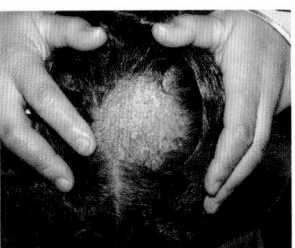

FIGURE 8.15

Tinea capitis. (From Cohen BA. *Atlas of Pediatric Dermatology.* 3rd ed. Mosby; 1993.)

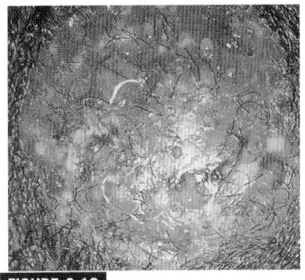

FIGURE 8.16

Kerion. (From Cohen BA. *Atlas of Pediatric Dermatology.* 4th ed. Elsevier Limited; 2013:218c.)

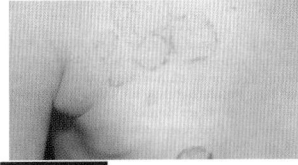

FIGURE 8.17

Tinea corporis. (From Cohen BA. *Atlas of Pediatric Dermatology.* 4th ed. Elsevier Limited; 2013:96.)

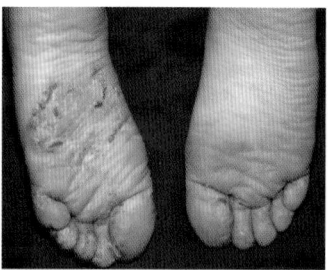

FIGURE 8.18

Tinea pedis. (From Cohen BA. *Dermatology Image Atlas*; 2001. http://www.dermatlas.org/)

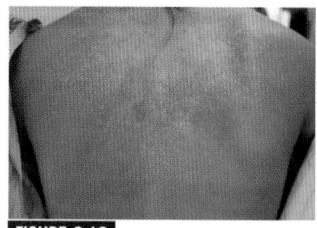

FIGURE 8.19

Tinea versicolor. (From Cohen BA. *Atlas of Pediatric Dermatology*. 4th ed. Elsevier Limited; 2013:99.)

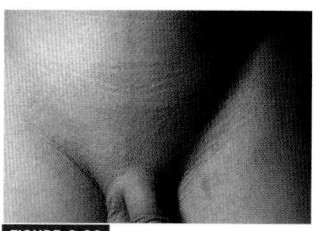

FIGURE 8.20

Scarlet fever. (From Cohen BA. *Dermatology Image Atlas*; 2001. http://www.dermatlas.org/)

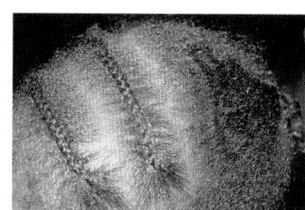

FIGURE 8.22

Traction alopecia. (From Cohen BA. *Atlas of Pediatric Dermatology*. 4th ed. Elsevier Limited; 2013:220.)

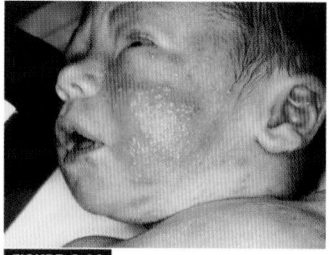

FIGURE 8.23

Erythema toxicum neonatorum. (From Cohen BA. *Pediatric Dermatology*. 2nd ed. Mosby; 1999:18.)

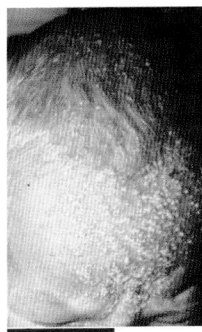

FIGURE 8.24
Transient neonatal pustular melanosis. (From Cohen BA. *Atlas of Pediatric Dermatology.* 4th ed. Elsevier Limited; 2013:20.)

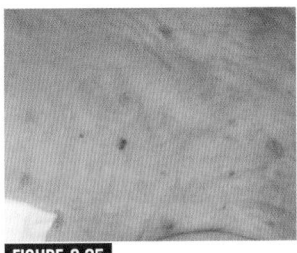

FIGURE 8.25
Hyperpigmentation from resolving transient neonatal pustular melanosis. (From Cohen BA. *Atlas of Pediatric Dermatology.* 4th ed. Elsevier Limited; 2013:20.)

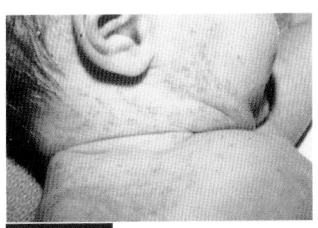

FIGURE 8.26
Miliaria rubra. (From Cohen BA. *Atlas of Pediatric Dermatology.* 4th ed. Elsevier Limited; 2013:21.)

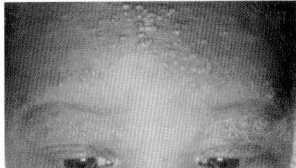

FIGURE 8.27
Milia. (From Cohen BA. *Atlas of Pediatric Dermatology.* 4th ed. Elsevier Limited; 2013:22.)

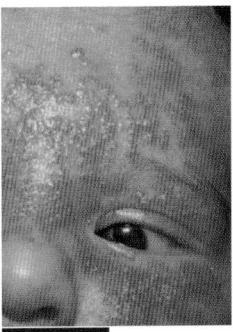

FIGURE 8.28
Neonatal acne. (From Cohen BA. *Atlas of Pediatric Dermatology.* 4th ed. Elsevier Limited; 2013:22.)

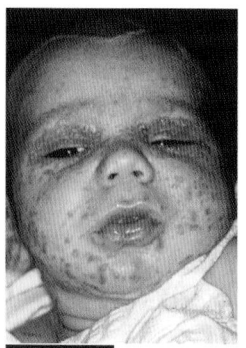

FIGURE 8.29

Seborrheic dermatitis. (From Cohen BA. *Atlas of Pediatric Dermatology*. 4th ed. Elsevier Limited; 2013:32.)

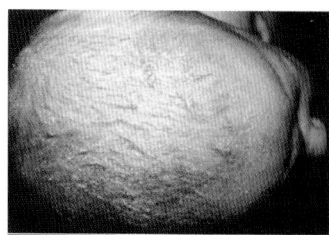

FIGURE 8.30

Seborrheic dermatitis. (From Cohen BA. *Atlas of Pediatric Dermatology*. 4th ed. Elsevier Limited; 2013:32.)

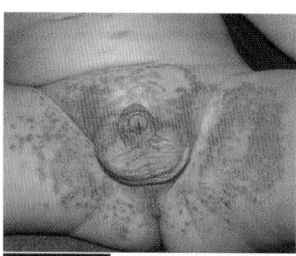

FIGURE 8.31

Diaper candidiasis. (From Cohen BA. *Atlas of Pediatric Dermatology*. 4th ed. Elsevier Limited; 2013:33.)

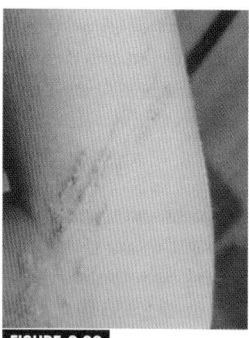

FIGURE 8.32

Poison ivy. (From Cohen BA. *Dermatology Image Atlas*; 2001. http://www.dermatlas.org/)

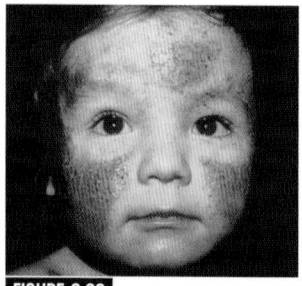

FIGURE 8.33

Infantile eczema. (From Cohen BA. *Atlas of Pediatric Dermatology*. 3rd ed. Mosby; 2005:79.)

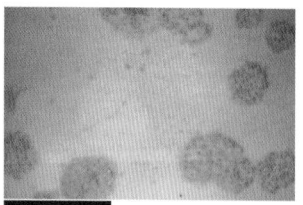

FIGURE 8.34

Nummular eczema. (From Cohen BA. *Atlas of Pediatric Dermatology*. 3rd ed. Mosby; 2005:80.)

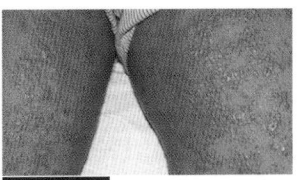

FIGURE 8.35

Follicular eczema. (From Cohen BA. *Atlas of Pediatric Dermatology*. 4th ed. Elsevier Limited; 2013:83.)

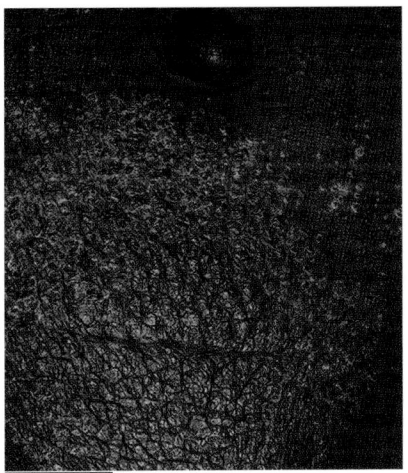

FIGURE 8.36

Childhood eczema with lesion in suprapubic area. (From Cohen BA. *Atlas of Pediatric Dermatology*. 3rd ed. Mosby; 2005.)

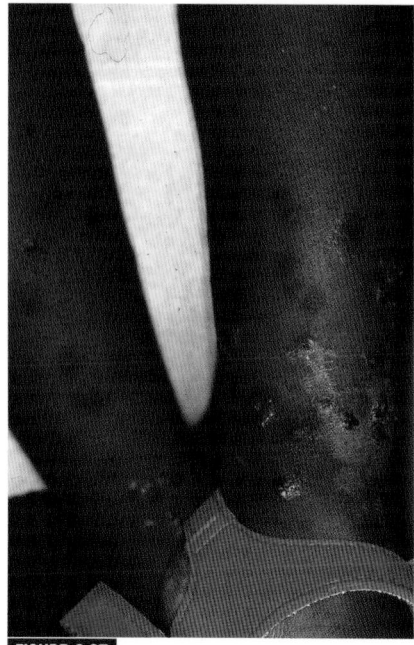

FIGURE 8.37

Papular urticaria from insect bite. (From Cohen BA. *Atlas of Pediatric Dermatology*. 5th ed. China: Elsevier Limited; 2021.)

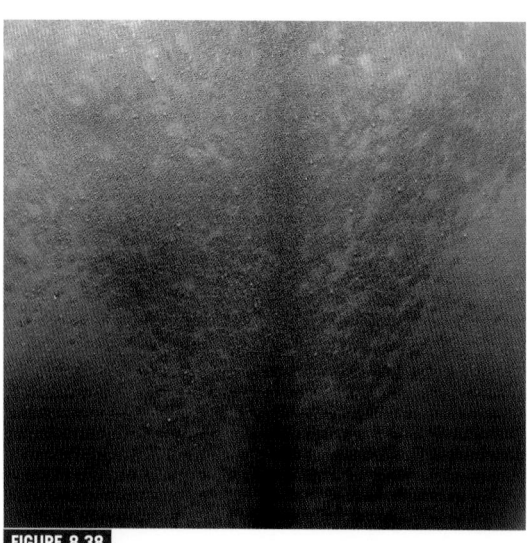

FIGURE 8.38

Confluent reticulated papillomatosis. (From Cohen BA. *Atlas of Pediatric Dermatology*. 5th ed. Elsevier Limited; 2021.)

severe hormonal acne (often on lower face, jawline) and have not responded to conventional first-line therapies. Should not be used as monotherapy. Combination oral contraceptives (see Chapter 5 for additional information) or spironolactone (antiandrogen)

6. **Oral isotretinoin:** Reserved for patients with severe nodular, cystic, or scarring acne who do not respond to traditional therapy or who cannot be weaned from oral antibiotics. Should be managed by a dermatologist. Most patients have complete resolution of their acne after 16 to 20 weeks of use.

   a. Side effects:

      (1) Teratogenicity: Patients and physicians are mandated by the FDA to comply with the iPledge program to eliminate fetal exposure to isotretinoin. Female patients with child-bearing potential must use two forms of birth control with routine pregnancy testing.

      (2) Hepatotoxicity, hyperlipidemia, and bone marrow suppression, a complete blood cell count, fasting lipid profile, and liver function tests should be obtained before initiation of therapy and repeated at 4 and 8 weeks.

VI. COMMON NEONATAL DERMATOLOGIC CONDITIONS (FIG. 8.21; FIGS. 8.23 TO 8.30, COLOR PLATES)

A. Erythema Toxicum Neonatorum (Fig. 8.23, Color Plates)

1. **Clinical presentation:** Most common rash of full-term infants; incidence declines with lower birth weight and prematurity. Appears as small erythematous macules and papules that evolve into pustules on erythematous bases. Rash most often occurs by 24 to 48 hours of life but can be present at birth or emerge as late as 2 to 3 weeks.

2. **Course:** Self-limited, resolves within 5 to 7 days; recurrences possible

B. Transient Neonatal Pustular Melanosis (Figs. 8.24 to 8.25, Color Plates)

1. **Clinical presentation:** More commonly affects full-term infants with darker pigmentation. At birth, appears as small pustules on nonerythematous bases that rupture and leave erythematous/hyperpigmented macules with a collarette of scale

2. **Course:** Self-limited macules fade over weeks to months.

C. Miliaria (Heat Rash) (Fig. 8.26, Color Plates)

1. **Clinical presentation:** Common newborn rash associated with warmer climates, incubator use, or occlusion with clothes/dressings. Appears as small erythematous papules or pustules usually on face, scalp, or intertriginous areas

2. **Course:** Rash resolves when infant is placed in cooler environment or tight clothing/dressings are removed.

D. Milia (Fig. 8.27, Color Plates)

1. **Clinical presentation:** Common newborn lesions. Appears as 1- to 3-mm white/yellow papules, frequently found on nose and face; due to retention of keratin and sebaceous materials in pilosebaceous follicles

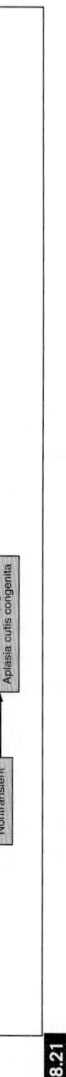

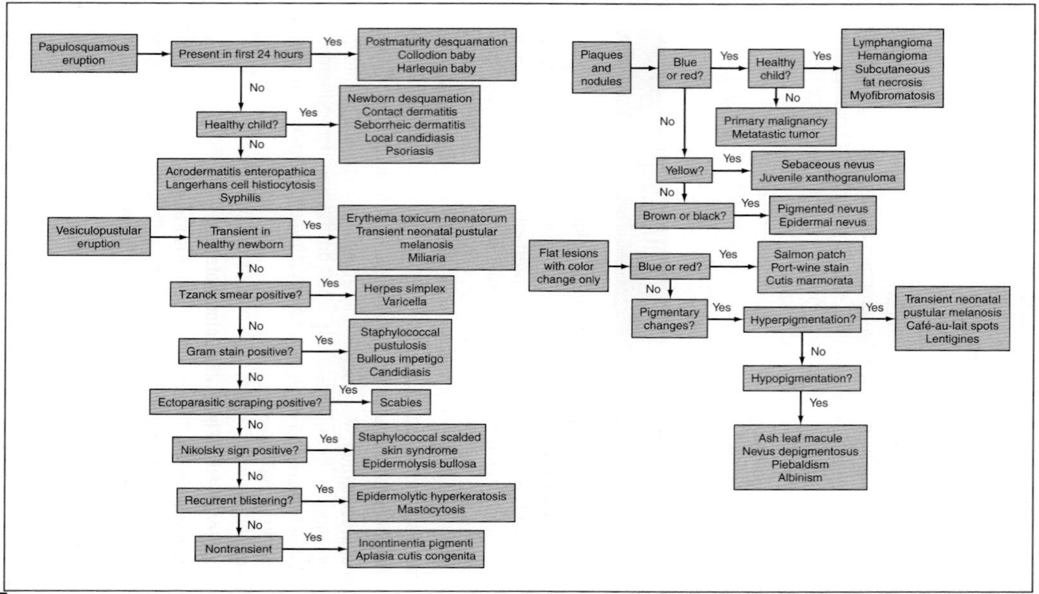

FIGURE 8.21

Evaluation of neonatal rashes. (Modified from Cohen BA. *Atlas of Pediatric Dermatology*. 5th ed. Elsevier Limited; 2021.)

2. **Course:** Self-limited, resolves within first few weeks to few months of life

E. Neonatal Acne (Fig. 8.28, Color Plates)

1. **Clinical presentation:** Seen in 20% of infants. Appears as inflammatory papules or pustules without comedones, usually on face and scalp. Secondary to effect of maternal and endogenous androgens on infant's sebaceous glands

2. **Course:** Peaks around 1 month, resolves within a few months, usually without intervention. Does not increase risk of acne as an adolescent

F. Seborrheic Dermatitis (Figs. 8.29 to 8.30, Color Plates)

1. **Clinical presentation:** Erythematous plaques with greasy yellow scales. Located in areas rich with sebaceous glands, such as scalp, cheeks, ears, eyebrows, intertriginous areas, diaper area. Unknown etiology. Can be seen in newborns, more commonly in infants aged 1 to 4 months. Can also be seen in older patients, particularly adolescents with chronic medical conditions

2. **Course:** Self-limited and resolves within a few weeks to months

3. **Treatment:** Can remove scales on scalp with an emollient (e.g., mineral or olive oil, or petroleum jelly) and a soft brush/fine comb. In more severe cases, antifungal shampoos or low-potency topical steroid can shorten the course, although no shampoos are FDA approved for children less than 2 years of age.

G. Congenital Dermal Melanocytosis

1. **Clinical presentation:** Most common pigmented lesion of newborns, usually seen in babies with darker skin tone. Appear as blue/gray macules without definite disappearance of dermal melanocytes. Can be mistaken for child abuse; thus accurate documentation at newborn and well-child visits is important

2. **Course:** Spots typically fade within first few years of life, with majority resolved or much improved by age 10 years.

3. **Other types:** Nevus of Ota involves the skin innervated by the first and second divisions of the trigeminal nerve and can cause neurocutaneous melanosis with up to 10% of patients developing sensorineural hearing loss or glaucoma ipsilateral to the skin lesion. Nevus of Ito involves the skin innervated by the posterior supraclavicular and lateral brachiocutaneous nerves.

H. Diaper Dermatitis[19]

1. **Clinical presentation:** Irritant contact dermatitis characterized by erythematous eruption on buttocks and genital areas with exclusion of other potential causes. Most commonly associated with increased loose stools from viral gastroenteritis, antibiotics, and other gastrointestinal disorders. Rarely associated with diaper candidiasis, characterized by a red, raised papular rash with small pustules at the periphery (Fig. 8.31). Tends to involve the skin prominences and spares the protected skin creases[19]

2. **Treatment:** Frequent diaper changes, air exposure, adequate drying, gentle cleaning, and judicious use of topical barrier preparations. If persistent, can use low-potency topical steroid until cleared no more than twice daily. For candidiasis, treatment with topical nystatin, miconazole, or clotrimazole is sufficient. Combination steroid/antifungal creams should be avoided due to steroid-related side effects and association with persistent fungal infections.[20]

VII. AUTOIMMUNE AND ALLERGIC DERMATOLOGIC CONDITIONS (FIGS. 8.32 TO 8.38, COLOR PLATES)

A. Contact Dermatitis

1. Irritant dermatitis: Exposure to physical, chemical, or mechanical irritants to the skin. Common irritants include frequent hand washing, hot water, lip-licking, thumb-sucking, and exposure to chemicals, paints, or certain foods like citrus fruits.
2. Allergic dermatitis
   a. **Pathogenesis:** Immune reaction to an environmental trigger that comes into contact with the skin. After initial sensitization period of 7 to 10 days in susceptible individuals, an allergic response occurs with subsequent exposures.
   b. **Common allergens:** *Toxicodendron* spp. (poison ivy, oak, sumac), nickel, cobalt, gold, dyes, fragrances, formaldehyde, latex, and acetophenone azine (found in shin guards and other sports equipment)
   c. Dermatitis that can progress to chronic scaling, lichenification, and pigment changes. Poison ivy (Fig. 8.32, Color Plates): Exposure to urushiol causes streaks of erythematous papules, pustules, and vesicles. Highly pruritic, can become edematous, especially if rash is on face or genitals. In extreme cases, anaphylaxis can occur.
   d. **Diagnosis:** Careful history taking and recognition of unusual shapes and locations suggesting an "outside job" allow for clinical diagnosis. Patch testing may also be helpful when trigger cannot be identified.
   e. **Treatment:**
      (1) Remove causative agent. Moisturize with ointment like Vaseline or Aquaphor twice per day. Use antihistamine and/or oatmeal baths as needed for itching, sedation, and sleeping, though they do not directly impact the rash.
      (2) Mild/moderate: Topical steroids twice a day for 1 week, then daily for 1 to 2 weeks
      (3) Widespread/severe: Systemic steroids for 2 to 3 weeks, with taper. There is no role for short courses of steroids because eruption will flare when drug is stopped.
      (4) For poison ivy contact, remove clothing and wash skin with mild soap and water as soon as possible.

B. Atopic Dermatitis (Eczema) (Figs. 8.33 to 8.36, Color Plates)

1. **Pathogenesis:** Due to inadequate skin barrier function from combination of genetic and environmental factors, resulting in transepidermal water loss and immunologically mediated inflammatory reaction. Can be associated with elevated serum IgE

2. **Epidemiology[21]:** Affects up to 20% of children in the United States, the vast majority with onset before age 5 years. Other comorbidities may follow, including asthma, allergic rhinitis, and food allergies. Eczema resolves or improves in over 75% of patients by adulthood.

3. **Clinical presentation:** Dry, pruritic skin with acute changes, including erythema, vesicles, crusting, and chronic changes, including scaling, postinflammatory hypo- or hyperpigmentation (eFigs. 8.1 and 8.2), and lichenification

    a. Infantile form: Erythematous, scaly lesions on the cheeks, scalp, and extensor surfaces. Covered areas (especially the diaper area) are usually spared.

    b. Childhood form: Lichenified plaques in flexural areas

    c. Adolescence: More localized and lichenified skin changes. Predominantly on skin flexures, hands, and feet

4. **Treatment[21]:** See Chapter 15.

    a. Lifestyle: Avoiding triggers (products with alcohol, fragrances, astringents, sweat, allergens, and excessive bathing). Avoid scratching (eczema is the "itch that rashes").

    b. Bathing: Should be less than 5 minutes in lukewarm water with a gentle bar soap and no washcloth or scrubbing. Skin should be patted dry (not rubbed) and followed by rapid application of an emollient ("soak and smear").

    c. To reduce the risk of secondary infection, consider diluted bleach baths once or twice a week (mix $\frac{1}{4}$ cup of bleach in full tub of lukewarm water and soak for 10 minutes, then rinse off with fresh water).

    d. Skin hydration: Frequent use of bland emollients with minimal water content (Vaseline or Aquaphor). Avoid lotions, as they have high water and low oil content, which worsens dry skin. Consider "wet dressings" in severe cases to increase absorption of medication and moisturization. After bathing, apply steroid ointment, then moisturizer, prior to clothing child in warm, damp pajamas. Follow with second layer of dry pajamas and remove after several hours or overnight.

    e. Oral antihistamines: There is little evidence that antihistamines improve skin lesions in atopic dermatitis. Nonsedating antihistamines can be used for environmental allergies and hives. Sedating antihistamines may be of transient benefit for sedation at bedtime.

    f. Treatment for inflammation:

        (1) **Mild disease: Topical steroids[22]** (Table 8.3): Low- and medium-potency steroid ointments once or twice daily for 7 days during a flare. Severe flares may require a high-potency steroid for a longer duration of therapy, followed by a taper to a low-potency

TABLE 8.3

RELATIVE POTENCIES OF TOPICAL CORTICOSTEROIDS

Class	Drug	Vehicle(s)	Strength (%)
I. VERY HIGH POTENCY	Augmented betamethasone dipropionate	Ointment	0.05
	Clobetasol propionate	Cream, foam, ointment	0.05
	Diflorasone diacetate	Ointment	0.05
	Halobetasol propionate	Cream, ointment	0.05
II. HIGH POTENCY	Amcinonide	Cream, lotion, ointment	0.1
	Augmented betamethasone dipropionate	Cream	0.05
	Betamethasone propionate	Cream, foam, ointment, solution	0.05
	Desoximetasone	Cream, ointment, gel	0.25 (C,O), 0.05 (G)
	Diflorasone diacetate	Cream	0.05
	Fluocinonide	Cream, gel, ointment, solution	0.05
	Halcinonide	Cream, ointment	0.1
	Mometasone furoate	Ointment	0.1
	Triamcinolone acetonide	Cream, ointment	0.5
III–IV. MEDIUM POTENCY	Betamethasone valerate	Cream, foam, lotion, ointment	0.1
	Clocortolone pivalate	Cream	0.1
	Desoximetasone	Cream	0.05
	Fluocinolone acetonide, Flurandrenolide	Cream, ointment	0.025 (C), 0.05 (O)
	Fluticasone propionate	Cream, ointment	0.05 (C), 0.005 (O)
	Triamcinolone acetonide, Mometasone furoate	Cream	0.1
V. LOWER-MEDIUM POTENCY	Hydrocortisone butyrate	Cream, ointment, solution	0.1
	Hydrocortisone probutate, Prednicarbate	Cream	0.1
	Hydrocortisone valerate	Cream, ointment	0.2
VI. LOW POTENCY	Alclometasone dipropionate	Cream, ointment	0.05
	Desonide	Cream, gel, foam, ointment	0.05
	Fluocinonide acetonide	Cream, solution	0.01
VII. LOWEST POTENCY	Dexamethasone	Cream	0.1
	Hydrocortisone	Cream, lotion	0.25
		Cream, ointment	0.5
		Cream, solution	1
	Hydrocortisone acetate	Cream, ointment	0.5–1

C, Cream; *G*, gel; *O*, ointment.

Modified from Eichenfield LF, Tom WL, Berger TG, et al. Guidelines of care for the management of atopic dermatitis. Section 2. Management and treatment of atopic dermatitis with topical therapies. *J Am Acad Dermatol.* 2014;71(1):116–132, Table 5.

steroid. Use of topical steroids in areas where skin is thin (groin, axilla, face, under breasts) should generally be avoided. Short durations of low-potency steroids may be used as needed in these areas. Ointments can be applied over steroid. Avoid overuse of steroids, as this can lead to chronic hyperpigmentation or hypopigmentation. Ensure that long-term eczema patients have frequent breaks from daily steroid use, such as week on and week off. Nonsteroidal topical agents may be used in sensitive areas; see below.

(2) **Moderate disease: Crisaborole** is a topical PDE4 inhibitor approved for mild to moderate eczema, with preliminary studies of the 2% ointment showing improvement in the majority of clinical signs and symptoms, particularly pruritus.[23] Topical calcineurin inhibitors (**tacrolimus ointment, pimecrolimus cream**) are second-line therapies that should only be used in consultation with a dermatologist due to FDA "black box" warnings on these medications for theoretical increased risk of cancer, although there are no data to confirm, and long-term safety studies are pending.[24,25]

(3) **Severe disease: Phototherapy** with narrowband UVB light is a treatment option for older children and adolescents. Low-dose **methotrexate** is a consideration before cyclosporine. For many dermatologists, low-dose oral methotrexate is the first oral option for severe disease unresponsive to aggressive topical therapy. Oral **cyclosporine** is only used in severe cases of older children and adolescents who have failed other treatments due to concern for renal compromise. **Dupilumab** is an IL-4 receptor α antagonist prescribed for refractory cases, starting at age six. A number of new agents, including topical and oral JAK and interleukin inhibitors, are in clinical trials.

5. **Complications[26]:**
   a. Bacterial superinfection: Usually *S. aureus*, sometimes group A *Streptococcus*. Depending on extent of infection, treat with topical mupirocin or systemic antibiotics.
   b. Eczema herpeticum superinfection with herpes simplex virus can cause severe systemic infection. Presents as vesiculopustular lesions with central punched-out erosions that do not respond to oral antibiotics. Must be treated systemically with acyclovir or valacyclovir. Should be evaluated by ophthalmologist if there is concern for eye involvement.
   c. Many children with eczema can develop decreased quality of life such as problems with sleeping due to discomfort and bullying due to scaring and disfigurement.

C. Papular Urticaria (Fig. 8.37, Color Plates)

1. **Pathogenesis:** Type IV hypersensitivity reaction to fleas, mosquitos, or bedbugs; also known as insect bite–induced hypersensitivity (IBIH)

2. **Clinical presentation/epidemiology:** Summarized by the SCRATCH principles[27]
   a. **S**ymmetric eruption: Exposed areas and scalp commonly affected. Spares diaper region, palms, and soles
   b. **C**luster: Appear as "meal clusters" or "breakfast, lunch, and dinner," which are linear or triangular groupings of lesions. Associated with bedbugs and fleas
   c. **R**over not required: A remote animal exposure or lack of pet at home does not rule out IBIH.
   d. **A**ge: Tends to peak by age 2. Not seen in newborn period. Most tend to develop tolerance by age 10.
   e. **T**arget lesions: Especially in darkly pigmented patients. **T**ime: Emphasize chronic nature of eruption and need for patience and watchful waiting.
   f. **C**onfused pediatrician/parent: Diagnosis often met with disbelief by parent and/or referring pediatrician
   g. **H**ousehold: Because of the nature of the hypersensitivity, usually only affects one family member in the household

3. **Management (3 Ps):**
   a. **P**revention: Wear protective clothing, use insect repellent when outside (AAP guidelines recommend up to 30% DEET- or 12% picaridin-containing repellents), launder bedding and mattress pads for bedbugs, and maximize flea control for pets.
   b. **P**ruritis control: Topical steroids or antihistamines may be of some benefit.
   c. **P**atience: Can be frustrating because of its persistent, recurrent nature. Assure patients that their symptoms will resolve and they will eventually develop tolerance.

D. Stevens-Johnson Syndrome and Toxic Epidermal Necrolysis

1. **Pathogenesis:**

Severe mucocutaneous reaction with partial to full epidermal necrosis due to keratinocyte necrosis. Stevens-Johnson syndrome (SJS) has less than 10% involvement of body surface area (BSA), whereas toxic epidermal necrolysis (TEN) has greater than 30% BSA involvement. BSA involvement between 10% to 30% is termed SJS/TEN. Overall mortality for pediatric patients is less than 8%. Commonly caused by medications initiated in previous 8 weeks, including sulfonamide antibiotics, lamotrigine, carbamazepine, phenobarbital, and several oncologic drugs. May also be caused by *Mycoplasma pneumonia* infections. Nearly one-third of cases have no identified trigger.

2. **Clinical presentation:**

Fever and flu-like prodrome for 1 to 3 days prior to mucocutaneous lesions. Ophthalmologic and oropharyngeal symptoms are often first sites of mucosal involvement. Urogenital mucosal involvement seen in two-thirds of patients may lead to urinary retention and have significant long-term anatomic changes in female patients. Epidermal lesions are described as exquisitely tender (with pain out of proportion), ill-defined, coalescing macules and patches of erythema with central purple-to-black areas. Lesions typically start on face and trunk then spread in a symmetric distribution sparing the scalp, palms, and soles. Bullae form with disease progression. Then, the epidermis sloughs with positive Nikolsky and Asboe-Hansen (lateral expansion of bullae with pressure) signs. Acute phase may last 8 to 12 days with reepithelization requiring up to four weeks.

3. **Diagnosis:**

Although usually not necessary, clinical diagnosis may be confirmed with a skin biopsy. Additional workup includes Complete blood count (CBC), comprehensive metabolic panel (CMP), erythrocyte sedimentation rate (ESR), C-reactive protein (CRP), bacterial and fungal cultures, *M. pneumoniae* PCR, and Chest x-ray (CXR).

4. **Treatment:**

Remove offending agent, supportive care, and close monitoring of all organ systems in the inpatient/ICU setting. There is controversy regarding IVIG and single dose of tumor necrosis factor alpha (TNF-alpha) inhibitor early in course. Systemic steroids probably should not be used.

5. **Complications:**

At risk for serious complications, including secondary bacterial infections (*Staphylococcus aureus* and *Pseudomonas aeruginosa*), septic shock, pneumonia, acute respiratory distress syndrome (ARDS), and epithelial necrosis of the GI tract. Most common complication in children is corneal scarring and dry eye.

VIII. NAIL DISORDERS[28]

1. Acquired nail disorders
   a. Paronychia: Red, tender, purulent swelling of proximal or lateral nail folds (eFigs. 8.3 and 8.4)
      (1) Acute form: Caused by bacterial invasion after trauma to cuticle
         (a) Clinical features: Exquisite pain, sudden swelling, and abscess formation around one nail
2. Congenital/hereditary nail disorders
   a. Isolated nail disorders (eFigs. 8.5 and 8.6)
      (1) Congenital nail dystrophy: Clubbing and spooning (koilonychia), may be autosomal dominant with no other anomalies

IX. DISORDERS OF PIGMENTATION[29]

1. Hyperpigmentation
   a. Congenital melanocytic nevi (CMN): Melanocytic nevi that are either present at birth or appear within the first few months of life in 1% to 3% of neonates[30]
      (1) Appearance: Black or tan with irregular borders and often dark terminal hairs
      (2) Risks:
         (a) Melanoma—At least 5% of large CMN greater than 20 cm with 70% of this cohort having cancerous transformation by 10 years

of age.[31] The presence of approximately 20 satellite nevi (smaller congenital nevi) also increases risk of melanoma.

   (b) Neurocutaneous melanosis—Children with large, multiple, satellite nevi, or lesions over the spine are at risk for leptomeningeal involvement with symptoms that may include hydrocephalus and seizures that may require evaluation by gadolinium contrast MRI.[32,33]

   b. Epidermal melanosis: Most lesions appear tan or light brown
      (1) Café-au-lait spots (eFig. 8.1): Discrete tan macules that appear at birth or during childhood in 10% to 20% of normal individuals, sizes vary from freckles to patches, may involve any site on skin. May be diagnostic marker for neurofibromatosis type 1 (≥6 lesions, each greater than 5 mm in diameter in prepubertal, or greater than 15 mm in postpubertal child) or other syndromes

2. Hypopigmentation and depigmentation
   a. Localized hypopigmentation
      (1) Hypopigmented macules (eFig. 8.7)
         (a) Epidemiology: 0.1% to 0.5% of normal newborns have a single hypopigmented macule, but it may be a marker for tuberous sclerosis as 70% to 90% of those affected have such macules on the trunk at birth.

3. Dyspigmentation
   a. Blaschkoid dyspigmentation[34]: Congenital hypopigmentation and hyperpigmentation along the lines of Blaschko (eFig. 8.8)
      (1) Patterns of hyper- or hypopigmentation: Whorl shape on trunk, V shape on the back, waves on the vertex scalp

X. RASHES OF UNKNOWN OR INFLAMMATORY ETIOLOGY

1. Pityriasis lichenoides et varioliformis acuta (PLEVA) and pityriasis lichenoides chronica (PLC)
   a. **Pathogenesis:** Spectrum of rare disorders known as the "pityriasis lichenoides" separated into acute and chronic forms. Pathogenesis theorized to involve T-cell dyscrasia and abnormal immune response to viral, bacterial, or protozoal infection
   b. **Presentation:** Typically affects children and young adults. PLEVA is an acute eruption of multiple erythematous macules, papules, and/or vesicles, which can become hemorrhagic or necrotic, affecting any cutaneous surface but without mucosal involvement. Lesions resolve over a few weeks, but new lesions develop as prior lesions fade. The rash may be asymptomatic, pruritic, or painful and last from a few weeks to 2 years. Some patients can go on to develop PLC, which is described as a more gradual development of red-brown papules that relapses and remits over months to years. In both conditions, hyper- or hypopigmentation commonly persists after resolution of lesions, but scarring may or may not occur.

   c. **Diagnosis:** Skin biopsy is required to confirm diagnosis with typical histopathologic findings. Immunohistochemistry may reveal CD8+ T-cell inflammatory infiltrate.

   d. **Treatment:** Usually benign and self-limiting and does not require treatment. If lesions are widespread, debilitating, or scarring, first-line therapies include systemic antibiotics and topical corticosteroids. Limited treatment data exist due to rarity of disorder and lack of clinical trials. Resistant cases may respond to phototherapy.

2. Confluent and reticulated papillomatosis (CARP) (Fig. 8.38, Color Plates)

   a. **Pathogenesis:** Unknown, but possibly related to disordered keratinization resulting in hyperproliferation. Reports also link CARP to *Malassezia* infection

   b. **Presentation:** Hyperpigmented, scaly macules and/or papillomatous papules that coalesce into patches in a reticular pattern. Lesions are typically most prominent in the intermammary, interscapular, neck, and axillary regions, and spare the mucosa. The rash can be mildly pruritic but is usually asymptomatic and can persist for up to 3 years if not treated.

   c. **Diagnosis:** Clinical diagnosis, but KOH scraping to rule out tinea may be necessary. Skin biopsy can be helpful, but there are no diagnostic histologic findings for CARP.

   d. **Treatment:** Systemic antibiotic therapy with doxycycline or minocycline is the mainstay of treatment. Benefits are attributed to the antiinflammatory properties, rather than antibacterial, as no specific bacterial cause has been identified.

3. Giannoti-Crosti syndrome, or popular acrodermatitis of childhood

   a. **Pathogenesis:** Possibly related to viral illness such as Epstein-Barr virus (most common trigger in the United States) or hepatitis B (most common trigger in Europe). There may be an association with IgE-mediated immunity and atopy.

   b. **Presentation:** Occurs primarily in children younger than 5 years old. Acute eruption of papules and vesicles involving the extensor surfaces of arms, legs, and feet, with involvement of face and buttocks. The trunk is relatively spared, and the mucosa is not involved. The lesions are flat-topped and typically either skin colored, pink, or brown. Symptoms of pruritis are variable. Occasionally, hemorrhagic lesions can occur, and Koebner phenomenon has been observed. Patients may experience concomitant malaise, fever, and diarrhea.

   c. **Diagnosis:** Clinical diagnosis, but skin biopsy may be used to exclude other diagnoses

   d. **Treatment:** Self-limited disease that resolves within 2 months. Antipruritic topical creams may be used for symptomatic relief but do not alter duration of disease.

H. Autoimmune Bullous Diseases: See Section XI, Online Content.

REFERENCES

A complete list of references can be found online.

Chapter 9

Development, Behavior, and Developmental Disability

Brenna M. Beck, MD, MEd and Christle Nwora, MD

🌐 See additional content online.

I. DEVELOPMENTAL DEFINITIONS[1,2]

A. Developmental Streams

1. **Gross motor skills:** Descriptions of posture and locomotion that involve the use of large proximal core muscle groups in the upper and lower extremities. Examples of gross motor skills include walking, running, and jumping.
2. **Fine motor skills:** Upper extremity distal muscle coordination and hand manipulative abilities and hand-eye coordination. Examples of fine motor skills include picking up small objects between the thumb and index finger (pincer grasp).
3. **Visual-motor problem-solving skills:** Integrated set of fine motor, eye-hand coordination, and cognitive skills. These require an intact motor substrate and a given level of nonverbal cognitive ability. Examples of visual-motor problem-solving skills include solving a puzzle or drawing shapes.
4. **Language:** The ability to understand and communicate with another person. This is the best predictor of intellectual performance in the absence of a communication disorder or significant hearing loss.
5. **Personal-social skills:** Communicative in origin; represent the cumulative use of language comprehension and expression and problem-solving skills to interact with others. Examples may include reciprocal play, sharing, and eye contact.
6. **Adaptive skills:** Skills concerned with self-help or activities of daily living. Examples of adaptative skills include toileting and brushing teeth.

B. Developmental Quotient

1. **A calculation that reflects the rate of development** in any given stream; represents the percentage of normal development present at the time of testing

$$\text{Developmental quotient (DQ)} = \frac{\text{Developmental age (DA)}}{\text{Chronological age (CA)}} \times 100\%$$

2. **Two separate developmental assessments** over time are more predictive of later abilities than a single assessment.[2]

3. In contrast to developmental quotient (DQ), intelligence quotient (IQ) **has greater statistical reliability and validity.** Biases may occur in IQ test results, which may be attributable to culture and environment.

C. Abnormal Development

1. **Delay:** Performance significantly below average in a given area of development. May occur in a single stream or several streams ("global developmental delay")

2. **Deviancy:** Atypical development within a single stream, such as developmental milestones occurring out of sequence. Deviancy does not necessarily imply abnormality but should alert one to the possibility that problems may exist. *Example*: An infant who rolls at an early age may have abnormally increased tone.

3. **Dissociation:** A substantial difference in the rate of development between two or more streams. *Example*: Increased motor delay relative to cognition seen in some children with cerebral palsy (CP)

4. **Two separate developmental assessments** over time are more predictive of later abilities than a single assessment.

II. GUIDELINES FOR NORMAL DEVELOPMENT AND BEHAVIOR

A. Developmental Milestones

Developmental assessment is based on the premise that milestone acquisition occurs at a specific rate in an orderly and sequential manner: See Table 9.1

B. Age-Appropriate Behavioral Issues in Infancy and Early Childhood: See Table 9.2

III. DEVELOPMENTAL SCREENING AND EVALUATION OF DEVELOPMENTAL DISORDERS

A. Developmental Screening and Screening Guidelines

1. **Developmental *surveillance* should be included in every well child visit, and any concerns should be addressed immediately with formal screening.** This includes direct observation of the child and eliciting and attending to the parent's concerns.

2. **Standardized developmental *screening* should be administered at 9-month, 18-month, and 30-month well child visits,** in the absence of developmental concerns. If a 30-month visit is not possible, this screening can be done at the 24-month visit.

3. See full American Academy of Pediatrics (AAP) guideline for developmental screening algorithm.[3]

B. Commonly Used Developmental Screening and Assessment Tools: See Table 9.3

C. Identification of Developmental "Red Flags": See Table 9.4

D. Evaluation of Abnormal Development

1. Referral to developmental and appropriate specialists

2. Referral to early intervention services for children aged 0 to 3 years (see Section V)

TABLE 9.1
DEVELOPMENTAL MILESTONES

Age	Social/Emotional Milestones	Language/Communication Milestones	Cognitive Milestones (learning, thinking, problem-solving)	Movement/Physical Development Milestones
2 months	Calms down when spoken to or picked up; looks at your face; seems happy to see you when you walk up to her; smiles when you talk to or smile at her	Makes sounds other than crying; reacts to loud sounds	Watches you as you move; looks at a toy for several seconds	Holds head up while on tummy; Moves both arms and both legs; Opens hands briefly
4 months	Smiles on his own to get your attention; chuckles (not yet a full laugh) when you try to make him laugh; looks at you, moves, or makes sounds to get or keep your attention	Makes cooing sounds ("ooo", "aahh"); makes sounds back when you talk to him; turns head toward the sound of your voice	If hungry, opens mouth when he sees breast or bottle; looks at her hands with interest	Holds head steady without support when you are holding him; holds a toy when you put it in his hand; uses his arm to swing at toys; brings hands to mouth; pushes up onto elbows-forearms when on tummy
6 months	Knows familiar people; likes to look at self in a mirror; laughs	Takes turns making sounds with you; blows "raspberries" (sticks tongue out and blows); makes squealing noises	Puts things in her mouth to explore them; reaches to grab a toy she wants; closes lips to show she doesn't want more food	Rolls from tummy to back; ushes up with straight arms when on tummy; leans on hands to support herself when sitting
9 months	Is shy, clingy, or fearful around strangers; shows several facial expressions, like happy, sad, angry, and surprised; looks when you call her name; reacts when you leave (looks, reaches for you, or cries); smiles or laughs when you play peek-a-boo	Makes a lot of different sounds like "mamamama" and "babababa"; lifts arms up to be picked up	Looks for objects when dropped out of sight (like his spoon or toy); bangs two things together	Gets to a sitting position by herself; moves things from one hand to her other hand; uses fingers to "rake" food towards himself; sits without support

12 months	Plays games with you, like pat-a-cake	Waves "bye-bye"; calls a parent "mama" or "dada" or another special name; understands "no" (pauses briefly or stops when you say it)	Puts something in a container, like a block in a cup; looks for things he sees you hide, like a toy under a blanket	Pulls up to stand; walks, holding on to furniture; drinks from a cup without a lid, as you hold it; picks things up between thumb and pointer finger, like small bits of food
15 months	Copies other children while playing, like taking toys out of a container when another child does; shows you an object she likes; claps when excited; hugs stuffed doll or other toy; shows you affection (hugs, cuddles, or kisses you)	Tries to say one or two words besides "mama" or "dada," like "ba" for ball or "da" for dog; looks at a familiar object when you name it; follows directions given with both a gesture and words (for example, he gives you a toy when you hold out your hand and say, "Give me the toy."); points to ask for something or to get help	Tries to use things the right way, like a phone, cup, or book; stacks at least two small objects, like blocks	Takes a few steps on his own; uses fingers to feed herself some food
18 months	Moves away from you, but looks to make sure you are close by; points to show you something interesting; puts hands out for you to wash them; looks at a few pages in a book with you; helps you dress him by pushing arm through sleeve or lifting up foot	Tries to say three or more words besides "mama" or "dada"; follows one-step directions without any gestures, like giving you the toy when you say, "Give it to me."	Copies you doing chores, like sweeping with a broom; plays with toys in a simple way, like pushing a toy care	Walks without holding on to anyone or anything; scribbles; drinks from a cup without a lid and may spill sometimes; feeds himself with his fingers; tries to use a spoon; climbs on and off a couch or chair without help

Continued

9

TABLE 9.1

DEVELOPMENTAL MILESTONES—CONT'D

Age	Social/Emotional Milestones	Language/Communication Milestones	Cognitive Milestones (learning, thinking, problem-solving)	Movement/Physical Development Milestones
24 months	Notices when others are hurt or upset, like pausing or looking sad when someone is crying; looks at your face to see how to react in a new situation	Points to things in a book when you ask, like "Where is the bear?"; says at least two words together, like "More milk."; points to at least two body parts when you ask him to show you; uses more gestures than just waving and pointing, like blowing a kiss or nodding yes	Holds something in one hand while using the other hand (for example, holding a container and taking the lid off); tries to use switches, knobs, or buttons on a toy; plays with more than one toy at the same time, like putting toy food on a toy plate	Kicks a ball; runs; walks (not climbs) up a few stairs with or without help; eats with a spoon
30 months	Plays next to other children and sometimes plays with them; shows you what she can do by saying, "Look at me!"; follows simple routines when told, like helping to pick up toys when you say, "It's clean-up time."	Says about 50 words; says two or more words together, with one action word, like "Doggie run"; names things in a book when you point and ask, "What is this?"; says words liek "I," "me," or "we"	Uses things to pretend, like feeding a block to a doll as if it were food; shows simple problem-solving skills, like standing on a small stool to reach something; follows two-step instructions like "Put the toy down and close the door."; shows he knows at least one color, like pointing to a red crayon when you ask, "Which one is red?"	Uses hands to twist things, like turning doorknobs or unscrewing lids; takes some clothes off by himself, like loose pants or an open jacket; jumps off the ground with both feet; turns book pages, one at a time, when you read to her

3 years	Calms down within within 10 minutes after you leave her, like at a childcare drop off; notices other children and joins them to play	Talks with you in conversation using at least two back-and-forth exchanges; asks "who," "what," "where," or "why" questions, like "Where is mommy/daddy?"; says what action is happening in a picture or book when asked, like "running," "eating," or "playing"; says first name, when asked; talks well enough for others to understand, most of the time	Draws a circle, when you show him how; avoids touching hot objects, like a stove, when you warn her	Strings items together, like large beads or macaroni; puts on some clothes by himself, like loose pants or a jacket; uses a fork
4 years	Pretends to be something else during play (teacher, superhero, dog); asks to go play with children if none are around, like "Can I play with Alex?"; comforts others who are hurt or sad, like hugging a crying friend; avoids danger, like not jumping from tall heights at the playground; likes to be a "helper"; changes behavior based on where she is (place of worship, library, playground)	Says sentences with four or more words; says some ewords from a song, story, or nursery rhyme; talks about at least one thing that happened during her day, like "I played soccer."; answers simple questions like "what is a coat for?" or "What is a crayong for?"	Names a few colors of items; tells what comes next in a well-known story; draws a person with three or more body parts	Catches a large ball most of the time; serves herself food or pours water, with adult supervision; unbuttons some buttons; holds crayon or pencil between fingers and thumb (not a fist)

Continued

9

TABLE 9.1

DEVELOPMENTAL MILESTONES—CONT'D

Age	Social/Emotional Milestones	Language/Communication Milestones	Cognitive Milestones (learning, thinking, problem-solving)	Movement/Physical Development Milestones
5 years	Follows rules or takes turns when playing games with other children; sings, dances, or acts for you; does simple chores at home, like matching socks or clearing the table after eating	Tells a story she heard or made up with at least two events (for example, a cat was stuck in a tree and a firefighter saved it); answers simple questions about a book or story after you read or tell it to him; keeps a conversation going with more than three back-and-forth exchanges; uses or recognizes simple rhymes (bat-cat, ball-tall)	Counts to 10; names some numbers between 1 and 5 when you point to them; uses words about time, like "yesterday," "tomorrow," "morning," or "night"; pays attention for 5 to 10 minutes during activities (for example, making arts and crafts – but screen time does not count); writes some letters in her name; names some letters when you point to them	Buttons some buttons; hops on one foot

CDC Developmental Milestones. National Center on Birth Defects and Developmental Disabilities, Centers for Disease Control and Prevention. Last Reviewed: Dec 29, 2022. Available at cdc.gov/ncddd/actearly/milestones/index.html. Jennifer M. Zubler, Lisa D. Wiggins, Michelle M. Macias, Toni M. Whitaker, Judith S. Shaw, Jane K. Squires, Julie A. Pajek, Rebecca B. Wolf, Karnesha S. Slaughter, Amber S. Broughton, Krysta L. Gerndt, Bethany J. Mlodoch, Paul H. Lipkin; Evidence-Informed Milestones for Developmental Surveillance Tools. Pediatrics March 2022; 149 (3): e2021052138. 10.1542/peds.2021-052138.

TABLE 9.2

AGE-APPROPRIATE BEHAVIORAL ISSUES IN INFANCY AND EARLY CHILDHOOD

Age	Behavioral Issue	Symptoms	Guidance
1—3 months	Colic	Paroxysms of fussiness/crying, ≥3 per day, ≥3 days/week, may pull knees up to chest, pass flatus	Crying usually peaks at 6 weeks and resolves by 3—4 months. Prevent overstimulation; swaddle infant; use white noise, swing, or car rides to soothe. Avoid medication and formula changes. Encourage breaks for the primary caregiver.
3—4 months	Trained night feeding	Night awakening	Comfort quietly, avoid reinforcing behavior (i.e., avoid night feeds). Do not play at night. Introducing cereal or solid food does not reduce awakening. Develop a consistent bedtime routine. Place baby in bed while drowsy and not fully asleep.
9 months	Stranger anxiety/separation anxiety	Distress when separated from parent or approached by a stranger	Use a transitional object (e.g., special toy, blanket). Use routine or ritual to separate from parent. May continue until 24 months but can reduce in intensity
	Developmental night waking	Separation anxiety at night	Keep lights off. Avoid picking child up or feeding. May reassure verbally at regular intervals or place a transitional object in crib
12 months	Aggression	Biting, hitting, kicking in frustration	Say "no" with negative facial cues. Begin time out (1 minute/year of age). No eye contact or interaction, place in a nonstimulating location. May restrain child gently until cooperation is achieved
	Need for limit setting	Exploration of environment, danger of injury	Avoid punishing exploration or poor judgment. Emphasize childproofing and distraction.
18 months	Temper tantrums	Occur with frustration, attention-seeking rage, negativity/refusal	Try to determine cause, react appropriately (i.e., help child who is frustrated, ignore attention-seeking behavior). Make sure child is in a safe location.

Continued

TABLE 9.2

AGE-APPROPRIATE BEHAVIORAL ISSUES IN INFANCY AND EARLY CHILDHOOD—CONT'D

Age	Behavioral Issue	Symptoms	Guidance
24 months	Toilet training	Child needs to demonstrate readiness: shows interest, neurologic maturity (i.e., recognizes urge to urinate or defecate), ability to walk to bathroom and undress self, desire to please/imitate parents, increasing periods of daytime dryness	Age range for toilet training is usually 2–4 years. Give guidance early; may introduce potty seat but avoid pressure or punishment for accidents. Wait until the child is ready. Expect some periods of regression, especially with stressors.
24–36 months	New sibling	Regression, aggressive behavior	Allow for special time with parent, 10–20 min daily of one-on-one time exclusively devoted to the older sibling(s). Child chooses activity with parent. No interruptions. May not be taken away as punishment
36 months	Nightmares	Awakens crying, may or may not complain of bad dream	Reassure child, explain that he or she had a bad dream. Leave bedroom door open, use a nightlight, demonstrate there are no monsters under the bed. Discuss dream the following day. Avoid scary movies or television shows.
	Night terrors	Agitation, screaming 1–2 hours after going to bed. Child may have eyes open but not respond to parent. May occur at same time each night	May be familial, not volitional. *Prevention:* For several nights, awaken child 15 min before terrors typically occur. Avoid overtiredness. *Acute:* Be calm; speak in soft, soothing, repetitive tones; help child return to sleep. Protect child against injury.

From Dixon SD, Stein MT. *Encounters With Children: Pediatric Behavior and Development.* Mosby; 2000.

3. Medical evaluation as outlined in Tables 9.5 through 9.7
4. Genetic evaluation (Table 9.8) is warranted for all children with developmental delay or intellectual disability (ID) if the cause is not known (e.g., previous traumatic brain injury or neurologic insult).

TABLE 9.3

DEVELOPMENTAL SCREENING TESTS BY DIAGNOSIS

Diagnosis Evaluated	Screening Test	Age	Completed by	Comments	Weblink
Cognitive and motor development	Ages and Stages Questionnaire (ASQ)	4–60 months	Parent	Increased time efficiency (can fill out while waiting) Documents milestones that are difficult to assess in the office	https://www.agesandstages.com
Developmental and behavioral problems	Parents' Evaluation of Developmental Status (PEDS)	0–8 years	Parent	May also be useful as a surveillance tool	https://www.pedstest.com
Language, problem-solving development	Capute Scales: Clinical Linguistic and Auditory Milestone Scale (CLAMS), Clinical Adaptive Test (CAT)	3–36 months	Clinician	Give quantitative DQs for language (CLAMS) and visual-motor/problem-solving (CAT) abilities	https://brookespublishing.com/product/the-capute-scales/
Autism spectrum disorders	Modified Checklist for Autism in Toddlers, Revised with Follow-Up (M-CHAT-R/F)	16–30 months	Parent	Positive screens require clinician follow-up	https://mchatscreen.com/
	Communication and Symbolic Behavior Scales and Developmental Profile (CSBS DP; Infant-Toddler Checklist)	6–24 months	Parent	The Infant Toddler Checklist is a one-page questionnaire that is part of a larger standardized screening tool (CSBS DP) Can be used in patients as young as 6 months	https://www.brookespublishing.com/checklist.pdf
	Childhood Autism Screening Test (CAST)	4–11 years	Parent	Only screening tool evaluated in preschool population	https://www.autismresearchcentre.com/tests/childhood-autism-spectrum-test-cast/

Modified from American Academy of Pediatrics. Identifying infants and young children with developmental disorders in the medical home: an algorithm for developmental surveillance and screening. *Pediatrics.* 2006;118:405–420; American Academy of Pediatrics. Identification and evaluation of children with autism spectrum disorders. *Pediatrics.* 2007;120:1183–1215; Robins DL, Casagrande K, Barton M, et al. Validation of the Modified Checklist for Autism in Toddlers, Revised with Follow-up (M-CHAT-R/F). *Pediatrics.* 2014;133:37–45.

9

TABLE 9.4

DEVELOPMENTAL "RED FLAGS"

Age of Patient	"Red Flag" Symptom
Any age	Loss of previously obtained developmental skills
	Parental or professional concerns about vision, including: vision fixing, following an object, or a confirmed visual impairment
	Hearing loss
	Persistently low muscle tone or floppiness
	Asymmetry of movements or other features suggestive of cerebral palsy, such as increased muscle tone
	Head circumference above the 99.6th percentile, below 0.4th percentile, or has crossed two major percentile lines (up or down)
5 months (corrected for gestation)	Not able to hold object placed in hand
6 months (corrected for gestation)	Not reaching for objects
12 months	Unable to sit unsupported
18 months	Not walking in male patients
	Not pointing at objects to share interest with others
24 months	Not walking in female patients
30 months and older	Unable to run
	Persistent toe walking

From Bellman M, Byrne O, Sege R. Developmental assessment of children. *BMJ.* 2013;346:31–36.

TABLE 9.5

DEVELOPMENTAL EVALUATION: PERTINENT HISTORY AND PHYSICAL

Prenatal and birth history	Prenatal genetic screening
	Perception of fetal movement
	Pregnancy complications
	Toxins/teratogens
	Gestational age
	Birthweight
	Days in hospital/NICU admission
	Newborn screen results
Past medical problems	Trauma
	Infection
	Medication
Developmental history	Timing of milestone achievement
	Delayed skills
	Loss of skills (regression)
Behavioral history	Social skills
	Eye contact
	Affection
	Hyperactivity, impulsivity, inattention, distractibility
	Self-regulation
	Perseveration
	Worries/avoidance
	Stereotypies, peculiar habits

TABLE 9.5

DEVELOPMENTAL EVALUATION: PERTINENT HISTORY AND PHYSICAL—CONT'D

Educational history	Need for special services
	Grade retention
	Established educational plans
Family history	History of developmental disabilities, ADHD, seizures, tics, stillbirths, neonatal death, congenital malformations, mental illness, or recurrent miscarriages
	Family members who were late talkers or walkers
	Family member school performance
	Family pedigree (see Chapter 13)
General exam	Height, weight, and head circumference
	Dysmorphic features or features with distinctive appearance
	Cardiac murmurs
	Midline defects
	Hepatosplenomegaly
	Skin exam
Age-directed neuro exam	Cranial nerves
	Tone and strength
	Postural reactions (eTable 9.1)
	Functional abilities
	Reflexes (including primitive reflexes for infants [Table 9.6])
In-clinic activities/tests	Goodenough—Harris Draw-a-Person Test
	Gesell figures (eFig. 9.1): Ask the child to copy various shapes.
	Gesell block skills (eFig. 9.2): Ask the child to reproduce block structures as built by the examiner.

TABLE 9.6

PRIMITIVE REFLEXES

Primitive Reflexes	Elicitation	Response	Timing
Moro reflex ("embrace" response) of fingers, wrists, and elbows	*Supine:* Sudden neck extension; allow head to fall back about 3 cm	Extension, adduction, and then abduction of UEs, with semiflexion	Present at birth; disappears by 3—6 months
Galant reflex (GR)	*Prone suspension:* Stroking paravertebral area from thoracic to sacral region	Produces truncal incurvature with concavity toward stimulated side	Present at birth; disappears by 2—6 months
Asymmetrical tonic neck reflex (ATNR, "fencer" response)	*Supine:* Rotate head laterally about 45—90 degrees	Relative extension of limbs on chin side and flexion on occiput side	Present at birth; disappears by 4—9 months

Continued

TABLE 9.6

PRIMITIVE REFLEXES—CONT'D

Primitive Reflexes	Elicitation	Response	Timing
Symmetrical tonic neck reflex (STNR, "cat" reflex)	*Sitting:* Head extension/flexion	Extension of UEs and flexion of LEs/flexion of UEs and LE extension	Appears at 5 months; not present in most normal children; disappears by 8—9 months
Tonic labyrinthine supine (TLS)	*Supine:* Extension of the neck (alters relation of the labyrinths)	Tonic extension of trunk and LEs, shoulder retraction and adduction, usually with elbow flexion	Present at birth; disappears by 6—9 months
Tonic labyrinthine prone (TLP)	*Prone:* Flexion of the neck	Active flexion of trunk with protraction of shoulders	Present at birth; disappears by 6—9 months
Positive support reflex (PSR)	*Vertical suspension:* Bouncing hallucal areas on firm surface	*Neonatal:* momentary LE extension followed by flexion *Mature:* extension of LEs and support of body weight	Present at birth; disappears by 2—4 months Appears by 6 months
Stepping reflex (SR, walking reflex)	*Vertical suspension:* Hallucal stimulation	Stepping gait	Disappears by 2—3 months
Crossed extension reflex (CER)	*Prone:* Hallucal stimulation of LE in full extension	Initial flexion, adduction, then extension of contralateral limb	Present at birth; disappears by 9 months
Plantar grasp	Stimulation of hallucal areas	Plantar flexion grasp	Present at birth; disappears by 9 months
Palmar grasp	Stimulation of palm	Palmar grasp	Present at birth; disappears by 9 months
Lower extremity placing (LEP)	*Vertical suspension:* Rubbing tibia or dorsum of foot against edge of tabletop	Initial flexion, then extension, then placing of LE on tabletop	Appears at 1 day
Upper extremity placing (UEP)	Rubbing lateral surface of forearm along edge of tabletop from elbow to wrist to dorsal hand	Flexion, extension, then placing of hand on tabletop	Appears at 3 months
Downward thrust (DT)	*Vertical suspension:* Thrusting LEs downward	Full extension of LEs	Appears at 3 months

LE, Lower extremity; *UE,* upper extremity.

TABLE 9.7

DEVELOPMENTAL EVALUATION: INITIAL LABS AND OTHER STUDIES

Hearing screening	Formal audiologic testing is indicated for all children with global developmental delay or any delay in communication or language
Neuroimaging	Consider if abnormal neurologic exam, concern about head circumference growth velocity, or global developmental delay present
Electroencephalogram	Consider if history of or concern for seizure disorder
Laboratory studies	Consider CBC, CMP, lead level, CK, TSH based on history and exam Confirm newborn screen results

CBC, Complete blood count; *CK*, creatine kinase; *CMP*, complete metabolic panel; *TSH*, thyroid stimulating hormone.

TABLE 9.8

DEVELOPMENTAL EVALUATION: GENETIC WORKUP

Chromosomal microarray (CMA)	Considered first-tier diagnostic test in *all* children with GDD/ID[33]
Fragile X testing	Should be performed in all boys *and* girls with GDD/ID of unknown cause. Of boys with GDD/ID of unknown cause, 2%—3% will have fragile X syndrome, as will 1%—2% of girls.
Testing for X-linked conditions	Consider genetic testing for X-linked genes in boys with GDD/ID after negative CMA and negative fragile X testing. Should be specifically in those patients whose pedigree is suggestive of an X-linked condition

The tests discussed above do not require referral to a genetic specialist and can be ordered by the patient's pediatrician as a part of the evaluation of global developmental delay/intellectual disability (GDD/ID). If unrevealing and severe DD/ID present, refer to genetic specialist for consideration of additional testing such as metabolic testing or whole exome sequencing.

From Moeschler JB, Shevell M. Comprehensive evaluation of the child with intellectual disability or global developmental delays. *Pediatrics*. 2014;134(3):e903—e918.

IV. SPECIFIC DISORDERS OF DEVELOPMENT

A. Overview

1. Mental and/or physical impairment(s) that cause significant limitations in functioning

2. **Developmental diagnosis** is a functional description; identification of an etiology is important to further inform treatment, prognosis, comorbidities, and future risk.

3. Individuals with disabilities represent 12%—30% of the US population. They are a heterogenous group that unfortunately are four times more likely to report fair to poor health when compared to those without a disability. Disability is categorized as a vulnerable population with health disparities.[4-6]

   a. Many children with disabilities also hold other marginalized identities, which means that providers must be cognizant of resource gaps and be intentional in addressing disparities.[7,8]

4. School- and home-based interventions for developmental disorders (see Section V)

B. Intellectual Disability (ID)

1. **Definition and epidemiology**
   a. Deficits in general cognitive and intellectual (problem-solving) and adaptive abilities
   b. Affects approximately 1% of population[9]
   c. Some communities prefer person-centered language (person with a disability), and others prefer identity-first language (disabled person). Adapt the use to the individual and family's preference.

2. **Clinical presentation**
   a. Delay in milestones (motor, language, social)
   b. Academic difficulty
   c. Identifiable features of known associated genetic syndrome (e.g., trisomy 21, fragile X, Rett syndrome)

3. **Diagnosis**
   a. Diagnostic criteria: (1) deficits in cognitive functioning, (2) deficits in adaptive functioning, (3) onset of these deficits during developmental period (before 18 years of age)
   b. Deficits in adaptive functioning must be in one or more domains of activities of daily living (ADLs).
   c. ID is further categorized as mild, moderate, severe, or profound (eTable 9.2).

4. **Interventions/treatment**
   Support, employment, and recreational programs through resources such as are available through local programs: The Arc (https://www.thearc.org), Parents' Place (https://www.ppmd.org/), or the Parent Center Hub (https://www.parentcenterhub.org)

C. Communication Disorders

1. **Definition**
   a. Deficits in communication, language, or speech
   b. Important to note that children who learn multiple languages may present with language differences that are not necessarily a language disorder[10,11]
   c. Can be subdivided into:
      (1) Receptive/expressive language disorder
      (2) Speech sound disorder
      (3) Childhood-onset fluency disorder (stuttering)
      (4) Social pragmatic communication disorder
   d. Differential diagnosis includes ID, hearing loss, significant motor impairment, or severe mental health difficulties.

2. **Interventions/treatment**
   a. Referrals to speech-language pathology (SLP), audiology

D. Learning Disability[9]

1. **Definition**
   A heterogenous group of deficits in an individual's ability to perceive and process information efficiently and accurately

2. **Diagnosis**
    a. Achievement on standardized tests that is substantially below expected for age, schooling and level of intelligence in one or more of the following areas: basic reading skills, reading comprehension, reading fluency skills, oral expression, listening comprehension, written expression, mathematic calculation, and mathematic problem solving
    b. There is no alternative diagnosis such as sensory impairment or ID
3. **Intervention/treatment**
    a. School-based services through IEP and 504 plans tailored to specific learning needs
    b. It is important to address the stigma associated with labeling a child as having a learning disability. This stigma may prevent families from engaging in care that can benefit the child.
    c. Black, non-Hispanic, and Hispanic children and children from other marginalized racial populations are less likely to be identified as having a learning disability than White, non-Hispanic children and are comparatively underrepresented in special education.[12] Ensure that all families know the resources that are available to them.
    d. Resources for families
        (1) https://www.idaamerica.org/
        (2) https://www.ncld.org/
        (3) International Dyslexia Association https://dyslexiaida.org/
        (4) https://espanol.ninds.nih.gov/es/trastornos/problemas-de-aprendizaje
        (5) https://catalog.ninds.nih.gov/

E. Cerebral Palsy (CP)

1. **Definition and epidemiology**
    a. A group of disorders of the development of movement and posture attributed to *nonprogressive* disturbances that occurred in the developing fetal or infant brain[13,14]
    b. Prevalence: 2 to 3/1000 live births[2]
    c. Disparities: Black children have an increase in prevalence of CP compared to White children, and this disparity was found only in children with greater functional limitations.[4] Following adjustment of socioeconomic status and perinatal factors, there was a paradoxical decreased risk of CP in Black children, indicating the influence of these factors on CP and their independent association in pregnant Black women.
2. **Clinical presentation**
    a. Delayed motor development, abnormal tone, atypical postures, persistent primitive reflexes past 6 months
    b. History of known or suspected brain injury
    c. Manifestations may change with brain maturation and development.
3. **Diagnosis**
    a. Classification is based on physiologic and topographic characteristics as well as severity (Table 9.9).[15]

TABLE 9.9

CLINICAL CLASSIFICATION OF CEREBRAL PALSY[15]

Type	Pattern of Involvement
I. SPASTIC (INCREASED TONE, CLASPED KNIFE, CLONUS, FURTHER CLASSIFIED BY DISTRIBUTION)	
Bilateral spasticity	Diplegia (legs primarily affected)
	Quadriplegia (all four extremities impaired; legs worse than arms)
Unilateral spasticity	Hemiplegia (ipsilateral arm and leg; arm worse than leg)
	Monoplegia (one extremity, usually upper; probably reflects a mild hemiplegia)
II. DYSKINETIC (LEAD-PIPE OR CANDLE-WAX RIGIDITY, VARIABLE TONE, ± CLONUS)	
Dystonic	Complex disorders often reflecting basal ganglia pathology, resulting in
Choreoathetoid	involuntary and uncontrolled movements. May be focal or generalized.
III. OTHER	
Ataxic	Movement and tone disorders often reflecting cerebellar origin
Hypotonic	Usually related to diffuse, often severe cerebral and/or cerebellar cortical dysfunction. May be axial, appendicular, or generalized
Rigid	Muscle contraction, seen in rare neurogenetic diseases

From Graham HK, Rosenbaum P, et al. Cerebral palsy. *Nat Rev Disease Primers.* 2016;2(15082).

   b. Brain imaging should be obtained with MRI; abnormal in 70%–90% of individuals with CP[16]

4. **Interventions/Treatment**

   a. Baseline and ongoing medical subspecialty care, including developmental pediatrics, neurology, orthopedics, and neurosurgery

   b. Interdisciplinary team involvement (see Section V)

   c. Equipment to promote mobility and communication, including augmentative and alternative communication—any form of communication other than oral speech (eTable 9.3)[17]

      (1) Augmentative communication: Communication supports/methods used by individuals who have some speech but limited use of their speech

      (2) Alternative communication: Communication supports/methods used by individuals who have no speech

   d. Pharmacotherapy for spasticity (e.g., botulinum toxin injections, baclofen), dyskinesia, hypersalivation (e.g., glycopyrrolate, scopolamine patch)[47]

   e. In carefully selected patients: intrathecal baclofen, selective dorsal rhizotomy, deep brain stimulation[48]

F. Autism Spectrum Disorder (ASD)

1. **Definitions and epidemiology**

   a. Encompasses previously named disorders of autistic disorder (autism), Asperger syndrome, childhood disintegrative disorder, and pervasive developmental disorder not otherwise specified (PDD-NOS)

    b. Increasing prevalence; 1 in 54 children in the United States had ASD in 2018[18,19]

    c. Almost five times more common in males than females[18]

2. **Screening**

    a. Formal screening for ASD recommended at the 18- and 24-month visits (see AAP practice guidelines for more detailed recommendations)[20]

    b. Recommendations upheld by the AAP despite a U.S. Preventive Services Task Force (USPSTF) draft recommendation statement citing insufficient evidence for screening.[21,22]

    c. Evaluate using screening tools such as **Modified Checklist for Autism in Toddlers (M-CHAT-R/F)** and **Childhood Autism Screening Test (CAST)** (see Table 9.3).

    d. There are racial and ethnic differences in the evaluation and diagnoses of ASD. Black and Hispanic children with ASD are noted to receive evaluations later than White children with ASD.[23]

3. **Diagnosis**

    a. Symptoms vary by age, developmental level, language ability, and supports in place.

    b. Diagnostic criteria include[9]:

        (1) **Impaired social communication and interaction**
           Examples: Lack of joint attention behaviors (e.g., showing toys, pointing for showing), diminished eye contact, no sharing of emotions, lack of imitation

        (2) **Restricted repetitive patterns of behavior, interests, or activities**
           Examples: Simple motor stereotypies (hand flapping, finger flicking), repetitive use of objects (spinning coins, lining up toys), repetitive speech (echolalia), resistance to change, unusual sensory responses

        (3) Presentation in early childhood and significant limitation of functioning

4. **Interventions/treatment**

    a. Applied behavior analysis (ABA)
        A treatment approach for young children with ASD is called applied behavior analysis (ABA). ABA has become widely accepted among healthcare professionals and is used in many schools and treatment clinics. ABA encourages positive behaviors and discourages negative behaviors while the child's progress is carefully tracked and measured.[49]

    b. Educational interventions, visual supports, naturalistic developmental behavioral interventions (integrating behavioral and child-responsive strategies to teach developmentally appropriate skills in a more natural and interactive setting)[21,22]

    c. Referral to SLP, OT/sensory-based interventions

    d. Family resources

        (1) https://www.autismspeaks.org/technology-and-autism

    (2) https://www.autism-society.org/living-with-autism/treatment-
        options/

    (3) https://www.nichd.nih.gov/health/topics/autism/conditioninfo/
        treatments

    (4) https://www.autismspeaks.org/tool-kit/atnair-p-parents-guide-
        applied-behavior-analysis

G. Attention Deficit/Hyperactivity Disorder (ADHD): See Chapter 24

V. LONGITUDINAL CARE OF CHILDREN WITH DEVELOPMENTAL DISORDERS AND DISABILITIES

A. Interdisciplinary Involvement

1. Neurodevelopmental pediatrician, child neurologist, developmental/
   behavioral pediatrician, other medical subspecialties as indicated (e.g.,
   orthopedics for CP can be very important)
2. Genetic counseling for families of children with a genetic condition
3. Psychologists for formal testing, counseling
4. Mental health support: People with disabilities reported approximately five
   times more mentally unhealthy days than those in the general
   population.[24,25]
5. Rehabilitation and therapists, including physical therapy (PT),
   occupational therapy (OT), and SLP
6. Educators and the school system
7. Community and parent advocacy organizations

B. Relevant Laws and Regulation

1. The **Individuals with Disabilities Education Act (IDEA)** sets forth regulations
   in the following areas for states that receive federal funding[26,27]:
   a. Entitles all children with qualifying disabilities to a free and
      appropriate public education in the least restrictive environment
   b. **Early intervention services:** Infants and toddlers younger than 3 years
      may be referred for evaluation to receive developmental service.
      Eligibility criteria vary by state; see The National Early Childhood
      Technical Assistance Center (https://www.ectacenter.org) for details.
   c. **Qualifying disabilities:** Children aged 3 to 21 years with autism
      spectrum disorder, ID, specific learning disability (LD), hearing or
      visual impairment, speech or language impairment, orthopedic
      impairment, traumatic brain injury, emotional disturbance, or other
      health impairment are eligible.
   d. **Individualized education program (IEP):** Written statement that
      includes a child's current capabilities, goals and how they will be
      measured, and services required. A comprehensive team is needed
      to develop and implement the IEP.
   e. **Transition services:** School systems must provide transition services
      that prepare students for postsecondary activities, and IEPs must
      include a statement of transition service needs starting no later than

age 14. The student must be included in the IEP process starting at age 14.

f. **Section 504 of the Rehabilitation Act of 1973 and the Americans with Disabilities Act (ADA):** Prohibits discrimination against individuals with any disability, more broadly defined as an impairment that limits function.[29] A Section 504 Plan can also be used to get reasonable accommodations for a child who has a disability but who does not meet criteria for special education and related services; for example, a quiet setting or extra time for testing, mobility assistance for a child who uses a wheelchair

C. Head Start and Early Head Start

Programs instituted by the federal government to promote school readiness of low-income children aged 3 to 5 years (Head Start) and younger than 3 years (Early Head Start) within their communities[28]

VI. TRANSITIONS FROM PEDIATRIC TO ADULT CARE FOR YOUTH WITH DEVELOPMENTAL DISABILITIES

A. The Need

Research reveals health disparities between adults with developmental disabilities and those without. Disparities include:

1. Increased ED utilization
2. Lack of identified adult provider
3. Worse self-perception of health[30]

B. The Role of the Pediatric Provider

1. AAP Consensus Statement on Transitions[31,32]
    a. Identify a health professional as point person to work with the youth and family on transition process.
    b. **Create healthcare transition plan by age 14** with the youth and family. **NOTE:** If a child's disability leaves them without capacity to make their own healthcare decisions, then parents must have court documents signed by two different physicians to have continued healthcare proxy (allowing parent to continue medical decision-making) established for after the child turns 18. This process should start before the child has turned 18 to avoid a lapse in the parent's ability to act as proxy for their child.
    c. Apply same guidelines for primary and preventive care for all adolescents and young adults.
    d. Ensure affordable, continuous insurance coverage.

C. Transition Domains

1. Transitions for young adults with disabilities occur across many domains of life and warrant support from an interdisciplinary team (Table 9.10).

TABLE 9.10

TRANSITION DOMAINS FOR YOUTH WITH DEVELOPMENTAL DISORDERS AND DISABILITIES

Transition Domain	Common Issues	Necessary Support Personnel/Services
Physical/emotional health	Difficulty identifying adult providers, retained in pediatric care, lost to follow-up, increased ED usage, insurance difficulties	Pediatrician, adult PCP, subspecialists
Education/ employment	Education services through IDEA end at 21 years old. Subsequent difficulty finding and engaging in postsecondary education and/or employment opportunities	Educational team members (teachers, therapists), vocational rehab specialists, college counselors, postsecondary education programs
Legal/financial	Difficulties with issues of SSI, guardianship, conservatorship	Attorney, legal counsel, family advocate
Housing/ transportation	Access to accessible housing and transportation, development and ongoing support of skills needs for independent living	Life skills courses, group homes, independent living supports/aides, resources through state departments of disability and the U.S. Department of Housing and Urban Development, state mobility services
Leisure pursuits/ respite care	Decreased structure of leisure pursuits with termination of school services at 21, increased burden on caregivers	Day programs, social engagement programs (e.g., Best Buddies, Special Olympics), respite care services for caregivers
Sexuality	Romantic and sexual relationships, vulnerability, reproductive rights, contraception, parenthood, access to appropriate screening and healthcare	Education team members (sexual education while in school), family members; OB/gyn providers, adult healthcare providers

ED, Emergency department; *IDEA,* Individuals with Disabilities Education Act; *OB/Gyn,* obstetrician/gynecologist; *PCP,* primary care physician; *SSI,* supplemental security income.

VII. SOCIAL DETERMINANTS OF HEALTH AND ADVERSITY SIGNIFICANTLY IMPACT CHILD DEVELOPMENT, ATTAINMENT OF DEVELOPMENTAL MILESTONES, AND/OR LONG-TERM HEALTH

A. Social Determinants of Health (SDOHs)

1. Definitions and epidemiology
   a. SDOHs are the conditions in which people are born, grow, work, live, and age, and the wider set of forces and systems shaping the conditions of daily life.[34]
2. Five key domains[35]:
   a. Economic stability (e.g., poverty and food insufficiency)

b. Education (e.g., high school graduate and early childhood education)
c. Social and community context (e.g., concerns about immigration status and social support)
d. Health and healthcare (e.g., health insurance status and access to a healthcare provider)
e. Neighborhood and built environment (e.g., neighborhood crime and quality of housing)

3. The role of the pediatric provider
   a. Considering SDOHs among children and youth is critical given that the physical, social, and emotional capabilities that develop early in life provide the foundation for life course health and well-being.[36]
   b. Screening for SDOHs has benefits such as improving diagnostic algorithms, identifying children and youth in need of more support, improving patient-provider relationships, and collecting data for epidemiological purposes.[33]
   c. Referral to clinic, community, or state resources when appropriate

B. Adverse Childhood Experiences (ACEs)

1. Definitions and epidemiology[3]
   a. All ACE questions refer to occurrences in the first 18 years of life. Studies indicate more than two-thirds of the population have experienced at least one ACE. The initial ACEs study only addressed those listed below, but there are likely many more ACEs that influence development and long-term health outcomes.
      (1) Abuse
          (a) Emotional abuse
          (b) Physical abuse
          (c) Sexual abuse
      (2) Household challenges
          (a) Mother treated violently
          (b) Substance abuse in the household
          (c) Mental illness in the household
          (d) Parental separation or divorce
          (e) Incarcerated household member
      (3) Neglect
          (a) Emotional neglect
          (b) Physical neglect
      (4) The Philadelphia ACE Project expanded the survey to include community adversity, factors that also impact development and long-term health.[38,39]
          (a) Experience of bullying
          (b) Discrimination
          (c) Witnessing violence
          (d) Being in the foster care system
          (e) Living through adverse neighborhood experiences or adverse community environments (the "other ACEs")

2. Mechanism by which ACEs influence health and well-being throughout the life span
   a. There is a dose-response relationship between ACEs and long-term negative physical and mental health outcomes in adults.
   b. Childhood ACEs may lead to toxic stress (see section 4a) and impact multiple biologic indices (e.g., brain development, immune function, stress response system, epigenetics).
3. Role of the pediatric provider
   a. Screening for ACEs and toxic stress with referral to resources and support can prevent long-term negative health outcomes throughout the life span.
   b. Supportive adult relationships are protective against toxic stress.[40]
      (1) Pediatricians have unique opportunity to support parent-child relationships.
4. Resources
   a. Safe Environment for Every Kid (https://www.seekwellbeing.org)
      (1) Stress
         (a) Definitions and epidemiology
            (i) **Positive stress:** Helps to guide growth
            (ii) **Tolerable stress:** Not helpful, but will not cause damage
            (iii) **Toxic stress:** Overcomes the child's undeveloped coping mechanisms and leads to long-term impairment and illness[40]
               (a) Results when a child experiences strong, frequent, or prolonged activation of the stress response systems in absence of protection from a supportive adult
               (b) Healthy brain development can be disrupted or impaired by prolonged, pathologic stress response with significant long-term implications for learning, behavior, health, and adult functioning.[41]
            (iv) **Traumatic stress:** The physical and emotional responses of a child to events that threaten the life or physical integrity of the child or of someone critically important to the child (e.g., parent, sibling). *Examples:* natural disaster, assault
               (a) There is a dose-response relationship to traumatic stress over time.
         (b) The role of the pediatric provider
            (i) Screening
            (ii) **Referral to effective treatments for children who have experienced trauma**
               (a) Trauma-focused cognitive-behavioral therapy[42]
               (b) Parent-child interactive therapy[43]
         (c) Resources
            (i) National Child Traumatic Stress Network (https://www.NCTSN.org)

(2) Resilience
    (a) Definitions and epidemiology
        (i) Resilience: The process by which a child moves through a traumatic event, using various protective factors for support, and returning to a "baseline" in terms of an emotional and physiologic response to the stressor[44]
    (b) Protective factors[45]
        (i) Cognitive capacity
        (ii) Healthy attachment relationships (especially with parents and caregivers)
        (iii) Motivation and ability to learn and engage with the environment
        (iv) Ability to regulate emotions and behavior
        (v) Supportive environmental systems, including education, cultural beliefs, and faith-based communities
    (c) Resources
        (i) Relational Health Framework: strengths-based approach to identifying and building safe, stable and nurturing relationships as a critical public health measure to promote resilience and counter toxic stress. https://www.aap.org/en/patient-care/early-childhood/early-relational-health/
        (ii) Protective Factors Framework: www.cssp.org/our-work/projects/protective-factors-framework/
        (iii) Strengthening Families: https://www.strengtheningfamiliesprogram.org
        (iv) The AAP Resilience Project: https://www.aap.org/en/patient-care/trauma-treatment-and-resilience/
        (v) Healthy Children: https://www.healthychildren.org

E. Relationship Between Adversity and Resilience

1. Traumatic event occurs (e.g., as broad as abuse to failing a test) → stress is experienced, which elicits emotional and physiologic responses → support is received (e.g., reassurance, identification of own internal strengths, connection with adult or social supports) → stability is reobtained and the individual is more skilled in identifying and using their own internal skills while maintaining awareness of and access to external supports. When the next traumatic event occurs, the individual draws on past experiences of support and stabilizes again.

F. Diversity and Equity in Adversity and Resilience

1. **Childhood adversity is common across all socioeconomic demographics.**
2. Certain populations have **increased risk of ACEs due to SDOHs and systemic barriers**[46]:
    a. Lower socioeconomic status
    b. Racial minorities or multiracial individuals
    c. Sexual minorities

VII. WEB RESOURCES

- Autism Speaks: https://www.autismspeaks.org
- Bright Futures: https://www.brightfutures.org
- Cerebral Palsy Foundation: https://yourcpf.org
- Disability Programs and Services: https://www.dol.gov/odep/topics/disability.htm
- Got Transition: https://www.gottransition.org
- Individuals With Disabilities Education Act (IDEA): https://idea.ed.gov
- Intellectual Disability: https://aaidd.org
- National Center for Learning Disabilities: https://www.ncld.org
- National Early Childhood Technical Assistance Center: https://www.ectacenter.org
- Reach Out and Read: https://www.reachoutandread.org

REFERENCES

A complete list of references can be found online.

Chapter 10

Endocrinology

Rashmi Pashankar, MD

See additional content online.

I. DIABETES

A. Diagnosis of Diabetes Mellitus[1-3]

Diagnostic criteria (must meet one of four):

1. Symptoms of diabetes (polyuria, polydipsia, weight loss, frequent yeast infections) and random blood glucose (BG)≥200 mg/dL
2. Fasting plasma glucose (FPG = no caloric intake for at least 8 hours)≥126 mg/dL
3. Oral glucose tolerance test (OGTT) with a 2-hour postload plasma glucose of≥200 mg/dL
4. Hemoglobin A_{1c} (HbA$_{1c}$)≥6.5% obtained via laboratory testing (POCT HbA1c is nondiagnostic)

NOTE: In the absence of symptoms of hyperglycemia, FPG or OGTT should be repeated on another day.

B. Definition of Increased Risk (Prediabetes)

1. FPG 100 to 125 mg/dL
2. 2-hour post-OGTT BG 140 to 199 mg/dL
3. HbA$_{1c}$ 5.7% to 6.4%

C. Interpreting Hemoglobin A_{1c}[1,2]

1. Estimates average BG for the past 3 months
2. HbA$_{1c}$ of 6% approximately equals an average BG of 130 mg/dL; each additional 1% $\approx$ 30 mg/dL more
3. Unreliable in patients with abnormal red cell life span or morphology (e.g., sickle cell disease, spherocytosis)
4. Although there are limited data supporting HbA$_{1c}$ for diagnosing type 2 diabetes in children and adolescents, the American Diabetes Association continues to recommend HbA$_{1c}$ for diagnosis of type 2 diabetes in this population.

D. Etiology: Distinguishing Between Types of Diabetes Mellitus[1,2]

1. Type 1 (T1DM) versus T2DM (most common types, polygenic; Table 10.1)
2. Other forms of diabetes[4,5]
   a. Monogenic diabetes: 1% to 2% of diabetes mellitus (DM). Due to single-gene mutations, typically relating to insulin production or release. Identifying gene can have clinical significance.

TABLE 10.1

CHARACTERISTICS SUGGESTIVE OF TYPE 1 VERSUS TYPE 2 DIABETES

Characteristic	Type 1	Type 2
Onset	As early as 1-year-old through adulthood	Usually postpubertal
Polydipsia and polyuria	Present for days to weeks	Absent or present for weeks to months
Weight	Weight loss	Obese (although weight loss is common in presentation with severe hyperglycemia)
Other physical findings		Acanthosis nigricans
Family history	Autoimmune diseases	Type 2 diabetes
Ketoacidosis	More common (1/3 at onset)	Less common (6% at onset)
Lab characteristics	Autoantibodies common; C-peptide generally should be unmeasurable >2 years after diagnosis	Autoantibodies less common, but sometimes present

(1) Suspect if autosomal dominant inheritance pattern of early-onset (<25 years) DM, insulin independence, absent T2DM phenotype (nonobese), or preservation of C-peptide

(2) Many well-described subtypes; some, such as MODY1 and MODY3 (due to mutations in transcription factors for insulin production) responsive to treatment with sulfonylureas

b. Neonatal diabetes (NDM): Defined as DM onset <6 months of age

(1) Rare: 1:160,000 to 260,000 live births, typically a de novo mutation

(2) May be transient (50% recur) or permanent

(3) Subset respond to sulfonylureas

c. Cystic fibrosis–related diabetes (CFRD): OGTT rather than HbA_{1c} is the recommended screening test.

d. Other causes of DM: Diseases of exocrine pancreas due to pancreatitis, trauma, infection, invasive disease (e.g., hemochromatosis)

E. Screening for Type 2 Diabetes Mellitus[1,6]

1. **Whom to screen:** Children who are overweight (body mass index [BMI] >85th percentile) *and* have one or more of the following risk factors:

a. Maternal history of diabetes or gestational diabetes mellitus during child's gestation

b. Family history of T2DM in a first- or second-degree relative

c. Race/ethnicity: African American, Native American, Hispanic, Asian, or Pacific Islander

d. Signs associated with insulin resistance (acanthosis nigricans, hypertension, dyslipidemia, polycystic ovarian syndrome, or small-for-gestational-age birth weight)

2. **How to screen:** Fasting plasma glucose, OGTT, or HbA$_{1c}$
3. **When to screen:** Begin at the age of 10 years or at the onset of puberty (whichever occurs first) and repeat at a minimum of every 3 years or more often if BMI is increasing.

F. Additional Testing in New-Onset Diabetes

1. **Diabetes autoantibodies**[1,2]**:** Recommended for all children with suspected T2DM or whose diabetes type is unclear
   a. Includes islet cell autoantibodies (ICAs) and antibodies to GAD (GAD65), insulin, tyrosine phosphatases IA-2, IA-2β, and β-cell–specific zinc transporter 8 (ZnT8)
   b. Confirmation of diagnosis of T1DM if 2 or more antibodies are present, though about 5% of T1DM will not have measurable ICAs, and some children with T2DM will have measurable ICAs
2. **Screening for autoimmune diseases in T1DM**[6]**:**
   a. Thyroid disease (present in 17% to 30% of patients with T1DM): Screen with TSH when clinically well and consider screening for thyroid antibodies. If TSH normal, recheck every 1 to 2 years or sooner if symptoms develop.
   b. Celiac disease (present in 1.6% to 16.4% of patients with T1DM): Screen with tissue transglutaminase (TTG) IgA antibody and total IgA. Repeat within 2 years of diabetes diagnosis and again after 5 years. Repeat more frequently if there are symptoms or a first-degree relative with celiac disease.

G. Management of Diabetes[6-8]

1. **Diabetes medications FDA approved for children:**
   a. Insulin: See Tables 10.2 and 10.3 for calculations. Insulin doses are subsequently adjusted based on actual blood sugars.
   b. Metformin: FDA approved in children ≥10 years old with type 2 diabetes, though sometimes used off label in younger children. Main side effects are gastrointestinal (GI) and are often transient. Extended-release option is available for patients with GI side effects.
   c. Glucagon-like peptide 1 (GLP-1) agonists (currently only liraglutide and exenatide): FDA approved in children ≥ 10 years old with T2DM. Main side effects include GI effects, pancreatitis, and hypoglycemia. Avoid if there is a family history of medullary thyroid cancer or personal history of pancreatitis.
2. **T1DM management:** The majority of children with T1DM should be treated with intensive insulin regimens via multiple daily injections, a continuous subcutaneous infusion via insulin pump, or an automated insulin delivery system.
3. **T2DM management:**
   a. Lifestyle modification therapy (nutrition and physical activity) and metformin should be initiated at time of diagnosis.
   b. Insulin therapy should be initiated if distinction between T1DM and T2DM is unclear, when HbA$_{1c}$ ≥8.5%, when random BG ≥250, in presence of diabetic ketoacidosis (DKA), or when patient with known

TABLE 10.2

SUBCUTANEOUS INSULIN DOSING

	Insulin	Dose Calculation	Sample Calculation for 24-kg Child	Dose
Total daily dose		0.5—1 unit/kg/day	$0.75 \times 24 = 18$ units/day	18 units
Basal	Glargine OR	1/2 daily total	$1/2 \times 18$ units $= 9$	9 units daily
	Detemir	1/2 daily total ÷ BID	$1/2 \times 18$ units $= 9$	4.5 units BID
Carbohydrate coverage ratio	Lispro, aspart OR	$500 ÷$ daily total	$500 ÷ 18 = 28$	1 unit: 28 g carbohydrate
	Regular	$450 ÷$ daily total	$450 ÷ 18 = 25$	1 unit: 25 g carbohydrate
Correction factor	Lispro, aspart OR	$1800 ÷$ daily total	$1800 ÷ 18 = 100$	1 unit expected to drop BG by 100 mg/dL
	Regular	$1500 ÷$ daily total	$1500 ÷ 18 = 83$	1 unit expected to drop BG by 83 mg/dL

T2DM is not meeting glycemic target with metformin and lifestyle modification alone. **NOTE:** If significant hyperglycemia (BG >600) or ketosis is present, patient should be evaluated for DKA or hyperosmolar hyperglycemic state

c. Consider addition of GLP-1 agonist therapy if glycemic targets are not met with metformin alone, or combined therapy with metformin and insulin.

TABLE 10.3

TYPES OF INSULIN PREPARATIONS AND SUGGESTED ACTION PROFILES FOR SUBCUTANEOUS ADMINISTRATION[54]

Insulin[a]	Onset	Peak	Effective Duration
Ultra-rapid—acting analog (faster aspart, lispro-aabc)	5—10 min	1—3 hr	3—5 hr
Rapid-acting (lispro, aspart, glulisine)	10—20 min	1—3 hr	3—5 hr
Short-acting (regular)	30—60 min	2—4 hr	5—8 hr
Intermediate acting (NPH)	2—4 hr	4—12 hr	12—24 hr
Long-acting			
Glargine	2—4 hr	8—12 hr	22—24 hr
Detemir	1—2 hr	4—7 hr	20—24 hr
Degludec	30—90 min	No peak	>42 hr

NOTE: Be aware that there are stronger concentrations of various types of insulin available (e.g., U-500 regular insulin, which is 5 times more concentrated than U-100 regular insulin; U-300 insulin glargine). There are also premixed combinations of rapid or short AND intermediate acting insulin (e.g., 70% NPH/30% regular [Humulin 70/30]).
[a]Assuming 0.1—0.2 U/kg per injection. Onset and duration vary significantly by injection site.
NPH, Neutral protamine Hagedorn.
Modified from The American Diabetes Association. *Practical Insulin: A Handbook for Prescribing Providers.* 2nd ed. American Diabetes Association; 2007.

4. **Goals of therapy:**
   a. HbA1c <7% (individualized to avoid excessive hypoglycemia)
   b. Assessment and management of complications: hypertension, dyslipidemia, nephropathy, retinopathy, neuropathy in all types of diabetes; additionally for obstructive sleep apnea, nonalcoholic fatty liver disease, and polycystic ovarian syndrome in type 2 diabetes
5. Interdisciplinary care team should include mental health provider and medical nutrition therapy with initial education and annual update. Regularly assess for eating disorders, disease-related coping, depression, and psychosocial stressors impacting diabetes management.

H. Diabetes Management Devices[9]

1. Technology is rapidly changing, but general principles are described below.
2. **Insulin pumps:** Contain rapid-acting insulin only and provide basal and bolus insulin. Doses can be programmed to vary throughout the day. Settings consist of:
   a. Basal rate—continuous insulin infusion
   b. Carbohydrate coverage—insulin-to-carbohydrate ratio
   c. Hyperglycemia correction—based on correction factor and target blood glucose
   NOTE: There is risk for DKA with interruptions in insulin delivery (e.g., pump malfunction) given lack of long-acting insulin.
3. **Continuous glucose monitors (CGMs):** Measure glucose concentration in interstitial fluid continuously and provide alerts for high and low glucose levels.
4. **Automated insulin delivery systems:** Use of continuous glucose monitor data and algorithms to automate insulin delivery to reduce hyperglycemia and hypoglycemia and increase time in target range.

I. Monitoring[6,8-10]

1. **Glycemic control:**
   a. Assessment of blood glucose using glucometer or CGM
      (1) Multiple times daily (e.g., before meals/snacks, at bedtime, prior to exercise, with symptoms of hypoglycemia, after treating for hypoglycemia, before driving)
      (2) CGM metrics over most recent 14 or more days: time in range (70–180 mg/dL), time below target (<70 and <54 mg/dL) and time above target (>180 mg/dL)
   b. HbA_{1c} every 3 months
2. Urine ketones should be checked with persistent hyperglycemia, any illness (regardless of blood glucose level), or with nausea/vomiting.
3. **Associated conditions or complications:** See Table 10.4.

J. Diabetic Emergencies[11,12]

1. **Diabetic ketoacidosis (DKA)**
   a. Definition: Hyperglycemia (or euglycemia in a patient with known diabetes), ketonemia, ketonuria, and metabolic acidosis (pH <7.30, bicarbonate <15 mEq/L)

TABLE 10.4

SCREENING FOR DIABETES-ASSOCIATED CONDITIONS AND COMPLICATIONS[6,10]

Type of Condition or Complication	Screening Test	Frequency
Hypertension	Blood pressure measurement	At every visit
Hyperlipidemia	Lipid profile	At diagnosis, then yearly if T2DM or T1DM, age 9—11 years and overweight or LDL>100; every 3 years if low-density lipoprotein (LDL) <100 mg/dL
Retinopathy	Dilated eye examination or retinal photography	T1DM: every 2 years after 3—5 years of diabetes, provided age >10 years T2DM: at diagnosis, yearly
Diabetic nephropathy	Random spot urine microalbumin-to-creatinine ratio	T1DM: yearly after 5 years of diabetes, provided age >10 years T2DM: at diagnosis, yearly
Neuropathy	Foot exam	T1DM: yearly after 5 years of diabetes, provided ≥ age 10 T2DM: at diagnosis, yearly
Nonalcoholic steatohepatitis (NASH)	ALT, AST	T2DM: at diagnosis, yearly
Obstructive sleep apnea (OSA)	Review of symptoms	T2DM: at every visit
Polycystic ovary syndrome (PCOS)	Menstrual history ± lab evaluation	T2DM: at every visit

ALT, Alanine amino transferase; *AST*, aspartate amino transferase; *T1DM*, type 1 diabetes mellitus; *T2DM*, type 2 diabetes mellitus.

  b. BG reflects hydration status, pH reflects DKA severity
  c. Symptoms: Nausea, emesis, abdominal pain, fruity breath, altered mental status, Kussmaul respirations
  d. Precipitating factors: New-onset DM, known diabetes with missed insulin doses, insulin pump/infusion site malfunction, or physiologic stress due to acute illness
  e. Management: See Fig. 10.1. Because the fluid and electrolyte requirements vary greatly from patient to patient, guidelines are only a starting point, and therapy must be individualized based on patient characteristics. **NOTE:** Initial insulin administration may cause transient worsening of the acidosis as potassium is driven into cells in exchange for hydrogen ions.
  f. Cerebral edema: Most severe complication of DKA. Overly aggressive hydration and rapid correction of hyperglycemia may play a role in its development. Risk factors include severe acidosis, evidence of renal insufficiency, young age and new onset, use of bicarbonate.
  g. Once DKA is resolved, transition to subcutaneous (SQ) insulin. See Tables 10.2 and 10.3 for calculations or resume home insulin doses.
2. **Hyperosmolar hyperglycemic state (HHS)**
  a. Definition: Extreme hyperglycemia (BG >600 mg/dL) and hyperosmolarity (>320 mOsm/kg), **without significant ketosis or acidosis**

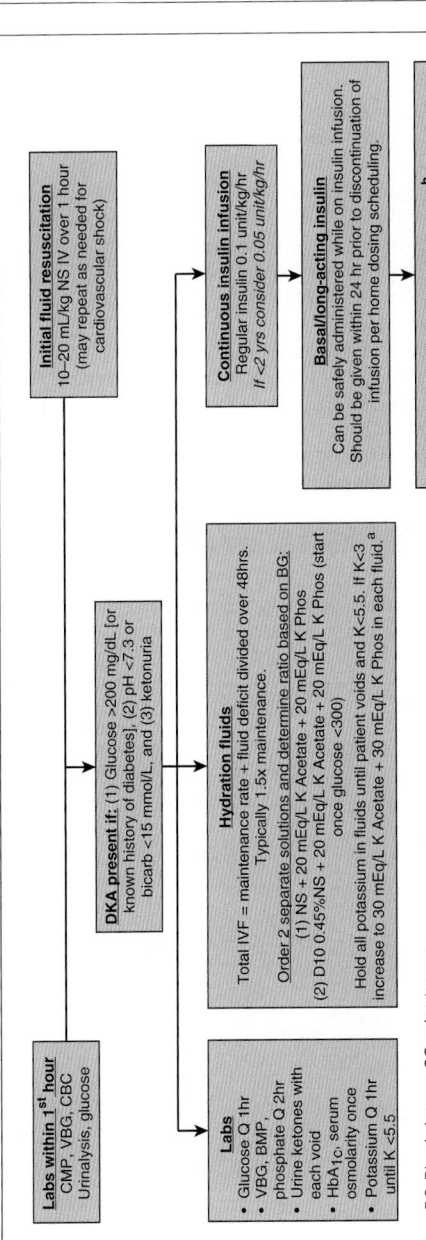

Labs within 1st hour
CMP, VBG, CBC
Urinalysis, glucose

Initial fluid resuscitation
10–20 mL/kg NS IV over 1 hour
(may repeat as needed for cardiovascular shock)

DKA present if: (1) Glucose >200 mg/dL [or known history of diabetes], (2) pH <7.3 or bicarb <15 mmol/L, and (3) ketonuria

Continuous insulin infusion
Regular insulin 0.1 unit/kg/hr
If <2 yrs consider 0.05 unit/kg/hr

Basal/long-acting insulin
Can be safely administered while on insulin infusion. Should be given within 24 hr prior to discontinuation of infusion per home dosing scheduling.

Transition to SC insulin[b]
(1) Administer rapid-acting insulin with meal to account for pre-meal BG and carbohydrates consumed.
(2) Stop insulin infusion and dextrose-containing fluids 30 minutes after rapid-acting insulin administered.

Hydration fluids
Total IVF = maintenance rate + fluid deficit divided over 48hrs.
Typically 1.5× maintenance.
Order 2 separate solutions and determine ratio based on BG:
(1) NS + 20 mEq/L K Acetate + 20 mEq/L K Phos
(2) D10 or 0.45%NS + 20 mEq/L K Acetate + 20 mEq/L K Phos (start once glucose <300)
Hold all potassium in fluids until patient voids and K<5.5. If K<3 increase to 30 mEq/L K Acetate + 30 mEq/L K Phos in each fluid.[a]

Labs
• Glucose Q 1hr
• VBG, BMP,
  phosphate Q 2hr
• Urine ketones with
  each void
• HbA1c: serum
  osmolarity once
• Potassium Q 1hr
  until K <5.5

BG, Blood glucose; *SC,* subcutaneous.
Note: This algorithm may need to be individualized depending on patient presentation.
a) Patients with DKA are total body K depleted and are at risk for severe hypokalemia during DKA therapy. However serum K levels may be normal or elevated as a result of the shift of K to the extracellular compartment in the setting of acidosis.
b) Appropriate to transition to SC insulin once pH >7.3, normal anion gap, normal physical exam, and patient ready to eat.

FIGURE 10.1

Management of diabetic ketoacidosis. (Modified from Cooke DW, Plotnick L. Management of diabetic ketoacidosis in children and adolescents. *Pediatr Rev.* 2008;29:431–436.)

b. Characteristics: Gradually increasing polyuria and polydipsia leading to profound dehydration, altered consciousness

c. Management:

(1) Fluids: Fluids alone will decrease BG due to dilution, promotion of glucosuria, and increased glucose uptake with improved circulation. Fluid replacement should be more rapid than in DKA with goal of gradual decline in serum sodium (about 0.5 mEq/dL/hr) and osmolality. Bolus ≥20 cc/kg 0.9% saline and repeat until perfusion improved. Then start maintenance fluids plus deficit replacement over 24 to 48 hours using 0.45% to 0.75% saline (if perfusion inadequate, consider isotonic fluids). Urine output should also be replaced.

(2) Insulin therapy: Start insulin (0.025 to 0.05 unit/kg/hr) when BG no longer declining at least 50 mg/dL/hr with fluids alone. Titrate insulin to decrease BG by 75 to 100 mg/dL/hr.

(3) Electrolytes: Potassium, phosphate, and magnesium deficits greater than in DKA; monitor every 2 to 4 hours. Start potassium replacement with 40 mEq/L once K <5 mEq/L.

II. THYROID GLAND[13-15]

A. Thyroid Tests[14,16,17]

1. **Normal thyroid function values:** See reference values for age (Table 10.5). Preterm infants have different ranges (Table 10.6).

TABLE 10.5

AGE-BASED NORMAL VALUES FOR ROUTINE THYROID FUNCTION TESTS

Test	Age	Normal Range	
TSH (mIU/L)	Birth—6 days	0.70—15.2	
	1 week—3 months	0.72—11.0	
	3 months—12 months	0.73—8.35	
	1—5 years	0.70—5.97	
	6—10 years	0.60—4.84	
	>10 years	0.45—4.50	
Free T_4 (ng/dL)	Birth—3 days	0.66—2.71	
	4—30 days	0.83—3.09	
	31 days—12 months	0.48—2.34	
	13 months—5 years	0.85—1.75	
	6—10 years	0.90—1.67	
	11—19 years	0.93—1.60	
	>19 years	0.82—1.77	
Total T_4 (mCg/dL)	<1 month	Male	Female
	1—23 months	4.5—17.2	4.5—17.2
	2—12 years	5.9—13.9	5.9—13.9
	13—20 years	5.7—11.6	5.7—11.6
	>20 years	5.1—10.3	5.3—11.7
		4.9—0.5	5.1—11.9

NOTE: If age-specific reference ranges are provided by the laboratory that is running the assay, please refer to those ranges.

T_4, Thyroxine; *TSH*, thyroid stimulating hormone.

TSH and Free T_4 reference ranges from Labcorp; Total T_4 reference range from Quest Diagnostics.

TABLE 10.6

MEAN TSH AND T₄ OF PRETERM AND TERM INFANTS 0–28 DAYS

Age ± SD	Cord (Day 0)	Day 7	Day 14	Day 28
T₄ (mCg/dL)				
23–27[a]	5.44 ± 2.02	4.04 ± 1.79	4.74 ± 2.56	6.14 ± 2.33
28–30	6.29 ± 2.02	6.29 ± 2.10	6.60 ± 2.25	7.46 ± 2.33
31–34	7.61 ± 2.25	9.40 ± 3.42	9.09 ± 3.57	8.94 ± 2.95
>37	9.17 ± 1.94	12.67 ± 2.87	10.72 ± 1.40	9.71 ± 2.18
FT₄ (ng/dL)				
23–27	1.28 ± 0.41	1.47 ± 0.56	1.45 ± 0.51	1.50 ± 0.43
28–30	1.45 ± 0.43	1.82 ± 0.66	1.65 ± 0.44	1.71 ± 0.43
31–34	1.49 ± 0.33	2.14 ± 0.57	1.96 ± 0.43	1.88 ± 0.46
>37	1.41 ± 0.39	2.70 ± 0.57	2.03 ± 0.28	1.65 ± 0.34
TSH (mIU/L)				
23–27[b]	2.1	2.2	2.4	2.6
28–30[b]	3.4	3.1	2.8	2.5
31–34	7.90 ± 5.20	3.60 ± 4.80	3.80 ± 9.30	3.50 ± 3.40
>37	6.70 ± 4.80	2.60 ± 1.80	2.50 ± 2.00	1.80 ± 0.90

[a]Weeks gestational age.
[b]Standard deviations unavailable in Kaluarachchi et al. reference. Percentile graphs present in reference.
FT₄, Free thyroxine; *T₄*, thyroxine; *TSH*, thyroid stimulating hormone.
Data modified from Williams FL, Simpson J, Delahunty C, et al. Collaboration from The Scottish Preterm Thyroid Group: Developmental trends in cord and postpartum serum thyroid hormones in preterm infants. *J Clin Endocrinol Metab.* 2004;89:5314–5320; Kaluarachchi DC, Allen DB, Eickhoff JC, Dawe SJ, Baker MW. Thyroid-stimulating hormone reference ranges for preterm infants. *Pediatrics.* 2019 Aug;144(2):e20190290. Epub 2019 Jul 16. PMID: 31311840. doi: 10.1542/peds.2019-0290

2. **Interpretation of abnormal thyroid function values:** See Table 10.7.
3. **Imaging studies:**
   a. Thyroid ultrasound: Most useful in assessing thyroid nodules for features suspicious for malignancy
   b. Thyroid uptake scan: Measures uptake of technetium (⁹⁹ᵐTc) pertechnetate or radioactive iodine by metabolically active thyroid tissue, helping to identify etiology of hyperthyroidism

TABLE 10.7

THYROID FUNCTION TESTS: INTERPRETATION

Disorder	TSH	T₄	Free T₄
Primary hyperthyroidism	L	H	High N to H
Primary hypothyroidism	H	L	L
Hypothalamic/pituitary hypothyroidism	L, N, H[a]	L	L
TBG deficiency	N	L	N
Euthyroid sick syndrome	L, N, H[a]	L	L to low N
TSH adenoma or pituitary resistance	N to H	H	H
Subclinical hypothyroidism[b]	H	N	N

[a]Can be normal, low, or slightly high.
[b]Treatment may not be necessary.
H, High; *L*, low; *N*, normal; *T₄*, thyroxine; *TBG*, thyroxine-binding globulin; *TSH*, thyroid stimulating hormone.

B. Hypothyroidism

1. **Types of hypothyroidism:** Can be either congenital or acquired and either primary or central. See Table 10.8 for details on identification and management.

2. **Subclinical hypothyroidism and obesity[18]:** Moderate elevations in thyroid stimulating hormone (TSH [4 to 10 mIU/L]), with normal or slightly elevated triiodothyronine (T_3) and thyroxine (T_4), are seen in 10% to 23% of obese children. There does not appear to be a benefit to treating these individuals. Values tend to normalize with weight loss. Could consider testing for thyroid antibodies to further clarify whether there is true thyroid dysfunction.

3. **Newborn screening for hypothyroidism[15-20]:** Mandated in all 50 states. Measures a combination of TSH and T_4, based on the particular state's algorithm; 1:25 abnormal tests are confirmed. Congenital hypothyroidism has prevalence of 1:3000 to 1:4000 US infants. If abnormal results are found, clinicians should follow recommendations of the American College of Medical Genetics ACT Sheets and Algorithm for confirmation testing.

C. Hyperthyroidism

1. **General features:**
   a. Epidemiology: Prevalence increases with age, rare before adolescence; female-to-male predominance
   b. Etiology: Most common cause is Graves disease, followed by subacute thyroiditis. Less common causes are Hashitoxicosis, autonomously functioning thyroid nodule, factitious hyperthyroidism (intake of exogenous hormone), TSH-secreting pituitary tumor (rare), and pituitary resistance to thyroid hormone. See Table 10.9 for comparison of Graves disease and Hashimoto thyroiditis.
   c. Laboratory findings: See Table 10.7. Further tests include TSH receptor—stimulating antibody, thyroid stimulating immunoglobulin (TSI), antithyroglobulin and antimicrosomal (thyroid peroxidase) antibodies.

2. **Thyroid storm[21]:**
   a. Presentation: Acute onset of hyperthermia, tachycardia, and restlessness. May progress to delirium, coma, and death
   b. Treatment: Admission to ICU. Emergent pediatric endocrinology consultation recommended. Therapy aimed at relieving symptoms (propranolol) and reducing peripheral conversion of T_4 to T_3 (hydrocortisone), thyroid hormone production (antithyroid drugs), release of hormone from thyroid gland (potassium iodide), and reabsorption from enterohepatic circulation (cholestyramine)

3. **Neonatal thyrotoxicosis:**
   a. Presentation: Microcephaly, frontal bossing, intrauterine growth restriction (IUGR), tachycardia, systolic hypertension leading to widened pulse pressure, irritability, failure to thrive, exophthalmos, goiter, flushing, vomiting, diarrhea, jaundice, thrombocytopenia, and cardiac failure or arrhythmias. Onset from immediately after birth to weeks

TABLE 10.8
HYPOTHYROIDISM[55,56]

Clinical Symptoms	Onset	Etiology	Management	Follow-up
PRIMARY/CONGENITAL				
Large fontanelles, lethargy, constipation, hoarse cry, hypotonia, hypothermia, jaundice. Most often picked up on newborn screen.	Symptoms usually develop by 2 weeks; almost always by 6 weeks. Some infants may be relatively asymptomatic if not caused by absence of thyroid gland.	**Primary:** Defect of fetal thyroid development most common. Other causes include TSH receptor mutation or thyroid dyshormonogenesis. *OR* **Central:** Deficiency of TSH or thyrotropin-releasing hormone (TRH).	Replacement with L-thyroxine once newborn screen is positive, pending results of confirmatory testing.[a] Goal T_4 in upper half of normal range. In primary hypothyroidism, TSH should be kept in normal range for age.	Monitor T_4 and TSH 1–2 weeks after initiation and then every 2 weeks until TSH normalizes. Once levels are adequate follow per schedule listed below. Treated patients are still at risk for developmental delay.
ACQUIRED				
Growth deceleration, coarse brittle hair, dry skin, delayed tooth eruption, cold intolerance.	Can occur as early as 2 years old.	**Primary:** Can be caused by Hashimoto thyroiditis (diagnosis supported by + antithyroglobulin or antimicrosomal antibodies), head/neck radiation. *OR* **Central:** Caused by pituitary/ hypothalamic insults including brain tumor.	Replacement with L-thyroxine.[a] Targets for TSH and T_4 same as for congenital hypothyroidism above.	Follow every 1–3 months during the first 12 months, every 2–4 months until 3 years, and then every 3–12 months until growth complete. Follow 4–6 weeks after any dose change.

NOTE: Thyroid hormone levels in premature infants are lower than those seen in full-term infants. Furthermore, the TSH surge seen at approximately 24 hours of age in full-term babies does not appear in preterm infants. In this population, lower levels are associated with increased illness; however, the effect of replacement therapy remains controversial.

[a]Because of the risk of inducing adrenal crisis if adrenocorticotropic hormone (ACTH) deficiency is present, the treatment of central hypothyroidism *should not be* started until normal ACTH/cortisol function is documented.

L-thyroxine, Levothyroxine; *TSH,* thyroid stimulating hormone.

10

TABLE 10.9
HYPERTHYROIDISM

Presentation	Distinguishing Imaging/Lab Findings	Management
GRAVES DISEASE		
Typical symptoms of hyperthyroidism plus diffuse goiter, eye symptoms, localized dermopathy, and lymphoid hyperplasia	TSH is often undetectable. ↑ ^{99m}Tc-pertechnate uptake. Positive TSI.	First-line treatment in children is methimazole. Radioactive iodine (^{131}I) or surgical thyroidectomy are options for initial treatment or refractory cases. Follow symptoms, T_4, and TSH levels.
HASHIMOTO THYROIDITIS		
± Initial hyperthyroidism, followed by eventual thyroid burnout and hypothyroidism	Often low but detectable TSH and less significant increase in T_4. ↓ ^{99m}Tc-pertechnate uptake. Significant elevation of thyroglobulin and/or microsomal antibody.	Hyperthyroid phase is usually self-limited; patient may eventually need thyroid replacement therapy. Propranolol if symptomatic during hyperthyroid phase.

^{99m}Tc, Technetium; T_4, thyroxine; TSH, thyroid stimulating hormone; TSI, thyroid stimulating immunoglobulin.

  b. Etiology: Occurs exclusively in infants born to mothers with Graves disease. Caused by transplacental passage of maternal TSI. Occasionally, mothers are unaware they have Graves. Even if a mother has received definitive treatment (thyroidectomy or radiation therapy), passage of TSI remains possible.
  c. Treatment and monitoring: Propranolol for symptom control. Methimazole to lower thyroxine levels. Digoxin may be indicated for heart failure. Disease usually resolves by 6 months of age.

III. PARATHYROID GLAND AND VITAMIN D[22-24]

A. Parathyroid Hormone Function
1. Increases serum calcium by increasing bone resorption
2. Increases calcium and magnesium reuptake and phosphorus excretion in the kidney
3. Increases 25-hydroxy vitamin D conversion to 1,25-dihydroxy vitamin D in order to increase calcium absorption in the intestine

B. Distinguishing Between Abnormalities Related to Parathyroid Hormone and Vitamin D
See Table 10.10.

C. Vitamin D Supplementation
Please see Chapter 21 for additional information.

IV. ADRENAL GLAND[25-29]

A. Adrenal Insufficiency
1. **Causes of adrenal insufficiency:**
   a. Impaired steroidogenesis, as in congenital adrenal hyperplasia

TABLE 10.10

DISTINGUISHING BETWEEN DISORDERS OF PARATHYROID GLANDS AND VITAMIN D REGULATION

	Hypoparathyroidism	Hyperparathyroidism	PTH Resistance/Pseudo-Hypoparathyroidism	Vitamin D Deficiency
PTH	↓ or inappropriately normal in the setting of hypocalcemia	↑	↑	-/↑
1,25-D	↓	↑	↓	↓
25-OHD	-	-/↓	-	↓
Calcium	↓	↑	↓	-/↓
Phosphorus	↑	↓	↑	-/↓
Alkaline phosphate	-/↓	-/↑	↑	↑
Common causes	DiGeorge, autoimmune (APS), iatrogenic	Primary: Adenoma, hyperplasia Secondary: Renal failure, rickets	Genetic mutations	Nutritional deficiency
First-line Rx	Calcium, calcitriol	Hydration with normal saline, surgical resection	Calcitriol	Vitamin D +/- calcium

1,25-D, 1,25 Dihydroxy vitamin D; *25-OHD,* 25-hydroxy vitamin D; *APS,* autoimmune polyendocrine syndrome; *MEN,* multiple endocrine neoplasia; *PTH,* parathyroid hormone; *Rx,* treatment.

10

    b. Adrenal destruction or dysfunction as in primary adrenal insufficiency (AI) (Addison disease), autoimmune polyendocrine syndrome, or adrenoleukodystrophy

    c. Secondary AI caused by impaired circulating adrenocorticotropic hormone (ACTH) due to hypothalamic or pituitary pathology

    d. Acquired insufficiency secondary to long-term corticosteroid use leading to HPA suppression. **NOTE:** This is the most common cause seen in clinical practice and may also occur in setting of chronic high-dose inhaled corticosteroids.

2. **Laboratory findings in adrenal insufficiency:**

    a. In primary AI, there is deficient mineralocorticoid and glucocorticoid production. In central AI, there is only deficient glucocorticoid production, and mineralocorticoid production is normal.

    b. Primary AI: Elevated ACTH, elevated plasma renin activity, low cortisol, low aldosterone, hypoglycemia, hyponatremia, hyperkalemia

    c. Central AI: Normal/low ACTH, normal plasma renin activity (no impairment of mineralocorticoid function), low cortisol, normal aldosterone, hyponatremia, hypoglycemia

    d. In infants with congenital adrenal hyperplasia (CAH), 17-hydroxyprogesterone (17-OHP) is increased (see Table 10.11 for normal values by age).

3. **Diagnosis of adrenal insufficiency:**

    a. Initial screening with AM cortisol level, which may be drawn concomitantly with an ACTH level

    b. See Table 10.12 for interpretation of AM cortisol results.

    c. Plasma ACTH elevation >100 pg/mL with concomitant hypocortisolemia <10 mCg/dL is consistent with glucocorticoid deficiency due to primary AI.

    d. Standard dose ACTH stimulation test is used to confirm diagnosis.

4. **ACTH stimulation test:**

    a. In brief, with ACTH deficiency or prolonged adrenal suppression, there is an inadequate rise in cortisol after a single ACTH dose.

    b. See Box 10.1 for interpretation of ACTH stimulation test.

5. **Congenital adrenal hyperplasia (CAH):**

    a. See Fig. 10.2.

    b. Group of autosomal recessive disorders characterized by a defect in one of the enzymes required in the synthesis of adrenal hormones

    c. The enzymatic defect results in impaired synthesis of adrenal steroids beyond the enzymatic block and overproduction of the precursors before the block.

    d. 21-hydroxylase deficiency accounts for 90% of cases.

    e. Most common cause of ambiguous genitalia in females

6. **Diagnosis of CAH on newborn screen:**

    a. The test measures 17-OHP and is 2% specific, resulting in a 98% false-positive rate due to artificial elevations from prematurity, sickness, stress.[27]

TABLE 10.11

17-HYDROXYPROGESTERONE, SERUM

Age	Baseline (ng/dL)
Premature (31–35 weeks)	≤405
Term infants (3 days)	<420
1–11 months	≤147
1 year	≤139
2–5 years	≤134
6 years	≤137
7 years	≤145
8 years	≤154
9 years	≤166
10 years	≤180
11 years	≤196
12 years	≤213
13 years	≤233
14 years	≤254
15 years	19–279
16 years	23–300
17 years	26–325
Males, Tanner II–III	12–130
Females, Tanner II–III	18–220
Males, Tanner IV–V	51–190
Females, Tanner IV–V	36–200
Male (18–30 years)	32–307
Adult female	
Follicular phase	23–102
Midcycle phase	67–349
Luteal phase	139–431

Reference ranges from Quest Diagnostics LC/MS assay (liquid chromatography/tandem mass spectroscopy).
For preterm infants or infants born small for gestational age, see Olgemöller B, Roscher AA, Liebl B, et al. Screening for congenital adrenal hyperplasia: adjustment of 17-hydroxyprogesterone cut-off values to both age and birth weight markedly improves the predictive value. *J Clin Endocrinol Metab.* 2003;88:5790–5794.

TABLE 10.12

CORTISOL, 8 A.M.

Interpretation	Cortisol (mCg/dL)
Suggestive of adrenal insufficiency	<5
Indeterminate	5–14
Adrenal insufficiency unlikely	>14

b. If 17-OHP is 40 to 100 ng/mL, repeat test.
c. If 17-OHP is higher than 100 ng/mL, obtain electrolytes and serum 17-OHP. If evidence of hyperkalemia or hyponatremia, initiate treatment with hydrocortisone.
d. In complete enzyme deficiency, adrenal crisis in untreated patients occurs at 1 to 2 weeks of age due to salt wasting.

BOX 10.1

PERFORMANCE AND INTERPRETATION OF ACTH STIMULATION TEST

Standard Dose ACTH Stimulation Test

Obtain initial baseline cortisol level
Give 250 mCg IV ACTH
Measure cortisol at 30 min
Measure cortisol at 60 min

Interpretation of Results

Cutoff for adequate cortisol response is highly variable depending on cortisol assay used and may be anywhere between 12.7 and 17.5 mCg/dL for both primary and central adrenal insufficiency. Cortisol reference ranges should be verified with the individual lab running the assay.

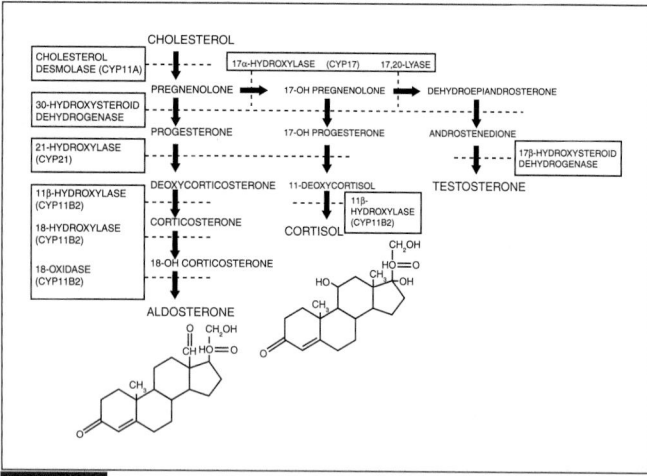

FIGURE 10.2

Biosynthetic pathway for steroid hormones.

7. **Diagnosis of CAH outside of newborn period:**
   a. Suspect partial enzyme deficiency if evidence of androgen excess (premature adrenarche, hirsutism, irregular menses, acne, advanced bone age).
   b. Morning 17-OHP levels may be elevated.
   c. Diagnosis may require an ACTH stimulation test. A significant rise in the 17-OHP level 60 minutes after ACTH injection is diagnostic. Cortisol response may be decreased.

8. **Addison disease[30]:**
   a. Primary AI due to autoimmune destruction of the adrenal glands

b. In children, it may be part of autoimmune polyendocrine syndrome type 1 (APS-1), which also includes hypoparathyroidism and chronic mucocutaneous candidiasis.

c. Individuals with autoimmune Addison disease should also be screened for other endocrinopathies (T1DM, celiac disease, hypothyroidism, hypoparathyroidism).

9. **Treatment of adrenal insufficiency:**
   a. See Table 10.13 for relative steroid potencies.
   b. See Table 10.14 for maintenance glucocorticoid and mineralocorticoid dosing.

TABLE 10.13

POTENCY OF VARIOUS THERAPEUTIC STEROIDS[a]

Steroid	Glucocorticoid Effect[b] (in mg of Cortisol per mg of Steroid)	Mineralocorticoid Effect[c] (in mg of Cortisol per mg of Steroid)
Cortisol (hydrocortisone)	1	1
Cortisone acetate (oral)	0.8	0.8
Cortisone acetate (intramuscular)	0.8	0.8
Prednisone	4	0.25
Prednisolone	4	0.25
Methylprednisolone	5	0.4
β-Methasone	25	0
Triamcinolone	5	0
Dexamethasone	30	0
9α-Fluorocortisone (fludrocortisone)	15	200
Deoxycorticosterone acetate	0	20
Aldosterone	0.3	200–1000

[a]Set relative to potency of cortisol.
[b]To determine cortisol equivalent of a given steroid dose, multiply dose of steroid by corresponding number in column for glucocorticoid or mineralocorticoid effect. To determine dose of a given steroid based on desired cortisol dose, divide desired hydrocortisone dose by corresponding number in the column.
[c]Total physiologic replacement for salt retention is usually 0.1 mg fludrocortisone, regardless of patient size.
Modified from Sperling MA. *Pediatric Endocrinology*. 3rd ed. Elsevier; 2008:476.

TABLE 10.14

MAINTENANCE DOSING STEROIDS

Adrenal Hormone	Dose
Glucocorticoid dosing	1. PO hydrocortisone 6–18 mg/m^2/day ÷ TID OR 2. PO prednisone 1.5–3.5 mg/m^2/day ÷ BID
Mineralocorticoid dosing[a]	1. PO fludrocortisone acetate 0.1 mg/m^2/day OR 2. If unable to take PO: IV hydrocortisone 50 mg/m^2/day[b] PLUS 3. Infants require an additional 1–2 g (17–34 mEq) of sodium supplementation daily

[a]Required in salt-losing forms of adrenal insufficiency.
[b]Synthetic steroids (e.g., prednisone, dexamethasone) do not have sufficient mineralocorticoid effect.

   c. Typically, lower doses are required for central AI, intermediate doses for primary AI, and higher doses for CAH in order to suppress excess androgen production.

10. **Stress dosing of steroids:**
   a. **Hydrocortisone and cortisone are the only glucocorticoids that provide the necessary mineralocorticoid effects;** prednisone and dexamethasone do not.
   b. See Table 10.15 for calculation of moderate and major stress dose steroid calculations.
   c. See Box 10.2 for rapid approximation of steroid dosing in the setting of acute adrenal crisis.

11. **Indications for stress dosing of steroids:**
   a. "Stress" is defined as systemic infection, febrile illness, diarrheal illness, trauma/fracture, burns, or surgery.
   b. Stress glucocorticoids should be given to patients:
     (1) With known primary or secondary AI
     (2) Following discontinuation of exogenous steroid (given for greater than 2 weeks at doses greater than physiologic replacement) until there is recovery of endogenous cortisol production (consider the need for 8 a.m. cortisol or ACTH stimulation test)
   c. Consider for hypotension refractory to fluid resuscitation in patients with suspicion for AI (even if not clinically diagnosed).

B. Adrenal Cortex Hormone Excess[29]

1. **Causes:**
   a. Hypercortisolism (Cushing syndrome):

TABLE 10.15

STRESS DOSING STEROIDS

Degree of Stress	Dose
Moderate stress (minor illness, fever)	1. PO hydrocortisone 30–50 mg/m²/day ÷ TID OR 2. PO prednisone 6–10 mg/m²/day ÷ BID
Severe stress (surgery, severe illness, compensated shock)	1. IV bolus of hydrocortisone 50 mg/m² then 50–100 mg/m²/day IV as continuous infusion or divided Q6 hr OR 2. IM injection of 25 mg/m²/dose Q6 hr

---

BOX 10.2

RAPID APPROXIMATION OF STRESS DOSE STEROID REQUIREMENT

Infant: 25 mg hydrocortisone
Small child: 50 mg hydrocortisone
Large child/adolescent: 100 mg hydrocortisone

    (1) Exogenous steroid use

    (2) Excess cortisol secretion from the adrenals

    (3) Excess ACTH production from ectopic ACTH–producing tumor

    (4) Excess ACTH production from a pituitary tumor (known as Cushing *disease*)

  b. Hyperaldosteronism:

    (1) Benign tumor of adrenal cortex (Conn syndrome)

    (2) Overproduction by both adrenal glands (idiopathic hyperaldosteronism)

    (3) Rarely glucocorticoid remediable aldosteronism

    (4) Less common in children than hypercortisolism

    (5) Lab findings include hypokalemia and hypernatremia

2. **Diagnosis of Cushing syndrome[31]:**

  a. Step 1: Demonstrate hypercortisolism with two separate measurements. Multiple screening tests are available; specificity increases when they are used in combination:

    (1) 24-hour urine cortisol (>90 mCg/24 hours consistent with hypercortisolism)

    (2) Midnight salivary cortisol level (>0.13 mCg/dL consistent with hypercortisolism)

    (3) Overnight low-dose dexamethasone suppression test: Give 1 mg dexamethasone at 11 p.m. followed by an 8 a.m. serum cortisol the next morning (normal suppression <1.8 mCg/dL).

  b. Step 2: Determine etiology of hypercortisolism (ACTH-dependent vs. independent)

    (1) Obtain plasma ACTH between 11 p.m. and 1 a.m.: >23 pg/mL in a patient with hypercortisolism (as diagnosed above) indicates ACTH dependency (Cushing disease vs. ectopic tumor).

    (2) If cause is Cushing disease (ACTH-dependent), ACTH level will be >100× elevated.

    (3) In ACTH-independent Cushing syndrome, level will be <5 pg/mL.

C. Adrenal Medulla Hormone Excess: Pheochromocytoma[32-34]

1. **Clinical findings:**

  a. Extreme, sustained elevations in blood pressure (accounts for <1% of pediatric hypertension)

  b. Associated with syndromes: multiple endocrine neoplasia (MEN) IIa and IIb, von Hippel-Lindau, neurofibromatosis (NF) 1, familial paraganglioma syndrome

2. **Diagnosis:**

  a. Urine metanephrines (see eTable 10.1 for age-specific normal values)

  b. Plasma metanephrines (see eTable 10.2 for age-specific normal values)

V. DISORDERS OF SODIUM AND WATER REGULATION[35]

A. Distinguishing Between Disorders of Sodium and Water Regulation: See Table 10.16

B. Correction of Hypo- and Hypernatremia: See Chapter 11

C. Conducting a Water Deprivation Test

1. Begin test after a 24-hour period of adequate hydration and stable weight.
2. Obtain a baseline weight after bladder emptying, as well as baseline urine and blood osmolality and electrolytes.
3. Restrict fluids (consider max 7 hours, 4 hours for infants).
4. Measure body weight and urine—specific gravity and volume hourly.
5. If urine specific gravity ≥1.014, or weight loss approaching 5%, terminate test and obtain urine and blood for osmolality and electrolytes.

D. Interpretation of Water Deprivation Test Results: See Table 10.17

E. Differentiating Between Central Versus Nephrogenic Causes of Diabetes Insipidus

1. Administer vasopressin subcutaneously at end of water deprivation test. Assess urine output, urine specific gravity, and water intake.

TABLE 10.16

DIFFERENTIATING BETWEEN DISORDERS OF SODIUM AND WATER REGULATION

	SIADH	Cerebral Salt Wasting	DI
Serum Na$^+$	<135 mEq/L	<135 mEq/L	>145 mEq/L[a]
Serum Osm	<280 mOsm/kg	<280 mOsm/kg	>300 mOsm/kg[a]
Urine Na$^+$	>40 mEq/L	>40 mEq/L	<40 mEq/L[b]
Urine Osm	>100 mOsm/kg (inappropriately concentrated)	>100 mOsm/kg (inappropriately concentrated)	<300 mOsm/kg (inappropriately dilute)
Volume status	Euvolemia	Hypovolemia	Hypovolemia
Urine output	Decreased	Increased	Increased
Other lab findings	High vasopressin	Low vasopressin	Central: low vasopressin (<0.5 pg/mL) Nephrogenic: high vasopressin
Causes	Nausea, CNS and pulmonary pathology, surgery, certain medications	CNS disorders, hypersecretion of atrial natriuretic peptide	Central: ↓ADH secretion from posterior pituitary Nephrogenic: ADH resistance at the nephron collecting duct
Treatment	Fluid restriction and correction of underlying cause Treatment with sodium will cause diuresis	Replacement of urine volume with IV solutions ± salt replacement	Central: Intranasal desmopressin acetate (DDAVP) Nephrogenic: Access to free water, salt restriction, consider thiazide diuretics, indomethacin

[a]Normal serum sodium and osmolality can be seen in compensated diabetes insipidus, and water deprivation test should be performed if clinical suspicion is high.

[b]Urine sodium generally low in diabetes insipidus; however, this depends on solute intake.

ADH, Antidiuretic hormone; *CNS,* central nervous system; *DI,* diabetes insipidus; *IV,* intravenous; *Na$^+$,* sodium; *Osm,* osmolarity; *SIADH,* syndrome of inappropriate ADH secretion.

TABLE 10.17

RESULTS OF WATER DEPRIVATION TEST IN NORMAL VERSUS CENTRAL/NEPHROGENIC DIABETES INSIPIDUS

	Normal (Psychogenic Polydipsia)	Central/Nephrogenic DI
Urine volume	Decreased	No change
Weight loss	No change	≤5%
Urine osmolality (mOsm/L)	500–1400 (>1000 generally excludes diagnosis of DI)	<150
Plasma osmolality (mOsm/L)	288–291	>290
Urine specific gravity	≥1.010	<1.005
Urine: plasma osmolality ratio	>2	<2

DI, Diabetes insipidus.

2. See Table 10.18 for interpretation of vasopressin test.

VI. GROWTH[35-37]

A. Assessing Height

1. **Mid-parental height and target height range:**
   a. Mid-parental height for boys: (Paternal height + maternal height + 5 in or 13 cm)/2
   b. Mid-parental height for girls: (Paternal height + maternal height − 5 in or 13 cm)/2
   c. Target height range: Mid-parental height ± 2 SD (1 SD = 2 in or 5 cm)
2. **Determining average growth velocity:** See Table 10.19.
3. See eFigs. 10.1 and 10.2 for normal growth velocity curves for American females and males, respectively.

TABLE 10.18

RESULTS OF VASOPRESSIN ADMINISTRATION IN EVALUATION OF DIABETES INSIPIDUS

	Psychogenic Polydipsia	Central[a]	Nephrogenic
Urine volume	↓	↓	No change
Urine specific gravity	≥1.010	≥1.010	No change
Oral fluid intake	No change	↓	No change

[a]In central diabetes insipidus, urine osmolality increases by 200% or more in response to vasopressin administration.

TABLE 10.19

ESTIMATED GROWTH VELOCITY IN CHILDREN BASED ON AGE

Age	Growth
Birth to 1 year old	25 cm/year
1 year old to 4 years old	10 cm/year
4 years old to 8 years old	5 cm/year
8 years old to 12 years old	5 cm/year[a]

[a]Rates may be considerably higher at later end of this age range when individuals have entered their pubertal growth spurt.

B. Short Stature

1. **Definition:**
   a. Short stature is height <2 SD below mean or <3rd percentile for age and sex.
   b. Growth failure is defined as height <2 SD below mid-parental height or height velocity <10th percentile for age resulting in a downward trend crossing height percentiles.
   c. Majority of children with short stature are healthy; true growth failure is typically pathologic and requires evaluation.

2. **Determining etiology:**
   a. See Table 10.20 for approach to differentiating between pathologic and nonpathologic causes of short stature.
   b. Bone age is determined by radiographs of left wrist and hand.
   c. See Fig. 10.3 for initial workup.
   d. A more extensive workup can be guided by history and physical exam and could include:
      (1) TTG and IgA (celiac disease)
      (2) CBC with differential (anemia, malignancy, inflammation)
      (3) CRP/ESR (inflammation, infection)
      (4) CMP (renal/liver disorders, malnutrition, calcium disorders)
      (5) TSH, free T_4 (hypothyroidism)
      (6) Karyotype or targeted gene testing (Turner syndrome, SHOX mutation)
      (7) IGF1, IGFBP-3 [proxy measurements for growth hormone (GH)]; IGFBP-3 has a higher specificity in children <10); see Table 10.21 and eTable 10.3 for normal values of IGF-1 and IGFBP-3, respectively.

3. **Indications for growth hormone use[38]:**
   The FDA has approved growth hormone for:
   a. Growth hormone deficiency

TABLE 10.20

PATHOLOGIC VERSUS NONPATHOLOGIC CAUSES OF SHORT STATURE

	Familial Short Stature	Constitutional Growth Delay	Pathologic Causes (e.g., Endocrine, Genetic)
Growth velocity	Normal	Normal	Decreased
Onset of puberty	Normal	Delayed	Depends on cause
Family history	Short stature	Delayed puberty	+/−
Bone age	Normal	Delayed	Usually delayed (may be normal in genetic causes)
Eventual adult height	Short, near mid-parental height	Normal	Depends on cause

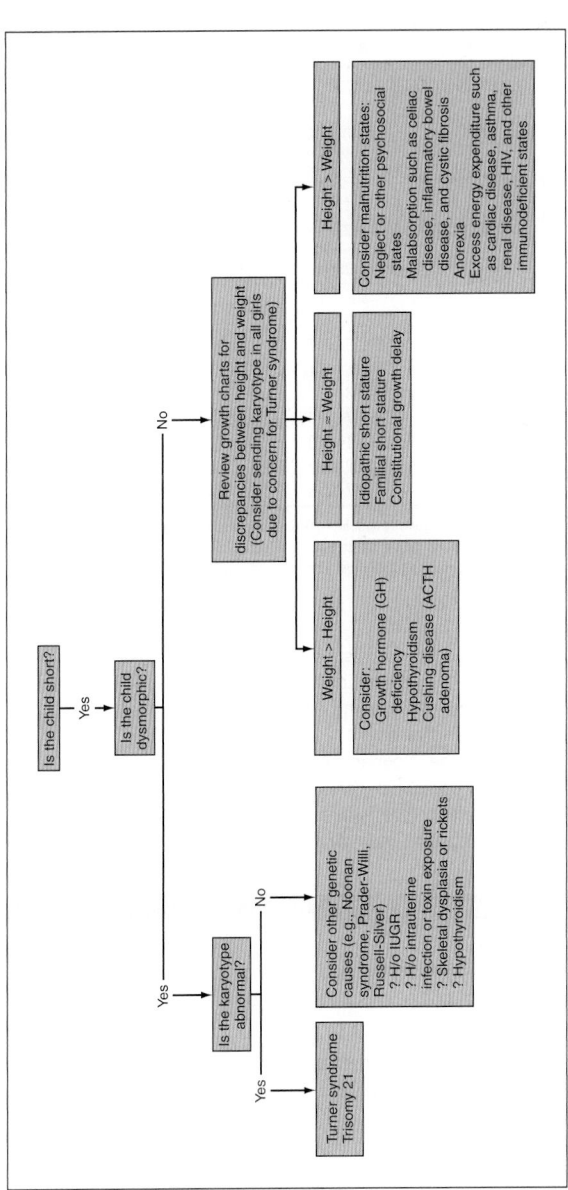

FIGURE 10.3

Differential diagnosis of short stature.

TABLE 10.21		
INSULIN-LIKE GROWTH FACTOR 1[a]		
Age (Years)	Male (ng/mL)	Females (ng/mL)
<1	14–142	17–185
1–1.9	12–134	15–175
2–2.9	12–135	16–179
3–3.9	30–155	38–214
4–4.9	28–181	34–238
5–5.9	31–214	37–272
6–6.9	38–253	45–316
7–7.9	48–298	58–367
8–8.9	62–347	76–424
9–9.9	80–398	99–483
10–10.9	100–449	125–541
11–11.9	123–497	152–593
12–12.9	146–541	178–636
13–13.9	168–576	200–664
14–14.9	187–599	214–673
15–15.9	201–609	218–659
16–16.9	209–602	208–619
17–17.9	207–576	185–551

[a]A clearly normal IGF-1 level argues against growth hormone (GH) deficiency, except in young children in whom there is considerable overlap between normal levels and those with GH deficiency.

Reference ranges from Quest Diagnostics LC/MS (liquid chromatography/tandem mass spectrometry) assay.

   b. Children born small-for-gestational-age (SGA) who, between 2 and 4 years of age, have shown inadequate catchup growth or evidence of normal growth velocity with height <2.5 SD below mean
   c. Chronic kidney disease
   d. Turner syndrome, Noonan syndrome, Prader-Willi syndrome
   e. Short stature homeobox containing gene (SHOX) deficiency
   f. Children with idiopathic short stature (height <2.25 SD below mean and unlikely to attain normal adult height)

VII. SEXUAL DEVELOPMENT[39-45]

A. Puberty

1. For normal pubertal stages, see Chapter 5.
2. For definitions of precocious and delayed puberty, see Table 10.22.

B. Lab Evaluation

1. LH, FSH, estradiol, and testosterone (free and total): see Tables 10.23 through 10.27 for normal values. **NOTE:** Early in puberty, LH production peaks overnight and is lower during the day, so consider obtaining levels in the early morning.
2. Gonadotropin (GnRH) stimulation test[46]:

TABLE 10.22

DEFINITIONS OF PRECOCIOUS AND DELAYED SEXUAL MATURATION

	Females	Males
Precocious	Before age 8 years: Thelarche (may be benign or progressive as seen in precocious puberty) Adrenarche (may be isolated or a feature of precocious puberty)	Before age 9 years: Testicular enlargement Adrenarche (may be isolated or a feature of precocious puberty)
Delayed	No thelarche by 13 years or >5 years between thelarche and menarche Primary amenorrhea: No menarche by age 16 years in the presence of secondary sexual characteristics, or no menarche and no secondary sexual characteristics by age 14 years	No testicular enlargement by 14 years

TABLE 10.23

LUTEINIZING HORMONE

Age	Males (mIU/mL)	Females (mIU/mL)
0–2 years	Not established	Not established
3–7 years	≤0.26	≤0.26
8–9 years	≤0.46	≤0.69
10–11 years	≤3.13	≤4.38
12–14 years	0.23–4.41	0.04–10.80
15–17 years	0.29–4.77	0.97–14.70

Tanner Stages	Males (mIU/mL)	Females (mIU/mL)
I	≤0.52	≤0.15
II	≤1.76	≤2.91
III	≤4.06	≤7.01
IV–V	0.06–4.77	0.10–14.70

Data from Quest Diagnostics immunoassay. For more information, see https://www.questdiagnostics.com.

TABLE 10.24

FOLLICLE-STIMULATING HORMONE

Age	Male (mIU/mL)	Female (mIU/mL)
0–4 years	Not established	Not established
5–9 years	0.21–4.33	0.72–5.33
10–13 years	0.53–4.92	0.87–9.16
14–17 years	0.85–8.74	0.64–10.98

Data from Quest Diagnostics immunoassay. For more information, see https://www.questdiagnostics.com.

TABLE 10.25

ESTRADIOL[a]

Age	Level (pg/mL)
Prepubertal children	<25
Males	6—44
Females	
Luteal phase	26—165
Follicular phase	None detected—266
Midcycle	118—355
Adult females on OCP	None detected—102

[a]Normal infants have elevated estradiol at birth, which decreases to prepubertal values during the first week of life. Estradiol levels increase again between age 1 and 2 months and return to prepubertal values by age 6—12 months.
OCP, Oral contraceptive pill.
Data from JHH Laboratories.

TABLE 10.26

TESTOSTERONE, TOTAL SERUM[a]

Age	Male (ng/dL)	Female (ng/dL)
Cord blood	17—61	16—44
1—10 days	≤187	≤24
1—3 months	72—344	≤17
3—5 months	≤201	≤12
5—7 months	≤59	≤13
7—12 months	≤16	≤11
1—5.9 years	≤5	≤8
6—7.9 years	≤25	≤20
8—10.9 years	≤42	≤35
11—11.9 years	≤260	≤40
12—13.9 years	≤420	≤40
14—17.9 years	≤1000	≤40
≥18 (adult)	250—1100	2—45
TANNER STAGE		
Stage I	≤5	≤8
Stage II	≤167	≤24
Stage III	21—719	≤28
Stage IV	25—912	≤31
Stage V	110—975	≤33

[a]Normal testosterone/dihydrotestosterone (T/DHT) ratio is <18 in adults and older children and <10 in neonates. A T/DHT ratio >20 suggests 5-α-reductase deficiency or androgen insensitivity syndrome.
Data from Quest Diagnostics LC/MS (liquid chromatography/tandem mass spectrometry) assay.

TABLE 10.27

TESTOSTERONE, FREE

Age	Male (pg/mL)	Female (pg/mL)
1—11 years	≤1.3	≤1.5
12—13 years	≤64.0	≤1.5
14—17 years	4.0—100.0	≤3.6
18—69 years	46.0—224.0	0.2—5.0

Data from Quest Diagnostics LC/MS (liquid chromatography/tandem mass spectrometry) assay.

a. Purpose: To evaluate for biochemical evidence of puberty when LH, FSH, and sex hormone testing is inconclusive.

b. Method: Give GnRH analog (leuprolide) SQ, and measure LH and FSH levels at 0 and 60 minutes.

c. Interpretation: Prepubertal children should show no or minimal increase in LH and FSH in response to GnRH. A rise of LH to >3.3 to 5.0 IU/L is evidence of central puberty.

3. **Delayed puberty**[41,45,47]: See Fig. 10.4 for information on evaluation and management of delayed puberty.

4. **Precocious puberty**[42,47]: See Fig. 10.5 for information on evaluation and management of precocious puberty.

C. Polycystic Ovarian Syndrome[48]

1. **Clinical features in adolescents:**

a. Diagnostic criteria (must have features of both):

   (1) Hyperandrogenism: Either clinical or biochemical

       (a) Clinical: Hirsutism, acne, male pattern alopecia

       (b) Biochemical characteristics: Elevated androgens including DHEA-S (see Table 10.28 for normal values), free or total testosterone

   (2) Menstrual abnormalities: Amenorrhea or oligomenorrhea (chronic anovulation)

NOTE: Appearance of multiple ovarian cysts is a diagnostic criterion for adults, but not for adolescents, as this can be a normal finding in adolescent females.

b. Common cause of female infertility

c. Often LH>FSH, but this is not required for diagnosis

d. Chronic anovulation and unopposed estrogen exposure increase risk for endometrial cancer.

e. Associated with insulin resistance and increased risk of type 2 diabetes

2. **Management:**

a. Combined oral contraceptives: First-line for management of menstrual abnormalities and hirsutism/acne. Increases SHBG (thus decreasing free testosterone), which may result in increased insulin sensitivity and restoration of ovulation

b. Anti-androgen therapy, such as spironolactone, to treat hirsutism

c. Weight reduction and other lifestyle changes

d. Metformin: Can be considered as possible treatment if goal is to treat insulin resistance

D. Ambiguous Genitalia[49]

1. **Clinical findings in a neonate suspicious for ambiguous genitalia:**

a. Apparent female with clitoromegaly (length >1 cm or width >6 mm in term infant), inguinal or labial mass, or posterior labial fusion

b. Micropenis (stretched penile length that is −2.5 SD below mean for age; see Table 10.29 for normal values)

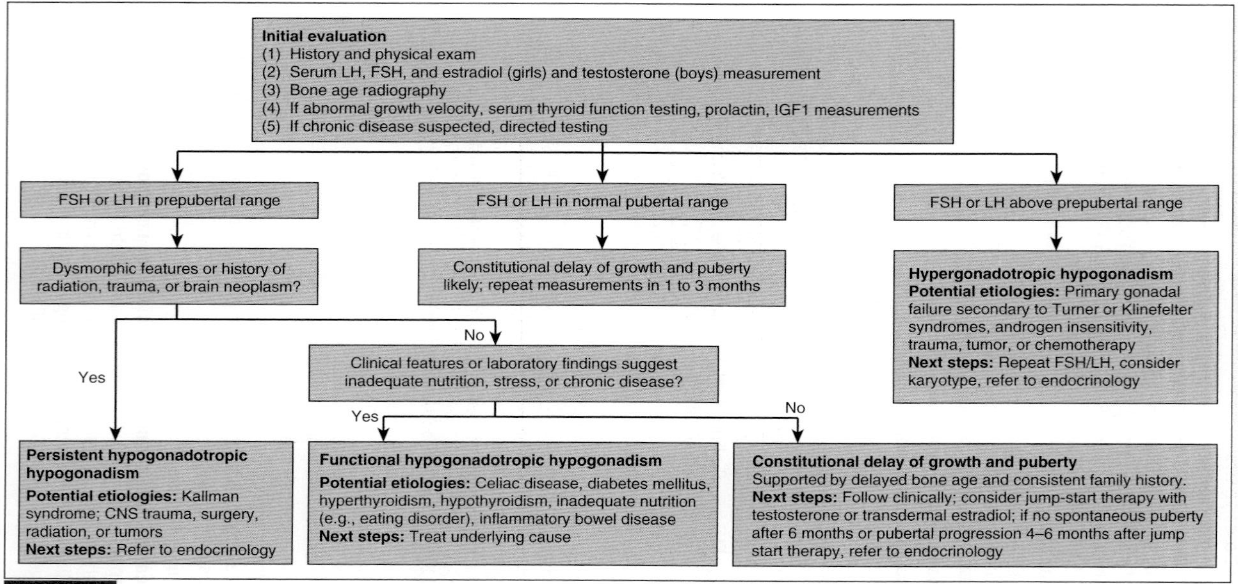
Initial evaluation
(1) History and physical exam
(2) Serum LH, FSH, and estradiol (girls) and testosterone (boys) measurement
(3) Bone age radiography
(4) If abnormal growth velocity, serum thyroid function testing, prolactin, IGF1 measurements
(5) If chronic disease suspected, directed testing
FSH or LH in prepubertal range
FSH or LH in normal pubertal range
FSH or LH above prepubertal range
Dysmorphic features or history of radiation, trauma, or brain neoplasm?
Constitutional delay of growth and puberty likely; repeat measurements in 1 to 3 months
Hypergonadotropic hypogonadism
Potential etiologies: Primary gonadal failure secondary to Turner or Klinefelter syndromes, androgen insensitivity, trauma, tumor, or chemotherapy
Next steps: Repeat FSH/LH, consider karyotype, refer to endocrinology
No
Yes
Clinical features or laboratory findings suggest inadequate nutrition, stress, or chronic disease?
Yes
No
Persistent hypogonadotropic hypogonadism
Potential etiologies: Kallman syndrome; CNS trauma, surgery, radiation, or tumors
Next steps: Refer to endocrinology
Functional hypogonadotropic hypogonadism
Potential etiologies: Celiac disease, diabetes mellitus, hyperthyroidism, hypothyroidism, inadequate nutrition (e.g., eating disorder), inflammatory bowel disease
Next steps: Treat underlying cause
Constitutional delay of growth and puberty
Supported by delayed bone age and consistent family history.
Next steps: Follow clinically; consider jump-start therapy with testosterone or transdermal estradiol; if no spontaneous puberty after 6 months or pubertal progression 4–6 months after jump start therapy, refer to endocrinology

FIGURE 10.4

An approach to the child presenting with delayed puberty. *CNS*, Central nervous system; *FSH*, follicle-stimulating hormone; *IGF1*, insulin-like growth factor 1; *LH*, luteinizing hormone; *MRI*, magnetic resonance imaging. (From Klein DA, Emerick JE, Sylvester JE, Vogt KS. Disorders of puberty. An approach to diagnosis and management. *Am Fam Physician*. 2017;96[9]:590–599.)

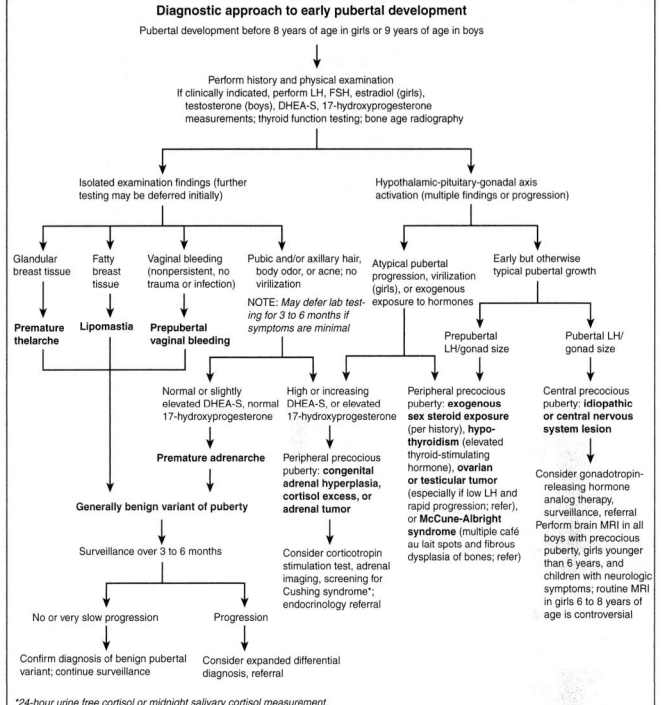

Diagnostic approach to early pubertal development

Pubertal development before 8 years of age in girls or 9 years of age in boys

↓

Perform history and physical examination
If clinically indicated, perform LH, FSH, estradiol (girls), testosterone (boys), DHEA-S, 17-hydroxyprogesterone measurements; thyroid function testing; bone age radiography

Isolated examination findings (further testing may be deferred initially)

Hypothalamic-pituitary-gonadal axis activation (multiple findings or progression)

Isolated examination findings:

- Glandular breast tissue → **Premature thelarche**
- Fatty breast tissue → **Lipomastia**
- Vaginal bleeding (nonpersistent, no trauma or infection) → **Prepubertal vaginal bleeding**
- Pubic and/or axillary hair, body odor, or acne; no virilization
  NOTE: May defer lab testing for 3 to 6 months if symptoms are minimal
  - Normal or slightly elevated DHEA-S, normal 17-hydroxyprogesterone → **Premature adrenarche** → **Generally benign variant of puberty** → Surveillance over 3 to 6 months → No or very slow progression → Confirm diagnosis of benign pubertal variant; continue surveillance / Progression → Consider expanded differential diagnosis, referral
  - High or increasing DHEA-S, or elevated 17-hydroxyprogesterone → Peripheral precocious puberty: **congenital adrenal hyperplasia, cortisol excess, or adrenal tumor** → Consider corticotropin stimulation test, adrenal imaging, screening for Cushing syndrome*; endocrinology referral

Hypothalamic-pituitary-gonadal axis activation:

- Atypical pubertal progression, virilization (girls), or exogenous exposure to hormones → Prepubertal LH/gonad size → Peripheral precocious puberty: **exogenous sex steroid exposure** (per history), **hypothyroidism** (elevated thyroid-stimulating hormone), **ovarian or testicular tumor** (especially if low LH and rapid progression; refer), or **McCune-Albright syndrome** (multiple café au lait spots and fibrous dysplasia of bones; refer)
- Early but otherwise typical pubertal growth → Pubertal LH/gonad size → Central precocious puberty: **idiopathic or central nervous system lesion** → Consider gonadotropin-releasing hormone analog therapy, surveillance, referral

Perform brain MRI in all boys with precocious puberty, girls younger than 6 years, and children with neurologic symptoms; routine MRI in girls 6 to 8 years of age is controversial

24-hour urine free cortisol or midnight salivary cortisol measurement.

FIGURE 10.5

An approach to the child presenting with early puberty. *DHEA-S*, Dehydroepiandrosterone sulfate; *FSH*, follicle-stimulating hormone; *LH*, luteinizing hormone; *MRI*, magnetic resonance imaging. (Reprinted with permission from Disorders of Puberty: An Approach to Diagnosis and Management, November 1, 2017, Vol 96, No 9, American Family Physician Copyright © 2017 American Academy of Family Physicians. All rights reserved.)

  c. Nonpalpable gonads in an apparent male
  d. Hypospadias associated with separation of scrotal sacs or undescended testis
  e. Discordance between prenatal karyotype and genital appearance

2. **Etiology:**
  a. Due to undervirilization of male genitalia or virilization of female genitalia
  b. Most common cause is CAH
  c. Other causes by male versus female karyotype:
     (1) 46,XY karyotype: Testicular regression, androgen insensitivity, testosterone biosynthesis disorders, rare forms of CAH, absence of SRY

TABLE 10.28

DEHYDROEPIANDROSTERONE SULFATE (DHEA-S)

Age	Male (mCg/dL)	Female (mCg/dL)
<1 months	≤316	15–261
1–6 months	≤58	≤74
7–11 months	≤26	≤26
1–3 years	≤15	≤22
4–6 years	≤27	≤34
7–9 years	≤91	≤92
10–13 years	≤138	≤148
14–17 years	38–340	37–307
TANNER STAGES (AGES 7–17)		
I	≤49	≤46
II	≤81	15–133
III	22–126	42–126
IV	33–177	42–241
V	110–370	45–320

Data from Quest Diagnostics assay. For more information see https://www.questdiagnostics.com.

TABLE 10.29

MEAN STRETCHED PENILE LENGTH (CM)[a]

Age	Mean ± SD	−2.5 SD
BIRTH		
30 weeks' gestation	2.5 ± 0.4	1.5
34 weeks' gestation	3.0 ± 0.4	2.0
Full term	3.5 ± 0.4	2.5
0–5 months	3.9 ± 0.8	1.9
6–12 months	4.3 ± 0.8	2.3
1–2 years	4.7 ± 0.8	2.6
2–3 years	5.1 ± 0.9	2.9
3–4 years	5.5 ± 0.9	3.3
4–5 years	5.7 ± 0.9	3.5
5–6 years	6.0 ± 0.9	3.8
6–7 years	6.1 ± 0.9	3.9
7–8 years	6.2 ± 1.0	3.7
8–9 years	6.3 ± 1.0	3.8
9–10 years	6.3 ± 1.0	3.8
10–11 years	6.4 ± 1.1	3.7
Adult	13.3 ± 1.6	9.3

[a]Measured from the pubic ramus to the tip of the glans while traction is applied along the length of the phallus to the point of increased resistance.

SD, Standard deviation.

Data from Feldman KW, Smith DW. Fetal phallic growth and penile standards for newborn male infants. *J Pediatr.* 1975;86:395.

(2) 46,XX karyotype: SRY+, classical (21-hydroxylase deficiency) or more rare forms of CAH

(3) Other: Sex chromosome mosaicism (e.g., 46,XY/46,xx, 46,XY/45,XO)

3. **Evaluation:**
   a. Labs: Timing of collection is important.
      (1) Initial testing (within first 24–48 hours of life): LH, FSH, testosterone, dihydrotestosterone (DHT, see eTable 10.4), anti-müllerian hormone (AMH) and expedited determination of sex chromosomes (ask that resulting lab rush results of sex chromosomes)
      (2) After 36 hours of life: 17-hydroxyprogesterone
      (3) Daily electrolytes until salt-wasting CAH is ruled out
      (4) Further testing as needed to evaluate for more rare forms of CAH: DHEA, 17-hydroxypregnenolone, 11-deoxycortisol, cortisol, ACTH
   b. Imaging: Options include genitogram (contrast study of the urogenital sinus and internal duct structures) or voiding cystourethrogram (VCUG), pelvic and abdominal ultrasound, and pelvic magnetic resonance imaging (MRI) to evaluate internal anatomy.
   c. Care should be taken to avoid premature gender/sex designation, completion of birth certificate, and naming of infant.

E. Cryptorchidism[50]

1. **Epidemiology and clinical course:**
   a. Can be present at birth (congenital) or after birth (acquired). Congenital rate is 1% to 4.6% of males born >2.5 kg.
   b. Increased risk with preterm birth or low birth weight.
   c. About $\frac{1}{3}$ to $\frac{1}{2}$ of cryptorchid testicles descend spontaneously, usually by age 3 months.
   d. Neoplasm more common in males with cryptorchidism and may occur in contralateral testis; early orchidopexy decreases risk of malignancy.
   e. Males with bilateral cryptorchidism have higher risk for reduced fertility.
   f. There is a higher risk of testicular torsion prior to repair.

2. **Evaluation:**
   a. Providers should palpate testes for quality and position in all males at each well child visit.
   b. Any phenotypic male newborn with bilateral, *nonpalpable* testes should undergo evaluation for CAH with karyotype and hormonal profile.
   c. In those without CAH, distinguish between cryptorchidism and anorchia (absent testes) with serum müllerian inhibiting substance and consider additional hormone testing (inhibin B, FSH, LH, and testosterone).

3. **Treatment:** Observe for 6 months, at which time if testis remains undescended, referral to specialist recommended. Orchidopexy between 6 and 18 months of age recommended.

VIII. NEONATAL HYPOGLYCEMIA EVALUATION[51,52]

A. Definition

1. Serum glucose level insufficient to meet metabolic requirements. For practical purposes, value is defined as a point-of-care glucose (POCG) <45 to 50 mg/dL within first 48 hours of life and <70 mg/dL beyond this period.

NOTE: Bedside glucometer is a convenient tool to screen for hypoglycemia but can be inaccurate by 10 to 15 mg/dL when in the range of hypoglycemia. STAT plasma glucose must be sent to establish diagnosis of hypoglycemia.

B. Treatment Goals

1. For neonates with suspected congenital hypoglycemia disorder and infants/children with confirmed hypoglycemia disorder, maintain plasma glucose >70 mg/dL.
2. For high-risk neonates without a suspected congenital hypoglycemia disorder, maintain plasma glucose >45 to 50 mg/dL for those <48 hours of age and >60 mg/dL for those aged >48 hours.

C. Management

See Chapter 18.

D. Further Workup

1. If serum glucose is consistently <70 mg/dL after 48 hours of life, at the time of hypoglycemia (serum glucose <45 to 50 mg/dL via glucometer), obtain STAT serum glucose, insulin, growth hormone, cortisol, free fatty acids, and β-hydroxybutyrate.
2. Consider **glucagon stimulation test:** Administer glucagon and obtain serum glucose levels Q10 min ×4. Repeat growth hormone and cortisol levels 30 minutes after documented hypoglycemia.

E. Interpretation of Results

1. A rise in glucose ≥30 mg/dL on glucagon stimulation test, along with elevated plasma insulin levels >2 μU/mL (absence of detectable insulin does not rule out hyperinsulinism, as insulin may be present below the lower limit of detection of the assay), low serum levels of free fatty acids (<1.5 mmol/L) and β-hydroxybutyrate (<2 mmol/L), and a persistent glucose requirement >8 mg/kg/min suggests a diagnosis of hyperinsulinemia.
2. Hypoglycemia with midline defects and micropenis in a male suggest hypopituitarism, supported by low serum levels of growth hormone and cortisol at the time of hypoglycemia.

F. Hyperinsulinemia

1. Hyperinsulinemia is the most common cause of neonatal hypoglycemia beyond the first 7 days of life and may be congenital or transient.

2. Congenital hyperinsulinism can be caused by dominant or recessive mutations in genes responsible for regulating insulin secretion from pancreatic β cells.
3. Transient hyperinsulinemia is commonly seen in infants of diabetic mothers and less commonly in the setting of perinatal asphyxia and intrauterine growth restriction.
4. Long-term management of persistent hyperinsulinism includes diazoxide, which inhibits pancreatic secretion of insulin by keeping β-cell ATP-sensitive potassium channels open; however, it has been rarely associated with pulmonary hypertension (black box warning[53]).

IX. ADDITIONAL NORMAL VALUES

Normal values may differ among laboratories because of variation in technique and type of assay used.

See the following tables for normal values:

eTable 10.1, Catecholamines, urine

eTable 10.2, Catecholamines, plasma

eTable 10.3, Insulin-like growth factor–binding protein

eTable 10.4, DHT

eTable 10.5, Androstenedione, serum

X. WEB RESOURCES

- **Children with Diabetes** (https://www.childrenwithdiabetes.com)
- **American Diabetes Association** (https://www.diabetes.org)
- **International Society for Pediatric and Adolescent Diabetes** (https://www.ispad.org)
- **Pediatric Endocrine Society** (https://www.lwpes.org)
- **The Endocrine Society** (https://www.endocrine.org)
- **American Thyroid Association** (https://www.thyroid.org)

REFERENCES

A complete list of references can be found online.

Chapter 11

Fluids and Electrolytes

Joniqua Ceasar, MD

See additional content online.

I. INTRODUCTION

Intravenous fluids (IVFs) should be thought of as a medication by those who prescribe them. Since the late 1950s, IVF choice has been largely guided by Holliday and Segar's estimations of sodium requirements. Using the electrolyte composition of human milk, they calculated that the average child requires 3 mEq sodium (Na) and 2 mEq potassium (K) per 100 to 120 mL water (H_2O).[1] According to their calculation, basic solute needs can be met by administering $^1/_4$ normal saline (NS), a hypotonic fluid. While this estimation led to a long-standing tradition in pediatric maintenance IVF (MIVF) therapy, evidence published over the past few decades culminated in new American Academy of Pediatrics (AAP) guidelines recommending isotonic fluids as the maintenance fluid of choice for the majority of hospitalized children.[2]

II. FLUID RESUSCITATION

A. Calculating Maintenance Fluid Volume

The Holliday-Segar method (Table 11.1 and Box 11.1) is the most widely used method to approximate maintenance fluid volume. This method estimates caloric expenditure in fixed-weight categories and assumes the average patient will require 100 mL of water for each 100 calories metabolized, with approximately 100 kcal burned per kg.[1] There is no evidence for a maximum rate, but experts recommend a maximum of 120 mL/hr in absence of any cardiac, hepatic, or renal pathology.[3-4] If concern exists, the maintenance fluid rate should be lowered to avoid volume overload.

NOTE: The Holliday-Segar method is not suitable for neonates <14 days old, because it generally overestimates fluid needs in neonates. (See Chapter 18 for neonatal fluid management.)

B. Calculating Fluid Loss

1. Total body water (TBW) is equal to 60% of a child's weight in kg (75% in infants).[5]

EQUATION 11.1: TBW^a = weight (kg) × 0.6

[a]TBW uses preillness weight; 1 L water = 1 kg water

TABLE 11.1

HOLLIDAY-SEGAR METHOD

	Fluid Volume	
Body Weight	mL/kg/day	mL/kg/hr
First 10 kg	100	≈ 4
Second 10 kg	50	≈ 2
Each additional kg	20	≈ 1

BOX 11.1

HOLLIDAY-SEGAR METHOD

Example: Determine the correct fluid rate for an 8-year-old child weighing 25 kg:

First 10 kg:	4 mL/kg/hr × 10 kg = 40 mL/hr	100 mL/kg/day × 10 kg = 1000 mL/day
Second 10 kg:	2 mL/kg/hr × 10 kg = 20 mL/hr	50 mL/kg/day × 10 kg = 500 mL/day
Each additional 1 kg:	1 mL/kg/hr × 5 kg = 5 mL/hr	20 mL/kg/day × 5 kg = 100 mL/day
	Answer: 65 mL/hr	Answer: 1600 mL/day

2. In a euvolemic child, 60% of TBW resides in the intracellular compartment (where potassium [K] concentration is 140 mEq/L and sodium [Na] is negligible), and 40% of TBW is in the extracellular compartment (where Na concentration is ~ 140 mEq/L and K is negligible).[6-8]

3. The most precise method of assessing fluid deficit uses weight loss:

EQUATION 11.2: Fluid deficit (L) = preillness weight (kg) − illness weight (kg)

4. Clinical assessment: If weight loss is not known, clinical observation may be used to approximate the percentage of dehydration (Table 11.2).[9,10]

EQUATION 11.3: % Dehydration[a] = $\dfrac{\text{fluid deficit}^{b}}{\text{preillness weight}} \times 100\%$

[a]1% dehydration = 10 mL/kg of fluid deficit;

[b]1 L of water = 1 kg of water

5. In a healthy child, insensible fluid volume loss is approximated as $\frac{1}{3}$ of the Holliday-Segar MIVF per day. **NOTE:** This calculation is based on fluid requirements of healthy children. Many hospitalized children have increased insensible losses (e.g., secondary to fever or

TABLE 11.2

CLINICAL OBSERVATIONS IN DEHYDRATION

	Older Child		
	3% (30 mL/kg)	6% (60 mL/kg)	9% (90 mL/kg)
	Infant		
	5% (50 mL/kg)	10% (100 mL/kg)	15% (150 mL/kg)
Dehydration classification	Mild	Moderate	Severe
Mental status	Alert		Lethargic/obtunded
Fontanelle	Flat	Soft	Sunken
Eyes	Normal	Deep set	Sunken
Tears	Present	Reduced	None
Buccal mucosa/lips	Normal/dry	Dry	Parched/cracked
Pulse rate	Normal	Slightly increased	Increased
Skin (touch)	Normal	Dry	Clammy
Skin turgor	Normal	Decreased	Tenting
Capillary refill	Normal	≈3–5 seconds	>5 seconds
Pulse quality	Normal	Weak	Feeble/impalpable
Urine output	Normal/mild oliguria	Mild oliguria	Severe oliguria/anuria

Data from Kliegman R, Geme SJ, eds. *Nelson Textbook of Pediatrics.* 21st ed. Elsevier; 2020; McMillan JA, DeAngelis CD, Feigin RD, Jones MD. *Oski's Pediatrics: Principles and Practice.* 4th ed. Saunders; 2006.

increased respiratory rate) that must be factored into fluid determinations.

C. Maintenance Fluid Choice in Hospitalized Children

Based on a growing body of evidence, the AAP recommends isotonic fluid as the most appropriate MIVF therapy for the vast majority of hospitalized children between the ages of 28 days and 18 years.[2] Neonates under 28 days of age should receive hypotonic fluids (e.g. D5 $\frac{1}{2}$ normal saline).[11]

1. See Table 11.3 for isotonic fluid options.
2. Various disease states can lead to an increased secretion of antidiuretic hormone (ADH), which promotes the retention of free water, leading to hyponatremia.[11,12] See Box 11.2 for examples.
3. Exceptions exist in certain patient populations, such as children with neurosurgical disorders, congenital or acquired cardiac disease, hepatic disease, cancer, acute kidney injury, chronic kidney disease, nephrotic syndrome, diabetes insipidus, and voluminous watery diarrhea or severe burns.[2]
4. See Tables 11.3 and 11.4 for electrolyte composition of various parenteral and enteral fluid replacement options.
5. Unless hyperkalemia is present or the child is in renal failure, maintenance potassium requirements (20 mEq/L of fluid) should be given.[14] Do not add potassium (K^+) to fluids until urine output has been established.[15,16]

TABLE 11.3

COMPOSITION OF FREQUENTLY USED PARENTERAL REHYDRATION FLUIDS

	D% CHO (g/100 mL)	Protein[a] (g/100 mL)	Cal/L	Na^{2+} (mEq/L)	K$^+$ (mEq/L)	Cl$^-$ (mEq/L)	HCO$_3^{-}$[b] (mEq/L)	Mg^{2+} (mEq/L)	Ca^{2+} (mEq/L)	mOsm/L
HYPOTONIC										
D$_5$W	5	—	170	—	—	—	—	—	—	252
D$_{10}$W	10	—	340	—	—	—	—	—	—	505
D$_5$ 1/4 NS (0.225% NaCl)	5	—	170	38.5	—	38.5	—	—	—	329
1/2 NS (0.45% NaCl)	—	—	—	77	—	77	—	—	—	154
ISOTONIC										
Lactated Ringer's	0–10	—	0–340	130	4	109	28	—	3	273
Plasmalyte	—	—	—	140	5	98	27	3	—	294
Bicarbonated Ringer's	0–10	—	0–340	147	4	155.5	—	—	≈4	—
NS (0.9% NaCl)	—	—	—	154	—	154	—	—	—	308
HYPERTONIC										
2% NaCl	—	—	—	342	—	342	—	—	—	684
3% NaCl	—	—	—	513	—	513	—	—	—	1027
8.4% sodium bicarbonate (1 mEq/mL)	—	—	—	1000	—	—	1000	—	—	2000
COLLOID										
Albumin 25% (salt poor)	—	25	1000	100–160	—	<120	—	—	—	300
Intralipid[c]	2.25	2.5	1100	2.5	0.5	4.0	—	—	—	258–284

[a]Protein or amino acid equivalent.

[b]Bicarbonate or equivalent (citrate, acetate, lactate).

[c]Values are approximate; may vary from lot to lot. Also contains <1.2% egg phosphatides.

CHO, Carbohydrate; *HCO$_3^-$,* bicarbonate; *NS,* normal saline.

BOX 11.2

CLINICAL SETTING OF INCREASED ADH RELEASE IN CHILDREN[9,29]

Hemodynamic Stimuli for ADH Release (Decreased Effective Volume)	Nonosmotic and Nonhemodynamic Stimuli for ADH Release
Hypovolemia	CNS disturbances (infection, brain tumors, head injury, thrombosis)
Nephrosis	Pulmonary disease (pneumonia, asthma, bronchiolitis, PPV)
Cirrhosis	
Congestive heart failure	Cancer
Hypoaldosteronism	Medications/drugs (Ecstasy, AEDs, cytoxan, vincristine, opiates, TCAs, SSRIs)
Hypotension	
Hypoalbuminemia	
	GI disturbances (nausea and emesis)
	Pain or stress
	Postoperative state

AEDs, antiepileptic drugs; *CNS,* central nervous system; *PPV,* positive pressure ventilation; *SSRIs,* selective serotonin reuptake inhibitors; *TCAs,* tricyclic antidepressants.

D. Volume Replacement Strategy[9,15,16]

1. Volume resuscitation and deficit replacement should generally be completed over 24 hours.
2. See Table 11.5 for a three-phase approach to fluid replacement.
3. Children with isonatremic hypovolemia can be repleted with isotonic fluid per AAP recommendations.[2] See Box 11.3 for sample calculations in isonatremic hypovolemia.
4. If ongoing losses can be measured directly, they should be replaced 1:1 concurrently with maintenance fluid administration. If the losses cannot be measured, an estimate of 10 mL/kg body weight for each watery stool and 2 mL/kg body weight for each episode of emesis should be administered.[5] See Table 11.6 for electrolyte composition of certain bodily fluids.
5. Oral intake is the preferred method for repletion and maintenance, if possible.

III. FLUID REMOVAL

A. Diuretics

1. Please see Chapter 19 for commonly used diuretics.
2. Maintenance fluids and diuretics should not be administered concurrently except in the following clinical scenarios:
   a. Needing to provide dextrose-containing fluids when there is also a concern for volume overload
   b. Treatment for hypercalcemia or hyperkalemia

TABLE 11.4
COMPOSITION OF ORAL REHYDRATION FLUIDS

	D% CHO (g/100 mL)	Na²⁺ (mEq/L)	K⁺ (mEq/L)	Cl⁻ (mEq/L)	HCO₃⁻ᵃ (mEq/L)	Ca²⁺ (mEq/L)	mOsm/L
ORAL FLUIDS							
Pedialyte	2.5	45	20	35	30	—	250
WHO solution	2	90	20	80	30	—	311
Rehydralyte	2.5	75	20	65	30	—	305
COMMONLY CONSUMED FLUIDS (NOT RECOMMENDED FOR ORAL REHYDRATION)ᵇ							
Apple juice	12	0.4	44	45	—	—	730
Coca-Cola	10.8	5.2	—	—	13.4	—	650
Gatorade	5.9	36	10	—	—	—	377
Ginger ale	9	3.5	0.1	—	3.6	—	565
Milk	4.9	22	36	28	30	—	260
Orange juice	10.4	0.2	49	—	50	—	654
Powerade	5.8	18	2.7	—	—	—	264

ᵃBicarbonate or equivalent (citrate, acetate, lactate).
ᵇElectrolyte values are approximate. Data will vary by brand.
CHO, Carbohydrate; *HCO₃⁻*, bicarbonate; *WHO*, World Health Organization.
Data from McMillan JA, DeAngelis CD, Feigin RD, Jones MD. *Oski's Pediatrics: Principles and Practice.* 4th ed. Saunders; 2006., and USDA website https://fdc.nal.usda.gov/index.html.

11

TABLE 11.5

VOLUME REPLACEMENT STRATEGY

Phase I	Phase II	Phase III
Initial Stabilization	**Deficit Repletion, Maintenance Volume, and Ongoing Losses**	**Recovery and Ongoing Losses**
Rapid fluid resuscitation with isotonic fluid[a]	Replace half of the remaining deficit over the first 8 hr (this includes any fluid given in the initial stabilization phase).	Continue maintenance fluid administration, taking ongoing losses into consideration.
20 mL/kg represents only a 2% volume replacement	Replace the second half of deficit over the following 16 hr, making sure to also include maintenance fluid volume during this time.	

[a]Should be used in patients in need of rapid volume expansion.
See Box 11.3 for sample calculation.

BOX 11.3

SAMPLE CALCULATIONS: ISONATREMIC DEHYDRATION

Example: A 15-kg (pre-illness weight) child with 10% dehydration and normal serum sodium

Requirement	Formula	Sample Calculation
Maintenance fluid requirements	Holliday–Segar formula	(100 mL/kg/day $\times$ 10 kg) + (50 mL/kg/day $\times$ 5 kg) = 1250 mL/24 hr = 52 mL/hr
Fluid deficit	Eq. 11.2 or Eq. 11.3	10 mL/kg $\times$ 15 kg $\times$ 10% = 1500 mL

FLUID REPLACEMENT RATE OVER 24 HR

$\frac{1}{2}$ fluid deficit replaced in first 8 hr   750 mL/8 hr = 94 mL/hr + 52 mL/hr maintenance = 146 mL/hr

$\frac{1}{2}$ fluid deficit replaced over 16 hr   750 mL/16 hr = 47 mL/hr + 52 mL/hr maintenance = 99 mL/hr

NOTE: If patient received an initial 20 mL/kg bolus (300 mL): 1500 mL − 300 mL = 1200 mL

$\frac{1}{2}$ fluid deficit in first 8 hr: 600 mL/8 hr = 75 mL + 52 mL/hr maintenance = 127 mL/hr

$\frac{1}{2}$ fluid deficit over next 16 hr: 600 mL/16 hr = 38 mL/hr + 52 mL/hr maintenance = 90 mL/hr

---

   c. Treatment for tubular toxins (e.g., rhabdomyolysis or nephrotoxic chemotherapy administration) when there is also a concern for volume overload

B. Indications for Acute Dialysis: Please refer to Chapter 19, Section IX.

IV. ELECTROLYTE MANAGEMENT

See Chapter 28 for age-specific normal values of electrolytes.

TABLE 11.6			
ELECTROLYTE COMPOSITION OF VARIOUS FLUIDS			
Source of Fluid	Na$^+$ (mEq/L)	K$^+$ (mEq/L)	Cl$^-$ (mEq/L)
Gastric	20–80	5–20	100–150
Pancreatic	120–140	5–15	90–120
Small bowel	100–140	5–15	90–130
Bile	120–140	5–15	80–120
Ileostomy	45–135	3–15	20–115
Diarrhea	10–90	10–80	10–110
Skin with burns[a]	140	5	110
Sweat			
Normal	10–30	3–10	10–35
Cystic fibrosis[b]	50–130	5–25	50–110

[a]3–5 g/dL of protein may be lost in fluid from burn wounds.
[b]Replacement fluid dependent on sodium content.
Modified from Kliegman RM, Stanton B, St. Gene J, et al. *Nelson Textbook of Pediatrics.* 19th ed. Saunders; 2011.

A. Serum Osmolality and Tonicity[2,9,17]

1. Fluids can be expressed in terms of their tonicity and their osmolality.
2. Serum osmolality (normally maintained at 285 to 295 mOsm/kg) is a measure of both permeable and nonpermeable solutes and is calculated using the following equation:

EQUATION 11.4: $\text{Osmolality} = 2\,\text{Na} + \dfrac{\text{glucose (mg/dL)}}{18} + \dfrac{\text{BUN (mg/dL)}}{2.8}$

3. Osmolality is measured as osmoles per weight (kg) versus osmolarity, which is measured as osmoles per volume (L).
4. Tonicity is effective osmolality. It is the net force on water across a semipermeable membrane (e.g., the cell membrane) based on the osmotic pressures. It is relative and determined largely by sodium content. Substances that flow freely across membranes, such as urea, are ineffective osmoles and influence osmolality but not tonicity.

B. Sodium

The equations within this section are **theoretical** and are not validated. They offer a starting point for calculation of electrolyte abnormalities, but clinical context is **ALWAYS** of the utmost importance and frequent monitoring is necessary. **Children with neurosurgical disorders, cardiac disease, hepatic disease, cancer, kidney disease, diabetes insipidus, and severe burns may require consultation with subspecialists before fluid choice and volume is administered.** When correcting dysnatremias, frequent lab monitoring (~2 to 4 hours) is indicated with adjustment of fluid type and rate as needed.

1. **Hyponatremia:** Excess Na loss (Na <135 mEq/L)
   a. Clinical manifestations and differential diagnosis (Table 11.7)

TABLE 11.7

HYPONATREMIA[7,14,9]

CLINICAL MANIFESTATIONS			
Related to rate of change: Nausea, headache, muscle cramps, weakness, confusion, apnea, lethargy, seizure, coma, hypothermia, depressed DTRs			

ETIOLOGIES			
Hypovolemic		**Euvolemic**	**Hypervolemic**
Renal Losses	**Extrarenal Losses**		
Salt-wasting nephropathy	GI losses	SIADH (see Chapter 10)	Nephrotic syndrome
Diuretic use	Skin losses	Excess salt-free infusions	Hypoalbuminemia
Juvenile nephronophthisis	Third spacing	Desmopressin acetate	Heart failure
Hypoaldosteronism (CAH, pseudohypoaldosteronism, UTI/obstruction)	Cystic fibrosis	Water intoxication	Cirrhosis
Cerebral salt-wasting syndrome		Hypothyroidism	Renal failure
Postobstructive diuresis		Sepsis	Glucocorticoid deficiency
ATN (polyuric phase)		Primary polydipsia[a]	
		Malnutrition[a]	

LABORATORY DATA			
↑ Urine Na (>20 mEq/L)	↓ Urine Na (<20 mEq/L)	↓ Urine volume	↓ Urine Na[b] (<20 mEq/L)
↑ Urine volume	↓ Urine volume	↑ Specific gravity	↓ Urine volume
↓ Specific gravity	↑ Specific gravity	↑ Urine osmolality (>100 mOsm/L)	
↓ Urine osmolality[c] (<100 mOsm/L)	↑ Urine osmolality (>100 mOsm/L)		

MANAGEMENT			
Replace losses (see hypovolemic hyponatremia)		Restrict fluids	
		Address the underlying cause	

[a]Urine osmolality is <100 mOsm/L.
[b]Urine Na may be appropriate for the level of Na intake in patients with SIADH and water intoxication.
[c]Minimum possible urine osmolality = 50 mOsm/kg.
ATN, Acute tubular necrosis; *CAH*, congenital adrenal hyperplasia; *DTR*, deep tendon reflex; *GI*, gastrointestinal; *SIADH*, syndrome of inappropriate antidiuretic hormone secretion; *UTI*, urinary tract infection.

---

   b. Causes of pseudohyponatremia:
     (1) Increased serum osmolality:
       (a) Hyperglycemia: Na decreased 1.6 mEq/L for each 100 mg/dL rise in glucose. The fluid shifts that cause the hyponatremia will partially correct on their own as the hyperglycemia normalizes.
     (2) Normal serum osmolality:
       (a) Hyperlipidemia: Na artificially decreased by $0.002 \times$ lipid (mg/dL)
       (b) Hyperproteinemia: Na artificially decreased by $0.25 \times$ [protein (g/dL) − 8]

   c. Management
     (1) The traditional equation used to calculate the excess sodium deficit in hyponatremia is:

EQUATION 11.5[3]:

Na deficit $(mEq)^a$ = [Desired Na (mEq/L) − Serum Na (mEq/L)] × TBW (L)

[a]This represents the *excess* sodium deficit in hyponatremic dehydration. It must be added to the daily sodium requirement for hospitalized patients of **~14 mEq/100 mL fluid given.**

     (2) Hyponatremia should be corrected **by no more than 10 to 12 mEq per 24 hr** to avoid rapid change of serum sodium, which can cause osmotic demyelination syndrome.[8,16,18]
     (3) Witnessed onset of hyponatremia over the course of hours does not pose as great of a risk and can be corrected in a similar amount of time to that in which it developed.[9]
     (4) If central nervous system (CNS) symptoms are present, hypertonic saline (HTS) should be administered over 3 to 4 hours to correct the hyponatremia by ~5 mEq/L.[7,8,14] Use Eq. 11.7 to determine rate of HTS.
     (5) To determine the sodium content of the fluid necessary for repletion:

EQUATION 11.6: Na content (mEq/L) =

$$\frac{\text{Na deficit} + (14 \text{ mEq}/100\text{mL} \times \text{maintenance fluid volume [mL]})}{\text{volume deficit}^a}$$

[a]Use daily maintenance volume requirements if euvolemic.

     (6) Once the fluid type is determined, the starting rate can be calculated using the following:

EQUATION 11.7:

$$\text{Fluid rate (mL/hour)} = \frac{\text{Na deficit (mEq)} \times 1000 \text{ mL}}{\text{infusate Na (mEq)} \times \text{hours IVF will run in a day}}$$

     (7) See Boxes 11.4 and 11.5 for sample calculations in hyponatremic dehydration.
2. **Hypernatremia:** Excess free water loss (Na >145 mEq/L)
   a. Clinical manifestations and differential diagnosis (Table 11.8)
   b. Management:
     (1) Hypernatremic hypovolemia occurs in scenarios in which free water is either unavailable/restricted or there is excessive loss of solute-free water (see Table 11.8).

BOX 11.4

SAMPLE CALCULATIONS: HYPONATREMIC DEHYDRATION

Example: A 15-kg (pre-illness weight) child with 10% dehydration and serum sodium 125 mEq/L without central nervous system symptoms

Requirement	Formula	Sample Calculation
Maintenance fluid requirements	Holliday-Segar formula	(100 mL/kg/d × 10 kg) + (50 mL/kg/d × 5 kg) = 1250 mL/24 hr = 52 mL/hr
Fluid deficit	Eq. 11.2 or Eq. 11.3	10 mL/kg × 15 kg × 10% = 1500 mL

FLUID REPLACEMENT RATE OVER 24 HRS

1500 mL/24 hr = 63 mL/hr + 52 mL/hr maintenance = 115 mL/hr

CALCULATIONS FOR FLUID SELECTION

Maintenance sodium requirements	3 mEq per 100 mL of maintenance fluid	3 mEq × (1250 mL/100 mL) = 38 mEq Na^+
Isotonic sodium deficit	8–10 mEq Na^+ per each 100 mL of fluid deficit	10 mEq × (1500 mL/100 mL) = 150 mEq Na^+
Sodium deficit	Eq. 11.5	(135 mEq − 125 mEq) × 9 = 90 mEq Na^+
Total sodium content	Eq. 11.6	90 mEq + (14 mEq/100 mL × 1250 mL) = 265 mEq
Sodium required per L	Divide total sodium by fluid deficit in L	265 mEq/1.5 L = 177 mEq

BOX 11.5

SAMPLE CALCULATIONS: SEVERE SYMPTOMATIC HYPONATREMIC DEHYDRATION

Initial Fluid Replacement for Neurologic Stabilization

Example: A 15-kg (pre-illness weight) child with altered mental status and serum sodium 110 mEq/L

Fluid to be used: 3% hypertonic saline (HTS)

Requirement	Formula	Sample Calculation
Sodium deficit	Eq. 11.5	5 mEq/L × 9 = 45 mEq Na^+
Rate of administration	Eq. 11.7	[(45 mEq × 1000 mL) /513 mEq × 4 hr] = 22 mL/hr of 3% HTS

TABLE 11.8

HYPERNATREMIA[7,6,9]

CLINICAL MANIFESTATIONS

With hypernatremic hypovolemia, there is better preservation of intravascular volume compared to hypovolemic hyponatremia. Lethargy, weakness, altered mental status, irritability, coma, and seizures. High-pitched cry, thrombosis, brain hemorrhage, muscle cramps, hyperpnea, and respiratory failure.

ETIOLOGIES

Low Urine Osmolality	Elevated Urine Osmolality[a,b]	
	↓ Urine Na (<20 mEq/L)	↑ Urine Na (>20 mEq/L)
Diabetes insipidus (central and nephrogenic) (see Chapters 10 and 19)	GI losses	Exogenous Na⁺ (meds, infant formula)
Postobstructive diuresis	Skin losses	Mineralocorticoid excess (e.g., hyperaldosteronism)
CKD	Respiratory	
Diuretic use	Increased insensible losses	
Polyuric phase of ATN	Adipsia	

MANAGEMENT

Timeline of onset can mirror timeline for correction.

[a]>1000 mOsm/kg in extrarenal water loss.

[b]This cause of hypernatremia is usually secondary to free water loss; therefore the fractional excretion of sodium may be decreased or normal.

ATN, Acute tubular necrosis; *CKD*, chronic kidney disease; *GI*, gastrointestinal; *Na*, sodium.

(2) Hypernatremia is dangerous because of complications from potential treatment sequelae, the most serious of which is cerebral edema.[6,9]

(3) Plan to correct the serum Na by no more than 10 mEq/24 hr and correct the free water deficit over 48 hours to minimize the risk of cerebral edema.[6,12,13,19]

(4) As with hyponatremia, witnessed onset of hypernatremia over the course of hours can be corrected rapidly; this is because the brain has not had time to produce idiogenic osmoles to adapt to the change in osmolality.[9,13]

(5) Expert opinion recommends starting with D5 ½ NS.[19] However, the sodium and fluid needs can also be calculated.

(6) The free water deficit is as follows:

EQUATION 11.8[4, 6]:

$$FWD \text{ (mL)} = TBW \text{ (mL)} \times \left[1 - \frac{Desired \ Na \ (mEq/L)}{Serum \ Na \ (mEq/L)}\right]^{a}$$

[a]The difference in desired and serum Na should be no more than 10 mEq/L/day.

(7) The FWD is used to calculate the solute fluid deficit (SFD) (i.e., the amount of fluid that contains electrolytes).

EQUATION 11.9: SFD = Fluid deficit[a] − FWD

$\qquad$ [a]See eq. 11.2 for fluid deficit calculations.

(8) Despite the hypernatremia, there is also a Na deficit that should be accounted for:

EQUATION 11.10:

$$\text{Na required (mEq)} = [\text{SFD (mL)} + \text{maintence fluid volume (mL)}] \times \frac{14 \text{ mEq}}{100 \text{mL}}$$

(9) The amount of sodium is then divided by the total fluid deficit in addition to the maintenance fluid volume. This will help approximate the fluid tonicity required.

EQUATION 11.11:

$$\text{Na content of fluid (mEq/L)} = \frac{\text{Na required (mEq)}}{\text{Fluid deficit (L)} + \text{maintence fluid volume (L)}}$$

(10) See Box 11.6 for sample calculations in hypernatremic dehydration.

BOX 11.6

SAMPLE CALCULATIONS: HYPERNATREMIC DEHYDRATION

Example: A 15-kg (pre-illness weight) child with 10% dehydration and serum sodium 155 mEq/L

Requirement	Formula	Sample Calculation
Maintenance fluid requirements	Holliday-Segar formula	(100 mL/kg/d × 10 kg) + (50 mL/kg/d × 5 kg) = 1250 mL/24 hr = 52 mL/hr
Total fluid deficit	Eq. 11.2 or Eq. 11.3	10 mL/kg × 15 kg × 10% = 1500 mL
Fluid Replacement Rate Over 24 hrs		
1500 mL/24 hr = 63 mL/hr + 52 mL/hr maintenance = 115 mL/hr		
Calculations for Fluid Selection		
Free water deficit	Eq. 11.8	9000 mL × [1 − (145 mEq/L/ 155 mEq/L)] = 585 mL (~600)
Solute fluid deficit	Eq. 11.9	1500 mL − 600 mL = 900 mL
Total sodium required	Eq. 11.10	(900 mL + 1250 mL) × 14 mEq/ 100 mL = 300 mEq Na$^+$
Na content of fluid	Eq. 11.11	300 mEq / (1.25 + 1.5 L) = 110 mEq/L Na

(11) If the fluid necessary contains >154 mEq of Na, then the following equation can be used to make a 1L bag at the desired tonicity[19]:

EQUATION 11.12:

$$\text{mL of 3\% saline} = 1000 \text{ mL} \times \frac{\text{desired Na (mEq/L)} - 154 \text{ (mEq/L)}}{513 \text{ (mEq/L)} - \text{desired Na (mEq/L)}}$$

(12) This equation can also be used to calculate rate to run HTS with NS bolus in a severely hypernatremic child. See Box 11.7.

3. Calculations pertaining to dysnatremias can be double-checked using the following equation:

EQUATION 11.13[4–6]:

$$\frac{\text{Change in Serum Na}}{\text{1L of parenteral fluid administration}} = \frac{(\text{Infusate Na} + \text{Infusate K}) - \text{Serum Na}}{\text{TBW} + 1}$$

BOX 11.7

SAMPLE CALCULATIONS: SEVERE HYPERNATREMIC DEHYDRATION

Initial Fluid Resuscitation Strategy to Avoid Rapid Sodium Correction When Serum Na$^+$ >175 mEq/L[16]

Example: A 3-kg (pre-illness weight) breastfed neonate appearing severely dehydrated with serum sodium 185 mEq/L and hemodynamic instability.

Resuscitation with normal saline (NS) may drop the serum Na$^+$ too quickly. Plan to simultaneously run NS and 3% hypertonic saline (HTS), given rapidly together (i.e., over 5 minutes), to effectively give resuscitation fluid with a concentration no more than 15 mEq/L below the child's serum Na$^+$. Repeat the boluses as needed to achieve hemodynamic stability.

Requirement	Formula	Sample Calculation
Ideal bolus fluid concentration	Serum sodium (in mEq/L) − 15 mEq/L	185 mEq/L − 15 mEq/L = 170 mEq/L
mL of HTS required per L of NS	Eq. 11.12	1000 mL × (170 mEq/L − 154 mEq/L) / (513 mEq/L − 170 mEq/L) = 47 mL
Bolus NS amount in mL	20 mL/kg × wt (in kg)	20 mL/kg × 3 kg = 60 mL
Bolus amount HTS in mL	mL HTS required per L of NS × NS bolus amount (in mL) / 1000 mL	47 mL × 60 mL / 1000 mL = 2.8 mL

C. Potassium

1. **Hypokalemia**
   a. Clinical manifestations and differential diagnosis (Table 11.9)
   b. The transtubular potassium gradient (TTKG) can help differentiate between etiologies of hypokalemia, as noted in Table 11.9:

EQUATION 11.14 [9]:

$$TTKG^a = \frac{[K]_{urine}}{[K]_{plasma}} \times \left(\frac{\text{plasma osmolality}}{\text{urine osmolality}} \right)$$

   [a] The urine osmolality must be greater than the serum osmolality for the calculation to be valid.

   c. Management: Potassium infusion rates generally should not exceed 1 mEq/kg/hr.[3]

2. **Hyperkalemia**
   a. Clinical manifestations and differential diagnosis (Table 11.10)
   b. Management (Fig. 11.1)

D. Calcium

1. **Hypocalcemia**
   a. Clinical manifestations and differential diagnosis (Table 11.11)
   b. Special considerations:
      (1) Albumin readily binds serum calcium. Correction for albumin: Δ of 1 g/dL changes the total serum calcium in the same direction by 0.8 mg/dL.
      (2) pH: Acidosis increases ionized calcium.
      (3) Symptoms of hypocalcemia refractory to calcium supplementation may be caused by hypomagnesemia.
      (4) Significant hyperphosphatemia should be corrected before the correction of hypocalcemia because renal calculi or soft-tissue calcification may occur if total $[Ca^{2+}] \times [PO_4^{3-}] \geq 70$.[9]

2. **Hypercalcemia:** Table 11.11

E. Magnesium

1. Hypomagnesemia: Table 11.12
2. Hypermagnesemia: Table 11.12

F. Phosphate

1. Hypophosphatemia: Table 11.13
2. Hyperphosphatemia: Table 11.13

V. ALGORITHM FOR EVALUATING ACID-BASE DISTURBANCES[9,20,21]

A. Determine the pH.

The body does not fully compensate for primary acid-base disorders; therefore the primary disturbance will shift the pH away from 7.40. See Chapter 28 for normal bicarbonate values by age.

TABLE 11.9

HYPOKALEMIA[9,28]

CLINICAL MANIFESTATIONS

Manifest at levels <2.5 mEq/L. Skeletal muscle weakness or ascending paralysis, muscle cramps, ileus, urinary retention, and cardiac arrhythmias. Electrocardiogram (ECG) changes: delayed depolarization, flat T waves, depressed ST segment, and U waves.

ETIOLOGIES

	Decreased Stores				
Metabolic Alkalosis					
Hypertensive	**Normotensive**	**Metabolic Acidosis**	**No Change in Serum pH**	**Extrarenal**	**Normal Stores[a]**
Renovascular disease	Gitelman syndrome	RTA (type I and II)	Meds (amphotericin, cisplatin,	Skin losses	Acute metabolic alkalosis
Excess renin	Bartter syndrome	DKA	aminoglycosides, penicillin or penicillin	GI losses/laxative	Hyperinsulinemia
Cushing syndrome	Hypoparathyroidism	Ureterosigmoidostomy	derivatives, diuretics)	abuse/enema abuse	Leukocytosis (if sample sits at room
CAH	Cystic fibrosis	Fanconi syndrome	Interstitial nephritis	Clay ingestion	temperature)
Adrenal adenoma	EAST syndrome			Malnutrition/anorexia	Meds (adrenergic agonists, theophylline,
Licorice ingestion	Loop and thiazide			nervosa	toluene, cesium chloride,
Liddle syndrome	diuretics				hydroxychloroquine, barium)
	Emesis				Familial hypokalemic periodic paralysis

LABORATORY DATA

TTKG >4				TTKG ≤4	~Urine K⁺

MANAGEMENT

Acute	Calculate deficit and replace with potassium acetate or potassium chloride. Enteral replacement is safer when feasible. Follow K⁺ closely. IV replacement generally should not exceed 1 mEq/kg given over 1 hr.
Chronic	Determine daily requirement and replace with potassium chloride or potassium gluconate.

[a]Blood pressure may vary.

CAH, Congenital adrenal hyperplasia; *DKA*, diabetic ketoacidosis; *GI*, gastrointestinal; *K⁺*, potassium; *RTA*, renal tubular acidosis; *EAST*, epilepsy, ataxia, sensorineural hearing loss, and tubulopathy; *TTKG*, transtubular potassium gradient.

11

TABLE 11.10

HYPERKALEMIA[9]

CLINICAL MANIFESTATIONS

Skeletal muscle weakness, fasciculations, paresthesias, and ascending paralysis. The typical ECG progression with increasing serum K^+ values:

1. Peaked T waves
2. Prolonged PR and widening of QRS
3. Loss of P waves
4. ST segment depression with further widening of QRS
5. Bradycardia, atrioventricular (AV) block, ventricular arrhythmias, torsades de pointes, and cardiac arrest

ETIOLOGIES

Increased Total Body K^+		Intracellular Shifts (No Change in Total Body K^+)
Increased Urine K^+	**Decreased Urine K^+**	
Transfusion with aged blood	Renal failure	Tumor lysis syndrome
Exogenous K^+	Hypoaldosteronism	Leukocytosis ($>200 \times 10^3/\mu L$)
Spitzer syndrome	Aldosterone insensitivity	Thrombocytosis ($>750 \times 10^3/\mu L$)[a]
	↓ Insulin causing hyperglycemia and/or DKA	Metabolic acidosis[b]
	Congenital adrenal hyperplasia	Blood drawing (hemolyzed sample)
	Type IV RTA	Rhabdomyolysis/crush injury
	Meds: ACE inhibitors, angiotensin II blockers, K^+-sparing diuretics, calcineurin inhibitors, NSAIDs, heparin, TMX, drospirenone	Malignant hyperthermia
		Theophylline intoxication

MANAGEMENT
See Fig. 11.1.

[a]For every platelet increase of 100,000/μL, there is a 0.15 mEq/L increase in serum K^+.

[b]For every 0.1-unit reduction in arterial pH, there is approximately a 0.2–0.4 mEq/L increase in plasma K^+.

ACE, Angiotensin-converting enzyme; *DKA*, diabetic ketoacidosis; *ECG*, electrocardiogram; K^+, potassium; *NSAIDs*, nonsteroidal antiinflammatory drugs; *RTA*, renal tubular acidosis; *TMX*, trimethoprim.

---

1. Acidemia (pH < 7.35):
   a. Respiratory acidosis: PCO_2 > 45 mmHg
   b. Metabolic acidosis: Arterial HCO_3 < 20 mmol/L
2. Alkalemia (pH > 7.45):
   a. Respiratory alkalosis: PCO_2 < 35 mmHg
   b. Metabolic alkalosis: Arterial HCO_3 > 28 mmol/L

B. Calculate the anion gap (AG).

1. **AG:** Represents anions other than bicarbonate and chloride required to balance the positive charge of Na. Normal: 12 mEq/L ± 2 mEq/L

$$\text{EQUATION 11.15: } AG = Na^+ - (Cl^- + HCO_3^-)$$

2. The majority of unmeasured anions contributing to the AG in normal individuals are albumin and phosphate. Correcting the AG for albumin concentration increases the utility of the traditional method.[22]

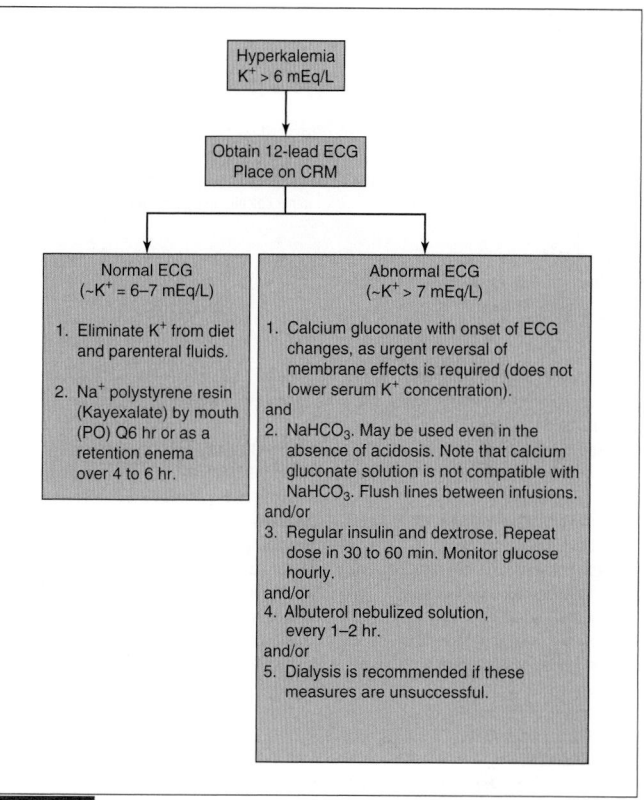

FIGURE 11.1

Algorithm for hyperkalemia. *CRM*, Cardiorespiratory monitor; *ECG*, electrocardiogram.

EQUATION 11.16: Corrected AG =

Observed AG + 2.5 × (Normal abumin − measured albumin)

AG > 15: Anion gap mtabolic acidosis (AGMA)

AG < 12: Nonelevated anion gap metabolic acidosis (NAGAMA)

AG > 20 mEq/L: Primary AGMA regardless of the pH or serum

HCO_3^- concentration

C. Calculate the delta gap (DG).[20]

If there is an AGMA, calculating the DG will help to determine if there is another, concurrent metabolic abnormality:

TABLE 11.11

HYPOCALCEMIA AND HYPERCALCEMIA

Hypocalcemia	Hypercalcemia
CLINICAL MANIFESTATIONS	
Signs and symptoms: Tetany, neuromuscular irritability with weakness, paresthesias, fatigue, cramping, altered mental status, seizures, laryngospasm, and cardiac arrhythmias	Signs and symptoms: Weakness, irritability, lethargy, seizures, coma, abdominal cramping, anorexia, nausea, vomiting, polyuria, polydipsia, renal calculi, and pancreatitis
Physical exam: • Trousseau sign (carpopedal spasm after arterial occlusion of an extremity for 3 minutes) • Chvostek sign (muscle twitching on percussion of the facial nerve)	
ECG changes: Prolonged QT interval	ECG changes: Shortened QT interval
ETIOLOGIES	
Hypoparathyroidism Vitamin D deficiency Hyperphosphatemia Pancreatitis Malabsorption (malnutrition) Drugs (anticonvulsants, cimetidine, aminoglycosides, calcium channel blockers) Hypomagnesemia/hypermagnesemia Maternal hyperparathyroidism (in neonates) Ethylene glycol ingestion Calcitriol (activated vitamin D) insufficiency Tumor lysis syndrome	Hyperparathyroidism Vitamin D intoxication Excessive exogenous calcium administration Malignancy Prolonged immobilization Thiazide diuretics Subcutaneous fat necrosis Williams syndrome Granulomatous disease (e.g., sarcoidosis) Hyperthyroidism Milk-alkali syndrome
MANAGEMENT	
Acute Consider IV replacement (calcium gluconate or calcium chloride [central access preferred]) Chronic Consider use of oral supplements of calcium carbonate, calcium gluconate, calcium glubionate, or calcium lactate	Increase UOP and Ca^{2+} excretion: 1. If the glomerular filtration rate and blood pressure are stable, give NS with maintenance K^+ at 2–3 times the maintenance rate 2. Diuresis with furosemide Consider hemodialysis for severe or refractory cases. Consider steroids in malignancy, granulomatous disease, and vitamin D toxicity to decrease vitamin D and Ca^{2+} absorption Severe or persistently elevated Ca^{2+}: Consider calcitonin or bisphosphonate

Ca^{2+}, Calcium; *ECG*, electrocardiogram; *UOP*, urine output.

EQUATION 11.17: $DG = (AG - 12) - (24 - HCO_3^-)$

DG > 6: combined AGMA and metabolic alkalosis

DG < −6: combined AGMA and NAGMA

TABLE 11.12

HYPOMAGNESEMIA AND HYPERMAGNESEMIA[9]

Hypomagnesemia				Hypermagnesemia
CLINICAL MANIFESTATIONS				
Prominent manifestations may be caused by concurrent hypocalcemia (see Table 11.11) Typically occur at levels <0.7 mg/dL: Anorexia, nausea, weakness, malaise, depression, nonspecific psychiatric symptoms, hyperreflexia, ECG changes: flattening of T wave and lengthening of ST segment				Typically occur at levels >4.5 mg/dL: Hypotonia, hyporeflexia, paralysis, lethargy, confusion, hypotension, and prolonged QT, QRS, and PR intervals. Respiratory failure and cardiac arrest at >15 mg/dL
ETIOLOGIES				
GI Disorders	Genetic	Medications	Miscellaneous	Renal Failure and Excessive Administration
Diarrhea	Gitelman syndrome	Amphotericin	Decreased intake	Status asthmaticus eclampsia/ preeclampsia, cathartics, enemas, phosphate binders, laxatives, lithium ingestions, milk-alkali syndrome
Malabsorption diseases	Bartter syndrome	Cisplatin	Hungry bone syndrome	
Short bowel	EAST syndrome	Cyclosporine	Exchange transfusion	
Malnutrition	AD hypoparathyroidism	Loop and thiazide diuretics	Diabetes mellitus	
Pancreatitis	Mitochondrial disorders	Mannitol	Steatorrhea	
	Miscellaneous disorders	Pentamidine	Hyperaldosteronism	
MANAGEMENT				
Acute		IV magnesium sulfate		Stop supplemental Mg^{2+}
Chronic		PO magnesium oxide or magnesium sulfate		Diuresis Ca^{2+} supplements, such as calcium chloride (central access preferred) or calcium gluconate

AD, Autosomal dominant; *Ca^{2+}*, calcium; *EAST*, epilepsy, ataxia, sensorineural hearing loss, and tubulopathy; *ECG*, electrocardiogram; *GI*, gastrointestinal; *IV*, intravenous; *Mg^{2+}*, magnesium ; *PO*, by mouth.

D. Calculate the osmolal gap.

> **EQUATION 11.18:** Serum osmolal gap = calculated serum osmolality −laboratory measured osmolality

TABLE 11.13

HYPOPHOSPHATEMIA AND HYPERPHOSPHATEMIA[9]

Hypophosphatemia	Hyperphosphatemia
CLINICAL MANIFESTATIONS	
Symptomatic only at very low levels (<1 mg/dL)	Symptoms of resulting hypocalemia and systemic calcification (i.e., deposition of phosphorus-calcium salts in tissues)
Acute: rhabdomyolysis, tremor, paresthesias, irritability, confusion, hemolysis, delirium, seizure, myocardial depression, and coma	
Chronic: Rickets, proximal muscle weakness	
ETIOLOGIES	
Refeeding syndrome	Tumor lysis syndrome
Insulin	Rhabdomyolysis
BMT	DKA/lactic acidosis
Hungry bone syndrome	Hemolysis
Decreased intake	Renal failure
Antacids	Hypoparathyroidism
Glucocorticoids	Hyperthyroidism
Rickets	Excessive intake (enemas/laxatives and cow's milk)
Hyperparathyroidism	Vitamin D intoxication
Increased renal losses (e.g., renal tubular defects, diuretic use)	Familial tumoral calcinosis
McCune-Albright syndrome	Acromegaly
Epidermal nevus syndrome	
Fanconi syndrome	
Metabolic acidosis/respiratory alkalosis	
Glycosuria	
Volume expansion	
Sepsis	
MANAGEMENT	
Acute IV potassium phosphate or sodium phosphate	Restrict dietary phosphate.
Chronic PO potassium phosphate or sodium phosphate	Phosphate binders (calcium carbonate, aluminum hydroxide)

BMT, Bone marrow transplant; *DKA*, diabetic ketoacidosis. *IV*, intravenous; *PO*, by mouth.

1. There is always a difference (<6) between calculated osmolality and measured osmolality.[24]
2. A markedly elevated osmolar gap (>10) in the setting of an AG acidosis is highly suggestive of acute methanol or ethylene glycol intoxication.[25-27]

E. Calculate expected compensatory response (Table 11.14).

1. Pure **respiratory** acidosis (or alkalosis): 10 mmHg rise (fall) in $PaCO_2$ results in an average 0.08 fall (rise) in pH.
2. Pure **metabolic** acidosis (or alkalosis): 10 mEq/L fall (rise) in HCO_3^- results in an average 0.15 fall (rise) in pH.

TABLE 11.14

CALCULATION OF EXPECTED COMPENSATORY RESPONSE[20,9]

Disturbance	Primary Change	Expected Compensatory Response
Acute respiratory acidosis	$\uparrow PaCO_2$	$\uparrow HCO_3^-$ by 1 mEq/L for each 10 mmHg rise in $Paco_2$
Acute respiratory alkalosis	$\downarrow PaCO_2$	$\downarrow HCO_3^-$ by 2 mEq/L for each 10 mmHg fall in $Paco_2$
Chronic respiratory acidosis	$\uparrow PaCO_2$	$\uparrow HCO_3^-$ by 4 mEq/L for each 10 mmHg rise in $Paco_2$
Chronic respiratory alkalosis	$\downarrow PaCO_2$	$\downarrow HCO_3^-$ by 4 mEq/L for each 10 mmHg fall in $Paco_2$
Metabolic acidosis	$\downarrow HCO_3^-$	$PaCO_2 = 1.5 \times [HCO_3^-] + 8 \pm 2$
Metabolic alkalosis	$\uparrow HCO_3^-$	$\uparrow PaCO_2$ by 7 mmHg for each 10 mEq/L rise in HCO_3^-

F. Determine the likely etiology.

Check for appropriate compensation. See Box 11.8 for helpful mnemonics.

G. If there is not appropriate compensation, consider an additional acid-base derangement (Fig. 11.2).

BOX 11.8

MNEMONICS FOR METABOLIC ACIDOSIS ETIOLOGIES

Anion Gap Metabolic Acidosis	Non–Anion Gap Metabolic Acidosis
Methanol	**D**iarrhea
Uremia	**U**reteral diversion
Diabetic ketoacidosis (or starvation ketosis)	**R**enal tubular acidosis
	Hyperalimentation
Paraldehyde, propylene glycol	**A**ddison's disease, **A**cetazolamide, **A**mmonium chloride
Isoniazid, iron, some IEMs	
Lactic acidosis (D and L)	**M**iscellaneous: amphotericin B, cholestyramine
Ethanol, ethylene glycol	
Rhabdomyolysis	
Salicylates (aspirin)	
Glycols (ethylene and propylene)	
Oxoproline	
L-lactate	
D-lactate	
Methanol	
Aspirin	
Renal failure	
Ketoacidosis	

IEM, Inborn error of metabolism.

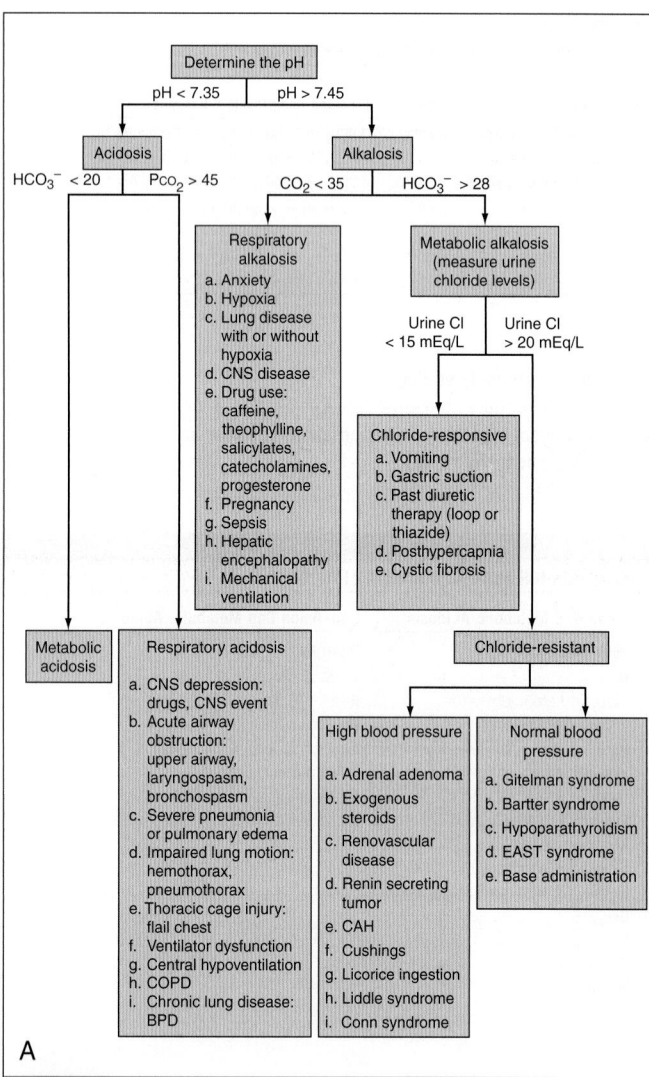

FIGURE 11.2

(A and B) Etiology of acid-base disturbances. *BPD*, Bronchopulmonary dysplasia; *CAH*, congenital adrenal hyperplasia; *CNS*, central nervous system; *COPD*, chronic obstructive pulmonary disease; *EAST*, epilepsy, ataxia, sensorineural hearing loss, and tubulopathy; *NSAID*, nonsteroidal antiinflammatory drug.

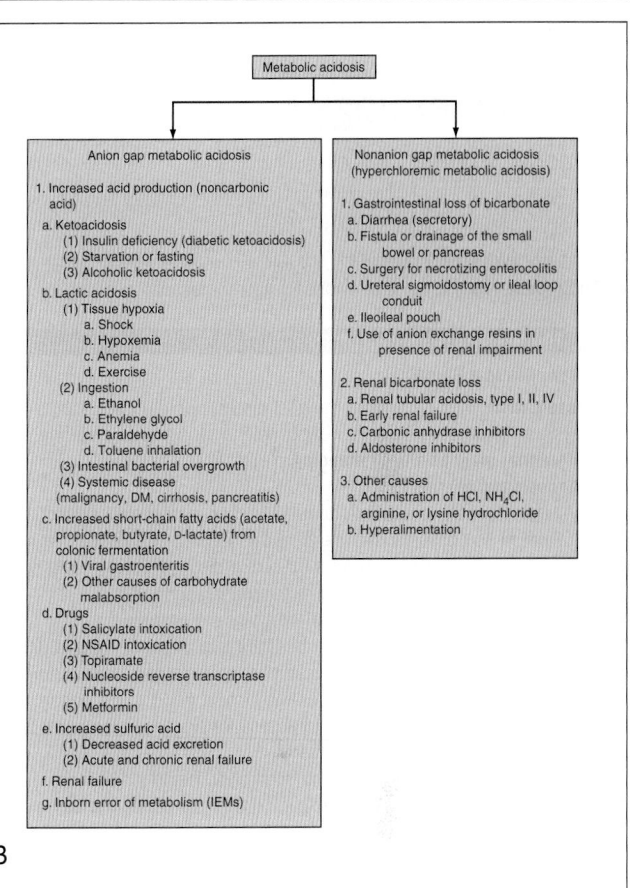

Metabolic acidosis

Anion gap metabolic acidosis

1. Increased acid production (noncarbonic acid)
   a. Ketoacidosis
      (1) Insulin deficiency (diabetic ketoacidosis)
      (2) Starvation or fasting
      (3) Alcoholic ketoacidosis
   b. Lactic acidosis
      (1) Tissue hypoxia
         a. Shock
         b. Hypoxemia
         c. Anemia
         d. Exercise
      (2) Ingestion
         a. Ethanol
         b. Ethylene glycol
         c. Paraldehyde
         d. Toluene inhalation
      (3) Intestinal bacterial overgrowth
      (4) Systemic disease
         (malignancy, DM, cirrhosis, pancreatitis)
   c. Increased short-chain fatty acids (acetate, propionate, butyrate, D-lactate) from colonic fermentation
      (1) Viral gastroenteritis
      (2) Other causes of carbohydrate malabsorption
   d. Drugs
      (1) Salicylate intoxication
      (2) NSAID intoxication
      (3) Topiramate
      (4) Nucleoside reverse transcriptase inhibitors
      (5) Metformin
   e. Increased sulfuric acid
      (1) Decreased acid excretion
      (2) Acute and chronic renal failure
   f. Renal failure
   g. Inborn error of metabolism (IEMs)

Nonanion gap metabolic acidosis (hyperchloremic metabolic acidosis)

1. Gastrointestinal loss of bicarbonate
   a. Diarrhea (secretory)
   b. Fistula or drainage of the small bowel or pancreas
   c. Surgery for necrotizing enterocolitis
   d. Ureteral sigmoidostomy or ileal loop conduit
   e. Ileoileal pouch
   f. Use of anion exchange resins in presence of renal impairment

2. Renal bicarbonate loss
   a. Renal tubular acidosis, type I, II, IV
   b. Early renal failure
   c. Carbonic anhydrase inhibitors
   d. Aldosterone inhibitors

3. Other causes
   a. Administration of HCl, NH_4Cl, arginine, or lysine hydrochloride
   b. Hyperalimentation

B

FIGURE 11.2, cont'd

REFERENCES

A complete list of references can be found online.

Chapter 12

Gastroenterology

Elshaddai Ephrem, MD

🜁 See additional content online.

🔊 **Audio Case File 12.1** A framework for gastrointestinal bleeding by age

I. GASTROINTESTINAL EMERGENCIES

A. Gastrointestinal Bleeding

1. **Presentation:** Blood loss from the gastrointestinal (GI) tract occurs in four ways: hematemesis, hematochezia, melena, and occult bleeding.
2. **Differential diagnosis of GI bleeding:** Table 12.1
3. **Diagnosis/management:**
    a. Assess airway, breathing, circulation, and hemodynamic stability.
    b. Perform full physical exam and verify bleeding with rectal examination and testing of stool or emesis for occult blood. Notable exam findings include abdominal tenderness, guarding, rebound, hepatosplenomegaly, perianal skin tags, or fissures.
    c. Obtain baseline laboratory tests: Complete blood cell count (CBC), coagulation studies, type and screen, reticulocyte count, complete metabolic panel (CMP), C-reactive protein (CRP), and erythrocyte sedimentation rate (ESR), and assess for disseminated intravascular coagulation (D dimer, fibrinogen).
    d. If concerned for hemodynamic instability, begin initial fluid resuscitation. Consider transfusion if there is continued bleeding, symptomatic anemia, and/or a hematocrit level <21%. Initiate intravenous (IV) proton pump inhibitor (PPI).
    e. Further evaluation and therapy based on the assessment and site of bleeding:
       (1) Upper GI bleeding: Consider esophagogastroduodenoscopy (EGD) and testing for *Helicobacter pylori*.[1] Gastric lavage via nasogastric (NG) tube or administration of IV erythromycin may increase visibility and diagnostic yield.[2-3]
       (2) Lower GI bleeding: Consider abdominal radiograph, upper GI study (± small bowel follow-through), air-contrast barium enema, colonoscopy, Meckel scan, tagged red cell scan, computed tomography (CT), and magnetic resonance enterography (MRE). Consider stool cultures, stool ova and parasites, *Clostridium difficile* toxin, and stool calprotectin.

TABLE 12.1		
DIFFERENTIAL DIAGNOSIS OF GASTROINTESTINAL BLEEDING		
Age	**Upper Gastrointestinal Tract**	**Lower Gastrointestinal Tract**
Newborns (0—30 days)	Swallowed maternal blood Gastritis NGT placement trauma	Necrotizing enterocolitis Malrotation with midgut volvulus Anal fissure Hirschsprung disease Food protein—induced allergic proctocolitis (FPIAP)
Infant (30 days—1 year)	Gastritis Esophagitis Peptic ulcer disease Pyloric stenosis Varices	Anal fissure Allergic proctocolitis Intussusception Meckel diverticulum Lymphonodular hyperplasia Intestinal duplication Infectious colitis Hirschsprung disease FPIAP (milk allergy)
Preschool (1—5 years)	Gastritis Esophagitis Peptic ulcer disease Esophageal varices Epistaxis Mallory-Weiss tear Foreign body ingestion	Juvenile polyps Lymphonodular hyperplasia Meckel diverticulum Hemolytic-uremic syndrome Henoch-Schönlein purpura Infectious colitis Anal fissure
School age and adolescence	Esophageal varices Peptic ulcer disease Epistaxis Gastritis Mallory-Weiss tear Drugs (NSAIDs, corticosteroids, alcohol)	Inflammatory bowel disease Infectious colitis Juvenile polyps Anal fissure Hemorrhoids

Modified from Baker RD, Baker SS. *Pediatrics in Review.* October 2021;42(10):546—557. https://doi.org/10.1542/pir.2020-000554

B. Acute Abdomen[4]

1. **Definition:** Severe abdominal pain that may require emergency surgical intervention
2. **Differential diagnosis:** Table 12.2
3. **Diagnosis:**
   a. **History:** Course and characterization of the pain, emesis, melena, hematochezia, diet, stool history, fever, travel history, menstrual history, vaginal/testicular symptoms, urinary symptoms, respiratory symptoms, and recent surgeries
   b. **Physical exam:** Rashes, arthritis, and jaundice. Abdominal tenderness on palpation, rebound/guarding, rigidity, masses, distention, or abnormal bowel sounds, rectal examination with stool hemoccult testing, pelvic examination (discharge, masses, adnexal/cervical motion tenderness), and genital examinations

TABLE 12.2

ACUTE ABDOMINAL PAIN

Gastrointestinal source	Appendicitis, pancreatitis, intussusception, malrotation with volvulus, inflammatory bowel disease, gastritis, bowel obstruction, mesenteric lymphadenitis, irritable bowel syndrome, abscess, hepatitis, perforated ulcer, Meckel diverticulitis, cholecystitis, choledocholithiasis, constipation, gastroenteritis, abdominal trauma, mesenteric ischemia, and abdominal migraine
Renal source	Urinary tract infection, pyelonephritis, and nephrolithiasis
Genitourinary source	Ectopic pregnancy, ovarian cyst/torsion, pelvic inflammatory disease, and testicular torsion
Oncologic source	Wilms tumor, neuroblastoma, rhabdomyosarcoma, and lymphoma
Other sources	Henoch-Schönlein purpura, pneumonia, sickle cell anemia, diabetic ketoacidosis, cannabinoid hyperemesis syndrome, juvenile rheumatoid arthritis, and incarcerated hernia

   c. **Labs:** CBC, CMP, coagulation studies, lactate, type and screen, urinalysis, amylase, lipase, gonorrhea/chlamydia testing, β-human chorionic gonadotropin (β-hCG), ESR, and CRP
   d. **Imaging:** Two-view abdominal radiographs to assess for obstruction, constipation, free air, gallstones, and kidney stones. Consider chest radiograph to evaluate for pneumonia, abdominal/pelvic ultrasonography, and abdominal CT with contrast or magnetic resonance imaging (MRI).
4. **Management:** Ensure patient is NPO and begin IV hydration. Consider nasogastric decompression, serial abdominal examinations, surgical/gynecologic/GI evaluation, pain control, and antibiotics as indicated.

II. CONDITIONS OF THE GASTROINTESTINAL TRACT

A. Vomiting

1. **Definition:** Forceful oral expulsion of gastric contents can be bilious or nonbilious.
2. **Differential diagnosis:** Table 12.3
3. **Diagnosis:**
   a. **History:** Diet, medications, drugs, timing (acute vs. chronic), exposures, character (bilious, bloody, projectile) and associated symptoms. Pay special attention to vomiting **without** concomitant diarrhea.
   b. **Physical exam:** HEENT and neurologic exam with specific attention to mucus membranes, skin and dentition, as well as a thorough abdominal exam
   c. **Labs:** Although not always necessary, consider CMP, CBC, UA, β-hCG, and lipase. Urine drug screen if suspect drug abuse.
   d. **Imaging:** Plain abdominal radiograph with upright view (to rule out obstruction or free air), abdominal ultrasound (US), upper GI series. Consider neurologic imaging if indicated.

TABLE 12.3

DIFFERENTIAL DIAGNOSIS OF VOMITING

Age	Typically Nonbilious	Typically Bilious
Newborn and infant (0 days—1 year)	Overfeeding, physiologic reflux, milk protein sensitivity, pyloric stenosis, necrotizing enterocolitis, metabolic disorder, infection (GU, respiratory, GI), esophageal/intestinal atresia/ stenosis, and Hirschsprung disease	Malrotation ± volvulus, intestinal atresia/stenosis, intussusception, pancreatitis
Preschool (1—5 years)	Cyclic vomiting, infectious (GI, GU), toxin ingestion, diabetic ketoacidosis (DKA), CNS mass effect, eosinophilic esophagitis, post-tussive, peptic disease, and appendicitis	Malrotation, intussusception, incarcerated hernia, pancreatitis, intestinal dysmotility
School age and adolescence	Eating disorders, pregnancy, CNS mass effect, eosinophilic esophagitis, DKA, peptic disease, cyclic vomiting, toxins/ drugs of abuse, infectious (GU, GI), and appendicitis	Peritoneal adhesions, malrotation, incarcerated hernia, pancreatitis, and intestinal dysmotility

CNS, Central nervous system; *DKA*, diabetic ketoacidosis; *GI*, gastrointestinal; *GU*, genitourinary.

4. **Management:** Hydration. Gastric decompression if GI obstruction suspected. Antiemetic therapy can be used in the acute setting; avoid chronic use (see Chapter 22 for discussion of antiemetic therapy). Consider surgical consultation if the vomiting is bilious.

B. Gastrointestinal Reflux Disease[5]

1. **Definition:** Gastroesophageal reflux (GER) is physiologic passage of gastric contents into the esophagus, and gastroesophageal reflux disease (GERD) is defined as troublesome symptoms or complications of GER.
2. **Differential diagnosis:** Dysmotility including achalasia, gastroparesis, ileus, and obstruction. Inflammatory conditions such as esophagitis, gastritis/dyspepsia, peptic ulcer disease. Anatomic abnormalities such as Zenker diverticulum, tracheoesophageal fistula, vascular ring, pyloric stenosis. Functional disorders including abdominal migraines and cyclical vomiting syndrome. Food allergies/intolerance in infants
3. **Diagnosis:**
   a. **History:** Recurrent regurgitation, choking, vomiting, heartburn, chest pain, dysphagia, stridor or wheezing, cough, recurrent aspiration pneumonia, dental erosions, and sleep disturbances. In infants, GERD may present as irritability, weight loss, feeding refusal, or Sandifer syndrome. History is typically sufficient for diagnosis and to initiate management.
   b. **Testing:** Esophageal pH monitoring and esophageal impedance monitoring if diagnosis unclear[6]

4. **Management:**
   a. **Lifestyle:** A prone or left-sided sleeping position and elevation of head of bed may improve GER symptoms in older children, but current studies for infants have been inconclusive. Infants up to 12 months should continue to sleep supine—risk of sleep-related infant death far outweighs benefit of prone or lateral sleeping in GERD. After feeds, infants should be kept upright and a trial of smaller more frequent feeds may be beneficial. Avoidance of secondhand smoke exposure.
   b. **Diet:** Milk-thickening agents can be beneficial for symptom relief. If severe and unresponsive to conservative management, consider 2- to 4-week trial of extensively hydrolyzed protein formula in infants or elimination of cow's milk in maternal diet to eliminate milk protein sensitivity as a cause of unexplained vomiting.
   c. **Pharmacotherapy:** Medication is not recommended for "happy spitters" or infants with uncomplicated GER. Both PPIs and H2 receptor antagonists (H2Ras) are effective in relieving symptoms and promoting mucosal healing.[7] There is insufficient evidence to support routine use of prokinetic therapies (metoclopramide and erythromycin).

C. Eosinophilic Esophagitis[8,9] (EOE)

1. **Definition:** A chronic, immune/antigen-mediated disease characterized by symptoms of esophageal dysfunction with ≥15 eosinophils/high-power field (hpf) on esophageal biopsy
2. **Diagnosis:**
   a. **History:** Dysphagia, food impaction, chest pain, food refusal or intolerance, GER symptoms, emesis, abdominal pain, and failure to thrive. Majority of patients with EoE have concurrent atopic disorder.
   b. **Diagnosis:** EGD with esophageal biopsies demonstrating at least 15 eos/hpf on histology with chronic symptoms of esophageal dysfunction. Must evaluate for other causes or contributions to esophageal eosinophilia. Importantly histologic evidence without clinical correlation is not diagnostic. Per the AGREE conference, a PPI trial is no longer needed for diagnosis. Consider obtaining allergy testing (see Chapter 15).
3. **Management[10]:**
   a. **Dietary therapy:** 6-food elimination diet (milk, wheat, eggs, soy, peanuts/tree nuts, seafood), elemental diet, or targeted elimination diet determined by allergy testing
   b. **Pharmacotherapy:** Topical swallowed steroids delivered via inhaler or budesonide are preferred as first-line therapy to induce remission with limited side effects (6- to 8-week course of fluticasone). PPI therapy can also be trialed for initial treatment. Systemic steroids for short-term use (e.g., dysphagia leading to dehydration or weight loss). No current evidence to support routine use of biologics
   c. **Complications:** Symptomatic strictures requiring esophageal dilation

D. Celiac Disease[11]

1. **Definition:** An immune-mediated inflammatory enteropathy caused by sensitivity to dietary gluten and related proteins (wheat, barley, and rye) in genetically susceptible individuals

2. **Diagnosis:**
   a. **History:** Presentation can be variable, and some patients are asymptomatic. Most common symptoms include diarrhea, vomiting, abdominal pain, constipation, distention, and failure to thrive. Non-GI symptoms include rash (dermatitis herpetiformis), osteoporosis, short stature, delayed puberty, and iron deficiency anemia that is resistant to oral iron. Increased occurrence in children with autoimmune disorders, Down syndrome, Turner syndrome, William syndrome, immunoglobulin A (IgA) deficiency, and in first-degree relatives of those with celiac disease
   b. **Labs:** First-line screening is IgA antibody to human recombinant tissue transglutaminase (TTG) and serum IgA. If known selective IgA deficiency with symptoms suggestive of celiac disease, testing with TTG IgG is recommended after 3 years of age.[12] CBC, iron studies, hepatic function panel, thyroid tests, calcium, and vitamin D are recommended. Additional antibody testing may be necessary for inconclusive clinical scenarios.
   c. **Procedures:** Biopsy is "gold standard" for diagnosis. Intestinal biopsies showing villous atrophy supports diagnosis. Results dependent on adequate consumption of gluten prior to testing; ensure 6 to 8 weeks of gluten ingestion prior to endoscopy.

3. **Management:** Lifetime gluten-free diet. Annual screening with TTG is recommended to monitor adherence to diet.

4. **Complications:** More often seen in adulthood but at risk for vitamin deficiencies and other autoimmune disorders. Higher risk of non-Hodgkin lymphoma, specifically enteropathy-associated T-cell lymphoma.

E. Inflammatory Bowel Disease[13,14]

1. **Classification:**
   a. **Crohn disease:** Transmural inflammatory process affecting any segment of the GI tract, most commonly terminal ileum. Commonly presents with abdominal pain, weight loss, diarrhea, and poor growth
   b. **Ulcerative colitis (UC):** Chronic, relapsing, inflammatory disease of the colon and rectum. Commonly presents with rectal bleeding and diarrhea

2. **Diagnosis:**
   a. **History:** Abdominal pain, weight loss, diarrhea, lethargy, nausea, vomiting, malnutrition, psychiatric symptoms, arthropathy, and rashes. Family history, exposure to infectious agents, or antibiotic treatment.
   b. **Physical exam:** Stomatitis, perianal skin tags, fissures, and fistulas. Assessment of hydration and nutritional status. Fever, orthostasis,

tachycardia, abdominal tenderness, distention, or masses suggest moderate to severe disease and need for hospitalization.

c. **Labs:** CBC, CMP, ESR, CRP. Fecal calprotectin has been shown to be elevated in inflammatory bowel disease (IBD) and may serve as a sensitive, noninvasive test.[15] IBD often associated with anemia, hypoalbuminemia, thrombocytosis, and elevated inflammatory markers. Stool studies to exclude infectious process are necessary.

d. **Imaging:** MRE is the preferred imaging modality for diagnosis of pediatric IBD due to high diagnostic accuracy and no radiation exposure. CT and fluoroscopy are other alternative strategies if MRE unavailable.

e. **Procedures:** Diagnostic endoscopy with biopsies used to confirm diagnosis

3. **Management**[16-19]**:**

a. **Induction of remission:**

(1) Crohn: Exclusive enteral formula-based nutrition (80%–100% caloric need by liquid formula), 5-aminosalicylates, antitumor necrosis factor (TNF) agents, and, if indicated, antibiotics or surgery. Corticosteroids can be used if necessary. Novel dietary options such as Crohn disease exclusion diet, specific carbohydrate diet (SCD), or any other low complex SCDs may be possible therapeutic options.[20,21]

(2) UC: Corticosteroids, 5-aminosalicylates, TNF agents, and if indicated, antibiotics or surgery. Therapy guided by severity of illness

b. **Maintenance of remission:** Immunosuppression includes thiopurines, methotrexate, cyclosporine, tacrolimus, and anti-TNF monoclonal antibodies. Avoid prolonged steroid use.

c. **Other:** Surgical intervention indicated only after medical management has failed in both Crohn disease and UC. In Crohn disease, surgery is indicated for localized disease (strictures), abscess, or disease refractory to medical management.

F. Constipation[22,23]

Normal stooling patterns by age: Infants 0 to 3 months, 2 to 3 bowel movements/day (breastfed infants may stool after every feed or go 5 to 7 days with no stool); 6 to 12 months, 1.8/day; 1 to 3 years, 1.4/day; >3 years, 1/day. If an exclusively breastfed <1 month old is not stooling regularly, it may be a sign of insufficient milk intake; monitor weight gain.

1. **Definitions:**

a. **Constipation:** Delay or difficulty in defecation for 2 or more weeks. Functional causes of constipation are the most common. History and physical exam are often sufficient for diagnosis.

(1) Functional: Consider Rome IV Criteria (eTable 12.1).

(2) Nonfunctional: See Table 12.4 for differential diagnosis.

TABLE 12.4	
DIFFERENTIAL DIAGNOSIS OF CONSTIPATION[a]	
Anatomic malformations	Anal stenosis, anterior displaced anus, imperforate anus, and pelvic mass (e.g., sacral teratoma)
Metabolic and gastrointestinal	Cystic fibrosis, diabetes mellitus, gluten enteropathy, hypercalcemia, hypokalemia, hypothyroidism, and multiple endocrine neoplasia type 2B
Neuropathic conditions	Neurofibromatosis, spinal cord abnormalities, spinal cord trauma, static encephalopathy, and tethered cord
Intestinal nerve or muscle disorders	Hirschsprung disease, intestinal neuronal dysplasia, visceral myopathies, and visceral neuropathies
Abnormal abdominal musculature	Down syndrome, gastroschisis, and prune belly
Connective tissue disorders	Ehlers-Danlos syndrome, scleroderma, and systemic lupus erythematosus
Drugs	Antacids, anticholinergics, antidepressants, antihypertensives, opiates, phenobarbital, sucralfate, and sympathomimetics
Other	Botulism, cow's milk protein intolerance, heavy metal ingestion (lead), and vitamin D intoxication

[a]Functional constipation remains the most common cause.

Constipation Guideline Committee of the North American Society for Pediatric Gastroenterology, Hepatology, and Nutrition. Evaluation and treatment of constipation in infants and children: Evidence-Based Recommendations from ESPGHAN and NASPGHAN. *J Pediatr Gastroenterol Nutr.* 2014;58(2):258–274.

2. **Diagnosis:**
   a. **History:** Age of onset, toilet training experience, frequency/consistency/size of stools, pain or bleeding with defecation, presence of abdominal pain, soiling of underwear, stool-withholding behavior, change in appetite, abdominal distention, allergies, dietary history, medications, developmental history, psychosocial history. Refer to Bristol Stool Form Scale for classification of stool history (Fig. 12.1). Delayed meconium, poor weight gain or weight loss, anorexia, nausea, vomiting, and family history (e.g., thyroid disorders, cystic fibrosis) would warrant further evaluation for nonfunctional causes.
   b. **Physical exam:** External perineum, perianal examination. Fecal impaction may be palpated on abdominal or digital rectal examination. Plain abdominal single view radiography can be considered when physical examination is unreliable.
3. **Management of functional constipation:** Box 12.1 and eTable 12.2
   a. **Disimpaction:**
      (1) Oral/nasogastric approach: Polyethylene glycol (PEG) solutions are effective for initial disimpaction. May also use other osmotic laxatives: magnesium citrate, lactulose
      (2) Rectal approach: Saline or mineral oil enemas effective. Avoid enemas in infants; glycerin suppositories may be used in infants less than 1 year.
   b. **Maintenance therapy** (usually 3 to 12 months): Goal is to prevent recurrence.

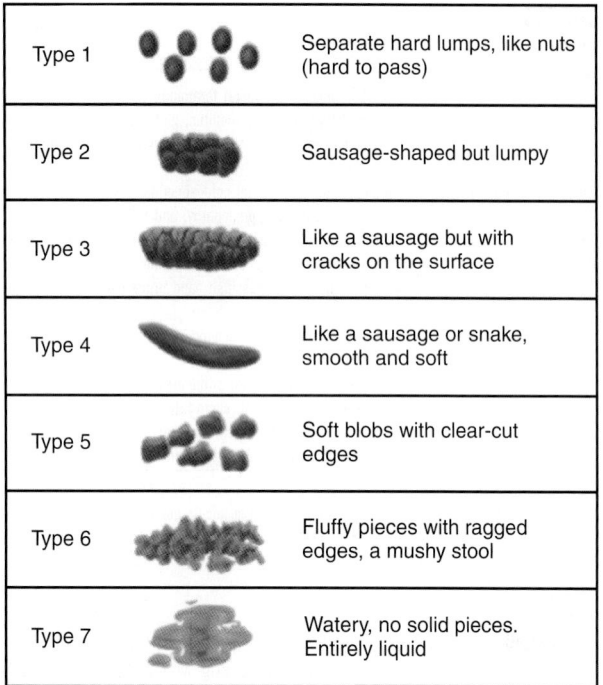

Type 1		Separate hard lumps, like nuts (hard to pass)
Type 2		Sausage-shaped but lumpy
Type 3		Like a sausage but with cracks on the surface
Type 4		Like a sausage or snake, smooth and soft
Type 5		Soft blobs with clear-cut edges
Type 6		Fluffy pieces with ragged edges, a mushy stool
Type 7		Watery, no solid pieces. Entirely liquid

FIGURE 12.1

Bristol Stool Form Scale. (From *Campbell-Walsh-Wein Urology*. 12th ed. Elsevier; 2020, Fig. 36.1.)

    (1) **Dietary changes:** Evidence supporting dietary intervention is weak; however, increased intake of fruits, vegetables, whole grains, and fluids other than milk is recommended.
    (2) **Behavioral modifications:** Regular toilet habits with positive reinforcement. Referral to a mental health specialist for motivational or behavioral concerns if soiling an issue
    (3) **Medications: Daily PEG.** Lactulose as second-line treatment. The use of stimulant laxatives and stool softeners may also be considered. Discontinue therapy gradually only after return of regular bowel movements with good evacuation. Evidence does not support use of probiotics.
  c. **Special considerations in infants aged <1 year:** 2 to 4 oz of 100% fruit juice (e.g., prune or pear) recommended in younger infants. Glycerin suppositories may be useful. While use is off label, PEG is routinely used in children <1 year of age. Avoid mineral oil, stimulant laxatives, and phosphate enemas.

BOX 12.1

MANAGEMENT OF CONSTIPATION

HOME CLEANOUT INSTRUCTIONS

Step 1: Take a stimulant laxative (bisacodyl, senna) with 8 oz of liquid, as per dosing instructions below.

Step 2: Drink polyethylene glycol (PEG). Mix with water or another clear non-carbonated liquid. Drink full amount in 2 hr. See below for dosing instructions.

Step 3: 1–2 hr after finishing PEG, should begin passing formed/thick brown stool. The stool should become thinner, and clearer stooling continues.

Step 4: If not stooling or passing very thick stools 4 hr after the PEG is finished, drink 1 capful of PEG in 8 oz of liquid every hour until stools are clear.

Step 5: Cleanout is finished when stool is mostly clear with very little sand-like material mixed in. Proceed to maintenance instructions below.

DOSING INSTRUCTIONS

Weight	Polyethylene Glycol (PEG) Dose	Stimulant Laxative Recommendation
8–10 kg	Mix 2.5 capfuls of PEG in 8 oz of clear drink	<2 years old: No stimulant laxative use
10.1–15 kg	Mix 3.5 capfuls of PEG in 16 oz of clear drink	2 years to <3 years old: Chewable senna (chocolate squares)[a]
15.1–20 kg	Mix 5 capfuls of PEG in 20 oz of clear drink	≥3 years old: Oral chewable senna
20.1–25 kg	Mix 6 capfuls of PEG in 24 oz of clear drink	(chocolate squares)
25.1–30 kg	Mix 7 capfuls of PEG in 28 oz of clear drink	until child can swallow pills, then oral bisacodyl
30.1–40 kg	Mix 9.5 capfuls of PEG in 40 oz of clear drink	laxative[a]
40.1–50 kg	Mix 12 capfuls of PEG in 48 oz of clear drink	
50.1 kg or more	Mix 14 capfuls of PEG in 56 oz of clear drink	

DAILY MAINTENANCE THERAPY

The day after colon cleanse, the patient should begin taking maintenance daily PEG for continued management of constipation.

Advise patient/family to mix PEG in clear noncarbonated drink or water at least once daily. See formulary for dosing. Advise to drink the entire solution in 30 min or less for it to work well. It is best to give the PEG after school and before dinner. Do not give PEG right before bedtime.

The goal of daily maintenance PEG is for the child to have 1 or 2 soft and easily passable bowel movements every day.

Advise to have child to sit on the toilet after every meal or whenever they feel the need to stool.

[a] See Formulary for dosing recommendations.

Modified from handout given to patients who visit the Johns Hopkins Children's Center Pediatric Chronic Constipation Center, as an example of constipation management; variations are found at other institutions.

G. Diarrhea[24]

1. **Definition:** Acute diarrhea is more than three loose or watery stools per day. Chronic diarrhea is diarrhea lasting more than 2 to 4 weeks.
2. **Pathogenesis:** It can be infectious or malabsorptive with an osmotic or secretory mechanism.
   a. **Osmotic diarrhea:** Water is drawn into intestinal lumen by maldigested osmotic compounds, as seen in celiac disease, pancreatic disease, or lactose intolerance. Stool volume depends on diet and decreases with fasting (stool osmolar gap ≥100 mOsm/kg).
   b. **Secretory diarrhea:** Water accompanies secreted or unabsorbed electrolytes into the intestinal lumen (e.g., excessive secretion of chloride ions caused by cholera toxin). Stool volume is increased and does not vary with diet (stool osmolar gap <50 mOsm/kg).
   c. Stool osmolar gap: The standard value is 290 mOsm/kg.[25]

$$\text{Stool osmolar gap} =$$
$$\text{Stool Osm} - \{2 \times [\text{stool (Na) mEq / L} + \text{stool (K) mEq / L}]\}$$

3. **Differential diagnosis:** Table 12.5
4. **Diagnosis:**
   a. **History:** Acute vs. chronic, travel history, recent antibiotic use, and immune status
   b. **Labs:** CMP, CBC, stool hemoccult testing, stool culture, *C. difficile* toxin, ova and parasites, and viral antigens (see Chapter 17 for common bacterial and viral pathogens)

TABLE 12.5

DIFFERENTIAL DIAGNOSIS OF COMMON CAUSES OF DIARRHEA

Diagnosis	Major Clinical Features
Infectious colitis (viral, bacterial, protozoal)	Blood or mucous in stool, possible exposure history (e.g., travel)
Lactose malabsorption	Bloating, flatulence, abdominal pain, and elevated breath hydrogen concentration postlactose ingestion
Small bowel bacterial overgrowth	Abdominal discomfort and increased risk if ileocecal valve removed
Irritable bowel syndrome	Constipation and/or diarrhea and absence of laboratory or imaging findings
Allergic enteropathy	Growth failure, hypoalbuminemia, anemia, and may have elevated serum IgE
Hirschsprung disease	Distended abdomen, abnormal barium enema, absent ganglion cells on rectal biopsy
Cystic fibrosis	Decreased fecal elastase, steatorrhea, and poor growth
IBD and celiac disease	See Sections III.D and III.E
Other: Hyperthyroidism, UTI, and encopresis	Dependent on etiology

IBD, Inflammatory bowel disease; *IgE*, immunoglobulin E; *UTI*, urinary tract infection.
Modified from Zella GC, Israel EJ. Chronic diarrhea in children. *Pediatr Rev.* 2012;33(5):207–218.

5. **Management:**
    a. **Oral rehydration therapy (ORT)[26]:** Enteral hydration has proven superior in reducing the length of hospital stay and adverse events.[21] Parenteral hydration is indicated in severe dehydration, hemodynamic instability, or failure of ORT.
    b. **Diet:** Restart regular diet as soon as tolerated.
    c. **Pharmacotherapy:** No supporting evidence for use of nonspecific antidiarrheal agents, antimotility agents (e.g., loperamide), antisecretory drugs, and toxin binders (e.g., cholestyramine). Consider evidence-based antimicrobial therapy for infectious diarrhea (see Chapter 17). If malabsorptive (e.g., celiac disease or IBD), therapy should be tailored to disease process.
    d. **Probiotics[27-29]:** Evidence supporting use of probiotics is limited; however, their efficacy has been demonstrated in the following circumstances: antibiotic-associated diarrhea, *C. difficile* diarrhea (severe recurrent disease only), hepatic encephalopathy, the prevention of atopic dermatitis, and possibly preventing necrotizing enterocolitis in premature infants.

III. CONDITIONS OF THE LIVER

A. Liver Laboratory Studies: Table 12.6

1. **Synthetic/metabolic function:** Albumin, prealbumin, international normalized ratio (INR), activated partial thromboplastin time (aPTT), gamma-glutamyl transferase (GGT), cholesterol levels, bilirubin, and ammonia
2. **Liver cell injury:** Aspartate aminotransferase (AST), alanine aminotransferase (ALT), and lactate dehydrogenase
3. **Biliary system:** Bilirubin (total and direct), urobilinogen, GGT, and alkaline phosphatase

B. Acute Liver Failure[30,31]

1. **Definition:** Laboratory evidence of liver injury with no known history of chronic liver disease, the presence of coagulopathy not corrected by vitamin K administration, and an INR >1.5 if patient has encephalopathy or >2.0 if patient does not have encephalopathy
2. **Differential diagnosis:** Table 12.7
3. **Diagnosis:**
    a. **History:** Fatigue, nausea, vomiting, irritability, confusion, drowsiness, skin changes, medications, ingestion, illicit drug use, family history, developmental delay, transfusion history
    b. **Physical exam:** Neurologic status, skin exam, hepatosplenomegaly, nutritional status, growth, bruising, petechiae. Slit lamp exam if concern for Wilson disease. Findings of chronic liver disease include clubbing, palmar erythema, cutaneous xanthoma, ascites, and prominent abdominal vessels.

TABLE 12.6

LIVER LABORATORY TESTS

Enzyme	Source	Increased	Decreased	Comments
AST/ALT	Liver, heart, skeletal muscle, pancreas, RBCs, and kidney	Hepatocellular injury, rhabdomyolysis, muscular dystrophy, hemolysis, and liver cancer	Vitamin B6 deficiency and uremia	ALT more specific than AST for liver, AST > ALT in hemolysis
Alkaline phosphatase	Osteoblasts, liver, small intestine, kidney, and placenta	Hepatocellular injury, bone growth, disease, trauma, pregnancy, and familial	Low phosphate, Wilson disease, zinc deficiency, hypothyroidism, and pernicious anemia	Highest in cholestatic conditions; must be differentiated from bone source
GGT	Renal tubules, bile ducts, pancreas, small intestine, and brain	Cholestasis, newborn period, and induced by drugs	Estrogen therapy, artificially low in hyperbilirubinemia	Not found in bone, increased in 90% of primary liver disease, specific for hepatobiliary disease in nonpregnant patient
Ammonia	Bowel flora and protein metabolism	Hepatic disease secondary to urea cycle dysfunction, hemodialysis, valproic acid therapy, urea cycle enzyme deficiency, organic acidemia, and carnitine deficiency		Converted to urea in liver

AST/ALT, Aspartate aminotransferase/alanine aminotransferase; *GGT,* γ-glutamyl transpeptidase; *RBCs,* red blood cells.

TABLE 12.7

DIFFERENTIAL DIAGNOSIS OF ACUTE LIVER FAILURE

Infection	Herpes simplex virus, hepatitis A, hepatitis B, adenovirus, cytomegalovirus, Epstein-Barr virus, enterovirus, human herpes virus 6, parvovirus B19, and dengue fever
Vascular	Budd-Chiari syndrome, portal vein thrombosis, venoocclusive disease, and ischemic hepatitis
Inherited/metabolic	Wilson disease, mitochondrial, tyrosinemia, galactosemia, hemochromatosis, fatty acid oxidation defect, and iron storage disease
Immune dysregulation	Natural killer cell dysfunction (hemophagocytic lymphohistiocytosis), autoimmune, and macrophage activation syndrome
Drugs/toxins	Acetaminophen, anticonvulsants, antimicrobials, chemotherapy, aflatoxins, herbal and dietary supplements
Other	Idiopathic and cancer/leukemia

  c. **Labs:** Liver synthetic/metabolic function, liver cell injury, and biliary
     system tests (see earlier). BMP, magnesium, phosphorus, CBC
     with peripheral smear, reticulocyte count, ammonia, lipase.
     Factors V, VII (depleted first in ALF), VIII, and fibrinogen. A urine
     toxicology screen and a serum acetaminophen level should be
     obtained (see Chapter 3). Viral hepatitis studies, autoantibodies,
     and evaluation for metabolic syndromes must be considered.

     NOTE: See Chapter 17 for interpretation of serologic markers of
     hepatitis B.

  d. **Imaging:** Abdominal US with Doppler flow. Consider head CT scan to
     exclude hemorrhage/edema and chest radiography.
  e. **Procedures:** Liver biopsy
  f. **Management:** Evaluate for underlying cause. Consider intensive care
     unit (ICU) level care with close monitoring of mental status, fluid
     balance, metabolic disturbances, hepatorenal syndrome, sepsis, and
     coagulopathies. Cerebral edema is life-threatening and may require
     intracranial pressure monitoring. Consider liver transplant when
     indicated.

C. Nonalcoholic Fatty Liver Disease[32]

1. **Definition:** Chronic liver disease from excessive fat accumulation in the
   liver, often secondary to insulin resistance and obesity. Most common
   liver disease in children in the United States
2. **Diagnosis:** Screen between 9 and 11 years for obese children and
   overweight children with risk factors. ALT is the recommended test. If ALT
   persistently elevated >2 times upper limit of normal for >3 months, further
   evaluation is warranted. Must exclude alternative etiologies
3. **Management:** Extensive lifestyle modifications, well-balanced healthy diet.
   No medications have proven benefit. Bariatric surgery can be considered
   if severe comorbidities. Screen for diabetes and other comorbid
   conditions.

D. Hyperbilirubinemia[33-35]

1. **Definition:** Bilirubin is the product of hemoglobin metabolism. There are two forms: direct (conjugated) and indirect (unconjugated). Hyperbilirubinemia is usually the result of increased hemoglobin load, reduced hepatic uptake, reduced hepatic conjugation, or decreased excretion. Direct hyperbilirubinemia is defined as a direct bilirubin >20% of the total bilirubin or a direct bilirubin of >2 mg/dL.

2. **Differential diagnosis:** Table 12.8

3. **Management:** Dependent upon etiology. Evaluation and diagnosis should be guided by history; however, liver laboratory studies (see earlier) and ultrasounds are warranted in many patients. Refer to Chapter 18 for evaluation and treatment of neonatal hyperbilirubinemia.

TABLE 12.8

DIFFERENTIAL DIAGNOSIS OF HYPERBILIRUBINEMIA

INDIRECT HYPERBILIRUBINEMIA	
Transient neonatal jaundice	Breast milk jaundice and physiologic jaundice
	Polycythemia and reabsorption of extravascular blood
Hemolytic disorders	Autoimmune disease, blood group incompatibility, hemoglobinopathies, microangiopathies, red cell enzyme deficiencies, and red cell membrane disorders
Enterohepatic recirculation	Cystic fibrosis, Hirschsprung disease, ileal atresia, and pyloric stenosis
Disorders of bilirubin metabolism	Acidosis, Crigler-Najjar syndrome, Gilbert syndrome, hypothyroidism, and hypoxia
Miscellaneous	Dehydration, drugs, hypoalbuminemia, sepsis, and panhypopituitarism

DIRECT HYPERBILIRUBINEMIA	
Biliary obstruction	Biliary atresia, choledochal cyst, fibrosing pancreatitis, gallstones or biliary sludge, inspissated bile syndrome, neoplasm, and primary sclerosing cholangitis
Infection	Cholangitis, cytomegalovirus, adenovirus, enterovirus, Epstein-Barr virus, herpes simplex virus, histoplasmosis, human immunodeficiency virus, leptospirosis, liver abscess, sepsis, syphilis, rubella, toxocariasis, toxoplasmosis, tuberculosis, urinary tract infection, varicella-zoster virus, and viral hepatitis
Genetic/metabolic disorders	α1-Antitrypsin deficiency, Alagille syndrome, Caroli disease, cystic fibrosis, Dubin-Johnson syndrome, galactokinase deficiency, galactosemia, glycogen storage disease, hereditary fructose intolerance, hypothyroidism, Niemann-Pick disease, progressive familial intrahepatic cholestasis (PFIC), Rotor syndrome, tyrosinemia, and Wilson disease
Chromosomal abnormalities	Trisomy 18, trisomy 21, and Turner syndrome
Drugs	Acetaminophen, aspirin, erythromycin, ethanol, iron, isoniazid, methotrexate, parenteral nutrition, oxacillin, rifampin, steroids, sulfonamides, tetracycline, and vitamin A
Miscellaneous	Neonatal hepatitis syndrome, parenteral alimentation, and Reye syndrome

IV. PANCREATITIS[36-38]

Definition: Inflammatory disease of the pancreas

A. Acute Pancreatitis[39]

1. **Diagnosis:**
   a. **History:** Abdominal pain, irritability, epigastric tenderness, nausea and vomiting. Multiple etiologies (Table 12.9). Per INSPPIRE criteria, diagnosis of acute pancreatitis requires at least two of the following:
      (1) Abdominal pain compatible with acute pancreatitis
      (2) Serum amylase and/or lipase values >3 times upper limit of normal
      (3) Imaging findings consistent with acute pancreatitis
   b. **Labs:** CMP, GGT, CBC, amylase, lipase, calcium, and triglycerides
   c. **Imaging:** Transabdominal US recommended. CT or MRI reserved for more complicated cases depending on etiology

TABLE 12.9	
CONDITIONS ASSOCIATED WITH ACUTE PANCREATITIS	
SYSTEMIC DISEASES	
Infections	Coxsackie, CMV, cryptosporidium, EBV, hepatitis, influenza A or B, leptospirosis, mycoplasma, mumps, rubella, typhoid fever, and varicella
Inflammatory and vasculitic disorders	Collagen vascular diseases, hemolytic uremic syndrome, Henoch-Schönlein purpura, IBD, and Kawasaki disease
Sepsis/peritonitis/shock	
IDIOPATHIC (UP TO 25% OF CASES)	
MECHANICAL/STRUCTURAL	
Trauma	Blunt trauma, child abuse, and ERCP
Anatomic anomalies	Annular pancreas, choledochal cyst, pancreatic divisum, stenosis, and other
Obstruction	Parasites, stones, and tumors
METABOLIC AND TOXIC FACTORS	
Drugs/toxins	Salicylates, cytotoxic drugs (l-asparaginase), corticosteroids, chlorothiazides, furosemide, oral contraceptives (estrogen), tetracyclines, sulfonamides, valproic acid, azathioprine, and 6-mercaptopurine
Cystic fibrosis	
Diabetes mellitus	
Hypercalcemia	
Hyperlipidemia	
Hypothermia	
Malnutrition	
Organic acidemia	
Renal disease	

CMV, Cytomegalovirus; *EBV,* Epstein-Barr virus; *ERCP,* endoscopic retrograde cholangiopancreatography; *IBD,* inflammatory bowel disease.

12

TABLE 12.10

PROPOSED ETIOLOGIES OF CHRONIC PANCREATITIS IN CHILDHOOD

Calcific	Cystic fibrosis, hereditary pancreatitis (e.g., PRSS1 and SPINK1 mutations), hypercalcemia, hyperlipidemia, idiopathic, and juvenile tropical pancreatitis
Obstructive (noncalcific)	Congenital anomalies, idiopathic fibrosing pancreatitis, renal disease, sclerosing cholangitis, sphincter of Oddi dysfunction, and trauma

Modified from Robertson MA. Pancreatitis. In: Walker WA et al, eds. *Pediatric Gastrointestinal Disease.* 3rd ed. BC Decker; 2000:1321–1344; Werlin SL. Pancreatitis. In: McMillan JA et al, eds. *Oski's Pediatrics.* Lippincott Williams & Wilkins; 2006:2010–2012.

2. **Management:**
   a. **Analgesia:** Acetaminophen or NSAIDs as first-line therapy; opiates for refractory pain
   b. **Nutrition:** Aggressive IV fluid hydration within initial 48 hours. Early enteral feeding recommended (within 72 hours of presentation and hemodynamically stable) and associated with shorter hospitalization and decreases comorbidity
   c. **Complications:** Multiorgan dysfunction, shock, pseudocysts, fluid collections, and necrosis. Antibiotics reserved for infected necrosis. Surgical consult as indicated

B. Chronic Pancreatitis[40,41]

1. **Diagnosis:**
   a. **History:** Abdominal pain consistent with pancreatic origin, pancreatic insufficiency; plus consistent imaging findings or biopsy with histopathologic features. Must be distinguished from acute recurrent pancreatitis (ARP), which is defined as at least two distinct episodes of pancreatitis with complete resolution of pain or normalization of laboratory levels
   b. **Labs:** Same as acute pancreatitis. Normal amylase/lipase does not exclude diagnosis of chronic pancreatitis or ARP. Fecal elastase to screen for exocrine function and fat-soluble vitamins assessment. Consider genetic testing.
   c. **Imaging:** Repeat imaging recommended with US and/or MRCP
   NOTE: See Table 12.10 for proposed etiologies of chronic pancreatitis in childhood.

2. **Management:** (For acute exacerbations) same as management of acute pancreatitis. Maintenance to focus on nonmedication strategies, adequate nutrition for growth, nonopioids, and planned opioids

V. WEB RESOURCES

- North American Society for Pediatric Gastroenterology, Hepatology, and Nutrition: https://www.naspghan.org
- Children's Digestive Health Information for Kids and Parents: https://www.gikids.org

- Celiac Disease Foundation: https://clinical.celiac.org
- Rome Foundation for Diagnosis and Treatment of Functional Gastrointestinal Disorders: https://www.theromefoundation.org
- Crohn's & Colitis Foundation: https://www.crohnscolitisfoundation.org

REFERENCES

A complete list of references can be found online.

Chapter 13

Genetics: Metabolism and Conditions With Distinctive Appearance

Jacqueline Wood, MD, MA *

🌐 See additional content online.

🔊 **Audio Case File 13.1** Newborn screening

I. METABOLISM[1-8]

A. Clinical Presentation of Metabolic Disease (Box 13.1)

1. Metabolic disease can be conceptualized into broad categories (Table 13.1).
2. When a particular diagnosis is considered, a complete patient history, including details of conception, pregnancy, prenatal screening and diagnostic studies, delivery, postnatal growth, development, and a three-generation family history in the form of a pedigree (eFig. 13.1) should accompany a comprehensive physical examination. The family history may be remarkable for close relatives who died of similar presentations (may be mistaken for "sepsis" or "SIDS").
3. A high index of suspicion is required, as routine investigations may be unrevealing. Be especially vigilant in a full-term baby presenting with "sepsis" who has no risk factors.

BOX 13.1
WHEN TO SUSPECT METABOLIC DISEASE[1-3]

Overwhelming illness in the neonatal period
Vomiting
Acute acidosis, anion gap
Massive ketosis
Hypoglycemia
Coagulopathy
Coma
Seizures, especially myoclonic
Hypotonia
Unusual odor of urine
Extensive dermatosis
Neutropenia, thrombocytopenia, or pancytopenia
Family history of siblings dying early

---

*The author would like to give special thanks to Shira G. Ziegler, MD PhD.

TABLE 13.1	
BROAD CLASSIFICATION OF METABOLIC DISEASE[1-6]	
Intoxication Disorders	See Table 13.2.
Toxic accumulation of small molecules upstream of a defective enzyme. Tend to present early in life with nonspecific symptoms that may include recurrent vomiting, irritability, lethargy progressing to coma, organ dysfunction. Symptoms may wax and wane with intercurrent illness.	Acidosis algorithm (Fig. 13.1) Hyperammonemia algorithm (Fig. 13.2)
Disorders of Reduced Fasting Tolerance	See Table 13.3.
Disorders in the body's ability to tolerate fasting, with early onset of hypoglycemia. Can present in infancy or later when trying to sleep through the night, including morning symptoms or seizures. Look for laboratory abnormalities and symptoms not usually found in typical fasting.	Hypoglycemia algorithm (Fig. 13.3)
Disorders of Complex Molecules	See Table 13.4.
These disorders have a broad phenotypic spectrum and typical biochemical screening can be unrevealing. Features can be present at birth and/or slowly progressive affecting multiple organ systems. Often enzymatic and/or broad molecular genetic testing is needed.	
Mitochondrial Disorders	See Table 13.5.
Defect in energy production through the electron transport chain. There is a broad spectrum of clinical manifestations, often involving high-energy organs including brain, muscle, and/or heart.	
Neurotransmitter Disorders	See Table 13.6.
Defect in neurotransmission which can present around birth with severe infantile epileptic encephalopathy, or later with parkinsonism-dystonia or, neurodevelopmental or psychiatric disorders.	

4. Routine newborn screening (see Section II) is meant to detect many metabolic disorders before onset of clinical symptoms, but the conditions screened vary by state and not all countries screen, so clinical suspicion should remain high if clinical picture is concerning.

B. Evaluation

1. **Initial laboratory tests:** Comprehensive metabolic panel, blood glucose, venous blood gas (VBG), ammonia (beware false-positives from prolonged tourniquet time, struggling children, lack of ice, or sample delay), complete blood cell count with differential, urinalysis
2. **Subsequent evaluation for metabolic disease:**
   a. Consult a geneticist.
   b. A basic metabolic workup includes plasma amino acids (PAA), urine organic acids (UOA), acylcarnitine profile, quantitative (free and total) plasma carnitine, lactate/pyruvate ratio. Further specialized biochemical testing is available.
3. **Additional labs given specific circumstances:**
   a. **Metabolic acidosis:** Ammonia, lactate, β-hydroxybutyrate, acetoacetate, UOA, urinalysis with urine pH, acylcarnitine profile, quantitative (free and total) plasma carnitine (Fig. 13.1)

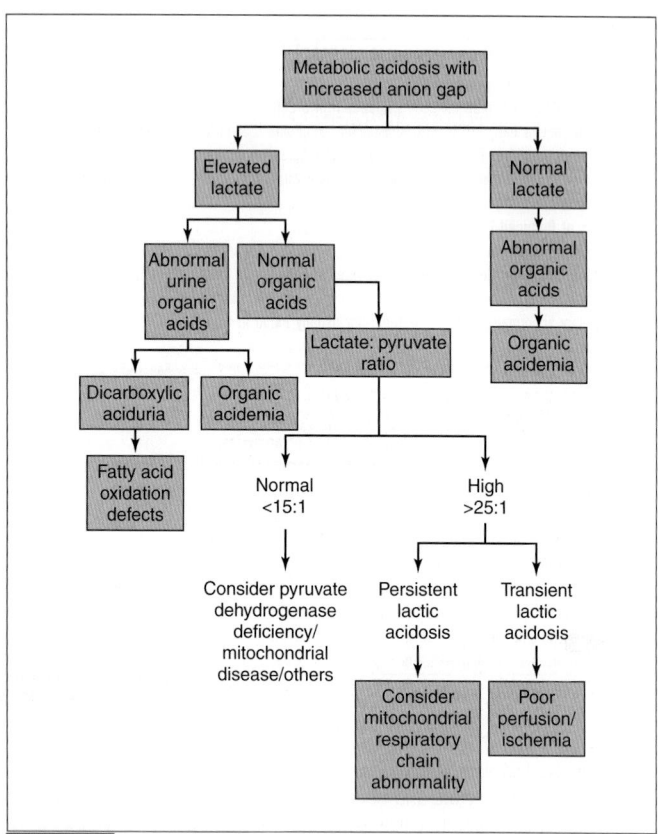

FIGURE 13.1

Evaluation of metabolic acidosis with increased anion gap. (From Burton B. Inborn errors of metabolism in infancy: a guide to diagnosis. *Pediatrics.* 1998;102:E69.)

   b. **Hyperammonemia:** VBG, UOA, PAA, acylcarnitine profile, urine orotic acid (Fig. 13.2)

   c. **Hypoglycemia:** Samples at time of hypoglycemia—glucose, insulin, growth hormone, cortisol, free fatty acids, β-hydroxybutyrate (see Chapter 10). Cortisol, fasting and postprandial lactate, urine ketones, creatine kinase, acylcarnitine profile, PAA, UOA (Fig. 13.3)

   d. **Neonatal seizures:** Cerebrospinal fluid (CSF) amino acids and PAA, CSF/serum glucose ratio, serum and CSF neurotransmitters, CSF and plasma lactate, plasma very-long-chain fatty acids, UOA, serum uric acid, urine sulfites. Consider trial of pyridoxine.

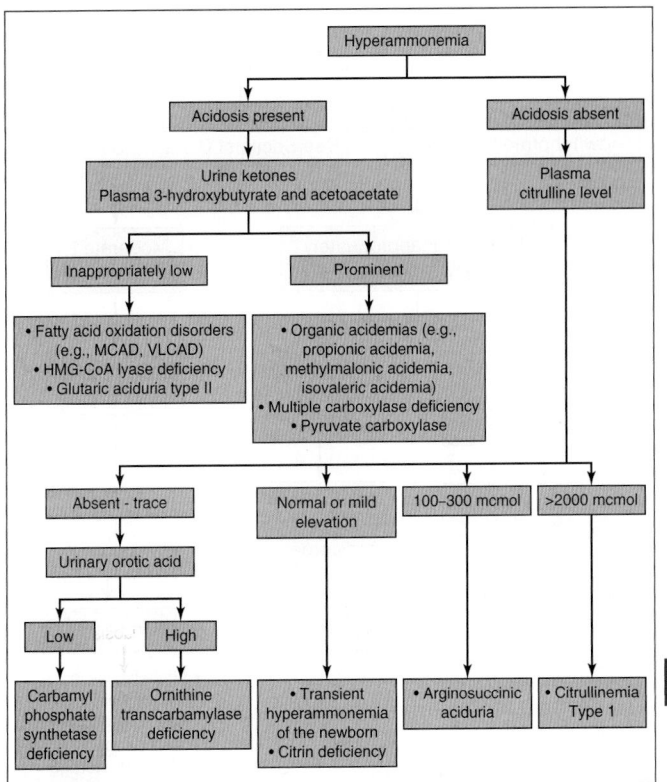

FIGURE 13.2

Evaluation of hyperammonemia. Indicates inappropriately low urinary ketones in the setting of symptomatic hypoglycemia. *HMG-CoA,* Hydroxymethylglutaryl-CoA; *MCAD,* medium-chain acyl-CoA dehydrogenase; *VLCAD,* very-long-chain acyl-CoA dehydrogenase. Whole exome sequencing can detect only single gene defects.

C. Categories of Metabolic Disorders

1. **Intoxication disorders** (Table 13.2)
2. **Disorders of reduced fasting tolerance** (Table 13.3)
3. **Disorders of complex molecules** (Table 13.4)
4. **Mitochondrial disorders** (Table 13.5)
5. **Neurotransmitter disorders** (Table 13.6)

D. Management of Metabolic Crisis

1. Specific acute management available in Tables 13.2–13.6

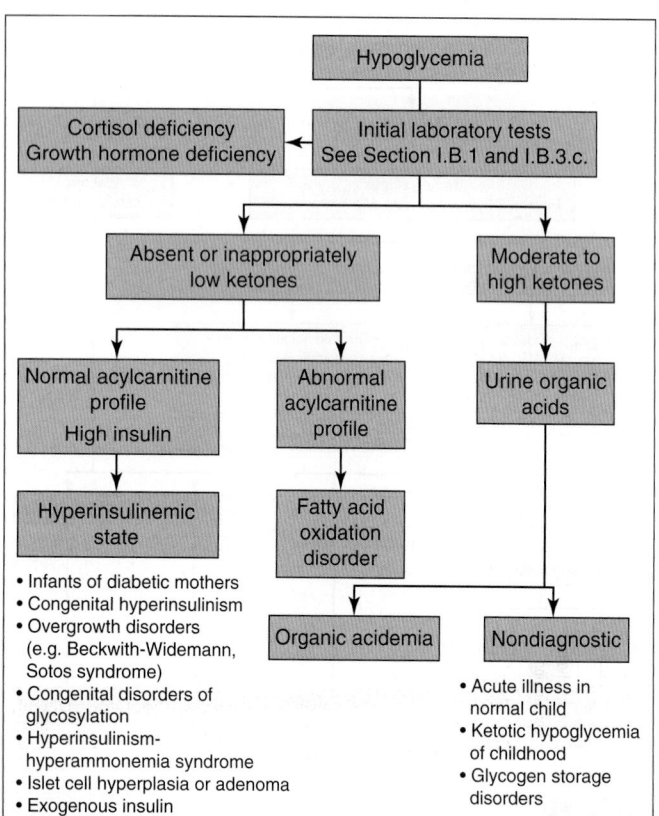

FIGURE 13.3

Evaluation of hypoglycemia. (Modified from Burton BK. Inborn errors of metabolism in infancy: a guide to diagnosis. *Pediatrics*. 1998;102:E69; Cox GF. Diagnostic approaches to pediatric cardiomyopathy of metabolic genetic etiologies and their relation to therapy. *Prog Pediatr Cardiol*. 2007;24:15–25.)

2. A general guiding principle is to provide hydration and enough glucose to meet the patient's caloric needs to stop catabolism.
   a. Use D10% + electrolytes for age at 1.5 to 2 times maintenance rate.
   b. Use caution in mitochondrial disorders (and do not use D10 in pyruvate dehydrogenase deficiency), because this may enhance lactic acidosis. If uncertain, measure lactate and acid-base status regularly.
3. For unknown/suspected metabolic disease, treatment should *not* be delayed during workup.

TABLE 13.2

INTOXICATION DISORDERS[1-6]

Disorders With Selected Examples	Etiology, Clinical Presentation	Acute Management[a]	Chronic Management[a]	Diagnostic Testing[a]
Urea Cycle Disorders OTC Deficiency CPS I Deficiency Citrullinemia	Unable to metabolize proteins to energy Acute intoxication episodes of hyperammonemia, ± respiratory alkalosis	**Reversal of Catabolism** Bolus if dehydration D10 + ¼ NS to NS at 1.5–2× maintenance **Stop Intake of Offending Agents** Stop protein intake (NPO). Resume within 24–48 hr to prevent deficiencies of essential nutrients **Toxin Removal** Removal of ammonia via sodium benzoate + sodium phenylacetate (Ammonul) with arginine IV or dialysis as indicated for ammonia >250 µmol/L	Protein-restricted diet Ammonia scavengers (e.g., sodium phenylbutyrate) Arginine supplementation (dependent on defect)	PAA Urine orotic acid Molecular testing OTC deficiency (most common, X-linked) and CPS I deficiency are not picked up on newborn screening
Organic Acidemias Propionic acidemia Methylmalonic acidemia Isovaleric acidemia	Unable to metabolize certain amino acids and fats Acute intoxication episodes of hyperammonemia with metabolic acidosis Bone marrow suppression, cardiomyopathy	**Reversal of Catabolism**, as above **Stop Intake of Offending Agents**, as above **Toxin Removal** Carnitine in propionic, methylmalonic, and isovaleric acidemia Glycine in isovaleric acidemia Bicarbonate if pH <7.1	Formula that restricts certain amino acids Carnitine	Acylcarnitine profile Quantitative (free and total) carnitine PAA UOA Molecular testing
Maple syrup urine disease	Unable to metabolize branched-chain amino acids (BCAAs) Acute intoxication with high leucine leads to intracranial edema and coma Inappropriate urinary ketones	**Reversal of Catabolism**, as above **Stop Intake of Offending Agents** Stop protein from food and continue BCAA-free formula, valine, and isoleucine **Toxin Removal** Dialysis in extreme situations	Diet and formula that restricts BCAAs Supplementation with isoleucine and valine	PAA UOA Molecular testing

Continued

13

TABLE 13.2

INTOXICATION DISORDERS[1-6]—CONT'D

Disorders With Selected Examples	Etiology, Clinical Presentation	Acute Management[a]	Chronic Management[a]	Diagnostic Testing[a]
Aminoacidopathies Phenylketonuria (PKU) Tyrosinemia (HT)	Unable to metabolize phenylalanine (PKU) or phenylalanine and tyrosine (HT) PKU: intellectual disability if untreated HT: liver failure, vomiting, pain crisis, hyponatremia, Fanconi syndrome	**Supportive.** Dextrose-based fluids are safe for use HT: Pain control and hydration during pain crisis	PKU: Phenylalanine-restricted diet; sapropterin effective in some HT: Tyrosine- and phenylalanine-restricted diet; Nitisinone	PAA HT: UOA for succinylacetone Molecular testing
Carbohydrate Disorders Galactosemia Hereditary fructose intolerance (HFI)	Unable to metabolize galactose (galactosemia) or fructose (HFI) Vomiting, diarrhea, liver failure, renal failure Galactosemia: risk of *Escherichia coli* sepsis	**Supportive.** Dextrose-based fluids are safe for use	Galactosemia: Avoidance of galactose (and lactose); soy-based formulas HFI: Avoidance of fructose (and sucrose)	Urine reducing substances Galactosemia: erythrocyte gal-1-phosphate, galactose-1-phosphate uridyltransferase activity Molecular testing
Metal Disorders Menkes Wilson disease hemochromatosis	Defects in the uptake or excretion of metals Liver disease + neurologic involvement (Menkes, Wilson) + cardiomyopathy (hemochromatosis)	Chelation therapy	Wilson: Copper avoidance, copper chelation Menkes: Copper supplementation Hemochromatosis: Phlebotomy, iron chelation	Serum copper Ceruloplasmin Iron Ferritin Transferrin Molecular testing

[a]Management and testing should be in partnership with a genetics physician, as comprehensive details are beyond the scope of this resource.

CPS, Carbamoyl phosphate synthetase; *D10*, dextrose 10%; *IV*, intravenous; *NPO*, nil per os; *NS*, normal saline; *OTC*, ornithine transcarbamylase; *PAA*, plasma amino acids; *UOA*, urine organic acids.

TABLE 13.3

DISORDERS OF REDUCED FASTING TOLERANCE[1-7,33]

Disorders With Selected Examples	Etiology, Clinical Presentation	Acute Management[a]	Chronic Management[a]	Diagnostic Testing[a]
Fatty Acid Oxidation (FAO) Disorders VLCAD deficiency LCHAD deficiency MCAD deficiency	Disorders of fat metabolism Hypoketotic hypoglycemia in fasting. Can also present with rhabdomyolysis, cardiomyopathy, liver disease	**Reversal of Fasting State** Bolus glucose if hypoglycemia $D10 + \frac{1}{2}$ NS to NS at $1-1.5\times$ maintenance **Stop Intake of Offending Agents** No IV lipids or long chain fats	Avoid prolonged fasting and supplement carbohydrates during illness; consider overnight feeds or uncooked cornstarch as needed for hypoglycemia. For VLCAD and LCHAD, maintain low-fat diet and supplement with medium-chain triglycerides or triheptanoin.	Acylcarnitine profile Quantitative (free and total) carnitine UOA Urine acylglycines
Glycogen Storage Disorders GSD1a, 1b GSD II GSD III GSD IV GSD V GSD VI GSD IX	Multisystem disorders resulting from defects in the synthesis and catabolism of glycogen *Hepatic glycogenoses* (GSD Ia [von Gierke], GSD VI, GSD IX): Hepatomegaly, fasting ketotic hypoglycemia, ± hyperlipidemia, uremia, lactic acidosis *Muscle glycogenoses* (GSD V [McArdle], GSD II [Pompe]): Skeletal and cardiac muscle involvement resulting in fatigue, elevations in creatine kinase *Mixed* (GSD III [Cori], GSD IV): Fasting ketotic hypoglycemia with myopathy	**Reversal of Fasting State**, as above	Prevent long periods of fasting with use of cornstarch. GSD II (Pompe): Enzyme replacement	Glucose Lactate Uric acid Lipid panel Transaminases CK Electrocardiogram Echocardiogram Enzyme activity Molecular testing

[a]Management and testing should be in partnership with a genetics physician, as comprehensive details are beyond the scope of this resource.

CK, Creatine kinase; D10, dextrose 10%; GSD, glycogen storage disease; IV, intravenous; LCHAD, long-chain L-3 hydroxyacyl-CoA dehydrogenase; MCAD, medium-chain acyl-CoA dehydrogenase; NS, normal saline; UOA, urine organic acids; VLCAD, very-long-chain acyl-CoA dehydrogenase.

13

TABLE 13.4

DISORDERS OF COMPLEX MOLECULES[1-6]

Disorders With Selected Examples	Etiology, Clinical Presentation	Management[a]	Diagnostic Testing[a]
Mucopolysaccharidoses MPS I (Hurler) MPS II (Hunter) MPS III (Sanfilippo) MPS IV (Morquio) MPS VI (Maroteaux-Lamy)	Chronic, progressive, multisystem disorders from glycosaminoglycan accumulation Coarse facial features and organomegaly: MPS I Hurler, MPS II Hunter, MPS III Sanfilippo Developmental delay: MPS III Sanfilippo Skeletal dysplasia: MPS IV Morquio	Acute management is supportive Stem cell transplantation: MPS I Enzyme replacement: MPS I, MPS II, MPS IV, MPS VI	Skeletal survey for dysostosis multiplex Urine glycosaminoglycans Urine oligosaccharides Enzyme activity Molecular testing
Sphingolipidoses Gaucher Niemann-Pick Type A, B Tay-Sachs Krabbe Fabry	Impaired degradation of sphingolipids Progressive psychomotor slowing and neurologic problems (e.g. epilepsy, ataxia, and spasticity), hepatosplenomegaly Normal intellect: Gaucher (+ bone crises), Niemann-Pick B (+ lung disease), Fabry (+ acroparesthesias, renal or cardiac disease)	Acute management is supportive Enzyme replacement: Gaucher, Fabry Stem cell transplant: Krabbe Substrate reduction with miglustat or eiglustat: Gaucher	Urine oligosaccharides Enzyme activity Molecular testing
Sterol Synthesis Disorders Smith-Lemli-Opitz Greenberg dysplasia	Multisystem disorders with dysmorphic features and variable skeletal dysplasia	Acute: Adrenal insufficiency may be present Chronic: Consider cholesterol supplementation and/or simvastatin for some disorders	Plasma sterols Serum cholesterol Molecular testing
Peroxisomal Disorders Zellweger Rhizomelic chondrodysplasia punctata (RCDP) X-linked adrenoleukodystrophy	Abnormal peroxisome function or synthesis Neurologic abnormalities such as hypotonia, encephalopathy, seizures, ocular findings Dysmorphic facial features: Zellweger Rhizomelia: RCDP Leukodystrophy: X-linked adrenoleukodystrophy	Acute: Stress dose corticosteroids if adrenal insufficiency for X-linked adrenoleukodystrophy Chronic: Stem cell transplant for X-linked adrenoleukodystrophy	Very-long-chain fatty acids including phytanic and pristanic Pipecolic acids Erythrocyte plasmalogen Molecular testing

[a]Management and testing should be in partnership with a genetics physician because comprehensive details are beyond the scope of this resource.

MPS, Mucopolysaccharidosis.

TABLE 13.5

MITOCHONDRIAL DISORDERS[1-6]

Disorders With Selected Examples	Clinical Presentation	Management[a]	Diagnostic Testing[a]
Mitochondrial Disorders MELAS MERRF Leigh Kearns-Sayre	Multisystemic disease which can include lactic acidosis, muscle weakness, cardiomyopathy, ataxia, ophthalmoplegia, neuropathy, chronic diarrhea	Acute: For MELAS, IV arginine may abort a neurologic crisis Chronic: Cocktail of antioxidants, vitamins, and cofactors	Serum and CSF lactate and pyruvate Plasma and CSF amino acids UOA Brain imaging Molecular testing Muscle biopsy

[a]Management and testing should be in partnership with a genetics physician, as comprehensive details are beyond the scope of this resource.

CSF, Cerebrospinal fluid; *IV,* intravenous; *MELAS,* mitochondrial encephalomyopathy, lactic acidosis, and stroke-like episodes; *MERRF,* myoclonic epilepsy with ragged red fibers; *UOA,* urine organic acids.

TABLE 13.6

NEUROTRANSMITTER DISORDERS[1-6,10]

Disorders With Selected Examples	Clinical Presentation	Management[a]	Diagnostic Testing[a]
Neurotransmitter Disorders Nonketotic hyperglycinemia (NKH) Sulfite oxidase deficiency B6-dependent seizures GABA receptor mutations or metabolism defects	Infantile epileptic encephalopathy	Acute: Consider trial of pyridoxine ± folinic acid Attenuated NKH: Administration of sodium benzoate and blockade of overstimulated NMDA receptors	CSF neurotransmitters CSF glucose Urine sulfite PAA UOA Molecular testing
Dopamine Disorders Dopa-responsive dystonia Tyrosine hydroxylase deficiency	Dystonia, dyskinesia	Dopamine	CSF biogenic amines

[a]Management and testing should be in partnership with a genetics physician, as comprehensive details are beyond the scope of this resource.

CSF, Cerebrospinal fluid; *GABA,* γ-aminobutyric acid; *PAA,* plasma amino acid; *UOA,* urine organic acid.

E. Commonly Used Medications

1. Carnitine 50 mg/kg/dose intravenous (IV) every 6 hours when ill, or 100 mg/kg/day orally (PO) divided every 8 hours when well. For dosing in primary carnitine deficiency, see Formulary.
2. Sodium phenylacetate (10%) + sodium benzoate (10%) (Ammonul) should be combined with arginine HCl in a 25 to 35 mL/kg 10% dextrose solution and administered through a central venous catheter to treat acute hyperammonemia in a urea cycle patient. Administration through a central venous catheter is preferred, however this medication can be administered peripherally.

a. For a child less than 20 kg, the dose is 250 mg/kg sodium phenylacetate and 250 mg/kg sodium benzoate.

b. For a child greater than 20 kg, the dose is 5.5 g/m^2 sodium phenylacetate and 5.5 g/m^2 sodium benzoate.

c. The dose of arginine HCl is 200 to 600 mg/kg for a child <20 kg, or 4–12 g/m^2 for a child or adult >20 kg, depending on the diagnosis.

   (1) 200 mg/kg or 4 g/m^2 for carbamylphosphate synthase (CPS) deficiency and ornithine transcarbamylase (OTC) deficiency.

   (2) 600 mg/kg or 12 g/m^2 for citrullinemia and argininosuccinate lyase (ASL) deficiency.

d. Administer as a loading dose over 90 to 120 minutes, followed by an equivalent dose as a maintenance infusion over 24 hours.

3. Arginine HCl for MELAS stroke-like episode: Treatment for MELAS is generally supportive. During the acute stroke-like episode, a bolus of intravenous arginine (500 mg/kg for children or 10 g/m^2 body surface area for adults) within three hours of symptom onset is recommended followed by the administration of a similar dosage of intravenous arginine as a continuous infusion over 24 hours for the next three to five days.[10](MELAS: mitochondrial encephalomyopathy, lactic acidosis, stroke-like episodes)

4. Sodium benzoate for nonketotic hyperglycinemia (NKH): Patients with attenuated NKH require a lower dose (200–550 mg/kg/day). For older children and adults, consider dosing based on body surface area (e.g., for attenuated NKH start at 5.5 g/m^2 BSA). Patients with severe NKH require a higher dose (550–750 mg/kg/day); for adults, maximum 16.5 g/m^2/day[10]

II. NEWBORN METABOLIC SCREENING[7]

A. Timing

1. First screen should be performed within the first 48 to 72 hours of life (at least 24 hours after initiation of feeding).

2. Second screen (requested in some states) should be performed after 7 days of age.

3. Preterm infants: Perform initial screen at birth (to collect sample before transfusions), another at age 48 to 72 hours, a third at age 7 days, and a final at age 28 days or before discharge (whichever comes first).

B. Abnormal Result

1. Requires immediate follow-up and confirmatory testing; consult a geneticist

2. ACT Sheets and Confirmatory Algorithms are available for more information on how to proceed with specific abnormalities: https://www.acmg.net/ACMG/Medical-Genetics-Practice-Resources/ACT_Sheets_and_Algorithms.aspx (search ACT sheets).

C. Results Affected by Transfusion

NOTE: Repeat newborn metabolic screen 3 months after last transfusion.

1. Biotinidase enzyme activity

2. Galactose-1-phosphate uridyltransferase (GALT) activity

3. Hemoglobinopathy evaluation

III. DYSMORPHOLOGY[7,11-14]

A. History

Pertinent history includes pregnancy course, prenatal exposures, type of conception (natural or assisted), perinatal history, developmental milestones, and review of systems.

B. Family History

1. Three-generation pedigree focused on both medical and developmental histories (see eFig. 13.1).
2. Helpful mnemonics include:
   a. SIDE mnemonic[15]: Anything SIMILAR in the family? Anything INHERITED through the family? Any premature, unexplained DEATHS? Any EXTRAORDINARY events?
   b. SCREEN mnemonic[16]: SOME CONCERNS about conditions running in the family? REPRODUCTION—any issues with pregnancy infertility, or birth defects? EARLY disease, death, or disability? ETHNICITY? NONGENETIC—any other risk factors?
   c. Rule of Too/Two[13]:
      (1) Too: tall? short? many? few? early? young? different?
      (2) Two: cancers? generations? in the family? birth defects?
3. **Patterns of inheritance:** See Online Content for discussion of different patterns of inheritance.

C. Physical Examination

1. **Major anomalies:** Structural anomalies that are found in less than 5% of the population and may cause significant cosmetic or functional impairment, often requiring medical or surgical management.
2. **Minor anomalies[11,12,14,17]:** Structural anomalies that are found in greater than 5% of the population with little or no cosmetic or functional significance to the patient.
3. Examples of major and minor anomalies (Table 13.7). Three or more minor anomalies may be a nonspecific indicator of occult or major anomaly.

D. Workup: Tailor to individual patient and existing information, including effective chart review, prior genetic testing, and genetic testing in the family

1. **Imaging to evaluate for major anomalies**
   a. Head ultrasound (US) or brain magnetic resonance imaging (MRI)
   b. Echocardiogram
   c. Complete abdominal US
   d. Skeletal survey with radiographs composed of: AP views of skull, chest/ribs, upper extremities and hands, lower extremities and feet; lateral views of skull, complete spine, chest, and odontoid view
2. **Dilated eye exam**
3. **Hearing evaluation**

TABLE 13.7

EXAMPLES OF DYSMORPHOLOGY EXAM FINDINGS[11-14,17]

	Major Anomalies	Minor Anomalies
General	Growth <3rd percentile	Short or tall stature
Head	Structural brain abnormalities (e.g., holoprosencephaly, schizencephaly), craniosynostosis	Asymmetric head shape, micrognathia, prominent metopic ridge, widows peak
Eyes	Anophthalmia, cataracts, coloboma	Palpebral fissures, epicanthal folds, hypertelorism or hypotelorism, telecanthus, epicanthus, ptosis
Ears, nose, throat	Cleft lip/palate, tracheal-esophageal fistula	Periauricular pits/tags, overfolded helix, everted ears, low-set ears, microtia, abnormal nasal bridge, branchial cleft cysts
Chest/lungs	Congenital diaphragmatic hernia, situs inversus	Inverted nipples, accessory nipples, pectus excavatum or carinatum
Heart	Congenital heart defects (e.g., tetralogy of Fallot, coarctation of aorta, atrial or ventricular septal defects)	Patent ductus arteriosus, valvular abnormalities
Abdomen	Omphalocele, gastroschisis, intestinal atresia	Umbilical hernia
Genitourinary	Ambiguous genitalia, horseshoe kidney	Hypogonadism, pelvic kidney, shawl scrotum, labial hypoplasia
Musculoskeletal	Skeletal dysplasia, spina bifida	Clubfeet, bowing, syndactyly of two digits, postaxial polydactyly, 5th finger clinodactyly, hypoplastic nails, short metacarpals or metatarsals
Skin	Cutis aplasia	Striae, café-au-lait spots, atypical skin creases, transverse palmar crease, nevus simplex, congenital dermal melanocytosis

4. **Genetic testing:** See Fig. 13.4 and Table 13.8. The patient should be referred to genetics for a dysmorphology evaluation and appropriate testing.

IV. PATTERNS OF GENETIC CONDITIONS WITH DISTINCTIVE APPEARANCE[11,14]

This section is not comprehensive; it covers some common reasons to seek a genetics consult. These conditions will often be managed by a multidisciplinary team.

A. Cardiac Conditions

1. **Congenital heart disease:** Investigation for co-occurring anomalies with abdominal US. Chromosome microarray testing indicated, including for 22q11 deletion syndrome (Table 13.9).

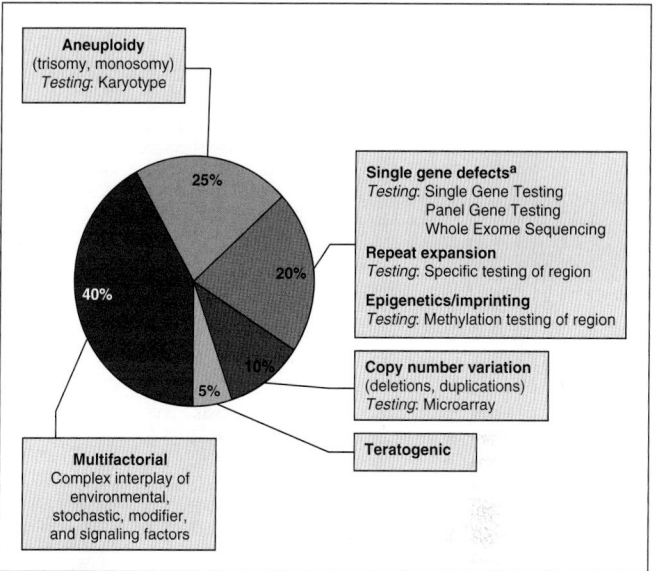

FIGURE 13.4

Etiologies of dysmorphic features.[29] [a]Whole exome sequencing can only reliably detect single base pair changes and insertions/deletions of less than 20 base pairs.

2. **Cardiomyopathy:** Can be from inborn errors of metabolism, channelopathies, mutations in genes important for sarcomere and desmosome production/function, or other single gene disorders.
3. **Long QT disorders:** Many single gene disorders

B. Ciliopathies

1. **Nonmotile ciliopathies:** Defects in primary (nonmotile) ciliary function. Cystic renal disease, brain malformations (molar tooth sign), retinal degeneration, congenital hepatic fibrosis, polydactyly, skeletal dysplasia, obesity. **Examples:** Cystic kidneys as a result of heritable polycystic kidney disease; neurodevelopmental ciliopathies such as Joubert syndrome or Bardet-Biedl syndrome
2. **Primary ciliary dyskinesias:** Defects in motile cilia. Recurrent respiratory infections (chronic sinopulmonary disease), infertility, situs inversus. **Examples:** More than 45 genes known to cause primary ciliary dyskinesia. When situs inversus is present, it is referred to as Kartagener syndrome.
3. **Evaluation:** Evaluation for potentially affected organ systems, including abdominal US, echocardiogram, brain MRI, and complete retinal evaluation with ophthalmology. Skeletal survey if limb defects. CMP to evaluate kidney and liver function. Unless a specific disorder is suspected, broad genetic testing is appropriate.

TABLE 13.8
DIAGNOSTIC GENETIC TESTING AND CLINICAL CONSIDERATIONS

Genetic Testing Technology	Description of Technology	Turnaround Time	Able to Detect	Specific Indications
Karyotype	Systematically arranged photomicrograph of chromosomes	1–2 weeks	Aneuploidy, larger deletions/ duplications (≥5 kb), translocation or balanced rearrangements	Indicated for suspected aneuploidy, recurrent miscarriage, looking for a balanced translocation
Fluorescence in situ hybridization (FISH)	Mapping a segment of DNA by molecular hybridization of a fluorescent probe	<1 week	Presence or absence of a specific site or chromosome	Not indicated, except in family studies and for rapid diagnosis of a suspected trisomy[32]
Microarray (a.k.a. Array CGH, SNP or oligochromosomal microarray)	Comparative genome hybridization using a high-density SNP profile or oligos (short segments of DNA) across the genome	2–4 weeks	Genomic gains or losses (copy number variation [CNV]), regions of homozygosity (consanguinity). Incidental findings unrelated to phenotype	First-line cytogenetic test for all patients with unexplained global developmental delay, intellectual disability, autism, and/or congenital anomalies
Single gene testing	Nucleotide-by-nucleotide Sanger sequencing of a single gene	~1 month	Mutations in specific gene of interest	Indicated when there is a strong clinical suspicion of a specific single gene disorder
Targeted mutation analysis	Detection of previously identified familial mutation or common population mutation	<1 month	Whether the patient has (or does not have) only the specific mutation tested	Confirmation of clinical diagnosis, presymptomatic genetic diagnosis, identification of carrier status, preimplantation genetic diagnosis, prenatal testing
Repeat expansion testing	Southern blot or triplet-repeat primed PCR	<1 month	The quantity of repeats in the specific gene tested	Indicated when there is a strong clinical suspicion of a triplet repeat disorder
Methylation analysis	Methylation multiplex ligation-dependent probe amplification	<1 month	Whether the region tested has normal or abnormal methylation	Indicated when there is a strong clinical suspicion of a specific methylation defect (e.g., Prader-Willi)

Next-generation sequencing (multiple gene panels)	Massively parallel sequencing of specific genes	1–2 months	Simultaneously identifies if there are any variants in multiple genes of interest	Used for syndromes with heterogeneity (mutations in different genes can cause the same phenotype, or the phenotypes are hard to distinguish clinically)
Whole exome sequencing (WES)	Massively parallel sequencing of almost all exons	2–6 months	Simultaneously identifies if there are any variants in the coding portions of genes that match the patient's phenotype. Incidental findings unrelated to phenotype	More comprehensive genomic test indicated in an otherwise negative workup, or when cost-benefit ratio of more targeted testing is in favor of WES
Whole genome sequencing (WGS)	Massively parallel sequencing of entire genome	Variable	More uniform coverage of exonic, intronic, and splice site mutations. Incidental findings unrelated to phenotype	Not widely clinically available; used mostly in research studies

CGH, Comparative genomic hybridization; *DNA,* deoxyribonucleic acid; *Kb,* kilobases; *PCR,* polymerase chain reaction; *SNP,* single nucleotide polymorphism.

13

TABLE 13.9

GENETIC SYNDROMES ASSOCIATED WITH CARDIAC DEFECTS[11]

Genetic Syndrome	Cardiac Defect	Other Features	Diagnostic Evaluation
Noonan syndrome[a]	Pulmonary valve stenosis, hypertrophic cardiomyopathy	Short stature, broad neck, lymphatic dysplasia, low ears and hypertelorism, coagulation defects	"RASopathy" gene panel including *PTPN11*
Williams syndrome (7q11.23 deletion)[a]	Supravalvular aortic stenosis	Periorbital fullness, broad nasal tip, large ears, thick lips, small teeth, hypercalcemia, renal artery stenosis, connective tissue abnormalities, overfriendliness	Microarray
Holt-Oram syndrome	ASD	Upper limb malformation, cardiac conduction disease	*TBX5* sequencing
Down syndrome[a]	VSD, AV canal defect	(See Section V)	Karyotype
Turner syndrome[a]	Coarctation of aorta	(See Section V)	Karyotype
22q11.2 Deletion syndrome[a]	Tetralogy of Fallot, interrupted aortic arch, VSD	(See Section V)	Microarray

[a]Published clinical management guidelines available.[20]
ASD, Atrial septal defect; *AV*, atrioventricular; *VSD*, ventricular septal defect.

C. Cleft Lip and Palate (CLP)

1. Can be isolated or part of a syndrome
2. **Risk factors:** Maternal smoking, heavy alcohol use, systemic corticosteroid use, folic acid and cobalamin deficiency[18]
3. Submucosal clefts may be indicated by a bifid uvula.
4. **Evaluation:** Children can have difficulties with feeding, speech, and hearing (chronic otitis or hearing loss as part of a syndrome). If not an isolated anomaly, may need further workup with ophthalmology and echocardiogram.
5. **Examples:** Autosomal dominant inheritance seen in Van der Woude syndrome (associated with lip pits) and Stickler syndrome (can have retinal detachment, hearing loss)

D. Connective Tissue Disorders

1. Consider when a patient has velvety skin, hyperextensible joints, abnormal scarring, poor healing, striae, pectus deformities, tall stature, myopia, lens dislocations, arachnodactyly
2. **Evaluation:** Some connective tissue disorders are associated with dilated aorta (echocardiogram), dysplastic vessels, or fragility of lens/retina (ophthalmology evaluation).

3. **Examples:** Dilated aorta with characteristic physical features in Marfan syndrome; vascular fragility in vascular Ehlers-Danlos (type IV); isolated hyperextensibility of joints in hypermobile Ehlers-Danlos (type III)

E. Developmental Delay, Intellectual Disability

1. All children should be offered genetic evaluation.
2. See Chapter 9 for information on evaluation.

Examples: Microarray is first tier test because it can detect microdeletion and microduplication syndromes, such as 1p36 deletion syndrome. *FMR1* repeat testing can detect fragile X syndrome and heterozygous females, who can also have developmental delays. The American College of Medical Genetics (ACMG) is currently reviewing the possibility of starting with whole exome sequencing (WES). If whole genome sequencing becomes the clinical standard, then chromosome microarray and even fragile X testing will no longer be indicated.

F. Deafness, Hard of Hearing

1. Approximately 60% of hearing loss is genetic. It can be syndromic or nonsyndromic.
2. Consider perinatal infectious causes (e.g., cytomegalovirus).
3. **Evaluation:** Consider connexin 26 and 30 gene testing as first step if nonsyndromic and/or broad gene panel testing. Individualize inner ear/ brain imaging. Ophthalmology assessment, ECG, and renal US should be considered for those with negative connexin testing.
4. **Examples:** Approximately half of nonsyndromic hearing loss is from *GJB2* (encodes connexin 26) gene mutations. Syndromic causes include Usher syndrome, which can also have gradual vision loss.

G. Hypotonia

1. **Central:** Abnormalities of brain function, normal strength or axial weakness, preserved/persistent newborn reflexes, normal CK, normal muscle bulk
   a. **Evaluation:** CK to differentiate. Evaluate for causes such as hypothyroidism (TSH); evaluate brain structure and function with MRI and EEG.
   b. **Examples:** Prader-Willi syndrome, peroxisomal disorders, many others
2. **Peripheral:** Alert, profound weakness that is often appendicular, absent reflexes, feeding difficulties, normal or increased CK
   a. **Evaluation:** Evaluate for causes such as hypothyroidism (TSH) or mitochondrial disease (lactate/pyruvate). Electromyography (EMG) to determine if muscle or nerve affected. Consider that cardiac muscle could be affected (echocardiogram).
   b. **Examples:** Spinal muscular atrophy (now included in newborn screening), myotonic dystrophy, muscular dystrophies

H. Limb and Stature Conditions

1. Can be defects in collagen formation, bone formation, or remodeling
2. **Evaluation:** Radiographic skeletal survey of all bones to localize dysplasia. Some conditions, including achondroplasia, can have narrowing at the

foramen magnum or cervical instability (flexion/extension C-spine films). There can be a risk of central or peripheral sleep apneas (sleep study). Karyotype for females with short stature to evaluate for Turner syndrome. Unless a specific condition is suspected, broad genetic testing is appropriate.

3. **Examples:** Rhizomelic limb shortening and narrow foramen magnum seen in achondroplasia. Cervical instability seen in *COL2A1* gene mutations (spondyloepiphyseal dysplasia congenita, Stickler syndrome). The presence of multiple congenital joint contractures is called arthrogryposis, which is seen in many conditions. Fractures can be seen in osteogenesis imperfecta and hypophosphatasia.

I. Liver Disease

1. Liver failure and/or direct and indirect hyperbilirubinemia can be a manifestation of a metabolic condition or the result of a genetic syndrome.

2. **Evaluation:** Metabolic workup, including PAA, UOA, urine succinylacetone, very-long-chain fatty acids, urine-reducing substances. Some syndromes have ocular features (ophthalmology evaluation). Unless a specific condition is suspected, broad genetic testing is appropriate.

3. **Examples:** Cholestasis found in progressive familial intrahepatic cholestasis (type 1, 2, and 3). Liver dysfunction can be seen in tyrosinemia. Indirect/unconjugated hyperbilirubinemia can be seen in Gilbert and Crigler-Najjar syndromes.

J. Oncologic Conditions[19]

1. Approximately 10% of pediatric oncology patients have a heritable cancer predisposition syndrome or germline mutation. This puts them and affected family members at risk for certain cancers and may affect their individualized treatments.

2. Obtain a thorough family history with specific cancer diagnoses and age of diagnosis.

3. **Evaluation:** Many cancers warrant referral. Genetic testing is tailored to each specific diagnosis. Examples include myelodysplastic syndrome, medulloblastoma, atypical teratoid rhabdoid tumor, sarcomas, pituitary blastoma, and many more.

4. **Examples:** Early onset of cancers in Li-Fraumeni syndrome (especially sarcoma) and von Hippel-Lindau syndrome (especially hemangioblastoma)

K. Overgrowth

1. Generalized overgrowth can result in macrosomia at birth or height and/or head circumference greater than the 98th percentile.

2. Hemihypertrophy may be the result of mosaicism from somatic changes.

3. Be aware that certain overgrowth syndromes have associated cancer risks and may require routine monitoring (e.g., abdominal US screening in Beckwith-Wiedemann syndrome).

4. **Evaluation:** Condition-specific genetic testing based on exam findings; may require skin biopsy. In some conditions, internal organs can be affected (echocardiogram, ECG, renal US).
5. **Examples:** Generalized overgrowth with developmental delays can be the result of Sotos syndrome, Beckwith-Wiedemann syndrome, or others. Segmental overgrowth/hemihypertrophy can result from somatic *PIK3CA* mutations affecting the brain (MCAP syndrome) or a limb (Klippel-Trénaunay syndrome).

L. Conditions Associated With Seizures

1. Consider genetics, especially with positive family history, intractable epilepsy, infantile onset, developmental regression, intellectual disability, dysmorphic features, autism, or brain malformations.
2. Can be the result of metabolic conditions or syndromic conditions
3. Increased recurrence risk in families even if no genetic cause identified
4. **Evaluation:** Consideration of microarray, epilepsy panels, or whole exome sequencing (particularly if dysmorphic features present); consider biochemical testing for inborn errors of metabolism; physical exam with Wood's lamp for cutaneous manifestations (e.g., hypopigmented macules).
5. **Examples:** Sodium channel defects (*SCN1A* mutations) can lead to a broad spectrum of seizures. Accompanying dermatologic findings can be characteristic for neurocutaneous conditions, including neurofibromatosis type 1 and tuberous sclerosis.

M. Skin Pigmentation Alterations

1. Can be the result of post-zygotic mosaicism. As a result, genetic variants may only be detectable in affected skin and not in blood.
2. Skin and the central nervous system are derived from the same neural crest lineage; many skin pigmentation anomalies have associated central nervous system abnormalities, including malformations or seizures. Often referred to as neurocutaneous conditions.
3. **Evaluation:** Examination with a Wood's lamp, ophthalmology evaluation
4. **Examples:** Multiple café-au-lait macules seen in neurofibromatosis type 1 and Legius syndrome. Genetic mosaicism in skin can lead to a pigmentation pattern called hypomelanosis of Ito.

N. Vascular Anomalies

1. Can involve arterial, vascular, and lymphatic systems. Can be caused by germline pathogenic variants or postzygotic somatic mutations (mosaicism). Some are associated with segmental overgrowth.
2. Vascular syndromes can cause clinically significant arteriovenous malformations and arteriovenous fistulas in the skin, internal organs, and brain/spine.
3. **Evaluation:** Examine mucosal membranes. Some conditions require evaluation for intraorgan arteriovenous malformations with abdominal US and/or MRI/magnetic resonance angiography (MRA) of brain and spine. Several conditions are autosomal dominant—obtain family history for vascular lesions.

4. **Examples:** Autosomal dominant history of multiple capillary malformations could be from *RASA1* mutations. Port-wine stains seen in Sturge-Weber syndrome. Telangiectasias on lips, nose, and hands seen in hereditary hemorrhagic telangiectasia

V. ETIOLOGIES OF DYSMORPHIC FEATURES (FIG. 13.4)[11,14,29]

A. Aneuploidy
Abnormal number of chromosomes

1. Aneuploidy syndromes are most commonly due to maternal nondisjunction and more rarely due to chromosomal translocation or mosaicism. Risk increases with maternal age.
2. The evaluation for aneuploidy often begins prenatally with a first trimester screen (nuchal translucency, nasal bone, free β-human chorionic gonadotropin [β-hCG], PAPP-A) or circulating cell-free fetal DNA analysis showing increased risk.
3. Prenatal diagnostic testing options include chorionic villus sampling in the first trimester or amniocentesis during or after the second trimester.
4. Fluorescence in situ hybridization (FISH) may be performed in the first 24 to 48 hours of life to indicate number of chromosomes but will not determine the morphology of the chromosomes (e.g., if a translocation is present). Therefore karyotype analysis is still indicated in aneuploidy syndromes, both to provide a diagnosis and to provide accurate genetic counseling.
5. **Specific aneuploidy syndromes:**
   a. **Down syndrome (Trisomy 21):**
      (1) **Features:** Hypotonia and characteristic facial features (brachycephaly, epicanthal folds, flat nasal bridge, upward-slanting palpebral fissures, Brushfield spots, small mouth and ears), excess skin at the nape of the neck, single transverse palmar crease, short fifth finger with clinodactyly, wide gap between the first and second toes. Intellectual disability present in all, but severity is variable.
      (2) Full health supervision guidelines from the American Academy of Pediatrics (AAP) are available (see Section VII).
      (3) In brief: In addition to karyotype, neonates should have echocardiogram to assess for congenital heart disease, ophthalmologic evaluation to assess for cataracts, hearing screen, complete blood count (CBC) to assess for transient myeloproliferative disease, thyroid studies to assess for hypothyroidism, and referral to early intervention services. Annual thyroid studies, CBC (add ferritin and CRP for any child at risk of iron deficiency), hearing and vision assessments. Cervical spine x-ray at age 3 years if asymptomatic (sooner imaging with immediate neurosurgical referral if symptomatic). Monitor for signs of obstructive sleep apnea and neurologic dysfunction.

b. **Edwards syndrome (Trisomy 18):**
   (1) **Features:** Intrauterine growth restriction and polyhydramnios, small for gestational age at birth, clenched hands with overlapping fingers, hypoplastic nails, short sternum, prominent occiput, low-set and structurally abnormal ears, micrognathia, rocker-bottom feet, congenital heart disease, cystic and horseshoe kidneys, seizures, hypertonia, significant developmental and cognitive impairments
   (2) Ninety percent die before 1 year of life.
c. **Patau syndrome (Trisomy 13):**
   (1) **Features:** Defects of forebrain development (holoprosencephaly), severe developmental disability, low-set malformed ears, cleft lip and palate (CLP), microphthalmia, aplasia cutis congenita, polydactyly (most frequently of the postaxial type), narrow hyperconvex nails, apneic spells, cryptorchidism, congenital heart defects
   (2) Ninety-five percent die before 6 months of life.
d. **Turner syndrome (45, X):**
   (1) **Features:** Short stature, gonadal dysgenesis with amenorrhea and lack of a pubertal growth spurt, broad chest with hypoplastic or inverted nipples, webbed neck. The diagnosis should be considered prenatally in a female fetus with hydrops, increased nuchal translucency, cystic hygroma, or lymphedema. Intelligence is usually normal, but patients are at risk for cognitive, behavioral, and social disabilities.
   (2) Full health supervision guidelines from the AAP are available (see Section VII).
   (3) In brief: Obtain baseline echocardiogram, renal US, ophthalmology and audiology evaluations. Routine thyroid testing, biochemical liver tests, Hemoglobin A_{1c}, vitamin D, TTG and immunoglobulin A (IgA), audiology, skin examinations, bone mineral density, and skeletal assessments.
e. **Klinefelter syndrome (47, XXY; 48, XXYY; 48, XXXY; and 49, XXXXY):**
   (1) **Features:** Primary hypogonadism, which may present in infancy with hypospadias or cryptorchidism or in adolescence/adulthood with infertility, gynecomastia, and small testes. Children may have expressive language delay.
   (2) There is an increased risk of breast carcinoma in 47, XXY.
   (3) Testosterone therapy is indicated at puberty for hypergonadotropic hypogonadism.

B. Copy Number Variation (Deletions and Duplications)
Partial loss or additional copies of genetic material on part of a chromosome

1. **22q11 Deletion syndrome (velocardiofacial syndrome, DiGeorge syndrome)**
   a. **Features:** Congenital heart disease (tetralogy of Fallot, interrupted aortic arch, ventricular septal defect [VSD], and truncus arteriosus most common), palatal abnormalities (velopharyngeal incompetence,

cleft palate), characteristic facial features in approximately two-thirds, developmental delays, learning disabilities, immunodeficiency, hypocalcemia, feeding problems, renal anomalies, hearing loss, laryngotracheoesophageal anomalies, growth hormone deficiency, autoimmune disorders, seizures (with or without hypocalcemia), and psychiatric disorders

b. **Diagnostic evaluation:** Microarray; FISH is no longer recommended. Assessments should include serum calcium, absolute lymphocyte count, B- and T-cell subsets, renal US, chest x-ray, cardiac examination, and echocardiogram

c. **Health supervision:** Hold live vaccines until immune function is assessed.

2. **5p− syndrome (cri-du-chat syndrome)**
   a. **Features:** High-pitched cry, delayed development, intellectual disability, microcephaly, low birth weight, hypotonia, hypertelorism, low-set ears, small jaw, round face, congenital heart disease (VSD, atrial septal defect [ASD], PDA)
   b. **Diagnostic evaluation:** Can be detected on karyotype or microarray

3. **1p36 Deletion syndrome**
   a. **Features:** Developmental delay, intellectual disability, delayed growth, hypotonia, seizures, speech delay, hearing and vision impairment, microcephaly, low ears with thick helices, congenital heart disease (structural defects or cardiomyopathy)
   b. **Diagnostic evaluation:** Microarray

C. Disorders of Methylation/Epigenetics

Heritable changes that affect gene activity and expression

1. **Prader-Willi syndrome**
   a. **Features:** Severe hypotonia and feeding difficulties in infancy, followed by an insatiable appetite in later infancy or early childhood. Developmental delays in motor and language abilities. All affected individuals have some degree of intellectual/learning disability. Short stature is common; males and females have hypogonadism, and in most, infertility.
   b. **Diagnostic evaluation:** Results from missing *paternally* contributed region. Methylation testing can detect almost all individuals—whether due to abnormal paternal-specific imprinting, a paternal deletion, or maternal uniparental disomy within the Prader-Willi/Angelman critical region of 15q. Follow up with further molecular testing.
   c. **Health supervision:** Full health supervision guidelines from the AAP are available (see Section VII). Monitor for feeding difficulties in infancy and close supervision beginning in childhood to prevent obesity. Evaluate for and treat hypothyroidism, sleep apnea (central and obstructive), central adrenal insufficiency,[21] and cryptorchidism.
   d. **Treatment:** Growth hormone can be beneficial, and hormone replacement therapy can aid in sexual development.

2. **Angelman syndrome**
   a. **Features:** Happy demeanor, hand-flapping, and fascination with water. Severe developmental delay, intellectual disability, severe speech impairment, gait ataxia, tremulous limbs, hypotonia, microcephaly, and seizures
   b. **Diagnostic evaluation:** Results from missing *maternally* contributed region. Methylation testing can detect almost all individuals—whether due to abnormal maternal-specific imprinting, a maternal deletion, or paternal uniparental disomy within the Prader-Willi/Angelman critical region of 15q. Some individuals can be detected through *UBE3A* sequence analysis.
   c. **Health supervision:** Monitor for seizures, behavior problems, feeding issues, sleep disturbance, scoliosis, strabismus, constipation, and gastroesophageal reflux disease.
   d. **Treatment:** Antiepileptic drugs for seizures; be careful not to overtreat, because Angelman syndrome also associated with movement abnormalities (*avoid* carbamazepine, vigabatrin, and tiagabine).[22] Speech therapy with a focus on nonverbal communication. Sedatives for nighttime wakefulness.
3. **Classic Rett syndrome:** X-linked condition present only in females because pathogenic *MECP2* variants are most often lethal in males who have only one X chromosome. Males who do survive with *MECP2* mutations have presentation different from Rett syndrome that often incudes neonatal encephalopathy.
   a. **Features:** Neurodevelopmental syndrome that presents after 6 to 18 months of typical development with acquired microcephaly, then developmental stagnation, followed by rapid regression. Gait ataxia or inability to ambulate; repetitive, stereotypical handwringing; fits of screaming or inconsolable crying; episodic breathing abnormalities (sighing, apnea, or hyperpnea); tremors; and generalized tonic-clonic seizures
   b. **Diagnostic evaluation:** Molecular testing of *MECP2*
   c. **Health supervision:** Regular ECG to evaluate QT interval,[23] monitor for scoliosis

D. Repeat Expansion

Pathogenic expansion of trinucleotide repeats during DNA replication

1. **Fragile X syndrome**
   a. Most common cause of inherited intellectual disability
   b. **Features:** Males have relative macrocephaly and prominent ears. Postpubertal macroorchidism and tall stature that slows in adolescence. Females have a range of intellectual disability due to the degree of inactivation of the affected X chromosome. Female premutation carriers (55 to 200 repeats) can develop primary ovarian insufficiency; males with 55 to 200 repeats can develop a tremor/ataxia phenotype.

   c. **Diagnostic evaluation:** Repeat expansion testing of *FMR1* gene to assess number of CGG trinucleotide repeats (typically >200 in fragile X syndrome).

   d. **Health supervision:** Full health supervision guidelines from the AAP are available (see Section VII). Symptom and supportive psychopharmacologic medications

2. Other examples include Huntington disease (CAG repeats), myotonic dystrophy (CTG repeats), and Friedrich ataxia (GAA repeats).

E. Mendelian/Single Gene Disorders

Mutation in a single gene causing a disorder

1. **Marfan syndrome**

   a. **Features:** Myopia, ectopia lentis, aortic dilatation with predisposition to rupture, mitral valve prolapse, pneumothorax, bone overgrowth and joint laxity, pectus carinatum or excavatum, scoliosis, pes planus

   b. **Diagnostic evaluation:** Clinical diagnosis based on the revised Ghent criteria (a "systemic score" system based on clinical features that can support a diagnosis if score is greater than or equal to 7). Sequencing of *FBN1* gene

   c. **Health supervision:** Annual ophthalmologic examination; annual echocardiography; intermittent surveillance of the entire aorta with computed tomography (CT) or MRA scans beginning in young adulthood. Avoid contact sports, competitive sports, isometric exercise. Full health supervision guidelines from the AAP are available (see Section VII).

   d. **Treatment:** β-blocker (atenolol) and/or an angiotensin-II type 1 receptor blocker (losartan) is current standard of care. Valve-sparing surgery to replace aortic root when diameter exceeds ∼4.5 cm in adults (or if rates of aortic dilation exceed ∼0.5 cm/year) and significant aortic regurgitation is present.[24]

2. **Ehlers-Danlos syndrome (EDS)**

   a. **Features:** Smooth, velvety, hyperextensible skin, widened scars, poor healing, easy bruising, joint hypermobility with recurrent dislocations, chronic joint or limb pain, and a positive family history. The vascular-type EDS is distinct and involves translucent skin, characteristic facies (pinched nose), as well as risk for arterial, intestinal, and uterine fragility or rupture.

   b. **Diagnostic evaluation:** Clinical evaluation and family history. There are more than thirteen types; for classical and vascular types, echocardiogram and DNA testing. Vascular type additionally needs CTA/MRA imaging of head to pelvis. Joint hypermobility can be scored with Beighton criteria. No known genetic cause of hypermobile type, which is most common

   c. **Treatment:** Physical therapy to improve joint stability, low-resistance exercise, and pain medications as needed; treat gastroesophageal reflux. Vascular EDS requires management in a clinic specializing in connective tissue disorders.

3. **Achondroplasia**
   a. **Features:** Short arms and legs (due to rhizomelia or shortening of the most proximal extremity segments: humerus and femur); bowing of the lower legs; large head with characteristic facial features including frontal bossing and midface retrusion. Infantile hypotonia is typical, followed by delayed motor development. Gibbus deformity of the thoracolumbar spine leads to exaggerated lumbar lordosis. Rarely, children have hydrocephalus and restrictive pulmonary disease. Stenosis at the foramen magnum in infancy increases the risk of death; lumbar spinal stenosis may present in childhood but is more common in adulthood. Intelligence and life span are usually normal. Average adult height for males and females is approximately 4 feet.
   b. **Diagnostic evaluation:** Clinical diagnosis based on characteristic physical exam. *FGFR3* mutation testing available if diagnostic uncertainty
   c. **Health supervision:** Full health supervision guidelines from the AAP are available (see Section VII). In brief: Use standard growth charts for achondroplasia. Baseline head CT including cervicomedullary junction in infancy, and precautions against uncontrolled head movement or neck manipulation. Monitor for signs of obstructive sleep apnea, middle ear complications (e.g., otitis media), or spinal stenosis (more common in adults). New treatments available and in clinical trials

F. Teratogen Exposure (Table 13.10)
G. In utero Forces[25]

1. Uterine compression:
   a. Can be intrinsic (oligohydramnios, multiple fetuses, uterine deformities) or extrinsic (small pelvis)
   b. Results in deformations, including craniofacial (plagiocephaly, flattened facies, crumpled ear, craniosynostosis), extremities (dislocated hips, equinovarus or calcaneovalgus feet, tibial bowing, contractures), torticollis, lung hypoplasia, scoliosis
2. Abnormal fetal muscular tone or posture can result in hyperextended knees, dislocated hips, contractures.
3. Placental compromise
4. Amniotic bands

VI. CONSENT AND DISCLOSURE OF GENETIC TESTING

A. Ethics of Genetic Testing in Pediatrics
Genetic testing in pediatric patients poses unique challenges given that children require proxies (most often parents) to give consent for testing. Several publications and statements have been released about genetic testing in children, including the "Ethical Issues with Genetic Testing in Pediatrics" statement made by the AAP.[26] Important considerations include:

TABLE 13.10

SELECTED TERATOGENS[11,30-31]

Exposure	Features
Intrauterine infections	See Chapter 17
Intrauterine substance exposure	Alcohol: Fetal alcohol spectrum disorder: microcephaly, small palpebral fissures with epicanthal folds, low nasal bridge with upturned nose, smooth philtrum and thin vermilion border, small chin, developmental delay, intellectual disability
	Cocaine: IUGR, developmental delay, learning disabilities, attention and behavioral challenges, occasional congenital anomalies
Intrauterine medication exposure *See Formulary for drug-specific information on risk in pregnancy.*	Phenytoin: Fetal hydantoin syndrome: growth deficiency, hypertelorism, flat nasal bridge, cleft lip and palate, long philtrum and thin bowed upper lip, digitalized thumbs, hypoplasia of distal phalanges
	Warfarin: Nasal hypoplasia, epiphyseal stippling, hypoplastic distal phalanges, Peters anomaly, brain malformations
	Valproate: High forehead, broad nasal bridge, small mouth and chin, cardiac defects, long/thin phalanges, developmental delay
	Retinoic acid: Microtia, depressed nasal bridge, hypertelorism, cardiac defects, brain malformations, intellectual disability
	ACE inhibitors: Oligohydramnios, renal tubular dysgenesis, poor ossification of calvaria, cardiac defects, brain malformations
	Methotrexate: Microcephaly, growth restriction, hypoplasia of skull bones, micrognathia, low-set ears, mesomelia, syndactyly
Maternal medical conditions	Diabetes mellitus: Polyhydramnios, macrosomia; variety of congenital anomalies including spina bifida, heart defects, skeletal anomalies, urinary/reproductive system anomalies
	Uncontrolled maternal PKU: Microcephaly, IUGR, hypertonia, cardiac defects, intellectual disability
Environmental exposures	High lead levels: Miscarriage, intrauterine growth restriction, learning and behavior problems
	High levels of radiation: Miscarriage, microcephaly, developmental delay; exposure of less than 5 rads (125 pelvic x-rays) not associated with increased risk of birth defects

This is not a comprehensive listing. Patient-oriented resource for exposures during pregnancy and breastfeeding: https://mothertobaby.org.[31]

ACE, Angiotensin-converting enzyme; *IUGR*, intrauterine growth restriction; *PKU*, phenylketonuria.

1. Testing and screening of a pediatric patient should be in his/her best interest and provide clear benefits.
2. If testing is performed for the interests of parents or other family members, it should not be to the detriment of the child.
3. Treatment and/or follow-up must be available after testing is sent.
4. Carrier testing or screening in children and adolescents is not broadly supported.
5. Predictive testing for late-onset disorders is discouraged until a patient is able to make an autonomous decision; in these cases, extensive pre-test counseling is recommended.

B. Informed Consent

Pretest counseling and informed consent are important prior to sending any genome-wide testing, and documentation of informed consent is recommended. Possible results from genetic testing include:

1. Positive: A causative/related variant is found.
2. Negative: Either no causative/related variant is present, *or* the available technology or scope of the test methodology was unable to detect the causative/related variant. A negative result does not guarantee the condition does not have a genetic etiology.
3. Variant(s) of uncertain significance: Variants for which the meaning is uncertain (could be variants without clinical significance or related to the patient's presentation but not previously reported)
4. Incidental or secondary finding(s): Variants anticipated to affect the patient's health that are unrelated to the indication for sending the test (and may be an adult-onset condition)
5. Discovery that parents are blood relatives and/or nonmaternity/ nonpaternity

C. Professional Disclosure of Familial Genetic Information

Pretest counseling should include the discussion that genetic testing may have implications for family members. With regard to disclosure of genetic testing results to at-risk family members when a patient or family member chooses not to disclose, the provider must weigh the duty to respect privacy and autonomy of the patient with the duty to prevent harm in another identifiable person. The ethical and legal duties of the physician are not well defined. The American Society of Human Genetics released a statement on professional disclosure of familial genetic information, which outlines "exceptional circumstances," which if all are present, disclosure may be permissible: (1) attempts to encourage disclosure by the patient have failed, (2) harm is "highly likely" to occur, (3) the harm is "serious and foreseeable," (4) either the disease is preventable/treatable or early monitoring will reduce risks, (5) the at-risk relative(s) are identifiable, and (6) the harm of failure to disclose outweighs the harm that may result from disclosure.[27]

D. Disclosure of Incidental Findings

Patients are sometimes given the option to be informed of any incidental or secondary findings when they pursue genetic testing, but in general, it is recommended that incidental findings should be reported when there is strong evidence of benefit to the patient. The minimal list of reportable incidental findings may be found in the ACMG March 2013 statement and related updates.[28]

VII. WEB RESOURCES

A. Specific Genetic Disorders

- Genetics Home Reference: https://ghr.nlm.nih.gov/ (patient-friendly information)
- GeneReviews: https://www.genereviews.org (expert-authored clinical descriptions including diagnosis and management recommendations)

- National Organization for Rare Disorders: https://www.rarediseases.org
- Online Mendelian Inheritance in Man (OMIM): https://omim.org (curated primary literature, can be used to search for clinical features to build a differential)

B. Guidelines for Genetic Conditions

- Newborn screening ACT Sheets and Confirmatory Algorithms: https://www.acmg.net/ACMG/Medical-Genetics-Practice-Resources/ACT_Sheets_and_Algorithms.aspx

C. Molecular Testing Resources

- Concert Genetics: https://www.concertgenetics.com
- Genetics Testing Registry: https://www.ncbi.nlm.nih.gov/gtr

D. Teratogen Evaluation

- LactMed: Drugs and lactation database available through the U.S. National Library of Medicine. https://www.ncbi.nlm.nih.gov/books/NBK501922/?report=classic
- Patient-oriented information on exposures during pregnancy: https://www.mothertobaby.org[31]

REFERENCES

A complete list of references can be found online.

Chapter 14

Hematology

Joan Park, MD

🜲 See additional content online.

🔊 **Audio Case File 14.1** Hemophilia/emicizumab

I. ANEMIA

A. Screening for Anemia

1. The American Academy of Pediatrics (AAP) recommends screening between 9 and 12 months with a repeat level in 6 months.
2. Screen yearly in high-risk children: history of prematurity or low birth weight, exposure to lead, exclusive breastfeeding without supplemental iron beyond 4 months, diet without iron-fortified cereals or foods naturally rich in iron, feeding problems, poor growth, inadequate nutrition[1]

B. Definition of Anemia

1. Anemia is defined as a reduction in hemoglobin (Hb) two standard deviations below the mean, based on age-specific norms.
2. See Table 14.1 at the end of the chapter for age-specific blood cell indices.

C. Causes of Anemia

1. See Fig. 14.1 for approach to anemia based on red blood cell (RBC) production, as measured by reticulocyte count and cell size. Note that normal ranges for Hb and mean corpuscular volume (MCV) are age dependent.
2. See Tables 14.2 and 14.3 for more details regarding specific causes of nonhemolytic and hemolytic anemia.

D. Evaluation of Anemia

1. Useful equations in the evaluation of anemia:
   a. **Mentzer index[2] = MCV/RBC**
      (1) Index >13 suggests iron deficiency anemia (IDA).
      (2) Index <13 suggests thalassemia trait.
   b. **Reticulocyte index = % reticulocytes × patient hematocrit/normal hematocrit[3]**
      (1) >2 is indicative of increased RBC production in appropriate response to anemia.
      (2) <2 is evidence of hypoproliferative anemia.
2. Other useful indices and tests
   a. **RBC distribution width (RDW):**
      (1) Normal RDW favors thalassemia but can also be elevated.

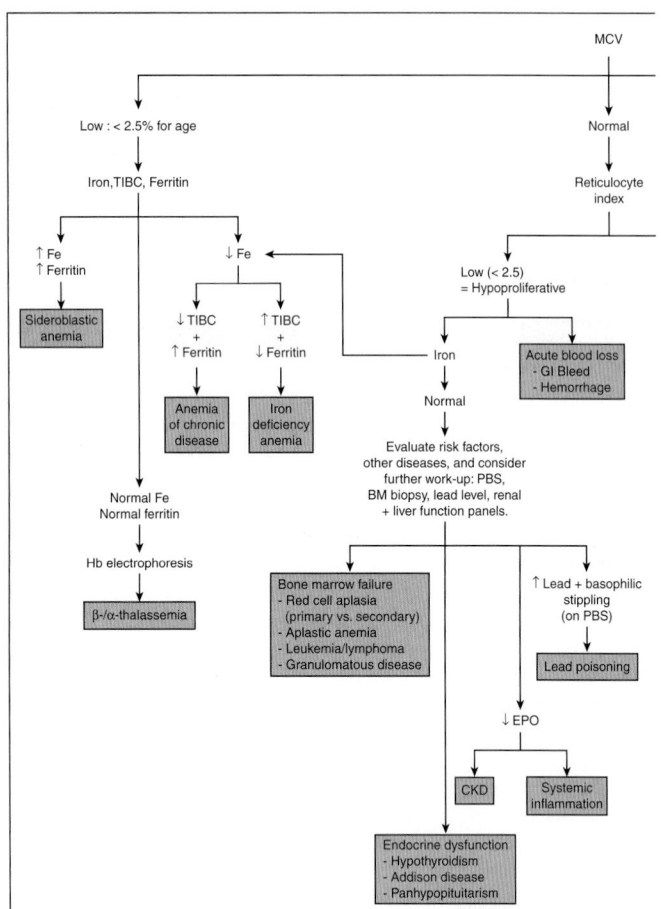

FIGURE 14.1

Approach to anemia. *AEDs,* Antiepileptic drugs; *BM,* bone marrow; *CKD,* chronic kidney disease; *DAT,* direct antiglobulin test; *EPO,* erythropoietin; *Fe,* iron; *G6PD,* glucose-6-phosphate dehydrogenase; *GI,* gastrointestinal; *HUS,* hemolytic uremic syndrome; *LDH,* lactate dehydrogenase; *MAHA,* microangiopathic hemolytic anemia; *MCV,* mean corpuscular volume; *MMA,* methylmalonic acid; *PBS,* peripheral blood smear; *PK,* pyruvate kinase; *SC,* sickle cell; *SD,* standard deviation; *TIBC,* total iron binding capacity; *TTP,* thrombotic thrombocytopenic purpura. (Data from Wang, M. Iron deficiency and other types of anemia in infants and children. *Am Fam Physician.* 2016:93[4]:270–278; Orkin SH, Nathan DG, Ginsburg D, et al. *Nathan and Oski's Hematology and Oncology of Infancy and Childhood.* 8th ed. Saunders; 2015.)

TABLE 14.2

NONHEMOLYTIC ANEMIA—CONT'D

Inherited Causes with Pancytopenia

Fanconi anemia	Autosomal recessive or X-linked disorder Presentation: Child with pancytopenia, radial and thumb abnormalities, renal anomalies, microcephaly, short stature, skin findings (hyperpigmentation, café-au-lait spots)
Shwachman-Diamond syndrome	Autosomal recessive mutation in *SBDS* gene Presentation: Young child with neutropenia ± thrombocytopenia and macrocytic anemia, exocrine pancreatic dysfunction, bony abnormalities
Dyskeratosis congenita	Mutation in gene encoding telomerase complex components Presentation: Anemia, thrombocytopenia, abnormal skin reticular hyperpigmentation, nail dystrophy, oral leukoplakia

ANC, Absolute neutrophil count; *CMV*, cytomegalovirus; *CRP*, C-reactive protein; *EBV*, Epstein Barr virus; *ESR*, erythrocyte sedimentation rate; *GI*, gastroenterology; *Hb*, hemoglobin; *HHV-6*, human herpesvirus 6; *HIV*, human immunodeficiency virus; *IBD*, inflammatory bowel disease; *JIA*, juvenile idiopathic arthritis; *MCHC*, mean corpuscular hemoglobin concentration; *NSAID*, nonsteroidal antiinflammatory drug; *RBC*, red blood cell; *SBDS*, Shwachman-Bodian-Diamond syndrome gene; *SLE*, systemic lupus erythematosus; *TIBC*, total iron binding capacity; *WBC*, white blood cell.

Data from Orkin SH, Nathan DG, Ginsburg D, et al. *Nathan and Oski's Hematology and Oncology of Infancy and Childhood.* 8th ed. Saunders; 2015. Camaschella, C. Iron-deficiency anemia. *N Engl J Med.* 2015;372(19):1832–1843. Weiss G, Goodnough LT. Anemia of chronic disease. *N Engl J Med.* 2005;352(10):1011–1023. Shimamura A, Alter BP. Pathophysiology and management of inherited bone marrow failure syndromes. *Blood Rev.* 2010;24(3):101–122. Hartung HD, Olson TS, Bessler M. Acquired aplastic anemia in children. *Pediatr Clin North Am.* 2013;60(6):1311–1336.

TABLE 14.3

HEMOLYTIC ANEMIA

EXTRINSIC HEMOLYTIC ANEMIA

14

DAT −

Microangiopathic hemolytic anemia (MAHA): HUS, TTP, DIC	Anemia due to RBC shearing with passage through microthrombi in microvasculature Diagnosis: Intravascular hemolysis, thrombocytopenia, schistocytes on peripheral smear
Hemoglobin disorders: Sickle cell disease, unstable hemoglobin	Denaturation of hemoglobin causes precipitation in RBC and reduces deformability. Diagnosis: Smear with Heinz bodies, bite or blister cells

DAT +

Warm autoimmune hemolytic anemia	Diagnosis: Jaundice ± splenomegaly, +anti-IgG and/or +anti-C3 Treatment: Corticosteroids (first line; prednisone), rituximab, IVIG, and other immunosuppressants, splenectomy Transfuse for severe anemia with cardiovascular compromise (i.e., Hb <5 g/dL) or reticulocytopenia
Cold autoimmune hemolytic anemia	Diagnosis: Acrocyanosis, hemoglobinuria, +anti-IgM autoantibodies Treatment: Cold avoidance

Continued

TABLE 14.3

HEMOLYTIC ANEMIA—CONT'D

Secondary autoimmune hemolytic anemia	Causes: Infections,[a] drug-associated,[b] malignancy (Hodgkin lymphoma), systemic lupus erythematosus, autoimmune lymphoproliferative syndrome, common variable immunodeficiency, posttransplant (stem cell or solid organ)
Transfusion reactions (ABO or Rh incompatibility)	See Table 14.19 for presentation of transfusion reactions.

INTRINSIC HEMOLYTIC ANEMIA

Membrane Disorders

Neonatal hemolytic disease	Maternal antibodies to incompatible fetal RBC antigens (Rh, A, B) cause hemolytic disease in utero and in neonatal period. Diagnosis: Mild anemia to hydrops fetalis, early jaundice Treatment: Intensive phototherapy, exchange transfusion
Hereditary spherocytosis	Inheritance: 75% AD. 25% spontaneous mutation or AR RBC membrane protein defect → membrane instability → RBC destruction via extravascular hemolysis Diagnosis: Family history with clinical suspicion and spherocytes on smear, osmotic fragility or EMA flow cytometry if unclear clinical picture Treatment: Folate supplementation if moderate-severe hemolysis, anticipatory guidance, splenectomy (for severe disease), cholecystectomy if needed for symptomatic cholelithiasis
Hereditary elliptocytosis	Inheritance: Typically AD Diagnosis: Elliptocytes on smear Treatment: Same as for hereditary spherocytosis

Enzyme Deficiencies

G6PD deficiency	Inheritance: X-linked disorder Enzyme deficiency predisposes to intravascular hemolysis with oxidative stress (e.g., with infections/illness, fava beans, medications) Diagnosis: G6PD assay when well (may be falsely elevated immediately after hemolytic episode) Treatment: Avoid oxidative triggers, transfuse for severe anemia.
Pyruvate kinase (PK) deficiency	Inheritance: AR disorder of *PKLR* or *PKM* genes causes chronic hemolysis. Diagnosis: Measure PK activity in RBCs. Treatment: Transfuse if symptomatic. Consider splenectomy if severe transfusion-dependent anemia.

[a]Infections include EBV, CMV, mycoplasma, pneumococcus, parvovirus.
[b]Causative drugs include penicillin, cephalosporins, quinine/quinidine, amphotericin B, NSAIDs, procainamide, IVIG.
ABO, Blood type; *AD,* autosomal dominant; *AR,* autosomal recessive; *CMV,* cytomegalovirus; *DAT,* direct antiglobulin test; *DIC,* disseminated intravascular coagulation; *EBV,* Epstein-Barr virus; *EMA,* eosin-5-maleimide; *G6PD,* glucose-6-phosphate dehydrogenase; *Hb,* hemoglobin; *HUS,* hemolytic uremic syndrome; *Ig,* immunoglobulin; *IVIG,* intravenous immunoglobulin; *NSAID,* nonsteroidal antiinflammatory drug; *RBC,* red blood cell; *Rh,* rhesus factor; *TTP,* thrombotic thrombocytopenic purpura.
Data from Noronha SA. Acquired and congenital hemolytic anemia. *Pediatr Rev.* 2016:37(6):235–246. Orkin SH, Nathan DG, Ginsburg D, et al. *Nathan and Oski's Hematology and Oncology of Infancy and Childhood.* 8th ed. Saunders; 2015.

(2) It is the first value to fall in early iron deficiency and is elevated with inflammation or infection.

d. **Coombs test[4]:**

  (1) Direct (direct antiglobulin testing [DAT]): Detects antibody/complement bound to patient's RBCs by mixing prepared nonspecific antihuman globulin with patient's blood. RBC agglutination = positive test

  (2) Indirect (indirect antiglobulin testing): Detects antibodies to RBC antigens in patient's plasma by mixing reagent RBCs with patient's serum. RBC agglutination = positive test

e. **Hemoglobin electrophoresis:**

  (1) Involves separation of Hb variants based on molecular charge and size. All positive sickle preparations and solubility tests for sickle Hb (e.g., Sickledex) should be confirmed with electrophoresis or isoelectric focusing (component of mandatory newborn screening in many states).

  (2) See Table 14.4 for neonatal Hb electrophoresis patterns.

  (3) See Fig. 14.2 for changes in Hb polypeptide over time in a normal fetus/infant.

TABLE 14.4	
NEONATAL HEMOGLOBIN ELECTROPHORESIS PATTERNS	
FA	Fetal Hb and adult normal Hb; the normal newborn pattern
FAV	Indicates presence of both HbF and HbA, but an anomalous band (V) is present that does not appear to be any of the common Hb variants
FAS	Indicates fetal Hb, adult normal HbA, and HbS, consistent with benign sickle cell trait
FS	Fetal and sickle HbS without detectable adult normal HbA. Consistent with clinically significant homozygous sickle Hb genotype (S/S) or sickle β^0-thalassemia, with manifestations of sickle cell disease during childhood
FC[a]	Designates presence of HbC without adult normal HbA. Consistent with clinically significant homozygous HbC genotype (C/C), resulting in a mild hematologic disorder presenting during childhood
FSC	HbS and HbC present. This heterozygous condition could lead to manifestations of sickle cell disease during childhood.
FAC	HbC and adult normal HbA present, consistent with benign HbC trait
FSA	Heterozygous HbS/β^+-thalassemia, a clinically significant sickling disorder
F[a]	Fetal HbF is present without adult normal HbA. May indicate delayed appearance of HbA, but is also consistent with homozygous β-thalassemia major or homozygous hereditary persistence of fetal HbF
FV[a]	Fetal HbF and an anomalous Hb variant (V) are present.
AF	May indicate prior blood transfusion. Submit another filter paper blood specimen when infant is 4 months of age, at which time the transfused blood cells should have been cleared.

[a]Repeat blood specimen should be submitted to confirm original interpretation.

Hemoglobin variants are reported in order of decreasing abundance; for example, FA indicates more fetal than adult hemoglobin.

NOTE: HbA: $\alpha_2\beta_2$; HbF: $\alpha_2\gamma_2$; HbA$_2$: $\alpha_2\delta_2$.

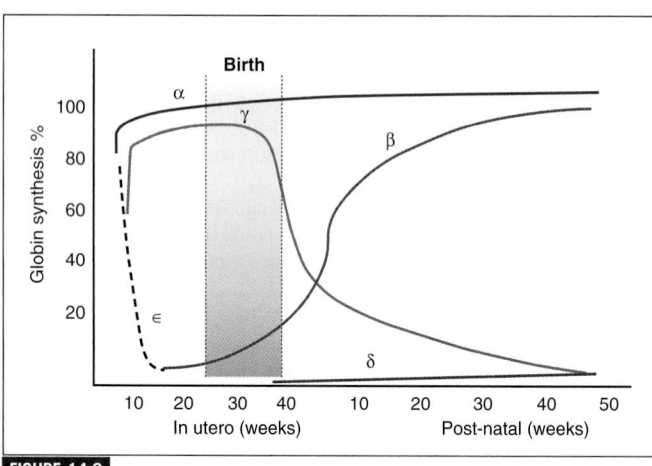

FIGURE 14.2

Neonatal hemoglobin electrophoresis patterns. (From Chandrakasan S, Kamat D. An overview of hemoglobinopathies and the interpretation of newborn screening results. *Pediatr Ann.* 2013:42[12]:502–508.)

f. **Blood smear interpretation[3]**
   (1) Howell-Jolly bodies = Impaired splenic function, postsplenectomy
   (2) Target cells = Hemoglobinopathies (HbSS, HbSC, HbC, thalassemias), liver disease, postsplenectomy
   (3) Bite cells, Heinz bodies = G6PD deficiency (during hemolysis)
   (4) Toxic granulation of neutrophils, bandemia, atypical lymphocytes = Infection
   (5) Pencil poikilocytes = IDA, thalassemia
   (6) Basophilic stippling = Lead poisoning, sideroblastic anemia
   (7) Pappenheimer bodies = Sideroblastic anemia
   (8) Hypersegmented neutrophils = Vitamin B_{12}, folate deficiencies
   (9) Blasts = Leukemia, lymphoma
   (10) Schistocytes (RBC fragments) = Microangiopathic hemolytic anemia (MAHA), burns, valve hemolysis
   (11) Spherocytes = Autoimmune hemolytic anemia, hereditary spherocytosis, ABO incompatibility/hemolytic disease of the newborn
   (12) Elliptocytes = Hereditary elliptocytosis, severe IDA
   (13) Teardrop cells = Myelofibrosis (and other bone marrow infiltrating processes), thalassemia
   (14) Echinocytes (burr cells) = Frequent artifact finding; uremia, pyruvate kinase deficiency

    (15) Acanthocytes (spur cells) = Liver disease, abetalipoproteinemia, hypothyroidism, vitamin E deficiency, severe malnutrition

    (16) See eFigs. 14.1 to 14.12 for examples of peripheral smears.

E. Management of Anemia

1. Iron deficiency anemia

a. Oral iron (ferrous sulfate)

    (1) Empirically treat children with microcytic anemia and history of poor dietary iron.[5]

    (2) In anemia of chronic disease, only use iron supplementation if evidence of absolute iron deficiency and ferritin <100 ng/mL.[5]

    (3) After initiation of iron supplementation, expect reticulocyte count to increase within the first week with a 1 g/dL increase in Hb in 4 weeks (if severe anemia with Hb <9 g/dL, a response should be seen in 2 weeks).[1]

b. Iron infusion (low-molecular-weight iron dextran[6] or iron sucrose[7]) is appropriate for children with iron malabsorption (PPI use, short bowel syndrome, primary malabsorption), poor response to oral iron therapy, inability to tolerate oral iron therapy, and hemodialysis-dependent patients receiving erythropoietin.

2. Sickle cell anemia

a. **Etiology:** Caused by a genetic defect in β-globin that leads to HbS polymerization and RBC sickling with deoxygenation, leading to hemolysis, adherence to blood vessel endothelium, and vaso-occlusive ischemia.

b. **Most common subtypes:** HbSS (sickle cell anemia) and HbSβ⁰ (sickle-β⁰-thalassemia) are most severe. HbSC (sickle-hemoglobin C disease) and HbSβ+ (sickle-β+-thalassemia) are often milder.

c. **Diagnosis:** Often made on newborn screen with Hb electrophoresis. The sickle preparation and Sickledex are rapid tests that are positive in all sickle hemoglobinopathies. False-negative test results may be seen in neonates and other patients with a high percentage of fetal Hb.

d. **Complications:** See Table 14.5. A hematologist should be consulted.

e. **Acute management of anemia in sickle cell disease[8]:**

    (1) Baseline lab values including CBC, reticulocyte, hemoglobin electrophoresis (percent HbF), creatinine, BUN, urinalysis, liver function tests, fractionated bilirubin should be collected to compare with those during acute illness.

    (2) RBC exchange transfusions: Indicated for patients with stroke, acute chest syndrome (ACS) with rapid progression or clinical deterioration, and multisystem organ failure. May be indicated for hepatic sequestration, intrahepatic cholestasis, and refractory priapism. Also indicated for children with prior stroke or transcranial Doppler reading >200 cm/sec.[8] Replace with HbS-negative cells. Follow Hct carefully with goal Hct <30% to avoid hyperviscosity.[9]

TABLE 14.5

SICKLE CELL DISEASE COMPLICATIONS

Complication	Presentation	Additional Testing	Disposition/Treatment
Fever	>101°F or 38.3°C	Blood cultures CXR Blood and urine cultures Throat and CSF cultures, if indicated	Admit if ill-appearing, temperature ≥40°C, infiltrate on CXR or abnormal SpO₂, WBCs >30,000/μL or <5,000/μL, platelets <100,000/μL, Hb <5 g/dL, history of sepsis. Antibiotics: Ceftriaxone, add IV Vancomycin if meningitis suspected or if severe illness. Clindamycin or levofloxacin if cephalosporin allergy.[47] Consider additional disease-specific coverage. If outpatient, return in 24 hr for second ceftriaxone dose.
Vaso-occlusive crisis	Dactylitis in <2 years old; unifocal or multifocal pain in >2 years old	Type and screen	Admit if signs of complications or pain not managed in outpatient setting. Recommendations for home pain control: • Mild-moderate pain: NSAIDs • Moderate-severe pain: Oxycodone, morphine, hydrocodone Recommendations for emergency department or inpatient pain control: • Use IV opioids (morphine, hydromorphone). Use fentanyl if renal or hepatic dysfunction. • Use PCA and provide as-needed doses for breakthrough pain. Schedule pain medication if not using PCA.[35] • Ketamine may be appropriate if poor response to opioids.[36] IV fluids as needed for dehydration. Evidence-based guidelines regarding amount or type of fluids are lacking.[37] Use incentive spirometry to reduce risk of ACS. Avoid transfusion unless other indication.
Acute chest syndrome	Fever, cough, chest pain, respiratory distress, hypoxia + new pulmonary infiltrate	CXR Type and screen Blood cultures	Admit IV antibiotics: IV cephalosporin + oral macrolide[32] O₂ as needed for goal SpO₂ >95%, incentive spirometry Analgesia, IV fluids (see above) Simple transfusion or partial exchange for moderate illness High-dose dexamethasone use is controversial.[33]

Splenic sequestration	Acutely enlarged spleen, Hb ≥2 g/dL below baseline	Type and screen	Admit for serial abdominal exams, IV fluid resuscitation. Simple transfusion if severe anemia.[a]
Aplastic crisis	Acute illness (often viral, commonly parvovirus B19) + Hb < baseline, low reticulocyte count	Type and screen, Parvovirus serology and PCR	Admit to isolated bed. IV fluids. Simple transfusion with RBCs
Stroke	Focal neurologic signs. May be precipitated by ACS, parvovirus, acute anemic events	MRI, TCD to detect increased velocities with stenosis	Emergency exchange transfusion preferable to simple transfusion, if possible[39]. Chronic transfusion to maintain sickle Hb to <30% in patients with abnormal TCD US findings or history of stroke
Acute renal failure	Hematuria, proteinuria, hypertension	Urine spot protein, 24-hr collection	Monitor renal function. Avoid nephrotoxic drugs/contrast. Consult nephrology and initiate renal replacement therapy (hemodialysis) if necessary.
Avascular necrosis	Pain at site that worsens with activity, reduced range of motion. Hip most commonly involved, then shoulder and other joints	XR of affected joint, MRI if necessary	Analgesics, physical therapy. Consult orthopedic surgery for assessment for possible decompression.
Priapism	Sustained painful erection lasting >4 hr	Not necessary	Oral and/or IV analgesia (as per VOC recommendations). Hydration with oral or IV fluids. Consider supplemental oxygen. Consult urology for possible aspiration and irrigation of corpus cavernosum (if does not self-resolve).

[a]Be cautious with transfused volume and use 5- to 10-mL/kg aliquots if hemodynamically stable as autotransfusion from spleen can cause rebound increase in Hb and viscosity.

ACS, Acute chest syndrome; *CSF,* cerebrospinal fluid; *CXR,* chest x-ray; *Hb,* hemoglobin; *IV,* intravenous; *MRI,* magnetic resonance imaging; *NSAIDs,* nonsteroidal antiinflammatory drugs; *PCA,* patient-controlled analgesia; *PCR,* polymerase chain reaction test; *PRN,* as needed; *RBCs,* red blood cells; SpO_2, peripheral oxygen saturation; *TCD,* transcranial Doppler; *US* = ultrasound; *VOC,* vaso-occlusive crisis; *WBC,* white blood cell; *XR,* X-ray.

Data from National Heart, Lung, and Blood Institute. *Evidence-Based Management of Sickle Cell Disease: Expert Panel Report,* 2014. National Heart, Lung, and Blood Institute; 2014.

14

(3) Do not transfuse for asymptomatic anemia unless concern for aplastic crisis (low reticulocyte count).

f. **Chronic management and health maintenance**[8]**:** See Table 14.6. Ongoing consultation and clinical involvement with a pediatric hematologist and/or sickle cell program are essential. Bone marrow transplant is the only current curative therapy.

3. **Thalassemia**

a. **Etiology:** Defects in α- or β-globin production lead to precipitation of excess chains, causing ineffective erythropoiesis and shortened survival of mature RBCs.

b. **α-Thalassemia:**

(1) Silent carriers ($\alpha-/\alpha\alpha$): Not anemic; Hb electrophoresis usually normal

(2) α-Thalassemia trait ($\alpha-/\alpha-$) or ($\alpha\alpha/--$): Causes mild microcytosis with or without mild anemia from birth; Hb electrophoresis usually normal. Hb Barts can be seen transiently in infancy (e.g., on state newborn screens) in patients with α-thalassemia trait.

(3) HbH disease (β_4) ($\alpha-/--$): Causes mild to moderate anemia from birth; higher levels of Hb Barts seen on newborn screen with transition to HbH (β-tetramer) on subsequent electrophoresis.

(4) Hb Barts/hydrops fetalis ($--/--$): Hb Barts (γ_4) cannot deliver oxygen; usually fatal in utero or in neonatal period.

c. **β-Thalassemia:** Ineffective erythropoiesis is more severe in β-thalassemia than α-thalassemia. Patients often develop more severe iron overload from increased enteral absorption and transfusions. Adult Hb electrophoresis with decreased Hb A, increased Hb A_2, and increased HbF.

(1) Thalassemia trait/thalassemia minor ($\beta/\beta+$) or ($\beta/\beta0$): Mildly decreased β-globin production. Usually asymptomatic with mild anemia.

(2) Thalassemia intermedia ($\beta+/\beta+$): Markedly decreased β-globin production. Presents by 2 years of age with moderate compensated anemia (Hb 7 to 10 g/dL). Wide variability in presentation that may include features noted in thalassemia major.

(3) Thalassemia major/Cooley anemia ($\beta0/\beta0$, $\beta+/\beta0$, or $\beta+/\beta+$): Minimal to no β-globin production. Presence of anemia within first 6 months of life requiring regular transfusions. Overstimulation of bone marrow, ineffective erythropoiesis, and iron overload results in jaundice, growth failure, hypersplenism, gallstones, skeletal abnormalities, liver cirrhosis, and cardiac impairment.

d. **Management**[10]

(1) Patients with thalassemia major are transfusion dependent. Patients with thalassemia intermedia may need occasional transfusions.

TABLE 14.6

SICKLE CELL DISEASE HEALTH MAINTENANCE

Medications	Penicillin	Twice daily in children with HbSS and HbSβ0 under 5 years old[a]
	Hydroxyurea[40]	Offer in children with HbSS or HbSβ0 >9 months.[b]
		Treatment goal: HbF >20%.[41]
		Maximum dose parameters: ANC ≥2000–4000/μL, Hb ≥8 g/dL without transfusion, platelet ≥80,000/μL, absolute reticulocyte count ≥80–100,000/μL
		Continue in acute hospitalization or illness.
		Discontinue in pregnant and breastfeeding women.
	Hormonal contraception	Progestin-only contraception (pills, injection, implant), levonorgestrel IUDs, and barrier methods preferred over estrogen-containing methods due to increased risk of blood clots
Immunizations[42]	Pneumococcal vaccine	13-valent conjugate vaccine per routine childhood schedule. 23-valent polysaccharide vaccine at 2 years old with second dose 5 years later
	Meningococcal vaccine	Give MenACWY-CRM (Menveo) at 2, 4, 6, 12 months.
		If over 2 years old, administer 2-dose series of MenACWY-CRM or MenACWY-D.
		Give meningococcal B vaccine in patients 10 years or older.
	Influenza vaccine	Yearly starting at 6 months
		Give to all household members and close contacts.
Imaging and labs	Transcranial doppler	Screen annually from 2 to 16 years old in HbSS or HbSβ0
		Not necessary to screen in HbSβ+ or HbSC
	Spot urine test	Screen for proteinuria by age 10; repeat annually. Refer those with microalbuminuria (>300 mg in 24 hr) to nephrologist.
Other	Ophthalmology	Annual exam starting at age 10 to evaluate for retinopathy

[a]Prophylaxis may be discontinued by age 5 years if patient has had no prior severe pneumococcal infections or splenectomy and has documented pneumococcal vaccinations, including second 23-valent vaccination. May be continued based on family preference. May be considered for children with HbSC/HbSβ+, especially after splenectomy.[8,34] Practice patterns vary.

[b]Increases levels of fetal Hb and decreases HbS polymerization in cells. Has been shown to significantly decrease episodes of vaso-occlusive crises, dactylitis, acute chest syndrome, number of transfusions, and hospitalizations. May decrease mortality in adults. Consider in HbSC/HbSβ+ if recurrent sickle cell-associated pain interfering with daily activities or quality of life.[40,43]

ANC, Absolute neutrophil count; HbF, hemoglobin F level; HbSβ+, sickle cell beta thalassemia disease; HbSC, Homozygous sickle cell disease; HbSS, Homozygous SC disease; IUD, intrauterine device.

Data from National Heart, Lung, and Blood Institute. *Evidence-Based Management of Sickle Cell Disease: Expert Panel Report, 2014.* National Heart, Lung, and Blood Institute; 2014. http://www.nhlbi.nih.gov/health-pro/guidelines/sickle-cell-disease-guidelines/

14

(2) Transfuse every 3 to 5 weeks to maintain Hb >9 to 10.5 mg/dL.
(3) Avoid hypertransfusion to Hb >14 to 15 g/dL due to risk of hyperviscosity-related symptoms, including stroke.
(4) Treat iron overload with chelation (deferasirox or deferiprone PO, deferoxamine SQ or rarely IV), which should be initiated in thalassemia major after 10 to 20 transfusions or when ferritin >1000 μg/L.
(5) Bone marrow transplant is curative.

II. ERYTHROCYTOSIS[12,48]

A. Definition of Erythrocytosis

1. Erythrocytosis is defined as number of RBCs (cells per volume) two standard deviations above the mean, based on age-specific norms.
2. See Table 14.1 at the end of the chapter for age-specific blood cell indices.
   a. Relative erythrocytosis: A reduction in plasma volume without an increase in RBC mass (e.g., dehydration due to diuretic use, vomiting, or diarrhea)
   b. Absolute erythrocytosis: An increase in RBC mass

B. Causes of Erythrocytosis

1. **Primary erythrocytosis:** Independently increased production of RBC (e.g., familial erythrocytosis, polycythemia vera)
2. **Secondary erythrocytosis:** Increased erythropoietin (EPO), with resultant increased RBC production
   a. Cardiopulmonary disease (e.g., congenital heart disease, chronic pulmonary disease, obstructive sleep apnea): Systemic hypoxia triggers increased EPO.
   b. Renal disease (e.g., renal artery stenosis): Kidneys sense less oxygen and produce EPO. Also seen after renal transplant.
   c. Tumors (e.g., renal, hepatic, CNS, or endocrine): Autonomous EPO synthesis by the tumor.
   d. Exposure to androgens (testosterone), anabolic steroids
   e. Congenital causes

C. Evaluation of Erythrocytosis

1. CBC ± blood smear should be obtained to evaluate RBC morphology and concurrent presence of leukocyte and platelet abnormalities.
2. Measure serum EPO, electrolytes, kidney and liver function tests, and urinalysis.

D. Management of Erythrocytosis

1. Treatment is directed at the underlying cause (e.g., hydration, addressing cardiopulmonary process) and consideration of hematocrit reduction (e.g. phlebotomy or partial exchange transfusion). Discuss use of a cytoreductive agent with a hematologist.
2. If patient has a stroke or chest pain, emergent hydration and/or phlebotomy is indicated.
3. Symptoms such as pruritus, erythromelalgia, bleeding, and gout should be managed accordingly.

III. NEUTROPENIA

A. Definition of Neutropenia

1. Neutropenia is defined as an absolute neutrophil count (ANC) <1500/μL. Severe neutropenia is defined as an ANC <500/μL.
2. See Table 14.7 at the end of the chapter for age-specific leukocyte differentials.
3. Repeat CBC 2 to 3 weeks later to determine if transient (e.g., secondary to a medication, infection) or persistent.[11]

B. Causes and Evaluation of Neutropenia[11]

1. CBC ± blood smear should be obtained to evaluate neutrophil morphology and concurrent presence of anemia or thrombocytopenia.
2. If pancytopenic, consider bone marrow aspiration and biopsy with cytogenetics.
3. If persistent neutropenia for more than 2 to 4 weeks, consider further workup based on potential etiologies (Table 14.8).

C. Management of Neutropenia

1. **Additional diagnostic testing[12]:**
   a. Repeat CBC 2×/week for 6 to 8 weeks for cyclic neutropenia.
   b. Reticulocyte index with anemia to differentiate between destructive processes and marrow failure
   c. Blood smear for morphologic abnormalities
   d. Immunologic testing (Coombs test, antineutrophil and antiplatelet antibodies) for autoimmune or alloimmune processes
   e. IgG, IgA, IgM for immunodeficiency
2. **Treatment:**
   a. Myeloid-specific cytokine granulocyte colony-stimulating factor (G-CSF; filgrastim)
      (1) Indications for continuous use: Severe congenital neutropenia, cyclic neutropenia, glycogen storage disease 1b, bone marrow failure (e.g., aplastic anemia, Shwachman Diamond-Oski syndrome)[12,13]
      (2) Indications for intermittent use: Life-threatening infection or history of recurrent or serious infections in patients with neutropenia[12]
      (3) Side effects: Bone pain, headache, rash
   b. Stem cell transplant: Indicated for bone marrow failure (e.g., Fanconi anemia), poor response to G-CSF, severe congenital neutropenia with high risk of myelodysplasia or acute myeloid leukemia[12]
3. **Complications:** See Chapter 22 for management of neutropenic fever and typhlitis.
4. **Anticipatory guidance[11]:**
   a. Maintain good oral hygiene and skin care to prevent local infections.
   b. Avoid rectal temperatures, rectal examinations, or rectal medications due to risk of mucosal trauma and bacteremia.
   c. No live or attenuated-live vaccines for patients with impaired T-/B-lymphocyte function.

TABLE 14.8

CAUSES OF NEUTROPENIA

	Cause	Mechanism	Presentation
ACQUIRED			
Infections	Viruses (EBV, CMV, parvovirus, HHV-6, HIV, viral hepatitis) Bacteria (typhoid fever, Brucellosis) Protozoa (Leishmania, malaria), Rickettsial infections, etc.	Bone marrow suppression, viral-induced immune neutropenia, redistribution to marginated pools	Occurs early in illness, persists 3–8 days and resolves spontaneously and/or with effective treatment of underlying illness
Medications	Many: Sulfasalazine, antipsychotics (clozapine, phenothiazines), thionamides, antimicrobials (TMP/SMX)	Direct marrow suppression (more common) or drug-induced immune-mediated destruction	Hypersensitivity reaction: fever, lymphadenopathy, rash. May have +ANA
Nutritional	Vitamin B_{12} deficiency Folic acid deficiency Copper deficiency	Ineffective hematopoiesis due to impaired DNA processing and nuclear maturation (with B_{12}/folate deficiency)	Mostly seen in chronically ill children, especially with malabsorption Hypersegmented neutrophils, megaloblastic anemia with B_{12}/folate deficiency High MMA and HcY in B_{12} deficiency vs. high HcY in folate deficiency
Hypersplenism	Inflammation, neoplasm, storage disorder, hemolytic anemia	Sequestration of WBCs in spleen	Concurrent anemia, thrombocytopenia. Rarely associated with infections

Autoimmune	Neonatal alloimmune neutropenia	Transfer of maternal IgG alloantibodies against fetus neutrophil antigens that were produced in response to fetal cells in maternal circulation
		Severe neutropenia with fever, infection. Transient, resolves after 6–8 weeks
	Primary autoimmune neutropenia	Antineutrophil antibodies cross-react with antigen on neutrophil surface resulting in neutrophil destruction
		Typically child 5–15 months old without recurrent infections despite severe neutropenia. +ANA. Marrow with myeloid hyperplasia and normal to increased mature neutrophils
	Secondary autoimmune neutropenia	Secondary to systemic disease: Systemic lupus erythematosus, Evans syndrome, rheumatoid arthritis/Felty syndrome, systemic sclerosis, infections (HIV, EBV)
		Presents with signs/symptoms of systemic autoimmune disease
	Pure white cell aplasia	Associated with thymoma, drug reactions, antiglomerular basement membrane antibody disease
		At risk of severe, recurrent infections. Disappearance of granulocytopoietic tissue from bone marrow. +Antibodies (e.g., GM-CFU inhibitory activity)
Acquired bone marrow disorders	Leukemia, lymphoma, solid tumor infiltration, myelofibrosis, granulomatous infections, aplastic anemia	Impaired production of all cell lines due to bone marrow infiltration
		Typically associated with anemia and/or thrombocytopenia. Bone marrow biopsy diagnostic
INHERITED[a]		
Severe congenital neutropenia	Severe congenital neutropenia	AD mutation in *ELANE* or *GFI1* genes results in rapid apoptosis of myeloid precursors, arrest at promyelocyte development stage
		Risk of myelodysplastic syndrome and acute myelogenous leukemia
		Recurrent infections: Mouth ulcers, gingivitis, otitis media, respiratory infections, skin cellulitis, abscesses
		Often with oncocytosis, eosinophilia, anemia, thrombocytosis
		Bone marrow: myeloid maturation arrest, normal/increased promyelocytes

Continued

14

TABLE 14.8

CAUSES OF NEUTROPENIA—CONT'D

Cause	Mechanism	Presentation
Kostmann syndrome	Severe form of SCN AR mutation in *HAX1* gene results in absent myeloid progenitors	Recurrent infections as above typically with monocytosis, eosinophilia
Cyclic neutropenia	AD mutation in *ELANE* gene	Periodic ~21-day cycles of neutropenia, typically associated with fever, oral ulcerations, ± gingivitis, pharyngitis, skin infections
Benign ethnic neutropenia	*DARC* gene polymorphism reducing Duffy antigen expression	Mild neutropenia in patient of West Indian, Yemenite, African, Greek, or Arab descent without increased infection incidence or severity
Bone marrow failure syndromes	Fanconi anemia	See Table 14.2	Pancytopenia
	Diamond-Blackfan anemia		

aThis is not an exhaustive list of all inherited causes of neutropenia.

AD, Autosomal dominant; *ANA,* antinuclear antibody; *AR,* autosomal recessive; *CMV,* cytomegalovirus; *DARC,* Duffy antigen/chemokine receptor; *EBV,* Epstein-Barr virus; *GM-CFU,* granulocyte-macrophage colony-forming unit; *HcY,* homocysteine; *HHV-6,* human herpesvirus 6; *HIV,* human immunodeficiency virus; *MMA,* methylmalonic acid; *SCN,* severe congenital neutropenia; *TMP/SMX,* trimethoprim-sulfamethoxazole; *WBC,* white blood cell.

Data from Segel GB, Halterman JS. Neutropenia in pediatric practice. *Pediatr Rev.* 2008;29(1):12–24. Moerdler S, LaTuga MS. Neonatal neutropenia. *NeoReviews.* 2018;19(1):e22–e28. Orkin SH, Nathan DG, Ginsburg D, et al. *Nathan and Oski's Hematology and Oncology of Infancy and Childhood.* 8th ed. Saunders; 2015.

d. Otherwise follow usual vaccination schedule.
e. If fever >38.4°C, seek emergent care for CBC, blood culture, and empiric antibiotics.
f. Children with mild-moderate neutropenia can attend school/daycare, if they avoid obviously ill children.

IV. LEUKOCYTOSIS[12]

A. Definition of Leukocytosis

1. Leukocytosis is defined as number of WBCs (cells per volume) two standard deviations above mean, based on age-specific norms.
2. See Chapter 22 for complications from hyperleukocytosis.
3. See Table 14.7 at the end of the chapter for age-specific leukocyte differentials.

B. Causes of Neutrophilia

1. Normal variation: Siblings and parents may also have neutrophilia.
2. Leukemoid reactions:
   a. Infection (bacteria, some viruses): May see increased neutrophil granule size, Döhle bodies, cytoplasmic vacuoles in neutrophils on blood smear
   b. Chronic inflammation (e.g. juvenile idiopathic arthritis, Kawasaki disease)
   c. Acute inflammation (e.g. stress, burns, massive trauma)
   d. Medications (e.g. catecholamines, glucocorticoids, myeloid growth factors, lithium, cyclophosphamide): Neutrophilia resolves soon after medication is stopped.
   e. Endocrine abnormalities (e.g. thyroid storm, hypercortisolism)
   f. Nonhematologic malignancy
   g. Genetic disorders (e.g. leukocyte adhesion deficiency, Down syndrome)

C. Causes of Eosinophilia

1. Premature birth: Eosinophilia may be seen in about 75% of low-birth-weight infants.
2. Infection (e.g. parasitic infections, infectious mononucleosis)
3. Allergic disorders (e.g. sensitization to mites and fungal infections, drug reaction, atopic dermatitis)
4. Pulmonary disorders (e.g. asthma, Loeffler syndrome, tropical pulmonary eosinophilia, polyarteritis nodosa, sarcoidosis)
5. Neoplasms
6. Other: Vascular occlusion of kidney, eosinophilic gastroenteritis, Addison disease

D. Causes of Monocytosis

1. Occasionally reported with tuberculosis, syphilis, subacute bacterial endocarditis. Noted early in course of infection and again on recovery, particularly if associated with granulocytopenia
2. Malignancy (e.g. juvenile myelomonocytic leukemia, lymphoma)

E. Causes of Basophilia

1. Allergic responses (along with eosinophilia), states of chronic inflammation (e.g. rheumatoid arthritis)
2. Has been reported in some chronic and acute infections

V. THROMBOCYTOPENIA AND IMPAIRED PLATELET FUNCTION

A. Definition of Thrombocytopenia

1. Defined as platelet count <150,000/μL
2. See Table 14.1 for age-specific values.

B. Bleeding Risk With Thrombocytopenia

1. Risk of clinically significant bleeding is related to both platelet function and number. Unlikely with platelet counts >30,000/μL in the absence of other complicating factors[14]
2. Risk of severe bleeding (CNS hemorrhage, gross hematuria, melena/hematochezia, hematemesis) increases with platelet counts <10,000/μL.[14]

C. Evaluation of Thrombocytopenia[15,16]

1. Platelet size: Large = mean platelet volume (MPV) >11 fL, normal = MPV 7 to 11 fL, small = MPV <7 fL
   a. Large platelets suggest increased marrow production in destructive processes (e.g., immune thrombocytopenia [ITP]) or some congenital disorders.
   b. Small platelets suggest production defects, typically seen in congenital disorders.
2. Peripheral blood smear: Confirm platelet count, evaluate size and morphology, and rule out pseudothrombocytopenia (i.e., spuriously low platelet count due to aggregation in EDTA tube only).
3. Immature platelet fraction: Correlates with measure of reticulated platelets, which reflects thrombopoiesis. Increases with peripheral destruction; is normal/low with bone marrow failure
4. Bone marrow aspiration: Obtain if systemic symptoms concerning for underlying malignancy, involvement of other cell lines, and/or blasts on smear. Differentiates decreased production versus increased destruction

D. Causes of Thrombocytopenia and Impaired Platelet Function

1. See Table 14.9 for an approach to the differential of thrombocytopenia.
2. See Table 14.10 for differential of abnormal platelet function.

E. Management of Thrombocytopenia

1. **ITP**[17]
   a. Pathophysiology: Immune-mediated destruction of circulating platelets
   b. Presentation: Otherwise healthy child with sudden bruising or bleeding after recent mild illness or vaccination, isolated thrombocytopenia (platelets <100,000/μL), and peripheral smear with thrombocytopenia and reticulated large platelets

TABLE 14.9

APPROACH TO THROMBOCYTOPENIA

ACQUIRED

Destructive • Smear: Large platelets • Increased IPF • Bone marrow: Normal-increased megakaryocytes	Immune-mediated	Immune thrombocytopenia (ITP) Evans syndrome: ITP + autoimmune hemolytic anemia Autoimmune disorders (antiphospholipid antibody syndrome, systemic lupus erythematosus) Drug-induced thrombocytopenia (heparin-induced thrombocytopenia) Neonatal alloimmune thrombocytopenia[a] Neonatal autoimmune thrombocytopenia[a]
	Platelet consumption	Thrombotic microangiopathies (TMAs; e.g., HUS, TTP) Disseminated intravascular coagulation (DIC) Kasabach-Merritt syndrome (giant cavernous hemangioma, other vascular malformation) Major surgery/trauma/burn
	Mechanical destruction	Extracorporeal membrane oxygenation (ECMO) Hemodialysis
	Sequestration	Hypersplenism (sickle cell disease, malaria)
Impaired platelet production • Smear: Normal-sized platelets • Low/normal IPF • Infiltration of bone marrow or reduced megakaryocytes	Infection	EBV, CMV, parvovirus, varicella, rickettsia, HIV, sepsis (DIC), congenital infection
	Nutritional deficiency	Folate, vitamin B_{12}, iron deficiency
	Acquired bone marrow failure	Aplastic anemia, myelodysplastic syndromes, medications (chemotherapy), radiation
	Inherited bone marrow failure	Fanconi anemia, Shwachman-Diamond syndrome
	Infiltrative bone marrow disease	Leukemia, lymphoma, infectious granulomas, storage diseases

CONGENITAL

Impaired platelet production	Small platelets	Wiskott-Aldrich syndrome[b] X-linked thrombocytopenia
	Large/giant platelets	Bernard-Soulier syndrome[b] Gray platelet syndrome[b] *MYH9*-related disorders[b] Type 2B von Willebrand disease[b] Paris-Trousseau-Jacobsen syndrome DiGeorge syndrome
	Normal platelets	Congenital amegakaryocytic thrombocytopenia (CAMT) Thrombocytopenia with absent radius (TAR) syndrome[b] Amegakaryocytic thrombocytopenia with radioulnar synostosis Autosomal dominant thrombocytopenia

[a]Neonatal alloimmune thrombocytopenia occurs when maternal IgG antiplatelet antibodies cross the placenta and destroy fetal platelets expressing a "foreign" antigen inherited from father. Neonatal autoimmune thrombocytopenia occurs in children of mothers with antiplatelet antibodies, often related to autoimmune disorders (e.g., immune thrombocytopenic purpura or systemic lupus erythematosus).

[b]These disorders typically also have disordered platelet function.

CMV, Cytomegalovirus; *EBV*, Epstein-Barr virus; *HIV*, human immunodeficiency virus; *HUS*, hemolytic uremic syndrome; *TTP*, thrombotic thrombocytopenic purpura.

Data from Buchanan GR. Thrombocytopenia during childhood: what the pediatrician needs to know. *Pediatr Rev.* 2005:26(11):401–409. Israels SJ, Kahr WH, Blanchette VS, et al. Platelet disorders in children: a diagnostic approach. *Pediatr Blood Cancer.* 2011:56(6):975–983.

TABLE 14.10

CAUSES OF PLATELET DYSFUNCTION

Medications	NSAIDs, Beta-lactam antibiotics, SSRIs
Underlying disease	Uremia, myeloproliferative disorders, myelodysplastic disorders
Inherited disorders	Glanzmann thrombasthenia
	von Willebrand disease
	Bernard-Soulier syndrome
	Storage pool diseases: Wiskott-Aldrich syndrome, thrombocytopenia with absent radii syndrome, Chediak-Higashi syndrome, Hermansky-Pudlak syndrome

NSAIDs, Nonsteroidal antiinflammatory drugs; *SSRIs,* selective serotonin reuptake inhibitors.

Data from Israels SJ, Kahr WH, Blanchette VS, et al. Platelet disorders in children: a diagnostic approach. *Pediatr Blood Cancer.* 2011:56(6):975–983.

---

c. Diagnostic testing: No additional testing needed if presentation consistent with ITP. If concerning features/risk factors present, consider evaluation for: infection [human immunodeficiency virus (HIV), hepatitis C, *Helicobacter pylori* infection], autoimmune disorders (lupus), immunodeficiencies (common variable immunodeficiency, DiGeorge syndrome). If a second autoimmune cytopenia is present (Evans syndrome), consider evaluation for autoimmune lymphoproliferative syndrome (ALPS).[18]

d. Management: Observation if no or mild bleeding (e.g., skin manifestations). Treat if mucosal or other significant bleeding or for situations with higher bleeding risk (e.g., perioperative, trauma) with intravenous immunoglobulin (IVIG), steroids, or anti-Rh (D) immune globulin in consultation with a hematologist.[18] Only transfuse platelets if life-threatening bleed, often with IVIG and high-dose steroids. May require emergent splenectomy. Second-line agents for chronic or refractory ITP include rituximab, thrombopoietin (TPO) mimetics, and other immunomodulatory agents.

2. **Thrombotic thrombocytopenic purpura (TTP)[19]**

a. Pathophysiology: Decreased ADAMTS13 activity results in impaired processing of von Willebrand factor (vWF) multimers, which causes microthrombi.

b. Presentation: Microangiopathic hemolytic anemia (MAHA), thrombocytopenia, acute kidney injury, fever, and fluctuating neurologic symptoms (headache, altered mental status, seizure, stroke).

c. Management: Early plasma exchange with fresh frozen plasma (FFP) and glucocorticoids. If high clinical suspicion, treat emergently before ADAMTS13 testing results.

3. **Hemolytic-uremic syndrome (HUS)**

a. Pathophysiology: Due to Shiga toxin–producing *Escherichia coli* O157:H7 or *Shigella* diarrhea; sometimes *Streptococcus pneumoniae,* HIV[20]

    b. Presentation: Early abdominal pain and bloody diarrhea, MAHA, late thrombocytopenia and renal failure

    c. Management: Supportive care with early/aggressive hydration, RBC/platelet transfusions as needed, antihypertensives, and neurologic monitoring[21]

4. **Complement-mediated ("atypical HUS," aHUS)**

    a. Pathophysiology: Uncontrolled activation of complement on cell membranes[21]

    b. Presentation: Same as HUS without associated above illnesses

    c. Diagnostic testing: Complement panel (not highly sensitive), complement factor H antibodies (seen in a subset of aHUS), consider genetic testing for complement protein gene variants

    d. Management: Eculizumab with or without concurrent plasma exchange and immunomodulating therapy (corticosteroids, cyclophosphamide, rituximab, mycophenolate mofetil, azathioprine)

5. **Drug-induced thrombocytopenia[22]**

    a. Presentation: Lightheadedness, chills, fever, nausea/vomiting, purpura, petechiae ~7 days after starting medication (onset variable)

    b. Diagnostic testing: For heparin-induced thrombocytopenia: +anti-PF4/heparin antibodies, +serotonin release assay. For other drugs: Flow cytometric detection of drug-dependent platelet antibodies

    c. Management: Discontinue medication permanently, transfuse if severe thrombocytopenia to prevent intracranial or intrapulmonary hemorrhage.

6. **Neonatal alloimmune thrombocytopenia[23]**

    a. Pathophysiology: Maternal IgG antibodies (usually against paternally inherited PLA-1/HPA-1a) cross placenta and cause neonatal platelet destruction.

    b. Presentation: Severe thrombocytopenia, intracranial hemorrhage (ICH)—most often occurring in utero

    c. Diagnostic testing: Identify antibodies to paternal platelet antigens in maternal or infant blood sample, or potential mismatch between mother and infant on platelet antigen typing.

    d. Management: Head ultrasound to screen for ICH, transfuse platelets if <30,000/μL or signs of bleeding, consider IVIG if poor response to platelet transfusion.

VI. THROMBOCYTOSIS[12]

A. Definition of Thrombocytosis

1. Thrombocytosis is defined as a platelet count greater than two standard deviations above mean, based on age-specific norms.

2. See Table 14.1 for age-specific values.

B. Causes of Thrombocytosis

1. See Table 14.11 for differential of thrombocytosis.

TABLE 14.11

ETIOLOGY OF THROMBOCYTOSIS

	Cause	Presentation
Secondary	Anemia	Iron deficiency
		Chronic hemolytic anemias
		Vitamin E deficiency
		Acute hemorrhage
		"Rebound" following thrombocytopenia
	Infection	Acute
		Chronic (e.g. TB, hepatitis, osteomyelitis)
	Inflammation	Rheumatoid arthritis
		Inflammatory bowel disease
		Ankylosing spondylitis
		Sarcoidosis
		Acute rheumatic fever
		Kawasaki syndrome
	Drug-induced	Vinca alkaloids
		Corticosteroids
		Epinephrine
	Neoplastic diseases	Lymphoma
		Neuroblastoma
		Solid tumors
	Asplenia	Surgical
		Congenital
		Afunctional
	Miscellaneous	Exercise
		Surgery (may persist for 1–2 weeks)
		Caffey disease
Primary (rare in pediatrics)		5q-syndrome
		Essential thrombocythemia
		Polycythemia vera
		Chronic myelogenous leukemia
		Primary myelofibrosis
		Acute megakaryoblastic leukemia
		Familial thrombocytosis

Adapted from Orkin SH, et al. *Nathan and Oski's Hematology and Oncology of Infancy and Childhood.* 8th ed. Philadelphia: Saunders; 2015.

C. Evaluation of Thrombocytosis

1. CBC and blood smear should be obtained to evaluate platelet morphology and concurrent presence of anemia, leukemic blasts, or leukoerythroblastic features.
2. Patients with unexplained vasomotor symptoms (erythromelalgia, flushing, pruritus), constitutional symptoms, thrombosis at unusual or multiple sites, and/or splenomegaly should be evaluated for potential myeloproliferative neoplasm.

D. Management of Thrombocytosis

1. Treatment is targeted at underlying etiology.

2. Patients with extreme thrombocytosis in the setting of myelodysplastic syndrome (MDS) or myeloproliferative neoplasms (MPN) are prone to both hemorrhage and thrombosis. Both should be managed according to the nature and severity of event.

VII. COAGULATION

A. Evaluation of Coagulation and Platelet Function

1. Coagulation
   a. See Fig. 14.3 for coagulation cascade.
   b. **Activated partial thromboplastin time (aPTT):** Measures intrinsic system (factors VIII, IX, XI, XII) and common pathway (fibrinogen, prothrombin, factors V and X)
   c. **Prothrombin time (PT):** Measures extrinsic pathway (factor VII) and common pathway
   d. **Thrombin time (TT):** Measures conversion of fibrinogen to fibrin. Prolonged with low or dysfunctional fibrinogen, anticoagulants (heparin, low-molecular-weight heparin, direct thrombin inhibitors), or specimen contamination from heparinized line, but not with common pathway abnormalities
   e. **Reptilase time (RT):** Normal with heparin or direct thrombin inhibitors, but prolonged with fibrinogen abnormalities
   f. **Mixing study:** Used in patients with abnormal clotting (i.e., prolonged PT, aPTT, or TT) to determine presence of factor deficiency (corrects with addition of normal plasma) or factor inhibitor (no correction would occur)
   g. **Dilute Russell viper venom time (dRVVT):** Russell viper activates factor X directly and is sensitive to inhibition by antiphospholipid antibodies. Prolonged dRVVT that corrects with addition of phospholipid to assay suggests presence of antiphospholipid antibodies (Lupus anticoagulant).[24]
   h. **Fibrinogen:** Low levels (<50 to 100 mg/dL) cause impaired clot formation and prolong PT and aPTT. Decreased in disseminated intravascular coagulation (DIC), liver disease, traumatic hemorrhage
   i. **D-dimer:** Fibrin degradation product increased with recent/ongoing fibrinolysis (e.g., deep vein thrombosis, pulmonary embolism, DIC, and many other clinical scenarios)
   j. **Thromboelastography (TEG):** Whole blood test that rapidly measures time parameters of clot formation and overall clot strength, detects increased fibrinolysis. Useful for identification of coagulopathy and to guide transfusion in cardiac surgery and trauma[25]
2. Platelet function[12]
   a. Always assess platelet number and use of platelet inhibitors (e.g., nonsteroidal antiinflammatory drugs [NSAIDs]) before platelet function testing.
   b. **Light transmission or whole blood impedance platelet aggregometry:** Measures platelet aggregation in vitro[16]

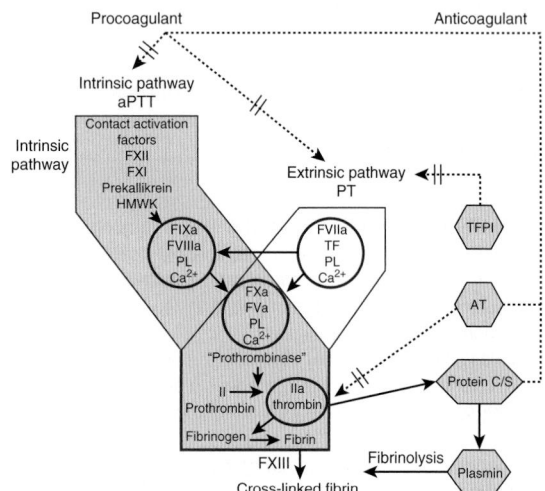

Normal PT and PTT
- von Willebrand disease (type 2B)
- Platelet dysfunction
- Thrombocytopenia
- Vascular abnormalities
- Factor XIII deficiency
- Fibrinolytic disorders

Prolonged aPTT and normal PT
- Factor VIII, IX, XI, XII
  deficiency or inhibitor
- Lupus anticoagulant
- von Willebrand disease
- Heparin

Prolonged PT and aPTT
- Normal TT:
  - Liver disease
  - Vitamin K deficiency (late)
  - Factor II/V/X deficiency or inhibitor
  - Combined factor deficiencies
  - Lupus anticoagulant
- Prolonged TT
  - DIC
  - Low fibrinogen
  - Dysfibrinogenemia

Prolonged PT and normal aPTT
- Factor VII deficiency or inhibitor
- Mild liver disease
- Vitamin K deficiency (early)
- Warfarin

FIGURE 14.3

Coagulation cascade and differential diagnosis of bleeding disorders. *aPTT,* Activated partial thromboplastin time; *AT,* antithrombin; *DIC,* disseminated intravascular coagulation; *PT,* prothrombin time; *TFPI,* tissue factor pathway inhibitor; *TT,* thrombin time. (Adapted from Rodriguez V, Warad D. Pediatric coagulation disorders. *Pediatr Rev.* 2016:37[7]:279–290. Adaptation courtesy James Casella and Clifford Takemoto.)

    c. **Platelet function analyzer-100 (PFA-100):** Measures primary hemostasis (platelet adhesion, activation, and aggregation) in vitro[16]

    d. **Bleeding time (BT):** Evaluates clot formation, including platelet number/function and vWF, in vivo. Technically challenging to perform and has been largely replaced by above-mentioned tests

B. Definition of Abnormal Coagulation

1. An incorrect anticoagulant-to-blood ratio (e.g., in under-filled lab tubes) will give inaccurate results.
2. Table 14.12 lists normal hematologic values for coagulation testing.

C. Causes and Management of Coagulopathy

1. **Medications**
   a. Heparin affects aPTT, thrombin time, dRVVT, and mixing studies.
   b. Warfarin affects PT, may mildly affect aPTT, and interferes with dRVVT by reducing the activity of vitamin K–dependent factors (II, VII, IX, X, protein C and S).
2. **Disseminated intravascular coagulation**
   a. Tissue damage (e.g., due to sepsis, trauma, malignancy) results in tissue factor release and systemic activation of coagulation system, consumption of coagulation factors and platelets, increased fibrin formation and fibrinolysis, MAHA, bleeding, and microthromboses.[26]
   b. Diagnosis: May have prolonged PT and aPTT, decreased fibrinogen, thrombocytopenia, increased D-dimer, increased fibrin degradation products, and/or presence of schistocytes on peripheral smear
   c. Treatment: Address underlying condition and supportive care. May require FFP, cryoprecipitate, and/or platelet transfusions if active bleeding or high bleeding risk
3. **Liver disease**
   a. The liver is the major site of synthesis of factors V, VII, IX, X, XI, XII, XIII.
   b. It is also involved in the synthesis of prothrombin, plasminogen, fibrinogen, proteins C and S, and antithrombin.
4. **Vitamin K deficiency**
   a. Often secondary to liver or biliary disease, pancreatic insufficiency, malabsorption, exclusive breastfeeding, prolonged antibiotic use, malignancy
   b. Necessary for synthesis of factors II, VII, IX, X, protein C, and protein S[12]
   c. Treatment: Parenteral vitamin K corrects PT in 2 to 6 hours (IV administration can be associated with hypersensitivity reactions). Oral form corrects in 6–8 hours.[27] Give FFP if evidence of severe bleeding. Prothrombin complex concentrate can be given in cases of life-threatening hemorrhage, including ICH.
5. **Hemophilia A (factor VIII deficiency) and hemophilia B (factor IX deficiency)[28]**
   a. Etiology: X-linked recessive disorders. Females can be symptomatic carriers.
   b. Diagnosis: Prolonged aPTT that corrects with mixing study, normal PT, low specific factor assays. Mild forms can have normal aPTT.
   c. Classification of disease severity[28]:
      (1) Severe: <1% factor activity; spontaneous bleeding (hemarthrosis, hematoma, bruising) without trauma

TABLE 14.12

AGE-SPECIFIC COAGULATION VALUES

Coagulation Test	Preterm Infant (30–36 Weeks), Day of Life 1[a]	Term Infant, Day of Life 1	Day of Life 3	1 Month–1 Year	1–5 Years	6–10 Years	11–16 Years	Adult
PT (s)	13.0 (10.6–16.2)	15.6 (14.4–16.4)	14.9 (13.5–16.4)	13.1 (11.5–15.3)	13.3 (12.1–14.5)	13.4 (11.7–15.1)	13.8 (12.7–16.1)	13.0 (11.5–14.5)
INR		1.26 (1.15–1.35)	1.20 (1.05–1.35)	1.00 (0.86–1.22)	1.03 (0.92–1.14)	1.04 (0.87–1.20)	1.08 (0.97–1.30)	1.00 (0.80–1.20)
aPTT (s)[b]	53.6 (27.5–79.4)	38.7 (34.3–44.8)	36.3 (29.5–42.2)	39.3 (35.1–46.3)	37.7 (33.6–43.8)	37.3 (31.8–43.7)	39.5 (33.9–46.1)	33.2 (28.6–38.2)
Fibrinogen (g/L)	2.43 (1.50–3.73)	2.80 (1.92–3.74)	3.30 (2.83–4.01)	2.42 (0.82–3.83)	2.82 (1.62–4.01)	3.04 (1.99–4.09)	3.15 (2.12–4.33)	3.1 (1.9–4.3)
Bleeding time (min)[a]	14 (11–17)	12 (10–16)[a]			6 (2.5–10)	7 (2.5–13)	5 (3–8)	4 (1–7)
Thrombin time (s)				17.1 (16.3–17.6)	17.5 (16.5–18.2)	17.1 (16.1–18.5)	16.9 (16.2–17.6)	16.6 (16.2–17.2)
Factor II (U/mL)	0.45 (0.20–0.77)	0.54 (0.41–0.69)	0.62 (0.50–0.73)	0.90 (0.62–1.03)	0.89 (0.70–1.09)	0.89 (0.67–1.10)	0.90 (0.61–1.07)	1.10 (0.78–1.38)
Factor V (U/mL)	0.88 (0.41–1.44)	0.81 (0.64–1.03)	1.22 (0.92–1.54)	1.13 (0.94–1.41)	0.97 (0.67–1.27)	0.99 (0.56–1.41)	0.89 (0.67–1.41)	1.18 (0.78–1.52)
Factor VII (U/mL)	0.67 (0.21–1.13)	0.70 (0.52–0.88)	0.86 (0.62–1.07)	1.28 (0.83–1.60)	1.11 (0.72–1.50)	1.13 (0.70–1.56)	1.18 (0.69–2.00)	1.29 (0.61–1.99)
Factor VIII (U/mL)	1.11 (0.50–2.13)	1.82 (1.05–3.29)	1.59 (0.83–2.74)	0.94 (0.54–1.45)	1.10 (0.36–1.85)	1.17 (0.52–1.82)	1.20 (0.59–2.00)	1.60 (0.52–2.90)
vWF (U/mL)[a]	1.36 (0.78–2.10)	1.53 (0.50–2.87)			0.82 (0.47–1.04)	0.95 (0.44–1.44)	1.00 (0.46–1.53)	0.92 (0.5–1.58)
Factor IX (U/mL)	0.35 (0.19–0.65)	0.48 (0.35–0.56)	0.72 (0.44–0.97)	0.71 (0.43–1.21)	0.85 (0.44–1.27)	0.96 (0.48–1.45)	1.11 (0.64–2.16)	1.30 (0.59–2.54)
Factor X (U/mL)	0.41 (0.11–0.71)	0.55 (0.46–0.67)	0.60 (0.46–0.75)	0.95 (0.77–1.22)	0.98 (0.72–1.25)	0.97 (0.68–1.25)	0.91 (0.53–1.22)	1.24 (0.96–1.71)
Factor XI (U/mL)	0.30 (0.08–0.52)	0.30 (0.07–0.41)	0.57 (0.24–0.79)	0.89 (0.62–1.25)	1.13 (0.65–1.62)	1.13 (0.65–1.62)	1.11 (0.65–1.39)	1.12 (0.67–1.96)
Factor XII (U/mL)	0.38 (0.10–0.66)	0.58 (0.43–0.80)	0.53 (0.14–0.80)	0.79 (0.20–1.35)	0.85 (0.36–1.35)	0.81 (0.26–1.37)	0.75 (0.14–1.17)	1.15 (0.35–2.07)
PK (U/mL)[a]	0.33 (0.09–0.57)	0.37 (0.18–0.69)			0.95 (0.65–1.30)	0.99 (0.66–1.31)	0.99 (0.53–1.45)	1.12 (0.62–1.62)
HMWK (U/mL)[a]	0.49 (0.09–0.89)	0.54 (0.06–1.02)			0.98 (0.64–1.32)	0.93 (0.60–1.30)	0.91 (0.63–1.19)	0.92 (0.50–1.36)

Factor XIIa (U/mL)[a]	0.70 (0.32–1.08)	0.79 (0.27–1.31)			1.08 (0.72–1.43)	1.09 (0.65–1.51)	0.99 (0.57–1.40)	1.05 (0.55–1.55)
Factor XIIIs (U/mL)[a]	0.81 (0.35–1.27)	0.76 (0.30–1.22)			1.13 (0.69–1.56)	1.16 (0.77–1.54)	1.02 (0.60–1.43)	0.97 (0.57–1.37)
D-dimer		1.47 (0.41–2.47)	1.34 (0.58–2.74)	0.22 (0.11–0.42)	0.25 (0.09–0.53)	0.26 (0.10–0.56)	0.27 (0.16–0.39)	0.18 (0.05–0.42)
FDPs[a]								Borderline titer = 1:25–1:50 Positive titer <1:50
COAGULATION INHIBITORS								
ATIII (U/mL)[a]	0.38 (0.14–0.62)	0.63 (0.39–0.97)			1.11 (0.82–1.39)	1.11 (0.90–1.31)	1.05 (0.77–1.32)	1.0 (0.74–1.26)
α_2-M (U/mL)[a]	1.10 (0.56–1.82)	1.39 (0.95–1.83)			1.69 (1.14–2.23)	1.69 (1.28–2.09)	1.56 (0.98–2.12)	0.86 (0.52–1.20)
C1-Inh (U/mL)[a]	0.65 (0.31–0.99)	0.72 (0.36–1.08)			1.35 (0.85–1.83)	1.14 (0.88–1.54)	1.03 (0.68–1.50)	1.0 (0.71–1.31)
α_1-AT (U/mL)[a]	0.90 (0.36–1.44)	0.93 (0.49–1.37)			0.93 (0.39–1.47)	1.00 (0.69–1.30)	1.01 (0.65–1.37)	0.93 (0.55–1.30)
Protein C (U/mL)	0.28 (0.12–0.44)	0.32 (0.24–0.40)	0.33 (0.24–0.51)	0.77 (0.28–1.24)	0.94 (0.50–1.34)	0.94 (0.64–1.25)	0.88 (0.59–1.12)	1.03 (0.54–1.66)
Protein S (U/mL)		0.26 (0.14–0.38)	0.36 (0.28–0.47)	0.49 (0.33–0.67)	1.02 (0.29–1.62)	1.01 (0.67–1.36)	1.09 (0.64–1.54)	0.75 (0.54–1.03)
FIBRINOLYTIC SYSTEM[a]								
Plasminogen (U/mL)	1.70 (1.12–2.48)	1.95 (1.60–2.30)			0.98 (0.78–1.18)	0.92 (0.75–1.08)	0.86 (0.68–1.03)	0.99 (0.7–1.22)
TPA (ng/mL)					2.15 (1.0–5.0)	2.42 (1.0–5.0)	2.16 (1.0–4.0)	4.90 (1.40–8.40)
α_2-AP (U/mL)	0.78 (0.4–1.16)	0.85 (0.70–1.0)			1.05 (0.93–1.17)	0.99 (0.89–1.10)	0.98 (0.78–1.18)	1.02 (0.68–1.36)
PAI (U/mL)					5.42 (1.0–10.0)	6.79 (2.0–12.0)	6.07 (2.0–10.0)	3.60 (0–11.0)

[a]Data from Andrew M, Paes B, Milner R, et al. Development of the human anticoagulant system in the healthy premature infant. *Blood.* 1987;70:165–172; Andrew M, Paes B, Milner R, et al. Development of the human coagulation system in the healthy premature infant. *Blood.* 1988;72(5):1651–1657; and Andrew M, Vegh P, Johnston M, et al. Maturation of the hemostatic system during childhood. *Blood.* 1992;8:1998–2005.

[b]aPTT values may vary depending on reagent.

α_2-AP, α_2-Antiplasmin; *α_1-AT,* α_1-antitrypsin; *α_2-M,* α_2-macroglobulin; *ATIII,* antithrombin III; *FDPs,* fibrin degradation products; *HMWK,* high-molecular-weight kininogen; *INR,* international normalized ratio; *PAI,* plasminogen activator inhibitor; *PK,* prekallikrein; *PT,* prothrombin time; *TPA,* tissue plasminogen activator; *VIII,* factor VIII procoagulant; *vWF,* von Willebrand factor.

Adapted from Monagle P, Barnes C, Ignjatovic V, et al. Developmental haemostasis. Impact for clinical haemostasis laboratories. *Thromb Haemost.* 2006;95;362–372.

14

      (2) Moderate: 1% to 5% factor activity; bleeding after minor trauma

      (3) Mild: 5% to 40% factor activity; bleeding with surgery or significant trauma

  d. Bleeding prophylaxis:

      (1) Home prophylaxis: Regular administration of intravenous (IV) factor replacement to maintain factor level >1 IU/dL to prevent spontaneous bleeds and preserve joint function. Initiate before onset of frequent bleeding, typically in 1- to 3-year-olds with severe hemophilia.[29] Emicizumab-kxwh is a bispecific antibody that is delivered subcutaneously (SQ) and can be used for prophylaxis in hemophilia A.

      (2) Surgical prophylaxis: Factor replacement to goal factor level 80 to 100 IU/dL (major procedure) or 50 to 80 IU/dL (minor procedure) preoperatively and through postoperative period of bleeding risk.[28] Consult hematologist before any diagnostic or therapeutic procedure, including dental, endoscopy with biopsy, arterial blood gas, etc.

  e. Treatment of acute bleeds:

      (1) Always remember: **"Factor first!"** Do not delay administration of first dose when suspicion for bleed or recent injury (e.g., do not wait for imaging or lab results).

      (2) Bolus dose factor VIII or factor IX concentrate. May require additional doses

      (3) Consult hematologist for all major bleeding.

      (4) See Table 14.13 for desired factor replacement level and dosing.

      (5) Half-life of factor VIII: 8 to 12 hours. Half-life factor IX: 18 to 24 hours[28]

TABLE 14.13

DESIRED FACTOR REPLACEMENT IN HEMOPHILIA

Dose calculation:

1. Units of factor VIII needed = weight (kg) × desired % replacement × 0.5
2. Units of factor IX needed = weight (kg) × desired % replacement × 1.0 or 1.2

Bleeding Site	Desired Level (%)
Minor soft tissue bleeding	20–30
Joint	40–70
Simple dental extraction	50
Major soft tissue bleeding	80–100
Serious oral bleeding	80–100
Head injury	100+
Major surgery (dental, orthopedic, other)	100+

NOTE: A hematologist should be consulted for all major bleeding and before surgery.

Round to the nearest vial; do not exceed 200%.

Dosing adapted from Nathan D, Oski FA. *Hematology of Infancy and Childhood.* WB Saunders; 1998.

(6) If suspected intracranial bleed, replete 100% factor level immediately on presentation and **before** additional diagnostic testing (e.g., CT scan).

(7) Alternative treatments:

(a) Desmopressin (DDAVP) can be used in mild hemophilia A only.

(b) Antifibrinolytic agents (tranexamic acid, aminocaproic acid) may be appropriate for minor mucosal bleeding.

(8) Cryoprecipitate (for hemophilia A only) or FFP are used in settings where no factor concentrate is available.

f. Factor inhibitors: IgG antibodies that develop with repeat factor exposure and complicate treatment. Patients with severe hemophilia A are at the highest risk.

(1) Screen for inhibitors with inhibitor assay if poor clinical response to factor. Consider screening during initiation of factor treatment and preoperatively.

(2) In the presence of inhibitors, patients may require higher doses of factor (only beneficial for low titer inhibitors), recombinant FVIIa concentrate, or activated prothrombin complex concentrates.

g. Healthcare maintenance

(1) Vaccinations: Given per routine schedule. Give prophylactic factor for intramuscular vaccines or give vaccine SQ with 23-gauge or smaller needle without factor prophylaxis and hold pressure at site for 2 minutes.[28]

(2) Physical activity: Avoid high-contact (e.g., soccer, hockey) and high-velocity (e.g., skiing) activities.[28]

(3) Medications to avoid: Aspirin, NSAIDs, anticoagulants

(4) Many younger children will need a central venous catheter for factor delivery and must therefore follow strict fever guidelines.

6. **von Willebrand disease (vWD)**

a. Pathophysiology: Most common inherited bleeding disorder. Abnormal platelet adhesion and aggregation, can have low factor VIII[30]

b. Diagnosis: Low circulating von Willebrand factor antigen (VWF:Ag) and/or low vWF function on ristocetin-based platelet aggregation study (VWF:RCo) or vW GP1bM binding assay, low or normal factor VIII activity, prolonged PFA-100. May require additional evaluation. Notably, the African American population may have an artifactually low ristocetin cofactor assay from a common D1472H von Willebrand polymorphism.

c. Classification[30]:

(1) Type 1 (75% to 80% cases): Partial quantitative deficiency of vWF

(2) Type 2 (20% to 25%): Qualitative dysfunction of vWF

(3) Type 3 (rare): Absence or near absence of vWF + markedly low factor VIII activity (can resemble hemophilia A patient on labs and presentation)

d. Treatment[30]:

(1) Desmopressin (DDAVP): Stimulates vWF release. Given IV, intranasal (1.5 mg/mL concentration only), or SQ (rarely). May be used as prophylaxis for minor surgeries or treatment for mild bleeding. Ineffective in type 3, variable effect in type 2. Patients should be tested for DDAVP response before using as prophylaxis.

(2) vWF-containing concentrates (Humate-P or Wilate): Replaces vWF and factor VIII, derived from blood donors. Recombinant vWF available (VONVENDI). Used for severe bleeding events and surgery

(3) Cryoprecipitate for life-threatening situations only if vWF concentrate unavailable

(4) Alternative therapies: IV or oral antifibrinolytic therapy (tranexamic acid and aminocaproic acid) can be used to prevent or treat mild mucocutaneous bleeding alone or in conjunction with other therapies.

D. Causes of Hypercoagulability

1. Most thrombotic events are due to an acquired condition; however, an inherited thrombophilia is more likely if there is a family history, an unusual thrombus location, absence of an inciting factor, and/or recurrent thromboses.
2. See Table 14.14 for etiologies and evaluation of hypercoagulable states.
3. Acquired conditions associated with venous thromboembolism include endothelial damage (vascular catheters, sepsis, smoking, diabetes, hypertension, surgery, hyperlipidemia), disturbed blood flow (central venous lines, congenital heart disease), hyperviscosity (macroglobulinemia, erythrocytosis, sickle cell disease), platelet activation (essential thrombocytosis, heparin-induced thrombocytopenia), malignancy, inflammatory bowel disease, parenteral nutrition, nephrotic syndrome, paroxysmal nocturnal hemoglobinuria, estrogen-containing hormonal therapy.

E. Thrombus Management

1. See Table 14.15 for anticoagulant use.
2. See Formulary for dosing and adjustment based on monitoring protocols.
3. **NOTE:** Children receiving anticoagulation therapy should be protected from trauma. The use of antiplatelet agents should be avoided.
4. See Table 14.16 for warfarin-reversal guidelines.
5. Consult a hematologist regarding interruption of anticoagulation for procedures and surgeries.

TABLE 14.14

HYPERCOAGULABLE STATES

Hypercoagulable Condition	Cause	Risk of VTE (Compared to General Population; Odds Ratio)	Associated Test
Factor V Leiden (activated protein C resistance)	AD Factor V Leiden mutation	3.77 (heterozygote)	Activated protein C resistance assay (screening test)
			Factor V Leiden (DNA-based PCR assay)
Factor VIII, IX, XI abnormalities[a]	Inherited or acquired elevated factor levels	6.7 (Factor VIII)	Factor VIII, IX, XI
Protein C and S deficiency[a]	AD. Homozygous more severe than heterozygous	7.72 (protein C); 5.77 (protein S)	Protein C and S activity
Antithrombin III deficiency[a]	AD. Type I: Low level and activity (homozygous not compatible with life). Type II: Low activity or dysfunction	9.44	Antithrombin III activity
Hyperhomocystinemia[a]	AR alteration in *MTHFR* gene	1.27	Homocysteine level (fasting)
			MTHFR genetic testing if homocysteine elevated
Prothrombin mutation	AD mutation in G20210A	2.64 (heterozygote)	DNR-based PCR assay
Antiphospholipid antibodies[a]	Rarely inherited. Typically sporadic: Spontaneous (primary) or secondary to autoimmune disorder (e.g., SLE) or infections	High	Phospholipid-based clotting assays (aPTT, dRVVT) that correct with phospholipid addition
			ELISA assays: cardiolipin and β2-glycoprotein antibodies
High lipoprotein(a)	Levels determined by genetics and environment	4.49	Lipoprotein(a) level
Plasminogen deficiency	Inherited hypoplasminogenemia (type I) or dysplasminogenemia (type II)		Plasminogen activity[b]

[a]These conditions may be inherited or acquired.

[b]Also consider testing tissue plasminogen activator (tPA) antigen and plasminogen activator inhibitor-1 (PAI-1) activity. Increased PAI-1 causes excess inhibition of tPA. Low tPA decreases fibrinolysis.

A hematologist should be consulted if initiating this workup.

AD, Autosomal dominant; *aPTT,* activated partial thromboplastin time; *AR,* autosomal recessive; *dRVVT,* dilute Russell viper venom time; *ELISA,* enzyme-linked immunosorbent assay, *PCR,* polymerase chain reaction, *SLE,* systemic lupus erythematosus, *VTE,* venous thromboembolism.

Data from Rodriguez V, Warad D. Pediatric coagulation disorders. *Pediatr Rev.* 2016;37(7):279–290. Young G, Albisetti M, Bonduel M, et al. Impact of inherited thrombophilia on venous thromboembolism in children: a systematic review and meta-analysis of observational studies. *Circulation.* 2008;118(13):1373–1382.

14

TABLE 14.15

ANTICOAGULANTS

Medication	Indication	Contraindications and Adverse Effects	Monitoring	Reversal
Heparin/UFH (IV)	Acute treatment for VTE, acute ischemic stroke (AIS), cerebral venous sinus thrombosis (CVST) without ICH Prevention of thrombosis with cardiac catheterization, cardiopulmonary bypass surgery, extracorporeal circuits	Heparin hypersensitivity, major active or high-risk bleeding, platelets <50,000, known/suspected HIT, concurrent epidural therapy Cautious use in patients with high bleeding risk or platelets <50,000/mm^3 Avoid IM injections and concurrent use of drugs affecting platelet function (NSAIDs, aspirin, clopidogrel).	Anti-Xa level (goal 0.3–0.7 U/mL) or aPTT (1.5–2.5 times the control aPTT) The aPTT range in seconds (~50–80 sec) should be calibrated to anti-Xa of 0.3–0.7 U/mL	Protamine sulfate
LMWH/enoxaparin (SQ)	Initial or ongoing therapy for VTE, CVST, AIS with cardioembolic source, recurrent AIS Patients with history or risks for HIT	HIT (lower risk than UFH) Chronic use (>6 months) may decrease bone density.	Anti-Xa activity (goal 0.5–1 U/ mL for thrombosis, 0.1–0.3 U/mL for prophylaxis)	Protamine sulfate (partial neutralization)
Warfarin (PO)	Long-term anticoagulation after bridge from UFH or LMWH for VTE, CVST, AIS Recurrent idiopathic VTE	Interactions with diet and medications (see eTable 14.1) Adjust dose in liver dysfunction, avoid in severe liver failure. Limited safety and efficacy data in newborns <3 months Warfarin-induced skin necrosis has been reported in patients initiated without bridging anticoagulation. Teratogenic	INR (2–3 with target 2.5, except with prosthetic cardiac valves) measured every 1–4 weeks	Vitamin K (see Table 14.18)

DIRECT THROMBIN INHIBITORS

Argatroban (IV)	Alternative to heparin in patients with HIT	Avoid or alter dose in patients with hepatic impairment.	aPTT 1.5–2.5× baseline	None
Bivalirudin (IV)	Inpatient treatment of VTE and prevention of thrombus during cardiac catheterization in patients with HIT	Adjust dose with renal impairment.	aPTT 1.5–2.5× baseline	None
Dabigatran (PO)[a]	Approved in adults to treat DVT/PE, reduce embolic risk in nonvalvular AF	*Studies ongoing for safety and efficacy in pediatric patients.*	None required	Idarucizumab

FACTOR XA INHIBITORS

Fondaparinux (SQ)[a]	Approved in adults to treat and prevent DVT/PE. Can be used in patients with HIT.	Adjust dose with renal impairment.	Anti-Xa level 0.5–1 mg/L	None
Apixaban (PO)[a]	Approved in adults to treat and prevent DVT/PE, reduce embolic risk in AF.	*Studies ongoing for safety and efficacy in pediatric patients.*	Can measure anti-Xa level	Andexanet alfa
Rivaroxaban (PO)[a]	Approved in adults to treat and prevent recurrent DVT/PE, prevent nonvalvular AF embolic complications.			

[a]These medications are undergoing Phase II/III trials for use in children and should not be used as first-line therapy.[44,45]

AF, Atrial fibrillation; *aPTT*, activated partial thromboplastin time; *DVT*, deep venous thrombosis; *HIT*, heparin-induced thrombocytopenia; *INR*, international normalized ratio; *IV*, intravenous; *LMWH*, low-molecular-weight heparin; *NSAID*, nonsteroidal antiinflammatory drug; *PE*, pulmonary embolism; *PO*, oral; *SQ*, subcutaneous; *UFH*, unfractionated heparin; *VTE*, venous thromboembolism.
Data from Monagle P, Chan AKC, Goldenberg NA, et al. Antithrombotic therapy in neonates and children: Antithrombotic therapy and prevention of thrombosis, 9th ed: American College of Chest Physicians evidence-based clinical practice guidelines. *CHEST.* 2012;141(2):e737S–e801s. Young G. Anticoagulation therapies in children. *Pediatr Clin North Am.* 2017;64(6):1257–1269.

14

TABLE 14.16

MANAGEMENT OF EXCESSIVE WARFARIN ANTICOAGULATION

INR and Bleeding	Intervention
INR 4–4.5 without serious bleeding	Hold or lower next warfarin dose. Recheck INR daily. For patients with high bleeding risk, consider standard dose of oral vitamin K.[a] When INR approaches therapeutic range, resume warfarin therapy.
INR ≥4.5 but <10 without serious bleeding	Hold warfarin. Recheck INR every 24 hr until <4. If high risk for bleeding, give standard dose of oral vitamin K.[a] When INR approaches therapeutic range, resume warfarin at a lower dose.
INR ≥10 without serious bleeding	Hold warfarin. Recheck INR every 12 hr. Give high-dose oral vitamin K every 12–24 hr as necessary.[b] When INR approaches therapeutic range, resume warfarin at a lower dose.
Minor bleeding at any INR elevation	Hold warfarin. Monitor INR every 12–24 hr depending on bleeding severity. Give standard-dose oral vitamin K and repeat as necessary if bleeding continues and INR not corrected at 24 hr.[a] Restart warfarin when INR approaches therapeutic range and when clinically appropriate at a lower dose.
Significant or life-threatening bleeding at any INR	Hold warfarin. Monitor INR every 4–6 hr. Administer high-dose vitamin K IV, repeat as needed.[b] Transfusion of FFP (10–15 mL/kg IV), consider prothrombin complex concentrate; consult blood bank and/or hematology for dosing. Restart warfarin when INR approaches therapeutic range and when clinically appropriate at a lower dose.

[a]Standard-dose vitamin K: 0.03 mg/kg PO for patients <40 kg in weight; 1–2.5 mg PO for patients ≥40 kg. For rapid reversal, 0.5–2.5 mg IV slow infusion over 30 minutes. Expect INR reduction at 24–48 hr with oral dosing, and at 12–14 hr with IV dosing.

[b]High-dose vitamin K: 0.06 mg/kg PO for patients <40 kg in weight; 5–10 mg for patients ≥40 kg. For emergent situations, 5–10 mg IV slow infusion over 30 minutes.

NOTE: Always evaluate for bleeding risks and potential drug interactions. Do not give intramuscular vitamin K to children on anticoagulants.

FFP, Fresh frozen plasma; *INR,* international normalized ratio; *IV,* intravenous; *PO,* by mouth.

The Johns Hopkins Hospital Children's Center pediatric policies, procedures, and protocols general care (Policy Number MDU043): Baltimore; 2019.

Adapted from Holbrook A, Schulman S, Witt DM, et al. *Evidence-Based Management of Anticoagulation Therapy. Antithrombotic Therapy and Prevention of Thrombosis,* 9th ed: American College of Chest Physicians evidence-based clinical practice guidelines. *CHEST.* 2012;141(2):e152S–e184S. Bolton-Maggs P, Brook L. The use of vitamin K for reversal of over-warfarinization in children. *Br J Haematol.* 2002;118:924–925.

TABLE 14.17	

ESTIMATED BLOOD VOLUME

Age	Total Blood Volume (mL/kg)
Preterm infants	90–105
Term newborns	78–86
1–12 months	73–78
1–3 years	74–82
4–6 years	80–86
7–18 years	83–90
Adults	68–88

Data from Nathan D, Oski FA. *Hematology of Infancy and Childhood.* WB Saunders; 1998.

VIII. BLOOD COMPONENT REPLACEMENT

A. Calculating Estimated Blood Volume (Table 14.17)

B. Indications for and Expected Response Following Blood Transfusions

1. See Table 14.18.
2. See Section X, Online Content, for information on directed-donor transfusions.

C. Diagnosis and Management of Transfusion Reactions (Table 14.19)

D. Infectious Risks of Blood Transfusion

1. Per-unit risk for transfusion recipients[31,32]
   a. HIV: 1 in 2,941,176
   b. Human T-lymphotropic virus (HTLV): 1 in 4,364,000
   c. Hepatitis B: 1 in 1,470,588
   d. Hepatitis C: 1 in 3,333,333
   e. Cytomegalovirus (CMV), Epstein-Barr virus (EBV), hepatitis A, parasites, and tickborne infections may also be transmitted by blood products.
2. Sepsis related to bacterial contamination
   a. Risk of transmission of bacteria in RBCs is 1 in 5 million units.
   b. Risk of transmission in platelets is 1 in 107,000 units.
   c. Risk is higher in platelets because they are stored at room temperature.

14

TABLE 14.18

BLOOD PRODUCTS

Product	Contains	Indications	Dose	Volume of 1 Unit (U)	Change in blood count
PRBCs	Concentrated RBCs w/Hct 55%–70%	Generally Hb <7 g/dL,[a] but consider clinical picture. Use typed and crossmatched products when possible. O– can be provided emergently without crossmatch if transfusion cannot be delayed. See Section X, Online Content, for specific types of PRBCs.	10–15 mL/kg (at max 2–4 mL/kg/hr) RBCs must be transfused within 4 hours of leaving blood bank.	300–350 mL after processing	To determine volume necessary for desired Hct: PRBC volume (mL) = {EBV [mL] × [desired Hct – actual Hct]/Hct of PRBCs[b]
Platelets		Severe (<10,000/μL) thrombocytopenia, symptomatic thrombocytopenia, to achieve platelets >50,000/μL before minor or >100,000/μL before major surgery or intracranial operation Transfusion indications for neonates: Platelets <20,000/μL; platelets <30,000/μL + weight <1 kg, age <1 week, clinically unstable, history major bleed (e.g., IVH), current bleed, coagulopathy/DIC, preprocedure; platelets >50,000/μL only if significant bleed	Children ≤30 kg[c]: 5–10 mL/kg or 1 equivalent unit per 5–10 kg Children >30 kg: 1 apheresis unit Transfuse as rapidly as able.	300 mL for 1 apheresis unit, 50 mL for 1 equivalent unit	10 mL/kg increases platelets by 50,000/μL.
FFP	Physiologic quantities all coagulation factors[d]	Treat severe clotting factor deficiencies with active bleeding (DIC, vitamin K deficiency with active bleeding, TTP) or before invasive procedure. Combine with vitamin K for emergency reversal of warfarin.	15 mL/kg; repeat PRN	250–300 mL	1 unit activity of all factors except V and VIII

| Cryoprecipitate | Enriched factors VIII and XIII, vWF, fibrinogen, fibronectin | For hypofibrinogenemia, dysfibrinogenemia | Children <5 kg: 1 single donor unit. Children 5–50 kg: 1 unit per 5–10 kg. Children >50 kg: 1–2 pools (5–10 units) | 10–15 mL for 1 unit, 50–100 mL for a pool | 1 unit contains approximately 80 units factor VIII, 150 mg fibrinogen.[e] |

[a]Restrictive transfusion protocol with Hb threshold 7 g/dL associated with fewer transfusions without differences in clinical outcomes.

[b]Hct of PRBCs is typically 55% to 70% depending on storage anticoagulant.

[c]1 unit of apheresis platelets is derived from a single donor and contains >3 × 10[11] platelets/mL. 1 equivalent unit is ~1/5th–1/6th an apheresis unit. Single-donor platelet concentrates are derived from a single donor and contain >5.5 × 10[10] platelets in approximately 50 mL. 4–6 equivalent units or platelet concentrates can be pooled to make equivalent of 1 apheresis unit.

[d]FFP does not include platelets or fibrinogen. Does include anticoagulant factors (antithrombin III, proteins C/S). **NOTE:** FFP unlikely to have significant effect when INR ≤1.6.[46]

[e]This is an estimation. 1 unit of cryoprecipitate is derived from 500 mL of blood from 1 donor. A pool is 5 individual donor units pooled together.

DIC, Disseminated intravascular coagulation; *EBV,* estimated blood volume; *FFP,* fresh frozen plasma; *Hb,* hemoglobin; *Hct,* Hb/hematocrit; *PRBCs,* packed red blood cells; *PRN,* as needed; *RBCs,* red blood cells; *TTP,* thrombotic thrombocytopenic purpura; *vWF,* von Willebrand factor.

Data from Bachowski G, Borge D, Brunker PAR, et al. *A Compendium of Transfusion Practice Guidelines.* 3rd ed. American Red Cross; 2017. Behrman RE, Kliegman RM, Jenson AH. *Nelson Textbook of Pediatrics.* 17th ed. Saunders; 2004.

14

TABLE 14.19

TRANSFUSION REACTIONS

Reaction	Timeline	Pathophysiology	Signs/Symptoms	Labs	Treatment
Acute hemolytic transfusion reaction	Immediate	Blood group incompatibility results in intravascular hemolysis, acute renal failure, DIC	Fevers, chills, flank pain, tachycardia, hypotension, shock, hematuria, bleeding	ABO, CBC hemolysis labs: DAT, haptoglobin, LDH, bilirubin +/− DIC labs: PT/aPTT, fibrinogen, D-dimer Urinalysis (evaluate for hemoglobinuria)	Stop transfusion. Notify blood bank. Supportive measures: IV normal saline to achieve UOP >1 mL/kg/hr, vasopressors as needed, nephrology consult if necessary for acute renal failure
Febrile nonhemolytic reaction	1–6 hr	Either cytokines from donor WBCs in product or recipient anti-neutrophil or anti-HLA antibodies against WBCs in donor product	Fever, chills, diaphoresis	Exclude alternative reactions (AHTR, sepsis)	Decreased incidence with leukoreduced products Stop transfusion. Notify blood bank. Antipyretics Consider future premedication with antipyretics (little evidence supporting practice).
Urticarial reaction	Immediate	Reaction to donor plasma proteins	Urticarial rash, respiratory distress	Possible formation IgE anti-IgA antibody	Stop transfusion. Notify blood bank. Epinephrine/steroids for respiratory compromise Antihistamines Resolved mild (cutaneous only) allergic reaction is the only time that a transfusion may be resumed with remainder of product.

| Delayed transfusion reaction | >24 hr posttransfusion (up to 30 days) | Minor blood group antigen incompatibility results in extravascular hemolysis | Fatigue, jaundice, dark urine | Anemia +DAT Evidence of hemolysis New RBC Abs | Monitor Hb level closely. Supportive care |

ABO, Blood type; *Abs*, antibodies; *AHTR*, acute hemolytic transfusion reaction; *aPTT*, activated partial thromboplastin time; *CBC*, complete blood count; *DAT*, direct antiglobulin test; *DIC*, disseminated intravascular coagulation; *Hb*, hemoglobin; *HLA*, human leukocyte antigen; *IV*, intravenous; *LDH*, lactate dehydrogenase; *PRBCs*, packed red blood cells; *PT*, prothrombin time; *RBC*, red blood cell; *UOP*, urine output; *WBCs*, white blood cells.

Data from Delaney M, Wendel S, Bercovitz RS, et al. Transfusion reactions: prevention, diagnosis, and treatment. *Lancet.* 2016;388(10061):2825–2836. Bachowski G, Borge D, Brunker PAR, et al. *A Compendium of Transfusion Practice Guidelines.* 3rd ed. American Red Cross; 2017.

14

TABLE 14.1

AGE-SPECIFIC BLOOD CELL INDICES

Age	Hb (g/dL)[a]	HCT (%)[a]	MCV (fL)[a]	MCHC (g/dL RBC)[a]	Reticulocytes	WBCs (×10³/mL)[b]	Platelets (10³/mL)[b]
26–30 weeks' gestation[c]	13.4 (11)	41.5 (34.9)	118.2 (106.7)	37.9 (30.6)	—	4.4 (2.7)	254 (180–327)
28 weeks	14.5	45	120	31.0	(5–10)	—	275
32 weeks	15.0	47	118	32.0	(3–10)	—	290
Term[d] (cord)	16.5 (13.5)	51 (42)	108 (98)	33.0 (30.0)	(3–7)	18.1 (9–30)[e]	290
1–3 days	18.5 (14.5)	56 (45)	108 (95)	33.0 (29.0)	(1.8–4.6)	18.9 (9.4–34)	192
2 weeks	16.6 (13.4)	53 (41)	105 (88)	31.4 (28.1)	—	11.4 (5–20)	252
1 month	13.9 (10.7)	44 (33)	101 (91)	31.8 (28.1)	(0.1–1.7)	10.8 (4–19.5)	—
2 months	11.2 (9.4)	35 (28)	95 (84)	31.8 (28.3)	—	—	—
6 months	12.6 (11.1)	36 (31)	76 (68)	35.0 (32.7)	(0.7–2.3)	11.9 (6–17.5)	—
6 months–2 years	12.0 (10.5)	36 (33)	78 (70)	33.0 (30.0)	—	10.6 (6–17)	(150–350)
2–6 years	12.5 (11.5)	37 (34)	81 (75)	34.0 (31.0)	(0.5–1.0)	8.5 (5–15.5)	(150–350)
6–12 years	13.5 (11.5)	40 (35)	86 (77)	34.0 (31.0)	(0.5–1.0)	8.1 (4.5–13.5)	(150–350)
12–18 YEARS							
Male	14.5 (13)	43 (36)	88 (78)	34.0 (31.0)	(0.5–1.0)	7.8 (4.5–13.5)	(150–350)
Female	14.0 (12)	41 (37)	90 (78)	34.0 (31.0)	(0.5–1.0)	7.8 (4.5–13.5)	(150–350)
ADULT							
Male	15.5 (13.5)	47 (41)	90 (80)	34.0 (31.0)	(0.8–2.5)	7.4 (4.5–11)	(150–350)
Female	14.0 (12)	41 (36)	90 (80)	34.0 (31.0)	(0.8–4.1)	7.4 (4.5–11)	(150–350)

[a]Data are mean (−2 SD).

[b]Data are mean (±2 SD).

[c]Values are from fetal samplings.

[d]Until 1 month of age, capillary hemoglobin exceeds venous: 1 hour: 3.6-g difference; 5 days: 2.2-g difference; 3 weeks: 1.1-g difference.

[e]Mean (95% confidence limits).

Hb, Hemoglobin; HCT, hematocrit; MCHC, mean cell hemoglobin concentration; MCV, mean corpuscular volume; RBC, red blood cell; WBC, white blood cell.

Data from Forestier F, Daffos F, Galacteros F, Bardakjian J, Rainaut M, Beuzard Y. Hematological values of 163 normal fetuses between 18 and 30 weeks of gestation. Pediatr Res 1986;20:342; Oski FA, Naiman JL. Hematological Problems in the Newborn Infant. WB Saunders; 1982; Nathan D, Oski FA. Hematology of Infancy and Childhood. WB Saunders; 1998; Matoth Y, Zaizor K, Varsano I, et al. Postnatal changes in some red cell parameters. Acta Paediatr Scand. 1971;60:317; and Wintrobe MM. Clinical Hematology. Williams & Wilkins; 1999.

TABLE 14.7

AGE-SPECIFIC LEUKOCYTE DIFFERENTIAL

Age	Total Leukocytes[a] Mean (Range)	Neutrophils[b] Mean (Range)	%	Lymphocytes Mean (Range)	%	Monocytes Mean	%	Eosinophils Mean	%
Birth	18.1 (9–30)	11 (6–26)	61	5.5 (2–11)	31	1.1	6	0.4	2
12 hr	22.8 (13–38)	15.5 (6–28)	68	5.5 (2–11)	24	1.2	5	0.5	2
24 hr	18.9 (9.4–34)	11.5 (5–21)	61	5.8 (2–11.5)	31	1.1	6	0.5	2
1 week	12.2 (5–21)	5.5 (1.5–10)	45	5.0 (2–17)	41	1.1	9	0.5	4
2 weeks	11.4 (5–20)	4.5 (1–9.5)	40	5.5 (2–17)	48	1.0	9	0.4	3
1 month	10.8 (5–19.5)	3.8 (1–8.5)	35	6.0 (2.5–16.5)	56	0.7	7	0.3	3
6 months	11.9 (6–17.5)	3.8 (1–8.5)	32	7.3 (4–13.5)	61	0.6	5	0.3	3
1 year	11.4 (6–17.5)	3.5 (1.5–8.5)	31	7.0 (4–10.5)	61	0.6	5	0.3	3
2 years	10.6 (6–17)	3.5 (1.5–8.5)	33	6.3 (3–9.5)	59	0.5	5	0.3	3
4 years	9.1 (5.5–15.5)	3.8 (1.5–8.5)	42	4.5 (2–8)	50	0.5	5	0.3	3
6 years	8.5 (5–14.5)	4.3 (1.5–8)	51	3.5 (1.5–7)	42	0.4	5	0.2	3
8 years	8.3 (4.5–13.5)	4.4 (1.5–8)	53	3.3 (1.5–6.8)	39	0.4	4	0.2	2
10 years	8.1 (4.5–13.5)	4.4 (1.5–8.5)	54	3.1 (1.5–6.5)	38	0.4	4	0.2	2
16 years	7.8 (4.5–13.0)	4.4 (1.8–8)	57	2.8 (1.2–5.2)	35	0.4	5	0.2	3
21 years	7.4 (4.5–11.0)	4.4 (1.8–7.7)	59	2.5 (1–4.8)	34	0.3	4	0.2	3

[a]Numbers of leukocytes are $\times 10^3/\mu L$; ranges are estimates of 95% confidence limits; percentages refer to differential counts.

[b]Neutrophils include band cells at all ages and a small number of metamyelocytes and myelocytes in the first few days of life.

Adapted from Cairo MS, Brauho F. Blood and blood-forming tissues. In: Randolph AM, ed. *Pediatrics*. 21st ed. McGraw-Hill; 2003.

IX. ADDITIONAL RESOURCES

A. Medications to Avoid With G6PD Deficiency: https://www.g6pd.org/en/G6PDDeficiency/SafeUnsafe.aspx

B. Medications Associated With Thrombocytopenia: https://www.ouhsc.edu/platelets/ditp.html

C. Anemia Algorithm App: Created for Adult Patients but Provides Useful Framework for Anemia Differential

REFERENCES

A complete list of references can be found online.

Chapter 15

Immunology and Allergy

Samantha E. Leong, MD, PhD

See additional content online.

I. ALLERGIC RHINITIS[1-6]

A. Epidemiology

1. Most common pediatric chronic medical condition: Prevalence in children up to 40%
2. Increases risk for recurrent otitis media, asthma, and acute and chronic sinusitis
3. Risk factors: Atopic family history, higher socioeconomic status, infant exposure to maternal smoking in utero and during early childhood, early personal history of atopic dermatitis and/or food allergy

B. Diagnosis

1. **History:**
   a. Allergen-driven mucosal inflammation leading to cyclical exacerbations or persistent symptoms
   b. Symptoms: Nasal (congestion, rhinorrhea, pruritus), ocular (pruritus, tearing), and postnasal drip (sore throat, cough)
   c. Patterns: Seasonal (depending on local allergens) versus perennial (year-round, often with seasonal peaks)
   d. Coexisting atopic diseases common (eczema, asthma, food allergy)
2. **Physical examination:**
   a. Allergic facies with shiners, mouth breathing, transverse nasal crease ("allergic salute"), accentuated lines below lower eyelids (Dennie-Morgan lines)
   b. May have swollen nasal turbinates
   c. Injected sclera with or without clear discharge, conjunctival cobblestoning
3. **Diagnostic studies:**
   a. Diagnosis can be made on clinical grounds; however, skin tests or allergen-specific IgE testing can identify specific sensitivities.
   b. Total IgE, peripheral blood eosinophil count, and imaging studies are not recommended due to poor specificity.

C. Differential Diagnosis

Vasomotor/nonallergic rhinitis (e.g., hypersensitivity to scents, alcohol, changes in climate), infectious rhinitis, adenoid hypertrophy, rhinitis medicamentosa (rebound rhinitis from prolonged use of nasal vasoconstrictors), sinusitis, nonallergic rhinitis with eosinophilia syndrome, nasal polyps

D. Management

1. **Allergen avoidance:**
   a. Relies on identification of triggers, most common of which are pollens, fungi, dust mites, insects, and animals
   b. High efficiency particulate air (HEPA) filter may be useful when animal allergens are a concern.
   c. Thorough housecleaning and allergy-proof bed coverings can be useful.

2. **Nasal irrigation with hypertonic saline:** Use distilled, sterile, or boiled water (at least 3 minutes) for homemade solutions.

3. **Pharmacotherapy** (Table 15.1)

TABLE 15.1

PHARMACOTHERAPY FOR MANAGEMENT OF ALLERGIC RHINITIS

Class of Agents (Examples)	Use	Adverse Effects
Oral antihistamines (e.g., cetirizine, levocetirizine, fexofenadine, loratadine, desloratadine)	First-line for mild or episodic symptoms or patients who cannot tolerate or refuse nasal sprays	Sedation and anticholinergic effects (second-generation preparations preferable to first-generation due to reduced central nervous system side effects)
Oral leukotriene inhibitors (e.g., montelukast)	Consider in patients not effectively treated with or intolerant of other therapies. More effective in combination with antihistamines	Serious neuropsychiatric events (e.g., suicidal thoughts and actions) have been reported.
Intranasal antihistamines (e.g., azelastine, olopatadine)	Effective for acute symptoms; faster onset of action than glucocorticoid nasal spray	Bitter taste, systemic absorption with potential for sedation
Intranasal corticosteroids (e.g., fluticasone, mometasone, budesonide, flunisolide, ciclesonide, and triamcinolone)	First-line for persistent or moderate-to-severe symptoms, as it is the most effective monotherapy for nasal congestion and ocular symptoms. Maximal therapeutic benefit when used over several days or weeks. No effect with as-needed use. Administration: Clear mucus crusting, point head slightly down, and direct nozzle away from septum aiming towards the side of the nostril.	Nasal irritation, sneezing, bleeding, and potential risk of reduced growth velocity and adrenal suppression at high doses, especially in patients on multiple steroid preparations. Growth monitoring recommended

15

Continued

TABLE 15.1

PHARMACOTHERAPY FOR MANAGEMENT OF ALLERGIC RHINITIS—CONT'D

Class of Agents (Examples)	Use	Adverse Effects
Intranasal combination agents (e.g., azelastine/ fluticasone)	Useful for moderate-to-severe allergic rhinitis. Additional efficacy in rapidity of onset and magnitude of symptom relief	As above for individual preparations
Ophthalmic agents: **Mast cell stabilizers** (e.g., cromolyn sodium, lodoxamide-tromethamine, nedocromil, pemirolast) **H1-antagonists and mast cell stabilizers** (e.g., alcaftadine, azelastine HCl, bepotastine, emedastine, epinastine, ketotifen fumarate, olopatadine)	Allergic conjunctivitis	Avoid use of steroids unless directed by an ophthalmologist.

4. **Immunotherapy:**
   a. Success rate is high when patients are chosen carefully and when performed by an allergy specialist.
   b. Consider when symptoms are inadequately controlled with medications and allergen avoidance.
   c. In addition to traditional subcutaneous immunotherapy, sublingual products have now been approved for several allergens.
   d. Not recommended for patients with poor adherence to therapy or those with poorly controlled asthma
   e. Not well studied in children younger than 5 years
   f. May reduce risk for future development of asthma, and treatment of allergic rhinitis may improve asthma control

II. FOOD ALLERGY[7-18]

A. Epidemiology

1. Prevalence is 6% to 8% in young children and 3% to 4% in adolescence with increasing worldwide prevalence.
2. Most common allergens in children: Milk, eggs, peanuts, tree nuts (e.g., cashew, walnut), soy, fish, shellfish, and wheat

B. Diagnosis (Fig. 15.1)

1. **History:**
   a. Identify specific foods and whether fresh vs. cooked.
   b. Establish timing and nature of reactions. Symptoms typically occur within minutes to hours of ingesting food.

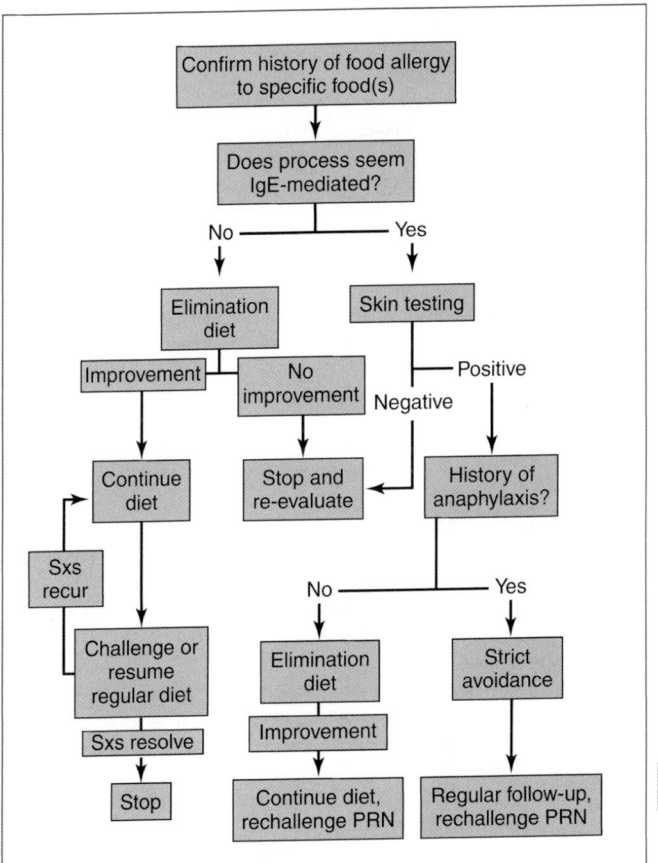

FIGURE 15.1

Evaluation and management of food allergy. *IgE,* Immunoglobulin E; *PRN,* as needed; *Sxs,* symptoms. (Data from Wood RA. The natural history of food allergy. *Pediatrics.* 2003;111:1631–1637.)

2. **Physical examination:**
   a. Often a combination of several syndromes
   b. **Anaphylaxis:** See Chapter 1.
   c. **Skin syndromes:**
      (1) **Urticaria/angioedema:**
         (a) Chronic urticaria is rarely related to food allergy.
         (b) Acute urticaria due to food allergy may be a risk factor for future anaphylaxis.
      (2) **Atopic dermatitis/eczema:**
         (a) Food allergy is more common in patients with atopic dermatitis.

      (b) Even if not apparent by history, at least one-third of children with moderate to severe atopic dermatitis have IgE-mediated food allergies.

  d. **Gastrointestinal syndromes:**

    (1) **Oral allergy syndrome:**

      (a) Pollen-associated food allergy caused by cross-reactivity of antibodies to pollens (e.g., apple and tree pollen)

      (b) Pruritus of oral mucosa after ingestion of certain fresh fruits and vegetables in patients with pollen allergies. Rarely results in edema of oral mucosa or progresses beyond mouth/throat

      (c) Inciting antigens are usually denatured by cooking.

    (2) **Allergic eosinophilic gastroenteritis, esophagitis:** See Chapter 12.

    (3) **Food protein–induced enterocolitis syndrome (FPIES):**

      (a) Presents in infancy

      (b) Vomiting and diarrhea (may contain blood); when severe, may lead to lethargy, dehydration, hypotension, acidosis

      (c) Most commonly associated with milk and soy but may occur with a wide variety of foods (e.g., rice, oat, fruits, and vegetables)

    (4) **Infantile proctocolitis:**

      (a) Confined to distal colon and can present with diarrhea or blood-streaked and mucus-containing stools

      (b) Symptoms usually resolve within 72 hours of stopping offending agent; rarely leads to anemia

3. **Diagnostic studies:**

  a. Testing can demonstrate sensitization (allergen-specific IgE). A positive result only means sensitization and not necessarily allergy (must correlate with clinical history and exam).

  b. **Skin testing:**

    (1) Skin-prick test has poor positive predictive value but very good negative predictive value.

    (2) Patient must not be taking antihistamines during week of testing.

    (3) Widespread skin conditions (e.g., dermatographism, urticaria, severe eczema) may limit ability to perform skin tests.

  c. **Measurement of allergen-specific IgE:**

    (1) Similar to skin tests, it has poor positive predictive value and excellent negative predictive value.

    (2) Levels above a certain range (variable among different antigens) have increasing positive predictive value.

    (3) Useful in patients with dermatologic conditions that preclude skin testing

    (4) Not affected by use of antihistamines

    (5) Component testing (measuring IgE to specific food proteins rather than crude extracts) may improve diagnostic accuracy for peanut, hazelnut, and possibly other foods.

  d. **Oral food challenges:**

    (1) Can verify clinical reactivity to a specific food allergen or document that a food allergy has been outgrown

    (2) Must be performed under close medical supervision with emergency medications readily available

    (3) Patient must not be taking antihistamines during week of testing

    (4) Most accurate when double-blinded using graded doses of disguised food

  e. **Trial elimination diet:**

    (1) Helpful if improvement with removal of food from diet

    (2) Especially useful in infants and essential for non-IgE-mediated food allergy

C. Differential Diagnosis

1. **Food intolerance:** Nonimmunologic, based on toxins or other properties of foods leading to adverse effects

2. **Malabsorption syndromes:**
   a. Cystic fibrosis, celiac disease (see Chapter 12), and lactase deficiency
   b. Gastrointestinal malformations

D. Management

1. **Allergen avoidance:**
   a. Most important intervention for all types of food allergy
   b. Patients must pay close attention to food ingredients. Implement an *"If you can't read it, you can't eat it"* approach to avoid risky unlabeled foods.
   c. Nutritional counseling and regular growth monitoring are recommended.

2. **Anaphylaxis:**
   a. See Chapter 1 for management of anaphylaxis.
   b. Prescribe epinephrine autoinjector for all at-risk patients.
   c. Counsel families to always have epinephrine autoinjectors readily available. Counsel to call 9-1-1 if using.
   d. Counsel on possibility of symptom recurrence after initial resolution, which may require a second dose. Autoinjector two-packs should not be divided between locations (e.g., households, school).
   e. Develop Anaphylaxis Action Plan indicating specific allergies, symptoms for which to observe, and medications to be administered.
   f. Make school aware of Anaphylaxis Action Plan and ensure they can administer lifesaving medications.

3. **Non-anaphylactic angioedema/urticaria:**
   a. Antihistamines or corticosteroids, based on severity and duration of symptoms
   b. Omalizumab approved for treatment of chronic urticaria

4. **Atopic dermatitis:** Symptomatic control (see Chapter 8)

5. **Food-specific immunotherapy:**
   a. Used to induce clinical desensitization to specific allergens
   b. Oral immunotherapy (OIT): Exposure to gradually increased quantity of ingested food (e.g., Palforzia is the first FDA-approved OIT for peanut allergy)
   c. Other strategies (sublingual, epicutaneous, use of monoclonal antibody drugs as adjuncts or monotherapy) are under investigation.

E. Natural History

1. About 50% of milk, egg, soy, and wheat allergies are outgrown by school age.
2. Peanut, tree nut, and shellfish allergies are outgrown only in 10% to 20%.
3. Skin tests and allergen-specific IgE may remain positive, even though symptoms resolve.

F. Prevention

1. For introducing new foods to infants with high-risk atopic disease, there is no evidence that delaying or avoiding common allergenic foods prevents atopic disease.
2. Based on studies that showed early, sustained introduction of peanut reduced peanut allergy frequency, AAP recommends early introduction of peanut-based foods (e.g., thinned peanut butter, peanut snacks, peanut flour, peanut butter powder) at 4 to 6 months in highest-risk infants (severe eczema and/or egg allergy) after testing.
3. Emerging evidence suggests that early introduction of other common allergenic foods may be protective against the development of food allergies.

III. DRUG ALLERGY[19-21]

A. Definition

1. **Drug allergy:** Immunologically mediated response to an agent in a sensitized person
2. **Drug intolerance:** Undesirable pharmacologic effect
3. Although 10% of patients report penicillin allergy, after evaluation, about 90% of these individuals can tolerate penicillin.

B. Diagnosis

1. Cutaneous manifestations are the most common presentation for drug allergic reactions.
2. **Diagnostic studies:** Penicillin is the only drug for which standardized skin testing reagents and procedures have been validated. Skin testing or supervised graded dose challenge may be done with caution for other medications, but results must be carefully considered in the context of the clinical picture, as both false positive and false negative results are common.

C. Management (Fig. 15.2)

1. **Avoidance:** When able, use alternative therapy.
2. **Desensitization:** Progressive administration of an allergenic substance to render immune system less reactive
3. **Graded challenge:** Administration of progressively increasing doses of a drug until full dose is reached; does not modify a patient's response to the drug but is used to optimize safety when the history and test results are not completely reassuring

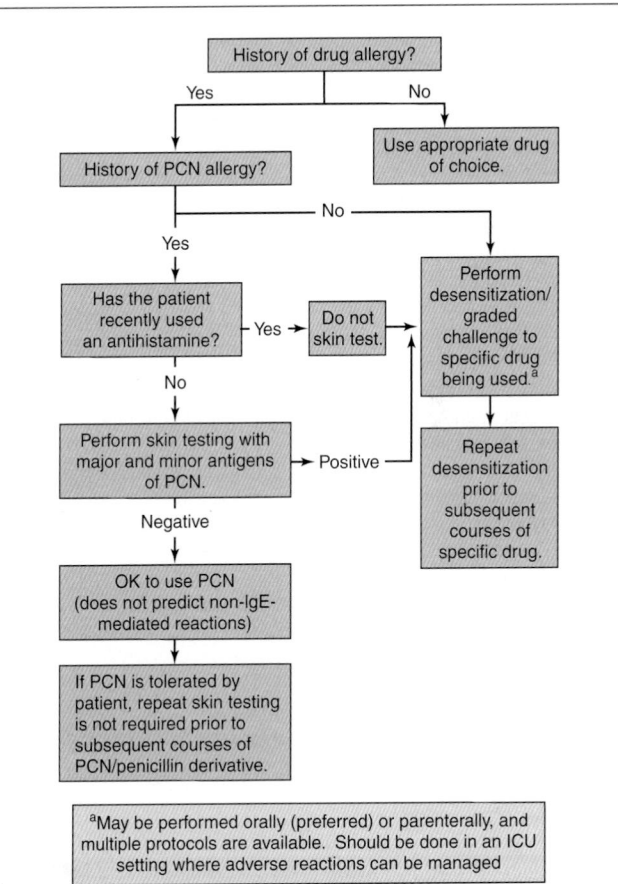

FIGURE 15.2

Evaluation and management of penicillin allergy. *ICU*, Intensive care unit; *IgE*, immunoglobulin E; *PCN*, penicillin. (Adapted from Mirakian R, Leech SC, Krishna MT, et al. Management of allergy to penicillins and other beta-lactams. *Clin Exp Allergy.* 2015;45:300.)

IV. IMMUNODEFICIENCY[22-27]

A. Clinical Presentation

1. Increased susceptibility to infection
   a. Chronic/recurrent infections
      (1) Four or more new ear infections within 1 year

    (2) Two or more serious sinus infections within 1 year

    (3) Two or more pneumonias within 1 year

    (4) Recurrent tissue or organ abscesses

    (5) Persistent thrush in mouth or fungal infection of skin

  b. Severe infections

    (1) Bacterial meningitis

    (2) Pneumonia with empyema

    (3) Sepsis in the absence of a known risk (e.g., indwelling vascular catheter)

    (4) Two or more months of antibiotics with little effect

    (5) Need for intravenous antibiotics to clear infections

  c. Opportunistic infections

    (1) *Pneumocystis jirovecii*

    (2) *Mycobacterium avium* cellulare

2. Autoimmune or inflammatory diseases

  a. Defects in immunity may also impair ability to discriminate self and non-self, manifesting as autoimmunity.

  b. May be limited to single target cells (e.g., hemolytic anemia, immune thrombocytopenia) or organs (e.g., thyroiditis)

  c. May involve multiple target organs or systems (e.g., systemic lupus erythematosus, vasculitis, arthritis)

3. Syndrome complex

  a. Wiskott-Aldrich syndrome: Thrombocytopenia, eczema

  b. DiGeorge syndrome: Congenital heart disease, facial dysmorphism, hypoparathyroidism

4. Other considerations

  a. Failure to gain weight or grow normally

  b. Family history of immunodeficiency or unexplained early deaths

  c. Lymphopenia in infancy

  d. Complications from a live vaccine

B. Evaluation (Table 15.2)

V. IMMUNOGLOBULIN THERAPY[28-34]

A. Intravenous Immunoglobulin (IVIG)

1. Indications:

  a. Replacement therapy for antibody-deficient disorders:

    (1) Children with severe hypogammaglobulinemia (<100 mg/dL) may benefit from a higher total *loading* dose in two separate doses a few days apart, followed by standard dosing every 3 to 4 weeks

    (2) Useful in human immunodeficiency virus (HIV), antibody deficiency (IgG concentration <400 mg/dL from failure to form antibodies to common antigens), recurrent serious bacterial infections, or prior to measles prophylaxis

EVALUATION OF SUSPECTED IMMUNODEFICIENCY

Suspected Functional Abnormality	Clinical Findings	Initial Tests	More Advanced Tests
Humoral (e.g., common variable immunodeficiency, X-linked agammaglobulinemia, IgA deficiency)	Sinopulmonary and systemic infections (pyogenic bacteria) Enteric infections (enterovirus, other viruses, *Giardia* spp.) Autoimmune diseases (immune thrombocytopenia, hemolytic anemia, inflammatory bowel disease)	Immunoglobulin levels (IgG, IgM, IgA) Antibody levels to T-cell-dependent protein antigens (e.g., tetanus or pneumococcal conjugate vaccines) Antibody levels to T-cell-independent polysaccharide antigens in a child ≥2 years (e.g., pneumococcal polysaccharide vaccine, such as Pneumovax)	B-cell enumeration Immunofixation electrophoresis
Cell-mediated immunity (e.g., severe combined immunodeficiency, DiGeorge syndrome)	Pneumonia (pyogenic bacteria, fungi, *Pneumocystis jiroveci*, viruses)	TRECs newborn screening[a] Total lymphocyte counts HIV ELISA/Western blot/PCR	T-cell enumeration (CD3, CD4, CD8) In vitro T-cell proliferation to mitogens, antigens, or allogeneic cells Chromosomal microarray or FISH 22q11 for DiGeorge deletion
Phagocytosis (e.g., chronic granulomatous disease (CGD), leukocyte adhesion deficiency, Chédiak-Higashi syndrome)	Cutaneous infections, abscesses, lymphadenitis (staphylococci, enteric bacteria, fungi, mycobacteria) Poor wound healing	WBC/neutrophil count and morphology	CGD: Nitroblue tetrazolium (NBT) test or dihydrorhodamine (DHR) reduction test Chemotactic assay Phagocytic assay
Spleen	Bacteremia/hematogenous infection (pneumococcus, other streptococci, *Neisseria* spp.)	Peripheral blood smear for Howell-Jolly bodies Hemoglobin electrophoresis (HbSS)	Technetium-99 spleen scan or sonogram
Complement	Bacterial sepsis and other bloodborne infections (encapsulated bacteria, especially *Neisseria* spp.) Lupus, glomerulonephritis Angioedema	CH50 (total hemolytic complement)	Alternative pathway assay (AH50) Mannose-binding lectin level Individual complement component assays

[a]Newborn screening using TRECs has now been implemented in multiple states. TRECs identify lymphopenia in children and prompt further testing for SCID or other immunodeficiencies associated with lymphopenia. *ELISA,* Enzyme-linked immunosorbent assay; *FISH,* fluorescent in situ hybridization; *HIV,* human immunodeficiency virus; *PCR,* polymerase chain reaction; *TRECs,* T-cell receptor excision circles; *WBC,* white blood cell.

From Lederman HM. Clinical presentation of primary immunodeficiency diseases. In: McMillan J, ed. *Oski's Pediatrics.* Lippincott Williams & Wilkins; 2006:2441–2444.

b. Immune thrombocytopenic purpura (see Chapter 14):
  (1) Initially given on a single day or in divided doses over 2 to 5 consecutive days
  (2) Maintenance dose given every 3 to 6 weeks based on clinical response and platelet count
c. Bone marrow transplantation:
  (1) Adjust dosing to maintain trough IgG level of at least 400 mg/dL.
  (2) May decrease incidence of infection and death but not acute graft-versus-host disease
d. Other indications:
  (1) Kawasaki disease (see Chapter 7).
  (2) Multi-system inflammatory syndrome in children (MIS-C) (see Chapter 7).
  (3) Guillain-Barré syndrome
  (4) Refractory dermatomyositis and polymyositis
  (5) Chronic inflammatory demyelinating polyneuropathy

2. **Precautions and adverse reactions:**
  a. Severe systemic symptoms (hemodynamic changes, respiratory difficulty, and anaphylaxis)
  b. Less-severe systemic reactions (headache, myalgia, fever, chills, nausea, and vomiting)
    (1) Decrease infusion rate and/or pre-medicate with intravenous corticosteroids and/or antipyretics.
    (2) Can progress to aseptic meningitis syndrome
  c. Acute renal failure (increased risk with preexisting renal insufficiency and with sucrose-containing IVIG)
  d. Acute venous thrombosis (increased risk with sucrose-containing IVIG)
  e. Use with caution in patients with confirmed undetectable IgA levels (e.g., patients with partial B-cell immunodeficiencies or familial IgA deficiency), as antibodies against IgA may trigger anaphylactic reaction.

B. Intramuscular Immunoglobulin (IMIG)

1. **Prophylaxis indications:** Hepatitis A, measles, rubella, rabies, and varicella-zoster (see Chapter 16)
2. **Administration:**
  a. No more than 5 mL should be given at one site in large child/adolescent, and 1 to 3 mL for smaller children/infants.
  b. Administration of greater than 15 mL at one time is essentially never warranted.
  c. Peak serum levels achieved by 48 hours; immune effect lasts 3 to 4 weeks.
3. **Precautions and adverse reactions:**
  a. Similar to IVIG (discussed previously)
  b. Local reaction at injection site increases with repeated use

c. Intravenous or intradermal use of IMIG is absolutely contraindicated due to high risk for anaphylactoid reactions.

C. Subcutaneous Immunoglobulin

1. **Indication:** Replacement therapy for antibody deficiency
2. **Administration:**
   a. See the Formulary for dosages and administration instructions.
   b. Larger doses can be given simultaneously in multiple sites or more frequently than once weekly.
   c. Using the same areas for injections improves tolerability.
   d. **Considerations:** Does not require venous access or special nursing (parents can administer), but may require multiple needlesticks in larger children, depending on the volume to be infused
3. **Precautions and adverse reactions:**
   a. Systemic side effects are rare because of the small volumes given and the slow absorption rate.
   b. Local redness and swelling are expected and generally decrease with every infusion.

D. Specific Immunoglobulins

1. Hyperimmune globulins:
   a. Prepared from donors with high titers of specific antibodies
   b. Includes hepatitis B immune globulin, varicella-zoster immune globulin, cytomegalovirus immune globulin, Rho(D) immune globulin, botulism immune globulin, and others
2. **Monoclonal antibody preparations** (rituximab, palivizumab, and others)

E. Vaccination Timing

See Chapter 16 for discussion of timing of routine vaccination after immunoglobulin administration.

VI. IMMUNOLOGIC REFERENCE VALUES

A. Serum IgG, IgM, IgA, and IgE Levels (Table 15.3)
B. Serum IgG, IgM, IgA, and IgE Levels for Low Birth Weight Preterm Infants (Table 15.4)
C. Lymphocyte Enumeration (Table 15.5)
D. Serum Complement Levels (Table 15.6)

TABLE 15.3

SERUM IMMUNOGLOBULIN LEVELS[a]

Age	IgG (mg/dL)	IgM (mg/dL)	IgA (mg/dL)	IgE (IU/mL)
Cord blood (term)	1121 (636—1606)	13 (6.3—25)	2.3 (1.4—3.6)	0.22 (0.04—1.28)
1 month	503 (251—906)	45 (20—87)	13 (1.3—53)	
6 weeks				0.69 (0.08—6.12)
2 months	365 (206—601)	46 (17—105)	15 (2.8—47)	
3 months	334 (176—581)	49 (24—89)	17 (4.6—46)	0.82 (0.18—3.76)
4 months	343 (196—558)	55 (27—101)	23 (4.4—73)	
5 months	403 (172—814)	62 (33—108)	31 (8.1—84)	
6 months	407 (215—704)	62 (35—102)	25 (8.1—68)	2.68 (0.44—16.3)
7—9 months	475 (217—904)	80 (34—126)	36 (11—90)	2.36 (0.76—7.31)
10—12 months	594 (294—1069)	82 (41—149)	40 (16—84)	
1 year	679 (345—1213)	93 (43—173)	44 (14—106)	3.49 (0.80—15.2)
2 years	685 (424—1051)	95 (48—168)	47 (14—123)	3.03 (0.31—29.5)
3 years	728 (441—1135)	104 (47—200)	66 (22—159)	1.80 (0.19—16.9)
4—5 years	780 (463—1236)	99 (43—196)	68 (25—154)	8.58 (1.07—68.9)[b]
6—8 years	915 (633—1280)	107 (48—207)	90 (33—202)	12.89 (1.03—161.3)[c]
9—10 years	1007 (608—1572)	121 (52—242)	113 (45—236)	23.6 (0.98—570.6)[d]
14 years				20.07 (2.06—195.2)
Adult	994 (639—1349)	156 (56—352)	171 (70—312)	13.2 (1.53—114)

[a]Numbers in parentheses are the 95% confidence intervals (CIs).

[b]IgE data for 4 years.

[c]IgE data for 7 years.

[d]IgE data for 10 years.

Data from Kjellman NM, Johansson SG, Roth A. Serum IgE levels in healthy children quantified by a sandwich technique (PRIST). *Clin Allergy.* 1976;6:51—59; Jolliff CR, Cost KM, Stivrins PC, et al. Reference intervals for serum IgG, IgA, IgM, C3, and C4 as determined by rate nephelometry. *Clin Chem.* 1982;28:126—128; Zetterström O, Johansson SG. IgE concentrations measured by PRIST in serum of healthy adults and in patients with respiratory allergy: a diagnostic approach. *Allergy.* 1981;36:537—547.

TABLE 15.4

SERUM IMMUNOGLOBULIN LEVELS FOR LOW BIRTH WEIGHT PRETERM INFANTS

Age (months)	Plasma Ig Concentrations in 25- to 28-Weeks' Gestation Infants				Plasma Ig Concentrations in 29- to 32-Weeks' Gestation Infants			
	IgG (mg/dL)[a]	IgM (mg/dL)[a]	IgA (mg/dL)[a]		IgG (mg/dL)[a]	IgM (mg/dL)[a]	IgA (mg/dL)[a]	
0.25	251 (114–552)	7.6 (1.3–43.3)	1.2 (0.07–20.8)		368 (186–728)	9.1 (2.1–39.4)	0.6 (0.04–1.0)	
0.5	202 (91–446)	14.1 (3.5–56.1)	3.1 (0.09–10.7)		275 (119–637)	13.9 (4.7–41)	0.9 (0.01–7.5)	
1.0	158 (57–437)	12.7 (3.0–53.3)	4.5 (0.65–30.9)		209 (97–452)	14.4 (6.3–33)	1.9 (0.3–12.0)	
1.5	134 (59–307)	16.2 (4.4–59.2)	4.3 (0.9–20.9)		156 (69–352)	15.4 (5.5–43.2)	2.2 (0.7–6.5)	
2.0	89 (58–136)	16.0 (5.3–48.9)	4.1 (1.5–11.1)		123 (64–237)	15.2 (4.9–46.7)	3.0 (1.1–8.3)	
3	60 (23–156)	13.8 (5.3–36.1)	3.0 (0.6–15.6)		104 (41–268)	16.3 (7.1–37.2)	3.6 (0.8–15.4)	
4	82 (32–210)	22.2 (11.2–43.9)	6.8 (1.0–47.8)		128 (39–425)	26.5 (7.7–91.2)	9.8 (2.5–39.3)	
6	159 (56–455)	41.3 (8.3–205)	9.7 (3.0–31.2)		179 (51–634)	29.3 (10.5–81.5)	12.3 (2.7–57.1)	
8–10	273 (94–794)	41.8 (31.1–56.1)	9.5 (0.9–98.6)		280 (140–561)	34.7 (17–70.8)	20.9 (8.3–53)	

[a]Geometric mean (numbers in parentheses are ±2 SD).

From Ballow M, Cates KL, Rowe JC, et al. Development of the immune system in very low birth weight (less than 1500 g) premature infants: concentrations of plasma immunoglobulins and patterns of infections. *Pediatr Res.* 1986;9:899–904.

15

TABLE 15.5

T AND B LYMPHOCYTES IN PERIPHERAL BLOOD

Age	CD3 (Total T Cell) Count[a] (%)[b]	CD4 Count[a] (%)[b]	CD8 Count[a] (%)[b]	CD19 (B Cell) Count[a] (%)[b]
0–3 months	2.50–5.50 (53–84)	1.60–4.00 (35–64)	0.56–1.70 (12–28)	0.30–2.00 (6–32)
3–6 months	2.50–5.60 (51–77)	1.80–4.00 (35–56)	0.59–1.60 (12–23)	0.43–3.00 (11–41)
6–12 months	1.90–5.90 (49–76)	1.40–4.30 (31–56)	0.50–1.70 (12–24)	0.61–2.60 (14–37)
1–2 years	2.10–6.20 (53–75)	1.30–3.40 (32–51)	0.62–2.00 (14–30)	0.72–2.60 (16–35)
2–6 years	1.40–3.70 (56–75)	0.70–2.20 (28–47)	0.49–1.30 (16–30)	0.39–1.40 (14–33)
6–12 years	1.20–2.60 (60–76)	0.65–1.50 (31–47)	0.37–1.10 (18–35)	0.27–0.86 (13–27)
12–18 years	1.00–2.20 (56–84)	0.53–1.30 (31–52)	0.33–0.92 (18–35)	0.11–0.57 (6–23)
Adult[c]	0.70–2.10 (55–83)	0.30–1.40 (28–57)	0.20–0.90 (10–39)	

[a]Absolute counts (number of cells per microliter $\times 10^{-3}$).

[b]Normal values (10th to 90th percentile).

[c]From Comans-Bitter WM, de Groot R, van den Beemd R, et al. Immunotyping of blood lymphocytes in childhood. Reference values for lymphocyte subpopulations. *J Pediatr.* 1997;130:388–393.

From Shearer WT, Rosenblatt HM, Gelman RS, et al. Lymphocyte subsets in healthy children from birth through 18 years of age: the Pediatric AIDS Clinical Trials Group P1009 study. *J Allergy Clin Immunol.* 2003;112:973–980.

TABLE 15.6

SERUM COMPLEMENT LEVELS[a]

Age	C3 (mg/dL)	C4 (mg/dL)
Cord blood (term)	83 (57–116)	13 (6.6–23)
1 month	83 (53–124)	14 (7.0–25)
2 months	96 (59–149)	15 (7.4–28)
3 months	94 (64–131)	16 (8.7–27)
4 months	107 (62–175)	19 (8.3–38)
5 months	107 (64–167)	18 (7.1–36)
6 months	115 (74–171)	21 (8.6–42)
7–9 months	113 (75–166)	20 (9.5–37)
10–12 months	126 (73–180)	22 (12–39)
1 year	129 (84–174)	23 (12–40)
2 years	120 (81–170)	19 (9.2–34)
3 years	117 (77–171)	20 (9.7–36)
4–5 years	121 (86–166)	21 (13–32)
6–8 years	118 (88–155)	20 (12–32)
9–10 years	134 (89–195)	22 (10–40)
Adult	125 (83–177)	28 (15–45)

[a]Numbers in parentheses are the 95% confidence intervals (CIs).

Modified from Jolliff CR, Cost KM, Stivrins PC, et al. Reference intervals for serum IgG, IgA, IgM, C3, and C4 as determined by rate nephelometry. *Clin Chem.* 1982;28:126–128.

REFERENCES

A complete list of references can be found online.

Chapter 16

Immunoprophylaxis

Lindsay Sheets, MD, MPH

🌐 See additional content online.

I. COMMON TYPES OF VACCINES ADMINISTERED TO CHILDREN[1]

A. Inactivated Vaccines
1. Killed version of pathogen
2. Do not provide immunity as robust or long-lasting as live vaccines, so may require several doses over time
3. Examples: Hepatitis A, influenza, injectable polio, rabies

B. Live, Attenuated Vaccines
1. Weakened (or attenuated) form of pathogen
2. Creates a robust and long-lasting immune response
3. Examples: Measles, mumps, rubella (MMR), rotavirus, smallpox, varicella, yellow fever, oral polio (no longer used in United States)

C. Subunit, Recombinant, Polysaccharide, and Conjugate Vaccines
1. Uses specific components of pathogen, such as protein, sugar, or capsid
2. Robust immune response but booster may be required for ongoing protection
3. Examples: *Haemophilus influenzae*, hepatitis B virus, human papillomavirus, *Bordetella pertussis* (pertussis), pneumococcal polysaccharide and conjugate vaccines, meningococcal polysaccharide and conjugate vaccines

D. Toxoid Vaccines
1. Use toxin from pathogen to create immunity to parts of pathogen that cause disease, instead of to entire pathogen itself.
2. May need booster shots
3. Examples: *Corynebacterium diphtheriae* (diphtheria), *Clostridium tetani* (tetanus)

E. mRNA Vaccines[2,3]
1. Messenger RNA enters host cell and is translated by ribosomes so that host cells produce proteins and subsequently induce antibody response.
   a. Example: Spike protein against SARS-CoV-2 virus
2. Noninfectious, nonintegrating platform. mRNA degrades quickly.

II. IMMUNIZATION SCHEDULES

A. Routine Vaccines for Children in the United States

1. Table 16.1: Routine Vaccines for Children and Adolescents in the United States[4]
2. All schedules: website—https://www.cdc.gov/vaccines/schedules/hcp/imz/child-adolescent.html; phone app—https://www.cdc.gov/vaccines/schedules/hcp/schedule-app.html#download
3. Schedules updated annually and put forth by Advisory Committee on Immunization Practices (ACIP)[5] and approved by Centers for Disease Control and Prevention (CDC) and American Academy of Pediatrics (AAP)
4. For the most recent guidelines on COVID-19 vaccination in pediatric patients, see: https://www.cdc.gov/coronavirus/2019-ncov/vaccines/recommendations/children-teens.html

B. Nonroutine Vaccines for Children in the United States[6]

1. For details on vaccines not routinely administered in the United States, including bacille Calmette-Guérin (BCG; tuberculosis vaccine), Japanese encephalitis, rabies, typhoid, and yellow fever, see Table 16.2.
2. For information on other vaccines licensed but not routinely distributed, including anthrax and smallpox, see https://emergency.cdc.gov/bioterrorism/

III. IMMUNIZATION GUIDELINES

A. Vaccine Informed Consent

1. The most recent Vaccine Information Statements (VISs) should be provided to patient (nonminor) or parent/guardian, with documentation of version date and date of administration.
2. VISs can be found at the following: https://www.cdc.gov/vaccines/hcp/vis/current-vis.html
3. Multi-vaccine VISs for DTaP, *Haemophilus influenzae* type b (Hib), HepB, polio, and PCV13 can be used when two or more of these vaccines are administered during the same visit.

B. Vaccine Administration

1. For information on vaccine storage, handling, and administration, see https://www.cdc.gov/vaccines/hcp/admin/
2. See Chapter 4 for details on intramuscular and subcutaneous administration procedures.
3. Simultaneous administration
   a. Routine childhood vaccines are safe and effective when administered simultaneously at different sites. There is no maximum number of vaccines that can be administered during the same visit.
   b. Spread them out in location on the body, at least 1 cm apart.
4. Combination vaccines reduce number of injections.

TABLE 16.1

ROUTINE VACCINES FOR CHILDREN AND ADOLESCENTS IN THE UNITED STATES

Disease	Vaccine Description	Dose and Administration	Side Effects[a]
Diphtheria, tetanus, pertussis	DTaP: Diphtheria and tetanus toxoids with acellular pertussis vaccine (preferred vaccine for children <7 years) DT: Diphtheria and tetanus toxoids without pertussis vaccine	0.5 mL IM × 5 doses (2, 4, 6, 15–18 months, and 4–6 years) • If at least 6 months have passed since dose #3, dose #4 may be given as early as 12 months of age. • If dose #4 inadvertently given ≥4 months but <6 months after dose #3 to a child ≥12 months old, it does NOT need to be repeated. • If dose #4 administered when child was ≥4 years old, dose #5 not necessary. Use DT for age <7 years if pertussis vaccine is contraindicated.	Mild: Injection site reaction (common), fever ≥38.0°C, drowsiness, fussiness/inconsolable crying, decreased appetite Severe: Allergic reactions, persistent crying >3 hours, hypotonic–hyporesponsive episode, seizures, and body temperature >40.5°C (all rare with DTaP)
	Tdap: Tetanus and diphtheria toxoids with acellular pertussis vaccine Td: Tetanus toxoid with reduced dose of diphtheria toxoid	0.5 mL IM Tdap × 1 dose at 11–12 years, then booster with Tdap or Td every 10 years after • Tdap may be administered regardless of interval since last tetanus and diphtheria toxoid–containing vaccine. • 1 dose during each pregnancy (ideally 27–36 weeks' gestation) Use Td for age ≥7 years if pertussis vaccine is contraindicated.	
Haemophilus influenzae type B (Hib)	Hib PRP-OMP: Capsular polysaccharide antigen conjugated to outer membrane protein of *Neisseria meningitidis* Hib PRP-T: Capsular polysaccharide antigen conjugated to tetanus toxoid	0.5 mL IM × 3–4 doses depending on which formulation used • Recommend 4 doses of PRP-T (2, 4, 6 and 12–15 months) or 3 doses of PRP-OMP (2, 4 and 12–15 months) • Should not be given prior to 6 weeks of age	Local injection site reaction (common), drowsiness, fussiness, restlessness, decreased appetite

Continued

16

TABLE 16.1

ROUTINE VACCINES FOR CHILDREN AND ADOLESCENTS IN THE UNITED STATES—CONT'D

Disease	Vaccine Description	Dose and Administration	Side Effects[a]
		• No need to use same formulation for entire series • See Section V.B.1 for children with high-risk conditions.	
Hepatitis A (HepA)	Inactivated virus purified from human fibroblast cultures	0.5 mL IM × 2 doses (12–23 months with minimum 6-month interval between doses) Use 1 mL IM per dose if age ≥19 years. Adolescents ≥18 years eligible for combination Hep A/Hep B vaccine series International travel for unvaccinated children: • Age 6–11 months: 1 dose before departure and revaccinate with 2 doses starting at 12 months • Age ≥12 months: 1 dose before departure	Local injection site reaction (common), fever ≥38.0°C, drowsiness, irritability, headache
Hepatitis B (HepB)	Produced by recombinant DNA technology; monovalent formulations may be used interchangeably	0.5 mL IM × 3 doses (birth, 1–2 months, 6–18 months) • All term newborns should receive monovalent HepB vaccine within 24 hours of birth. • 4 doses acceptable if combined vaccines used after birth dose • See Section V.C for details regarding preterm infants. Use 1 mL IM per dose if age ≥20 years or giving 2-dose adolescent series (age 11–15 years). • Adolescents ≥18 years eligible for combination Hep A/Hep B vaccine series	Pain at injection site, fatigue, fever ≥38.0°C

Human papilloma virus (HPV)	HPV9: Protects against HPV types 6, 11, 16, 18, 31, 33, 45, 52, and 58 HPV4 and bivalent HPV vaccines not distributed in United States	0.5 mL IM × 2 doses (separated by 6–12 months) at age 11–12 years • Series may be started at age 9; consider if history of sexual abuse or assault. • If first dose at age ≥15 years or immunocompromised, give 3 doses at intervals of 0, 1–2, and 6 months.	Pain and local injection site reaction (common), headache. Recommended to observe for syncope for 15 min after administration
Influenza NOTE: Influenza vaccine recommendations change annually; see CDC for up-to-date recommendations.[42]	LAIV4: Intranasal live, attenuated quadrivalent vaccine for healthy children age ≥2 years IIV4: Subvirion or purified surface-antigen quadrivalent vaccines for age ≥6 months ccIIV4: Cell culture-based quadrivalent vaccine for age ≥4 years RIV4: Recombinant quadrivalent vaccine for age ≥18 years	0.2 mL intranasally (0.1 mL per nare) 0.25–0.5 mL IM if age 6–35 months (see manufacturer recommendations) 0.5 mL IM if age ≥3 years • Give annually starting at age 6 months • Children ≤8 years who have not previously received ≥2 total doses (regardless of interval) should receive 2 doses separated by ≥4 weeks.	Local injection site reaction, fever within 24 hr after immunization in children <2 years, drowsiness, irritability, myalgia, headache, GI symptoms Possible association with GBS (rare: 1–2 cases per million doses)
Measles, mumps, rubella (MMR)	Combination vaccine composed of live, attenuated viruses	0.5 mL SQ × 2 doses (12–15 months, 4–6 years) • Required minimum 4-week interval between doses • Children >12 years old not eligible for vaccine International travel: • Age 6–11 months: 1 dose prior to departure, then revaccinate with 2 doses—dose #1 at 12–15 months, dose #2 ≥4 weeks later • Age ≥12 months (and unvaccinated): 2 doses at least 4 weeks apart prior to departure	High fever (>39.4°C) usually 6–12 days after immunization, and may last ≤5 days; febrile seizures may occur 5–12 days after the first dose (rare) Other reactions include transient rash transient thrombocytopenia (1 in 22,000–40,000), encephalitis, and encephalopathy (<1 in 1 million)

Continued

16

TABLE 16.1

ROUTINE VACCINES FOR CHILDREN AND ADOLESCENTS IN THE UNITED STATES—CONT'D

Disease	Vaccine Description	Dose and Administration	Side Effects[a]
N. meningitidis (Meningococcal)	MenACWY-D (Menactra): Quadrivalent (serogroups A, C, Y, W) polysaccharide diphtheria toxoid conjugate for age ≥9 months MenACWY-CRM (Menveo): Quadrivalent (serogroups A, C, Y, W) oligosaccharide diphtheria conjugate for age ≥2 months	0.5 mL IM × 2 doses (11–12 years, 16 years) • If dose #1 not given until age ≥16 years, dose #2 not needed • See Section V.B.2 for children with high-risk conditions. International travel: See CDC website for recommendations based on vaccine formulation and age of patient.	Local injection site reaction, sleepiness, malaise, headache, nausea, diarrhea
	MenB-4C (Bexero): Serogroup B vaccine for age 10–25 years MenB-FHbp (Trumemba): Serogroup B vaccine for age 10–25 years	0.5 mL IM × 2 doses (preferred age 16–18 years) • Recommend shared decision-making for adolescents aged 16–23 years who are not at increased risk. • Dose intervals (vaccines not interchangeable): MenB-4C—1 month; MenB-FHbp—6 months • See Section V.B.2 for children with high-risk conditions.	Local injection-site reaction, headache, myalgia, arthralgia, nausea
Polio	IPV: Inactivated injectable vaccine containing 3 types of poliovirus NOTE: OPV, a live, attenuated oral vaccine, is no longer available in the United States; see Table 16.2	0.5 mL IM/SQ × 4 doses (2, 4, 6–18 months, 4–6 years) • If 4 or more doses of IPV are administered before the fourth birthday due to use of combination vaccines, it is still recommended that an additional dose be given after the fourth birthday ≥6 months after the previous dose.	Local injection site reaction, fever ≥38.0°C, irritability, tiredness, loss of appetite

Rotavirus	RV5: Pentavalent live, attenuated oral vaccine containing five reassortant human and bovine rotavirus strains	2 mL PO × 3 doses (2, 4, 6 months) • If any dose RV5 (RotaTeq) or unknown, 3 doses should be given • First dose must be given before 15 weeks. Cannot give final dose after 8 months old. • Do NOT readminister if infant spits out or vomits dose.	Diarrhea, vomiting, irritability, otitis media, nasopharyngitis, and bronchospasm (uncommon) Small risk of intussusception (1 excess case per 30,000–100,000 vaccinated infants), usually within 1 week of vaccination
	RV1: Monovalent live, attenuated oral vaccine	1 mL PO × 2 doses (2, 4 months) • First dose must be given before 15 weeks. Cannot give final dose after 8 months old. • If infant spits out or vomits dose, 1 replacement dose can be given at same visit.	
Streptococcus pneumoniae (Pneumococcal)	PCV13: Pneumococcal conjugate vaccine containing 13 purified capsular polysaccharides of *S. pneumoniae*, each coupled to a variant of diphtheria toxin: PCV7 serotypes (4, 6B, 9V, 14, 18C, 19F, and 23F) + additional serotypes (1, 3, 5, 6A, 7F, and 19A) for age ≥6 weeks	0.5 mL IM × 4 doses (2, 4, 6, 12–15 months) • See Section V.B.3 for children with high-risk conditions. • PCV13 and PPSV23 should not be administered during the same visit.	Local injection site reaction, irritability, decreased appetite, decreased sleep, increased sleep, fever
	PPSV23: Purified capsular polysaccharide from 23 serotypes (1, 2, 3, 4, 5, 6B, 7F, 8, 9N, 9V, 10A, 11A, 12F, 14, 15B, 17F, 18C, 19A, 19F, 20, 22F, 23F, and 33F) for age ≥2 years	0.5 mL IM/SQ • See Section V.B.3 for children with high-risk conditions. • When both PCV13 and PPSV23 are indicated, administer PCV13 first.	

Continued

16

TABLE 16.1

ROUTINE VACCINES FOR CHILDREN AND ADOLESCENTS IN THE UNITED STATES—CONT'D

Disease	Vaccine Description	Dose and Administration	Side Effects[a]
Varicella	Cell-free live, attenuated varicella virus vaccine for age ≥12 months	0.5 mL SQ × 2 doses (12–15 months, 4–6 years) • Dose #2 may be given as early as 3 months after dose #1. • If dose #2 inadvertently given <3 months but ≥4 weeks after dose #1, it is still valid.	Local injection site reaction, fever Mild varicelliform rash within 5–26 days of vaccine administration may occur, though not all postimmunization rashes are attributable to vaccine; vaccine rash is often mild, but patient may be infectious.

[a]Unless otherwise indicated, side-effect profiles for vaccines are derived from vaccine-specific package inserts. Prevalence of each potential side effect differs depending on which vaccine formulation used. More information available at https://www.immunize.org/fda/.[43]

CDC, Centers for Disease Control and Prevention; DT, Diphtheria and tetanus vaccine; DTaP, diphtheria, tetanus, acellular pertussis vaccine; GBS, Guillain-Barré syndrome; Hib, Haemophilus influenzae type b; IIV, inactivated influenza vaccine; IM, intramuscular; IPV, inactivated polio vaccine; LAIV, live, attenuated influenza vaccine; OPV, oral polio vaccine; PO, per os; PCV13, pneumococcal 13-valent conjugate vaccine; PPSV23, pneumococcal 23-valent polysaccharide vaccine; SQ, subcutaneous; Td, tetanus and diphtheria vaccine; Tdap, tetanus, diphtheria, acellular pertussis vaccine.

TABLE 16.2

NONROUTINE VACCINES FOR CHILDREN AND ADOLESCENTS

Disease	Indication	Type	Dose and Administration	Side Effects[a]
Japanese encephalitis (JE)	≥1-month travel in endemic areas (most rural areas of Asia) during the JE season May also be considered for shorter-term travel with higher exposure risk (i.e., during epidemic or time outdoors in rural areas)	JE-VC: inactivated cell culture–derived JE vaccine for age ≥2 months	0.25 mL IM × 2 doses for age 2 months–2 years 0.5 mL IM × 2 doses for age ≥3 years • For children <18 years, 4-week interval between doses • For adolescents ≥18 years, can reduce interval between doses to 7 days • If exposure ongoing, annual booster recommended	Fever, irritability, and diarrhea in young children; injection site pain and headache in adolescents and adults
Polio	Oral polio vaccine not available in the United States but is used worldwide Trivalent vaccine: Protective against all 3 poliovirus types in >95% of recipients In 2016 most countries switched to the bivalent vaccine.	Bivalent (bOPV): Live, attenuated vaccine against wild types 1 and 3, but not 2 Trivalent (tOPV): Live, attenuated vaccine against wild types 1, 2, and 3	3 doses at minimum 4-week intervals starting at age 6 weeks • Give additional OPV at birth in countries with endemic polio or high risk of importation. • Give ≥1 IPV dose, starting at 14 weeks (can be administered with OPV).	Rare vaccine-associated paralytic poliomyelitis occurs for ~ 1 in 2.4 million doses.
Rabies	High-risk groups: Veterinarians, animal handlers, laboratory workers, children living in high-risk environments, those traveling to high-risk areas, spelunkers Postexposure prophylaxis (see Table 16.5)	HDCV: Inactivated virus cultured in human diploid cells PCECV: Inactivated virus cultured in purified chicken embryo cells	Pre-exposure: 1 mL IM × 3 doses (Days 0, 7, and 21 or 28) Postexposure: 1 mL IM × 4 doses (Days 0, 3, 7, 14) • Administer in deltoid (children and adolescents) or anterolateral thigh (small children and infants), NOT in gluteal area.	Uncommon in children; in adults, local injection site reactions, mild systemic reactions Arthus-like reaction (urticaria, arthralgia, angioedema, vomiting, fever, malaise)

Continued

16

TABLE 16.2

NONROUTINE VACCINES FOR CHILDREN AND ADOLESCENTS—CONT'D

Disease	Indication	Type	Dose and Administration	Side Effects[a]
			• Should be administered to body part distant from where RIG was injected • Follow serum Ab titers at 6-month intervals for those at continuous risk and at 2-year intervals for those at risk of frequent exposure. • Give booster doses only if titers are nonprotective.	prophylaxis recipients at 2–21 days after booster.
Respiratory Syncytial Virus (RSV)[36]	Preterm infants: • Born <29 WGA and <12 months at the start of RSV season • Chronic lung disease of prematurity in first year of life or requiring ongoing medical support in second year of life Children <12 months with: • Anatomic pulmonary abnormality or neuromuscular disorder impairing upper airway clearance • Moderate-to- severe pulmonary hypertension • Hemodynamically significant heart disease (discuss with cardiologist) Children <2 years with: • Cardiac transplant • Profound immunocompromise	Palivizumab: Humanized mouse IgG1 monoclonal antibody to RSV	15 mg/kg IM Give every 28–30 days during RSV season for up to 5 doses • First dose should be given prior to the beginning of RSV season • Children who develop an RSV infection should discontinue use of Palivizumab	Fever and rash (local skin reaction)

(IB)	United States if a child is frequently exposed to someone with pulmonary TB that is untreated, ineffectively treated, or resistant to treatment, and the child cannot be given long-term primary preventive therapy. Children should be HIV-negative and those ≥2 months should have a negative purified protein derivative (PPD).	prepared from *Mycobacterium bovis* About ≤80% effective	sterile water (2 mL if age <1 month) Give 0.2–0.3 mL of reconstituted vaccine percutaneously with a multiple puncture device in the deltoid region.	lymphadenopathy and pustule formation at injection site can occur.
Typhoid	Travel to areas with risk of exposure to *Salmonella* serotype Typhi, people with frequent close contact with a documented carrier, laboratory workers in contact with *Salmonella* serotype Typhi, and people living in areas with endemic infection	ViCPS: Vi capsular polysaccharide vaccine for age ≥2 years Ty21a: Oral live, attenuated vaccine for age ≥6 years	0.5 mL IM Give 1 dose ≥2 weeks prior to exposure; booster every 2 years 1 capsule by mouth every other day for a total of 4 doses ≥1 week prior to exposure; booster every 5 years	Local injection site reaction, subjective fever, decreased activity Mild reactions including abdominal pain, nausea, diarrhea, vomiting, fever, or headache
Yellow fever	Travel to endemic areas including parts of sub-Saharan Africa and South America Required by some countries as a condition of entry	YF-Vax: Live, attenuated (17D strain) vaccine approved for age ≥9 months	0.5 mL SQ Give 1 dose ≥10 days prior to travel. No booster doses indicated unless immunocompromised or at increased risk due to location or duration of exposure (e.g., prolonged travel or lab workers)	Rare viscerotropic disease (multiple-organ system failure) and neurotropic disease (encephalitis, meningitis) Increased risk of adverse events in adults >65 years and persons with thymic dysfunction; increased risk of postvaccine encephalitis in ages <9 months

^aUnless otherwise indicated, side-effect profiles for vaccines are derived from vaccine-specific package inserts: https://www.immunize.org/fda/43

Ab, Antibody; *BCG*, bacille Calmette-Guérin; *HDCV*, human diploid cell vaccine; *IM*, intramuscular; *IPV*, inactivated polio vaccine; *PCECV*, purified chick embryo cell vaccine; *RIG*, rabies immune globulin; *SQ*, subcutaneous;

16

a. MMR-Varicella (ProQuad)[7] can be used for children 12 months to 12 years of age. There is increased risk of febrile seizures if ProQuad is used as first dose for ages 12 to 47 months.

C. Live, Attenuated Vaccines

1. Certain vaccines have live components that must replicate to produce immunity: influenza (intranasal), MMR, oral polio vaccine (OPV), BCG, typhoid (oral), varicella, yellow fever.
2. Systemic adverse reactions following these vaccines are usually mild and usually occur 3 to 21 days after vaccine administration.
3. Special consideration must be taken when administering these vaccines to patients with certain underlying medical conditions (see Section V).

D. Timing and Spacing of Vaccine Doses

1. For information on recommended timing and spacing of vaccines, see https://www.cdc.gov/vaccines/hcp/acip-recs/general-recs/timing.html
2. If patient is "behind" on a vaccine series, there is no maximum interval between doses that would require restarting entire series, except for oral typhoid vaccine.
3. Combination vaccines
   a. Minimum age for administration of vaccine is oldest age required for administration of any of vaccine's individual components.
      Example: For DTaP/HepB/IPV vaccine, HepB series starts at birth, but DTaP and IPV start at 6–8 weeks, so this combination vaccine should not be administered to children <6 weeks. In fact, all HepB-containing[8] combination vaccines should not be administered to infants <6 weeks because of other components.
   b. Minimum interval between doses is equal to greatest required interval of any vaccine's individual components.
4. Live, attenuated vaccines
   a. If live vaccines are not administered at the same visit, they should be separated by interval of 28 days.

E. Contraindications and Precautions

1. Contraindication: A condition, often temporary, that increases likelihood of vaccine recipient having serious adverse reaction to vaccine; vaccination should not occur while contraindication is present
2. Precaution: A condition that may increase likelihood or severity of adverse reaction in vaccine recipient, may cause diagnostic confusion, or may compromise vaccine's ability to induce immunity. Vaccination usually should be deferred when precaution present, unless benefit of protection from vaccine outweighs vaccine risk.
3. Table 16.3: Contraindications and precautions to select vaccines
4. Table 16.4: Conditions incorrectly perceived as contraindications or precautions to vaccination (vaccines may be administered under these conditions)
5. For full details, see https://www.cdc.gov/vaccines/hcp/acip-recs/general-recs/contraindications.html

TABLE 16.3

CONTRAINDICATIONS AND PRECAUTIONS TO SELECT VACCINES[9-11,44,45]

Vaccine	Contraindication	Precaution
All vaccines	Severe (life-threatening) allergic reaction after 1 dose or to any vaccine component (see package inserts)	Moderate-severe acute illness (wait until after recovery, if possible) Latex allergy: https://www.cdc.gov/vaccines/pubs/pinkbook/downloads/appendices/B/latex-table.pdf
Live vaccines	Most forms of altered immunocompetence (see Section V.A for exceptions) Solid organ transplant Pregnancy: Wait until after pregnancy; avoid becoming pregnant for ≥1 month after vaccine.	Patients on corticosteroids: See Table 16.6 HSCT patients: Delay ≥3 months after immunosuppressive therapy has been discontinued. See Table EC 16.2 Patients on biologic response modifier therapies: Contraindicated during therapy and for weeks to months after its discontinuation or if patient has received other live vaccines in past 4 weeks.
Diphtheria, tetanus, pertussis	Encephalopathy (including coma or status epilepticus) within 7 days of administration of prior dose of DTaP/Tdap not attributable to another identifiable cause	Evolving/progressive neurologic disorder, including uncontrolled seizures: Defer DTaP/Tdap temporarily until disorder stabilized; use DT or Td instead in children age ≥1 year, reconsider pertussis immunization at each visit (i.e., if condition stabilized) GBS within 6 weeks of previous dose History of Arthus-type hypersensitivity reaction (including severe pain or swelling) after tetanus or diphtheria toxoid–containing vaccine: Defer vaccination for 10 years after last administration.
Hepatitis A	Anaphylaxis to neomycin	
Hepatitis B	Anaphylaxis/hypersensitivity to yeast	Defer for infants <2000 g if mother HBsAg negative; see Fig. 16.1 for details
HPV	Anaphylaxis to yeast	Pregnancy: Delay vaccination until after pregnancy.
Influenza (IIV)		History of GBS within 6 weeks after a previous dose Egg allergy other than hives (administer in a supervised medical setting)[46]
Influenza (LAIV)	Contacts of severely immunocompromised patients requiring care in protective environment Children <5 years with existing diagnosis of asthma or history of wheezing in past 12 months Receiving aspirin or aspirin-containing products Persons with active communications/leaks	History of GBS within 6 weeks after a previous dose Asthma in children ≥5 years Medical conditions that might be at higher risk of complications from influenza Egg allergy other than hives (administer in a supervised medical setting)[46]

Continued

TABLE 16.3

CONTRAINDICATIONS AND PRECAUTIONS TO SELECT VACCINES[9-11,44,45]**—CONT'D**

Vaccine	Contraindication	Precaution
	between CSF and oropharyngeal space Presence of cochlear implant (consult specialist if no other influenza vaccine available) Use of influenza antiviral therapy in past 2–17 days, depending on which antiviral used (may interfere with immunogenicity)	
Japanese encephalitis	Anaphylaxis to protamine sulfate	
MenACWY	Anaphylaxis to yeast	History of preterm birth
MenB		Pregnancy Latex sensitivity
MMR		History of thrombocytopenia or TTP Recent blood product administration (within 3–11 months, depending on product and dose). See Table EC 16.4 Need for TB testing (PPD or interferon-γ release assay testing may be done on day of immunization but otherwise should be postponed 4–6 weeks) Personal or family history of seizures (MMRV only)
Pneumococcal	PCV13: Anaphylaxis to any vaccine containing diphtheria toxoid or yeast	
Polio[47]	IPV: Anaphylaxis to neomycin, streptomycin, polymyxin B, 2-phenoxyethanol, and formaldehyde OPV: Immunocompromised patients and close/household contacts	Pregnancy: No evidence of harm, but avoid or give prior to pregnancy if possible
Rabies	Severe allergic reaction to prior dose—switch to PCECV if there is a reaction to HDCV (and vice versa)	
Rotavirus	SCID History of intussusception	Concern for immunocompromise, pre-existing chronic gastrointestinal disease, spina bifida, or bladder exstrophy
Tuberculosis (BCG)[48]	Immunocompromised, including HIV infection, or likelihood that patient will receive immunosuppressive therapy soon	

		Pregnancy: No evidence of harm, but avoid or give prior to pregnancy if possible
Typhoid (Ty21a only)[43]		Certain antibiotics or antimalarials that would be active against *Salmonella* serovar Typhi or interfere with immunogenicity
Varicella[49]	Anaphylaxis to neomycin or gelatin	On aspirin or aspirin-containing products; avoid using salicylates for 6 weeks after vaccination
		Recent blood product administration (within 3–11 months, depending on product and dose, see Table EC 16.4)
		Other live vaccines in past 4 weeks
		Receipt of antiviral drugs (acyclovir, famciclovir, or valacyclovir) 24 hours before vaccination; avoid for 14 days after vaccination
Yellow fever[43,50]	Anaphylaxis to eggs	Age 6–8 months: Risk of vaccine-associated encephalitis
	Symptomatic HIV infection or $CD4^+$ count <200/mm³ (or <15% for age <6 years)	Pregnant or breastfeeding: Rare cases of in utero or breastfeeding transmission of the vaccine virus
	Age <6 months	Asymptomatic HIV infection with $CD4^+$ count 200–499/mm³ (or 15%–24% for age <6 years)
	Thymus disorder	

BCG, bacille Calmette-Guérin; *CSF*, cerebral spinal fluid; *DT*, Diphtheria and tetanus vaccine; *DTaP*, diphtheria, tetanus, acellular pertussis vaccine; *GBS*, Guillain-Barré syndrome; *HBsAg*, Hepatitis B surface antigen; *HDCV*, human diploid cell vaccine; *HIV*, human immunodeficiency virus; *HPV*, human papilloma virus; *HSCT*, hematopoietic stem cell transplant; *IIV*, inactivated influenza vaccine; *IPV*, inactivated poliovirus vaccine; *LAIV*, live, attenuated influenza vaccine; *MMR*, measles, mumps, rubella; *MMRV*, measles, mumps, rubella, varicella; *OPV*, oral poliovirus vaccine; *PCECV*, purified chick embryo cell vaccine; *PPD*, purified protein derivative; *SCID*, severe combined immunodeficiency; *Td*, tetanus and diphtheria vaccine; *Tdap*, tetanus, diphtheria, acellular pertussis vaccine; *TTP*, thrombotic thrombocytopenic purpura.

Modified from Table 4.1, Centers for Disease Control and Prevention. "Contraindications and Precautions." Vaccine Recommendations and Guidelines of the ACIP. Last updated October 18, 2022 https://www.cdc.gov/vaccines/hcp/acip-recs/general-recs/contraindications.html

16

IV. POSTEXPOSURE PROPHYLAXIS (TABLE 16.5)

V. SPECIAL PATIENT POPULATIONS[9]

A. Altered Immunocompetence[10,11]

1. For full details, see https://www.cdc.gov/vaccines/hcp/acip-recs/general-recs/immunocompetence.html
2. General principles
   a. Primary immunodeficiency: Congenital and usually inherited conditions defined by inherent absence or deficiency in cellular or humoral components that provide immunity
   b. Secondary immunodeficiency: Acquired loss or deficiency in cellular or humoral immune components as a consequence of disease process or its therapy

---

TABLE 16.4

CONDITIONS INCORRECTLY PERCEIVED AS CONTRAINDICATIONS OR PRECAUTIONS TO VACCINATION[9-11,44,45]

Vaccine	NOT Contraindication/Precaution
All vaccines	Mild acute illness with or without fever
	Mild-moderate local reaction (i.e., swelling, redness, soreness); low-grade or moderate fever after previous dose
	Recent exposure to an infectious disease
	Current antimicrobial therapy (Exceptions: oral typhoid, varicella)
	Convalescent phase of illness
	Breastfeeding
	Preterm birth (Exception: hepatitis B vaccine in specific circumstances; see Fig. 16.1)
	History of penicillin allergy, other nonvaccine allergies, relatives with allergies, or receiving allergen extract immunotherapy
	History of GBS (Exception: within 6 weeks of influenza or tetanus toxoid–containing vaccine)
COVID-19 (SARS-CoV-2)	Pregnancy
	HIV or other altered immunocompetence
DTaP/TDap	Fever within 48 hours of previous dose of DTaP/DTP
	Personal or family history of seizures, including seizures after previous dose of DTaP: Consider antipyretic use for 24 hours after vaccination.
	Collapse or shock-like state within 48 hours of a previous dose
	Persistent, inconsolable crying lasting ≥3 hours within 48 hours of a previous dose
	Stable neurologic conditions (e.g., cerebral palsy, well-controlled seizures, or developmental delay)
Hepatitis B	Autoimmune disease
HPV	Evidence of active or prior HPV infection, such as abnormal Pap smear, history of genital warts, or positive HPV DNA test
Influenza (IIV)	Non-severe allergy to egg or latex
	Pregnancy: Give regardless of trimester
	Use of warfarin or aminophylline
Influenza (LAIV)	Contacts of persons with chronic disease or altered immunocompetence not requiring care in protected environment
	Breastfeeding
MMR	Family member or household contact who is pregnant or immunodeficient
	Patient female of child-bearing age
	Positive tuberculin skin test or interferon-γ release assay
	Anaphylaxis to egg
Polio (IPV)	Previous receipt of ≥1 dose of OPV
PPSV23	History of invasive pneumococcal disease or pneumonia
Rotavirus	Prematurity (give at hospital discharge)
Varicella	Family member or household contact who is pregnant or immunodeficient

(Exception: If patient experiences presumed vaccine-related rash 7–25 days after vaccination, patient should avoid direct contact with immunocompromised persons for duration of rash.)

Humoral immunodeficiency (e.g., agammaglobulinemia)

DNA, Deoxyribonucleic acid; *DTaP*, diphtheria, tetanus, acellular pertussis vaccine; *GBS*, Guillain-Barré syndrome; *HPV*, human papilloma virus; *IIV*, inactivated influenza vaccine; *IPV*, inactivated polio vaccine; *LAIV*, live, attenuated influenza vaccine; *OPV*, oral polio vaccine; *PPD*, purified protein derivative; *PPSV23*, pneumococcal 23-valent polysaccharide vaccine; *RA*, rheumatoid arthritis; *SLE*, systemic lupus erythematosus.

Modified from Table 4.2, Centers for Disease Control and Prevention. "Contraindications and Precautions." Vaccine Recommendations and Guidelines of the ACIP. Last updated August 5, 2021. https://www.cdc.gov/vaccines/hcp/acip-recs/general-recs/contraindications.pdf

     (1) In general, inactivated vaccines should be administered at least 2 weeks and live vaccines at least 4 weeks before initiation of immunosuppression or transplantation.

  c. See Chapter 15 for specific information about immunodeficiencies.

  d. See Table EC 16.1 for specific vaccine recommendations and contraindications in patients with immunodeficiency.

3. Primary immunodeficiency

  a. Live vaccines generally contraindicated, except for most complement deficiencies

  b. Non-live vaccines should be administered according to routine schedule. Immune response may vary.

  c. For immunodeficiencies that cause increased incidence/severity of some vaccine-preventable diseases, additional vaccination(s) may be recommended.

  d. Passive immunoprophylaxis with immunoglobulin therapy may be indicated.

     (1) See Chapter 15 for specific details.

     (2) See Table 16.5 for postexposure prophylaxis guidelines.

  e. Routine immunization of household contacts recommended

4. **Functional or anatomic asplenia (including sickle cell disease)**

  a. Penicillin prophylaxis: See Chapter 14 for details.

  b. See Section V.B for Hib, meningococcal, and pneumococcal vaccination recommendations.

  c. Do not administer live attenuated influenza vaccine (LAIV).

  d. Children ≥2 years undergoing elective splenectomy

     (1) Administer pneumococcal and meningococcal vaccines ≥2 weeks before surgery for optimal immune response.

     (2) If Hib immunization not previously completed, administer 1 dose ≥2 weeks before surgery.

5. **Known or suspected human immunodeficiency virus (HIV) disease**

  a. See Section V.B for Hib, meningococcal, and pneumococcal vaccination recommendations.

  b. CD4 count-dependent vaccines: Give to all HIV-infected children without evidence of severe immunocompromise (i.e., age 1–13 years

TABLE 16.5

POSTEXPOSURE PROPHYLAXIS (PEP)

Disease	Prophylaxis Type	Indication/Administration Details[a]
COVID-19 (SARS CoV-2)	Monoclonal Ab	For the latest information on agents available and criteria to qualify, visit the U.S. Food and Drug Administration website.
Hepatitis A	Vaccine[37] IMIG[51]	Indicated for children ≥12 months if ≤2 weeks since exposure OR if >2 weeks since exposure and exposure ongoing For children <12 months if ≤2 weeks since exposure Immunocompromised children with exposure Children with chronic liver disease with exposure Dosing: 0.1 mL/kg IM
Hepatitis B See Table 16.7 for details on percutaneous exposure to blood.	Vaccine HBIG: Prepared from plasma containing high-titer anti-HBsAg antibodies	Give series to any previously unimmunized person with percutaneous/mucosal exposure to HBsAg-positive bodily fluids. Give within 12 hours after birth to any infant with maternal HBsAg status positive/unknown. Give within 12 hours after birth to infants with maternal HBsAg status positive; see Fig. 16.1 for guidance when maternal HBsAg unknown. Give to any previously unimmunized person or known nonresponder with percutaneous/mucosal exposure to HBsAg-positive blood/bodily fluids. Dosing: • 0.5 mL IM for infants <12 months • 0.06 mL/kg IM for children ≥12 months
Hib (invasive)	Vaccine Chemoprophylaxis	Invasive Hib ≤24 months: Initiate 1 month after acute illness and continue immunization series as if previously unimmunized Not required if invasive Hib disease develops in children >24 months For any child who contracts invasive Hib disease after completing immunization series, consider immunologic workup. Exposure only: Rifampin prophylaxis recommended for household contacts in certain circumstances (see Table 3.9 of the 2021 Red Book for details[52])

Influenza NOTE: Recommendations vary by season; see CDC for up-to-date recommendations[42]	Chemoprophylaxis	Most commonly used: Neuraminidase inhibitors (e.g., oseltamivir) given the high resistance to adamantanes (e.g., amantadine) For the following groups, give within 7 days of exposure: • Unimmunized high-risk children, including those for whom the vaccine is contraindicated or children immunized <2 weeks before exposure • Unimmunized individuals in close contact with high-risk individuals • Immunodeficient individuals unlikely to have protective response to vaccine • Control of outbreaks in a closed setting • Immunized high-risk individuals if vaccine strain different from circulating strain Delay for ≥2 weeks if LAIV has been given Not a substitute for immunization
Measles	Vaccine	Intervention of choice for measles outbreak; prevents or modifies disease if given within 72 hours of exposure
	IMIG	Indicated in children <1 year or nonimmune individuals who cannot receive the vaccine Prevents or modifies disease if given within 6 days of exposure
	IVIG	Recommended for nonimmune pregnant women and severely immunocompromised hosts (including HIV-infected children) regardless of immunization status Additional therapy not required if given within 3 weeks before exposure
Mumps	Vaccine	Persons ≥12 months who previously received ≤2 doses of MMR and are identified by public health authorities to be at increased risk during a mumps outbreak should receive 1 dose of MMR[53]
Meningococcal	Vaccine	Adjunct to chemoprophylaxis when an outbreak is caused by a vaccine-preventable serogroup
	Chemoprophylaxis	Indications: • Direct exposure to an infected person's oral secretions (including unprotected healthcare workers) • Close contact in the 7 days prior to onset of disease (e.g., child care, preschool, and household contacts and passengers seated next to the index patient during airline flights ≥8 hours) Initiate within 24 hours of index patient diagnosis See Table 3.36 of the *2021 Red Book* for details.[52]

Continued

16

TABLE 16.5

POSTEXPOSURE PROPHYLAXIS (PEP)—CONT'D

Disease	Prophylaxis Type	Indication/Administration Details[a]
Pertussis	Vaccine	Immunize all unimmunized or partially immunized close contacts based on the recommended schedule.
	Chemoprophylaxis	Azithromycin, erythromycin, or clarithromycin recommended for household contacts and other close contacts. Alternatives include TMP-SMX (see Table 3.44 of the *2021 Red Book* for details[52]).
Rabies See Table 16.8 for details based on type of exposure. NOTE: PEP indicated for bites, scratches, or contamination of open wound or mucous membrane with infectious material of potentially rabid animal or human	Vaccine	If unimmunized: give vaccine on Days 0, 3, 7, and 14 with 1 × RIG on day 0. If immunosuppressed, give a fifth dose on day 28, and monitor response by checking neutralizing Ab levels 714 days after series completion. If RIG is unavailable, give vaccine alone. If previously immunized: booster doses on days 0 and 3
	RIG: Antirabies Ig prepared from plasma of donors hyperimmunized with rabies vaccine	If unimmunized: • Give 1 × RIG on day 0 with vaccine • If no vaccine, give RIG alone • May be given within 7 days after initiating immunization Do not give RIG if previously immunized. Dosing: 20 units/kg; infiltrate around the wound, give remainder IM
	Other management	Consider tetanus prophylaxis and antibiotics, if indicated. General wound management: • Clean immediately with soap and water and flush thoroughly. • Avoid suturing wound unless indicated for functional or cosmetic reasons. Report all patients suspected of rabies infection to public health authorities.
Rubella	Rubella Ig	Does not prevent infection or viremia Routine use of rubella Ig in susceptible pregnant individuals with known exposure is not recommended.
Tetanus	Vaccine	See Table 16.9 for details.
	TIG	Give to any child with HIV infection or other severe immunodeficiency for any tetanus-prone wound, regardless of vaccination status. Dosing: 1 × 250 units IM

Varicella[b]	Vaccine	Vaccinate immunocompetent, nonimmune people ≥12 months as soon as possible after exposure, preferably within 5 days. Do not give vaccine concurrently with or for 5 months after VariZIG. Avoid antivirals for 21 days after vaccination.
	VariZIG: Prepared from plasma containing high-titer antivaricella antibodies	Give as soon as possible within 10 days of significant exposure in individuals with no immunity and a high likelihood of complications from infection, including: • Immunocompromise • Pregnant women • Certain newborn infants Dosing (weight-based, IM, 125 units = 1 vial): • 62.5 units for ≤2 kg • 125 units for 2.1–10 kg • 250 units for 10.1–20 kg • 375 units for 20.1–30 kg • 500 units for 30.1–40 kg • 625 units for >40 kg May be used if VariZIG is not available
	IVIG	Dosing: 400 mg/kg IV
	Chemoprophylaxis	If VariZIG or IVIG are not available, consider prophylaxis with 7 days of acyclovir or valacyclovir beginning 7–10 days after exposure in immunocompromised, nonimmune patients.

[a] Unless otherwise indicated, postexposure prophylaxis recommendations are derived from pathogen-specific chapters in Section 3 of American Academy of Pediatrics. *Red Book: 2021-2024 Report of the Committee on Infectious Diseases.* 32nd ed. AAP; 2021.

[b] See Fig 3.17 of the 2021 *Red Book* for specifics[52]

CDC, Centers for Disease Control and Prevention; *HBIG*, hepatitis B immune globulin; *HBsAg*, hepatitis B surface antigen; *Hib*, *Haemophilus influenzae* type b; *HIV*, human immunodeficiency virus; *Ig*, immunoglobulin; *IM*, intramuscular; *IMIG*, intramuscular immunoglobulin; *IVIG*, intravenous immunoglobulin; *LAIV*, live, attenuated influenza vaccine; *MMR*, measles, mumps, rubella; *RIG*, rabies immune globulin; *TIG*, tetanus immune globulin; *TMP-SMX*, trimethoprim-sulfamethoxazole; *VariZIG*, varicella zoster immune globulin.

16

with CD4$^+$ ≥15% for ≥6 months OR age ≥14 years with CD4$^+$ count ≥200 cells/mm for ≥6 months).

    (1) Varicella

    (2) MMR

  c. Do not administer the following vaccines:

    (1) MMR-varicella combined vaccine

    (2) LAIV

    (3) OPV and/or BCG, unless in areas where infection risk outweighs possibility of vaccine-associated disease

  d. Consider passive immunoprophylaxis or chemoprophylaxis after exposures (see Table 16.5).

6. **Malignancy**

  a. Recommendations vary based on patient's specific treatment regimen. Always consult with patient's oncologist first.

  b. General strategies include the following:

    (1) Defer routine immunization, except for Inactivated influenza vaccine (IIV), during chemotherapy.

    (2) Presume loss of immunity with chemotherapy, and revaccinate per CDC catch-up immunization schedule after treatment completion.

  c. Timing of resumption of immunization varies based on patient's specific treatment regimen (from 3 months to ≥24 months).

    (1) Inactivated vaccines and live vaccines are generally delayed until ≥3 months postcompletion of chemotherapy. However, if regimen included anti-B cell antibodies, all vaccines should be delayed until ≥6 months postcompletion of chemotherapy.

    (2) Inactivated influenza vaccine (IIV) should be given annually, even during chemotherapy (except during treatment with intensive chemotherapy or anti-B-cell antibodies).

7. **Hematopoietic stem cell transplant (HSCT) recipients**

  a. After transplant, HSCT recipients are considered to no longer have immunity to previously received vaccines. Reimmunize against all vaccine-preventable illnesses.

    (1) Inactivated vaccines are safe to administer 6 to 12 months after HSCT. Reasonable to consider pneumococcal series at 6 months and remainder at 12 months.

    (2) Give IIV 6 months post-HSCT.

      NOTE: During community outbreak, IIV may be given as early as 4 months post-HSCT.

    (3) Do not administer live vaccines during first 24 months posttransplant.

    (4) Do not administer live vaccines to patients with graft-versus-host-disease or ongoing immunosuppression, even if 24 months posttransplant.

    (5) For specific vaccine recommendations, see Table EC 16.2.

  b. Consider passive immunoprophylaxis or chemoprophylaxis after exposures (see Table 16.5).

   c. Household contacts should receive routine immunizations. Only exception is LAIV if the HSCT recipient's level of immunocompromise is severe (e.g., HSCT in last 3 months). HSCT recipients should avoid contact with body fluids or skin eruptions of household contact who received rotavirus or varicella vaccines, respectively.

8. **Solid organ transplant recipients**
   a. See Section V.B.3 for pneumococcal vaccination recommendations.
   b. Before transplant: Give all routinely recommended vaccines. Give live vaccines ≥4 weeks prior to transplantation.
      (1) Children 6–11 months can receive MMR if not immunosuppressed and if transplant is ≥4 weeks away.
      (2) Children 6 to 11 months (or without evidence of varicella immunity) can receive varicella vaccine if not immunosuppressed and if transplant is ≥4 weeks away.
   c. After transplant: Inactivated vaccines, including those indicated for immunocompromised hosts, should resume 2 to 6 months after transplant. Live vaccines are generally not administered after transplant. For specific vaccine recommendations, see Table EC 16.3.

9. **Patients on corticosteroids**
   a. Only live vaccines are potentially contraindicated.
   b. See Table 16.6 for details.

10. **Patients on biologic response modifiers**
   a. See Table 1.18 of the *2021 Red Book* for details.
   b. Antibodies to proinflammatory cytokines or proteins that bind to cytokine receptors (e.g., tumor necrosis factor [TNF]-α inhibitors) are considered highly immunosuppressive.
   c. Prior to initiating therapy:
      (1) Perform serologic testing for hepatitis B virus and vaccinate/revaccinate if hepatitis B surface antibody (HBsAb) is <10 mIU/mL.
      (2) Give inactivated vaccines (including IIV) ≥2 weeks prior to starting therapy.
      (3) Give live-virus vaccines ≥4 weeks prior, unless contraindicated by condition or other therapies.
   d. During/after therapy:
      (1) Live-virus vaccines: Contraindicated during therapy. Interval after therapy for safe administration has not been established.
      (2) Inactivated vaccines (including IIV): Administer according to schedule.

11. **Patients treated with immunoglobulin or other blood products**
   a. See Table EC 16.4 for suggested intervals between blood product and MMR or varicella administration.

B. Disease-Specific Considerations

1. **Children at high risk of Hib**[12,13]

TABLE 16.6

LIVE VACCINE IMMUNIZATION FOR PATIENTS RECEIVING CORTICOSTEROID THERAPY

Steroid Dose	Recommended Guidelines
Topical, inhaled, or local injection of steroids Low-dose steroids (<2 mg/kg/day or <20 mg/day of prednisone equivalent[a]) Physiologic maintenance doses	Live vaccines can generally be given unless there is clinical evidence of immunosuppression.
High-dose steroids (≥2 mg/kg/day or ≥20 mg/day of prednisone equivalent[a]), duration of therapy <14 days	Live vaccines may be given immediately after cessation of therapy (but consider 2-week delay).
High-dose steroids (≥2 mg/kg/day or ≥20 mg/day of prednisone equivalent[a]), duration of therapy ≥14 days	Delay live vaccines until 4 weeks after discontinuation of therapy.
Systemic or local steroids in patients with underlying disease affecting immune response (e.g., lupus) or receiving other immunosuppressant medication	Do not administer live vaccines.

[a]20 mg/day cutoff for children weighing more than 10 kg.
Adapted from pages 81–82 of the *2021 Red Book*.[52]

TABLE 16.7

HEPATITIS B VIRUS PROPHYLAXIS FOR NON-HEALTHCARE PROVIDERS AFTER PERCUTANEOUS EXPOSURE TO BLOOD

Exposed Person	HBsAg Status of Source of Blood		
	Positive	Negative	Unknown
Unimmunized	HBIG and HBV series	HBV series	HBV series
Previously immunized	Give 1 dose HBV booster.	No treatment	No treatment

HBIG, hepatitis B immune globulin; *HBsAg*, hepatitis B surface antigen; *HBV*, hepatitis B vaccine.
Adapted from Table 16.6 in Prevention of hepatitis B virus infection in the United States: recommendations of the Advisory Committee on Immunization Practices. *MMWR Recomm Rep.* 2018;67(1):1–31.[8]

    a. Indications: Functional or anatomic asplenia (including sickle cell disease), HIV infection, immunoglobulin deficiency, early component complement deficiency, or chemotherapy/radiation

    b. Age <12 months: Administer primary series.

    c. Age 12–59 months:

        (1) Received 0–1 dose(s) <12 months: Administer 2 doses at 8-week intervals.

        (2) Received ≥2 doses <12 months: Administer 1 additional dose at least 8 weeks after previous dose.

        (3) If patient undergoing chemotherapy or radiation, only readminister vaccine posttreatment if most recent dose was given <2 weeks prior to starting chemotherapy or radiation.

    d. Age ≥5 years with asplenia or HIV and not fully immunized: Administer 1 dose at least 8 weeks after previous dose.

2. **Children at high risk of meningococcal disease**[14-18]

TABLE 16.8

RABIES POSTEXPOSURE PROPHYLAXIS BASED ON ANIMAL

Animal Type	Evaluation and Disposition of Animal	Postexposure Prophylaxis Recommendations
Dog, cat, ferret	Healthy and available for 10 days' observation	Do not begin prophylaxis unless animal develops signs of rabies.
	Rabid or suspected rabid: euthanize animal and test brain	Provide immediate immunization and RIG.[a]
	Unknown (escaped)	Consult public health officials.
Skunk, raccoon, bat,[b] fox, woodchuck, most other carnivores	Regard as rabid unless geographic area is known to be free of rabies or until animal is euthanized and proven negative by testing	Provide immediate immunization and RIG.[a]
Livestock, rodents, rabbit, other mammals	Consider individually	Consult public health officials; these bites rarely require treatment.

[a]Treatment may be discontinued if animal fluorescent antibody is negative.

[b]In the case of direct contact between a human and a bat, consider prophylaxis even if a bite, scratch, or mucous membrane exposure is not apparent.

RIG, Rabies immune globulin.

Adapted from Table 3.49 of the *2021 Red Book.*[52]

TABLE 16.9

INDICATIONS FOR TETANUS PROPHYLAXIS

Prior Tetanus Toxoid Doses	Clean, Minor Wounds		All Other Wounds	
	Tetanus Vaccine[a]	TIG	Tetanus Vaccine[a]	TIG
Unknown or <3	Yes	No	Yes	Yes
≥3, last <5 years ago	No	No	No	No
≥3, last 5–10 years ago	No	No	Yes	No
≥3, last ≥10 years ago	Yes	No	Yes	No

[a]DTaP preferred under age 7 years; Tdap preferred over Td for children ≥7 years if patient is underimmunized or hasn't received Tdap previously; otherwise, either one is acceptable. DT or Td if pertussis is contraindicated.

DT, Diphtheria and tetanus vaccine; *DTaP,* diphtheria, tetanus, acellular pertussis vaccine; *Td,* tetanus and diphtheria vaccine; *Tdap,* tetanus, diphtheria, acellular pertussis vaccine; *TIG,* tetanus immune globulin.

Adapted from Table 3.68 of the *2021 Red Book.*[52]

16

    a. Indications: Functional or anatomic asplenia, HIV infection, persistent complement deficiency (including eculizumab use), travel to or residence in areas with hyperendemic or epidemic meningococcal disease, or residence in community with meningococcal outbreak

    b. Age <2 years:

      (1) MenACWY-CRM (Menveo): If age 8 weeks–6 months, administer 4 doses at 2, 4, 6, and 12 months. If age 7–23 months and unvaccinated, administer 2 doses, with second dose ≥12 weeks after first dose and after first birthday.

      (2) MenACWY-D (Menactra): Before age 2 years, can use for persistent complement component deficiency or travel but

not for anatomic/functional asplenia, sickle cell disease, or HIV infection before. If age 9–23 months, give two doses 12 weeks apart.

c. Age ≥2 years:
  (1) Administer two doses of Menactra or Menveo (minimum 8-week interval) to children at increased risk due to medical condition.
  (2) Only one dose is needed for children at increased risk due to traveling, living in hyperendemic regions, or outbreak.
  (3) Administer Menactra ≥4 weeks after completing PCV13 series.

d. Age ≥10 years with asplenia or persistent complement deficiency:
  (1) Administer MCV4 series.
  (2) Administer two-dose MenB-4C (Bexsero) series or three-dose MenB-FHbp (Trumenba) series. The two MenB vaccines are **not** interchangeable; use the same product for all doses in series.

e. Boosters:
  (1) MCV4 series
    (a) Most recent dose administered when child <7 years old: Administer one booster dose 3 years after completion of primary series, then every 5 years thereafter.
    (b) Most recent dose administered when child ≥7 years old: Administer one booster dose every 5 years.
  (2) MenB series
    (a) Ongoing risk due to disease process: Administer one booster dose 1 year after completion of primary series, then every 2–3 years thereafter.
    (b) Ongoing risk due to outbreak: Consider one booster dose 1 year after completion of primary series.

3. **Children at high risk for pneumococcal disease**[19-21]
  a. Indications:
    (1) Immunocompromised: Functional or anatomic asplenia (including sickle cell disease), primary immunodeficiencies, HIV infection, malignancy, immunosuppressive or radiation therapy, solid organ transplant, chronic renal failure, or nephrotic syndrome
    (2) Other chronic conditions: Chronic heart disease, chronic lung disease, diabetes mellitus, cerebrospinal fluid leak, cochlear implant, chronic liver disease, or alcoholism
  b. See Fig. 16.2 for recommendations.

C. Preterm Infants

1. **Immunize according to chronologic age, using regular vaccine dose.**
  NOTE: Due to limited evidence regarding risk for nosocomial transmission of rotavirus following vaccine in hospitalized patients, individual institutions may decide whether to administer rotavirus vaccine to infants during hospitalization. Otherwise, administer at time of discharge.

2. **Hepatitis B:** See Fig. 16.1.

3. **Respiratory syncytial virus (RSV)** immunoprophylaxis: See Table 16.2.

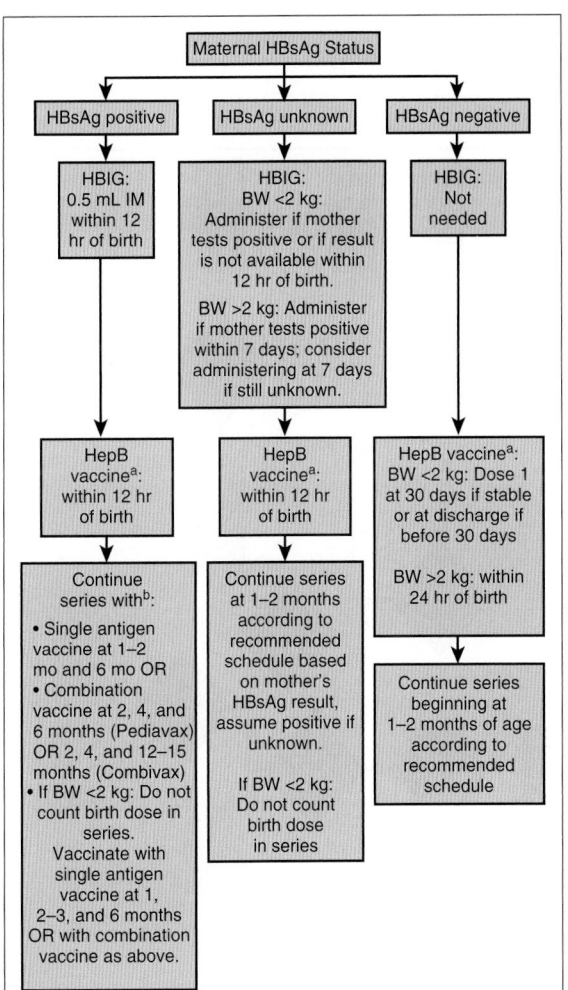

FIGURE 16.1

Management of neonates born to mothers with unknown or positive hepatitis B surface antigen *(HBsAg)* status. [a]Only single antigen vaccine should be used. [b]Reimmunization may be required based on anti-HBs; test for HBsAg and anti-HBs at age 9 to 12 months or 1 to 2 months after completion of HepB series if delayed. HBsAg-negative infants with anti-HBs levels ≥10 mIU/mL are protected. HBsAg-negative infants with anti-HBs levels <10 mIU/mL should be reimmunized with a fourth dose and retested. If still <10 mIU/mL, two additional doses should be given. If after six doses the levels are <10 mIU/mL, no additional doses of HepB vaccine are indicated. *BW*, Birth weight; *HBIG*, hepatitis B immune globulin; *HepB*, hepatitis B. (Modified from American Academy of Pediatrics. *Red Book: 2021-2024 Report of the Committee on Infectious Diseases.* 32nd ed. AAP; 2021.)

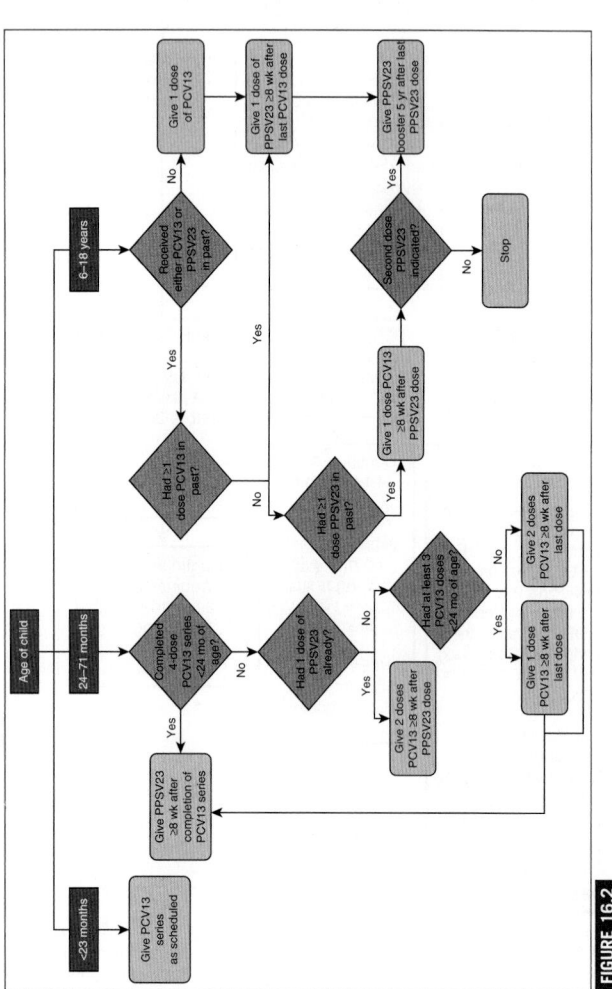

FIGURE 16.2

Pneumococcal immunization recommendations for children at high risk of pneumococcal disease. (Adapted from Table 3.65 in American Academy of Pediatrics. *Red Book: 2021-2024 Report of the Committee on Infectious Diseases.* 32nd ed. AAP; 2021.)

D. Pregnant Women

1. **Tdap (tetanus, diphtheria, acellular pertussis):** Give during each pregnancy, preferably at 27–36 weeks' gestation, regardless of prior immunization status.
2. **Give IIV** regardless of trimester. Do not administer LAIV.
3. **Other inactivated vaccines:** Considered precautionary and generally deferred until after the pregnancy, unless specific disease-risk/indication for vaccine present.
4. **Live vaccines:** Generally contraindicated during pregnancy

E. Immigration, Emigration, and Travel

1. **Travelers:**
   a. See CDC's Travelers' Health site for destination-specific recommendations: https://www.cdc.gov/travel/destinations/list
   b. Consider referral to a travel clinic.
2. **Immigrants from outside the United States:** See CDC's Immigrant and Refugee Health site for recommendations for immigrants, refugees, and international adoptees: https://www.cdc.gov/immigrantrefugeehealth/

VI. COUNSELING AND COMMUNICATION ABOUT VACCINES[22-34]

A. Vaccine Hesitant versus Vaccine Refusal[33]

1. **Vaccine hesitant:** Not dichotomous, but a continuum. For example, parents may delay but eventually accept vaccines or accept some vaccines and refuse others. 20% of children in United States have a vaccine-hesitant parent.
2. **Vaccine refusal:** Parents refuse all or some vaccines. 1.3% of toddlers in United States are completely unvaccinated; there has been increased vaccine refusal in last decade.
3. AAP recommends continued engagement with vaccine-hesitant/refusal parents while providing other health services and attempting to modify opposition to vaccines.[26]
4. **Determinants of vaccine acceptance**
   a. The 3C Model: Confidence, Complacency, Convenience. Key determinants of vaccine acceptance in global populations as determined by the World Health Organization SAGE Working Group on Vaccine Hesitancy.[25] See Section VIII, Online Content, for more details.
   b. Parental concerns about vaccines, including concerns about vaccine safety, vaccine necessity, and freedom of choice. See eBox 16.1 for details.

B. Countering Vaccine Hesitancy[26]

1. General principles
   a. Factor with greatest influence on parental decision to vaccinate is one-on-one conversation with child's pediatrician.
   b. Acknowledge and address parent and/or patient-specific concerns, while correcting misconceptions in nonconfrontational manner. Emphasize mutual desire to do what is best for the child.

16

BOX 16.1

COMMUNICATION STRATEGIES TO INCREASE VACCINE UPTAKE

- Presumptive > Participatory Approach[26]
  - Participatory: Would you like to vaccinate your child today? What do you think about vaccines?
  - Presumptive: Your child is due for three vaccines, so we will plan to give those during today's visit.
- CASE Approach[41]
  - Example statement of patient/guardian vaccine hesitancy: I've heard the MMR vaccine causes autism, so I don't want my child to get that one.
  - **Corroborate:** Acknowledge parental concern and find a point on which you can agree to set tone for respectful, successful discussion.
    - Example: That makes sense! There's lots of buzz on the news and internet about vaccines and autism. If the MMR vaccine caused autism, I wouldn't want your child to get it either.
  - **About Me:** Describe efforts you have made to build knowledge base and expertise. Consider including personal anecdotes, narratives, etc.
    - Example: I've been studying this claim for many years and have read many studies about the MMR vaccine, as well as about autism. I always want to make sure I have the most up-to-date information on this topic to give families.
  - **Science:** Present data (i.e., autism, Tdap in pregnancy, safety of ingredients)
    - Example: Dozens of studies have looked for a connection between the vaccine and autism, but no association has been identified. In fact, studies on autism show that children with autism display signs long before they receive the MMR vaccine. On the other hand, the MMR vaccine prevents measles, and I have seen how serious measles can be: one in three children become so sick they have to be hospitalized. Some even die.
  - **Explain/Advise:** Based on information you have presented, then give your strong recommendation.
    - Example: Choosing not to vaccinate will not protect your child from autism, but choosing to vaccinate will protect her from multiple dangerous diseases so that she can live a long and healthy life. I strongly recommend your child receive these vaccines today.

---

c. Present vaccination as default practice (opt-out, **not** opt-in).

d. Effective approaches to counseling on vaccine hesitancy include aspects of storytelling, anecdotes, and science-based messaging. Storytelling/anecdotes often play larger role in parents' decision to vaccinate, rather than data.[34]

e. Gain versus loss: framed messaging[34]

  (1) Though fear-based messaging has been effective in anti-vaccination movement, studies show it is ineffective for promoting vaccines.

  (2) Emphasize what patients/families will gain from vaccination, rather than what they might lose from not vaccinating.

  (3) Explain that vaccines benefit individual children and communities through herd immunity.

2. Specific strategies and resources
   a. See Box 16.1 for examples of specific communication strategies.
   b. See Section VIII, Online Content, and eBox 16.2 for more information on interventions and online provider resources.

VII. WEB RESOURCES[35-40]

- Advisory Committee on Immunization Practices (ACIP) Vaccine Recommendations and Guidelines: https://www.cdc.gov/vaccines/hcp/acip-recs/index.html
- Epidemiology and Prevention of Vaccine-Preventable Diseases (Pink Book): https://www.cdc.gov/vaccines/pubs/pinkbook/index.html
- AAP Report of the Committee on Infectious Diseases (Red Book): https://redbook.solutions.aap.org/
- CHOP Vaccine Education Center: https://www.chop.edu/centers-programs/vaccine-education-center
- WHO Immunization, Vaccines and Biologicals: https://www.who.int/teams/immunization-vaccines-and-biologicals
- VaxView: https://www.cdc.gov/vaccines/vaxview/index.html
- Data for ACIP-recommended vaccine coverage across the United States
- Vaccine Adverse Event Report System: https://vaers.hhs.gov/
  National vaccine safety surveillance program run by the CDC and U.S. Food and Drug Administration that collects information about postvaccination adverse events
- Vaccines for Children Program: https://www.cdc.gov/vaccines/programs/vfc/about/index.html
  Provides vaccines to children whose parents/guardians may not be able to afford them
- Centers for Disease Control and Prevention Vaccine Shortages and Delays: https://www.cdc.gov/vaccines/hcp/clinical-resources/shortages.html

16

REFERENCES

A complete list of references can be found online.

Chapter 17

Microbiology and Infectious Disease

Amali Gunawardana, MD and Ashley Wallace Wu, MD

🜚 See additional content online.

🔊 **Audio Case File 17.1** Resistance mechanisms in gram-negative rods

I. COMMON NEONATAL AND PEDIATRIC INFECTIONS: GUIDELINES FOR DIAGNOSIS AND INITIAL MANAGEMENT

Tables 17.1 to 17.6 and Figs. 17.1 to 17.3 present the most common neonatal and pediatric infections, organized by site of infection or by organism, when applicable. These recommendations are based on national guidelines and recent literature. They are not meant to replace clinical judgment.

For recommendations on preliminary identification of bacteria and antibiotic selection based on spectrum of activity for commonly used antibiotics, please see Sections II and III. Please note that local resistance patterns should guide antibiotic selection. Follow published institutional guidelines and culture results for individual patients and infections. When possible, always use the agent with the narrowest spectrum of activity, particularly when organism susceptibilities are known.

A. **Congenital, Perinatal, and Neonatal Infections (Table 17.1)**
B. **Pediatric Infections by System (Table 17.2)**
C. **Pediatric Viral Illnesses (Table 17.3)**
D. **Pediatric Tickborne Diseases (Table 17.4)**
E. **Pediatric Parasitic Infections (Table 17.5)**
F. **Pediatric Fungal Infections (Table 17.6)**
G. **Febrile Infants**

1. Etiology
   a. Bacterial infections (urinary tract infection [UTI], bacteremia, meningitis) should be considered in all febrile infants. Risk is significant even if well-appearing without a clear source. Most bacterial infections in age <90 days are UTIs.
   b. 0–28 days: *Escherichia coli*, group B streptococcal (GBS) disease. Rarely, *Listeria* spp.
   c. 29+ days: Invasive infections resulting from *Haemophilus influenzae* type B and *Streptococcus pneumoniae* have declined significantly since the introduction of conjugate vaccines.

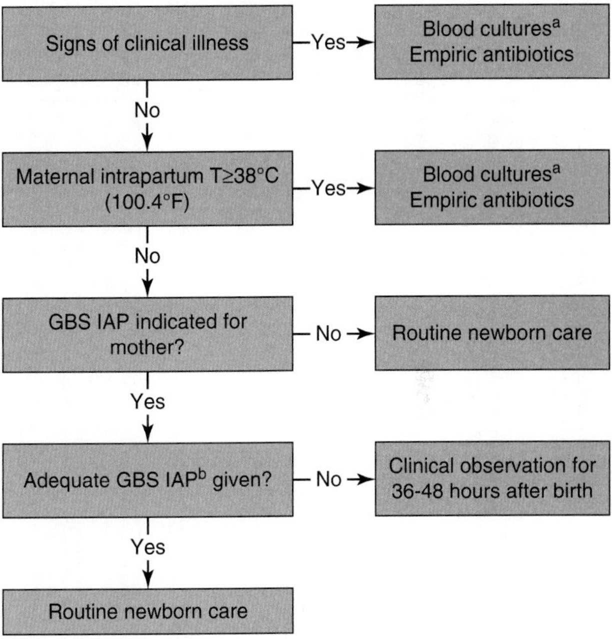

Figure flowchart:

Signs of clinical illness —Yes→ Blood cultures[a] Empiric antibiotics

↓ No

Maternal intrapartum T≥38°C (100.4°F) —Yes→ Blood cultures[a] Empiric antibiotics

↓ No

GBS IAP indicated for mother? — No → Routine newborn care

↓ Yes

Adequate GBS IAP[b] given? — No → Clinical observation for 36-48 hours after birth

↓ Yes

Routine newborn care

[a] Consider lumbar puncture and CSF culture before initiation of empiric antibiotics for infants who are at the highest risk of infection, especially those with critical illness. Lumbar puncture should not be performed if the infant's clinical condition would be compromised, and antibiotics should be administered promptly and not deferred because of procedure delays.

[b] Adequate GBS IAP is defined as the administration of penicillin G, ampicillin, or cefazolin ≥4 hours before delivery.

FIGURE 17.1

Example of categorical risk factor assessment for infants ≥35 weeks' gestation. The risk of infection is highly variable among newborn infants, depending on the gestational age, duration of membrane rupture, and timing and content of administered intrapartum antibiotics. This approach likely results in empiric treatment of many relatively low-risk infants. Newer, multivariate approaches are available online. (From Puopolo KM, Lynfield R, Cummings JJ. Committee on Infectious Diseases. Management of infants at risk for Group B streptococcal disease. *Pediatrics*. 2019;144[2]:e20191881.)

   d. *Staphylococcus aureus* is a significant cause of infection in the neonatal intensive care unit population.
   e. Fever following immunization is common (40% chance of fever within 48 hours).[1]
2. Workup and initial therapy *(continued on page 491)*

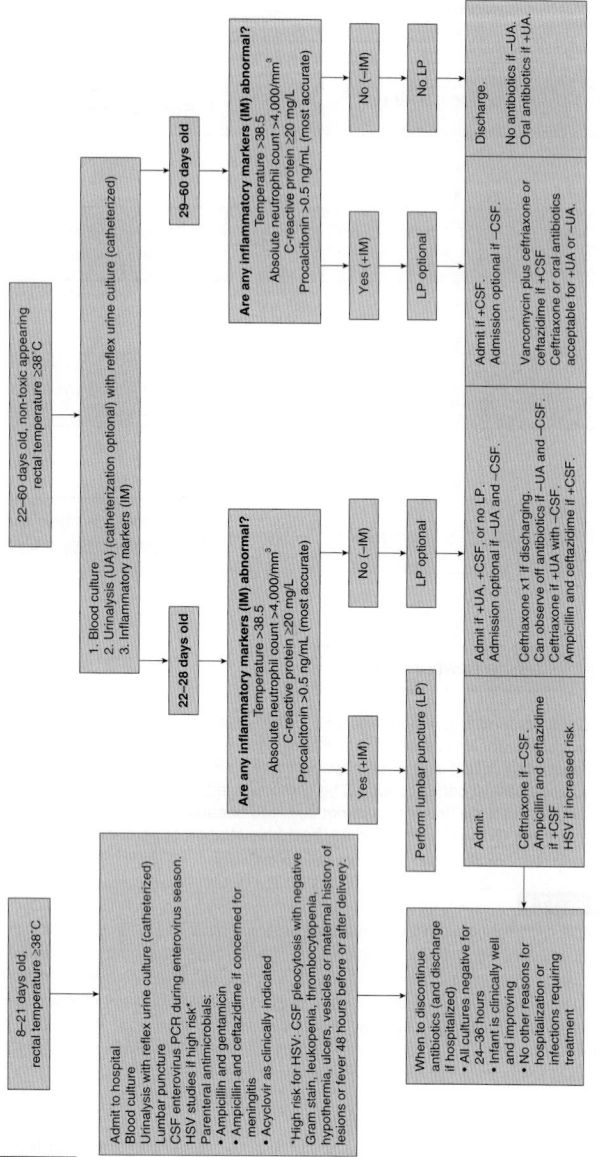

FIGURE 17.2

Algorithm for management of a previously healthy term infant 8 to 60 days with a fever without localizing signs. This algorithm is a suggested but not exhaustive approach. *CSF*, Cerebrospinal fluid; *HSV*, herpes simplex virus; *IM*, inflammatory marker; *LP*, lumbar puncture; *UA*, urinalysis. (Based on Pantell RH, Roberts KR, Adams WG, et al. Evaluation and management of well-appearing febrile infants 8 to 60 days old. *Pediatrics.* 2021;148[2].)

CONGENITAL, PERINATAL, AND NEONATAL INFECTIONS

	Presentation	Etiology	Diagnosis	Treatment
Cytomegalovirus (CMV)[2]	**Congenital:** 90% asymptomatic at birth. Diagnosed within 3 weeks of birth. IUGR, jaundice, thrombocytopenia, petechiae, hepatosplenomegaly, transaminitis, microcephaly, intracranial calcifications, sensorineural hearing loss, and retinitis **Postnatal:** Sepsis-like syndrome, thrombocytopenia, pneumonitis, hepatitis, typically in preterm and very-low-birth-weight infants	Human herpesvirus. Congenital infection is transmitted in utero. Postnatal infection may be acquired via birth canal or breastmilk. Persists in leukocytes and tissue	PCR or rapid viral culture of saliva, urine, blood, or CSF Variable practices for screening infants (urine or saliva). May target those who fail newborn hearing screen or those with low birth weight	Congenital: IV ganciclovir or PO valganciclovir for 6 months if symptomatic Hearing tests at regular intervals Postnatal: IV ganciclovir for 2–3 weeks. Follow CMV serum viral load and ANC during treatment.
Chlamydia trachomatis[2]	Ophthalmia (onset 5–12 days), afebrile pneumonia (onset 2–19 weeks), nasal stuffiness and otitis media, asymptomatic colonization	Obligate intracellular bacteria Affects 50% of infants born vaginally to affected moms	NAAT (gold standard), culture, or DFA of conjunctival cells and nasopharynx Test for gonorrhea.	Oral erythromycin ×14 days or oral azithromycin ×3 days Saline irrigation Erythromycin ointment NOT effective for ophthalmia prophylaxis
Gonorrhea[2]	Ophthalmia (onset 2–5 days), scalp abscess at electrode site, disseminated disease (sepsis, arthritis, meningitis)	Intracellular gram-negative diplococcus	Culture and Gram stain of exposed sites (conjunctiva, vagina, rectum, oropharynx) NAAT superior but not approved for conjunctival swab Gonococcal ophthalmia warrants hospitalization and workup for disseminated disease. Test for Chlamydia trachomatis.	Ceftriaxone or cefotaxime (if available) (single dose for ophthalmia, 7 days for scalp abscess/disseminated, 10–14 days for meningitis) Erythromycin ointment effective for ophthalmia prophylaxis

Continued

17

TABLE 17.1

CONGENITAL, PERINATAL, AND NEONATAL INFECTIONS—CONT'D

	Presentation	Etiology	Diagnosis	Treatment
Group B streptococcal disease (GBS)[27]	**Early onset (0–6 days):** 95% present within 48 hours. Most commonly pneumonia, bacteremia, or meningitis. 2% case fatality in term infants, 20% in preterm infants **Late onset (7–89 days):** Typically presents between 3–4 weeks. Most commonly bacteremia or meningitis. Also septic arthritis, osteomyelitis, UTI, and cellulitis.	Transmitted by mother with genitourinary GBS colonization OR maternal infection (bacteremia, endometritis, chorioamnionitis) Intrapartum antibiotics decrease transmission (at least 1 dose ≥4 hr prior to delivery) and early-onset disease.	Multiple accepted approaches for risk assessment among infants born >35 weeks of gestation. Example of common, categorical approach shown in Fig. 17.1. Newer, multivariate risk assessment (Neonatal Early-Onset Sepsis Calculator) is available at: https://neonatalsepsiscalculator.kaiserpermanente.org/. Diagnosis made by culture	**Intrapartum antibiotic prophylaxis:** Penicillin G preferred, ampicillin as alternative **Presumptive early-onset GBS sepsis:** ampicillin and gentamicin **Empiric treatment for late-onset GBS meningitis:** ampicillin and ceftazidime (or cefotaxime, if available) Ceftriaxone if >30 days. Consider inclusion of vancomycin for drug-resistant *Streptococcus pneumoniae* meningitis.
Hepatitis B virus (HBV)[2]	90% of infants infected perinatally or in first year of life develop chronic HBV infection, leading to: 1. Chronic low-grade hepatitis 2. Progression to cirrhosis and hepatocellular carcinoma 3. Risk of reactivation and acute hepatitis	Hepadnavirus usually transmitted perinatally (rather than in utero), from mother with acute or active chronic infection. 95% of transmission prevented with appropriate immunoprophylaxis at birth[29]	If mother HBsAg-positive, test infant for HBsAg and anti-HBsAg between 9 and 12 months (or 1–2 months after final HBV vaccine). Monitor HBV DNA and ALT in chronic HBV. Infection cleared at ~1% per year. See Table 17.7 for interpretation of serologies.	See Chapter 16 for immunoprophylaxis with HBV vaccine and hepatitis B immunoglobulin (HBIG). Breastfeeding is safe with appropriate immunoprophylaxis. Refer for treatment if active HBV replication with elevated ALT for 6 months.
Hepatitis C virus (HCV)[2]	80% of acute infections become chronic. Syndrome less pronounced than in hepatitis B	Flavivirus transmitted in utero or perinatally from about 5% of infected (RNA-positive) mothers	HCV antibody at 18 months for definitive diagnosis (maternal HCV antibodies persist 12+ months). Monitor ALT every 6 months.	Rapidly evolving field New oral antiviral regimens approved for age >3 years old. Breastfeeding safe. Consider pausing if nipples bleeding.

virus (HSV)[2]	1. Localized to skin, eyes, and mouth (45%) 2. Localized to CNS (30%) 3. Disseminated (25%) with sepsis, pneumonitis, hepatitis, consumptive coagulopathy, and CNS involvement	commonly via maternal genital tract with active HSV lesions. Less commonly ascending (in utero) and postnatal (via caregivers) transmission. >75% of cases born to mothers without known history of HSV	vesicles, mouth, nasopharynx, conjunctivae, and anus PCR or culture of blood and CSF LFTs Viremia can be seen in nondisseminated disease.	mouth disease; 21 days for CNS or disseminated disease. CSF clearance must be proven. Treat eye involvement with additional topical antiviral. All types receive 6 months PO acyclovir prophylaxis.
Parvovirus[2]	Fetal hydrops, IUGR, isolated pleural/ pericardial effusions, death in 2%– 6%, highest risk in 1st half of pregnancy	Small single-stranded DNA virus, replicates in erythrocyte precursors	IgM for diagnosis of acute infection PCR aids in diagnosis of hydrops fetalis.	Supportive care. Some success with intrauterine blood transfusion for hydrops fetalis
Rubella[2]	IUGR, cataracts, glaucoma, cardiac anomalies (patent ductus arteriosus and peripheral pulmonic stenosis), deafness, "blueberry muffin rash"	Togavirus transmitted via primary maternal infection (85% chance of transmission if maternal infection before 12 weeks gestation)	IgM at birth. Level typically would increase within first 6 months of life. Diagnosis can be confirmed by stable or increasing IgG level over first 7 to 11 months. RNA PCR and viral culture also used.	Supportive care, with evaluation by ophthalmology and cardiology Safe to vaccinate breastfeeding moms
Syphilis[2]	May be asymptomatic at birth Oro/nasopharyngeal secretions ("snuffles"), mucocutaneous lesions, maculopapular rash, hepatosplenomegaly, hemolytic anemia, thrombocytopenia If untreated, late disease affects CNS, bones/joints/teeth, eyes, and skin	*Treponema pallidum* is a spirochete transmitted in utero at any stage of maternal syphilis or at delivery.	If maternal nontreponemal serology positive (RPR or VDRL), obtain maternal serum treponemal test and screen infant using nontreponemal tests. Reverse sequence testing is also practiced. Full evaluation includes: CBC with differential, transaminases, CSF analysis, chest x-ray, long-bone x-rays, abdominal US, neuroimaging,	**Proven or highly probable** (abnormal exam, RPR or VDRL titer fourfold greater than maternal titer, or positive darkfield or PCR test): IV aqueous penicillin G or IM procaine penicillin G for 10 days. **If possible** (normal exam, RPR/VDRL ≤ fourfold maternal titer, AND one of the following: 1) mother not treated, inadequately treated, not documented, 2) mother treated with non-penicillin

Continued

TABLE 17.1

CONGENITAL, PERINATAL, AND NEONATAL INFECTIONS—CONT'D

	Presentation	Etiology	Diagnosis	Treatment
			ophthalmologic exam, auditory brainstem response testing. Refer to Red Book for interpretation of screening tests, diagnostic approach, and treatment algorithms.	regimen, or 3) mother treated <4 weeks before delivery): IV aqueous penicillin G for 10 days. **If less likely** (normal exam, RPR/VDRL ≤ fourfold maternal titer, mother adequately treated >4 weeks before delivery, and no evidence of reinfection/relapse): IM benzathine penicillin G single dose. **If unlikely** (normal exam, RPR/VDRL ≤ fourfold maternal titer, mother treated before pregnancy, and maternal titer low and stable before and throughout pregnancy): ensure titer returns to negative. Some experts give benzathine penicillin G single dose. Breastfeeding is safe in absence of breast chancre.
Toxoplasmosis[2]	May be asymptomatic at birth. Severe manifestations: chorioretinitis, cerebral calcifications, hydrocephalus. Other: IUGR, microcephaly, seizures, hearing loss, strabismus, petechial rash, cytopenias	Intracellular parasite transmitted via primary infection during pregnancy (contracted from cat feces or undercooked meat)	Serologies and PCR. Positive IgM after 5 days or IgA after 10 days or IgG after 12 months is diagnostic. Positive PCR in CSF, blood, or urine is diagnostic. Eye exam for chorioretinitis. CT is most sensitive for cerebral	Pyrimethamine + sulfadiazine with folinic acid for at least 12 months. Monitor ANC. Regular eye exams every 3–6 months

| Varicella | **Congenital infection:** varicella embryopathy (limb hypoplasia, cutaneous scarring, eye/CNS damage) **Perinatal infection:** Disseminated infection. Highest risk with maternal disease onset at 5 days before through 2 days after delivery. High mortality because of lack of sufficient maternal antibodies | Herpesvirus transmitted via primary maternal infection, most commonly during 1st or early 2nd trimester. Also via active lesions peripartum | PCR of vesicle or scab contents is gold standard. PCR of saliva is less sensitive | Acyclovir ×10 days in disseminated disease. Immunoprophylaxis with VariZIG (or IVIG) when: 1. Mother develops primary varicella between 5 days prepartum and 2 days postpartum. 2. Hospitalized preterm infants with known exposure[30] |
| Zika virus[31] | Microcephaly, CNS or ocular anomalies, deafness, congenital contractures | Flavivirus transmitted in utero after primary maternal infection | Workup: RNA PCR of blood/urine, IgM in serum, and neuroimaging. If obtaining CSF, can check RNA PCR and IgM. Test if: 1. Clinical findings with possible maternal infection in pregnancy based on stay in endemic areas 2. Lab-proven maternal infection in pregnancy, even without clinical findings | Supportive. Head ultrasound, audiology evaluation, and full ophthalmologic exam by 1 month. See Red Book and latest WHO/CDC algorithms. |

ALT, Alanine aminotransferase; *ANC,* absolute neutrophil count; *CBC,* complete blood count; *CDC,* Centers for Disease Control and Prevention; *CNS,* central nervous system; *CRP,* C-reactive protein; *CSF,* cerebrospinal fluid; *CT,* computed tomography; *DFA,* direct fluorescent antibody; *DNA,* deoxyribonucleic acid; *FNA,* fine needle aspiration; *HBsAg,* hepatitis B surface antigen; *Ig,* immunoglobulin; *IM,* intramuscular; *IUGR,* intrauterine growth restriction; *IV,* intravenous; *IVIG,* intravenous immunoglobulin; *NAAT,* nucleic acid amplification test; *PCR,* polymerase chain reaction; *PO,* by mouth; *RNA,* ribonucleic acid; *RPR,* rapid plasma regain; *UTI,* urinary tract infection; *VDRL,* venereal disease research laboratory test; *WHO,* World Health Organization.

17

TABLE 17.2

PEDIATRIC INFECTIONS BY SYSTEM

	Presentation	Etiology	Diagnosis	Treatment
CENTRAL NERVOUS SYSTEM				
Meningitis[32,33]	**Infant:** Ill-appearing, fever, hypothermia, lethargy, vomiting, poor feeding, seizures, bulging fontanelle **Child and adolescent:** Fever, headache, altered mental status, nuchal rigidity, photophobia, nausea, vomiting. Can be progressive or acute and fulminant	**<1 month:** Group B Streptococcus, Escherichia coli, Listeria **1–23 months:** Streptococcus pneumoniae, Neisseria meningitidis, S. agalactiae (GBS), Haemophilus influenzae **2+ years:** S. pneumoniae, N. meningitidis, Haemophilus influenzae Brain abscess: Streptococcus anginosus, other Streptococcus spp., anaerobes, Staphylococcus aureus	Indication for head CT prior to LP: immunocompromised, known CNS disease, papilledema, focal neurologic deficit LP for Gram stain, culture, and CSF analysis. See Table 17.8.	Initiate antibiotics as soon as the possibility of bacterial meningitis is considered; do not delay antibiotics for head CT or LP. **<1 month:** ampicillin + ceftazidime (or cefotaxime, if available) **1+ month:** vancomycin + ceftriaxone Adjunctive dexamethasone (administered at the initiation of antibiotic treatments) may reduce hearing loss in children >6 weeks with H. influenzae type B meningitis; has also been found to improve mortality, decrease hearing loss, and decrease neurologic complications in adults with pneumococcal meningitis; therefore, some experts recommend adjunctive dexamethasone in children/adolescents with pneumococcal meningitis. Brain abscess: vancomycin + ceftriaxone + metronidazole
CNS hardware infection[33]	Similar to meningitis	Staphylococcus epidermidis, S. aureus, gram-negative bacilli including Pseudomonas spp., Cutibacterium acnes	MRI with gadolinium CSF analysis, Gram stain, and culture (shunt sampling/tap or LP)	Vancomycin and cefepime Removal of all infected hardware with placement of an external ventriculostomy preferred over shunt externalization

Continued

HEAD AND NECK

Conjunctivitis[34]	Foreign body sensation, itching, burning, photophobia, hyperemia	Infectious: Most commonly viral (especially adenovirus). *S. pneumoniae*, *H. influenzae*, *Neisseria* spp., *Chlamydia trachomatis*, *Staphylococcus* spp. Noninfectious: allergic, toxic, inflammatory, dry eyes	Clinical diagnosis is nonspecific, and individual symptoms are unreliable. Allergic: Watery, pruritic Viral: Fever, bilateral conjunctivitis, lymphadenopathy Bacterial: Fever, purulent discharge, pain, adherence of eyelids upon awakening, lack of itching	**Viral:** Supportive care. **Bacterial:** Ophthalmic polymyxin B/TMP drops for bacterial infection. Ointments preferred in young children. Conjunctivitis secondary to gonorrhea/chlamydia requires systemic antibiotic treatment in addition to topical therapy. Conjunctivitis in contact lens wearers should always be treated. Ophthalmology consult if photophobia, vision loss, severe pain, recurrent episodes, or suspected gonorrhea
Acute otitis media[35]	Nonspecific symptoms and signs, including fever, irritability, apathy, poor feeding, vomiting, and diarrhea. May have ear pain and/or rubbing	*S. pneumoniae*, *H. influenzae*, *Moraxella catarrhalis*	Moderate-to-severe bulging of the tympanic membrane, mild bulging with signs of inflammation, or new-onset otorrhea	High-dose amoxicillin × 10 days if <2 years old OR if severe symptoms regardless of age; 7 days if 2–5 years old, 5 days if 6 years or older If received amoxicillin in past 30 days, give amoxicillin/clavulanate. Consider watchful waiting if: 6–23 months—unilateral AOM without otorrhea or severe symptoms (toxic-appearing, T ≥39°C, otalgia >48 hr) 24+ months—unilateral or bilateral AOM without otorrhea or severe symptoms If treatment failure after 48–72 hr: amoxicillin-clavulanate × 10 days or IM ceftriaxone × 1–3 days

17

TABLE 17.2

PEDIATRIC INFECTIONS BY SYSTEM—CONT'D

	Presentation	Etiology	Diagnosis	Treatment
Mastoiditis[36]	Complication of acute otitis media Tender mastoid, protruding auricle	*S. pneumoniae, Streptococcus pyogenes, S. aureus, H. influenzae*	Clinical. Contrast CT or MRI if complications suspected (CNS signs, ill-appearing, treatment failure)	Empiric ceftriaxone and vancomycin Often requires surgical management
Otitis externa[37]	Ear pain, pruritus, discharge, auricle and tragus tenderness and erythema	*Pseudomonas* spp., *S. aureus*	Culture in severe cases.	Otic drops × 7 days: ciprofloxacin or polymyxin-neomycin Wick if outer canal swollen.
Group A streptococcal pharyngitis[19]	Classic signs: Fever, tonsillar exudates, lymphadenopathy, absence of cough Higher concern between age 3 and 15 Scarlet fever (from exotoxin production) involves diffuse, finely papular, erythematous rash 24–48 hr after onset of symptoms	*S. pyogenes*	Rapid antigen detection test or nucleic acid test (NAT). If negative, confirm with culture. IDSA recommends testing if 3+ years old, without viral symptoms (cough, rhinorrhea, hoarseness, oral ulcers).	Amoxicillin × 10 days or benzathine penicillin IM × 1 dose Nonsevere PCN allergy: cephalexin × 10 days PCN-allergic: clindamycin × 10 days Second line: azithromycin × 5 days
Peritonsillar abscess[38,39]	Sore throat, trismus, uvular deviation Can be bilateral Most common in adolescents	Often polymicrobial: *S. pyogenes*, viridans group streptococci, *S. aureus, Haemophilus* spp., oral anaerobes	Clinical. Consider imaging if diagnosis unclear.	Ampicillin/sulbactam or ceftriaxone/ cefotaxime (if available) + clindamycin Often requires aspiration or I&D
Retropharyngeal/ parapharyngeal abscess[38,39]	Sore throat, fever, dysphagia, neck stiffness, medial deviation of wall of oropharynx (parapharyngeal abscess)	Often polymicrobial: *S. pyogenes*, viridans group streptococci, *S. aureus, Haemophilus* spp., oral anaerobes	Clinical. Consider imaging if diagnosis unclear.	Ampicillin/sulbactam or ceftriaxone/ cefotaxime (if available) + clindamycin If no airway compromise, can trial antibiotics × 48–72 hr, prior to obtaining CT and surgical management

Condition	Clinical features	Microbiology	Diagnosis	Treatment
Ludwig angina (submandibular cellulitis)[40]	Rapidly progressive, bilateral cellulitis, often originating as dental infection Causes elevation of the tongue, risk of airway compromise	Often polymicrobial: viridans group Streptococci, S. aureus, oral anaerobes	Clinical. Consider imaging if diagnosis unclear.	Ampicillin/sulbactam or ceftriaxone + metronidazole (if PCN allergic: levofloxacin + metronidazole) Add vancomycin to above regimens if concern for MRSA. Consider surgical drainage.
Lemierre syndrome[41]	Thrombophlebitis of internal jugular vein seeded from primary oropharyngeal infection, bacteremia, or distant site(s) of infection. High-grade fever (>39.5C), neck swelling/tenderness, exudative tonsillitis, or grayish pseudomembranes	Fusobacterium necrophorum, oral Streptococci	WBC count, CRP, and ESR often are markedly elevated. CT with contrast is most useful imaging modality An unremarkable oropharyngeal appearance at the time of septicemia does not rule out Lemierre syndrome.	Aqueous penicillin G AND metronidazole Surgical management often required
Preseptal cellulitis[42]	May follow external trauma, spread from sinuses or hematogenous infection	S. aureus, Streptococcus spp.	Clinical	Amoxicillin/clavulanate × 7 days
Orbital cellulitis[42]	Proptosis, ophthalmoplegia, pain on extraocular movements, and blurred vision	Streptococcus spp., S. aureus, H. influenzae, M. catarrhalis Most commonly extension of rhinosinusitis Immunocompromised or diabetic—consider fungal (e.g. Mucorales)	CT with contrast; ophthalmology and ENT consultation	Ceftriaxone or cefotaxime (if available) + vancomycin OR ampicillin/sulbactam + vancomycin (if no concern for CNS involvement) Often requires abscess drainage

Continued

TABLE 17.2

PEDIATRIC INFECTIONS BY SYSTEM—CONT'D

	Presentation	Etiology	Diagnosis	Treatment
Sinusitis (bacterial)[43]	Rhinorrhea, inflammation of septum and turbinates, tenderness over sinuses	*S. pneumoniae, H. influenzae* (nontypeable), *M. catarrhalis* If chronic, also *S. aureus*, anaerobes	Clinical: Persistent sinusitis 10+ days without improvement, worsening course after initial improvement, or severe symptoms (purulent discharge, fever ≥39°C) for 3+ days	Amoxicillin/clavulanate × 10–14 days. Some experts recommend only 7 days of antibiotic treatment. If mild but persistent symptoms >10 days, can opt to observe with close follow-up. In chronic sinusitis, consider culture to guide antibiotics.
Cervical lymphadenitis[2,44-46]	Distinguished from reactive lymphadenopathy by fluctuance, warmth, overlying erythema	**Acute (<2 weeks): Unilateral:** most commonly *S. aureus*, *S. pyogenes* **Bilateral:** Consider EBV, CMV. **Chronic (>2 weeks):** Consider *Bartonella henselae* (cat scratch disease), nontuberculous mycobacterium (NTM), Toxoplasmosis, HIV, TB	Consider ultrasound if diagnosis unclear. Consider FNA and culture if no improvement in 48–72 hr. If >2 weeks, consider tuberculin skin test.	PO: Cephalexin or amoxicillin/clavulanate or clindamycin empirically. Definitive treatment is based on culture and susceptibility. Duration × 7–14 days If no response to PO/severe disease: cefazolin, clindamycin, or vancomycin Bartonella: Azithromycin × 5 days shown to have mild effect. Needle aspiration as needed for relief of symptoms only, because disease is self-limited and spontaneously resolves in 2–4 months. NTM: Curative management-surgical excision, if incomplete or recurrence, antibiotics can be used (macrolide + rifampin)
Oral candidiasis (thrush)	White plaques on tongue, buccal mucosa, and/or palate	*Candida albicans* is most common.	Clinical	Nystatin swish and swallow or clotrimazole troches for 7–14 days. Nystatin for infants

Community-acquired pneumonia[47]	Fever, respiratory distress, cough On exam, tachypnea, hypoxia, diminished breath sounds, crackles, asymmetric breath sounds	Bacterial: *S. pneumoniae,* nontypeable *H. influenzae, M. catarrhalis.* *Mycoplasma pneumoniae* and *Chlamydophila pneumoniae* may be considered in subacute presentations. Viral: Influenza, parainfluenza, human metapneumovirus, adenovirus	Clinical diagnosis for mild disease. Chest x-ray if hypoxic, respiratory distress, or hospitalized. CBC or inflammatory markers (CRP, ESR, procalcitonin) are not reliable to differentiate bacterial vs viral pneumonia. Blood culture not required for mild disease	**Outpatient:** High-dose amoxicillin × 5 days. **Inpatient:** Ampicillin × 5 days. **ICU:** Ceftriaxone plus coverage for MRSA empirically (e.g., TMP/SMX, vancomycin, clindamycin). Vancomycin not preferred due to poor lung penetration. Some experts discontinue MRSA coverage based on negative MRSA nares screening. Small parapneumonic effusions treated with antibiotics alone
Pertussis[2]	Mild URI symptoms (catarrhal stage). Progresses to whooping cough (paroxysmal stage) Duration 6–10 weeks Atypical presentation in neonates with cyanosis, gasping and posttussive emesis	*Bordetella pertussis.* Droplet transmission. Incubation 7–10 days	NAAT performed on posterior nasopharynx specimen	Azithromycin × 5 days. Alternative: TMP-SMX. Treatment during paroxysmal stage unlikely to affect clinical course but reduces transmission. Postexposure prophylaxis recommended for household and other close contacts (including children in daycare) = also azithromycin × 5 days
Tuberculosis	See Section I.H			
GASTROINTESTINAL				
Appendicitis[48]	Right lower quadrant pain, anorexia, fever More difficult to diagnose in females or those <3 years of age	Enteric pathogens + anaerobes	Clinical diagnosis Imaging (ultrasound, otherwise CT with contrast or MRI)	Ceftriaxone + metronidazole + source control Nonoperative management only considered if symptoms <48 hr and no abscess or fecalith

Continued

17

TABLE 17.2

PEDIATRIC INFECTIONS BY SYSTEM—CONT'D

	Presentation	Etiology	Diagnosis	Treatment
Gastroenteritis[2,49,50]	Typically mild disease that does not require hospitalization. Worrisome signs include: age <3 months, underlying disease, persistent vomiting, high-output diarrhea (>8×/day), family reported signs of severe dehydration.	Etiologies without treatment: toxin-mediated *S. aureus*, *Bacillus cereus*, *Clostridium perfringens*; viral: norovirus, rotavirus, astrovirus, adenovirus	If suspect inflammatory bacterial enteritis: stool culture or bacterial NAAT panel. Depending on exposures and chronicity, consider stool for ova and parasites.	Enteral rehydration is preferred to intravenous rehydration regardless of etiology.
		Nontyphoid *Salmonella* spp.[51]		If <3 months, immunocompromised, hemoglobinopathy, or severe disease, treat with ceftriaxone or azithromycin. Optimal treatment duration unknown, range 3–14 days. Consider longer duration (7 days) in immunocompromised hosts, infants, and those with invasive disease (bacteremia), where evaluating for focal infection is often warranted to guide management and treatment duration.
		Shigella spp.		If <3 months, immunocompromised, or severe disease, treat with ceftriaxone × 2–5 days, azithromycin × 3 days, or ciprofloxacin × 3 days.

Campylobacter spp.		If severe disease, age <3 months, relapse, immunocompromised: azithromycin × 3 days or erythromycin × 5 days or ciprofloxacin × 3–5 days. Most patients do not require antimicrobial therapy.
E. coli		In most cases there is no need for antibiotics. Azithromycin × 3 days or fluoroquinolone × 3 days if severe or prolonged (>14 days); no antibiotics for STEC O157:H7, as antibiotics may increase risk of hemolytic uremic syndrome[52]
Clostridioides difficile colitis[53]	Diarrhea, pseudomembranous colitis with fever and abdominal pain. Fulminant disease can present with shock, ileus, or megacolon. Asymptomatic colonization is common in infants <12 months old.	Stool *C. difficile* toxin gene NAAT Do not test unless ≥3 unformed stools within 24 hr. Make sure patient is not receiving laxatives.	Discontinue antibiotics if possible. **Non-severe:** PO vancomycin (preferred) or PO metronidazole **Severe:** PO vancomycin or PO fidaxomicin **Fulminant** (shock, ileus, or toxic megacolon): PO vancomycin + IV metronidazole If ileus: rectal vancomycin + IV metronidazole
Giardia[?]	Intermittent cramps, watery diarrhea that becomes foul-smelling, greasy, fatty Can be asymptomatic, acute, or chronic	Flagellate protozoan Fecal-oral transmission of cysts Incubation period 1–3 weeks	Stool EIA or DFA Stool NAAT panel if available	Metronidazole × 5–7 days Alternatives: nitazoxanide × 3 days or tinidazole × 1 dose, paromomycin preferred in pregnancy

17

Continued

TABLE 17.2

PEDIATRIC INFECTIONS BY SYSTEM—CONT'D

	Presentation	Etiology	Diagnosis	Treatment
Helicobacter pylori[54,55]	Chronic gastritis, duodenal ulcer. Can often be asymptomatic. Warning signs include severe chronic abdominal pain, anorexia and failure to thrive, occult blood in stool, nighttime wakening with pain, or persistent vomiting. Associations: iron deficiency anemia, short stature, and chronic immune thrombocytopenia	Fecal-oral transmission Up to 90% prevalent in resource-poor countries	Diagnosis should aim to find the underlying cause of symptoms and not solely look for H. pylori infection. Diagnostic testing for H. pylori not recommended in children with functional abdominal pain. Gold standard: gastric biopsy with culture (also yields susceptibilities). Test of cure (stool EIA or urea breath test) 4–6 weeks after treatment	Regimen selection should preferentially be guided by susceptibilities. If unknown susceptibilities, the following regimens may be initiated: Triple therapy options: PPI + amoxicillin + clarithromycin × 14 days or PPI + amoxicillin + metronidazole × 14 days Quadruple therapy options: PPI + bismuth + amoxicillin + metronidazole (if <8 years old) × 14 days or PPI + bismuth + metronidazole + tetracycline (if at least 8 years old) × 14 days
GENITOURINARY				
Cystitis (UTI)[56,57]	Dysuria, urgency, frequency, new-onset enuresis, suprapubic pain Foul-smelling urine is not sensitive for UTI.	E. coli (>80%), Klebsiella spp., Enterococcus spp. The following are not considered pathogens in healthy children: Lactobacillus spp., coagulase-negative staphylococci, and Corynebacterium spp.	Diagnosis requires pyuria (≥10 WBCs/hpf) and culture demonstrating ≥50,000 CFU/mL of a uropathogen for catheterized specimens or ≥100,000 CFU/mL of a uropathogen for clean-catch samples	PO cephalexin, cefadroxil, or nitrofurantoin: 3 days

| Pyelonephritis[56,58] | Symptoms of cystitis, plus fever, flank pain, nausea/vomiting

All nonverbal infants and toddlers presenting with systemic symptoms and evidence of UTI are considered to have pyelonephritis. Risk factors for infants less than 2 years:
Temp >39°C
Fever >2 days
Young age (<12 mo)
Uncircumcised male
Risk factors for all ages: bladder-bowel dysfunction, congenital anomalies of the kidney and urinary tract (including vesicoureteral reflux) | See cystitis. | See cystitis.
In infants, bagged urine specimen can be used for screening urinalysis, and if positive, should send catheterized sample for culture and repeat urinalysis. | If tolerating PO, not ill-appearing, and no concerns regarding adherence, PO can be considered. Cephalexin or cefadroxil is reasonable first line.
If not tolerating PO or ill-appearing, IV cefazolin or ceftriaxone
Pseudomonal coverage if history of prior pseudomonas or catheter dependent
Transition to oral antibiotics once clinically improving. Consider renal US if no improvement/persistent fever after 72 hours of antibiotics.
Duration: 7 days. Longer treatment up to 14 days can be considered in certain circumstances.
In young (<2 years) patients with 1st time febrile UTI: renal bladder ultrasound; VCUG if abnormal. If US normal and recurrent UTI occurs, obtain VCUG.[59] |
| Sexually transmitted infections | See Chapter 5. | | | |

Continued

TABLE 17.2

PEDIATRIC INFECTIONS BY SYSTEM—CONT'D

	Presentation	Etiology	Diagnosis	Treatment
OSTEOARTICULAR				
Osteomyelitis[60,61]	Majority in long bones: Pain, limping, swelling, erythema, fever Spinal infection in infants involving the discs: Gradual irritability, refusal to crawl/sit Spinal infection involving vertebra in adolescents: Back pain	Hematogenous spread S. aureus (>80% cases), GAS, S. pneumoniae, GBS (<3 months), Kingella kingae (<5 years), Salmonella spp. (if history of sickle cell disease)	Blood cultures, consider bone cultures. Inflammatory markers: CRP Imaging: x-ray, MRI If feasible, withhold antibiotics prior to obtaining invasive diagnostic testing (Gram stain/culture of fluid/aspirate/bone). If patient is ill appearing, do not withhold antibiotics.	Consider empiric coverage based on local resistance patterns. For children <5 years: (cefazolin or oxacillin) ± (TMP/SMX or clindamycin if concern for MRSA) For children >5 years: Cefazolin (TMP/SMX or clindamycin if concern for MRSA). If unstable or ill-appearing, IV vancomycin preferred. Switch to oral therapy when clinically improved. Duration 3–4 weeks for acute infection
Hardware-associated bone infection[60]	Pain, limping, swelling, erythema, fever	Coagulase-negative staphylococci, S. aureus, C. acnes, gram-negative bacilli including Pseudomonas spp.	Same as osteomyelitis	Cefepime and vancomycin empirically; add rifampin if S. aureus, but need to confirm susceptibility. Prolonged duration of treatment
Septic arthritis[2,62]	Pain, swelling of joint, inability to bear weight, gait abnormality, fever	S. aureus (>80% cases) GAS, S. pneumoniae, K. kingae (<5 years), Salmonella (if history of sickle cell disease) Borrelia burgdorferi (Lyme arthritis; if subacute	Kocher criteria used to differentiate septic joint from transient synovitis. Designed for hips, but often applied to knee/ankle If 3 of 4 criteria met, 93% chance of septic joint:	Early drainage relieves discomfort, prevents synovial damage. Consider empiric coverage based on local resistance patterns. For children <5 years: Cefazolin ± (TMP/SMX or clindamycin if concern for MRSA.

	presentation involving large joint). *Neisseria gonorrhoeae* (adolescents with migratory arthritis)	1. Non–weight bearing 2. Fever 3. ESR >40 mm/hr 4. WBC >12,000/mm³ If criteria met or high-risk: Knee—x-ray Hip—ultrasound Joint aspiration suggests septic arthritis if >50,000 WBC/mm³. For Lyme arthritis: two-tier test with serology and confirmation western blot and/or PCR from joint fluid	For children >5 years: cefazolin or clindamycin or TMP/SMX If unstable or ill-appearing, IV vancomycin preferred Lyme arthritis: Ceftriaxone, then step down to amoxicillin or doxycycline *N. gonorrhoeae*: ceftriaxone. Should also treat for chlamydia and test for other STIs. Duration 3–4 weeks for acute infection. Switch to oral therapy when clinically improved.

SKIN AND SOFT TISSUE

Nonpurulent cellulitis/ erysipelas[63]	Intact skin, erythema, warmth, swelling, tenderness, nonpurulent	Beta-hemolytic *streptococci*. Less common *S. aureus*	Clinical Blood or wound culture not routinely recommended	Cephalexin or Cefadroxil × 5 days
Purulent cellulitis/abscess[63]	Erythema, warmth, fever, tenderness, fluctuance, induration, history of purulent drainage	*S. aureus*	Clinical Ultrasound can confirm drainable collection. Wound cultures for hospitalized or immunocompromised children	**Mild** (no systemic signs of infection): I&D. One study demonstrated benefit of TMP/SMX or clindamycin regardless of abscess size, but must weigh with side effects.[64] **Moderate** (systemic signs of infection: fever, tachycardia, tachypnea, abnormal WBC count): I&D + antibiotics (cefazolin, clindamycin, TMP/SMX, or doxycycline) **Severe** (systemic signs of infection with failed I&D + antibiotics, immunocompromised): I&D + vancomycin

Continued

17

TABLE 17.2

PEDIATRIC INFECTIONS BY SYSTEM—CONT'D

	Presentation	Etiology	Diagnosis	Treatment
Animal/human bites[63]	Higher-risk injury with puncture wounds	Often polymicrobial: S. aureus, streptococci, Pasteurella multocida (animal), Capnocytophaga spp. (animal), oral anaerobes, Eikenella corrodens (human)	Clinical: Puncture vs. nonpuncture	Antibiotic prophylaxis is indicated if moderate/severe wound especially of hand or face, immunocompromise, possible penetration of periosteum or joint capsule, or edema of the area. Prophylaxis: amoxicillin/clavulanate × 5 days. See Chapter 2 for additional management. See Chapter 16 for postexposure prophylaxis recommendations for tetanus and rabies.
Dermatophyte (tinea) infections[2]	**Tinea capitis:** Multiple scaly patches with alopecia and patches of alopecia with black dots at follicular orifices that represent broken hairs. May also present with widespread scaling, kerion, or favus **Tinea pedis** (athlete's foot): Interdigital hyperkeratotic or vesiculopustular eruption **Tinea cruris** (jock itch): Involving the inguinal fold, groin, pubic/perianal area, or upper thighs **Tinea corporis:** Dermatophyte infection occurring in sites other than feet, groin, face,	Dermatophytes	Tinea capitis, pedis, cruris, corporis: Clinical Can confirm with skin scrapings in 10% potassium hydroxide (KOH) or fungal culture	Tinea capitis: Oral griseofulvin or terbinafine × 4–8 weeks or 2 weeks after clinical resolution Fungal shedding decreased with selenium sulfide or ketoconazole shampoo Tinea pedis, cruris, corporis: Topical antifungal Tinea pedis: 2–4 weeks Tinea cruris: 4–6 weeks Tinea corporis: 4–6 weeks

Tinea unguium (onychomycosis): White or yellow discoloration of finger- or toenail, often with thickening, splitting, or deformity		nail clippings in 10% KOH or culture/staining.	topical ciclopirox 5/6 twice daily for 4–48 weeks preferred (no lab monitoring) Alternative: Oral terbinafine 6 weeks if fingernail; 12 weeks if toenail

BLOODSTREAM

Catheter-related bloodstream infections[65]	Fever, erythema around catheter site; pain or hemodynamic instability with infusion	S. aureus, gram-negative bacilli including Pseudomonas spp., coagulase-negative staphylococci (usually requires two positive cultures to exclude contaminant), Enterococcus spp.	Two sets of cultures (one peripheral, one from suspected catheter) prior to antibiotics If unable to draw peripheral culture, draw two sets from lumen(s) several minutes apart.	Vancomycin and cefepime Remove line whenever possible. If line removal is not possible, infection is uncomplicated, and no sign of exit site or tunnel infection, can consider central line lock therapy with antibiotics or HCl to salvage line. Should be used in conjunction with systemic antimicrobial therapy. If candidemia, line removal is indicated. Refer to IDSA guidelines for further management. Consultation with infectious disease specialist is recommended.
Malaria[2,66]	Paroxysmal fevers and malaise Severe malaria: 5 + % parasitemia, CNS involvement, shock, hypoglycemia, anemia, thrombocytopenia, acidosis	Plasmodium falciparum, vivax, ovale, malariae, knowlesi P. vivax and ovale form hypozoites in liver, difficult to eradicate. Incubation period 7 to 30 days P. vivax and ovale can recur weeks to years later because of reemergence of hepatic hypnozoites.	Thick and thin blood smears If high suspicion with negative smears, repeat every 12–24 hr for 72 hr (minimum 3 smears). Rapid antigen detection tests exist. Speciation is performed by microscopy, with	Severe: IV artesunate, followed by full course of oral regimen Nonsevere (chloroquine-resistant or unknown resistance): artemether-lumefantrine × 3 days or atovaquone-proguanil × 3 days or mefloquine Nonsevere (chloroquine-sensitive) or P. malariae/knowlesi: chloroquine or hydroxychloroquine

Continued

17

TABLE 17.2

PEDIATRIC INFECTIONS BY SYSTEM—CONT'D

	Presentation	Etiology	Diagnosis	Treatment
			confirmation by PCR in specialized labs.	*P. vivax* or *P. ovale*: Add anti-relapse treatment with primaquine phosphate × 14 days; perform G6PD testing prior to initiation. Travel prophylaxis varies by region due to chloroquine resistance. See CDC Yellow Book for resistance info and specific regimens.
OTHER				
Fever of unknown origin[67,68]	Defined as temperature greater than 38°C for >8 days without a clear source	Localized or systemic infections are most commonly identified etiology. Other etiologies include: rheumatologic, neoplastic, collagen vascular disease (e.g., juvenile idiopathic arthritis), drug fever, and Kawasaki disease. Often an uncommon presentation of a common disease	No specific guidelines exist; stepwise approach is recommended. First line: CBC, BMP, LFTs, UA, urine and blood cultures. Further studies targeted per history and physical/initial workup.	Consider discontinuing all nonessential medications to aid in diagnosis. Treatment depends on etiology identified.

AAP, American Academy of Pediatrics; *ANA,* antinuclear antibody; *AOM,* acute otitis media; *AUA,* American Urologic Association; *BMP,* basic metabolic panel; *CBC,* complete blood count; *CDC,* Centers for Disease Control and Prevention; *CFU,* colony-forming unit; *CMV,* cytomegalovirus; *CN,* cranial nerve; *CNS,* central nervous system; *CRP,* C-reactive protein; *CSF,* cerebrospinal fluid; *CT,* computed tomography; *DFA,* direct fluorescent antibody; *EBV,* Epstein-Barr virus; *EIA,* enzyme immunoassay; *ENT,* ear-nose-throat physician (otolaryngologist); *ESR,* erythrocyte sedimentation rate; *FNA,* fine-needle aspiration; *GBS,* group B streptococcus; *HIV,* human immunodeficiency virus; *hpf,* high-power field; *ICU,* intensive care unit; *I&D,* incision and drainage; *IDSA,* Infectious Disease Society of America; *IM,* intramuscular; *IV,* intravenous; *LFTs,* liver function tests; *LP,* lumbar puncture; *MRI,* magnetic resonance imaging; *MRSA,* methicillin-resistant *Staphylococcus aureus*; *NAAT,* nucleic acid amplification test; *PCN,* penicillin; *PCR,* polymerase chain reaction; *PO,* by mouth; *RIVUR,* randomized intervention for children with vesicoureteral reflux; *STEC,* Shiga toxin–producing *Escherichia coli*; *T,* temperature; *TB,* tuberculosis; *TMP,* trimethoprim; *TMP/SMX,* trimethoprim sulfamethoxazole; *UA,* urinalysis; *URI,* upper respiratory infection; *UTI,* urinary tract infection; *VCUG,* voiding cystourethrography; *VP,* ventriculoperitoneal; *WBC,* white blood cell.

TABLE 17.3

PEDIATRIC VIRAL ILLNESSES

	Presentation	Transmission and Incubation	Diagnosis	Treatment
Cytomegalovirus (CMV)[2]	Children: most commonly asymptomatic. Adults/adolescents: infectious mononucleosis-like syndrome with fever and hepatitis. Immunocompromised: pneumonia, retinitis, colitis, leukopenia, thrombocytopenia. See Table 17.1 for congenital CMV.	Primary infection from respiratory droplets or vertical transmission. Can also be transmitted via non-leukodepleted blood transfusion, solid organ transplant, or hematopoietic stem cell transplant. Persists after primary infection with intermittent shedding	CMV DNA PCR to determine presence of infection (i.e., viral replication)—quantitative preferred. Histopathology required for definitive diagnosis of tissue invasive disease. IgG to screen for risk of reactivation (e.g., organ transplant donors and recipients); not useful for diagnosing active infection/disease	Immunocompetent children: no treatment. Immunocompromised children (e.g., HSCT, SOT): preemptive therapy for CMV viremia to prevent CMV disease OR treatment of CMV disease: Preferred: ganciclovir IV or valganciclovir PO. Alternatives: foscarnet IV or cidofovir IV (more nephrotoxic). Universal prophylaxis in serodiscordant SOT recipients with valganciclovir PO
Dengue[2]	Febrile phase (2–7 days) with myalgias, arthralgias, retro-orbital headache. Critical phase (24–48 hr) follows defervescence with increased vascular permeability. Convalescent phase with gradual improvement. Severe dengue (hemorrhagic fever): severe abdominal pain, bleeding, shock	Four virus subtypes; severe dengue more common with second or subsequent infections. Transmitted by *Aedes* mosquitoes. Incubation period 3–14 days	RT-PCR or anti-dengue virus IgM EIA	Supportive. Avoid NSAIDs (bleeding risk)

Continued

17

TABLE 17.3

PEDIATRIC VIRAL ILLNESSES—CONT'D

	Presentation	Transmission and Incubation	Diagnosis	Treatment
Epstein-Barr virus (EBV)[2]	Infectious mononucleosis: Fever, pharyngitis with petechiae or exudates, hepatosplenomegaly, atypical lymphocytosis. Variable presentation in young children. Associated with post-transplant lymphoproliferative disease, Burkitt lymphoma, nasopharyngeal carcinoma, and other malignancies	Transmitted via oral secretions or sexual contact. Incubation period 30–50 days	Heterophile antibody positive by 2 weeks postexposure; though low sensitivity in children under 4 years. IgM/IgG to viral capsid antigen if heterophile negative and suspicion high. See Fig. 17.3.	Supportive. No strenuous activity or contact sports × 21 days, or until symptoms and splenomegaly resolve. Steroids if tonsillar swelling threatens airway, massive splenomegaly, myocarditis, hemolytic anemia, or HLH
Human immunodeficiency virus (HIV)[2]	See Section I. I.			
Influenza[2]	Often abrupt onset of systemic symptoms (fever, myalgias, chills, headache, malaise, anorexia) with URI, croup, bronchiolitis, pneumonia Complications include AOM, secondary bacterial pneumonia (especially *Staphylococcus aureus* and *Streptococcus pneumoniae*); rarely myositis, myocarditis, or CNS complications, including encephalitis, myelitis, Guillain-Barré syndrome	Incubation 1–4 days	Clinical diagnosis; lab confirmation should be performed given overlapping presentation with SARS-CoV-2. Multiple rapid antigen and PCR tests exist.	Oseltamivir for 5 days. Alternatives include inhaled zanamivir, IV peramivir, and PO baloxavir. Most effective within 48 hr of onset of symptoms Treat all patients who are hospitalized, have severe illness, or are at high risk for complications. Consider treating patients who could transmit to elderly or unvaccinated contacts. Counsel families on influenza vaccination.

Measles[2]	Fever, cough, coryza, conjunctivitis, Koplik spots, descending maculopapular rash. At risk for acute encephalitis and subacute sclerosing panencephalitis	Droplet and airborne precautions. Incubation period 8–12 days	RT-PCR from throat swab or urine or serum IgM (ideally, obtain all 3, as this will increase likelihood of achieving a diagnosis)	Supportive. Counsel families on measles vaccination. Vitamin A reduces morbidity and mortality. Avoid aspirin/salicylate-containing products due to risk of Reye syndrome. Recommendations change yearly. See http://www.cdc.gov/flu.
Mumps[2]	Swelling of 1+ salivary glands, often parotid. Orchitis more common after puberty	Droplet precautions until 5 days after onset of parotid swelling. Incubation period 12–25 days	RT-PCR from buccal swab. Serum IgM	Supportive
Parvovirus B19 (Fifth disease)[2]	Mild viral syndrome followed by slapped cheek rash with circumoral pallor. Symmetric, macular, reticular rash on trunk, spreads peripherally. Polyarthropathy. Transient aplastic crisis. Can cause chronic infection and anemia in immunocompromised	Droplet precautions. Incubation period 4–14 days	Serum IgM. PCR required if immunocompromised	Supportive. RBC transfusion in aplastic crisis. IVIG used in infections of immunodeficient patients

Continued

17

TABLE 17.3

PEDIATRIC VIRAL ILLNESSES—CONT'D

	Presentation	Transmission and Incubation	Diagnosis	Treatment
Rubella[2]	Descending, erythematous, maculopapular rash, lymphadenopathy, low-grade fever. Often asymptomatic See Table 17.1 for congenital rubella.	Droplet precautions until 7 days after onset of the rash Incubation period 12–23 days	Serum IgM	Supportive
Severe acute respiratory syndrome coronavirus 2 (SARS-CoV-2)[69]	Many children with SARS-CoV-2 may be asymptomatic or with mild to moderate symptoms including fever, cough, and pharyngeal erythema.[28] In contrast with infected adults, most infected children appear to have a milder clinical course.[70]	Aerosol and respiratory droplet transmission. Shedding can start 1–2 days prior to symptoms and continue >2 weeks. Incubation period: 5 days (2–14) Virus detected in stool with implications for fecal-oral transmission.	Nasopharyngeal swab for PCR per CDC criteria Respiratory tract specimen NAAT, antigen tests also available but less sensitive[73,74]	Recommendations for SARS-CoV-2 are constantly evolving as new data become available; refer to https://www. covid19treatmentguidelines.nih. gov/ for most up-to-date recommendations. Refer to website above for currently recommended therapeutics for non-hospitalized children at risk for progression to severe disease. Prophylaxis: Vaccination is recommended for those eligible and is currently authorized for use in children ages 6 months and older.

| Varicella zoster virus (VZV)[2] | Primary varicella (chickenpox): pruritic macules that progress to vesicles, plus fever and malaise. Herpes zoster: painful, vesicular, dermatomal rash. See Table 17.1 for congenital VZV. | Airborne spread or direct contact. Incubation period 10–21 days. Reactivation of latent VZV from sensory ganglia. | Clinical. PCR of vesicular fluid | Supportive care if healthy host. Treat with acyclovir/valacyclovir if chronic skin or lung disease, unvaccinated and 12+ years old, or immunocompromised. |

DNA, Deoxyribonucleic acid; *EIA,* enzyme immunoassay; *HLH,* hemophagocytic lymphohistiocytosis; *Ig,* immunoglobulin; *IVIG,* intravenous immunoglobulin; *NSAIDs,* nonsteroidal antiinflammatory drugs; *RBC,* red blood cell; *RT-PCR,* reverse-transcriptase polymerase chain reaction.

17

TABLE 17.4

PEDIATRIC TICKBORNE DISEASES

	Presentation	Etiology	Diagnosis	Treatment
Lyme disease[2,75]	Early localized: <1 month after tick bite. Erythema migrans Early disseminated: 3–10 weeks after bite. Secondary erythema migrans with multiple smaller target lesions, cranioneuropathy (especially facial nerve palsy), systemic symptoms, rarely carditis with heart block or aseptic meningitis Late disease: 2–12 months after bite. Pauciarticular arthritis of large joints, peripheral neuropathy, encephalopathy	Spirochete *Borrelia burgdorferi* (*B. afzelii* and *B. garinii* in Europe and Asia) Requires 24–48 hr of tick attachment Incubation 3–32 days (median 11 days) Most common in New England and mid-Atlantic. Less common in upper Midwest and Northwest Can have coinfection with *Borrelia miyamotoi*, Babesiosis, Anaplasma	Early: Clinical. No testing indicated. Early disseminated and late disease: EIA or IFA for antibodies. If positive, Western blot to confirm IgM detectable for first 30 days. (Consider false positive if >4 wk after symptom onset) IgG detectable by week 4–6. False positives occur with viral infections, other spirochetes, and autoimmune disease. Perform LP as clinically indicated for CNS involvement.	Erythema migrans/early Lyme disease: amoxicillin (14 days) or cefuroxime (14 days) or doxycycline (10 days). Lyme carditis: ceftriaxone or doxycycline or amoxicillin or cefuroxime × 14–21 days Lyme arthritis: doxycycline or amoxicillin × 28 days Lyme facial nerve palsy: doxycycline × 14–21 days Lyme meningitis (neuroborreliosis): ceftriaxone or doxycycline × 14–21 days (in patients with parenchymal involvement of the brain or spinal cord, IV ceftriaxone therapy is preferred over PO doxycycline therapy) In high-risk areas, can consider one-time dose of prophylactic doxycycline following removal of engorged tick for children of any age. Doxycycline traditionally avoided in children <8 years old; however, evidence suggests low risk of teeth staining.

Disease	Clinical	Organism/Epidemiology	Diagnosis	Treatment
Rocky Mountain spotted fever[2]	Initial symptoms can be nonspecific. Rash initially erythematous and macular, progresses to maculopapular and petechial. Classically spreads proximally from ankles and wrists, involves palms and soles. Peripheral and periorbital edema, anemia, leukopenia, thrombocytopenia, elevated LFTs, hyponatremia. Can progress to meningismus, AMS, DIC, digital necrosis, shock	*Rickettsia rickettsii* Incubation 3–12 days Widespread; most common in South Atlantic, Southeastern, and South Central United States Case fatality 20%–80%	Clinical, with lab confirmation. Gold standard is indirect fluorescent antibody; IgG and IgM increase around 7–10 days. Serum PCR if available. Negative result (PCR or antibody testing) does not rule out the diagnosis.	Doxycycline recommended for children of any age. Should be started as soon as the diagnosis is suspected. Duration: Continue until patient is afebrile for ≥3 days, with clinical improvement.
Ehrlichiosis[2]	Systemic febrile illness. Rash common around day 5. Leukopenia, thrombocytopenia, elevated LFTs, CSF pleocytosis. More severe disease: Pulmonary infiltrates, bone marrow hypoplasia, respiratory failure, encephalopathy, meningitis, DIC, spontaneous hemorrhage, and renal failure	*Ehrlichia chaffeensis* and *Ehrlichia ewingii* Incubation period 5–14 days Southeastern, south central, East Coast, and midwestern United States Coinfection with *Anaplasma* and other tickborne diseases common	Identification of DNA by PCR from whole blood is highly sensitive and specific. Paired acute and convalescent indirect fluorescent antibody are most commonly used tests. Peripheral smear with morulae	Doxycycline for at least 3 days after defervescence, for a minimum total course of 7–14 days.
Anaplasmosis[2]	Same as *Ehrlichia*	*Anaplasma phagocytophilum* Incubation 5–21 days Upper Midwest and Northeastern United States, northern California	Same as *Ehrlichia*	Same as *Ehrlichia*

Continued

17

TABLE 17.4

PEDIATRIC TICKBORNE DISEASES—CONT'D

	Presentation	Etiology	Diagnosis	Treatment
Babesiosis [2,76]	>50% children asymptomatic or mild presentation [77] Systemic febrile illness, hemolytic anemia Severe cases with ARDS, DIC, shock, splenic rupture	*Babesia microti* (less commonly *B. duncani* or *divergens*) Vector-borne (tick) or blood transfusion Incubation 1–5 wk for vector-borne. Can be longer for transfusion related Northeast and upper midwestern US Half are coinfected with *B. burgdorferi*.	Blood smear (Giemsa or Wright stain). Monitor smears during/after treatment.	Oral Atovaquone + Azithromycin for 7–10 days. Longer course of IV antibiotics if immunocompromised Limited data for exchange transfusion; may be of benefit in severe disease.

CDC, Centers for Disease Control and Prevention; *CNS,* central nervous system; *DIC,* disseminated intravascular coagulation; *DNA,* deoxyribonucleic acid; *EIA,* enzyme immunoassay; *hr,* hour; *IFA,* immunofluorescent assay; *IgG,* immunoglobulin G; *IgM,* immunoglobulin M; *LFTs,* liver function tests; *LP,* lumbar puncture; *PCN,* penicillin; *PCR,* polymerase chain reaction.

TABLE 17.5

PEDIATRIC PARASITIC INFECTIONS: UNITED STATES

	Presentation	Transmission and Incubation	Diagnosis	Treatment
American trypanosomiasis (Chagas disease)[2]	Acute period (2–3 months). Most asymptomatic or mild febrile illness. Can have rash, myalgia, lymphadenopathy, hepatosplenomegaly, meningoencephalitis, acute myocarditis, unilateral eye edema (Romaña sign), or local inflammatory reaction of the skin (chagoma). In chronic course, 20%–40% develop complications: cardiomyopathy with conduction abnormalities, colonic or esophageal dilation. Congenital presentation includes prematurity, low birth weight, hepatosplenomegaly, fever, neurologic abnormalities, anasarca, and petechiae.	*Trypanosoma cruzi* parasite Transmitted in feces of the Triatome ("kissing") bug. Vector-borne spread primarily in Mexico and Central/South America Incubation 1–2 wk Transmission rate 50% in acute Chagas, congenitally (transmission rate 50% in acute Chagas, 2%–5% in chronic disease), solid organ transplant or transfusion.	Acute: Giemsa Chronic: IgG (check two different assays for improved sensitivity) Direct microscopy or PCR available	Benznidazole (age >2 year old) or Nifurtimox (birth to 18 years old) Treatment not recommended for cardiomyopathy due to adverse drug profile without clinical benefit. Donated blood is screened.
Cyclosporiasis[2]	Profuse, protracted watery diarrhea. Low-grade fevers in 50%. Biliary disease Affects immunocompetent and immunocompromised hosts	*Cyclospora cayetanensis*, protozoan Spread via fecal oral route via oocysts, which become infectious after days/ weeks in cool moist environment. Incubation period 2–14 days	Oocyst identification in stool, intestinal fluid aspirate, or intestinal biopsy. Variably acid fast PCR available	Trimethoprim-sulfamethoxazole for 7–10 days. Alternative is nitazoxanide.

Continued

TABLE 17.5

PEDIATRIC PARASITIC INFECTIONS: UNITED STATES—CONT'D

	Presentation	Transmission and Incubation	Diagnosis	Treatment
Cysticercosis[2]	Neurocysticercosis can manifest as seizures, headaches, obstructive hydrocephalus, other neurologic signs. In endemic areas, it is responsible for up to 30% of epilepsy cases.	*Taenia solium.* Fecal-oral spread or undercooked pork containing larval cysts Prevalent in parts of Latin America, Asia, and sub-Saharan Africa Incubation period is typically several years.	Neuroimaging: (CT) identifies calcifications, MRI identifies extraparenchymal cysts and parasites Antibody assays to confirm diagnosis (poor sensitivity and specificity).	Albendazole (>1 year old) +/– praziquantel (off label) and corticosteroids (for host inflammatory response with cysticercidal medications) Anticonvulsant until radiographic and symptomatic resolution May require surgical management
Toxocariasis	Most infections are asymptomatic with persistent eosinophilia. Visceral disease (often age 2–7 years old) includes fever, cough, wheezing, abdominal pain, rash, myocarditis. Ocular disease (older children and adolescents) with isolated unilateral vision loss Neurotoxocariasis can present with seizures secondary to meningoencephalitis, space occupying lesions, cerebral vasculitis, etc.	*Toxocara canis* or *Toxocara catis,* roundworms of dogs and cats 5% seroprevalence in US. More common in southern US Unclear incubation period	ELISA (CDC laboratory). Cannot distinguish past and present infections. Less sensitive for ocular disease Liver imaging for visceral disease	Albendazole (>1 year old) or mebendazole Add corticosteroids for myocarditis, CNS involvement, or ocular disease.
Toxoplasmosis[2] See Table 17.1 for perinatal disease.	>50% of children asymptomatic Immunocompetent children present with mono-like illness.	*Toxoplasma gondii,* an obligate intracellular parasite Many infectious forms. Tachyzoites cause symptoms;	IgG peaks at 3–5 months, remains positive indefinitely. IgM detectable by 1 week, peaks at 1 month, undetectable by 6–9 months.	Treat if immunocompromised, pregnant, infant, ocular involvement, or severe/persistent symptoms.

More severe manifestations include chorioretinitis, meningoencephalitis, myocarditis, myositis, ADEM. Brain abscess and shock may occur in immunocompromised, particularly in seropositive HSCT (R+) and seronegative cardiac transplant recipients (D+/R−).	tissue cysts form latent infections in brain, eye, cardiac, skeletal muscle tissue. Seropositivity in US is 11%. Half of infected individuals do not have identified risk factor. Incubation period 4–21 days	PCR for body fluid/tissue. Cannot differentiate between acute, reactivation, and latent infection	Pyrimethamine + folinic acid + sulfadiazine Add prednisone for chorioretinitis. Prophylaxis with trimethoprim-sulfamethoxazole for children with HIV, recurrent chorioretinitis, or other high-risk immunocompromising conditions
Trichomoniasis	See Chapter 5.		

This table includes parasitic infections denoted by Centers for Disease Control and Prevention (CDC) to be present in the United States.

ADEM, acute disseminated encephalomyelitis; *CDC,* Centers for Disease Control and Prevention; *CNS,* central nervous system; *CT,* computed tomography; *ELISA,* enzyme-linked immunosorbent assay; *HSCT,* hematopoietic stem cell transplant; *Ig,* immunoglobulin; *MRI,* magnetic resonance imaging; *PCR,* polymerase chain reaction.

17

TABLE 17.6

PEDIATRIC FUNGAL INFECTIONS

	Presentation	Transmission and Incubation	Diagnosis	Treatment
Aspergillosis[2,78]	Ubiquitous in environment Immunocompromised patients at risk for invasive pulmonary aspergillosis, sinusitis, and CNS disease. Can be complicated by angioinvasion, dissemination, thrombosis, and hemorrhage Allergic bronchopulmonary aspergillosis (ABPA) in children with asthma or cystic fibrosis: wheezing, productive cough, fever, eosinophilia, pulmonary infiltrates	*Aspergillus fumigatus* (>75%), *flavus, terreus, nidulans, niger* Inhalation of spores from environment Incubation period unknown	Characteristic hyphae on KOH or silver nitrate stain of tissue or BAL fluid. Fungal biomarker (serum or BAL galactomannan) can aid in early diagnosis. Serum galactomannan is less sensitive in non-neutropenic hosts (solid organ transplant and immunodeficiency) when compared to neutropenic hosts (hematologic malignancy and HSCT).	**Invasive aspergillosis:** Voriconazole is drug of choice, alternatives include isavuconazole, posaconazole, and polyenes. Highly variable voriconazole pharmacokinetics in children, monitor troughs, goal 1–6 mcg/mL Serial serum galactomannan can aid in monitoring progression of disease. **ABPA:** Steroids are the primary treatment. For steroid-refractory ABPA, add itraconazole.
Blastomycosis[2,79]	Asymptomatic in 50%. Productive cough with variable radiographic appearance (consolidation, pneumonitis, infiltrate, nodules). Dissemination in 25% of symptomatic cases (cutaneous lesions common, CNS infection less common)	*Blastomyces* spp. Inhalation of infectious conidia from environment Ohio and Mississippi river region, southeastern US, Great Lakes region	Characteristic broad-based budding yeast on KOH or silver stain of sputum, tracheal aspirate, BAL, CSF, urine, or biopsy Urine antigen testing more useful than serologic testing	All cases in children should be treated. **Severe:** Amphotericin B (1–2 weeks) + itraconazole (6–12 months) **CNS infection:** Amphotericin B (4–6 weeks) + Itraconazole (12 months) **Mild/moderate:** Itraconazole (6–12 months)

| Candidiasis[2,80] | Mucocutaneous disease in immunocompetent patients. Concern for immunodeficiency if recurrent/chronic Esophageal/laryngeal plaque in immunocompromised Disseminated/candidemia in preterm neonates, immunocompromised and ICU patients with central lines | *Candida* species. *Candida albicans* most common, but other species account for >50% of invasive infections and have different resistance patterns. Budding yeast with pseudohyphae. Incubation period unknown | Mucocutaneous: clinical diagnosis. Yeast and pseudohyphae on KOH or Gram, calcofluor white, or fluorescent antibody stains Imaging and endoscopy can support diagnosis. Culture 70% sensitive for detecting candidemia and 50% sensitive for detecting invasive candidiasis without candidemia. Once positive culture identified, rapid tests available (PNA FISH probes and PCR). Beta-D-glucan not recommended to be sent in children; poor sensitivity and specificity. LP, brain imaging, dilated retinal exam for neonate with candidemia or candiduria | Mucocutaneous: oral (mucosal) or topical (cutaneous) nystatin, clotrimazole, miconazole. If refractory or immunocompromised host, use fluconazole. Breastfeeding should be continued. **Vulvovaginal:** See Chapter 5. **Esophagitis:** Oral fluconazole **Asymptomatic candiduria:** Remove catheter. **Neonatal invasive disease:** Amphotericin B for >3 weeks. Avoid lipid formulation due to poor urinary penetration. **Child with invasive disease or candidemia:** Echinocandin or fluconazole (if susceptible) × 14 days from first negative blood culture |
| Cryptococcus[2,81] | Often asymptomatic/mild. Cough, chest pain, constitutional symptoms, pulmonary masses, consolidation, or interstitial changes. Severe manifestations include ARDS, meningitis, fungemia. Patients with defects in T-lymphocyte mediated immunity most at risk (e.g., patients with HIV/AIDS) | *Cryptococcus neoformans* and *gattii.* Inhalation from environment (soil, bird droppings) British Columbia, Canada, Pacific Northwest US, Australia, Papua New Guinea Incubation 8–13 months | Cryptococcal antigen testing of serum or CSF Definitive diagnosis with isolation of encapsulated yeast on India ink (best for BAL fluid) Mass spectrometry and PCR | Amphotericin B and oral flucytosine for >2 weeks, then fluconazole for >8 weeks Follow up LP at 2 weeks. Treat increased ICP and immune reconstitution inflammatory syndrome as needed. |

Continued

17

TABLE 17.6

PEDIATRIC FUNGAL INFECTIONS—CONT'D

	Presentation	Transmission and Incubation	Diagnosis	Treatment
Histoplasmosis[2,82]	95% asymptomatic Pulmonary or disseminated, acute or chronic, primary or reactivation Acute pulmonary presentation with fever, chills, dry cough, hilar/mediastinal adenopathy. Resolves in 2–3 weeks Severe infection can cause hypoxemia ARDS, airway compromise, pericarditis. Disseminated presentation (typically age <2 years old or immunocompromised) with prolonged fever, failure to thrive, hepatosplenomegaly, pancytopenia, DIC, GI bleeding, CNS involvement	*Histoplasma*, a dimorphic fungi Transmitted primarily via inhalation of conidia from environment, vertically, or horizontally (transplant, exposure to cutaneous lesion) Present in most of world, particularly central/eastern US Incubation 1–3 weeks	Antigen testing of serum, urine, BAL is used for diagnosis and monitoring of treatment response. Antibody testing for subacute/chronic disease and CNS involvement Definitive diagnosis with culture	**Mild acute infection** often self-limited. If no improvement in 4 weeks, give itraconazole for 6–12 weeks. **Disseminated infection** requires amphotericin B +/− steroids for 1–2 weeks, then 12 weeks of itraconazole. **Chronic pulmonary infection** treated with 1–2 years of itraconazole
Pneumocystis pneumonia	In immunocompromised host, dyspnea, tachypnea, hypoxemia, cough, fever/chills. Diffuse interstitial/alveolar changes on CXR. Mortality 5%–40% when untreated, 100% when treated	*Pneumocystis jirovecii*, an atypical fungus. No latency/reactivation. Airborne transmission. Incubation unknown (~53 days in transplant recipients)	Evaluation of BAL fluid (stain for cysts, sporozoites, and trophozoites). PCR sensitive but not FDA approved. Beta-D-glucan may be useful if bronchoscopy not able to be performed.	IV trimethoprim-sulfamethoxazole × 21 days. Alternative is pentamidine. Other drug combinations studied in adults. First-line prophylaxis with trimethoprim-sulfamethoxazole. Alternative is atovaquone, dapsone, or aerosolized pentamidine.

ARDS, acute respiratory distress syndrome; *BAL*, bronchoalveolar lavage; *CNS*, central nervous system; *CSF*, cerebrospinal fluid; *CXR*, chest X-ray; *DIC*, disseminated intravascular coagulation; *FDA*, Food and Drug Administration; *GI*, gastrointestinal; *HIV/AIDS*, human immunodeficiency virus/acquired immunodeficiency syndrome; *ICP*, intracranial pressure; *ICU*, intensive care unit; *LP*, lumbar puncture; *PCR*, polymerase chain reaction; *PNA FISH*, Fluorescence in

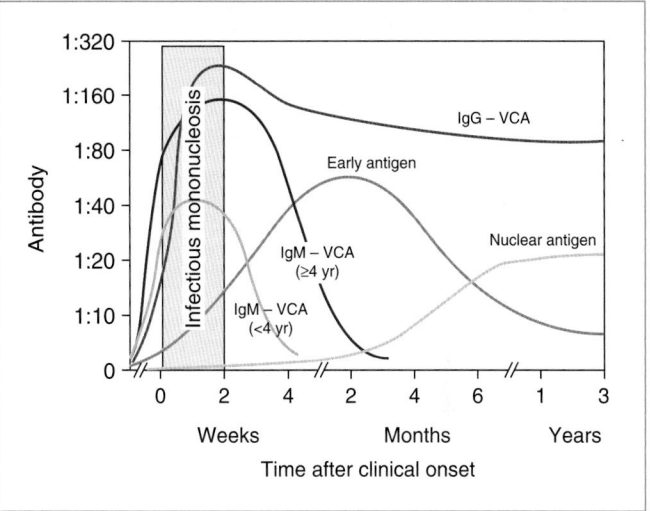

FIGURE 17.3

Graphic representation of the development of antibodies to Epstein-Barr virus antigens as a function of time from infection. Antibody titers are calculated as geometric mean values expressed as reciprocals of the serum dilution. The immunoglobulin M *(IgM)* response to viral capsid antigen *(VCA)* varies according to age of the patient. *IgG,* Immunoglobulin G. (From Jenson HB. Epstein-Barr virus. In: Kliegman RE, Stanton B, St Geme J, et al, eds. *Nelson Textbook of Pediatrics.* 20th ed. Elsevier; 2016.)

    a. Any ill-appearing or otherwise high-risk infant requires a full sepsis workup. Unimmunized infants, premature infants, infants with complicated neonatal courses, or infants who received antibiotics recently are at higher risk for serious bacterial infection.

    b. For well-appearing febrile infants, there are many established approaches, including the Rochester, Philadelphia, and Boston criteria and the Step-by-Step approach. In 2021 the AAP released guidelines for febrile infants 8–60 days. An adapted approach is outlined in Fig. 17.2.

H. Tuberculosis: Diagnosis and Treatment[2,3]

1. Diagnosis

    a. See Box 17.1 for screening guidelines and Box 17.2 for information on interpretation of tuberculin skin tests (TSTs). Interferon gamma release assays (IGRAs, namely T-SPOT-TB and QuantiFERON-TB Gold In-Tube) offer high specificity and can be used in children ≥2 years old.[4]

    b. If positive screening test, obtain chest x-ray.

BOX 17.1

TUBERCULOSIS SCREENING GUIDELINES[2]

The American Academy of Pediatrics recommends treatment for at-risk individuals. Clinicians should complete at-risk assessment questionnaire at first well-child visit, then every 6 months in 1st year of life, and then routine care (at least annually). Screening to identify at-risk individuals:

- Born outside the United States in countries with endemic infection
- Traveled outside United States in countries with endemic infection[84]
- Family member with positive tuberculin skin test (TST)
- Exposed to someone who had tuberculosis disease
- Children on immunosuppressive therapies (e.g., tumor necrosis factor blockers/antagonists)
- Depending on local epidemiology: children who spend time with individuals who have spent time in jail/prison/shelter, use illegal drugs, or are HIV positive, children who consume unpasteurized milk/products, household members who were born or have recently traveled/arrived from countries with endemic infection (outside the United States)

BOX 17.2

DEFINITIONS OF POSITIVE TUBERCULIN SKIN TESTING[2]

Induration ≥5 mm

- Children in close contact with known or suspected contagious cases of TB disease
- Children suspected to have active or previous TB disease based on clinical or radiographic findings
- Children on immunosuppressive therapy or with immunosuppressive conditions (including HIV infection)

Induration ≥10 mm

- Children at increased risk for dissemination based on young age (<4 years) or with other medical conditions (cancer, diabetes mellitus, chronic renal failure, or malnutrition)
- Children with increased exposure: Those born in or with travel to endemic countries; those exposed to HIV-infected adults, homeless persons, those with substance use disorder, nursing home residents, or incarcerated or institutionalized persons

Induration ≥15 mm

- Children ≥4 years without any risk factors

HIV, Human immunodeficiency virus: *TB,* tuberculosis.

---

 c. If symptoms indicate active tuberculosis (TB) disease, determine source.
  (1) Consider pediatric protocol chest CT over x-ray when available.[5]
  (2) Specimen sources include sputum, bronchial washings, gastric aspirates (morning aspirate before feeding/ambulation × 3

TABLE 17.7

INTERPRETATION OF THE SEROLOGIC MARKERS OF HEPATITIS B IN COMMON SITUATIONS

Serologic Marker

HBsAg	Total HBcAb	IgM HBcAb	HBsAb	Interpretation
−	−	−	−	No prior infection, not immune
−	−	−	+	Immune after hepatitis B vaccination (if concentration ≥10 IU/mL) or passive immunization from HBIG administration
−	+	−	+	Immune after recovery from HBV infection
+	+	+	−	Acute HBV infection
+	+	−	−	Chronic HBV infection

HBcAb, antibody to hepatitis B core antigen; *HBsAb*, antibody to hepatitis B surface antigen; *HBsAg*, Hepatitis B surface antigen; *HBIG*, hepatitis B immune globulin; *HBV*, hepatitis B virus; *IgM*, immunoglobulin M.
From Davis AR, Rosenthal P. Hepatitis B in children. *Pediatr Rev.* 2008;29(4):111–120.

specimens), pleural fluid, cerebrospinal fluid, urine, tissue biopsy.

(3) Acid-fast smear and/or nucleic acid amplification testing may provide rapid diagnosis. The latter may also detect rifampin resistance. Solid media culture can take as long as 10 weeks, liquid media 1 to 6 weeks.

d. Lumbar puncture is recommended in children less than 12 months with confirmed TB. In children older than 12 months, lumbar puncture should be considered only if neurologic signs and symptoms are present.

2. Treatment of latent TB infection

a. Rule out active TB.

b. Treatment regimens:
   (1) Rifampin is preferred, especially for children ≤5 years
   (2) 12 weeks of weekly isoniazid and rifapentine (preferred regimen if ≥2 years of age)
   (3) Rifampin daily for 4 months (preferred regimen if isoniazid-resistant)
   (4) Isoniazid plus rifampin daily for 3 months
   (5) 6 or 9 months of isoniazid daily (twice-weekly dosing regimen available)

c. Treat all children <5 years or immunocompromised if exposed to an individual with TB disease, even if testing (TST/IGRA) is negative. Some experts would discontinue treatment in immunocompetent children if repeat testing is negative at 8–10 weeks.

3. Treatment of active TB

a. High rates of resistance in endemic countries. Treatment should be initiated in consultation with an infectious disease specialist.

b. Drug-susceptible pulmonary TB: 6-month regimen, including 2 months RIPE (rifampin, isoniazid, pyrazinamide, ethambutol), followed by 4 months of rifampin/isoniazid. Rifampin is preferred, especially for children ≤5 years.

c. Extrapulmonary or drug-resistant TB: Consult infectious disease specialist.

d. Pyridoxine supplementation if breastfed, meat-/milk-deficient diet, symptomatic HIV, or pregnant

I. Human Immunodeficiency Virus and Acquired Immunodeficiency Syndrome[6]

Please see the National Institutes of Health (NIH) guidelines on the diagnosis and management of children with HIV infection at https://www.aidsinfo.nih.gov/ for the most up-to-date recommendations.

1. Diagnosis
   a. Perinatal: See Table 17.9 for diagnosis in perinatal period.[7,8]
   b. Infants and children[8,10]: HIV nucleic acid testing must be used under 18 months to avoid confounding from maternal antibodies. Antigen/antibody testing can be performed after 18 months. If concern for breastmilk exposure, test immediately, then at 4 to 6 weeks, 3 months, and 6 months after breastfeeding is discontinued.
   c. Adolescents[10]: Fourth-generation HIV antigen/antibody assay with opt-out consent as part of routine clinical care. If positive, confirm with HIV-1/HIV-2 differentiation immunoassay; if indeterminate, HIV-1 nucleic acid testing.
2. Management[7,11]
   a. See Table 17.9 for management during perinatal period.
   b. Initiation of therapy for all children with HIV is recommended by the Department of Health and Human Services (HHS) Panel on Antiretroviral Guidelines for Adults and Adolescents and the World Health Organization (WHO).

TABLE 17.8

CEREBROSPINAL FLUID ANALYSIS IN SUSPECTED MENINGITIS

	Bacterial Meningitis	Viral Meningitis	No CNS Infection
WBC (cells/mm^3)	>10; typically >100, but wide range	10–100	<10
Cell type	PMN predominance (80+%)	Mononuclear	Mononuclear
Protein (mg/dL)	>100	60–100	<60
Glucose (mg/dL)	<40	40–80	40–80

CNS, Central nervous system; *PMN*, polymorphonuclear neutrophil; *WBC*, white blood cell.

Modified from Tunkel AR, Hartman BJ, Kaplan SL, et al. Practice guidelines for the management of bacterial meningitis. *Clin Infect Dis.* 2004;39(9):1267-1284. doi:10.1086/425368. Analysis of cerebrospinal fluid is necessary to differentiate various types of meningitis. Initial studies such as cell counts and Gram stain can be helpful, but culture of cerebrospinal fluid remains diagnostic. Opening pressure is generally in the range of 200 to 500 mm H$_2$O, although values may be lower in neonates, infants, and children with acute bacterial meningitis. Neonates tend to have higher baseline WBC and protein in the CSF. For additional data on normal WBC and protein concentrations in infants <60 days old, please reference Table 2 in Thompson J, et al. Cerebrospinal fluid reference values for young infants undergoing lumbar puncture. *Pediatrics.* 2018;141(3). or Table 2 in Pantell, Robert H, et al. Evaluation and management of well-appearing febrile infants 8 to 60 days old. *Pediatrics.* 2021;148:2.

TABLE 17.9

DIAGNOSIS AND MANAGEMENT FOR INFANTS WITH *IN UTERO* HIV EXPOSURE[B]

Age	Laboratory Tests[a]	Next Steps
Prenatal/labor	Opt-out testing of all pregnant women HIV antibody testing in first trimester, with repeat testing before 36 weeks' gestation preferred if high risk Rapid HIV testing with confirmation if unknown HIV status during labor	Start ART in mother. If viral load RNA >1000 copies/mL or unknown at labor, start IV zidovudine (ZDV) and consider cesarean section if greater than 38 weeks' gestation.
Newborn	HIV nucleic acid test (DNA and RNA) if maternal status unknown, or high risk of infection Baseline CBC with differential	Start ZDV within 6 hr of delivery. If low risk (mother who received ART during pregnancy with viral load <50 near delivery), continue ZDV for 4 weeks. If high risk, presumptive HIV therapy using zidovudine, lamivudine, and either nevirapine or raltegravir from birth to 6 weeks; expert consultation recommended. Two-drug ARV prophylaxis with zidovudine and nevirapine can be considered on a case-by-case basis but should be in consultation with a pediatric infectious disease specialist. In the US, HIV+ mothers should be counseled against breastfeeding. If breastfeeding is desired, an HIV specialist should be consulted.[15]
2–3 weeks	HIV nucleic acid test (DNA > RNA) CBC with differential	Check ZDV dosing and administration. Assess psychosocial needs, consider case management referral.
4–6 weeks	HIV nucleic acid test (DNA or RNA) CBC with differential	Discontinue ZDV monotherapy regardless of PCR result (ZDV monotherapy is used during first 6 weeks for prophylaxis only). If positive, start ART according to guidelines, and start *Pneumocystis jirovecii* pneumonia prophylaxis, such as TMP-SMX. Presumptively exclude HIV infection if results of ≥2 weeks PCR and ≥4 weeks PCR both negative.

Continued

17

TABLE 17.9

DIAGNOSIS AND MANAGEMENT FOR INFANTS WITH *IN UTERO* HIV EXPOSURE[a]—CONT'D

Age	Laboratory Tests[a]	Next Steps
2 months		Discontinue TMP-SMX if DNA or RNA testing negative.
4–6 months	HIV nucleic acid test (DNA or RNA)	Definitively exclude HIV infection: two negative PCRs at ≥1 month and ≥4 months OR two negative HIV-antibody tests from separate specimens obtained at ≥=6 months of age, as long as no signs/symptoms of HIV infection.
18–24 months	Antibody testing may be performed to confirm clearance of maternal HIV antibodies. If present, need to use nucleic acid testing.	

[a]Any abnormal result requires prompt pediatric HIV specialist consultation.

ART, Antiretroviral therapy; *CBC,* complete blood cell count; *DNA,* deoxyribonucleic acid; *HIV,* human immunodeficiency virus; *IV,* intravenous; *PCR,* polymerase chain reaction; *RNA,* ribonucleic acid; *TMP-SMX,* trimethoprim–sulfamethoxazole; *ZDV,* zidovudine.

Modified from Department of Health and Human Services guidelines for pediatric and perinatal HIV infection (see https://www.aidsinfo.nih.gov for more detailed information). National Perinatal HIV Hotline: 1-888-448-8765.

   c. Therapy: Combination antiretroviral therapy (ART) of at least three drugs from at least two different classes. Consider consultation with an infectious disease specialist.

3. Monitoring[6,9]

   a. At diagnosis: CD4 count, plasma HIV RNA viral load, genotype resistance. If starting therapy, HLA-B*5701 (screening for hypersensitivity to abacavir), tropism testing, hepatitis B serology (HBsAb, HBsAg, HBcAb total), hepatitis C screening (HCV Ab, or, if indicated, HCV RNA), basic chemistry, ALT, AST, total bilirubin, CBC with differential, lipid profile, glucose, urinalysis (UA), pregnancy test if applicable

   b. Follow-up: At 1 to 2 weeks to evaluate for adverse effects and provide support for adherence. At 2 to 4 weeks after initiation or switching therapy: CD4, viral load, and labs according to possible toxicities of ART. Then similar testing as above every 3 to 6 months

   c. Once viral suppression achieved, CD4 improved, good adherence, and otherwise stable for 2 to 3 years, can space labs to every 6 to 12 months

   d. Children infected with HIV should have latent TB skin testing starting at age 3 to 12 months, and then annually.

   e. Vaccines[2] (see Chapter 16 and Red Book for details)

4. Preexposure prophylaxis (PrEP)[15]

   a. Common indications

     (1) Men who have sex with men: HIV-positive partner, bacterial sexually transmitted infection (STI, e.g. gonorrhea, chlamydia, syphilis) in past 6 months, history of inconsistent or condomless anal intercourse with an unknown status or nonmonogamous partner, commercial (or exchange) sex, history of high number of sex partners

     (2) Heterosexual men and women: HIV-positive partner, bacterial STI in past 6 months, history of inconsistent condom use, commercial (or exchange) sex, history of high number of sex partners, living in a high HIV prevalence setting

   b. Initiation

     (1) Labs: Fourth-generation HIV test, syphilis, gonorrhea, chlamydia, hepatitis B virus (HBV), hepatitis C virus (HCV, if history of IV drug use), urinalysis, and renal function. Pregnancy test if indicated. Counsel on condom use.

     (2) Use emtricitabine/tenofovir alafenamide (Descovy) for biological males. Effective only after 7 days. Emtricitabine/tenofovir disoproxil (Truvada) for biological females and males. Effective only after 21 days. Consult infectious disease specialist for initiation of PrEP unless provider has extensive experience.

     (3) Descovy and Truvada are FDA approved for adolescents >35 kg. Descovy is not approved to prevent transmission via vaginal intercourse.

   c. Follow-up
     (1) Every 3 months: HIV test; renal function (if normal at 3 months, can be spaced to every 6 months); syphilis/gonorrhea/chlamydia testing if patient is symptomatic, engaging in anal intercourse, has prior history of STIs, or has multiple partners. Counsel on condom use at every visit.
     (2) Every 6 months: Same as above, plus routine STI screening (including oral and/or anal testing, if applicable)

5. Postexposure prophylaxis (PEP)[13-15]
   a. Indications for occupational PEP: Consider with percutaneous, mucosal, or skin exposure to blood or bodily fluids from a patient with known HIV or in whom there is high suspicion. See Section IV for further information.
   b. Indications for nonoccupational PEP (nPEP): Unprotected vaginal/anal intercourse, oral sex with ejaculation or blood exposure, needle sharing, or injuries with blood exposure from an individual with known HIV or unknown status
   c. Labs: Fourth-generation HIV test, HBV surface antigen and antibody, HCV antibody, renal function, liver enzymes. Consider tetanus prophylaxis, STI testing, and pregnancy testing, if applicable.
   d. Regimen: Initiate as soon as possible (lower likelihood of efficacy after 72 hours); three-drug (or more) ART regimen for 28 days. Regimens for children >2 years old and adolescents: tenofovir and emtricitabine in combination with one of the following integrase inhibitors: bictegravir, elvitegravir, dolutegravir, raltegravir. Regimen for infants/children <2 years old: zidovudine and lamivudine in combination with one of the following integrase inhibitors: raltegravir, dolutegravir. Consult infectious disease expert for any initiation of PEP.
   e. Follow-up testing can occur at 6 weeks, 12 weeks, and 6 months; for occupational exposures, if fourth-generation testing available, follow-up testing can be done at 6 weeks and 4 months.
   f. Clinicians' PEP Line: 1-888-448-4911

II. MICROBIOLOGY

A. Collection of Specimens for Blood Culture

1. Preparation: To minimize contamination, clean venipuncture site with 70% isopropyl ethyl alcohol. Apply tincture of iodine or 10% povidone-iodine and allow skin to dry for at least 1 minute, or scrub site with 2% chlorhexidine for 30 seconds and allow skin to dry for 30 seconds. Clean blood culture bottle injection site with alcohol only.
2. Collection: Two sets of cultures from two different sites of equal blood volume should be obtained for each febrile episode, based on patient weight: less than 8 kg, 1 to 3 mL; 8 to 13 kg, 4 to 5 mL; 14 to 25 kg, 5 to 6 mL; greater than 25 kg, 10 mL. Peripheral sites preferred. If concern for central line infection, collect one from central access site, second from peripheral. Consider anaerobic blood cultures if concern for the following:

head and neck infections, intra-abdominal infections, immunodeficiency, trauma, or pressure sore.[16,17]

B. Rapid Microbiologic Identification of Common Aerobic Bacteria (Fig. 17.4) and Anaerobic Bacteria (Fig. 17.5)

NOTE: Molecular assays for identification of bacteria and antibiotic resistance are increasingly available.

III. ANTIBIOTIC THERAPY AND STEWARDSHIP

A. Spectra of Activity for Commonly Used Antibiotics (Fig. 17.6)

REFERENCES

A complete list of references can be found online.

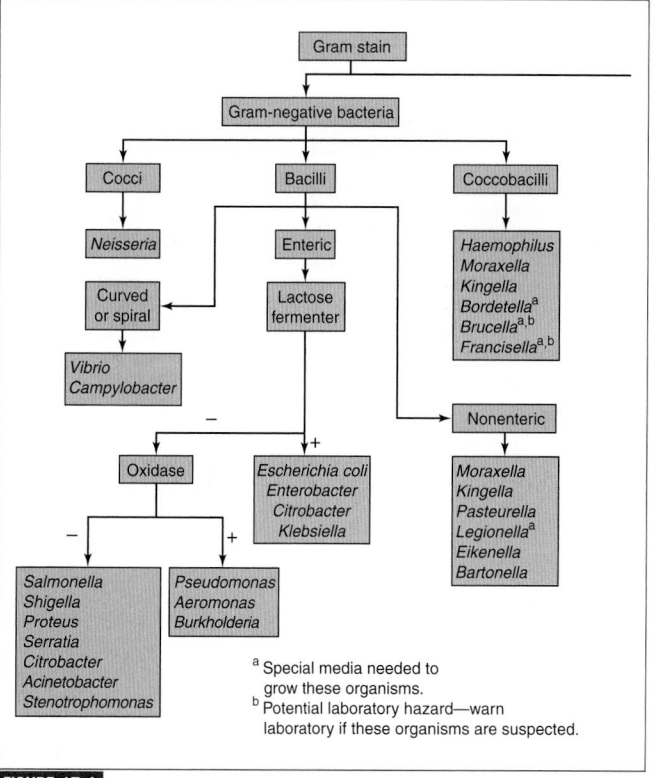

FIGURE 17.4

Algorithm demonstrating identification of aerobic bacteria.

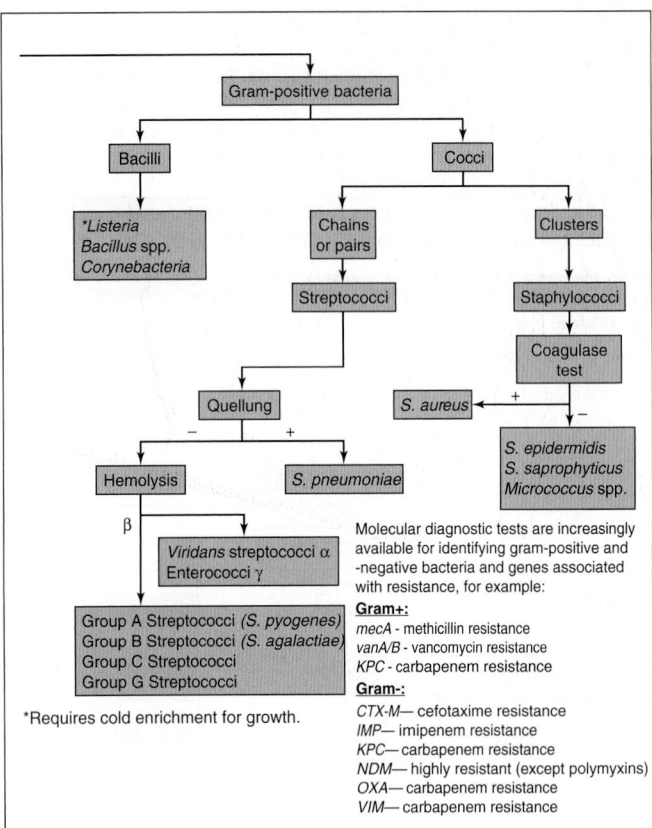

Molecular diagnostic tests are increasingly available for identifying gram-positive and -negative bacteria and genes associated with resistance, for example:

Gram+:
mecA - methicillin resistance
vanA/B - vancomycin resistance
KPC - carbapenem resistance

Gram-:
CTX-M— cefotaxime resistance
IMP— imipenem resistance
KPC— carbapenem resistance
NDM— highly resistant (except polymyxins)
OXA— carbapenem resistance
VIM— carbapenem resistance

FIGURE 17.4
cont'd.

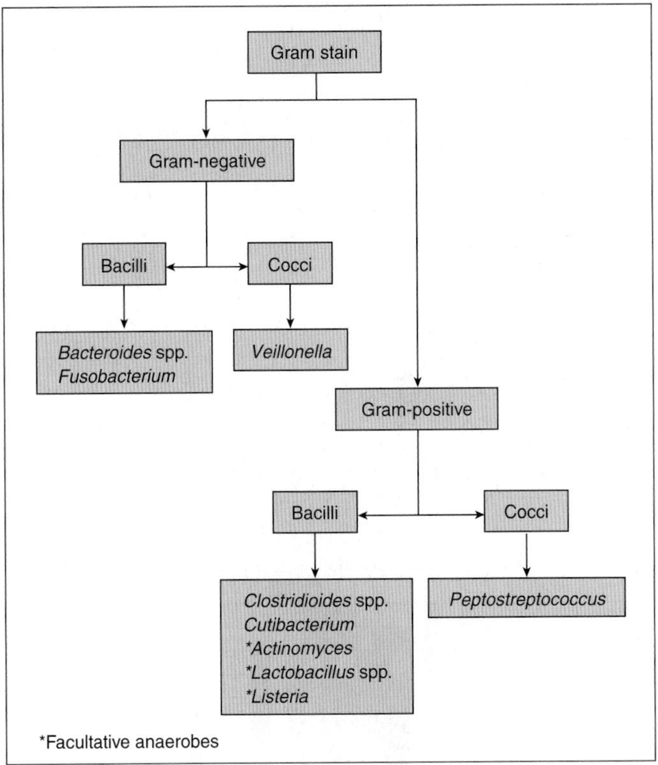

```
                    ┌─────────────┐
                    │ Gram stain  │
                    └─────────────┘
                          │
              ┌───────────┴───────────┐
              │                       │
      ┌───────────────┐               │
      │ Gram-negative │               │
      └───────────────┘               │
          │                           │
   ┌──────┴──────┐                    │
┌─────────┐  ┌─────────┐              │
│ Bacilli │◄─►│ Cocci  │              │
└─────────┘  └─────────┘              │
     │            │                   │
┌──────────────┐ ┌──────────────┐     │
│Bacteroides   │ │ Veillonella  │     │
│spp.          │ └──────────────┘     │
│Fusobacterium │                      │
└──────────────┘                      │
                          ┌───────────────┐
                          │ Gram-positive │
                          └───────────────┘
                                │
                      ┌─────────┴─────────┐
                  ┌─────────┐        ┌─────────┐
                  │ Bacilli │◄──────►│  Cocci  │
                  └─────────┘        └─────────┘
                       │                  │
          ┌──────────────────┐  ┌────────────────────┐
          │Clostridioides spp.│  │Peptostreptococcus │
          │Cutibacterium      │  └────────────────────┘
          │*Actinomyces       │
          │*Lactobacillus spp.│
          │*Listeria          │
          └──────────────────┘
```

*Facultative anaerobes

FIGURE 17.5

Algorithm demonstrating identification of anaerobic bacteria.

17

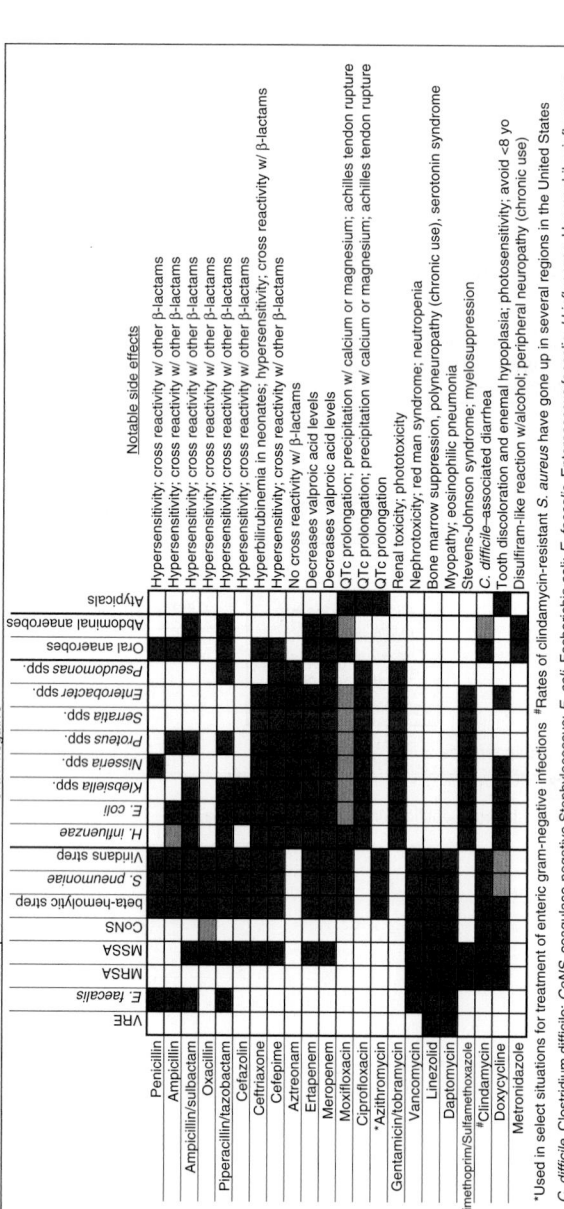

FIGURE 17.6

Approximation for the spectrum of activity for commonly used antibiotics and common pediatric infections. Exact sensitivities will change with different local resistance patterns. For antibiotic recommendations for specific infections, refer to relevant part of Section I.

*Used in select situations for treatment of enteric gram-negative infections. #Rates of clindamycin-resistant *S. aureus* have gone up in several regions in the United States

C. difficile, Clostridium difficile; *CoNS,* coagulase-negative Staphylococcus; *E. coli,* Escherichia coli; *E. faecalis,* Enterococcus faecalis; *H influenzae,* Haemophilus influenzae; *MRSA,* methicillin-resistant Staphylococcus aureus; *MSSA,* methicillin-sensitive Staphylococcus aureus; *S. pneumoniae,* Streptococcus pneumoniae; *VRE,* vancomycin-resistant Enterococcus

Chapter 18

Neonatology

Elizabeth Lee, MD

⊘ See additional content online.
🔊 **Audio Case File 18.1** Ventilation strategies in the neonatal ICU

I. NEWBORN RESUSCITATION

A. Algorithm for Neonatal Resuscitation (Fig. 18.1)

1. Essential functional equipment: Radiant warmer, prewarmed blankets, hat, bag-mask/NeoPIP ventilator, appropriately sized laryngoscope, appropriately sized endotracheal tube (ETT) ± stylet, suction device and bulb syringe, emergency medications, and vascular access supplies
2. Meconium-stained fluids: Routine intrapartum oropharyngeal/nasopharyngeal suctioning and endotracheal intubation are not recommended for vigorous and nonvigorous infants.[1]
3. Cord clamping should be delayed for at least 30 to 60 seconds for vigorous term and preterm infants, given no maternal or fetal indications for immediate clamping. See eBox 18.1 for exclusions. Cord milking should NOT be used for infants less than 28 weeks of gestation given link with intraventricular hemorrhage. There is insufficient evidence to support or refute use of umbilical cord milking for infants born at 32 weeks of gestation or more, including term.[2]

B. Endotracheal Tube Size and Depth of Insertion (Table 18.1)

1. Quick estimations:
   a. ETT size: 2.5 mm for infants <30 weeks gestational age (wGA); 3.0 mm for 30 to 34 wGA; 3.5 mm for >35 wGA.
   b. ETT depth: Infant's weight (kg) + 6 cm

C. Vascular Access (See Chapter 4 for Umbilical Venous/Artery Catheter Placement)

NOTE: During emergent placement, an umbilical venous catheter (UVC) may be inserted just far enough to obtain blood return; no measurement or verified placement is needed prior to emergent use.

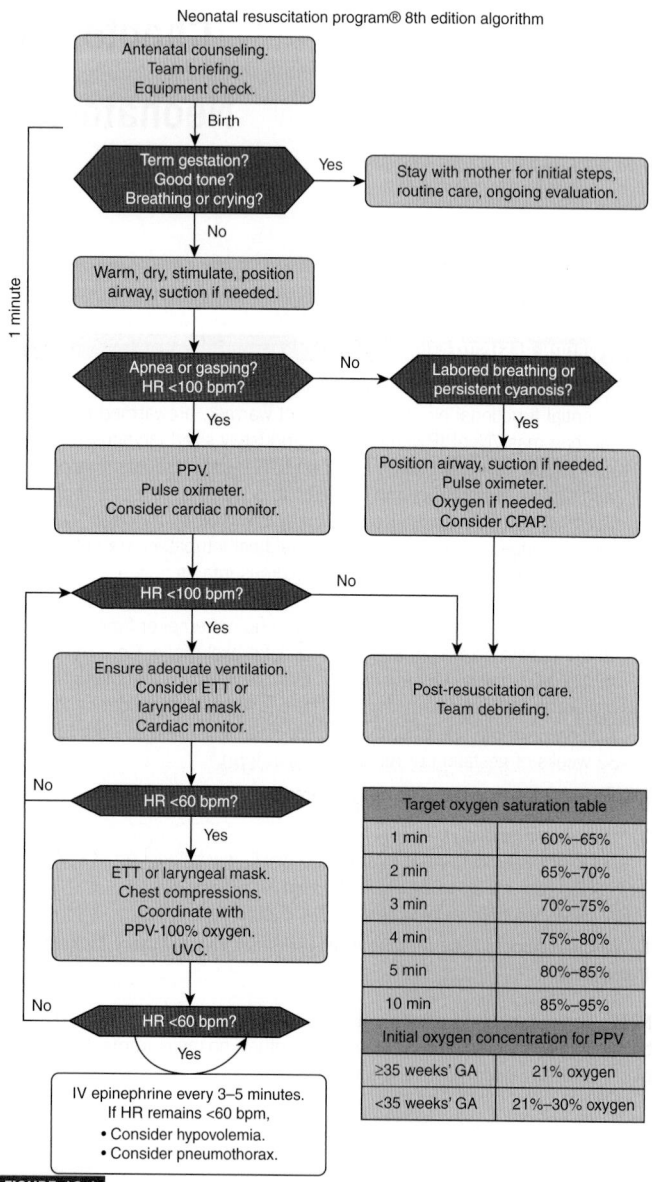

Neonatal resuscitation program® 8th edition algorithm

FIGURE 18.1

Overview of resuscitation in the delivery room. *CPAP*, Continuous positive airway pressure; *HR*, heart rate; *IV*, intravenous; *PPV*, positive pressure ventilations. (From American Academy of Pediatrics [AAP], American Heart Association. *Textbook of Neonatal Resuscitation [NRP]*. 8th ed. American Academy of Pediatrics; 2021.)

TABLE 18.1

PREDICTED ENDOTRACHEAL TUBE SIZE AND DEPTH BY BIRTH WEIGHT AND GESTATIONAL AGE

Gestational Age (Weeks)	Weight (g)	ETT Size (mm)	ETT Depth of Insertion (cm From Upper Lip)
23–24	500–600	2.5	5.5
25–26	700–800	2.5	6
27–29	900–1000	2.5	6.5
30–32	1100–1400	2.5–3.0	7
33–34	1500–1800	3.0	7.5
35–37	1900–2400	3.0–3.5	8
38–40	2500–3100	3.5	8.5

ETT, Endotracheal tube.

Data from Peterson J, Johnson N, Deakins K, et al. Accuracy of the 7-8-9 rule for endotracheal tube placement in the neonate. *J Perinatol.* 2006;26:333–336.

II. ROUTINE NEWBORN CARE OF A TERM INFANT

A. General Care for the Full-Term Healthy Newborn With Uncomplicated Delivery

NOTE: Protocols vary by hospital.

1. Drying, removal of wet blankets. Then, preferably, skin-to-skin contact with mother[3] or otherwise placed under warmer
2. Feeding: Breastfeeding soon after birth and on demand thereafter. Breastfed newborns should feed 8 to 12 times daily. Formula-fed newborns should be offered a bottle soon after birth.
3. Vitamin K IM injection for prevention of hemorrhagic disease of the newborn.
4. Antibiotic ophthalmic ointment for prophylaxis against gonococcal infection.
5. Monitor clinically for jaundice, accounting for newborn's risk factors for hyperbilirubinemia. Transcutaneous bilirubin monitoring may be useful as a screening tool but does not replace plasma level.[4] Obtain plasma total bilirubin level if warranted. See Section IX for further management.
6. Consider blood glucose monitoring if infant is at increased risk or is symptomatic of hypoglycemia (see Fig. 18.2 for management).
7. Monitor for stool/urine output. Most infants should have 1 void and 1 meconium stool within first 24 hours.[5]
8. Monitor for excessive weight loss (>10% loss).

B. Prior to Discharge[6]

1. Newborn metabolic screening: First screen typically performed within first 72 hours of life, at least 24 hours after initiation of feeding (see Chapter 13)
2. Vaccinations: Hepatitis B vaccine (see Chapter 16)
3. Critical congenital heart disease screening: Measure pre- and/or postductal oxygen saturation (see Chapter 7).
4. Newborn hearing screening
5. Document bilateral ophthalmic red reflex.
6. Establish primary care.

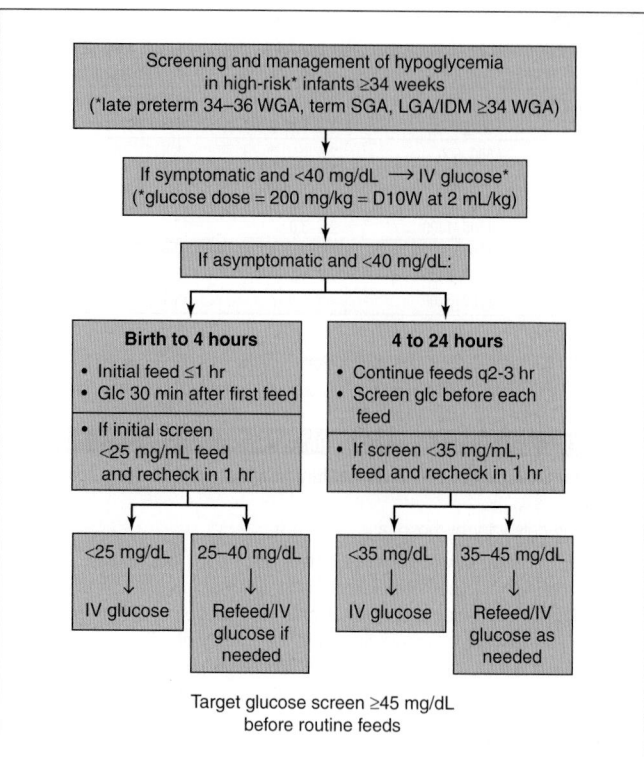

FIGURE 18.2

Screening for and management of postnatal glucose homeostasis. *D10W*, 10% Dextrose in water; *glc*, glucose; *IDM*, infant of diabetic mother; *IV*, intravenous; *LGA*, large for gestational age; *SGA*, small for gestational age; *WGA*, weeks' gestational age. (Modified from Adamkin D, Committee on the Fetus and Newborn. Postnatal glucose homeostasis in late-preterm and term infants. *Pediatrics.* 2011;127:575–579.)

III. NEWBORN ASSESSMENT

A. Vital Signs and Birth Weight

1. **Mean arterial blood pressure (MAP):** Related to birth weight, gestational age
2. **Birth weight:**
   a. Extremely low birth weight (ELBW): <1000 g, very low birth weight (VLBW): <1500 g, low birth weight (LBW): <2500 g
   b. Small for gestational age (SGA): <10% for gestational age
   c. Large for gestational age (LGA): >90% for gestational age

B. APGAR Scores (Table 18.2)

Assess at 1 and 5 minutes. Repeat at 5-minute intervals if score at 5 minutes is <7.[7]

TABLE 18.2

APGAR SCORES

Score	0	1	2
Heart rate	Absent	<100 bpm	>100 bpm
Respiratory effort	Absent, irregular	Slow, crying	Good
Muscle tone	Limp	Some flexion of extremities	Active motion
Reflex irritability (nose suction)	No response	Grimace	Cough or sneeze
Color	Blue, pale	Acrocyanosis	Completely pink

Data from Apgar V. Proposal for a new method of evaluation of the newborn infant. *Anesth Analg.* 1953;32:260.

C. Gestational Age Estimation

If obstetric dating by Ultrasound (US) or Last Menstrual Period (LMP) is not available, Ballard scoring can be utilized for gestational age estimation. The Ballard score is most accurate at approximately 24 hours and estimates gestational age based on neuromuscular and physical maturity ratings (eFig. 18.1).

1. Posture: Observe infant quiet and supine. Score 0 for arms, legs extended; 1 for starting to flex hips and knees, arms extended; 2 for stronger flexion of legs, arms extended; 3 for arms slightly flexed, legs flexed and abducted; and 4 for full flexion of arms and legs.
2. Square window: Flex infant's hand on forearm enough to obtain fullest possible flexion without wrist rotation. Measure angle between hypothenar eminence and ventral aspect of forearm.
3. Arm recoil: With infant supine, flex infant's forearms for 5 seconds, fully extend by pulling on hands, then release. Measure the angle of elbow flexion to which arms recoil.
4. Popliteal angle: Hold infant supine with infant's pelvis flat, infant's thigh held in knee-chest position. Extend infant's leg by gentle pressure and measure popliteal angle.
5. Scarf sign: With infant supine, pull infant's hand across the neck toward opposite shoulder. Determine how far elbow will reach across. Score 0 if elbow reaches opposite axillary line, 1 if past midaxillary line, 2 if past midline, and 3 if elbow unable to reach midline.
6. Heel-to-ear maneuver: With baby supine, draw infant's foot as near to head as possible without forcing it. Observe distance between foot and head and degree of extension at knee.

D. Birth Trauma

1. **Extradural fluid collections:** See Table 18.3 and Fig. 18.3.
2. **Fractured clavicle:** Possible crepitus/deformity/decreased movement on day 1 ± swelling/discomfort on day 2.
3. **Brachial plexus injuries:** See Section XI.

E. Selected Anomalies, Syndromes, and Malformations (see Chapter 13 for genetic disorders)

1. **Infant of a diabetic mother:** Frequently at risk of hypoglycemia, polycythemia, transient tachypnea of the newborn (TTN). Other associated defects include sacral agenesis, femoral hypoplasia, cardiac

TABLE 18.3

BIRTH-RELATED EXTRADURAL FLUID COLLECTIONS

	Caput Succedaneum	Cephalohematoma	Subgaleal Hemorrhage
Location	At point of contact; can extend across sutures	Usually over parietal bones; does not cross sutures	Beneath epicranial aponeurosis; may extend to orbits or nape of neck
Findings	Vaguely demarcated; pitting edema, shifts with gravity	Distinct margins; initially firm, more fluctuant after 48 hr	Firm to fluctuant, ill-defined borders; may have crepitus or fluid waves
Timing	Maximal size/firmness at birth; resolves in 48–72 hr	Increases after birth for 12–24 hr; resolution over weeks	Progressive after birth; resolution over weeks
Severity	Minimal	Rarely severe	May be severe, especially in the setting of associated coagulopathy

Data from Davis DJ. Neonatal subgaleal hemorrhage: diagnosis and management. *CMAJ*. 2001;164:1452.

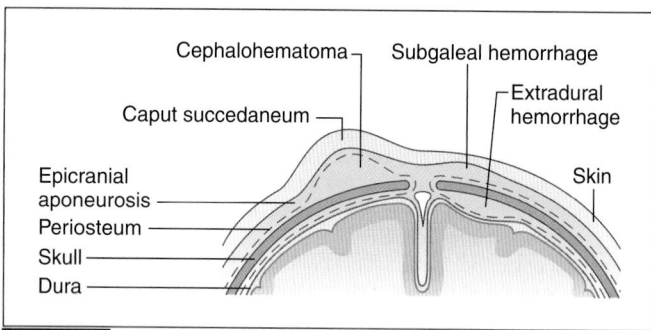

FIGURE 18.3

Types of extradural fluid collections seen in newborn infants.

defects, cleft palate/lip, preaxial radial defects, microtia, microphthalmia, holoprosencephaly, microcephaly, anencephaly, spina bifida, cauda equina, hemivertebrae, urinary tract defects, and polydactyly.

2. **VACTERL association: V**ertebral defects, **A**nal atresia, **C**ardiac defects, **T**racheo-**E**sophageal fistula, **R**enal anomalies, and **L**imb abnormalities

3. **CHARGE syndrome: C**oloboma, **H**eart disease, choanal **A**tresia, **R**etarded growth and development (may include central nervous system anomalies), **G**enital anomalies (may include hypogonadism), and **E**ar abnormalities or deafness

IV. FLUIDS, ELECTROLYTES, AND NUTRITION

A. Fluids

1. **Fluid requirements of newborns** (Table 18.4). Of note, insensible water loss increases with greater degree of prematurity through immature skin and renal losses.

TABLE 18.4

ESTIMATED MAINTENANCE FLUID REQUIREMENTS OF NEWBORNS

Birth Weight (g)	Fluid Requirements (mL/kg/24 hr) by Age			
	Day 1	Day 2	Days 3–6	Days 7+
<750	100–140	120–160	140–200	140–160
750–1000	100–120	100–140	130–180	140–160
1000–1500	80–100	100–120	120–160	150
>1500	60–80	80–120	120–160	150

Data from Gleason CA, Juul SE, eds. *Avery's Diseases of the Newborn.* 10th ed. Elsevier; 2018.

B. Glucose

1. **Glucose infusion rate (GIR):** Preterm neonates require approximately 5 to 6 mg/kg/min of glucose (40 to 100 mg/dL).[8] Term neonates require approximately 3 to 5 mg/kg/min of glucose. Calculate as follows:

$$\text{GIR}\,(\text{mg/kg/min}) = 0.167 \times [\text{dextrose concentration}]\left[\text{infusion rate}\left(\frac{\text{mL}}{\text{hr}}\right)\right]/[\text{Weight (kg)}]$$

2. **Management of hyperglycemia and hypoglycemia:** Table 18.5 and Fig. 18.2 (see Chapters 1 and 10).

C. Electrolytes, Minerals, and Vitamins

1. **Electrolyte requirements** (Table 18.6)
2. **Mineral and vitamin requirements:**
   a. Infants born at <34 weeks' gestation have higher calcium, phosphorus, sodium, iron, and vitamin D requirements and require breastmilk fortifier or special preterm formulas with iron. Fortifier is generally added to breastmilk after the second week of life.
   b. Iron: Preterm infants tolerating full enteral feeds require an elemental iron supplement of 2 to 6 mg/kg/day. Timing of initiation remains controversial, generally after age 10–14 days.[9]
   c. Vitamin D: 400 IU/day is recommended for all infants from birth to 12 months of age regardless of mode of feeding.[10]
   d. ADEK: Indicated for infants with malabsorption and/or cholestasis tolerating full enteral feeds.

D. Nutrition

1. **Growth and caloric requirements:** Table 18.7
2. **Total parenteral nutrition** (see Chapter 21)

V. CYANOSIS IN THE NEWBORN

A. Differential Diagnosis

1. **General:** Hypothermia, hypoglycemia, sepsis
2. **Cardiac:** Congestive heart failure, congenital cyanotic heart disease
3. **Respiratory:** Persistent pulmonary hypertension of the newborn (PPHN), diaphragmatic hernia, pulmonary hypoplasia, choanal atresia,

18

TABLE 18.5

MANAGEMENT OF HYPERGLYCEMIA AND HYPOGLYCEMIA

	Hypoglycemia	Hyperglycemia
Definition	Serum glucose <40 mg/dL in term and late preterm infants	Serum glucose >125 mg/dL in term infants, >150 mg/dL in preterm infants
Differential diagnosis	Insufficient glucose delivery Decreased glycogen stores Increased circulating insulin (e.g., infant of a diabetic mother, maternal drugs, Beckwith-Wiedemann syndrome, tumors) Endocrine and metabolic disorders Sepsis or shock Hypothermia, polycythemia, or asphyxia	Excess glucose administration Sepsis Hypoxia Hyperosmolar formula Neonatal diabetes mellitus Medications
Evaluation	Assess for symptoms and calculate glucose delivery to infant. Confirm bedside glucose with laboratory serum glucose. Consider other laboratory evaluations: Complete blood cell count with differential; electrolytes; blood, urine, ± cerebrospinal fluid cultures; urinalysis; insulin and C-peptide levels	
Management	See Fig. 18.2. If glucose <40 and symptomatic, treat with intravenous glucose (dose = 200 mg/kg, which is equivalent to dextrose 10% at 2 mL/kg). Change dextrose infusion rates gradually. Generally, no more than 2 mg/kg/min in a 2-hr interval (see Chapter 1) Monitor glucose levels every 30–60 min until normal.	Gradually decrease glucose infusion rate if receiving >5 mg/kg/min. Monitor glucosuria. Consider insulin infusion for persistent hyperglycemia.

Modified from Paul S, et al. Recommendations from the Pediatric Endocrine Society for evaluation and management of persistent hypoglycemia in neonates, infants, and children. *J Pediatr.* 2015;167(2):238–245.

TABLE 18.6

ELECTROLYTE REQUIREMENTS

	Before 24 hr of Life	Transitional, After 24 hr of Life[a]	Growing Premature Infant	Growing Term Infant
Sodium (mEq/kg/day)	0–1	2–5	3–5	2–4
Potassium (mEq/kg/day)	0	0–2	2–3	2–3

[a]Pending postnatal diuresis has been established. Period to physiologic and metabolic stability generally occurring between 2 and 7 days.

pneumothorax, respiratory distress syndrome (RDS), TTN, pneumonia, meconium aspiration

4. **Neurologic:** Central apnea, central hypoventilation, intraventricular hemorrhage (IVH), meningitis

TABLE 18.7

AVERAGE CALORIC REQUIREMENTS AND GROWTH FOR PRETERM AND TERM INFANTS

	Preterm Infant	Term Infant
Caloric requirements (kcal/kg/day) [parental/enteral]	PN: 85–110 EN: 105–130 Up to 150 for infants with cardiac conditions or BPD[a]	PN: 90–100 EN: 100–120
Growth after 10 days of life	<2 kg: 15–20 g/kg/day >2 kg: 25–35 g/day	20–30 g/day

[a]Signifies an exception for infants with cardiac conditions or BPD.

BPD, Bronchopulmonary dysplasia; *EN*, enteral nutrition or feeds into stomach; *PN*, parenteral nutrition or IV nutrition.

5. **Hematologic:** Polycythemia, methemoglobinemia
6. **Medications:** Respiratory depression from maternal medications (e.g., magnesium sulfate, narcotics, general anesthesia)

B. Evaluation

1. **Physical examination:** Note central vs. peripheral and persistent vs. intermittent cyanosis, respiratory effort, single vs. split S_2, presence of heart murmur. Acrocyanosis is a normal finding in newborns.
2. **Clinical tests:** Preductal/postductal arterial blood gases or pulse oximetry to assess for right-to-left shunt, and transillumination of chest for possible pneumothorax, hyperoxia test (see Chapter 7).
3. **Other data:** Complete blood cell count (CBC) with differential, serum glucose, lactate, chest radiograph, echocardiography. Consider blood, urine, and cerebrospinal fluid cultures if sepsis is suspected.

VI. RESPIRATORY DISEASES

A. General Respiratory Considerations

1. **Exogenous surfactant therapy:**
   a. Indications: RDS in preterm infants. Consider in meconium/blood/ amniotic fluid aspiration, pneumonia, persistent pulmonary hypertension of newborn (PPHN).
   b. Administration: If newborn is gestational age (GA) ≤26 weeks, first dose is typically given in delivery room or as soon as stabilized in NICU; repeat dosing can be considered based on oxygen requirements and level of respiratory support.
   c. Complications: Pneumothorax, pulmonary hemorrhage
2. **Supplemental O$_2$:** Adjust inspired oxygen to maintain O_2 saturation. Ideal target oxygen saturations vary based on factors such as gestational age, chronologic age, and underlying conditions, and aim to minimize adverse outcomes from hypoxemia and hyperoxemia. Higher targets (>94%) can be used when the retinas are mature (see Section XIII) and in cases of pulmonary hypertension.[11]

18

B. Respiratory Distress Syndrome (RDS)

1. **Etiology:** Deficiency of pulmonary surfactant resulting in increased surface tension and alveolar collapse. Surfactant is produced in increasing quantities after 32 weeks' gestation.
2. **Prevention:**
   a. Antenatal maternal steroids have been shown to decrease neonatal morbidity and mortality.[12]
   b. Optimal timing: First course at >24 hours and <7 days prior to anticipated preterm delivery
   c. Repeat course: Considered in women at gestational age (GA) <34 weeks and whose prior steroid course was administered >14 days prior. Serial courses not currently recommended.
3. **Incidence:** Table 18.8
4. **Risk factors:** Prematurity, maternal diabetes, cesarean section without antecedent labor, perinatal asphyxia, second twin, previous infant with RDS. Of note, certain maternal factors may accelerate lung maturity including: hypertension, sickle cell disease, narcotic addiction, intrauterine growth retardation, prolonged rupture of the membranes, and fetal stress.
5. **Clinical presentation:**
   a. Respiratory distress (e.g., increased work of breathing, desaturations) worsens during first few hours of life, progresses over 48 to 72 hours, and subsequently improves.
   b. Recovery is accompanied by brisk diuresis.
   c. CXR consistent with hypoinflation along with diffuse and symmetric "ground glass" appearance See Chapter 26 for imaging findings.
6. **Management:**
   a. Ventilatory and oxygenation support
   b. Surfactant therapy

C. Persistent Pulmonary Hypertension of the Newborn (PPHN)

1. **Etiology:** Idiopathic or secondary to conditions leading to increased pulmonary vascular resistance, vasoconstriction, and right-to-left shunting

---

TABLE 18.8

INCIDENCE OF RESPIRATORY DISTRESS SYNDROME BY GESTATIONAL AGE AND ANTE-NATAL STEROID ADMINISTRATION[12,32-34]

Gestational Age (Week)	Antenatal Steroids Administered	Antenatal Steroids Not Administered
<30	35%	60%
30–34	10%	25%
34–36	1.4%[a]; 5.5%	2.3%[a]; 6.4%
>37	2.6%	5.4%

[a]Neonates with severe respiratory distress syndrome.

NOTE: The use of antenatal corticosteroids in >34 weeks' gestational age is controversial because of inconsistent data regarding efficacy and limited data regarding long-term effects.

2. **Risk factors:** Most commonly seen in term or postterm newborns, those born by cesarean section, and newborns with a history of fetal distress and low APGAR scores. Other risk factors are: hypoxemia and acidosis leading to vasoconstriction, interstitial pulmonary disease (meconium aspiration syndrome, pneumonia), hyperviscosity syndrome (polycythemia), and pulmonary hypoplasia, either primary or secondary to congenital diaphragmatic hernia or renal agenesis

3. **Diagnostic features: PPHN usually presents within 12 to 24 hours of birth**
   a. Severe hypoxemia (Pao_2 <35 to 45 mmHg in 100% O_2) disproportionate to radiologic changes
   b. Structurally normal heart with right-to-left shunt at foramen ovale and/or ductus arteriosus; pre/postductal oxygenation gradient (≥7 to 15 mmHg is significant)
   c. Critically important to distinguish from cyanotic heart disease. If little to no improvement in oxygenation with oxygen therapy, perform detailed cardiac exam and hyperoxia test (see Chapter 7 for interpretation), and consider echocardiogram.

4. **Principles of therapy:**
   a. **Improve oxygenation:** Supplemental oxygen administration and optimization of oxygen-carrying capacity with blood transfusions as indicated
   b. **Minimize pulmonary vasoconstriction:**
      (1) Minimal handling of infant or noxious procedures. Sedation and occasionally paralysis of intubated neonates may be necessary.
      (2) Avoid severe hyperventilation-associated hypocarbia (PCO_2 <30 mmHg), which can be associated with myocardial ischemia and decreased cerebral blood flow. Hyperventilation may result in barotrauma and predispose to chronic lung disease. Consider high-frequency ventilation.
   c. **Maintenance of systemic blood pressure and perfusion:** Reversal of right-to-left shunt through volume expanders and/or inotropes
   d. **Consider pulmonary vasodilator therapy:** see Chapter 1
      (1) Inhaled nitric oxide (iNO): Reduces pulmonary vascular resistance (PVR). Typical starting dose is 20 parts per million (ppm), though research suggests lower doses in premature neonates (10 ppm) may be sufficient. Unlikely to have additional benefit at >40 ppm. Complications include methemoglobinemia (reduce NO dose for methemoglobin >4%), NO_2 poisoning (reduce NO dose for NO_2 concentration >1 to 2 ppm).
      (2) Prostacyclin analog (e.g., epoprostenol): Pulmonary vasodilator, normally produced by lung when lung vessels are constricted
      (3) Sildenafil: Cyclic cGMP-specific phosphodiesterase type 5 (PDE5) inhibitor; results in pulmonary vasodilation
   e. **Consider extracorporeal membrane oxygenation (ECMO):** Reserved for cases of severe cardiovascular instability, oxygenation index (OI) >40 for >3 hour, or alveolar-arterial gradient (A-aO_2) ≥610 for 8 hours (see Chapter 1 for OI and A-a gradient equations). Infants typically need to

be >2000 g and at gestation >34 weeks to be ECMO candidates. Obtain head ultrasound and consider EEG before initiating ECMO.

D. Transient Tachypnea of the Newborn

1. **Etiology:** Incomplete or delayed resorption of amniotic fluid from the lungs
   a. Immaturity of respiratory epithelial Na^+ transport
2. **Risk factors:** Birth by cesarean section, male sex, macrosomia, lower gestational age, maternal diabetes, maternal asthma, maternal smoking
3. **Diagnostic features:**
   a. Symptoms present within first 6 hours of delivery and resolve within first postnatal week, usually within 72 hours.
   b. Tachypnea: Greater than 60 breaths/min, often in the range of 80 to 100 breaths/min
   c. Retractions, grunting, or nasal flaring may be present. Cyanosis and hypoxia are rare.
   d. CXR consistent with retained fluid: Congestion, perihilar streaking, fluid in the interlobar fissure
   e. Exclusion of other diagnoses: For example, pneumonia, aspiration, congenital malformations, subarachnoid hemorrhage, hypoxic-ischemic encephalopathy (HIE), pneumothorax, acidosis, RDS
4. **Management:**
   a. NPO with gavage feedings or 10% dextrose-containing fluids via IV for persistent tachypnea
   b. Supplemental oxygen and/or CPAP as indicated
   c. No proven benefit of adjuncts, including diuretics or racemic epinephrine

E. Pneumothorax

1. Seen in 1% to 2% of normal newborns
2. Associated with use of high ventilatory pressures and underlying diseases such as RDS, meconium aspiration, and pneumonia
3. Consider monitoring in a neonatal intensive care unit (NICU).
4. If concern exists for tension pneumothorax, consider needle thoracostomy and/or chest tube placement (see Chapter 4).

VII. APNEA AND BRADYCARDIA

A. Apnea

1. **Definition:** Respiratory pause >20 seconds or a shorter pause associated with cyanosis, pallor, hypotonia, or bradycardia <100 bpm. May be central (no diaphragmatic activity), obstructive (upper airway obstruction), or mixed
2. **Etiology:** See Fig. 18.4. Apnea of prematurity occurs in most infants born at <28 weeks' gestation, ~20% of infants born at 34 weeks' gestation, and <10% of infants born beyond 34 weeks' gestation. Usually resolves by 34 to 36 weeks postmenstrual age but may persist after term in infants born at <25 weeks' gestation.[13]

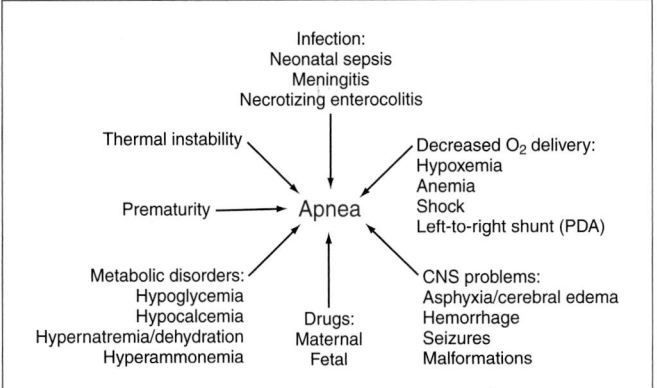

FIGURE 18.4

Causes of apnea in the newborn. *CNS*, Central nervous system; *PDA*, patent ductus arteriosus. (From Klaus MH, Fanaroff AA. *Care of the High-Risk Neonate.* 5th ed. WB Saunders; 2001:268.)

3. **Management:**
   a. Consider pathologic causes for apnea (e.g., meningitis, seizures).
   b. Pharmacotherapy with caffeine or other stimulants
   c. Continuous positive airway pressure or mechanical ventilation (see Chapter 1).

B. Bradycardia Without Central Apnea

Etiologies include obstructive apnea, mechanical airway obstruction, gastroesophageal reflux, increased intracranial pressure, increased vagal tone (defecation, yawning, rectal stimulation, and placement of nasogastric [NG] tube), electrolyte abnormalities, heart block

VIII. CARDIAC DISEASES

A. Patent Ductus Arteriosus

1. **Definition:** Failure of ductus arteriosus to close in first 72 hours of life or reopening after functional closure. Typically results in left-to-right shunting of blood once PVR has decreased. If PVR remains high, blood may be shunted right to left, resulting in hypoxemia.

2. **Diagnosis:**
   a. Examination: Systolic murmur may be continuous and best heard at the left upper sternal border or left infraclavicular area. Bounding peripheral pulses with widened pulse pressure if large shunt. Hyperactive precordium and palmar pulses may be present.
   b. Chest radiograph: May show cardiomegaly and increased pulmonary vascular markings, depending on size of shunt
   c. Echocardiogram
   d. ECG: Normal to moderate left ventricular hypertrophy in small to moderate patent ductus arteriosus (PDA); biventricular hypertrophy in large PDA

3. **Management:**
   a. Indications for treatment, timing of intervention, and best management strategy remain controversial.[14]
   b. Current treatment options: ibuprofen, indomethacin, acetaminophen, watchful waiting
      (1) Ibuprofen is as effective as indomethacin but fewer renal adverse effects and risk of necrotizing enterocolitis.[14]
      (2) Complications
         (a) Renal: Transient decrease in glomerular filtration rate and decreased urine output
         (b) GI: Transient gastrointestinal bleeding (no increased incidence of necrotizing enterocolitis [NEC]). Spontaneous isolated intestinal perforations (SIP) are seen with indomethacin use. Rates are higher with concomitant hydrocortisone use.
         (c) Heme: Prolonged bleeding time, and disturbed platelet function for 7 to 9 days independent of platelet count (no increased incidence of intracranial hemorrhage)
   c. Acetaminophen is emerging as a newer treatment modality with continued evolving research. It appears to be as similarly effective as oral ibuprofen without above effects on kidneys and platelets.[14]
   d. Surgical ligation of the duct
   e. Transcatheter closure of PDA

B. **Cyanotic Heart Disease (See Chapter 7)**

IX. HEMATOLOGIC DISEASES

A. **Unconjugated Hyperbilirubinemia in the Newborn[15,16]**

1. **Overview:**
   a. During first 3 to 4 days of life, total serum bilirubin (TSB) increases to 6.5 ± 2.5 mg/dL.
   b. Maximum rate of bilirubin increase for normal infants with nonhemolytic hyperbilirubinemia: 5 mg/dL/24 hr or 0.2 mg/dL/hr
   c. Always consider clinical jaundice or TSB >5 mg/dL in first 24 hours as pathologic.
   d. Risk factors: Birth weight <2500 g, exclusive breastfeeding, prematurity, ABO incompatibility, cephalohematoma or significant bruising, predischarge total bilirubin in high-risk zone, observed jaundice in first 24 hours, infant of a diabetic mother, previous sibling requiring phototherapy, low albumin, infection, race

2. **Evaluation:**
   a. Maternal prenatal testing: ABO and Rh (D) typing and serum screen for isoimmune antibodies
   b. Infant or cord blood: Blood and Rh typing (if maternal blood type is O or Rh negative, or prenatal blood typing was not performed). Consider hemoglobin, reticulocyte count, blood smear, glucose-6-phosphate dehydrogenase (G6PD) testing, direct Coombs test.

3. **Management:**
    a. Phototherapy: Ideally, intensive phototherapy produces a TSB decline of 1 to 2 mg/dL within 4 to 6 hours, with further subsequent decline. Guidelines:
        (1) Preterm newborn (Table 18.9)
        (2) Term newborn (Fig. 18.5)
    b. Intravenous immunoglobulin (IVIG): In isoimmune hemolytic disease, IVIG administration (0.5 to 1 g/kg over 2 hours) is recommended if TSB is rising despite intensive phototherapy or TSB is within 2 to 3 mg/dL of exchange transfusion level (see Chapter 15 for discussion of IVIG).

TABLE 18.9

GUIDELINES FOR MANAGEMENT OF HYPERBILIRUBINEMIA IN PRETERM INFANTS AGED <1 WEEK

Gestational Age (Weeks)	Phototherapy (mg/dL)	Consider Exchange Transfusion (mg/dL)
<28 0/7	5–6	11–14
28 0/7–29 6/7	6–8	12–14
30 0/7–31 6/7	8–10	13–16
32 0/7–33 6/7	10–12	15–18

Data from Maisels MJ, Watchko JF, Bhutani V. An approach to the management of hyperbilirubinemia in the preterm infant less than 35 weeks of gestation. *J Perinatol.* 2012;32(9):660–664.

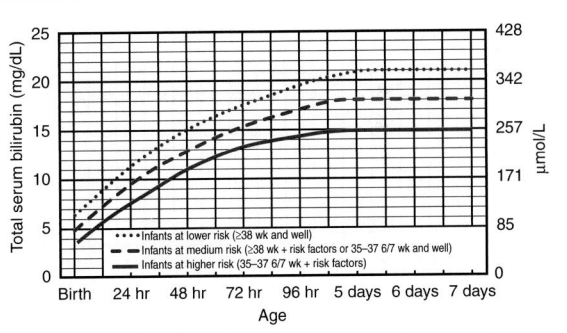

- Use total bilirubin. Do not subtract direct reacting or conjugated bilirubin.
- Risk factors: Isoimmune hemolytic disease, G6PD deficiency, asphyxia, significant lethargy, temperature instability, sepsis, acidosis, or albumin <3.0 g/dL (if measured)
- For well infants 35–37 6/7 wk, can adjust TSB levels for intervention around the medium risk line. It is an option to intervene at lower TSB levels for infants closer to 35 wk and at higher TSB levels for those closer to 37 6/7 wk.
- It is an option to provide conventional phototherapy in hospital or at home at TSB levels 2–3 mg/dL (35–50 mmol/L) below those shown, but home phototherapy should not be used in any infant with risk factors.

FIGURE 18.5

Guidelines for phototherapy in infants born at 35 weeks of gestation or more. *G6PD*, Glucose-6-phosphate dehydrogenase; *TSB*, total serum bilirubin.

18

c. Neonatal double-volume exchange transfusion (see Table 18.9 and Fig. 18.6):

   (1) Volume: Exchange volume is generally twice the infant's blood volume, generally 160 mL/kg for full-term infant, 200 mL/kg for preterm infant. Can consider single volume based on clinical stability

   (2) Route: During exchange, blood is removed through umbilical arterial catheter (UAC) and an equal volume is infused through UVC. If UAC is unavailable, use a peripheral arterial line or single venous catheter.

   (3) Procedure: Replaces up to 85% of infant's circulation. Exchange in 15-mL aliquots for full-term infants. Exchange at 2 to 3 mL/kg/min in premature/less stable infants to avoid hemolysis.

   (4) Complications: Emboli, thromboses, hemodynamic instability, electrolyte disturbances (e.g. hypocalcemia), coagulopathy, infection, death

   NOTE: CBC, reticulocyte count, peripheral smear, bilirubin, Ca^{2+}, glucose, total protein, infant blood type, Coombs test, and newborn screen should be performed on a preexchange sample of blood; they are of no diagnostic value with postexchange blood. **If indicated, save preexchange blood for serologic or genetic studies.**

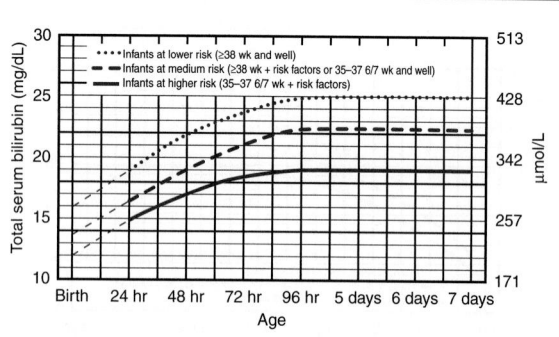

- The dashed lines for the first 24 hours indicate uncertainty due to a wide range of clinical circumstances and a range of responses to phototherapy.
- Immediate exchange transfusion is recommended if infant shows signs of acute bilirubin encephalopathy (hypertonia, arching, retrocollis, opisthotonos, fever, high-pitched cry) or if TBS is ≥5 mg/dL (85 μmol/L) above these lines.
- Risk factors: Isoimmune hemolytic disease, G6PD deficiency, asphyxia, significant lethargy, temperature instability, sepsis, acidosis.
- Measure serum albumin and calculate B/A ratio.
- Use total bilirubin. Do not subtract direct reacting or conjugated bilirubin.
- If infant is well and 35–37 6/7 wk (median risk), can individualize TSB levels for exchange based on actual gestational age.

FIGURE 18.6

Guidelines for exchange transfusion in infants born at 35 weeks of gestation or more. *B/A*, Bilirubin/albumin; *G6PD*, glucose-6-phosphate dehydrogenase; *TSB*, total serum bilirubin.

B. Conjugated Hyperbilirubinemia (See Chapter 12)

1. **Definition:** Direct bilirubin >2.0 mg/dL and >10% of TSB
2. **Etiology:** Biliary obstruction/atresia, choledochal cyst, hyperalimentation, α_1-antitrypsin deficiency, hepatitis, sepsis, infections (especially urinary tract infections), hypothyroidism, inborn errors of metabolism, cystic fibrosis, red blood cell abnormalities
3. **Management:** Ursodiol for infants on full feeds; consider supplementation with fat-soluble vitamins (A, D, E, K); otherwise depends on etiology. Phototherapy is not contraindicated but poses the risk for "bronze baby" syndrome or transient dark, gray-brown discoloration of the skin, serum, and urine. This transient effect should be weighed against risk of continued rise and need for exchange transfusion.

C. Polycythemia

1. **Definition:** Venous hematocrit >65% confirmed on two consecutive samples. May be falsely elevated when obtained by heel stick or falsely lower when obtained by arterial stick[17]
2. **Etiologies:** Twin-twin transfusion, maternal-fetal transfusion, intrauterine hypoxia, maternal diabetes, delayed cord clamping, neonatal thyrotoxicosis, congenital adrenal hyperplasia, trisomies, Beckwith-Wiedemann syndrome
3. **Clinical findings:** Plethora, respiratory distress, tachypnea, hypoglycemia, irritability, lethargy, seizures, apnea, jitteriness, poor feeding, thrombocytopenia, hyperbilirubinemia, cardiac failure
4. **Complications:** Hyperviscosity predisposes to venous thrombosis and CNS injury. Hypoglycemia may result from increased erythrocyte utilization of glucose.
5. **Management:** Partial-volume exchange transfusion for symptomatic infants, with isovolemic replacement (80 mL/kg at term, or 100 mL/kg for preterm) of blood with isotonic fluid. Blood is exchanged in 10- to 20-mL increments with goal to reduce hematocrit to <55%.

X. GASTROINTESTINAL DISEASES

A. Necrotizing Enterocolitis

1. **Definition:** Serious intestinal inflammation and injury thought to be multifactorial, including bowel ischemia, immaturity, and infection. Occurs principally in infants who have been fed
2. **Risk factors:** Prematurity, RDS, hypoxic ischemic encephalopathy (HIE), polycythemia–hyperviscosity syndrome, umbilical vessel catheterization, exchange transfusion, bacterial and viral pathogens, enteral feeds, PDA, congestive heart failure, cyanotic heart disease, intrauterine cocaine exposure
3. **Clinical findings:** See eTable 18.1.
   a. Systemic: Temperature instability, apnea, bradycardia, metabolic acidosis, hypotension, disseminated intravascular coagulopathy

   b. Intestinal: Blood in stool, absent bowel sounds, and/or abdominal tenderness or mass. Elevated pregavage residuals in the absence of other clinical symptoms rarely raise a suspicion of NEC.
   c. Radiologic: Ileus, intestinal pneumatosis, portal vein gas, ascites, pneumoperitoneum (see Chapter 26)
4. **Management:** Nothing by mouth, NG tube decompression, maintain adequate hydration and perfusion, broad spectrum antibiotics for 7 to 10 days based on hospital antibiogram, surgical consultation. Surgery is performed for signs of perforation or necrotic bowel.
5. **Minimizing risk of NEC:**
   a. The exclusive use of human milk, including donor breastmilk, has been shown to decrease the risk of NEC and associated mortality.[18]
   b. Several studies link the use of probiotics and a decreased risk of NEC.[19] However, variations among formulations of probiotics, dosing, and lack of long-term studies on outcome have prevented the standard use of probiotics in the NICU.[20]
   c. There have been additional studies on supplements including L-arginine, glutamine, and lactoferrin,[21] but data remain insufficient to support a practice recommendation.[22]

B. Bilious Emesis
See eTable 18.2 and Chapter 12.

1. **Etiologies:**
   a. **Proximal:** Duodenal atresia, annular pancreas, malrotation with or without volvulus, jejunal obstruction/atresia; generally abdominal distention not prominent
   b. **Distal:** Ileal atresia, meconium ileus, colonic atresia, meconium plus, hypoplastic left colon syndrome, Hirschsprung disease; generally with abdominal distention
   c. **Functional (i.e., poor motility):** NEC, electrolyte abnormalities, sepsis
2. **Workup:** Abdominal x-ray, upper gastrointestinal series, contrast enema, sweat test, mucosal rectal biopsy

   NOTE: Must eliminate malrotation as an etiology because volvulus is a surgical emergency
C. Abdominal Wall Defects (Table 18.10)
D. Gastroesophageal Reflux Disease (See Chapter 12)

XI. NEUROLOGIC DISEASES

A. Neonatal Hypoxic-Ischemic Encephalopathy
1. **Initial management:** Passive cooling, detailed Sarnat exam[23]
2. **Therapeutic hypothermia (TH):** Infants with evidence of hypoxic-ischemic encephalopathy (HIE) shortly after birth who are at gestation >35 weeks should be considered for therapeutic hypothermia. TH protocol should be initiated within 6 hours of delivery.

3. **Criteria for hypothermia include one or more of the following:**
   a. Cord gas or blood gas in the first hour of life with a pH <7.0 or base deficit >16
   b. For newborns with a pH 7.01 to 7.15 or base deficit 10 to 15.9, additional criteria should be met (e.g., significant perinatal event).
      (1) 10-minute APGAR ≤5
         (a) Evidence of moderate to severe encephalopathy
      (2) Need for assisted ventilation at birth for at least 10 minutes
4. **Severity and outcome of HIE in full-term neonate:** Table 18.11.

B. **Intraventricular Hemorrhage**

1. **Definition:** IVH usually arises in the germinal matrix and periventricular regions of the brain.
2. **Incidence**[24,25]:
   a. 30% to 40% of infants <1500 g; 50% to 60% of infants <1000 g
   b. Highest incidence within first 72 hours of life: 50% within 24 hours, 90% within 96 hours

TABLE 18.10

DIFFERENCES BETWEEN OMPHALOCELE AND GASTROSCHISIS

	Omphalocele	Gastroschisis
Position	Central abdominal	Right paraumbilical
Hernia sac	Present	Absent
Umbilical ring	Absent	Present
Umbilical cord insertion	At the vertex of the sac	Normal
Herniation of other viscera	Common	Rare
Extraintestinal anomalies	Frequent	Rare
Intestinal infarction, atresia	Less frequent	More frequent

TABLE 18.11

SEVERITY AND OUTCOME OF HYPOXIC-ISCHEMIC ENCEPHALOPATHY IN FULL-TERM NEONATE

	Mild	Moderate	Severe
Level of consciousness	Increased irritability, hyperalert	Lethargic	Stupor or coma
Seizures	Rare	Common	Uncommon
Primitive reflexes	Exaggerated	Suppressed	Absent
Brain stem dysfunction	Rare	Rare	Common
Elevated intracranial pressure	Rare	Rare	Variable
Duration	<24 hr	>24 hr (variable)	>5 days
Poor outcome (%)[a]	0	20–40	100

[a]Poor outcome is defined by presence of intellectual disability, cerebral palsy, or seizures.

Data from MacDonald M, Mullett M. Severity and outcome of hypoxic-ischemic encephalopathy in full term neonate. In: *Avery's Neonatology.* 6th ed. Lippincott Williams & Wilkins; 2005.

3. **Diagnosis and classification[25]:**
   a. Ultrasonography; grade is based on maximum amount of hemorrhage seen by age 2 weeks:
      (1) Grade I: Hemorrhage in germinal matrix only
      (2) Grade II: IVH without ventricular dilation
      (3) Grade III: IVH with ventricular dilation
      (4) Grade IV: Periventricular hemorrhagic infarct with or without IVH

      NOTE: Many institutions use descriptive data (as opposed to the grading system) to denote severity of IVH.
4. **Screening:** Indicated in infants <32 weeks' gestational age or birth weight <1500 g within 72 hours of birth; repeat in 1 to 2 weeks
5. **Outcome:** Increased risk for neurodevelopmental (ND) disabilities and posthemorrhagic hydrocephalus follows grade III–IV IVH. More subtle learning/ND disabilities may occur with grade II IVH.

C. **Periventricular White Matter Injury[24]**

1. **Definition and ultrasound findings:** Ischemic necrosis of periventricular white matter, characterized by CNS depression within first week of life and later findings of cysts on ultrasound with or without ventricular enlargement (caused by cerebral atrophy) or noncystic white matter injury visualized by MRI
2. **Incidence:** More common in preterm infants but also occurs in term infants
3. **Etiology:** Primarily ischemia-reperfusion injury, infectious, hypoxia, acidosis, acute hypotension, low cerebral blood flow, hypoglycemia
4. **Outcome:** Commonly associated with cerebral palsy with or without sensory and cognitive deficits

D. **Neonatal Seizures (See Chapter 20)**

E. **Neonatal Abstinence Syndrome[26]**

1. Assess in utero drug exposure (IUDE) to maternal substance use and medications; consider potential polypharmacy.
2. Onset of symptoms usually occurs within first 24 to 72 hours from birth (methadone may delay symptoms until 96 hours or later). Symptoms may last weeks to months. Box 18.1 shows signs and symptoms of opioid withdrawal.
3. Treatment:
   a. Nonpharmacologic: Includes rooming in, breastfeeding, skin-to-skin, swaddling, and environmental controls such as decreased disruptions
   b. Pharmacologic: Target to known IUDE

F. **Peripheral Nerve Injuries**

1. **Etiology:** Result from lateral traction on shoulder (vertex deliveries) or head (breech deliveries)
2. **Clinical features** (Table 18.12)
3. **Management:** Evaluate for associated trauma (clavicular and humeral fractures, shoulder dislocation, facial nerve injury, cord injuries). Full recovery is seen in 85% to 95% of cases in first year of life.

BOX 18.1

SIGNS AND SYMPTOMS OF OPIOID WITHDRAWAL

W	Wakefulness
I	Irritability, insomnia
T	Tremors, temperature variation, tachypnea, twitching (jitteriness)
H	Hyperactivity, high-pitched cry, hiccups, hyperreflexia, hypertonia
D	Diarrhea (explosive), diaphoresis, disorganized suck
R	Rub marks, respiratory distress, rhinorrhea, regurgitation
A	Apnea, autonomic dysfunction
W	Weight loss
A	Alkalosis (respiratory)
L	Lacrimation (photophobia), lethargy
S	Seizures, sneezing, stuffy nose, sweating, sucking (nonproductive)

TABLE 18.12

BRACHIAL PLEXUS INJURIES

Plexus Injury	Spinal Level Involved	Clinical Features
Erb-Duchenne palsy (90% of cases)	C5–C6 Occasionally involves C4	Adduction and internal rotation of arm. Forearm is pronated; wrist is flexed. Diaphragm paralysis may occur if C4 is involved.
Total palsy (8%–9% of cases)	C5–T1 Occasionally involves C4	Upper arm, lower arm, and hand involved. Horner syndrome (ptosis, anhidrosis, and miosis) exists if T1 is involved.
Klumpke paralysis (<2% of cases)	C7–T1	Hand flaccid with little control. Horner syndrome if T1 is involved.

XII. UROLOGIC DISORDERS

A. Lower Urinary Tract Obstruction

1. **Definition:** Rare birth defects caused by partial or complete blockage of the urethra. Common causes include posterior urethral valves (PUV), urethral atresia, and triad syndrome (constricted narrowing in mid-portion of urethra). More common in males

2. **Diagnosis and evaluation:** Fetal anatomy ultrasound (18 to 24 weeks) with visualization of markedly distended bladder, often with a thickened wall (2 mm).[27,28] A "keyhole" sign representing dilation of the PUV proximal to the obstruction may be seen but is not specific.

   a. Other tests include fetal MRI, echocardiogram, vesicocentesis, and karyotype to rule out coexisting abnormalities and determine gender.

18

3. **Clinical findings:** Pulmonary hypoplasia, renal dysplasia, oligohydramnios, ureterectasis, caliectasis, hydronephrosis, clubfeet, Potter facies
4. **Management:** Consultation with pediatric urology and nephrology to review prenatal and postnatal options. Prenatally, elective termination or expectant management should be offered for fetuses with poor prognostic profiles. Postnatal interventions include dialysis, vesicostomy, and transplantation.

B. Bladder Exstrophy-Epispadias-Cloacal Exstrophy Complex

1. **Definition:** Anomalies involving urinary tract eversion; with genitourinary, musculoskeletal, and occasionally gastrointestinal malformations. See eTable 18.3 for comparison.
2. **Diagnosis:** Fetal anatomy ultrasound showing abnormality of bladder filling, low-set umbilical cord, abdominal mass that increases in size throughout pregnancy, separation of pubic bones and small genitals
3. **Management:** Reconstructive surgery that aims to establish bladder continence, preserve renal function, repair epispadias and genitalia, and close the pelvic bones

XIII. RETINOPATHY OF PREMATURITY[29]

A. Definition
Interruption of normal progression of retinal vascularization

B. Etiology
Exposure of the immature retina to high oxygen concentrations can result in vasoconstriction and obliteration of the retinal capillary network, followed by abnormal vasoproliferation. Risk is correlated to degree of prematurity.

C. Diagnosis
Dilated funduscopic examination should be performed in the following patients:

1. All infants born ≤30 weeks' gestation or with birth weight <1500 g
2. Infants born >30 weeks' gestation with unstable clinical course, including those requiring cardiorespiratory support

D. Timing of Screening[30]

1. All infants born ≤27 weeks' gestation, initial retinopathy of prematurity (ROP) screening examination performed at 31 weeks' postmenstrual age
2. All infants born ≥28 weeks' gestation, initial ROP screening examination performed at 4 weeks' chronologic age
3. Infants born before 25 weeks' gestation, consider earlier screening at 6 weeks' chronologic age (even if before 31 weeks' postmenstrual age) based on the severity of comorbidities to enable earlier detection and treatment of aggressive posterior ROP (a severe form of rapidly progressive ROP).

E. Classification

1. **Stage** of ROP (Fig. 18.7)

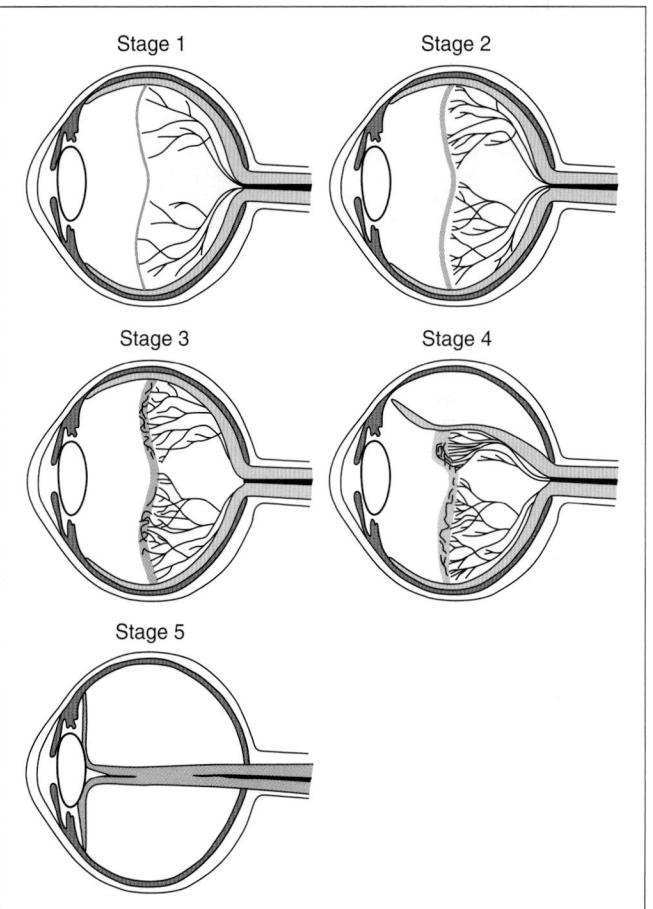

FIGURE 18.7

Retinopathy of prematurity: Stages and plus disease. (From Hellström A, Smith L EH, Dammann O. Retinopathy of prematurity. *Lancet.* 2013;382[9902]:1445–1457. Copyright 2013, Elsevier.)

a. Stage 1: Demarcation line separates avascular from vascularized retina.
b. Stage 2: Ridge forms along demarcation line.
c. Stage 3: Extraretinal, fibrovascular proliferation tissue forms on ridge.
d. Stage 4: Partial retinal detachment
e. Stage 5: Total retinal detachment

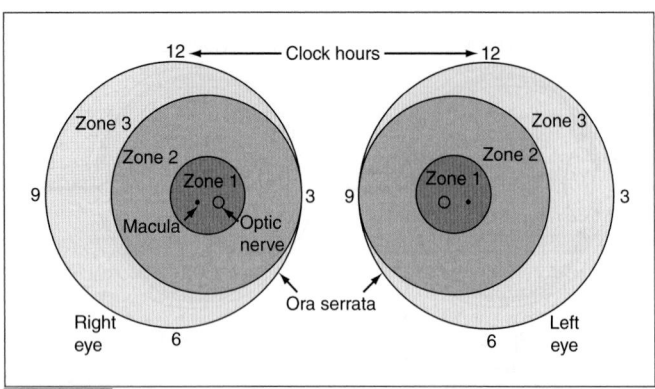

Zones of the retina. (From American Academy of Pediatrics. Screening examination of premature infants for retinopathy of prematurity, AAP policy statement. *Pediatrics*. 2018 [6];142:1–9.)

NOTE: Stage 0 is equivalent to no evidence of ROP on fundoscopic exam.

2. **Zone of retina** (Fig. 18.8)
3. **Plus disease:** Abnormal dilation and tortuosity of posterior retinal blood vessels in two or more quadrants of retina; may be present at any stage
4. **Number of clock hours or 30-degree sectors involved**

F. Management[29-30]

1. **Type 1 ROP:** Peripheral retinal ablation should be considered. Anti-VEGF treatment may be as effective for Zone I disease. Type 1 ROP classified as:
   a. Zone I: Any stage ROP with plus disease
   b. Zone I: Stage 3 ROP without plus disease
   c. Zone II: Stage 2 or 3 ROP with plus disease
2. **Type 2 ROP:** Serial examinations rather than retinal ablation should be considered. Type 2 ROP classified as:
   a. Zone I: Stage 1 or 2 ROP without plus disease
   b. Zone II: Stage 3 ROP without plus disease
3. **Follow-up (eTable 18.4):** Serial fundoscopic exams through at least term-corrected age and based on degree of ROP disease present

---

XIV. COMMONLY USED MEDICATIONS IN THE NEONATAL INTENSIVE CARE UNIT

See Table 18.13. For neonatal specific drug dosing, refer to Chapter 30, Formulary.

TABLE 18.13

DOSING OF COMMONLY USED ANTIMICROBIALS IN THE NEONATAL INTENSIVE CARE UNIT, BASED ON POSTMENSTRUAL AND POSTNATAL AGE

Drug	Dosing (IV)
Acyclovir	HSV infection: 20 mg/kg/dose
Ampicillin	Typical dosing: 25–50 mg/kg/dose; GBS meningitis: ≤7 postnatal days: 300 mg/kg/day divided Q8 hr ≥8 postnatal days: 300 mg/kg/day divided Q6 hr
Cefotaxime	Sepsis/meningitis: 50 mg/kg/dose Gonococcal infections: 25 mg/kg/dose
Ceftazidime	Sepsis/meningitis: 30–50 mg/kg/dose Consider use of ceftazidime for neonatal sepsis in the absence of cefotaxime due to drug shortages, and in whom ceftriaxone is contraindicated.
Fluconazole[a]	Invasive candidiasis: Loading 12–25 mg/kg/dose; maintenance 6–12 mg/kg/dose
Gentamicin	See chart below. See Formulary for recommendations for therapeutic monitoring.
Metronidazole	Loading dose: 15 mg/kg/dose; maintenance dose: see chart below
Oxacillin	25–50 mg/kg/dose; use higher dose for meningitis
Piperacillin/tazobactam	100 mg/kg/dose
Vancomycin	Bacteremia: 10 mg/kg/dose; meningitis: 15 mg/kg/dose See Formulary for recommendations for therapeutic monitoring.

Dosing Interval Chart: Ampicillin, Oxacillin

PMA (Weeks)	Postnatal (Days)	Interval (Hours)
≤29[a]	0–28	12
	>28	8
30–36	0–14	12
	>14	8
37–44	0–7	12
	>7	8
≥45	All	6

Dosing Interval Chart: Vancomycin

PMA (Weeks)	Postnatal (Days)	Interval (Hours)
≤29	0–14	18
	>14	12
30–36	0–14	12
	>14	8
37–44	0–7	12
	>7	8
≥45	All	6

Dosing Interval Chart: Metronidazole

PMA (Weeks)	Maintenance Dose (mg/kg)	Interval (Hours)
24–25	7.5	24
26–27	10	24
28–33	7.5	12
34–40	7.5	8
>40	7.5	6

Dosing Interval Chart: Gentamicin

PMA (Weeks)	Postnatal (Days)	Dose (mg/kg)	Interval (Hours)
≤29	0–7	5	48
	8–28	4	36
	≥29	4	24
30–34	0–7	4.5	36
	≥8	4	24
≥35	All	4	24[e]

Dosing Interval Chart: Fluconazole

Gest. Age (Weeks)	Postnatal (Days)	Interval (Hours)
≤29	0–14	48
	>14	24
≥30	0–7	48
	>7	24

Dosing Interval Chart: Acyclovir

PMA (Weeks)	Postnatal (Days)	Interval (Hours)
	All	
<30		8–12
≥30	All	8

TABLE 18.13

DOSING OF COMMONLY USED ANTIMICROBIALS IN THE NEONATAL INTENSIVE CARE UNIT, BASED ON POSTMENSTRUAL AND POSTNATAL AGE—CONT'D

Dosing Interval Chart: Piperacillin/Tazobactam, Ceftazidime		
PMA (weeks)	Postnatal (Days)	Interval (Hr)
≤29	0–28	12
	>28	8
30–36	0–14	12
	>14	8
37–44	0–7	12
	>7	8
≥45	All	8

Dosing Interval Chart: Cefotaxime	Sepsis		Meningitis[b,c]	
GA (Weeks)	Postnatal (Days)	Interval (Hr)	Postnatal (Days)	Interval (Hr)
All weeks	<7	12	0–7	8–12
<32	≥7	8	>7	6–8
≥32	≥7	6		

[a]Thrush = 6 mg/kg/dose on day 1, then 3 mg/kg/dose orally (PO) Q24 hr, regardless of gestational or postnatal age.
[b]Consider smaller doses and longer intervals for very low–birth-weight neonates (less than 2 kg).
[c]Usual dose same for bone and joint, genitourinary, intraabdominal, lower respiratory tract, or skin and skin structure infections.
[d]Use every 36 hr dosing for patients undergoing therapeutic hypothermia.
See Online NeoFax: http://neofax.micromedexsolutions.com/neofax/neofax.php?strTitle=NeoFax&area=1&subarea=0
GBS, Group B *Streptococcus*; *GA*, gestational age; *GC*, gonococcus; *IV*, intravenous; *PDA*, patent ductus arteriosus; *PMA*, postmenstrual age.

XV. WEB RESOURCES

- Extremely Preterm Birth Outcomes Tool: https://www.nichd.nih.gov/research/supported/EPBO/use
- Premature growth chart and calculator: http://peditools.org/fenton2013
- Bilitool (for gestational age (GA) >35 weeks): https://bilitool.org
- Premie BiliRecs (GA 27–34 weeks): https://pbr.stanfordchildrens.org
- NeoFax: https://neofax.micromedexsolutions.com/neofax
- Neonatal sepsis calculator: https://neonatalsepsiscalculator.kaiserpermanente.org/
- 8th edition, Neonatal Resuscitation Program (NRP) algorithm: https://nrplearningplatform.com/instructor-toolkit/assets/Instructor_ToolKit/RESOURCES/DocumentsAndForms/resources/NRP%208th-Ed%20ITK%20Algorithm%20w%20logos.pdf

REFERENCES

A complete list of references can be found online.

Chapter 19

Nephrology

Ryan Handoko, MD

See additional content online.

I. URINALYSIS[1]: SEE TABLE 19.1

A. Common indications include infectious workup (urinary tract infection [UTI], pyelonephritis), abdominal trauma, suspected diabetes or renal disease, rhabdomyolysis, edema, failure to thrive.

B. Best if urine specimen is evaluated within 1 hour of voiding, otherwise should be kept at 4°C

C. Annual screening urinalysis (UA) is not recommended by the American Academy of Pediatrics (AAP), unless patient is at high risk of chronic kidney disease.

II. KIDNEY FUNCTION TESTS

A. Tests of Glomerular Function

1. **Glomerulogenesis is complete at 36 weeks' gestation.** Glomerular filtration rate (GFR) increases over the first 2 years of life related to glomerular maturation.

2. **Normal GFR values**, as measured by inulin clearance (gold standard), are shown in Table 19.2.

3. **Creatinine clearance (CCr):** Closely approximates inulin clearance in the normal range of GFR. When GFR is low, CCr overestimates GFR. May be inaccurate in children with obstructive uropathy or problems with bladder emptying secondary to challenges getting complete timed urine collections.

$$CCr\,(mL\,/\,min\,/\,1.73\,m^2) = [U \times (V\,/\,P)] \times 1.73/BSA$$

where U (mg/dL) = urinary creatinine concentration; V (mL/min) = total urine volume (mL) divided by the duration of the collection (min) (24 hours = 1440 minutes); P (mg/dL) = serum creatinine concentration (may average two levels); and BSA (m²) = body surface area.

4. **Estimated GFR (eGFR) from plasma creatinine:** Varies related to body size/ muscle mass. If body habitus is markedly abnormal or a precise measurement of GFR is needed, consider other methods. Creatinine must be in steady state to estimate GFR; use caution in the setting of acute kidney injury. Three methods to calculate estimated GFR:

TABLE 19.1

URINALYSIS COMPONENTS

Test	Purpose	Normal Findings	Special Notes
Appearance	General impression	Colorless to amber. Cloudy/turbid urine can be normal.	Causes of turbid urine: <ul><li>Uric acid crystals in acidic urine</li><li>Phosphate crystals in alkaline urine</li><li>Cellular and infectious material</li></ul>Causes of red/orange urine: Foods, drugs (propofol, chlorpromazine, thioridazine, rifampin), hemoglobinuria, porphyrias
Specific gravity	Correlates with kidney's ability to concentrate urine; surrogate of osmolality and hydration status	Between 1.003 and 1.030	Isosthenuria: Urine with osmolality equal to plasma (specific gravity of 1.010). May indicate disease affecting ability to concentrate/dilute urine Falsely elevated by: Glucose, high protein, iodine-based contrast, ketoacids
pH	Evaluate renal tubule hydrogen ion maintenance	pH 4.5–8, average range of 5–6	Influenced by serum pH Alkaline urine may indicate UTI with urea-splitting organisms or certain types of stones
Protein	Evaluate for proteinuria	Dipstick values: Negative Trace 1+ ($\sim$30 mg/dL) 2+ ($\sim$100 mg/dL) 3+ ($\sim$300 mg/dL) 4+ (>1000 mg/dL)	Confirm and quantify significant proteinuria with random urine protein/creatinine ratio or 24-hr urine collection Evaluate for postural proteinuria with first morning void Concentrated urine can lead to false-positive result.
Glucose	Detect glucose in urine	Glucosuria is always abnormal	Glucosuria typically seen when blood glucose >160–180 mg/dL Consider diabetes mellitus, proximal renal tubular disease, pregnancy Dipstick only measures glucose; reduction tests (Clinitest) will detect other sugars for suspected inborn errors of metabolism

Ketones	Detect breakdown of fatty acids	Negative to trace	Suggests diabetes mellitus or starvation-induced catabolism Neonatal ketoacidosis may indicate inborn error of metabolism
Nitrite	Detect Gram-negative bacterial metabolism	Negative	Specific (90%–100%), but not sensitive (15%–82%) for UTI False-positive from phenazopyridine
Leukocyte esterase	Detect presence of WBCs	Negative	Indicates pyuria Sensitive (67%–84%), but less specific (64%–92%) for UTI
Hemoglobin	Detect presence of RBCs or hemoglobin	Negative	Indicates hematuria or hemoglobinuria False-positive on dipstick: Myoglobin (e.g., crush injury, rhabdomyolysis, vigorous exercise), contamination with blood outside the urinary tract
Bilirubin, urobilinogen	Evaluate for hyperbilirubinemia	Negative	Positive with indirect hyperbilirubinemia Urobilinogen may be present in low amounts; increased in all cases of hyperbilirubinemia
Red blood cells	Differentiate hemoglobinuria from intact RBCs	Centrifuged urine normally contains <5 RBCs/hpf	RBC morphology suggests location of bleeding; dysmorphic RBCs suggest a glomerular origin, normal RBCs suggest lower tract bleeding
White blood cells	Detect inflammation/infection	Centrifuged urine normally contains <5 WBCs/hpf	Consider UTI, sterile pyuria, inflammatory disorders (e.g., Kawasaki).
Epithelial cells	Index of possible contamination	<5 squamous epithelial cells/hpf	15–20 squamous epithelial cells/hpf suggests contamination, although any amount may indicate contamination
Sediment	Investigate for formed elements: casts, cells, crystals	None	Hyaline casts: may be normal (e.g., dehydration). Other possibly pathologic casts include RBC, WBC, tubular epithelial, and granular casts.

RBC, Red blood cell; *UTI*, urinary tract infection; *WBC*, white blood cell.

TABLE 19.2

NORMAL VALUES OF GLOMERULAR FILTRATION RATE

Age (Sex)	Mean GFR ± SD (mL/min/1.73 m^2)
1 week (M and F)	41 ± 15
2–8 weeks (M and F)	66 ± 25
>8 weeks (M and F)	96 ± 22
2–12 years (M and F)	133 ± 27
13–21 years (M)	140 ± 30
13–21 years (F)	126 ± 22

F, Female; *M*, male; *SD*, standard deviation.
Modified from Hogg RJ, Furth S, Lemley KV, et al. National Kidney Foundation's Kidney Disease Outcomes Quality Initiative Clinical Practice Guidelines for Chronic Kidney Disease in Children and Adolescents: evaluation, classification, and stratification. *Pediatrics.* 2003;111:1416.

a. **Bedside chronic kidney disease in children (CKiD) cohort:** Only
   applicable if creatinine measured by enzymatic assay.
   Recommended for eGFR determination in children aged 1 to 16
   years. Estimated GFRs of ≥75 mL/min/1.73 m^2 determined by this
   equation likely represent normal kidney function; clinical correlation is
   recommended with GFR estimation.[2]

$$eGFR(mL / min / 1.73 m^2) = 0.413 \times (L / Pcr)$$

where *0.413* is the proportionality constant, *L* = height (cm), and
Pcr = plasma creatinine (mg/dL).

b. **Schwartz equation:** Historical equation for eGFR in children. However,
   laboratories are increasingly shifting to enzymatic assays to determine
   creatinine; use of enzymatically determined creatinine (vs. Jaffe
   method) with the Schwartz equation leads to overestimation of GFR
   and should be considered when applying clinically:

$$eGFR(mL / min / 1.73 m^2) = kL/Pcr$$

where *k* = proportionality constant (Table 19.3); *L* = height (cm); and
Pcr = plasma creatinine (mg/dL).

TABLE 19.3

PROPORTIONALITY CONSTANT FOR CALCULATING GLOMERULAR FILTRATION RATE

Age	*k*-Values
Low birth weight during first year of life	0.33
Term AGA during first year of life	0.45
Children and adolescent girls	0.55
Adolescent boys	0.70

AGA, Appropriate for gestational age.
Data from Schwartz GJ, Brion LP, Spitzer A. The use of plasma creatinine concentration for estimating glomerular filtration rate in infants, children, and adolescents. *Pediatr Clin North Am.* 1987;34:571.

c. **Modification of diet in renal disease (MDRD) and chronic kidney disease epidemiology collaboration (CKD-EPI):** Used to calculate GFR in those >18 years old, recently updated in 2021 to omit race.[3] Available at National Kidney Disease Education Program (NKDEP) website and National Kidney Foundation (NKF) website (see Section XII).

5. **Other measurements of GFR:** May be used when more precise determination of GFR is needed (e.g., dosing of chemotherapy). These methods include iothalamate, diethylenetriaminepentaacetic acid (DTPA), and iohexol. Cystatin C is a low molecular protein that can also be used to estimate GFR and is more accurate than serum creatinine in individuals with conditions that significantly impact muscle mass, the source of creatinine.

B. Tests of Kidney Tubular Function

1. **Proximal tubule and solute handling:**

   a. **Proximal tubule reabsorption:** Proximal tubule is responsible for reabsorption of electrolytes, glucose, and amino acids. Studies to evaluate proximal tubular function compare urine and blood levels of specific compounds, arriving at a percentage of tubular reabsorption (Tx):

   $$Tx = 1 - [(Ux / Px)/(UCr / PCr)] \times 100$$

   where Ux = concentration of compound in urine; Px = concentration of compound in plasma; Ucr = concentration of creatinine in urine; and Pcr = concentration of creatinine in plasma. This formula can be used for amino acids, electrolytes, calcium, and phosphorus. It is commonly used to calculate tubular reabsorption of phosphate (TRP). In a patient with hypophosphatemia and preserved proximal tubular function, the tubular reabsorption of phosphate would be expected to be near 100%.

   b. **Fractional excretion of sodium (FENa)[4]:** Commonly used to assess tubular function. Must consider sodium and volume status. May be inaccurate with recent diuretic use.

   $$FENa = [(UNa / PNa) / (UCr / PCr)] \times 100$$

   where UNa = concentration of sodium in urine; and PNa = concentration of sodium in plasma. FENa is usually <1% in prerenal azotemia or glomerulonephritis, and >1% (usually >3%) in acute tubular necrosis (ATN) or postrenal azotemia. Infants have diminished ability to reabsorb sodium; FENa in volume-depleted infants is <3%.

   (1) **Fractional excretion of urea (FEurea):** May be useful in certain clinical scenarios, including patients on diuretics. Use FENa equation above, substituting urea for sodium. FEurea is usually <35% in prerenal azotemia and >50% in ATN.[4]

(2) **Fractional excretion of bicarbonate (FHCO₃):** May help differentiate the types of renal tubular acidosis (RTA). The majority of bicarb reabsorption occurs in proximal tubule.

$$FeHCO_3 = [(UHCO_3 / PHCO_3) / (UCr / PCr)] \times 100$$

Normal FEHCO₃ is <5%. Distal RTA is usually <5%. >15% suggests proximal (type II) RTA.

2. **Distal tubule and pH balance:**
   a. **Urine anion gap (UAG):** Used as an indirect measure of ammonium production in the distal nephron.

   $$UAG = UNa + UK - UCl$$

   where UNa = concentration of sodium in urine; UK = concentration of potassium in urine; and UCl = concentration of chloride in urine. Positive UAG (usually >20) suggests a distal RTA. Negative UAG (usually <−20) suggests high urinary NH4+ (e.g., secondary to diarrhea).

   b. **Urine pH:** A urine acidification defect (distal RTA) should be suspected when random urine pH values are >6 in the presence of moderate systemic metabolic acidosis. Confirm acidification defects by simultaneous venous or arterial pH, plasma bicarbonate concentration, and determination of the pH of fresh urine.

   c. **Urine osmolality:** Urine is concentrated distally in the kidney tubules. Urine osmolality, ideally on a first morning urine specimen, may be used to evaluate capacity to concentrate urine. If osmolality is >600 mOsm/L, then tubular dysfunction, including disease states such as diabetes insipidus leading to inappropriate water loss, is unlikely. For more formal testing, see the water deprivation test in Chapter 10.

   d. **Urine calcium:** Hypercalciuria may be seen with distal RTA, vitamin D intoxication, hyperparathyroidism, immobilization, excessive calcium intake, use of steroids or loop diuretics, or an idiopathic cause. Diagnosis is as follows:
      (1) 24-hour urine: Calcium >4 mg/kg/24 hr (gold standard)
      (2) Spot urine: Determine calcium/creatinine (Ca/Cr) ratio. Normal urine Ca/Cr ratio does not rule out hypercalciuria. Correlate clinically and follow elevated spot urine Ca/Cr ratio with a 24-hr urine calcium determination if indicated (Table 19.4).[5]

TABLE 19.4

AGE-ADJUSTED CALCIUM/CREATININE RATIOS

Age	Ca^{2+}/Cr Ratio (mg/mg) (95th Percentile for Age)
<7 months	0.86
7–18 months	0.60
19 months to 6 years	0.42
Adults	0.22

From Sargent JD, Stukel TA, Kresel J, et al. Normal values for random urinary calcium-to-creatinine ratios in infancy. *J Pediatr.* 1993;123:393.

III. BLOOD PRESSURE (BP) AND CHRONIC HYPERTENSION[6-11]

NOTE: See Chapter 1 for the management of acute hypertension.

See Tables 19.5 and 19.6 for normal BP values (systolic blood pressure [SBP], diastolic blood pressure [DBP]) by age.[9,11]

A. Definition

Hypertension is defined as the sustained elevation of BP at or above the 95th percentile for those <13 years or ≥130/80 for those ≥13 years. Any BP that is >90th percentile or ≥120/80 should be repeated at a clinic visit; if persistently elevated when confirmed by manual auscultation, the child should return for a repeat measurement for confirmation (see Section III.E for management).

B. Measurement of Blood Pressure in Children

1. All children ≥3 years should have BP measured annually. Children ≥3 years should have BP measured at **all** visits if at increased risk for hypertension: obesity, taking medications known to increase BP, renal disease, history of aortic arch obstruction/coarctation, diabetes.
2. Children aged <3 years with risk factors should have BP measured at all well child care visits. Risk factors include history of prematurity <32 weeks' gestation or small for gestational age, very low birth weight, congenital heart disease, kidney/urologic disease or family history of kidney disease, recurrent UTIs, malignancy, solid organ or bone marrow transplant, taking medications known to increase BP, systemic illness associated with hypertension, and evidence of increased intracranial pressure.
3. BP should be measured in a seated position in an upper extremity after 5 minutes of rest with feet/back/arm supported and mid-cuff at heart level; auscultation is preferred. Appropriate cuff size has a bladder width at least 40% of upper arm circumference at midway point. Bladder length should cover 80% to 100% of arm circumference. Cuffs that are too small may result in falsely elevated BPs. Choose a larger-sized cuff if there is a choice between two.

C. Etiologies of Hypertension in Neonates, Infants, and Children (Table 19.7)

Drugs causing hypertension include glucocorticoids, calcineurin inhibitors, sympathomimetics, oral contraceptives, stimulants (methylphenidate), ephedrine, erythropoietin, NSAIDs, caffeine, tobacco, ethanol, cocaine, and amphetamines.

D. Evaluation of Chronic Hypertension

1. Rule out factitious causes of hypertension (improper cuff size or measurement technique [e.g., manual vs. oscillometric]), nonpathologic causes of hypertension (e.g., fever, pain, anxiety, muscle spasm), and iatrogenic mechanisms (e.g., medications, excessive fluid administration).
2. **History:** Headache, blurred vision, dyspnea on exertion, edema, obstructive sleep apnea symptoms (including poor sleep quality or duration), endocrine symptoms (e.g., diaphoresis, flushing, constipation, weakness), history of neonatal intensive care unit stay; rule out

TABLE 19.5

BLOOD PRESSURE LEVELS FOR THE 50TH, 90TH, 95TH, AND 99TH PERCENTILES OF BLOOD PRESSURE FOR GIRLS AGED 1–17 YEARS BY PERCENTILES OF HEIGHT

Age (years)	BP Percentile	SBP (mmHg) Height Percentile or Measured Height							DBP (mmHg) Height Percentile or Measured Height						
		5%	10%	25%	50%	75%	90%	95%	5%	10%	25%	50%	75%	90%	95%
1	Height (in)	29.7	30.2	30.9	31.8	32.7	33.4	33.9	29.7	30.2	30.9	31.8	32.7	33.4	33.9
	Height (cm)	75.4	76.6	78.6	80.8	83	84.9	86.1	75.4	76.6	78.6	80.8	83	84.9	86.1
	50th	84	85	86	86	87	88	88	41	42	42	43	44	45	46
	90th	98	99	99	100	101	102	102	54	55	56	56	57	58	58
	95th	101	102	102	103	104	105	105	59	59	60	60	61	62	62
	95th + 12 mmHg	113	114	114	115	116	117	117	71	71	72	72	73	74	74
2	Height (in)	33.4	34	34.9	35.9	36.9	37.8	38.4	33.4	34	34.9	35.9	36.9	37.8	38.4
	Height (cm)	84.9	86.3	88.6	91.1	93.7	96	97.4	84.9	86.3	88.6	91.1	93.7	96	97.4
	50th	87	87	88	89	90	91	91	45	46	47	48	49	50	51
	90th	101	101	102	103	104	105	106	58	58	59	60	61	62	62
	95th	104	105	106	106	107	108	109	62	63	63	64	65	66	66
	95th + 12 mmHg	116	117	118	118	119	120	121	74	75	75	76	77	78	78
3	Height (in)	35.8	36.4	37.3	38.4	39.6	40.6	41.2	35.8	36.4	37.3	38.4	39.6	40.6	41.2
	Height (cm)	91	92.4	94.9	97.6	100.5	103.1	104.6	91	92.4	94.9	97.6	100.5	103.1	104.6
	50th	88	89	89	90	91	92	93	48	48	49	50	51	53	53
	90th	102	103	104	104	105	106	107	60	61	61	62	63	64	65
	95th	106	106	107	108	109	110	110	64	65	65	66	67	68	69
	95th + 12 mmHg	118	118	119	120	121	122	122	76	77	77	78	79	80	81
4	Height (in)	38.3	38.9	39.9	41.1	42.4	43.5	44.2	38.3	38.9	39.9	41.1	42.4	43.5	44.2
	Height (cm)	97.2	98.8	101.4	104.5	107.6	110.5	112.2	97.2	98.8	101.4	104.5	107.6	110.5	112.2
	50th	89	90	91	92	93	94	94	50	51	51	53	54	55	55
	90th	103	104	105	106	107	108	108	62	63	64	65	66	67	67
	95th	107	108	109	109	110	111	112	66	67	68	69	70	70	71
	95th + 12 mmHg	119	120	121	121	122	123	124	78	79	80	81	82	82	83

Age (years)	BP Percentile	SBP (mmHg) Height Percentile or Measured Height							DBP (mmHg) Height Percentile or Measured Height						
		5%	10%	25%	50%	75%	90%	95%	5%	10%	25%	50%	75%	90%	95%
5	Height (in)	40.8	41.5	42.6	43.9	45.2	46.5	47.3	40.8	41.5	42.6	43.9	45.2	46.5	47.3
	Height (cm)	103.6	105.3	108.2	111.5	114.9	118.1	120	103.6	105.3	108.2	111.5	114.9	118.1	120
	50th	90	91	92	93	94	95	96	52	52	53	55	56	57	57
	90th	104	105	106	107	108	109	110	64	65	66	67	68	69	70
	95th	108	109	109	110	111	112	113	68	69	70	71	72	73	73
	95th + 12 mmHg	120	121	121	122	123	124	125	80	81	82	83	84	85	85
6	Height (in)	43.3	44	45.2	46.6	48.1	49.4	50.3	43.3	44	45.2	46.6	48.1	49.4	50.3
	Height (cm)	110	111.8	114.9	118.4	122.1	125.6	127.7	110	111.8	114.9	118.4	122.1	125.6	127.7
	50th	92	92	93	94	96	97	97	54	54	55	56	57	58	59
	90th	105	106	107	108	109	110	111	67	67	68	69	70	71	71
	95th	109	109	110	111	112	113	114	70	71	72	72	73	74	74
	95th + 12 mmHg	121	121	122	123	124	125	126	82	83	84	84	85	86	86
7	Height (in)	45.6	46.4	47.7	49.2	50.7	52.1	53	45.6	46.4	47.7	49.2	50.7	52.1	53
	Height (cm)	115.9	117.8	121.1	124.9	128.8	132.5	134.7	115.9	117.8	121.1	124.9	128.8	132.5	134.7
	50th	92	93	94	95	97	98	99	55	55	56	57	58	59	60
	90th	106	106	107	109	110	111	112	68	68	69	70	71	72	72
	95th	109	110	111	112	113	114	115	72	72	73	73	74	74	75
	95th + 12 mmHg	121	122	123	124	125	126	127	84	84	85	85	86	86	87
8	Height (in)	47.6	48.4	49.8	51.4	53	54.5	55.5	47.6	48.4	49.8	51.4	53	54.5	55.5
	Height (cm)	121	123	126.5	130.6	134.7	138.5	140.9	121	123	126.5	130.6	134.7	138.5	140.9
	50th	93	94	95	97	98	99	100	56	56	57	59	60	61	61
	90th	107	107	108	110	111	112	113	69	70	71	72	72	73	73
	95th	110	111	112	113	115	116	117	72	73	74	74	75	75	75
	95th + 12 mmHg	122	123	124	125	127	128	129	84	85	86	87	87	87	87

TABLE 19.5

BLOOD PRESSURE LEVELS FOR THE 50TH, 90TH, 95TH, AND 99TH PERCENTILES OF BLOOD PRESSURE FOR GIRLS AGED 1–17 YEARS BY PERCENTILES OF HEIGHT—CONT'D

Age (years)	BP Percentile	SBP (mmHg) Height Percentile or Measured Height							DBP (mmHg) Height Percentile or Measured Height						
		5%	10%	25%	50%	75%	90%	95%	5%	10%	25%	50%	75%	90%	95%
9	Height (in)	49.3	50.2	51.7	53.4	55.1	56.7	57.7	49.3	50.2	51.7	53.4	55.1	56.7	57.7
	Height (cm)	125.3	127.6	131.3	135.6	140.1	144.1	146.6	125.3	127.6	131.3	135.6	140.1	144.1	146.6
	50th	95	95	97	98	99	100	101	57	58	59	60	60	61	61
	90th	108	108	109	111	112	113	114	71	71	72	73	73	73	73
	95th	112	112	113	114	116	117	118	74	74	75	75	75	75	75
	95th + 12 mmHg	124	124	125	126	128	129	130	86	86	87	87	87	87	87
10	Height (in)	51.1	52	53.7	55.5	57.4	59.1	60.2	51.1	52	53.7	55.5	57.4	59.1	60.2
	Height (cm)	129.7	132.2	136.3	141	145.8	150.2	152.8	129.7	132.2	136.3	141	145.8	150.2	152.8
	50th	96	97	98	99	101	102	103	58	59	59	60	61	61	62
	90th	109	110	111	112	113	115	116	72	73	73	73	73	73	73
	95th	113	114	114	116	117	119	120	75	75	76	76	76	76	76
	95th + 12 mmHg	125	126	126	128	129	131	132	87	87	88	88	88	88	88
11	Height (in)	53.4	54.5	56.2	58.2	60.2	61.9	63	53.4	54.5	56.2	58.2	60.2	61.9	63
	Height (cm)	135.6	138.3	142.8	147.8	152.8	157.3	160	135.6	138.3	142.8	147.8	152.8	157.3	160
	50th	98	99	101	102	104	105	106	60	60	60	61	62	63	64
	90th	111	112	113	114	116	118	120	74	74	74	74	74	75	75
	95th	115	116	117	118	120	123	124	76	77	77	77	77	77	77
	95th + 12 mmHg	127	128	129	130	132	135	136	88	89	89	89	89	89	89

Age (years)	BP Percentile	SBP (mmHg) Height Percentile or Measured Height							DBP (mmHg) Height Percentile or Measured Height						
		5%	10%	25%	50%	75%	90%	95%	5%	10%	25%	50%	75%	90%	95%
12	Height (in)	56.2	57.3	59	60.9	62.8	64.5	65.5	56.2	57.3	59	60.9	62.8	64.5	65.5
	Height (cm)	142.8	145.5	149.9	154.8	159.6	163.8	166.4	142.8	145.5	149.9	154.8	159.6	163.8	166.4
	50th	102	102	104	105	107	108	108	61	61	61	62	64	65	65
	90th	114	115	116	118	120	122	122	75	75	75	76	76	76	76
	95th	118	119	120	122	124	125	126	78	78	78	78	79	79	79
	95th + 12 mmHg	130	131	132	134	136	137	138	90	90	90	90	91	91	91
13	Height (in)	58.3	59.3	60.9	62.7	64.5	66.1	67	58.3	59.3	60.9	62.7	64.5	66.1	67
	Height (cm)	148.1	150.6	154.7	159.2	163.7	167.8	170.2	148.1	150.6	154.7	159.2	163.7	167.8	170.2
	50th	104	105	106	107	108	108	109	62	62	63	64	65	65	66
	90th	116	117	119	121	122	123	123	75	75	75	76	76	76	76
	95th	121	122	123	124	126	126	127	79	79	79	79	80	80	81
	95th + 12 mmHg	133	134	135	136	138	138	139	91	91	91	91	92	92	93
14	Height (in)	59.3	60.2	61.8	63.5	65.2	66.8	67.7	59.3	60.2	61.8	63.5	65.2	66.8	67.7
	Height (cm)	150.6	153	156.9	161.3	165.7	169.7	172.1	150.6	153	156.9	161.3	165.7	169.7	172.1
	50th	105	106	107	108	109	109	109	63	63	64	65	66	66	66
	90th	118	118	120	122	123	123	123	76	76	76	76	77	77	77
	95th	123	123	124	125	126	127	127	80	80	80	80	81	81	82
	95th + 12 mmHg	135	135	136	137	138	139	139	92	92	92	92	93	93	94
15	Height (in)	59.7	60.6	62.2	63.9	65.6	67.2	68.1	59.7	60.6	62.2	63.9	65.6	67.2	68.1
	Height (cm)	151.7	154	157.9	162.3	166.7	170.6	173	151.7	154	157.9	162.3	166.7	170.6	173
	50th	105	106	107	108	109	109	109	64	64	64	65	66	67	67
	90th	118	119	121	122	123	123	124	76	76	76	77	78	78	78
	95th	124	124	125	126	127	128	128	80	80	80	81	82	82	82
	95th + 12 mmHg	136	136	137	138	139	139	140	92	92	92	93	94	94	94

Continued

TABLE 19.5

BLOOD PRESSURE LEVELS FOR THE 50TH, 90TH, 95TH, AND 99TH PERCENTILES OF BLOOD PRESSURE FOR GIRLS AGED 1–17 YEARS BY PERCENTILES OF HEIGHT—CONT'D

Age (years)	BP Percentile	SBP (mmHg) Height Percentile or Measured Height							DBP (mmHg) Height Percentile or Measured Height						
		5%	10%	25%	50%	75%	90%	95%	5%	10%	25%	50%	75%	90%	95%
16	Height (in)	59.9	60.8	62.4	64.1	65.8	67.3	68.3	59.9	60.8	62.4	64.1	65.8	67.3	68.3
	Height (cm)	152.1	154.5	158.4	162.8	167.1	171.1	173.4	152.1	154.5	158.4	162.8	167.1	171.1	173.4
	50th	106	107	108	109	109	110	110	64	64	65	66	66	67	67
	90th	119	120	122	123	124	124	124	76	76	76	77	78	78	78
	95th	124	125	125	127	127	128	128	80	80	80	81	82	82	82
	95th + 12 mmHg	136	137	137	139	139	140	140	92	92	92	93	94	94	94
17	Height (in)	60.0	60.9	62.5	64.2	65.9	67.4	68.4	60.0	60.9	62.5	64.2	65.9	67.4	68.4
	Height (cm)	152.4	154.7	158.7	163.0	167.4	171.3	173.7	152.4	154.7	158.7	163.0	167.4	171.3	173.7
	50th	107	108	109	110	110	110	111	64	64	65	66	66	66	67
	90th	120	121	123	124	124	125	125	76	76	77	77	78	78	78
	95th	125	125	126	127	128	128	128	80	80	80	81	82	82	82
	95th + 12 mmHg	137	137	138	139	140	140	140	92	92	92	93	94	94	94

BP, Blood pressure; *DBP*, diastolic blood pressure; *SBP*, systolic blood pressure.

From Clinical practice guideline for screening and management of high blood pressure in children and adolescents. *Pediatrics.* 2017;e20171904; https://doi.org/10.1542/peds.2017-1904

TABLE 19.6

BLOOD PRESSURE LEVELS FOR THE 50TH, 90TH, 95TH, AND 99TH PERCENTILES OF BLOOD PRESSURE FOR BOYS AGED 1 TO 17 YEARS BY PERCENTILES OF HEIGHT

Age (years)	BP Percentile	SBP (mmHg) Height Percentile or Measured Height							DBP (mmHg) Height Percentile or Measured Height						
		5%	10%	25%	50%	75%	90%	95%	5%	10%	25%	50%	75%	90%	95%
1	Height (in)	30.4	30.8	31.6	32.4	33.3	34.1	34.6	30.4	30.8	31.6	32.4	33.3	34.1	34.6
	Height (cm)	77.2	78.3	80.2	82.4	84.6	86.7	87.9	77.2	78.3	80.2	82.4	84.6	86.7	87.9
	50th	85	85	86	86	87	88	88	40	40	40	41	41	42	42
	90th	98	99	99	100	100	101	101	52	52	53	53	54	54	54
	95th	102	102	103	103	104	105	105	54	54	55	55	56	57	57
	95th + 12 mmHg	114	114	115	115	116	117	117	66	66	67	67	68	69	69
2	Height (in)	33.9	34.4	35.3	36.3	37.3	38.2	38.8	33.9	34.4	35.3	36.3	37.3	38.2	38.8
	Height (cm)	86.1	87.4	89.6	92.1	94.7	97.1	98.5	86.1	87.4	89.6	92.1	94.7	97.1	98.5
	50th	87	87	88	89	89	90	91	43	43	44	44	45	46	46
	90th	100	100	101	102	103	103	104	55	55	56	56	57	58	58
	95th	104	105	105	106	107	107	108	57	58	58	59	60	61	61
	95th + 12 mmHg	116	117	117	118	119	119	120	69	70	70	71	72	73	73
3	Height (in)	36.4	37	37.9	39	40.1	41.1	41.7	36.4	37	37.9	39	40.1	41.1	41.7
	Height (cm)	92.5	93.9	96.3	99	101.8	104.3	105.8	92.5	93.9	96.3	99	101.8	104.3	105.8
	50th	88	89	89	90	91	92	92	45	46	46	47	48	49	49
	90th	101	102	102	103	104	105	105	58	58	59	59	60	61	61
	95th	106	106	107	107	108	109	109	60	61	61	62	63	64	64
	95th + 12 mmHg	118	118	119	119	120	121	121	72	73	73	74	75	76	76

Continued

TABLE 19.6

BLOOD PRESSURE LEVELS FOR THE 50TH, 90TH, 95TH, AND 99TH PERCENTILES OF BLOOD PRESSURE FOR BOYS AGED 1 TO 17 YEARS BY PERCENTILES OF HEIGHT—CONT'D

Age (years)	BP Percentile	SBP (mmHg) Height Percentile or Measured Height							DBP (mmHg) Height Percentile or Measured Height						
		5%	10%	25%	50%	75%	90%	95%	5%	10%	25%	50%	75%	90%	95%
4	Height (in)	38.8	39.4	40.5	41.7	42.9	43.9	44.5	38.8	39.4	40.5	41.7	42.9	43.9	44.5
	Height (cm)	98.5	100.2	102.9	105.9	108.9	111.5	113.2	98.5	100.2	102.9	105.9	108.9	111.5	113.2
	50th	90	90	91	92	93	94	94	48	49	49	50	51	52	52
	90th	102	103	104	105	105	106	107	60	61	62	62	63	64	64
	95th	107	107	108	108	109	110	110	63	64	65	66	67	67	68
	95th + 12 mmHg	119	119	120	120	121	122	122	75	76	77	78	79	79	80
5	Height (in)	41.1	41.8	43.0	44.3	45.5	46.7	47.4	41.1	41.8	43.0	44.3	45.5	46.7	47.4
	Height (cm)	104.4	106.2	109.1	112.4	115.7	118.6	120.3	104.4	106.2	109.1	112.4	115.7	118.6	120.3
	50th	91	92	93	94	95	96	96	51	51	52	53	54	55	55
	90th	103	104	105	106	107	108	108	63	64	65	65	66	67	67
	95th	107	108	109	109	110	111	112	66	67	68	69	70	70	71
	95th + 12 mmHg	119	120	121	121	122	123	124	78	79	80	81	82	82	83
6	Height (in)	43.4	44.2	45.4	46.8	48.2	49.4	50.2	43.4	44.2	45.4	46.8	48.2	49.4	50.2
	Height (cm)	110.3	112.2	115.3	118.9	122.4	125.6	127.5	110.3	112.2	115.3	118.9	122.4	125.6	127.5
	50th	93	93	94	95	96	97	98	54	54	55	56	57	57	58
	90th	105	105	106	107	109	110	110	66	66	67	68	68	69	69
	95th	108	109	110	111	112	113	114	69	70	70	71	72	72	73
	95th + 12 mmHg	120	121	122	123	124	125	126	81	82	82	83	84	84	85
7	Height (in)	45.7	46.5	47.8	49.3	50.8	52.1	52.9	45.7	46.5	47.8	49.3	50.8	52.1	52.9
	Height (cm)	116.1	118	121.4	125.1	128.9	132.4	134.5	116.1	118	121.4	125.1	128.9	132.4	134.5
	50th	94	94	95	97	98	98	99	56	56	57	58	58	59	59
	90th	106	107	108	109	110	111	111	68	68	69	70	70	71	71
	95th	110	110	111	112	114	115	116	71	71	72	73	73	74	74

Age (years)	BP Percentile	SBP (mmHg) Height Percentile or Measured Height							DBP (mmHg) Height Percentile or Measured Height						
		5%	10%	25%	50%	75%	90%	95%	5%	10%	25%	50%	75%	90%	95%
8	Height (in)	47.8	48.6	50	51.6	53.2	54.6	55.5	47.8	48.6	50	51.6	53.2	54.6	55.5
	Height (cm)	121.4	123.5	127	131	135.1	138.8	141	121.4	123.5	127	131	135.1	138.8	141
	50th	95	96	97	98	99	99	100	57	57	58	59	59	60	60
	90th	107	108	109	110	111	112	112	69	70	70	71	72	72	73
	95th	111	112	112	114	115	116	117	72	73	73	74	75	75	75
	95th + 12 mmHg	123	124	124	126	127	128	129	84	85	85	86	87	87	87
9	Height (in)	49.6	50.5	52	53.7	55.4	56.9	57.9	49.6	50.5	52	53.7	55.4	56.9	57.9
	Height (cm)	126	128.3	132.1	136.3	140.7	144.7	147.1	126	128.3	132.1	136.3	140.7	144.7	147.1
	50th	96	97	98	99	100	101	101	57	58	59	60	61	62	62
	90th	107	108	109	110	112	113	114	70	71	72	73	74	74	74
	95th	112	112	113	115	116	118	119	74	74	75	76	76	77	77
	95th + 12 mmHg	124	124	125	127	128	130	131	86	86	87	88	88	89	89
10	Height (in)	51.3	52.2	53.8	55.6	57.4	59.1	60.1	51.3	52.2	53.8	55.6	57.4	59.1	60.1
	Height (cm)	130.2	132.7	136.7	141.3	145.9	150.1	152.7	130.2	132.7	136.7	141.3	145.9	150.1	152.7
	50th	97	98	99	100	101	102	103	59	60	61	62	63	63	64
	90th	108	109	111	112	113	115	116	72	73	74	74	75	75	76
	95th	112	113	114	116	118	120	121	76	76	77	77	78	78	78
	95th + 12 mmHg	124	125	126	128	130	132	133	88	88	89	89	90	90	90
11	Height (in)	53	54	55.7	57.6	59.6	61.3	62.4	53	54	55.7	57.6	59.6	61.3	62.4
	Height (cm)	134.7	137.3	141.5	146.4	151.3	155.8	158.6	134.7	137.3	141.5	146.4	151.3	155.8	158.6
	50th	99	99	101	102	103	104	106	61	61	62	63	63	63	63
	90th	110	111	112	114	116	117	118	74	74	75	75	75	76	76
	95th	114	114	116	118	120	123	124	77	78	78	78	78	78	78
	95th + 12 mmHg	126	126	128	130	132	135	136	89	90	90	90	90	90	90

TABLE 19.6

BLOOD PRESSURE LEVELS FOR THE 50TH, 90TH, 95TH, AND 99TH PERCENTILES OF BLOOD PRESSURE FOR BOYS AGED 1 TO 17 YEARS BY PERCENTILES OF HEIGHT—CONT'D

Age (years)	BP Percentile	SBP (mmHg) Height Percentile or Measured Height							DBP (mmHg) Height Percentile or Measured Height						
		5%	10%	25%	50%	75%	90%	95%	5%	10%	25%	50%	75%	90%	95%
12	Height (in)	55.2	56.3	58.1	60.1	62.2	64	65.2	55.2	56.3	58.1	60.1	62.2	64	65.2
	Height (cm)	140.3	143	147.5	152.7	157.9	162.6	165.5	140.3	143	147.5	152.7	157.9	162.6	165.5
	50th	101	101	102	104	106	108	109	61	62	62	62	62	63	63
	90th	113	114	115	117	119	121	122	75	75	75	75	75	76	76
	95th	116	117	118	121	124	126	128	78	78	78	78	78	79	79
	95th + 12 mmHg	128	129	130	133	136	138	140	90	90	90	90	90	91	91
13	Height (in)	57.9	59.1	61	63.1	65.2	67.1	68.3	57.9	59.1	61	63.1	65.2	67.1	68.3
	Height (cm)	147	150	154.9	160.3	165.7	170.5	173.4	147	150	154.9	160.3	165.7	170.5	173.4
	50th	103	104	105	108	110	111	112	61	60	61	62	63	64	65
	90th	115	116	118	121	124	126	128	74	74	74	75	76	77	77
	95th	119	120	122	125	128	130	131	78	78	78	78	80	81	81
	95th + 12 mmHg	131	132	134	137	140	142	143	90	90	90	90	92	93	93
14	Height (in)	60.6	61.8	63.8	65.9	68.0	69.8	70.9	60.6	61.8	63.8	65.9	68.0	69.8	70.9
	Height (cm)	153.8	156.9	162	167.5	172.7	177.4	180.1	153.8	156.9	162	167.5	172.7	177.4	180.1
	50th	105	106	109	111	112	113	113	60	60	62	64	65	66	67
	90th	119	120	123	126	127	128	129	74	74	75	77	78	79	80
	95th	123	125	127	130	132	133	134	77	78	79	81	82	83	84
	95th + 12 mmHg	135	137	139	142	144	145	146	89	90	91	93	94	95	96

Age (years)	BP Percentile	SBP (mmHg) Height Percentile or Measured Height							DBP (mmHg) Height Percentile or Measured Height						
		5%	10%	25%	50%	75%	90%	95%	5%	10%	25%	50%	75%	90%	95%
15	Height (in)	62.6	63.8	65.7	67.8	69.8	71.5	72.5	62.6	63.8	65.7	67.8	69.8	71.5	72.5
	Height (cm)	159	162	166.9	172.2	177.2	181.6	184.2	159	162	166.9	172.2	177.2	181.6	184.2
	50th	108	110	112	113	114	114	114	65	64	64	65	66	67	68
	90th	123	124	126	128	129	130	130	78	76	78	79	80	81	81
	95th	127	129	131	132	134	135	135	81	79	81	83	84	85	85
	95th + 12 mmHg	139	141	143	144	146	147	147	93	91	93	95	96	97	97
16	Height (in)	63.8	64.9	66.8	68.8	70.7	72.4	73.4	63.8	64.9	66.8	70.7	70.7	72.4	73.4
	Height (cm)	162.1	165	169.6	174.6	179.5	183.8	186.4	162.1	165	169.6	174.6	179.5	183.8	186.4
	50th	111	112	114	115	115	116	116	63	64	66	67	68	69	69
	90th	126	127	128	129	131	131	132	77	78	79	80	81	82	82
	95th	130	131	133	134	135	136	137	80	81	83	84	85	86	86
	95th + 12 mmHg	142	143	145	146	147	148	149	92	93	95	96	97	98	98
17	Height (in)	64.5	65.5	67.3	69.2	71.1	72.8	73.8	64.5	65.5	67.3	69.2	71.1	72.8	73.8
	Height (cm)	163.8	166.5	170.9	175.8	180.7	184.9	187.5	163.8	166.5	170.9	175.8	180.7	184.9	187.5
	50th	114	115	116	117	117	118	118	65	66	67	68	69	70	70
	90th	128	129	130	131	132	133	134	78	79	80	81	82	82	83
	95th	132	133	134	135	137	138	138	81	82	84	85	86	86	87
	95th + 12 mmHg	144	145	146	147	149	150	150	93	94	96	97	98	98	99

BP, Blood pressure; *DBP*, diastolic blood pressure; *SBP*, systolic blood pressure.

From Clinical practice guideline for screening and management of high blood pressure in children and adolescents. *Pediatrics.* 2017;e20171904; https://doi.org/10.1542/peds.2017-1904

TABLE 19.7

CAUSES OF HYPERTENSION BY AGE GROUP

Age	Most Common	Less Common
Neonates/infants	Renal artery thrombosis after umbilical artery catheterization Coarctation of aorta Renal artery stenosis Bronchopulmonary dysplasia or chronic lung disease	Medications Patent ductus arteriosus Intraventricular hemorrhage
1–10 years	Renal parenchymal disease Coarctation of aorta Bronchopulmonary dysplasia or chronic lung disease Essential hypertension	Renal artery stenosis Hypercalcemia Neurofibromatosis Neurogenic tumors Pheochromocytoma Mineralocorticoid excess Hyperthyroidism Transient hypertension Immobilization-induced Sleep apnea Essential hypertension Medications
11 years to adolescence	Renal parenchymal disease Coarctation of aorta Essential hypertension	All diagnoses listed in this table

Modified from Sinaiko A. Hypertension in children. *N Engl J Med.* 1996;335:26; Viera AJ, Neutze D. Diagnosis of secondary hypertension: an age-based approach. *Am Fam Physician.* 2010;82:12; Gupta-Malhotra M, Banker A, Shete S, et al. Essential hypertension vs. secondary hypertension among children. *Am J Hypertens.* 2015;28:1.

pregnancy, history of UTIs, history of medications and supplements, illicit drug use, or any family history of kidney dysfunction or hypertension.

3. **Physical examination:** Four-extremity pulses and BP, endocrine disease stigmata, edema, hypertrophied tonsils, skin lesions, abdominal mass, or abdominal bruit

4. **Clinical evaluation of confirmed hypertension:**
   a. Laboratory studies:
      (1) All patients: Urinalysis (UA), serum electrolytes, creatinine, blood urea nitrogen (BUN), lipid profile
      (2) Obese patients: Hgb A1c, AST/ALT, fasting lipid panel
      (3) Consider on basis of history and exam: Fasting serum glucose, thyroid stimulating hormone, drug screen, polysomnography, complete blood count
   b. Clinical practice guidelines recommend 24-hour ambulatory blood pressure monitoring (ABPM) be conducted in all children with persistently elevated blood pressure to confirm the diagnosis of hypertension. Other at-risk populations (e.g., coarctation of the aorta status–post repair, CKD, history of hypertension) should also have this monitoring done yearly regardless of clinic blood pressure.

c. Imaging:
   (1) Renal ultrasound in patients <6 years old or those with abnormal UA or renal function
   (2) Echocardiography to evaluate for left ventricular hypertrophy if pharmacologic treatment considered
   (3) Consider renovascular imaging if renal artery stenosis is suspected.
d. Patients ≥6 years of age do not require extensive evaluation for secondary causes if they have a strong family history of hypertension (HTN), are overweight, and do not have any evidence of secondary causes on history and physical exam.

E. Classification and Treatment of Hypertension (Table 19.8)
Target: SBP and DBP to <90th percentile and <130/80 mmHg in adolescents ≥13 years old. Consider target 50th percentile in those with CKD.

1. **Nonpharmacologic:** Aerobic exercise, sodium restriction, smoking cessation, and weight loss indicated in all patients with hypertension. Reevaluate BP after lifestyle interventions, and begin pharmacologic therapy if hypertension persists.
2. **Pharmacologic:** Indications include secondary hypertension, symptomatic hypertension, stage 2 hypertension without a clearly modifiable factor (e.g., obesity), diabetes mellitus, and persistent hypertension despite nonpharmacologic measures.
3. **Treatment monitoring:** Repeat echocardiogram every 6 to 12 months in those with cardiac end organ damage or those at high risk. Repeated 24-hour ABPM can be used to assess treatment effectiveness as needed.

F. Antihypertensive Drugs for Outpatient Management of Primary Hypertension in Children 1 to 17 Years of Age
Clinical guidelines recommend angiotensin-converting-enzyme inhibitors, angiotensin II receptor blockers, thiazide diuretics, or long-acting calcium channel blockers as first-line medications for management of chronic hypertension in children.[9] Medication choice may be impacted by underlying comorbidities, contraindications, and side effects. Providers should familiarize themselves with existing guidelines, medication contraindications, and side effects. A list of medications and common side effects is found in Table 19.9.

IV. URINARY TRACT INFECTIONS[12-17]

A. History
Highly dependent on patient age. Inquire about fever, dysuria, frequency, urgency, and back/abdominal pain. Obtain voiding history (stool, urine), stream characteristics in toilet-trained children, sexual activity, sexual abuse, circumcision status, prolonged/bubble baths or swimming, evaluation of growth curve, recent antibiotic use, and family history of vesicoureteral reflux (VUR), recurrent UTIs, or chronic kidney disease.

B. Physical Examination
Vital signs, abdominal examination for tenderness, flank masses, bowel distention, evidence of impaction, meatal stenosis or circumcision in males,

---

TABLE 19.8

CLASSIFICATION OF HYPERTENSION IN CHILDREN AND ADOLESCENTS AND MANAGEMENT RECOMMENDATIONS

	Ages 1–13 Years	Ages ≥13 Years	Frequency of BP Measurement	Pharmacologic Therapy (in Addition to Lifestyle Modifications)
Normal BP	<90th percentile	<120/<80	Annually (or sooner if at increased risk; see Section III.B)	None
Elevated BP	90th to <95th percentile *OR* 120/80 to <95th percentile, whichever is lower	120/<80 to 129/<80	Recheck in 6 months; if persistent over 2 additional visits, conduct ABPM and diagnostic evaluation	None, unless compelling indications: CKD, DM
Stage 1 hypertension	95th to 95th percentile plus 12 mmHg *OR* 130/80 to 139/89, whichever is lower	130/80 to 139/89	Recheck in 1–2 weeks; if persistently elevated over 2 additional visits, conduct ABPM and diagnostic evaluation	Initiate therapy, especially if symptomatic, end-organ damage is present, CKD, DM, persistent hypertension despite nonpharmacologic measures
Stage 2 hypertension	≥95th percentile plus 12 mmHg *OR* ≥140/90, whichever is lower	≥140/90	Evaluate and refer within 1 week, or immediately if the patient is symptomatic	Initiate therapy

All blood pressures expressed in mmHg.

ABPM, Ambulatory blood pressure monitoring; *CKD*, chronic kidney disease; *DBP*, diastolic blood pressure; *DM*, diabetes mellitus; *SBP*, systolic blood pressure.

Modified from Flynn JT, Kaelber DC, Baker-Smith CM, et al, and AAP Subcommittee on Screening and Management of High Blood Pressure in Children. Clinical practice guideline for screening and management of high blood pressure in children and adolescents. *Pediatrics*. 2017;140(3):e20171904.

vulvovaginitis or labial adhesions in females, neurologic examination of lower extremities, perineal sensation and reflexes, and rectal and sacral examination (for anteriorly placed anus).

C. Risk Factors

2011 AAP guidelines,[12] reaffirmed in 2016,[13] for children 2 to 24 months provide resources to help clinicians stratify the risk of UTI in the absence of

TABLE 19.9

ANTIHYPERTENSIVE DRUGS FOR OUTPATIENT MANAGEMENT OF HYPERTENSION IN CHILDREN 1 TO 17 YEARS OF AGE

Class	Drug	Comments
Angiotensin-converting enzyme (ACE) inhibitor	Benazepril Captopril Enalapril Fosinopril Lisinopril Ramipril Quinapril	Blocks conversion of angiotensin I to angiotensin II Decreases proteinuria while preserving renal function **Contraindicated:** Pregnancy, compromised renal perfusion (e.g., renal artery stenosis) Check serum potassium and creatinine periodically to monitor for hyperkalemia and uremia. Monitor for cough and angioedema.
Angiotensin-II receptor blocker (ARB)	Candesartan Irbesartan Losartan Olmesartan Valsartan	**Contraindicated:** Pregnancy Check serum potassium and creatinine periodically to monitor for hyperkalemia and uremia.
α- and β-blockers	Labetalol Carvedilol	Cause decreased peripheral resistance and decreased heart rate **Contraindicated:** Asthma, heart failure, insulin-dependent diabetes Heart rate is dose-limiting. May impair athletic performance
β-blocker	Atenolol Esmolol Metoprolol Propranolol	Decreases heart rate, cardiac output, and renin release Noncardioselective agents (e.g., propranolol) are contraindicated in asthma and heart failure. Metoprolol and atenolol are β_1 selective. Heart rate is dose-limiting. May impair athletic performance Should not be used in insulin-dependent diabetics
Calcium channel blocker	Amlodipine Felodipine Isradipine	Acts on vascular smooth muscles Renal perfusion/function is minimally affected; generally few side effects Amlodipine and isradipine can be compounded into suspensions.
	Extended-release nifedipine	May cause tachycardia
Central α-agonist	Clonidine	Stimulates brainstem α_2 receptors and decreases peripheral adrenergic drive May cause dry mouth and/or sedation (↓ opiate withdrawal) Transdermal preparation also available Sudden cessation of therapy can lead to severe rebound hypertension.
Loop diuretics	Furosemide Bumetanide	Side effects are hyponatremia, hypokalemia, and ototoxicity.
Thiazide diuretics	Hydrochlorothiazide Chlorthalidone Chlorothiazide	Side effects are hypokalemia, hypercalcemia, hyperuricemia, and hyperlipidemia.

Continued

TABLE 19.9

ANTIHYPERTENSIVE DRUGS FOR OUTPATIENT MANAGEMENT OF HYPERTENSION IN CHILDREN 1 TO 17 YEARS OF AGE—CONT'D

Class	Drug	Comments
Potassium-sparing diuretics	Spironolactone Triamterene Amiloride	Useful as add-on therapy in patients being treated with drugs from other drug classes Potassium-sparing diuretics are modest antihypertensives. They may cause severe hyperkalemia, especially if given with ACE inhibitor or ARB.
Peripheral α-antagonist	Doxazosin Prazosin Terazosin	May cause hypotension and syncope, especially after first dose
Vasodilator	Hydralazine	Directly acts on vascular smooth muscle and is very potent Tachycardia, sodium retention, and water retention are common side effects.
	Minoxidil	Used in combination with diuretics or β-blockers Minoxidil is usually reserved for patients with hypertension resistant to multiple drugs.

Modified from Flynn JT, Kaelber DC, Baker-Smith CM, et al, and AAP Subcommittee on Screening and Management of High Blood Pressure in Children. Clinical practice guideline for screening and management of high blood pressure in children and adolescents. *Pediatrics.* 2017;140(3):e20171904.

another source of infection in a febrile child. (This was reassessed in 2021[14] for improper use of race as a factor in disease risk; new AAP guidance forthcoming.)

1. Females are at higher risk for UTI than males.
2. Uncircumcised males are at higher risk than circumcised males.
3. Other risk factors include fever ≥39°C and fever >1 to 2 days.

D. Methods of Urine Collection

1. **If a child is 2 months to 2 years old, has a fever, and appears sufficiently ill to warrant immediate antibiotics,** obtain UA and urine culture by transurethral catheterization. **Suprapubic percutaneous aspiration** may be useful in critically ill children, is generally very safe, and is similar to bladder catheterization in sensitivity and specificity.
2. **If a child is 2 months to 2 years old, has a fever, and does not appear ill enough to warrant immediate antibiotics,** obtain urine by catheterization or the most convenient method available. **Bag or absorbent pad** may be helpful when UTI is unlikely (to rule out infection), but both have very high false-positive rates (>75% of cultures positive) and should not be sent for culture.[12] If UA does not suggest UTI, it is reasonable to avoid antimicrobial therapy. If UA does suggest UTI, urine culture should be obtained by catheterization.
3. **If a child is >2 years old and toilet trained,** may provide midstream clean-catch urine specimen.

E. Diagnosis

To establish the diagnosis of UTI, both UA results suggestive of infection and positive urine culture are recommended.

1. Nitrite test:
   a. Detects products of reduction of dietary nitrates by urinary Gram-negative bacterial species (especially *Escherichia coli*, *Klebsiella*, and *Proteus*)
   b. Sensitivity 15% to 82% and specificity 90% to 100% for UTI[12]
   c. Special circumstances: False-negative (low sensitivity) results commonly occur with insufficient time (<4 hours) for conversion of urinary nitrates to nitrites (age-dependent voiding frequency) and inability of bacteria to reduce nitrates to nitrites (many Gram-positive organisms such as *Enterococcus*, *Mycobacterium* spp., and fungi).
2. Leukocyte esterase test:
   a. Detects esterase released from leukocyte lysis
   b. Sensitivity 67% to 84% and specificity 64% to 92% for UTI[12]
3. Pyuria is defined at a threshold of ≥5 WBCs/hpf. Absence of pyuria is rare if a true UTI is present.
4. Urine culture:
   a. Transurethral catheterization or suprapubic aspiration: >50,000 colony-forming units (CFU) per mL diagnostic of UTI. Some sources suggest >10,000 CFU/mL in the presence of fever, symptoms, and pyuria may also be diagnostic.[15]
   b. Clean catch: >100,000 CFU/mL necessary to diagnose a UTI
   c. Bagged specimen: Should not be used to collect urine culture
   d. Catheter-associated (indwelling urethral or suprapubic): No specific data for pediatric patients. Adult Infectious Diseases Society of America guidelines define it as presence of symptoms and signs compatible with UTI and >1000 CFU/mL of one or more bacterial species in a single catheter urine specimen or in a midstream voided urine specimen from a patient whose catheter has been removed within previous 48 hours.[16]

F. Classification

Pyelonephritis (upper UTI), rather than cystitis (lower UTI), is suggested by fever ≥38.5°C (especially if lasting >48 hours after initiating appropriate antibiotics), systemic symptoms, costovertebral angle tenderness, elevated C-reactive protein (CRP), leukocytosis.

G. Imaging

1. **Renal and bladder ultrasound (RBUS):** Evaluates for anatomic abnormalities and abscesses. Indications include children 2 to 24 months with first UTI, recurrent or atypical UTIs, or if no response to treatment within 48 hours. If there is clinical improvement <48 hours and follow-up is reliable, RBUS should be done after full recovery. If there is no response to treatment or follow-up is uncertain, then RBUS during illness is indicated.

2. **Voiding cystourethrography (VCUG):** Evaluates bladder anatomy, emptying, and looks for signs of vesicoureteral reflux (VUR). Should not be obtained routinely after first febrile UTI. Indications include children 2 to 24 months with abnormal RBUS findings (hydronephrosis, scarring, or other findings suggestive of either high-grade VUR or obstructive uropathy), complicated or recurrent pyelonephritis.[12] Consider if family history of VUR. Optimal time is 2 to 6 weeks after infection.

H. Treatment of Culture-Positive Urinary Tract Infection

For empiric therapy, see Chapter 17.

1. **Organisms:**
    a. *E. coli* is the most common cause of pediatric UTI.
    b. Other common pathogens: *Klebsiella, Proteus* spp., *Staphylococcus saprophyticus*, and *Staphylococcus aureus*.
    c. Neonatal UTI: Group B streptococci and other bloodborne pathogens
    d. *Enterococcus* and *Pseudomonas* are more prevalent in abnormal hosts (e.g., recurrent UTI, abnormal anatomy, neurogenic bladder, hospitalized patients, or those with frequent bladder catheterizations). Consider blood cultures if urine grows uncommon organism or *Staphylococcus*.
2. **Treatment considerations and duration:**
    a. Route: Parenteral antibiotics for children who are toxic, dehydrated, or unable to tolerate oral medication because of vomiting or noncompliance
    b. Duration: 3 to 5 days for uncomplicated cases[17]; 7 to 14 days for toxic children and those with pyelonephritis
3. **Inadequate response to therapy:** Consider renal abscess or urinary obstruction; RBUS and repeat urine culture is indicated. Repeat cultures should also be considered in patients with recurrent UTIs to rule out persistent bacteriuria.
4. **Management of VUR:**
    a. Classification of VUR: Fig. 19.1
    b. Antibiotic prophylaxis: Evidence suggests that prophylactic trimethoprim-sulfamethoxazole reduces the risk of UTI recurrence by 50%, but with no significant difference in renal scarring. Some experts suggest that recent studies are insufficiently powered to detect a difference in the relatively rare outcomes of renal scarring and thus recommend shifting guideline recommendations from "no prophylaxis" to "selective prophylaxis" in certain groups of patients.[18]
    c. Surgical intervention: Monitor persistence/grade of VUR annually, often in consultation with a pediatric urologist. Spontaneous resolution may occur, although less likely with higher grade. Higher-grade VUR that persists as the child grows may ultimately require surgical intervention.
5. **Asymptomatic bacteriuria:** Defined as bacteria in urine on microscopy and Gram stain in an afebrile, asymptomatic patient without pyuria. Antibiotics not necessary if voiding habits and urinary tract are normal.

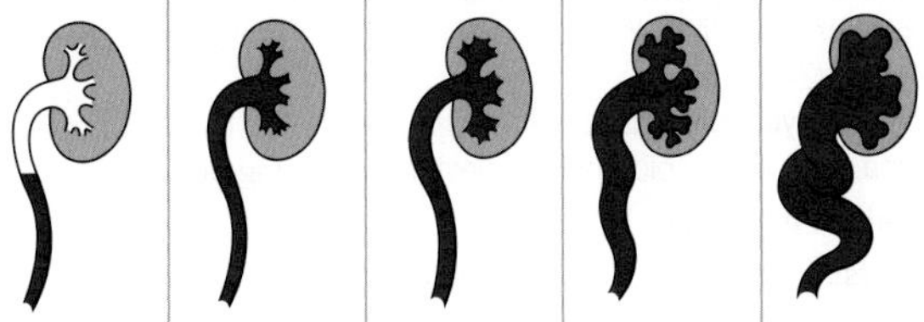

Grade I	Grade II	Grade III	Grade IV	Grade V
Ureter only	Ureter, pelvis, calyces; no dilatation, normal calyceal fornices	Mild or moderate dilatation and/or tortuosity of ureter; mild or moderate dilatation of the pelvis, but no or slight blunting of the fornices	Moderate dilatation and/or tortuosity of the ureter; mild dilatation of renal pelvis and calyces; complete obliteration of sharp angle of fornices, but maintenance of papillary impressions in majority of calyces	Gross dilatation and tortuosity of ureter; gross dilatation of renal pelvis and calyces; papillary impressions are no longer visible in majority of calyces

FIGURE 19.1

International classification of vesicoureteral reflux. (Modified from Rushton H. Urinary tract infections in children: epidemiology, evaluation, and management. *Pediatr Clin North Am.* 1997;44:5; International Reflux Committee. Medical vs. surgical treatment of primary vesicoureteral reflux: report of the International Reflux Study Committee. *Pediatrics.* 1981;67:392.)

6. **Referral to pediatric urology:** Consider in children with abnormal voiding patterns based on history or imaging, neurogenic bladder, abnormal anatomy, recurrent UTI, or poor response to appropriate antibiotics.

V. PROTEINURIA[19-21]

A. Definitions

1. **Orthostatic proteinuria:** Excretion of significant amounts of protein while in the upright position. A benign condition and common cause of proteinuria in children and adolescents

2. **Fixed proteinuria:** Proteinuria found on first morning urine void over several consecutive days. Suggestive of kidney disease

3. **Microalbuminuria:** Presence of albumin in urine below detectable range of dipsticks. In adults, defined as 30 to 300 mg/g creatinine. Most often used in screening for kidney disease secondary to diabetes

4. **Significant proteinuria:** Urine protein to urine creatinine (UPr:UCr) ratio 0.2 to 2.0 mg/mg or 4 to 40 mg/m^2/hr in a 24-hour collection

5. **Nephrotic-range proteinuria:** UPr:UCr ratio >2 mg/mg or >40 mg/m^2/hr in a 24-hour collection. In adults, 24-hour urine protein excretion of 3000 mg/24 hours

6. **Nephrotic syndrome:** Nephrotic-range proteinuria, hypoalbuminemia, edema, and hyperlipidemia (cholesterol >200 mg/dL)

B. Methods of Detection

1. **Urinalysis** (see Table 19.1): Proteinuria on a urine dipstick should be verified by a urine protein/creatinine ratio in an appropriately collected first morning urine specimen. Urine samples collected immediately upon rising in the morning help distinguish the contribution of benign orthostatic proteinuria to the proteinuria detected on dipstick or randomly timed spot urine collection.

2. **First morning urine protein/creatinine ratio:**
   a. Approximates 24-hour urine collections well
   b. Appropriate collection is essential for accurate results. A child must empty the bladder before going to bed. If the child gets up during the night, the bladder should be emptied before returning to bed. When the child wakes up in the morning, the urine sample should be provided immediately.
   c. Normal ratios:
      (1) <2 years old: <0.5 mg/mg
      (2) >2 years old: <0.2 mg/mg
   d. Abnormal ratios (mg/mg): Significant proteinuria detected on a first morning protein/creatinine ratio should prompt verification of appropriate collection. Repeat specimen should be analyzed within 1 to 2 weeks, or sooner based on clinical scenario (e.g., edema, hypertension, or symptom of concern would prompt a more expedited workup).

3. **24-hour urine protein:** May have a contribution from benign orthostatic proteinuria, which cannot be ruled out without a fractional urine collection. Protein level >4 mg/m^2/hr is considered significant.

C. Etiologies (Box 19.1)

D. Evaluation[20]

Further evaluation is necessary if proteinuria is significant/symptomatic and not secondary to orthostatic proteinuria (Box 19.2).

E. Nephrotic Syndrome[21]

1. **Epidemiology:** Idiopathic nephrotic syndrome of childhood is the most common form, representing approximately 90% of cases in children between the ages of 1 and 10 years. *Minimal change disease* is the most common renal pathology found among children with idiopathic nephrotic

BOX 19.1

CAUSES OF PROTEINURIA

Transient proteinuria: Fever, exercise, dehydration, cold exposure, congestive heart failure, seizure, stress, recent use of epinephrine

Orthostatic proteinuria

Glomerular diseases characterized by isolated proteinuria: Idiopathic (minimal change) nephrotic syndrome, focal segmental glomerulosclerosis, secondary causes of nephrotic syndrome, mesangial proliferative glomerulonephritis, membranous nephropathy, membranoproliferative glomerulonephritis, amyloidosis, diabetic nephropathy, sickle cell nephropathy

Glomerular diseases with proteinuria as a prominent feature: Acute postinfectious glomerulonephritis (streptococcal, endocarditis, hepatitis B or C virus, HIV), immunoglobulin A nephropathy, Henoch-Schönlein purpura nephritis, lupus nephritis, serum sickness, Alport syndrome, vasculitic disorders, reflux nephropathy

Tubular disease: Cystinosis, Fanconi syndrome, Wilson disease, Lowe syndrome, Dent disease (X-linked recessive nephrolithiasis), galactosemia, tubulointerstitial nephritis, acute tubular necrosis, renal dysplasia, polycystic kidney disease, reflux nephropathy, renal transplant rejection, drugs (aminoglycosides, cisplatin, penicillamine, lithium, NSAIDs, cyclosporine), heavy metals (lead, gold, mercury)

Modified from Kliegman RM, St. Geme JW III, Blum NJ, et al. *Nelson Textbook of Pediatrics.* 21st ed. Elsevier; 2020.

BOX 19.2

BASIC EVALUATION OF SIGNIFICANT (NEPHROTIC AND NONNEPHROTIC) PROTEINURIA

Complete metabolic panel with phosphorus
C3 and C4
Erythrocyte sedimentation rate (ESR), C-reactive protein (CRP)
Antinuclear antibody, anti–double-stranded DNA antibody
Hepatitis B, C, and HIV in high-risk populations
Antineutrophil antibodies (c- and p-ANCA)
Lipid panel
Renal and bladder ultrasonography
Referral to nephrologist

---

syndrome in this age group. Nephrotic syndrome may be a manifestation of a primary kidney disease, a systemic disorder resulting in glomerular injury, or rarely medication.

2. **Clinical manifestations:** Hypoalbuminemia and decrease in oncotic pressure results in generalized edema. Initial swelling commonly occurs on the face (especially periorbital), as well as in the pretibial area. Eye swelling is often mistaken for allergic reactions or seasonal allergies (Box 19.3).

3. **Etiologies:** See Table 19.10.

BOX 19.3

FACTORS SUGGESTING DIAGNOSIS OTHER THAN IDIOPATHIC MINIMAL CHANGE NEPHROTIC SYNDROME

Age <1 year or >10 years
Family history of kidney disease
Extrarenal disease (arthritis, rash, anemia)
Chronic disease of another organ or systemic disease
Symptoms due to intravascular volume expansion (hypertension, pulmonary edema)
Kidney failure
Active urine sediment (red blood cell casts)

TABLE 19.10

ETIOLOGIES OF NEPHROTIC SYNDROME

Primary Causes (90%)	Secondary Causes (10%)
Minimal change nephrotic syndrome (MCNS): 85% of idiopathic causes in children	Infections (HIV, hepatitis B, hepatitis C)
Focal segmental glomerulosclerosis (FSGS)	Systemic lupus erythematosus
Membranous nephropathy	Diabetes mellitus
IgA nephropathy	Drugs
Genetic disorders involving the slit diaphragm	Malignancy (leukemias, lymphomas)

4. **Investigations at first presentation:** UA and microscopy (microhematuria present in 30% and is not prognostic); urine P/Cr ratio; serum albumin, total protein, cholesterol, creatinine; infectious workup (consider tuberculosis, HIV, hepatitis B, hepatitis C, as indicated)
5. **Management of idiopathic nephrotic syndrome of childhood:** Empirical corticosteroid treatment without kidney biopsy is recommended for children without atypical features. Hospitalization recommended for children with overwhelming edema or infection. Home monitoring of proteinuria would include frequent first-morning dipsticks, with duration determined by provider.
   a. Steroid-responsive: Approximately 95% of patients with minimal change disease (MCD) and 20% with focal segmental glomerulosclerosis (FSGS) achieve remission within 4 to 8 weeks of starting prednisone. Response to corticosteroids is the best prognostic indicator, including the likelihood of underlying MCD.
      (1) Although duration of therapy varies, one common regimen includes prednisone 60 mg/m^2 daily or 2 mg/kg/day (maximum dose 60 mg/day) for 6 weeks, followed by 40 mg/m^2 or 1.5 mg/kg on alternate days for 6 weeks.[21,22]

(2) Relapses of idiopathic nephrotic syndrome are treated with a shorter duration of corticosteroids, which also vary according to the center and the consensus body. Commonly, prednisone 60 mg/m^2 or 2 mg/kg/day (maximum dose 60 mg/day) until urine protein is negative for 3 consecutive days, followed by 40 mg/m^2 or 1.5 mg/kg on alternate days for 4 weeks

b. Frequently relapsing: Defined as two or more relapses within 6 months of initial response, or four or more relapses in any 12-month period

c. Steroid-dependent: Defined as two consecutive relapses during tapering or within 14 days of cessation of steroids. Some patients can be managed with low-dose steroids, given daily or on alternate days, but many will relapse. Second-line treatments for frequently relapsing and steroid-dependent nephrotic syndrome: Cyclophosphamide, mycophenolate mofetil (MMF), calcineurin inhibitors, levamisole, or rituximab

d. Steroid-resistant: Lack of remission or partial remission after 8 weeks of corticosteroids. Second-line agents, including calcineurin inhibitors or MMF, are often introduced once steroid resistance is confirmed.

e. Indications for renal biopsy: Macroscopic hematuria, age <12 months or >12 years, systemic or syndromic findings, persistent creatinine elevation >1 to 2 weeks, low complement levels, and persistent proteinuria after 4 to 8 weeks of adequate steroid treatment[23]

6. **Complications:**
   a. AKI; thromboembolic disease; potentially life-threatening infection. See Chapter 16 for vaccine recommendations.
   b. Chronic systemic steroids: Cushingoid skin changes, cataracts, accelerated atherosclerosis, osteoporosis, gastric ulcer, mood swings, insomnia, insulin resistance, immunosuppression

VI. HEMATURIA[19,24]

A. Definition

1. **Microscopic hematuria:** >5 RBCs/hpf on centrifuged urine. Not visible to the naked eye
2. **Macroscopic (gross) hematuria:** Visible blood in urine
3. **Acute nephritic syndrome:** Classically tea or cola-colored urine, facial or body edema, hypertension, and oliguria

B. Etiologies: See Table 19.11

C. Evaluation (Fig. 19.2)

Differentiate glomerular and extraglomerular hematuria: Examine urine sediment, looking for RBC casts and protein.

1. Glomerular hematuria
   a. Usually hypertensive; dysuria usually absent; edema, fever, pharyngitis, rash, and arthralgia may suggest glomerular disease

TABLE 19.11

CAUSES OF HEMATURIA IN CHILDREN

Upper urinary tract disease	Isolated renal disease	IgA nephropathy; Alport syndrome; thin glomerular basement membrane nephropathy; postinfectious/poststreptococcal glomerulonephritis; membranous nephropathy; membranoproliferative glomerulonephritis; rapidly progressive glomerulonephritis; focal segmental glomerulosclerosis; antiglomerular basement membrane disease; hereditary angiopathy with nephropathy, aneurysms, muscle cramps (HANAC)
	Multisystem disease	Systemic lupus erythematosus nephritis, Henoch-Schönlein purpura nephritis, granulomatosis with polyangiitis, polyarteritis nodosa, Goodpasture syndrome, hemolytic-uremic syndrome, sickle cell glomerulopathy, HIV nephropathy
	Tubulointerstitial disease	Pyelonephritis, interstitial nephritis, papillary necrosis, acute tubular necrosis
	Vascular disorders	Arterial or venous thrombosis, malformations (aneurysms, hemangiomas), nutcracker syndrome, hemoglobinopathy (sickle cell trait/disease), crystalluria
	Anatomic disorders	Hydronephrosis, cystic-syndromic kidney disease, polycystic kidney disease, multicystic dysplasia, tumor (Wilms tumor, rhabdomyosarcoma, angiomyolipoma, medullary carcinoma), trauma
Lower urinary tract disease		Inflammation (infectious and noninfectious) Cystitis Urethritis Urolithiasis Trauma Coagulopathy Heavy exercise Bladder tumor Factitious syndrome, factitious syndrome by proxy

Data from Kliegman RM, St. Geme JW III, Blum NJ, et al. *Nelson Textbook of Pediatrics.* 21st ed. Elsevier; 2020.

b. Laboratory: Dysmorphic RBCs and casts on UA, complete blood cell count (CBC) with differential and smear, serum electrolytes with calcium, BUN/creatinine, serum protein/albumin, and other testing driven by history and exam, including ANA, hepatitis B and C serologies, HIV, audiology screen, if indicated

c. Consider other studies to determine underlying diagnosis: C3/C4, antineutrophil antibody (c- and p-antineutrophil cytoplasmic antibodies), anti–double-stranded DNA

2. Extraglomerular hematuria

a. Rule out infection: Urine culture, gonorrhea, chlamydia

b. Rule out trauma: History, consider imaging of abdomen/pelvis

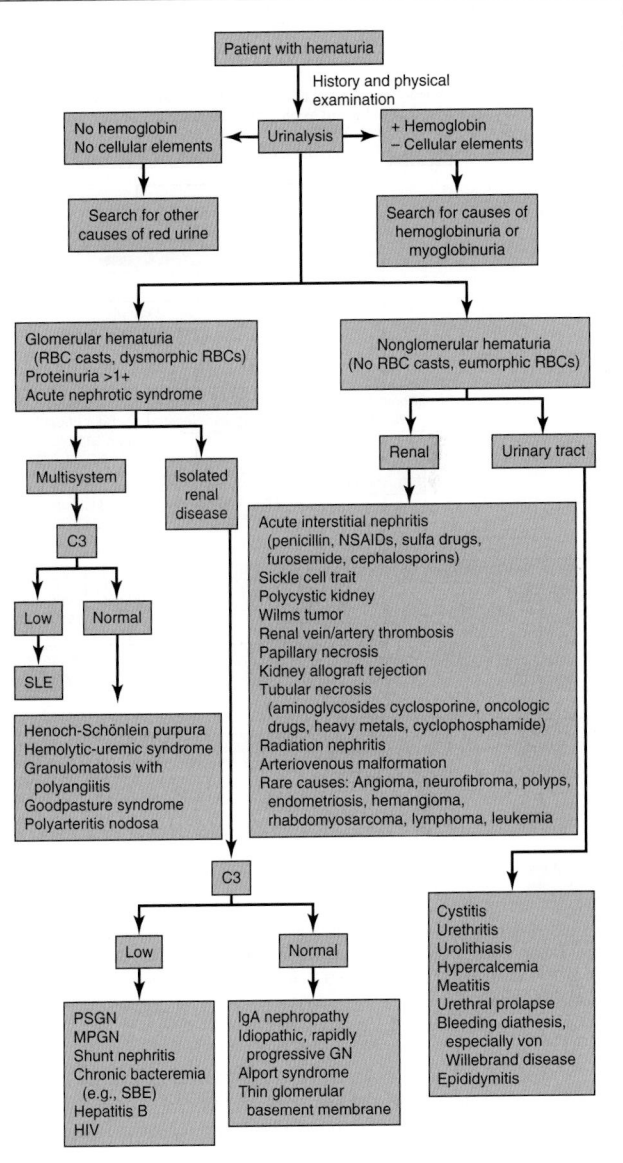

FIGURE 19.2

Diagnostic strategy for hematuria. *GN*, Glomerulonephritis; *HIV*, human immunodeficiency virus; *MPGN*, membranoproliferative glomerulonephritis; *NSAIDs*, nonsteroidal antiinflammatory drugs; *PSGN*, poststreptococcal glomerulonephritis; *RBC*, red blood cell; *SBE*, subacute bacterial endocarditis; *SLE*, systemic lupus erythematosus.

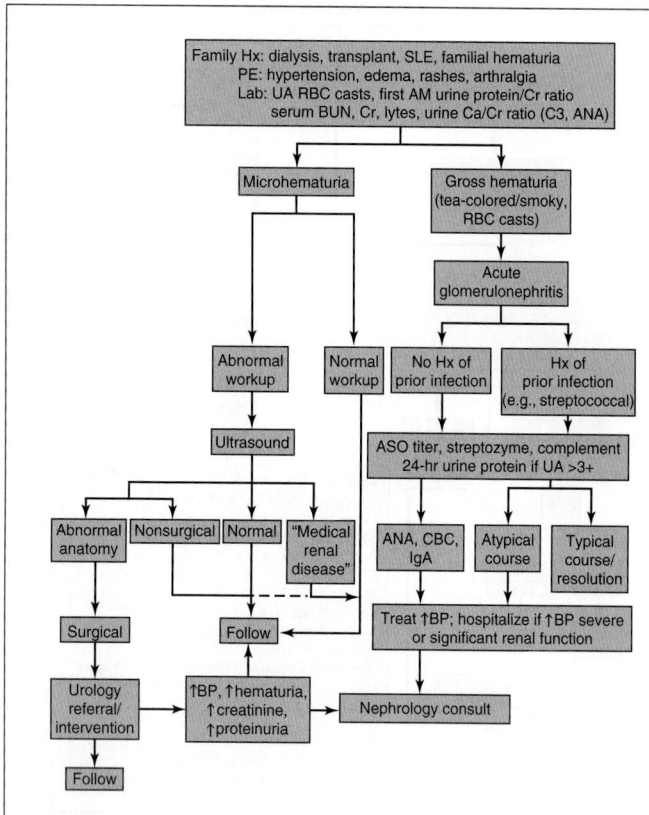

FIGURE 19.3

Management algorithm for hematuria. *ANA*, antinuclear antibody; *BP*, blood pressure; *ASO*, antistreptolysin O; *BUN*, blood urea nitrogen; *CBC*, complete blood count; *PE*, physical exam; *SLE*, systemic lupus erythematosus. (Data from Hay WM, Levin MJ, Deterding RR, et al. *CURRENT Diagnosis & Treatment Pediatrics.* 21st ed. https://www.accessmedicine.com, Fig. 24.1.)

   c. Investigate other potential causes: Urine Ca/Cr ratio or 24-hour urine for kidney stone risk analysis, sickle cell screen, renal/bladder ultrasound. Consider serum electrolytes with calcium, coagulation studies.

D. Management (Fig. 19.3)

VII. ACUTE KIDNEY INJURY[25,26]

A. Definition
Sudden decline in kidney function; clinically represented by rising creatinine, with or without changes in urine output

B. Etiology (Table 19.12)

Causes are generally subdivided into three categories:

1. **Prenal:** Impaired perfusion of kidneys, the most common cause of acute kidney injury (AKI) in children. Volume depletion is a common cause of prerenal AKI.

2. **Renal:**
   a. Parenchymal disease due to vascular or glomerular lesions
   b. Acute tubular necrosis: Diagnosis of exclusion when no evidence of renal parenchymal disease is present and prerenal and postrenal causes have been eliminated, if possible

3. **Postrenal:** Obstruction of the urinary tract, commonly resulting from inherited anatomic abnormalities in children

TABLE 19.12

ETIOLOGIES OF ACUTE KIDNEY INJURY

Prerenal	**Decreased true intravascular volume:** Hemorrhage, volume depletion, sepsis, burns **Decreased effective intravascular volume:** Congestive heart failure, hepatorenal syndrome **Altered glomerular hemodynamics:** NSAIDs, ACE inhibitors (when renal perfusion is already low)
Intrinsic renal	**Acute tubular necrosis:** Hypoxic/ischemic insults Drug-induced—aminoglycosides, amphotericin B, acyclovir, chemotherapeutic agents (ifosfamide, cisplatin) Toxin-mediated—endogenous toxins (myoglobin, hemoglobin); exogenous toxins (ethylene glycol, methanol) **Interstitial nephritis:** Drug-induced—β-lactams, NSAIDs (may be associated with high-grade proteinuria), sulfonamides, PPIs Idiopathic **Uric acid nephropathy:** Tumor lysis syndrome **Glomerulonephritis:** In most severe degree, presents as rapidly progressive glomerulonephritis (RPGN) **Vascular lesions:** Renal artery thrombosis, renal vein thrombosis, cortical necrosis, hemolytic uremic syndrome **Hypoplasia/dysplasia:** Idiopathic or exposure to nephrotoxic drugs in utero
Postrenal	Obstruction in a solitary kidney Bilateral ureteral obstruction Urethral obstruction Bladder dysfunction

ACE, Angiotensin-converting enzyme; *NSAIDs,* nonsteroidal antiinflammatory drugs; *PPIs,* proton pump inhibitors.
Data from Andreoli SP. Acute kidney injury in children. *Pediatr Nephrol.* 2009;24:253–263.

C. Clinical Presentation

Pallor, decreased urine output, systemic and pulmonary edema, hypertension, vomiting, and lethargy. The hallmark of early kidney failure is often oliguria.

1. **Oliguria:** Urine output <0.5 mL/kg/hr (for at least 6 hours). May reflect intrinsic or obstructive kidney disease. Always interpret urine output in the context of physical exam, clinical scenario, and fluid delivery. For example, low urine output may be appropriate (physiologic response to water depletion in a prerenal state) and "normal" urine output may be inappropriate in a volume-depleted patient (potentially representing kidney tubular damage or another pathologic state). Laboratory differentiation of oliguria is found in Table 19.13.
2. **Blood urea nitrogen/creatinine (BUN/Cr) ratio (both in mg/dL):** Interpret ratios with caution in small children with low serum creatinine.
   a. 10 to 20 (normal ratio): Suggests intrinsic renal disease in the setting of oliguria
   b. >20: Suggests volume depletion, prerenal azotemia, or gastrointestinal bleeding
   c. <5: Suggests liver disease, starvation, or inborn error of metabolism

D. Acute Tubular Necrosis

Clinically defined by three phases:

1. **Oliguric phase:** Period of severe oliguria that may last days. If oliguria or anuria persists for longer than 3 to 6 weeks, kidney recovery from ATN is less likely.
2. **High urine output phase:** Begins with increased urine output and progresses to passage of large volumes of isosthenuric urine containing sodium levels of 80 to 150 mEq/L
3. **Recovery phase:** Signs and symptoms usually resolve rapidly, but polyuria may persist for days to weeks.

E. Treatment Considerations

1. Careful monitoring of volume status (daily weights, strict input/output). Consider placement of indwelling catheter to monitor urine output.
2. Prerenal and postrenal factors should be addressed or excluded.
3. Intravascular volume resuscitation and maintenance with appropriate fluids in consultation with a pediatric nephrologist

TABLE 19.13

LABORATORY DIFFERENTIATION OF OLIGURIA

Test	Prerenal	Renal
FENa	≤1%	>3%
BUN/Cr ratio	>20:1	<10:1
Urine specific gravity	>1.015	<1.010

BUN, Blood urea nitrogen; *Cr,* creatinine; *FENa,* fractional excretion of sodium.

4. Monitor metabolic/electrolyte abnormalities, discontinue unnecessary nephrotoxic medications and follow drug levels closely when available, adjust dosing of medications based on creatinine clearance (see Chapter 31), monitor blood pressure closely, and maintain appropriate nutrition (low phosphorus, low potassium).

5. See Section IX for indications for acute dialysis.

F. Complications

1. Dependent on clinical severity
2. Usually includes fluid overload (hypertension, congestive heart failure [CHF], or pulmonary edema), electrolyte disturbances (hyperkalemia), metabolic acidosis, hyperphosphatemia, and uremia

G. Radiographic Imaging Considerations in AKI/CKD

1. Clinical significance of contrast-induced nephropathy (CIN) is uncertain in both adults and children, including those with mild-moderate CKD. Postcontrast AKI should be used instead of CIN when cause of AKI postcontrast exposure is uncertain.[27,28]

2. If patient at high risk for CIN, such as those with AKI or CKD, consider radiographic studies that do not require administration of radiographic iodinated contrast media (RICM), weighing risks and benefits.

3. If RICM is required, use of low or iso-osmolality contrast media is preferred.[28]

4. Recent trial suggests no hydration to be noninferior to hydration in adult CKD patients with eGFR 30 to 59 mL/min per 1.73 m^2.[29]

5. Recent trial suggests no benefit to either sodium bicarbonate or acetylcysteine in preventing CIN.[30]

6. Gadolinium and nephrogenic systemic fibrosis: Newer group II gadolinium-based contrast agents (GBCAs) are thought to have minimal or negligible risk of causing nephrogenic systemic fibrosis, unlike older group I agents, which are contraindicated in patients with GFR <30 mL/min per 1.73 m^2. Thus, screening of renal function prior to administration of a group II GBCA is optional.[31]

VIII. CHRONIC KIDNEY DISEASE[32,33]

A. Definition

Kidney damage for >3 months, as defined by structural or functional abnormalities, with or without decreased GFR. Classified as:

Stage I: Kidney injury with normal or increased GFR

Stage II: GFR 60 to 89 mL/min/1.73 m^2

Stage III: GFR 30 to 59 mL/min/1.73 m^2

Stage IV: GFR 15 to 29 mL/min/1.73 m^2

Stage V: GFR <15 mL/min/1.73 m^2 or dialysis

B. Etiology

1. Children <5 years: Most commonly due to congenital anomalies of the kidney and urinary tract (see Chapter 18, Section XII).

2. Older children: More commonly acquired glomerular diseases (e.g., glomerulonephritis, FSGS) or hereditary disorders (e.g., Alport syndrome).

C. Clinical Manifestations (Table 19.14)

D. General Management

1. **Nutrition:** Growth should be monitored closely; supplemental nutrition should be considered if not reaching caloric goals, which are higher in children with CKD. Potassium and sodium restriction may be required in advanced CKD. Growth hormone therapy may be considered in consultation with pediatric nephrology/endocrinology.

2. **Anemia:** Evaluate with CBC and iron studies. Iron deficiency is common and should be treated with oral (preferred) or IV iron. Consider erythropoietin-stimulating agents in consultation with pediatric nephrology.

3. **CKD–mineral and bone disorder:** Characterized by phosphate retention, decreased free calcium, and decreased 1,25 hydroxyvitamin D. Serum calcium, phosphate, alkaline phosphatase, vitamin D, and parathyroid hormone should be regularly monitored. Control phosphate with phosphate binders, supplement with calcium and vitamin D, as indicated.

4. **Cardiovascular:** Regularly monitor blood pressure and lipid panel. Treating hypertension slows the progression of CKD.

IX. DIALYSIS[34-36]

A. Indications for Acute Dialysis

Acute dialysis is indicated when metabolic or fluid derangements are not controlled by aggressive medical management alone. Should be initiated in consultation with a nephrologist. Generally accepted criteria include the following:

1. **Acidosis:** Intractable metabolic acidosis
2. **Electrolyte abnormalities:** Hyperkalemia >6.5 mEq/L despite restriction of delivery and medical management; calcium and phosphorus imbalance (e.g., hypocalcemia with tetany, seizures in the presence of a very high serum phosphate level); derangements implicated in neurologic abnormalities
3. **Ingestion or accumulation of dialyzable toxins or poisons:** Lithium, ammonia, alcohol, barbiturates, ethylene glycol, isopropanol, methanol, salicylates, theophylline. Consult poison control experts when available.
4. **Volume overload:** Evidence of pulmonary edema or hypertension
5. **Uremia:** BUN >150 mg/dL (lower if rising rapidly), uremic pericardial effusion, neurologic symptoms, platelet dysfunction

B. Techniques

1. **Peritoneal dialysis (PD):** Requires catheter to access peritoneal cavity, as well as adequate peritoneal perfusion. May be used acutely or chronically. Contraindications: Abdominal wall defects (omphalocele,

TABLE 19.14

CLINICAL MANIFESTATIONS OF CHRONIC KIDNEY DISEASE

Manifestation	Mechanisms
Edema	Accumulation of Na+ and water
	Decreased oncotic pressure
	Reduced cardiac output
	Mineralocorticoid excess
Uremia	Decline in GFR
Acidosis	Urinary bicarbonate wasting
	Decreased excretion of NH_4 and acid
Sodium wasting	Solute diuresis, tubular damage
	Aldosterone resistance
Sodium retention	Nephrotic syndrome
	CHF
	Reduced GFR
Urinary concentrating defect	Solute diuresis, tubular damage
	ADH resistance
Hyperkalemia	Decline in GFR, acidosis
	Aldosterone resistance
Renal osteodystrophy	Impaired production of 1,25(OH) vitamin D
	Decreased intestinal calcium absorption
	Impaired phosphorus excretion
	Secondary hyperparathyroidism
Growth retardation	Protein-calorie deficiency
	Renal osteodystrophy
	Acidosis
	Anemia
	Inhibitors of insulin-like growth factors
Anemia	Decreased erythropoietin production
	Low-grade hemolysis
	Bleeding, iron deficiency
	Decreased erythrocyte survival
	Inadequate folic acid intake
	Inhibitors of erythropoiesis
Bleeding tendency	Thrombocytopenia
	Defective platelet function
Infection	Defective granulocyte function
	Glomerular loss of immunoglobulin/opsonins
Neurologic complaints	Uremic factors
Gastrointestinal ulceration	Gastric acid hypersecretion/gastritis
	Reflux
	Decreased motility
Hypertension	Sodium and water overload
	Excessive renin production
Hypertriglyceridemia	Diminished plasma lipoprotein lipase activity
Pericarditis and cardiomyopathy	Unknown
Glucose intolerance	Tissue insulin resistance

ADH, Antidiuretic hormone; *CHF,* congestive heart failure; *GFR,* glomerular filtration rate; *NH₄,* ammonium.
Modified from Brenner BM. *Brenner and Rector's The Kidney.* 11th ed. Elsevier; 2019.

gastroschisis, bladder exstrophy, diaphragmatic hernia), severe inflammatory bowel disease, or infectious source in the abdomen[34]

2. **Intermittent hemodialysis (HD):** Requires placement of special vascular access catheters. May be method of choice for certain toxins (e.g., ammonia, uric acid, poisons) or when there are contraindications to peritoneal dialysis

3. **Continuous arteriovenous hemofiltration/hemodialysis (CAVH/D) and continuous venovenous hemofiltration/hemodialysis (CVVH/D):** Requires special vascular access catheter. Lower efficiency of solute removal compared with intermittent hemodialysis, but higher efficiency is not necessary because of the continuous nature of this form of dialysis. Sustained nature of dialysis allows for more gradual removal of volume/ solutes, which is ideal for patients with hemodynamic or respiratory instability.

C. **Complications (Table 19.15)**

TABLE 19.15

COMPLICATIONS OF DIALYSIS

PD	HD	CAVH/D, CVVH/D
PD catheter leaks: Confirm leakage of PD fluid with glucose dipstick. Discontinue PD for 7 to 10 days or lower dialysate volume.	Intradialytic hypotension: Causes include rapid fluid removal, predialysis antihypertensive medication, bradykinin release, hypotonic dialysate. Reduce or pause ultrafiltration.	Intradialytic hypotension
PD associated peritonitis (PDAP): Acute clouding of dialysate, abdominal pain/distention, vomiting. Culture peritoneal fluid and start empiric intraperitoneal antibiotics in consultation with nephrology. Refer to published ISPD Consensus Guidelines for treatment recommendations.[35]	HD fistula complications include vascular stenosis and thrombosis.	Use of citrate for anticoagulation can cause citrate overload (metabolic alkalosis), citrate accumulation (metabolic acidosis), hypocalcemia, and hypomagnesemia.

CAVH/D, continuous arteriovenous hemofiltration/hemodialysis; *CVVH/D*, continuous venovenous hemofiltration/ hemodialysis; *HD*, hemodialysis; *ISPD*, International Society of Peritoneal Dialysis; *PD*, peritoneal dialysis
Modified from Warady BA, Bakkaloglu S, Newland J, et al. Consensus guidelines for the prevention and treatment of catheter-related infections and peritonitis in pediatric patients receiving peritoneal dialysis: 2012 update. *Perit Dial Int.* 2012;32:S29–S86; Sigwalt F, Bouteleux A, Dambricourt F, et al. Clinical complications of continuous renal replacement therapy. *Contrib Nephrol.* 2018;194:109–117.

X. TUBULAR DISORDERS

A. **Renal Tubular Acidosis (Table 19.16)[37]**

1. A group of transport defects resulting in abnormal urine acidification; result of defects in reabsorption of bicarbonate (HCO_3-), excretion of hydrogen ions (H^+), or both

TABLE 19.16

RENAL TUBULAR ACIDOSIS BIOCHEMICAL AND CLINICAL CHARACTERISTICS

	Type 1 (Distal)	Type 2 (Proximal)	Type 4 (Hypoaldosteronism)
Mechanism	Impaired distal acidification	Impaired bicarbonate absorption	Decreased aldosterone secretion or aldosterone effect
Etiology	Hereditary Sickle cell disease Toxins/drugs Cirrhosis Obstructive uropathy Connective tissue disorder	Hereditary Metabolic disease Fanconi syndrome Prematurity Toxins/heavy metals Amyloidosis PNH	Absolute mineralocorticoid deficiency Adrenal failure CAH DM Pseudohypoaldosteronism Interstitial nephritis
Minimal urine pH	>5.5	<5.5 (urine pH can be >5.5 with a bicarbonate load)	<5.5
Fractional excretion of bicarbonate (FeHCO₃)	↓ (<5%)	↑ (>15%)	↓ (<5%)
Plasma K⁺ concentration	Normal or ↓	Usually ↓	↑
Urine anion gap	Positive	Positive or negative	Positive
Nephrocalcinosis/ nephrolithiasis	Common	Rare	Rare
Treatment	1–3 mEq/kg/day of HCO₃ (5–10 mEq/kg/day if bicarb wasting)	5–20 mEq/kg/day of HCO₃	1–5 mEq/kg/day of HCO₃ May add fludrocortisone and potassium binders

CAH, Congenital adrenal hyperplasia; *DM*, diabetes mellitus; *PNH*, paroxysmal nocturnal hemoglobinuria.
Modified from Avner ED, Harmon WE, Niaudet P, et al. *Pediatric Nephrology*. Springer-Verlag Berlin Heidelberg; 2016.

2. Results in a persistent normal anion gap hyperchloremic metabolic acidosis
3. RTA syndromes have a normal GFR and often do not progress to kidney failure.
4. Clinical presentation may be characterized by failure to thrive, polyuria, constipation, vomiting, and dehydration.
5. **Fractional excretion of bicarbonate (FeHCO₃) should be checked after a HCO₃ load.** Can help differentiate the types of RTA. See Section II.B for equation.
6. **Urine anion gap (UAG) is also useful;** however, it should not be used when a patient is volume depleted or has an anion-gap metabolic acidosis. See Section II.B for equation.

B. Fanconi Syndrome

1. Generalized dysfunction of the proximal tubule resulting not only in bicarbonate loss but also in variable wasting of phosphate, glucose, and amino acids

2. May be hereditary, as in cystinosis and galactosemia, or acquired through toxin injury and other immunologic factors
3. Clinically characterized by rickets and impaired growth

C. Nephrogenic Diabetes Insipidus

1. **Water conservation is dependent on antidiuretic hormone (ADH) and its effects on the distal renal tubules.** Polyuria (urine output >5 mL/kg/hr or >2 L/day), a hallmark of nephrogenic diabetes insipidus (NDI), is due to diminished or lack of response of the ADH receptor in the distal renal tubules. Hereditary defects of ADH receptor or acquired insults (e.g., interstitial nephritis, sickle cell disease, lithium toxicity, CKD) may underlie NDI.
2. **Must be differentiated from other causes of polyuria:** Central diabetes insipidus (ADH deficiency that may be idiopathic or acquired through infection or pituitary trauma; see Chapter 10), diabetes mellitus, psychogenic polydipsia, cerebral salt wasting

XI. NEPHROLITHIASIS[38-44]

A. Risk Factors
Male sex; history of UTI (especially those <5 years); congenital and structural urologic abnormalities (urinary stasis), neurogenic bladder, hypercalciuria, hyperoxaluria/oxalosis, hypocitraturia, other metabolic abnormalities; family history of stones, renal failure, consanguinity

B. Presentation
1. Microscopic hematuria (90%), flank/abdominal pain (50% to 75%), gross hematuria (30% to 55%), and concomitant UTI in up to 20%
2. Have higher likelihood than adults of having asymptomatic stones, especially younger children

C. Diagnostic Imaging
1. Ultrasonography is an effective and preferred modality, particularly at centers with expertise, given benefit of avoiding radiation exposure (75% sensitive for renal stones).[40]
2. Noncontrast CT may be preferred to improve diagnostic sensitivity (e.g., with radiolucent stones such as uric acid stones, ureteral stones, lack of ultrasonographic expertise).

D. Management
1. **Pain control, urine culture, hydration.** Some centers initiate α-blockers to facilitate stone passage, although evidence of benefit in children is equivocal.[41-43]
2. **Antibiotics:** Should be considered in treatment of all stones, especially if fever and/or pyuria present, because of the high association with UTI
3. **Urologic intervention** (e.g., extracorporeal shock wave lithotripsy, ureteroscopy, percutaneous nephrolithotomy): Consider with unremitting pain, urinary obstruction, increasing stone size, size ≥7 mm, or cystine/struvite stone, especially in the setting of AKI or at-risk patients (e.g., solitary kidney, anatomic anomalies).[43]

4. **Strain urine to collect stone; analyze stone composition to aid in prevention of future stones.**

E. Workup

1. Up to 75% of children with a kidney stone will have a metabolic abnormality (e.g., hypercalciuria, hyperoxaluria, hyperuricosuria, cystinuria).
2. Workup should include analysis of the stone (if possible); UA; basic metabolic panel; and serum calcium, phosphate, magnesium, and uric acid levels. If evidence of elevated calcium or phosphate, obtain parathyroid hormone (PTH) level and consider checking 25- and 1,25(OH) vitamin D levels.
3. After symptoms have resolved, a 24-hour urine collection should be obtained. Risk factors for stone formation should be analyzed: urine volume, osmolarity, sodium, calcium, urate, oxalate, citrate, and cystine. This test is also referred to as a "stone risk analysis."

F. Prevention

1. **All children with history of stones should increase fluid intake** (e.g., at least 2 L/day in those aged >10 years old).
2. **Targeted interventions of any identified metabolic abnormalities** (e.g., low-sodium diet in those with hypercalciuria). Pharmacologic interventions are also available in certain scenarios (e.g., citrate supplementation).
3. **Dietary modifications:** Long-term adherence (5 years) to normal calcium, low-sodium diet may decrease recurrence of stones in people with idiopathic hypercalciuria with recurrent nephrolithiasis.[44]

XII. WEB RESOURCES

- International Pediatric Nephrology Association: https://theipna.org/
- National Kidney Disease Education Program: https://www.niddk.nih.gov/health-information/communication-programs/nkdep
- National Kidney Foundation: https://www.kidney.org/professionals/kdoqi/gfr_calculator

REFERENCES

A complete list of references can be found online.

Chapter 20

Neurology

Hannah E. Edelman, MD, PhD and Maera J. Stratton, MD

See additional content online.

🔊 **Audio Case File 20.1** Seizure mimics: an age-based approach

I. NEUROLOGIC EXAMINATION

A. Mental Status: Alertness, Orientation (Person, Place, Time, Situation), Language, Cognition

1. Infants: Observe "cuteness" and ability to dynamically engage caretakers.
2. Toddlers: Bring toys. Observe and engage in play.
3. School age: Ask children to draw or describe school or friends.

B. Cranial Nerves (eTable 20.1)

1. For a quick assessment of cranial nerves for all patients, observe:
   a. (II) Visual response to objects in each visual quadrant
   b. (III, IV, VI) Conjugate gaze at full lateral and vertical positions, nystagmus, ptosis
   c. (VII) Symmetry and expressiveness of face at rest and with emotive activation
   d. (VIII) Finger rub, or response to and localization of sound for infants
   e. (IX, X, XII) Quality of phonation and articulation; ask about feeding, chewing, swallowing

C. Motor

1. **Muscle bulk:** Atrophy or pseudohypertrophy is a red flag.
2. **Tone:** Spasticity, rigidity, hypotonia
   a. Infants: Observe infant undressed to assess resting posture (varies with age). Active tone: Traction response, axillary stability (slip-through), posture in horizontal suspension. Passive tone (resistance of movements of the joints): Flap hands/feet, scarf sign
   b. Red flags: Scissoring, toe-walking, inability to supinate hand, clasped thumb or grasp
3. **Strength:**
   a. Younger children: Observe ease of normal functions: rising from floor, standing broad jump, running, climbing onto chair or exam table. Note presence of accommodations child is making to execute movements (e.g., shoulder shrug or trunk tilt to raise arm).
   b. Older children: Confrontation testing, pronator drift
   c. For conventional rating scale, see Box 20.1.
4. **Involuntary movements:** Fasciculations, tics, dystonia, chorea, athetosis, myoclonus, tremor

BOX 20.1

STRENGTH RATING SCALE

0/5: No movement (i.e., no palpable tension at tendon)
1/5: Flicker of movement
2/5: Movement in a gravity-neutral plane
3/5: Movement against gravity but not resistance
4/5: Subnormal strength against resistance (requires accommodation to execute movement)
5/5: Normal strength against resistance (motion is smooth, comfortably executed, without accommodation)

D. Sensory

1. Primarily important if any concern for spinal cord defect or peripheral nerve injury
2. Focus initial investigation along three axes for meaningful lesion localization:
   a. Distal deficit with preserved (or less impaired) proximal sensation suggests **polyneuropathy.**
      (1) Pain/temperature deficit: Small fiber polyneuropathy/anterior spinal cord
      (2) Position/vibration deficit: Large fiber polyneuropathy/posterior spinal cord
   b. Lower body more affected than upper body suggests **spinal cord injuries.**
      (1) See Fig. 20.1 for dermatomes.
      (2) Ask about continence, assess rectal tone.
   c. If difference between left and right, concern for **unilateral brain or spinal cord lesion**

E. Reflexes

1. **Tendon reflexes:** Gradation (Box 20.2) and localization (eTable 20.2). Helpful in localizing abnormalities including upper versus lower motor neuron pathology, especially in presence of weakness or asymmetry (eTable 20.3). Compare right to left, upper to lower extremities, and distal to proximal reflexes. Generalized high or low reflexes are of little significance in the setting of normal strength and coordination.
2. **Primitive reflexes:** Expected during specific time windows (Table 20.1)

F. Coordination and Gait

1. **Evaluate coordination while watching age-appropriate activities.**
2. **Tests for cerebellar function:** Rapid alternating movements, finger-to-nose, heel-to-shin, walking, running

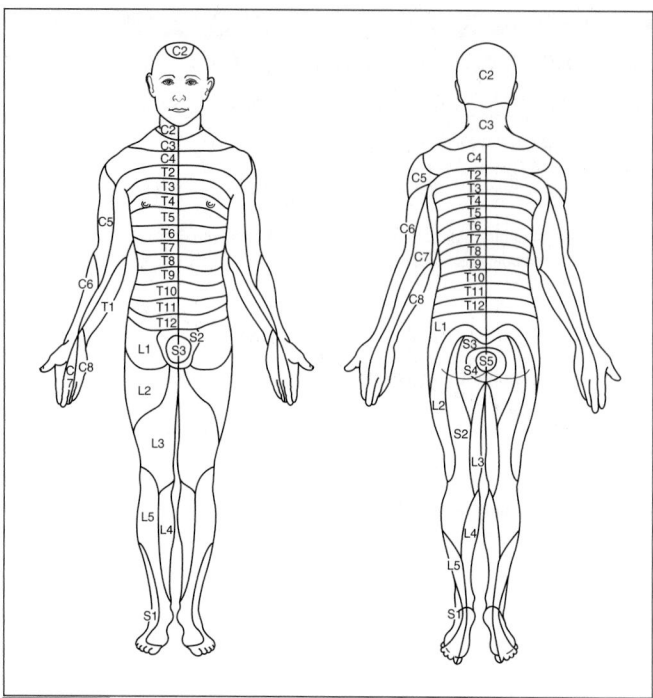

FIGURE 20.1

Dermatomes. (From Athreya BH, Silverman BK. *Pediatric Physical Diagnosis.* Appleton-Century-Crofts; 1985:238–239.)

BOX 20.2
REFLEX RATING SCALE

0: None
1+: Diminished (need use of clasped hands/gritting teeth to engage reflex)
2+: Normal
3+: Increased (reflexes cross neighboring joint or cross to other side)
4+: Hyperactive with clonus

II. NEUROLOGIC EMERGENCIES

A. Stroke[1-4]

1. Presentation and etiology
   a. 50% ischemic, 50% hemorrhagic overall in pediatric stroke, but approximately 80% ischemic in perinatal stroke. Strokes have many mimics which are more common, which means strokes themselves are frequently missed (Box 20.3). Perinatal stroke

TABLE 20.1

PRIMITIVE REFLEXES

Reflex	Appears	Extinguishes
Palmar grasp	28 WGA	2–3 months
Moro	28 WGA	5–6 months
Rooting	32 WGA	1 month
Tonic neck	35 WGA	6–7 months
Parachute	7–8 months	Remains for life

WGA, Weeks' gestational age.

Modified from Schor NF. Neurologic evaluation, Chapter 608. In: Kliegman RM, St. Geme J, ed. *Nelson Textbook of Pediatrics.* 21st ed. Elsevier; 2020.

BOX 20.3

STROKE MIMICS PRESENTING WITH ACUTE-ONSET FOCAL NEUROLOGIC DEFICIT

1. Migraine
2. Seizure ± postictal (Todd) paralysis
3. Functional disorders
4. Mass lesion
5. Infection
6. Drug toxicity (e.g., methotrexate)
7. Posterior reversible encephalopathy syndrome (PRES)
8. Metabolic abnormality
9. Demyelinating lesion

(28 weeks' gestational age to 28 days postnatal) rarely presents with focal symptoms; presentation most likely to include seizures, altered level of consciousness, feeding difficulties, early handedness. Even in childhood stroke (28 days to 18 years), seizure and headache are far more common presenting symptoms than in adults. It is important to consider stroke on the differential for acute neurologic changes.
   b. Etiologies vary by age (eTable 20.4).[1] Patients with increased risk of recurrent stroke: history of cardiac disease and cardiac surgery, cerebral arteriopathy, sickle cell disease, thrombophilias
2. Management
   a. **Stroke team activation** (where available) or **urgent neurology consultation,** along with transfer to a tertiary care center with expertise in childhood stroke.
   b. **Supportive care and neurologic monitoring:** Maintain normoglycemia, maintain normothermia (avoid fevers), maintain oxygenation, prompt seizure treatment. Monitor for signs of increased intracranial pressure.
   c. **Optimize cerebral perfusion pressure:** Ensure adequate fluid volume and maintenance of median blood pressure (BP) for age, allow permissive hypertension in cases of ischemic stroke.
   d. **Reperfusion therapies:** Thrombolytic therapy with intravenous tissue plasminogen activator (tPA) or mechanical thrombectomy may be considered under appropriate circumstances in centers with extensive

pediatric stroke experience, although not recommended in the perinatal period for arterial ischemic stroke (American Heart Association guidelines).

e. **Early rehabilitation** with physical, occupational, and speech therapy as needed.

f. **Children with sickle cell disease:** Consult a hematologist. Hydration and emergent exchange transfusion to reduce sickle hemoglobin (see Chapter 14)

B. Status Epilepticus and Breakthrough Seizures

1. **Definition[5,6]:** Status epilepticus is defined as continuous clinical or electrographic seizure activity lasting ≥5 minutes or two or more discrete seizures without return of consciousness between them. See Chapter 1 for management algorithm.

2. **Breakthrough seizures (ED assessment):** Assess for missed medications or significant weight gain, lack of sleep, stress, drugs/alcohol, physical exertion, illness, dehydration, flickering lights, menses, and drug interactions that can lower seizure threshold (e.g. tricyclic antidepressants, certain antibiotics, over-the-counter cold preparations, diphenhydramine, herbal supplements). Consider antiseizure medication levels (see Table 20.2 for therapeutic drug levels).

C. Encephalopathy[7-10]

1. **Definitions:**
   a. Encephalopathy: Diffuse neuronal dysfunction manifesting as acute or chronic altered mental status
   b. Encephalitis: Inflammation of brain parenchyma secondary to infection or inflammatory response

2. **Selected causes of encephalopathy:** Box 20.4

3. **Diagnosis:** Targeted based on clinical scenario and associated symptoms. See Chapter 1 for possible etiologies and workup considerations. May require serum and/or CSF studies for infectious/inflammatory/metabolic markers, EEG, neuroimaging (e.g., MRI or PET)

4. **Treatment:** Dependent on etiology. See Chapter 1 for emergency management of acute altered level of consciousness. See Chapter 17 for treatment of meningitis.

D. Hydrocephalus with Increased Intracranial Pressure[11-13]

1. **Etiology:** Communicating (abnormal CSF reabsorption) versus noncommunicating (obstruction of CSF flow); congenital versus acquired (postinfectious, posthemorrhagic, mass lesions)

2. **Diagnosis**
   a. Clinical signs: Macrocephaly, increasing head circumference (HC), bulging/tense fontanelle, splayed sutures, headaches, blurry/spotty vision, diplopia, decreased level of consciousness, "setting-sun" eye sign due to upward gaze paresis, vomiting, Cushing's triad (hypertension, bradycardia, irregular respirations), papilledema, CN palsies (III, IV, VI)

TABLE 20.2

COMMONLY USED ANTISEIZURE MEDICATIONS

Antiseizure Medication (Trade Name)	Standard Therapeutic Levels[a]	IV Preparation Available?	Side Effects
Brivaracetam (Briviact)	–	–	Somnolence/sedation, dizziness, fatigue, nausea/vomiting
Cannabidiol (Epidiolex)	–	–	Hepatotoxicity, somnolence, decreased appetite, diarrhea, fatigue, insomnia, infections. Can interact with other antiseizure drugs (e.g. clobazam)
Carbamazepine (Tegretol/Carbatrol)	4–12 mg/L	–	Black box: TEN/SJS in patients with HLA-B*1502 allele, aplastic anemia, agranulocytosis. Other: sedation, ataxia, diplopia, hyponatremia, hepatotoxicity, may worsen generalized seizures
Clobazam (Onfi)	30–300 mCg/L	–	Sedation, dizziness
Clonazepam (Klonopin)	20–70 mCg/L	–	Sedation, drooling, dependence
Diazepam (Diastat, Valium)	–	Yes, 1:1 conversion	Sedation, dry mouth, respiratory depression
Eslicarbazepine acetate (Aptiom)	10–35 mg/L	–	Hyponatremia, dizziness, somnolence, vomiting, headache, diplopia, vertigo, ataxia, tremor
Ethosuximide (Zarontin)	40–100 mg/L	–	GI upset
Felbamate (Felbatol)	30–60 mg/L	–	Black box: aplastic anemia (rare), liver failure. Other: sleep disturbances, weight loss
Fenfluramine (Fintepla)	–	–	Risk of cardiac valve abnormalities (recommend echo every 6 months), weight loss
Gabapentin (Neurontin)	2–20 mg/L	–	Weight gain, leg edema, dizziness
Lacosamide (Vimpat)	5–10 mg/L	Yes, 1:1 conversion	Sedation, reduced benefit with sodium channel drugs, increased PR interval
Lamotrigine (Lamictal)	2.5–15 mg/L	–	Black box: SJS/TEN (risk greater in pediatric patients, increased risk in combination with valproate). OCPs significantly decrease level. Other: fatigue, ataxia, diarrhea
Levetiracetam (Keppra)	12–46 mg/L	Yes, 1:1 conversion	Abnormal behavior, irritability, rare psychosis
Oxcarbazepine (Trileptal)	3–35 mg/L (10-hydroxycarbazepine level)	–	Hyponatremia, weight gain, dizziness

Continued

TABLE 20.2

COMMONLY USED ANTISEIZURE MEDICATIONS—CONT'D

Antiseizure Medication (Trade Name)	Standard Therapeutic Levels[a]	IV Preparation Available?	Side Effects
Perampanel (Fycompa)	-	-	Black box: psychiatric/behavioral reactions (hostility). Other: dizziness, headache
Phenobarbital (Luminal)	10–40 mg/L	Yes, 1:1 conversion	Somnolence, syncope, erythroderma
Phenytoin (Dilantin)	10–20 mg/L	Yes, 1:1 conversion	Ataxia, hirsutism, gingival hyperplasia, teratogenicity, morbilliform rash, purple-glove syndrome with infusion
Pregabalin (Lyrica)	2–5 mg/L	-	Peripheral edema, weight gain, constipation, dizziness, ataxia, sedation
Rufinamide (Banzel)	5–30 mg/L	-	Shortened QT interval, nausea, dizziness, sedation, headache. Interacts with other antiseizure drugs
Tiagabine (Gabitril)	20–200 mCg/L	-	Can worsen generalized seizures
Topiramate (Topamax)	5–20 mg/L	-	Cognitive side effects, weight loss, renal stones, metabolic acidosis, glaucoma
Valproic acid (Depakote, Depakene)	50–100 mg/L	Yes, 1:1 conversion (Use total PO daily dose divided Q6 hr, see Formulary)	Black box: hepatotoxicity. Other: thrombocytopenia, weight gain, alopecia, pancreatitis, PCOS, teratogenicity
Vigabatrin (Sabril)	0.8–36 mg/L	-	Black box: permanent peripheral visual field defects. Other: rash, weight gain, irritability, dizziness, sedation
Zonisamide (Zonegran)	10–40 mg/L	-	Renal stones, weight loss; rare: SJS, aplastic anemia

[a]Draw level immediately before an oral dose for ideal sampling time.

GI, gastrointestinal; *HLA,* human leukocyte antigen; *IV,* intravenous; *mCg,* microgram; *MhD,* 10-monohydroxy metabolite; *OCP,* oral contraceptive pill; *PCOS,* polycystic ovarian syndrome; *SJS,* Stevens-Johnson syndrome; *TEN,* toxic epidermal necrolysis.

Data from Patsalos PN, Berry DJ, Bourgeois BFD, et al. Antiepileptic drugs—best practice guidelines for therapeutic drug monitoring: a position paper by the Subcommission on Therapeutic Drug Monitoring, ILAE Commission on Therapeutic Strategies. *Epilepsia.* 2008;49(7):1239–1276; Jacob S, Nair AB. An updated overview on therapeutic drug monitoring of recent antiepileptic drugs. *Drugs R D.* 2016;16(4):303–316.

BOX 20.4

DIFFERENTIAL DIAGNOSIS OF ENCEPHALOPATHY

1. Infectious and parainfectious: meningitis, encephalitis, ADEM
2. Autoimmune: NMDAR, VGKC-complex, Hashimoto's thyroiditis-associated
3. Trauma
4. Seizure-related: status epilepticus, postictal, epileptic encephalopathy
5. Toxins: medications, drugs, heavy metals, carbon monoxide
6. Metabolic: uremia, hyperammonemia, hyper- or hypoglycemia, lactic acidosis
7. Hypertension, posterior reversible encephalopathy syndrome (PRES)
8. Hypoxic-ischemic: neonatal, drowning, cardiorespiratory arrest, vascular
9. Intracranial hemorrhage
10. Malignancy
11. Genetic: leukoencephalopathy, mitochondrial, ADANE

ADANE, Autosomal-dominant acute necrotizing encephalitis; *ADEM,* acute disseminated encephalomyelitis; *NMDAR,* N-methyl-D-aspartate receptor; *VGKC,* voltage-gated potassium channel.

---

  b. In infants, obtain serial measurements of HC. Obtain neuroimaging if significant increase in HC percentile or if patient is symptomatic.
  c. Imaging: Ultrafast MRI (or similar protocol) preferred to CT where available; can consider venous imaging if high suspicion of cerebral sinus venous thrombosis

3. **Treatment**
   a. **Medical:**
      (1) Emergently manage acute increase of intracranial pressure (ICP; see Chapter 1).
      (2) Slowly progressive hydrocephalus: Acetazolamide and furosemide may provide temporary relief by decreasing the rate of CSF production.
   b. **Surgical:** CSF shunting versus endoscopic third ventriculostomy (ETV)
      (1) Ventriculoperitoneal shunts used most commonly.
      (2) Patients with shunt dysfunction often present with signs of increased ICP. Causes include infection, obstruction (clogging or kinking), disconnection, migration of proximal or distal tips, valve programming.
      (3) Evaluation of shunt integrity: See Chapter 26 for discussion of imaging. Consult pediatric neurosurgery (if available).

E. Weakness

1. **Botulism[14,15]**
   a. **Etiology:** May result from colonization of the colon by *Clostridium botulinum* bacteria, ingestion of botulinum toxin in food, or by wound colonization and toxin production. Botulinum toxin irreversibly cleaves the protein complex necessary for acetylcholine vesicle release into the neuromuscular junction. Predominantly affects those <1 year of age (most commonly <6 months) secondary to immaturity of the gut flora; however, foodborne botulism affects children of all ages.
   b. **Clinical features and diagnosis:** Subacute onset weakness of skeletal muscles diffusely, concentrating in eye, face, and bulbar muscles early. Dilated and poorly reactive pupils are common and specific when

present (note that normal pupil size in infants is smaller than in older children; ≤4 mm). Presenting symptoms in infants may be constipation for days to weeks before onset of weakness, poor feeding, and weak cry. At high risk for respiratory failure secondary to respiratory and bulbar muscle weakness. Tachycardia is common. Confirm diagnosis by toxin assay of stool (not culture) performed by state lab or CDC; may use sterile saline enema for specimen collection. Electromyography and nerve conduction studies can help confirm diagnosis.

c. **Treatment:** Assess and stabilize airway; approximately 25% of children require intubation/advanced airway. Treat with one-time dose of human botulism immune globulin (BabyBIG or BIG-IV), available through Infant Botulism Treatment and Prevention Program (http://www.infantbotulism.org/). Prompt treatment is key—do not wait for confirmatory testing. With appropriate treatment, prognosis for full recovery is excellent. See Chapter 16 for recommended interval before measles or varicella vaccination after botulism immune globulin administration.

2. **Guillain-Barré syndrome (GBS)**[16-18]
   a. **Etiology:** Presumed immune attack against peripheral nerve myelin. In some cases, triggered by illness (e.g., *Campylobacter jejuni* infection, Zika virus, SARS-CoV2 virus)
   b. **Clinical features:** Ascending weakness and sensory loss with rapid decline reaching greatest disability often less than 2 weeks after onset. Respiratory status can be compromised, ~20% of patients require mechanical ventilation. Often with autonomic instability. Poorly localized pain, ataxia often prominent in children
   c. **Diagnosis:** Elevated spinal fluid protein without cellular infiltrate ("albuminocytologic dissociation") present in 50% to 70% of patients. Nerve conduction studies and MRI (nerve root enhancement) can be helpful.
   d. **Treatment:** Patients should be hospitalized at presentation to monitor respiratory stability. Acute phase treatment with IVIG (0.4 g/kg daily for 5 days), or plasmapheresis (200–250 mL plasma/kg for 5 sessions) helpful if initiated early. Combined or repeat treatments do not offer additional benefit. Supportive care. Recovery tends to require months to years.
   e. **Variants or differential diagnosis of GBS**
      (1) Acute: Miller Fisher syndrome (ataxia, ophthalmoplegia, and areflexia), acute motor axonal neuropathy (AMAN)
      (2) Chronic: Chronic inflammatory demyelinating polyneuropathy (CIDP) is a similar but slower progressive autoimmune disorder that often requires chronic immunosuppressive therapy.

F. Ataxia[19,20]

1. Impaired coordination of movement and balance; broad-based gait
2. Differential diagnosis of acute ataxia (Box 20.5)
3. Evaluation (Box 20.6)

20

BOX 20.5

DIFFERENTIAL DIAGNOSIS OF ACUTE ATAXIA (IN NO PARTICULAR ORDER)

1. Ingestion (e.g., antiseizure medications, antipsychotics, sedatives, hypnotics) or intoxication (e.g., alcohol, hydrocarbon fumes, heavy metals)
2. Postinfectious: acute cerebellar ataxia, cerebellitis (e.g., viral causes), acute disseminated encephalomyelitis
3. Head trauma: cerebellar contusion or hemorrhage, posterior fossa hematoma, vertebrobasilar dissection, postconcussion syndrome
4. Basilar migraine
5. Benign paroxysmal vertigo
6. Intracranial mass lesion: tumor, vascular malformation
7. Opsoclonus–myoclonus ataxia syndrome: Chaotic eye movements combined with ataxia and myoclonus. Postinfectious or paraneoplastic (neuroblastoma/neural crest tumors) etiology
8. Hydrocephalus
9. Infection: labyrinthitis, abscess
10. Seizure: ictal or postictal
11. Vascular events: cerebellar hemorrhage or stroke
12. Guillain-Barré syndrome or Miller-Fisher variant (ataxia, ophthalmoplegia, and areflexia). Warning: If bulbar signs present, patient may lose ability to protect airway.
13. Rare inherited paroxysmal ataxias
14. Inborn errors of metabolism
15. Multiple sclerosis
16. Somatic symptom/functional neurologic disorder

BOX 20.6

CONSIDERATIONS FOR INITIAL EVALUATION OF ACUTE ATAXIA

1. Complete blood cell count, electrolytes, urine and serum toxicology
2. Imaging (CT or MRI)
3. Lumbar puncture
4. EEG
5. If neuroblastoma is suspected (opsoclonus–myoclonus ataxia syndrome), obtain urine vanillylmandelic acid and homovanillic acid, as well as MRI or CT of chest and abdomen.

CT, Computed tomography; *EEG*, electroencephalogram; *MRI*, magnetic resonance imaging.

III. CHRONIC OR GRADUALLY PROGRESSIVE CONDITIONS

A. Headaches[21-33]

1. **Classification of headaches**
   a. **Primary headaches:** Migraine, tension type, cluster, trigeminal autonomic cephalalgias (TACs), other primary headache disorders
   b. **Secondary headaches:** Trauma, infection, substance use or withdrawal, vascular disorder, neurologic disorder, increased intracranial pressure

    c. **Differential diagnosis:** Acute (Box 20.7) and chronic (Box 20.8)
2. **Evaluation of headaches**
    a. Obtain history (Box 20.9) and physical exam (eTable 20.5)
    b. Evaluate for red flags (Box 20.10).
    c. If red flags are present, obtain appropriate imaging (CT for hemorrhage, MRI/MRA/MRV for vascular abnormalities).
    d. Perform lumbar puncture (LP) if concern for infection or increased intracranial pressure (Box 20.11). *If no red flags are present and normal neurologic exam, imaging and LP are not recommended.*
3. **Migraine headache**
    a. Migraines can be throbbing, pulsatile, or pressure-like in children. Usually bifrontal in children and unilateral in adolescents and adults. There are many potential triggers (e.g., stress, caffeine, menses, sleep disruption). See Box 20.12 for diagnostic criteria.

BOX 20.7

DIFFERENTIAL DIAGNOSIS OF ACUTE HEADACHE

Evaluation of the first acute headache should consider pathologic causes listed here on the differential along with more common etiologies.
1. Increased intracranial pressure (ICP): Trauma, hemorrhage, tumor, hydrocephalus, idiopathic intracranial hypertension, abscess, arachnoid cyst, cerebral edema
2. Decreased ICP: Ventriculoperitoneal shunt placement, lumbar puncture, cerebrospinal fluid leak
3. Meningeal inflammation: Meningitis, leukemia, subarachnoid or subdural hemorrhage
4. Vascular: Vasculitis, arteriovenous malformation, hypertension, cerebrovascular accident
5. Bone, soft tissue: Referred pain from scalp, eyes, ears, sinuses, nose, teeth, pharynx, cervical spine, temporomandibular joint
6. Infection: Systemic, encephalitis, sinusitis
7. Medication or intoxicant exposure (e.g., stimulants, steroids, drugs of abuse)
8. First primary headache

BOX 20.8

DIFFERENTIAL DIAGNOSIS OF RECURRENT OR CHRONIC HEADACHES

1. Migraine (with or without aura)
2. Tension
3. Analgesic rebound
4. Caffeine withdrawal
5. Sleep deprivation or chronic hypoxia (e.g., sleep apnea)
6. Tumor
7. Psychogenic: Conversion disorder, malingering, depression, acute stress, mood disorder
8. Cluster headache
9. New daily persistent headache

BOX 20.9

IMPORTANT HISTORICAL INFORMATION IN EVALUATING HEADACHE

1. When did the headaches begin?
2. How did the headache begin? Associated trauma, social stressors (school, home)?
3. What is the frequency and duration of the headaches?
   a. Headache pattern (e.g., intermittent, progressive, chronic)
   b. Time of day
4. Where is the pain, what is it like, and does it radiate? Focal occipital pain is concerning for secondary headaches.
5. Associated symptoms? What do you do during the headache?
   a. Aura or prodrome
   b. Constitutional symptoms (weight changes), vision changes, or any other neurologic symptoms (weakness, tingling, photophobia, phonophobia)
   c. Triggers and alleviating/exacerbating factors
6. Other history (e.g., health problems, medications, family history of migraine)
7. How do the headaches affect your ability to function? Ask about school absences.

b. **Classification[21]:** With or without aura. An aura is any neurologic symptom that occurs prior to onset of a migraine (e.g., visual aberrations, paresthesias, numbness, dysphasia).
c. **Precursors to migraines and close associations:** Cyclic vomiting, abdominal migraines, recurrent abdominal pain, paroxysmal vertigo of childhood, paroxysmal torticollis of infancy, and motion sickness
d. **Treatment:** Combination of acute and prophylactic treatment
   (1) **Symptomatic treatment:** Avoid medication overuse as it can lead to rebound headaches. Optimal acute therapy can prevent progression to chronic migraines.
      (a) Outpatient setting:
         (i) Dark, quiet room and sleep
         (ii) Nonsteroidal antiinflammatory drugs (NSAIDs; e.g., naproxen, ibuprofen, ketorolac) and/or acetaminophen. Limit to 3 days per week or 14 days per month.
         (iii) Caffeine (e.g., coffee, tea, soda)
         (iv) Triptans. Only effective at migraine onset. Limit to 9 days per month.
         (v) Antidopaminergics have antiemetic properties, and may be effective even if nausea is not a prominent symptom. Prochlorperazine shown to be superior to metoclopramide[22]
      (b) Emergency department (ED)/inpatient setting:
         (i) Often helpful to combine medications and administer intravenous (IV) "migraine cocktail" (see Fig. 20.2 for example ED algorithm)
         (ii) Steroids (e.g., methylprednisolone) may be useful in intractable cases, although evidence is lacking.
         (iii) Dihydroergotamine may be considered.

BOX 20.10

RED FLAGS IN HEADACHE EVALUATION

1. Progressively worsening headaches
2. "Thunderclap" headache (less than 5 minutes from onset to maximal intensity)
3. Altered mental status
4. New-onset focal neurologic symptoms
5. Optic nerve edema
6. Nuchal rigidity
7. Seizures
8. Visual symptoms not typical of migraines (e.g., colorful, hallucinatory, short duration), diplopia, decreased visual acuity, visual field deficits
9. Concurrent fever (especially if accompanied by other red flags)
10. Headache worse with supine position or Valsalva (cough, straining)
11. Association with persistent emesis
12. Immunocompromised or on anticoagulation
13. Signs of endocrine pathology (e.g., short stature, obesity, polyuria, sluggishness, constipation, virilization)

BOX 20.11

LUMBAR PUNCTURE

1. See Chapter 4 for indications, contraindications, and procedure.
2. Standard tests: Cell counts + differential, Gram stain, cerebrospinal fluid (CSF) culture, protein, glucose. Consider viral studies (e.g., herpes simplex virus, enterovirus).
3. Manometer for opening pressure (OP) if concern for increased intracranial pressure. Performed in a lateral decubitus position. OP of <28 cm H_2O generally considered normal; however, interpret results in conjunction with other clinical and examination findings.
4. There is inconsistent evidence regarding correction factors for CSF white blood cell counts in the setting of blood-contaminated CSF from a traumatic lumbar puncture.
5. Xanthochromia: Yellow or pink discoloration of CSF due to breakdown of hemoglobin. Suspect subarachnoid hemorrhage.

Data from Fishman RA. *Cerebrospinal Fluid in Diseases of the Nervous System.* 2nd ed. Saunders; 1992:190; Avery RA. Interpretation of lumbar puncture opening pressure measurements in children. *J Neuro Ophthalmol.* 2014;34(3):284–287.

(2) **Preventative treatment:**
    (a) Lifestyle modification is a mainstay[23]:
        (i) adequate sleep[30]
        (ii) meals
        (iii) hydration
        (iv) regular
        (v) exercise

BOX 20.12

DIAGNOSTIC CRITERIA FOR PEDIATRIC MIGRAINE WITHOUT AURA[21,24,25]

At least five attacks fulfilling the following criteria:
1. Headache 2–72 hours in children younger than 18 years (untreated or unsuccessfully treated)
2. At least two of the following characteristics:
   a. Unilateral or bilateral
   b. Pulsating quality
   c. Moderate to severe in intensity
   d. Aggravated by or causing avoidance of routine physical activities
3. At least one of the following occurs during the headache:
   a. Nausea and/or vomiting
   b. Photophobia and phonophobia (which may be inferred from behavior)
4. Not better accounted for by another diagnosis

   (vi) weight loss if overweight
   (vii) Avoid triggers, stress, caffeine withdrawal, tobacco exposure
   (b) Consider prophylactic medications (eTable 20.6) in any of the following situations:
   (i) Migraines occur more than once per week or affect quality of life.
   (ii) Frequent ED visits
   (iii) Complicated migraines
   (iv) Migraines not responsive to abortive medications
 (2) **Alternative/complementary therapies:**
   (a) Cognitive behavioral therapy
   (b) Biofeedback
   (c) Physical therapy
   (d) Acupuncture

Clinicians may use PedMIDAS scale[31] to determine disability associated with migraine. Recent systematic review of migraine prophylaxis in children suggests that preventative medication may be no more effective than placebo.[23] New biologic (anti-calcitonin gene-related peptide or CGRP)[32,33] was approved in adults in 2018; there are no studies yet in the pediatric population.

B. Seizures[5,6,34-48]

1. **Differential diagnosis of recurrent events that mimic epilepsy in childhood** (Table 20.3)
2. **Seizures: First and recurrent**
   a. **Definition:** Paroxysmal, transient, synchronized discharge of cortical neurons resulting in alteration of function (motor, sensory, cognitive)
   b. **Causes of seizures**
   (1) Diffuse brain dysfunction: Fever, metabolic compromise, toxin or drugs, hypertension

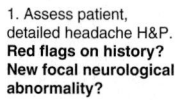

1. Assess patient, detailed headache H&P. **Red flags on history? New focal neurological abnormality?**

Yes

2. Further evaluation for underlying cause: Neuroimaging, labs.

No

2. **Phase 1:** Allow to rest in dark quiet area.

Intravenous pathway:	Oral pathway:
Normal saline bolus (20 mL/kg, max 1 L)	Oral fluids
Ketorolac (0.5 mg/kg, max 30 mg)	Ibuprofen (10 mg/kg, max 600 mg)
Prochlorperazine (0.15 mg/kg, max 10 mg)	Prochlorperazine (0.15 mg/kg, max 10 mg)

Only give diphenhydramine (1 mg/kg, max 50 mg) if history of dystonic reaction to prochlorperazine.

3. Reassess hourly: **Pain resolved or sufficiently resolved?** — Yes → 4. Discharge home.

No

4. After <u>2 hours</u> with insufficient response, proceed to **phase 2:**

Normal saline bolus (20 mL/kg, max 1 L)
Valproic acid (IV/PO: 10–15 mg/kg, max 1000 mg)
+/– Magnesium (25–75 mg/kg, max 2 g)

5. Reassess hourly: **Pain resolved or sufficiently resolved?** — Yes → 6. Discharge home.

No

6. After 2 additional hours with insufficient response, consult neurology service (if available); consider admission for inpatient management.

FIGURE 20.2

Emergency department management of migraine headaches at Johns Hopkins Children's Center. H&P, history and physical.

    (2) Focal brain dysfunction: Stroke, neoplasm, focal cortical dysgenesis, trauma

  c. **Febrile seizure**[34-36]

    (1) Simple febrile seizure: Primary generalized seizure associated with fever in a child 6 to 60 months of age that is nonfocal, lasts for <15 minutes, and does not recur in a 24-hour period

      (a) Management: Identify the source of fever. No further workup (neuroimaging, EEG, or bloodwork) or antiseizure medications are necessary for a simple febrile seizure in a well-appearing, fully immunized child with a normal neurologic examination and no meningeal signs

20

TABLE 20.3

DIFFERENTIAL DIAGNOSIS OF RECURRENT EVENTS THAT MIMIC EPILEPSY IN CHILDHOOD

Event	Differentiation From Epilepsy
SYNCOPE AND ANOXIC EVENTS	
Breath-holding spells (18 mo–3 yr)	Loss of consciousness and generalized convulsions, always provoked by an event that makes child upset
Vasovagal syncope	Triggers: Postural change, heat, emotion. Preceded by dizziness, diaphoresis, nausea, and vision changes. Slow collapse, rapid return to awareness; may have associated convulsions and brief confusion after event
Cardiogenic syncope	Triggers: Exercise, strong emotion, water immersion. Abnormal ECG/Holter monitor finding. No consistent convulsive movements
Cough syncope	Prolonged cough spasm during sleep in asthmatic, leading to loss of consciousness, often with urinary incontinence
BEHAVIORAL, PSYCHOLOGICAL, AND PSYCHIATRIC DISORDERS	
Psychogenic nonepileptic seizure (PNES)	Also known as pseudoseizures. No EEG changes except movement artifact during event. Thrashing, proximal truncal movements. Eye closure with resistance to opening. Guards face with hand drop. Brief/absent postictal period. Often exacerbated by psychological stressor
SLEEP-RELATED CONDITIONS	
Narcolepsy	Excessive daytime sleepiness, cataplexy (sudden atonia triggered by emotion), sleep paralysis, sudden-onset REM on EEG
PAROXYSMAL MOVEMENT DISORDERS	
Tics	Involuntary, nonrhythmic, repetitive movements not associated with impaired consciousness. Strong urge to perform movement but temporarily suppressible
Stereotypies (mannerisms)	Repetitive movements or vocalizations (e.g., rocking, head banging)
Paroxysmal dyskinesias	Dystonia, choreoathetosis in response to specific triggers (e.g., startle, movement). Often familial
MIGRAINE-ASSOCIATED DISORDERS	
Migraine	Headache or visual changes that may precede attack. Autonomic or sensory changes can mimic focal seizure. Family history of migraines. EEG with regional area of slowing during attack
Paroxysmal vertigo (toddler)	Episode of vertigo, vomiting, staggering, and falling in a child. May become anxious, no loss of awareness; may have associated nystagmus
MISCELLANEOUS EVENTS	
Sandifer syndrome	GER in infancy. Paroxysmal dystonic posturing (back arching) associated with meals
Myoclonus	Involuntary muscle jerking or twitch

ECG, Electrocardiography; *EEG,* electroencephalography; *GER,* gastroesophageal reflux; *REM,* rapid eye movement.
Data from Fine A, Wirrell EC. Seizures in children. *Pediatr Rev.* 2020;41(7):321–347. doi:10.1542/pir.2019-0134; Glauser TA, Loddenkemper T. Management of childhood epilepsy. *Continuum.* 2013;19(3, Epilepsy):656–681; *Epilepsy imitators.* ILAE 2018: https://www.epilepsydiagnosis.org/epilepsy-imitators.html

      (b) Indications for lumbar puncture: Meningeal signs, incomplete or unknown *Haemophilus influenzae* or *Streptococcus pneumoniae* immunization status, or if pretreated with antibiotics (which can mask signs and symptoms of meningitis)

   (2) Complex febrile seizure: Seizure associated with a fever that is focal, lasts for >15 minutes, or recurs within 24 hours

      (a) Management: Identify the source of fever; treat as per status epilepticus guidelines if seizure continues (see Chapter 1). Obtain EEG. Consider nonemergent MRI (to evaluate for associated focal lesion), LP if concern for CNS infection. Consider prescribing rectal diazepam for home emergency use. Slightly increased risk of developing epilepsy at a later age

d. **Evaluation of unprovoked seizure**[37,38]

   (1) Rule out provocative factors: Obtain vitals. Consider obtaining glucose, electrolytes, blood urea nitrogen, creatinine, complete blood cell count, toxicology screen.

   (2) EEG is recommended in all children with first unprovoked seizure to evaluate for an epilepsy syndrome; however, it does not have to be emergently obtained.[37] Interictal EEGs may be normal, particularly in children with focal seizures. Repeat EEGs, prolonged EEG monitoring with video as clinically indicated

   (3) Imaging: High-resolution MRI can assist with identification of underlying brain malformation, although it is not routinely indicated when evaluating a first-time seizure. CT is not recommended.

e. **Epilepsy:** Recurrent, unprovoked seizures, a single seizure with an abnormal EEG, *or* diagnosis of genetic syndrome characterized by recurrent seizures. Assess seizure type, epilepsy classification (eTable 20.7),[38-42] and severity of disorder. See Table 20.4 for selected epilepsy syndromes of childhood.

f. **Treatment**[38,43,44,46-48]

   (1) First seizure, nonfocal, and with return to baseline: No antiseizure medication typically indicated. Overall recurrence rate approximately 50% in 2 to 5 years. Epileptiform abnormalities on EEG indicate a higher chance of recurrence; clinician can consider antiseizure therapy after first seizure if EEG abnormalities.

   (2) Educate parents and patient regarding seizure safety.[44] Review seizure first aid and precautions, including supervision during bathing or swimming. Be aware of driver's license laws in the state (https://www.epilepsy.com/driving-laws). Advocate for teacher and school awareness; provide seizure plan. Consider home abortive therapy.

   (3) Pharmacotherapy (see Table 20.2): Initiate if known etiology of seizure (diagnosis of epilepsy syndrome), recurrent unprovoked seizure (risk of recurrent seizure >80% after second unprovoked

TABLE 20.4

SELECTED EPILEPSY SYNDROMES[38,40,42-44]

Syndrome	Etiology	Evaluation	Treatment	Comments
Neonatal seizures (broad category encompassing a spectrum from benign to morbid syndromes)	Brain malformation, HIE, intracranial hemorrhage, inborn errors of metabolism, CNS infection, cerebral infarction, hypoglycemia, hypocalcemia, hypomagnesemia. Consider benign neonatal seizures ("fifth day fits").	Screen for electrolyte and metabolic abnormalities, pyridoxine deficiency, and sepsis. Obtain LP, head ultrasound, CT or MRI, EEG.	Treat underlying abnormality, consider pyridoxine ± EEG, phenobarbital, levetiracetam (± additional agents). No treatment needed for benign neonatal seizures	Occur within first 28 days of life; may be myoclonic, tonic, clonic, or subtle Presents as blinking, chewing, bicycling, or apnea Distinguished from jitteriness by vital sign changes and inability to provoke or suppress movements
Early infantile epileptic encephalopathy (Ohtahara syndrome) and early myoclonic encephalopathy	Structural malformations, metabolic disorders (glycine encephalopathy, pyridoxine dependent epilepsy, mitochondrial mutations), genetic mutations	EEG with burst suppression pattern	Trial of pyridoxine, antiseizure medications, ketogenic diet Seizures are difficult to control. If due to metabolic disorder, treat appropriately.	Tonic and myoclonic seizures with onset in neonatal period Can progress to infantile spasms and/or Lennox-Gastaut Poor neurodevelopmental outcome

Continued

TABLE 20.4

SELECTED EPILEPSY SYNDROMES[38,40,42-44]**—CONT'D**

Syndrome	Etiology	Evaluation	Treatment	Comments
Infantile spasms	Unclear; often early insult (HIE, postnatal hemorrhage), structural, genetic (tuberous sclerosis complex, Down syndrome), or metabolic abnormalities	EEG with interictal hypsarrhythmia, MRI	High-dose steroids (oral prednisolone) or ACTH; vigabatrin (particularly for tuberous sclerosis), ketogenic diet	Onset after age 2 mos, peak onset 4–6 mos Highly variable appearance (flexor, extensor, mixed) often upon awakening and in clusters Overall poor long-term outcomes, especially if known etiology. Early recognition and treatment can improve this.
Lennox-Gastaut syndrome	Multifactorial etiology. Often progression from other epileptic encephalopathy	EEG with slow spike-wave discharges and intermittent runs of multiple spikes or fast activity	Clobazam, felbamate, lamotrigine, rufinamide, topiramate, valproic acid, ketogenic diet, cannabidiol	Multiple seizure types, cognitive impairment, and characteristic EEG findings Significant secondary morbidity associated with atonic seizures
Childhood absence seizures	Suspected to be genetic	EEG with sudden generalized 3–4 Hz spike-and-wave discharges Hyperventilation precipitates seizure.	Ethosuximide, lamotrigine, valproic acid	Onset 4–10 years Staring spells with diminished awareness, ± automatisms (eye blinking, mouth movements) Often resolves by adolescence, with good neurologic outcome
Childhood epilepsy with centrotemporal spikes (BECTS, benign Rolandic epilepsy)	Suspected to be genetic	EEG with spike wave discharges in centrotemporal regions, increased with sleep	Treatment is not always necessary. If frequent or distressing, may use levetiracetam or oxcarbazepine	Onset 4–11 years Seizures often nocturnal and upon awakening, with paresthesia of mouth or tongue, motor phenomena of ipsilateral face occasionally with generalization Seizure remission typically by puberty

20

Dravet syndrome	Most cases associated with *SCN1A* mutation	Genetic testing, EEG nonspecific	Clobazam, levetiracetam, stiripentol, valproate, fenfluramine, cannabidiol	Seizures starting in infancy or early childhood, often associated with heat Developmental regression, prolonged (often myoclonic) seizures
Juvenile myoclonic epilepsy	Suspected to be genetic	Clinical history, sleep-deprived EEG (reveals generalized spike and wave discharges with normal background activity)	Lamotrigine, levetiracetam, valproate, zonisamide	Adolescent onset often with absence seizures Develop myoclonus upon awakening and GTCs. Triggers: sleep deprivation, excessive alcohol intake, photic stimulation Full remission rare, majority require lifelong antiseizure medications.
Panayiotopoulos syndrome (early onset childhood occipital epilepsy)	Unknown	EEG with shifting multifocal spikes (often occipital spikes)	Often not treated Occasionally intermittent benzodiazepines, levetiracetam, oxcarbazepine	Onset 3–6 years Characteristic autonomic component (e.g., vomiting, pallor, hypersalivation, thermoregulatory or cardiorespiratory irregularities) Typically resolves 2–3 years after onset or by puberty

BECTS, Benign epilepsy with centrotemporal spikes; *CNS,* central nervous system; *CT,* computed tomography; *EEG,* electroencephalography; *GTC,* generalized tonic-clonic; *HIE,* hypoxic-ischemic encephalopathy; *LP,* lumbar puncture; *MRI,* magnetic resonance imaging.

seizure). Choose therapy according to seizure type. Consider rectal diazepam (children older than 2), diazepam nasal spray (children >6), midazolam nasal spray (children >12) if seizures are prolonged (>5 minutes) or if there is hemodynamic instability.

(4) Ketogenic diet[48]:

  (a) High-fat, low-carbohydrate therapy typically used for intractable seizures
  (b) Should be managed by trained providers
  (c) Urine/serum ketones can be monitored to assess compliance.
  (d) Side effects include transient GI upset and hyperlipidemia, chronic metabolic acidosis, kidney stones, decreased growth.
  (e) Factor in carbohydrate content of formulations when prescribing medications to a child on a ketogenic diet.
  (f) Avoid dextrose-containing intravenous fluids.

(5) Surgical therapies considered for children with identified seizure focus located in noneloquent cortex and/or those who have failed antiseizure medications.

  (a) Device implantation: Vagus nerve stimulation, deep brain stimulation, responsive neurostimulation (NeuroPace; not yet approved in children)
  (b) Resections: Hemispherectomy, focal resection (e.g., temporal lobectomy), corpus callosotomy

C. Neuromuscular Disorders[49-57]

1. Spinal muscular atrophy (SMA)[49,50]

a. **Etiology:** Motor neuron degeneration caused by autosomal recessive mutations in *SMN1* gene with resulting insufficient levels of SMN protein. Severity correlates inversely with copy number of *SMN2*.

b. **Clinical features:** Varying degrees of symmetric and progressive muscle weakness (proximal > distal) with preserved cognition. Diaphragm preserved. Patients with severe forms do not survive past early childhood without treatment; cause of death is generally respiratory failure. May be identified on newborn screening

c. **Treatment:** Evaluation of weak/hypotonic infant for possible SMA is urgent, as effective treatment (nusinersen [Spinraza], onasemnogene abeparvovec-xioi [Zolgensma], risdiplam [Evrysdi]) is possible, but magnitude of benefit decreases with time.

2. Duchenne or Becker muscular dystrophies (DMD/BMD)[51-53]

a. **Etiology:** X-linked mutation in *DMD* gene, encoding dystrophin, causes disruption of muscular cytoskeleton. Primarily affects males. Duchenne form is more severe and caused by complete disruption of dystrophin; partial function causes milder Becker form.

b. **Clinical features:** Delayed motor milestones and progressive proximal symmetric muscle weakness starting in early childhood leading to wheelchair use for mobility by age 13. Elevated serum CK levels

c. **Treatment:** Corticosteroids (prednisone or deflazacort [Emflaza]) are mainstay.[52] Exon-skipping therapies for patients with susceptible *DMD* mutations (eteplirsen [Exondys 51], viltolarsen [Viltepso], golodirsen [Vyondys 53], casimersen [Amondys 45]).[53] Patients require multidisciplinary management: At high risk for cardiomyopathy, respiratory, and orthopedic complications

3. **Myasthenia gravis**[54-58]

   a. **Etiology:** Autoantibodies binding the acetylcholine receptor (AChR) or muscle-specific kinase (MuSK) impair neuromuscular junction function. Subtypes include transient neonatal myasthenia (resulting from transplacental transfer of maternal antibodies from mother with myasthenia), congenital myasthenic syndrome (genetic defects of neuromuscular junction proteins), and juvenile myasthenia gravis (classic autoimmune disease in children).

   b. **Clinical features:** A key feature is fatigable, variable weakness. Often concentrates in orbital muscles (double vision, ptosis, ophthalmoplegia), or bulbar weakness (slurred/nasal voice, difficulty chewing, swallowing, talking). Can also manifest with generalized weakness of limbs and trunk. Triggers include illness, fever, heat, and some medications. Weakness can worsen with illness and compromised respiratory status. A good bedside test for respiratory function is the single breath count. Ask the patient to count as high as possible in a single breath; the result correlates with vital capacity and <20 suggests impairment.[57] For bedside assessment of bulbar muscle fatigue, use the "slurp test."[58] Ask patient to drink 4 ounces of water through a straw quickly: if slows after 1 or 2 ounces, at risk of bulbar decompensation; if marked slowing or times especially prolonged, at risk for respiratory failure.

   c. **Treatment:** Refer to/consult specialist for management.
      (1) Myasthenic crisis/rapid onset of symptoms: plasmapheresis, IVIG, and IV neostigmine. Evaluate the need to secure definitive airway.
      (2) Obtain thymic imaging nonemergently.
      (3) Avoid use of common medications that can exacerbate myasthenia gravis (Box 20.13).[54,56]
      (4) Chronic management:
         (a) Cholinesterase inhibitor (e.g., pyridostigmine)
         (b) Prednisolone (caution about paradoxical worsening with large initial dose)
         (c) Immunosuppressive, steroid-sparing medications (e.g., azathioprine, mycophenolate, rituximab)
         (d) Consider thymectomy in patients with AChR antibodies

D. Functional Neurologic Disorders (FNDs)[59-62]

1. **Definition:** The DSM-5 defines functional neurologic disorders (FNDs; previously known as conversion disorders) as:
   a. One or more symptoms of altered voluntary motor or sensory function

---

BOX 20.13

MEDICATIONS TO AVOID IN MYASTHENIA GRAVIS

1. Anesthetic: succinylcholine
2. Antibiotic: aminoglycosides (e.g., amikacin, gentamycin, streptomycin), fluoroquinolones (e.g., ciprofloxacin, levofloxacin), and tetracyclines (e.g., doxycycline, minocycline, tetracycline)
3. Antimalarial: chloroquine, hydroxychloroquine
4. Antipsychotic: chlorpromazine, risperidone
5. Cardiac: beta-blocker (e.g., propranolol, sotalol, metoprolol), calcium-channel blocker (e.g., verapamil, amlodipine), antiarrhythmic (e.g., procainamide, quinidine)
6. Immunotherapy: checkpoint inhibitor
7. Other: botulinum toxin, desferrioxamine, magnesium, penicillamine

---

    b. Clinical findings provide evidence of incompatibility between the symptom and recognized neurologic or medical conditions.

    c. The symptom or deficit is not better explained by another medical or mental disorder.

    d. The symptom or deficit causes clinically significant distress or impairment in social, occupational, or other important areas of functioning or warrants medical evaluation.

2. **Etiology:** FNDs can present as changes in sensory, motor, or cognitive function but without a known physiologic cause (e.g., negative imaging, LP, and EEG; and/or nonfocal or inconsistent neurologic exam). Although the etiology is currently unknown, recent research using functional MRIs and other imaging modalities has found differences in neural networks, brain connections, and levels of brain activity during tasks between those with and without FNDs.

3. **Diagnosis:** Once thought to be a diagnosis of exclusion, *FNDs do not necessarily need negative imaging or EEG to confirm.* If there are localizing signs, concern for true seizure, or concern for infection, imaging, EEG, and LP respectively should be obtained as functional overlay is common with other neurologic syndromes. Otherwise, many signs can lead to the diagnosis of FND without further diagnostic studies:

    a. Hoover's sign: weakness of hip extension that returns to normal with contralateral hip flexion against resistance

    b. Breakaway/give-way weakness

    c. Variability in frequency of tremor

    d. No falls, even with excessive swaying or imbalance

    e. Forced closure of eyes during seizure-like activity

    f. Dystonia with fixed-jaw deviation in one direction

4. **Discussions with family:** See eTable 20.8 for examples of ways to explain FNDs and their treatment to patients and families.

5. **Management:** Current mainstays of treatment include physical therapy rehabilitation and cognitive behavioral therapy in either an inpatient or comprehensive outpatient setting. When treating FNDs, use a

multidisciplinary approach involving PT, OT, speech therapy, psychology, psychiatry, and neurology and tailor the treatment to the individual's specific needs.

IV. WEB RESOURCES

- American Academy of Neurology Practice Guidelines: https://www.aan.com/Guidelines
- American Migraine Foundation: https://www.americanmigrainefoundation.org
- Child Neurology Foundation: https://www.childneurologyfoundation.org
- Child Neurology Society: https://www.childneurologysociety.org
- Epilepsy Diagnosis (with videos): https://www.epilepsydiagnosis.org
- Epilepsy Foundation: https://www.epilepsy.com
- Headache resource (from Children's Mercy Kansas): https://www.headachereliefguide.com
- International League Against Epilepsy: https://www.ilae.org
- Muscular Dystrophy Association: https://www.mda.org

REFERENCES

A complete list of references can be found online.

Chapter 21

Nutrition and Growth

Audrey Companiony Hopkins, MD

⊘ See additional content online.
🔊 **Audio Case File 21.1** Pediatric food insecurity

I. ASSESSMENT OF GROWTH

A. Types of Growth Charts

1. Child <24 months: World Health Organization (WHO) international growth charts[1]
2. Child ≥2 years: Centers for Disease Control and Prevention (CDC) growth charts[1]
3. Growth charts for premature infants
   a. Corrected age = infant's chronologic age − number of weeks of prematurity (using 40 weeks as full-term gestation) and should be used up to 3 years[2,3]
   b. Chronologic age should be used if child's growth "catches up" before 3 years.[4]
   c. Oslen, Bertino, and Fenton growth charts can be used to assess growth in premature infants up to 41 weeks (Oslen) to 50 weeks (Fenton).[5] After 4 to 8 weeks postterm, the WHO growth chart can be used.[6]
   d. The choice of growth chart has some variability across practice sites and preferences.[6]
4. Special populations[7,8]
   a. WHO or CDC growth charts are recommended in all cases due to limited reference data for condition-specific growth charts.
   b. Condition-specific growth charts can show families how a specific condition can alter growth potential.
   c. Growth charts have been created for Down syndrome, Prader-Willi syndrome, Williams syndrome, Cornelia de Lange syndrome, Turner syndrome, and Marfan syndrome.

B. Interpretation of Growth Charts[9,10]

1. Stunting/short stature: Length or height <5th percentile
2. Underweight:
   a. Children <2 years: Weight for length/height <5th percentile
   b. Children ≥2 years: Body mass index (BMI) for age <5th percentile or BMI <18.5 kg/m^2

3. Healthy weight: BMI for age 5th percentile to <85th percentile or BMI 18.5 to 24.9 kg/m^2
4. Overweight:
   a. Children <2 years: Weight for length/height >95th percentile
   b. Children ≥2 years: BMI for age ≥85th to <95th percentile or BMI 25 to 29.9 kg/m^2
5. Obese:
   a. Children <2 years: No consensus definition exists.
   b. Children ≥2 years: BMI for age ≥95th percentile or BMI ≥30 kg/m^2
   c. Extended growth charts have been created for children with obesity. These growth charts track modified z-scores (BMI z and %BMI p95) that are based on a fixed SC (one-half the distance between 0 and 2 z-scores), which eliminate the failure of the BMI z-score to track the BMI of children who are persistently greater than the 95th percentile.[11]

C. General Guidelines Regarding Appropriate Growth[12,13]

1. Term infants usually lose approximately 5% to 10% of their birth weight but regain the weight within 2 weeks.
2. Infants should gain 20 to 30 g/day from birth to 3 months, 15 to 22 g/day from 3 to 9 months, and 6 to 11 g/day from 9 to 12 months.
3. Term infants double their birth weight in 4 to 5 months and triple it by 1 year of age.
4. Height doubles from birth to age 3 to 4 years of age.
5. The average size of a 4-year-old is 40 inches and 35 lb.
6. From age 3 to 10 years of age, children grow an average of 2.5 inches per year.

II. MANAGEMENT OF OVERWEIGHT AND OBESE CHILDREN

A. AAP Recommendations for the Prevention of Obesity[14-16]

1. Exclusive breastfeeding until 6 months of age and then breastfeeding maintenance until at least 12 months
2. Daily breakfast and family mealtimes
3. Limit sugary beverages, fast food, and energy-dense foods, and encourage fruits and vegetables.
4. Develop a family media plan with limits and technology-free zones. For infants less than 18 months, no media other than video chatting. If media used with toddlers 18 to 24 months, parents should watch and engage with children during use. For children 2 to 5 years, a max of 1 hour of high-quality programming a day with co-viewing when possible
5. Recommend 60 minutes of moderate-to-vigorous exercise per day.

B. Prevention and Management of Obesity in the Primary Care Setting (Table 21.1)

C. Conditions Associated With Obesity[14]

1. Endocrine:
   a. Polycystic ovarian syndrome

TABLE 21.1

MANAGEMENT AND MONITORING STRATEGIES FOR CHILDREN BASED ON BODY MASS INDEX

BMI	Initial Management	Monitoring—Follow-up
Normal BMI	• Praise child and family. • Screen for genetic dyslipidemia with nonfasting lipid profile between ages 9–11 and 18–21. • Maintain weight velocity.	Next well child visit
Normal BMI that is increasing percentiles (crossing two percentile lines is a risk factor for obesity)	• Screen for genetic dyslipidemia as above • Patient education	Next well child visit
Overweight BMI	• Patient education • If health risk factors, obtain fasting glucose, hemoglobin A1c or oral glucose tolerance test, lipid profile, ALT, and AST.	2–4 weeks
Obese BMI	• Patient education • Obtain fasting glucose, hemoglobin A1c or oral glucose tolerance test, lipid profile, ALT, and AST. • Some specialist clinics screen for vitamin D deficiency and insulin resistance (i.e., measure fasting insulin), but their clinical utility and cost effectiveness is unclear. • No guidelines on which age to start laboratory screening, but some experts start at 2 years of age • Consider other labs (e.g., thyroid studies, cortisol) based on clinical picture.	2–4 weeks

Further follow-up and management for those who are overweight or obese:

(a) At each follow-up, record weight, measure blood pressure, and use an empathetic and empowering counseling style (e.g., motivational interviewing).

(b) Establish goals: Positive behavior change, weight maintenance, or decrease in BMI velocity. Children aged 2 to 5 years who have obesity should not lose more than 1 pound/month; children and adolescents with obesity should not lose more than an average of 2 pounds/week.

(c) If no improvement after 3 to 6 months, refer to structured weight management program. If no improvement after 3 to 6 months, the next step is a comprehensive, multidisciplinary approach. If no improvement, refer for evaluation at a tertiary care center for medication management and weight reduction surgery.

ALT, Alanine aminotransferase; *AST*, aspartate aminotransferase; *BMI*, body mass index.

b. Precocious puberty
   c. Prediabetes/type 2 diabetes
2. Gastrointestinal:
   a. Cholelithiasis
   b. Gastroesophageal reflux
   c. Nonalcoholic fatty liver disease
3. Neurologic: Pseudotumor cerebri
4. Orthopedic:
   a. Blount disease
   b. Slipped capital femoral epiphysis (SCFE)
5. Behavioral health:
   a. Anxiety
   b. Binge eating disorder
   c. Depression

III. MALNUTRITION IN INFANTS AND CHILDREN

A. Defining Malnutrition[15]

NOTE: Also called growth failure or under-nutrition; previously called failure to thrive

1. Condition of under-nutrition generally identified in the first 3 years of life
2. Can be described by the following growth scenarios:
   a. Primary indicators when single data point available:
      (1) Weight for length/height z-score
      (2) BMI for age z-score
      (3) Length/height for age z- score
      (4) Wasting or mid-upper arm circumference (MUAC)
      (5) Presence of nutritional edema
   b. Primary indicators when two or more data points available:
      (1) Weight gain velocity (<2 years old)
      (2) Degree of weight loss (2 to 20 years of age)
      (3) Deceleration in weight for length/height z-score
      (4) Inadequate nutrient intake

B. Classifying the Degree to Which a Patient Is Malnourished (Table 21.2)[16]

1. Acute (duration <3 months)
2. Chronic or stunting (duration >3 months); suggested by height/length for age

C. Resources for Determining Z-scores[17]

1. PediTools (https://www.peditools.org)
2. Standardized height and weight calculator (https://www.quesgen.com/BMIPedsCalc.php)
3. CDC website (https://www.cdc.gov/growthcharts/zscore.htm)
4. WHO website (https://www.who.int/childgrowth/standards/chart_catalogue)

TABLE 21.2

DEFINITIONS FOR CATEGORY OF MALNUTRITION

	Mild	Moderate	Severe
Weight for height and BMI	−1 to −1.9 z-score	−2 to −2.9 z-score	−3 or greater z-score
Mid-upper arm circumference z-score[a]	≥ −1 to −1.9	≥ −2 to −2.9	≥ −3
Weight gain velocity (<2 years)	Less than 75% of the norm for expected weight gain	Less than 50% of the norm for expected weight gain	Less than 25% of the norm for expected weight gain
Weight loss (2–20 years)	5% usual body weight	7.5% usual body weight	10% usual body weight
Deceleration in weight for length/height z-score	Decline of 1 z-score	Decline of 2 z-scores	Decline of 3 z-scores
Inadequate nutritional intake	51%–75% estimated energy/protein need	26%–50% estimated energy/protein need	<26% estimated energy/protein need

[a]See Section IIIC for how to calculate z-score.

BMI, Body mass index.

Modified from Becker P, Carney LN, Corkins MR, et al. Primary indicators when 2 or more data points available. Consensus statement of the Academy of Nutrition and Dietetics/American Society for Parenteral and Enteral Nutrition: indicators recommended for the identification and documentation of pediatric malnutrition. *Nutr Clin Pract*. 2015;30(10):147–161.

D. Differential Diagnosis of Malnutrition[18]

1. Secondary to disease/injury
2. Decreased intake (e.g., fluid restriction, cardiac failure, anorexia nervosa, food insecurity, food aversions)
3. Increased requirement/hypermetabolism (e.g., burns, malignancy, diabetes mellitus, inborn errors of metabolism)
4. Excessive loss (e.g., chronic diarrhea, burn, proteinuria)
5. Malabsorption (e.g., Crohn disease, cystic fibrosis)

E. Physical Exam Findings Consistent With Malnutrition[19-21]

1. Fat loss (e.g., orbital, buccal, triceps, ribs)
2. Muscle wasting (e.g., temporalis, pectoralis, deltoid, latissimus dorsi, quadriceps)
3. Edema
4. Functional limitations (e.g., hand grip strength)
5. Micronutrient deficiencies
   a. Iron
      (1) Exam findings: Koilonychias, pale conjunctiva and nail beds
      (2) Risk factors: Low birth weight, feeding problems, poor growth, exclusive breastfeeding >6 months
   b. Vitamin C
      (1) Exam findings: Perifollicular hemorrhage, scorbutic tongue, bleeding gum, bruising

      (2) Risk factors: Limited diet, infant on cow's milk, dialysis, malabsorption

  c. Vitamin A

      (1) Exam findings: Bitot spot, follicular hyperkeratosis

      (2) Risk factors: Limited diet, fat malabsorption, alcoholism, cystic fibrosis, short bowel

  d. Vitamin B_6

      (1) Exam findings: Seborrheic dermatitis, angular palpebritis, hypertrophied papillae

      (2) Risk factors: Dialysis, sickle cell disease, malabsorption; diuretic, anticonvulsant, contraceptive, and isoniazid use

  e. Zinc

      (1) Exam findings: Dermatitis, vesicobullous lesions, diaper rash

      (2) Risk factors: Prematurity, parenteral nutrition (PN), cholestasis, diarrhea, high phytate intake, celiac or Crohn disease, AIDS, liver or renal disease, alcoholism, trauma, burn, sleeve gastrectomy, diuretic and valproate use

  f. Vitamin D[22]

      (1) Exam findings: Widening of the wrists and ankles, genu varum or valgum, prominence of the costochondral junctions (rachitic rosary), delayed closure of fontanelles, craniotabes, and frontal bossing

      (2) Risk factors: Exclusive breastfeeding beyond 3 to 6 months, prematurity, maternal vitamin D deficiency, strict vegetarian diets/cult diets, malabsorption disorders (cystic fibrosis, Crohn disease, cholestatic hepatopathies)

F. Diagnostic Evaluation of Malnutrition[23-26]

1. There is no consensus on workup algorithm.
2. Routine labs and imaging are often low yield and generally not recommended; workup should be guided by clinical suspicion.
3. If warranted, reasonable initial testing could include complete blood count, complete metabolic panel, urinalysis, and erythrocyte sedimentation rate.
4. If the child's length has decelerated and is below 50%, can screen for hypothyroidism and growth hormone deficiency
5. If recurrent or severe upper respiratory or opportunistic infections, consider testing for human immunodeficiency and tuberculosis and measuring immunoglobulin and complement levels.
6. Based on clinical suspicion, can consider celiac screening, sweat chloride testing, echocardiogram, hepatitis serology, stool studies
7. Consider hospitalization for observed feeding if the child fails outpatient management, suspicion for abuse/neglect or traumatic injury, severe psychological caregiver impairment, serious malnutrition, or at risk for re-feeding.

G. Red Flags That Suggest a Medical Cause of Malnutrition[27]

1. Developmental delay or dysmorphic features

2. Cardiac findings (e.g., murmur, edema, jugular venous distention)
3. Failure to gain weight despite adequate calories
4. Organomegaly or lymphadenopathy
5. Recurrent or severe respiratory, mucocutaneous, or urinary infections
6. Recurrent vomiting, diarrhea, or dehydration

H. Approach to the Management of Malnourished Patients[28,29] (Box 21.1)

1. Address the etiology of malnutrition.
2. Approximately 20% to 30% more energy may be required to achieve catch-up growth in children. This should continue until the previous growth percentiles are regained.
3. Catch-up linear growth may lag several months behind weight.
4. See Box 21.1 for instructions on the calculation of catch-up growth requirements.
5. Screen for food insecurity and offer social work and community resources.
6. Pharmacotherapy (e.g., cyproheptadine, megestrol) may be helpful for patients with significant underlying diseases (e.g., cancer, cystic fibrosis).

IV. RE-FEEDING SYNDROME

A. Patients at Risk of Developing Re-feeding Syndrome[19]

1. Chronic malnutrition (e.g., prolonged fasting ≥5 days, malignancy)
2. Renal/endocrine (e.g., chronic diuretic use, diabetic hyperglycemic hyperosmolar syndrome)
3. Gastrointestinal loss (e.g., inflammatory bowel disease, chronic pancreatitis, short bowel)
4. Infectious (e.g., AIDS, tuberculosis)
5. Cardiac (e.g., congenital heart disease)
6. Pulmonary (e.g., cystic fibrosis)

BOX 21.1

DETERMINING CATCH-UP GROWTH REQUIREMENTS

1. Plot the child's height and weight on the appropriate growth charts.
2. Determine recommended calories required for age [recommended dietary allowances (RDA)].
3. Determine the ideal weight (50th percentile) for child's height.
4. Multiply the RDA calories by ideal body weight for height (kg).
5. Divide this value by the child's actual weight (kg). For example, for a 12-month-old boy whose weight is 7 kg and length is 72 cm, RDA for age would be 98 kcal/kg/day, and ideal body weight for height is 9 kg (50th percentile weight for height); thus his catch-up growth requirement would be as follows:

$$98 \text{ kcal/kg/day} \times (9 \text{ kg}\,/\,7 \text{ kg}) = 126 \text{ kcal/kg/day}$$

Modified from Nestle Health Science. Calorie and protein requirements. Pediatric nutrition helpful hints: Specialized nutrition for your most vulnerable patients. https://www.nestlehealthscience.us/asset-library/documents/resources/pediatric%20helpful%20hints.pdf; and Corrales KM, Utter SL. Failure to thrive. In: Samour PQ, Helm KK, Lang CE, eds. *Handbook of Pediatric Nutrition.* 2nd ed. Aspen Publishers; 1999:406.

7. Psychiatric (e.g., anorexia nervosa, chronic alcohol use)
8. Social (e.g., child abuse/neglect, homelessness, food insecurity)

B. Management of Re-feeding Syndrome[20]

1. Maintain continuous cardiorespiratory monitoring or check vital signs every 4 hours, depending on level of concern.
2. Ensure strict intake and output monitoring with calorie count and daily weights.
3. Obtain at least daily basic metabolic panel with phosphorous and magnesium. Obtain more frequently if electrolyte replacement needed, or if there are concerning trends.
4. Measure pre-albumin, albumin, zinc.
5. Consider giving thiamine 100 to 300 mg PO daily (or 50 to 100 mg IV) × 3 days before feeding. There is some debate whether this is required.
6. Give a multivitamin daily.
7. Feeding should not proceed without appropriate supplementation.
8. Recommendations vary, but start at $\frac{1}{4}$ to $\frac{1}{2}$ of estimated caloric needs depending on degree of risk.
9. Dietary advancement over 3 to 7 days with caloric increases of 10% to 25% per day until recommended caloric goals achieved.
10. Enteral feeding is preferred over parenteral feeding.

V. NUTRITIONAL NEEDS OF HEALTHY CHILDREN

A. Dietary Allowances for Carbohydrates and Protein (Table 21.3)
B. Fat Requirements (Table 21.4)
C. Vitamin Requirements (Tables 21.5 and 21.6)

1. Vitamin D[21-23]

TABLE 21.3

RECOMMENDED DIETARY ALLOWANCES: CALORIE AND PROTEIN REQUIREMENTS[a]

Category	Age (years)	kcal/kg	Protein g/kg
Infants	0–0.5	108	2.2
	0.5–1	98	1.6
Children	1–3	102	1.2
	4–6	90	1.1
	7–10	70	1.0
Males	11–14	55	1.0
	15–18	45	0.9
	19–24	40	0.8
Females	11–14	47	1.0
	15–18	40	0.8
	19–24	38	0.8

[a]This recommended dietary allowance (RDA) by definition meets the needs of 97% of healthy children. This is a quick reference to estimate calorie and protein needs, but further estimation may be required, using various other energy and protein need equations and factors, typically used by a registered dietitian.
Data from Nestle Health Science. Calorie and protein requirements. Pediatric nutrition helpful hints: Specialized nutrition for your most vulnerable patients. https://www.nestlehealthscience.us/asset-library/documents/resources/pediatric%20helpful%20hints.pdf; and National Academy of Sciences. *Recommended Dietary Allowances.* 10th ed. National Academy Press; 1989:33–36.

TABLE 21.4

FAT REQUIREMENTS: ADEQUATE INTAKE[a]

Age	Total Fat (g/day)	Linoleic Acid (g/day)	α-Linolenic Acid (g/day)
0–6 months	31	4.4 (n-6 PUFA)	0.5 (n-3 PUFA)
7–12 months	30	4.6 (n-6 PUFA)	0.5 (n-3 PUFA)
1–3 years	[b]	7	0.7
4–8 years	[b]	10	0.9
9–13 years, boys	[b]	12	1.2
9–13 years, girls	[b]	10	1.0
14–18 years, boys	[b]	16	1.6
14–18 years, girls	[b]	11	1.1
Pregnancy	[b]	13	1.4
Lactation	[b]	13	1.3

[a]If sufficient scientific evidence is not available to establish a recommended dietary allowance (RDA), an adequate intake (AI) is usually developed. For healthy breastfed infants, the AI is the mean intake. The AI for other life stage and gender groups is believed to cover the needs of all healthy individuals in the group, but a lack of data or uncertainty in the data prevents specifying with confidence the percentage of individuals covered by this intake.

[b]No AI, estimated average requirement (EAR), or RDA established.

PUFA, Polyunsaturated fatty acid.

From Otten JJ, Hellwig JP, Meyers LD, eds. *Dietary Reference Intakes: The Essential Guide to Nutrient Requirements.* National Academies Press; 2006.

    a. Breastfed and partially breastfed infants should be supplemented with 400 international units (IU) per day beginning in the first few days of life until 12 months.

    b. Formula-fed infants should be supplemented until the infant is taking 34 oz of formula per day.

    c. For preterm infants tolerating full enteral feeds and weighing >1500–2000 g, supplement with 400 IU/day. Supplement with 200–400 IU/day for infants <1500 g.

    d. Supplement children and adolescents with 600 IU/day if the child is ingesting <1000 mL (34 oz) per day of vitamin D fortified milk or not taking that amount through fortified foods.

    e. At-risk children (e.g., cystic fibrosis) and those with laboratory confirmed vitamin D insufficiency/deficiency should also be supplemented.

    f. See Table 21.6 for interpreting vitamin D levels.

2. Folate[24,25]

    a. All women capable of becoming pregnant should consume 400 mCg from supplements or diet.

    b. This should continue as women enter prenatal care.

    c. If a woman had a prior pregnancy with a neural tube defect and is planning another pregnancy, she should consume 4 mg of folic acid daily (requires a prescription) at least 4 weeks before becoming pregnant and continue through the first 12 weeks of pregnancy.

D. Mineral Requirements (Table 21.7)

1. Iron[26]

TABLE 21.5

DIETARY REFERENCE INTAKES: RECOMMENDED INTAKES FOR INDIVIDUALS—VITAMINS

Life Stage	Vit. A[a] (IU)	Vit. C (mg/day)	Vit. D[b,c] (IU)	Vit. E[d] (IU)	Vit. K (mCg/day)	Thiamin (mg/day)	Riboflavin (mg/day)	Niacin[e] (mg/day)	Vit. B$_6$ (mg/day)	Folate[f] (mCg/day)	Vit. B$_{12}$ (mCg/day)	Pantothenic Acid (mg/day)	Biotin (mCg/day)	Choline[g] (mg/day)
INFANTS														
0–6 months	1333	40*	400*	4*	2.0	0.2*	0.3*	2*	0.1*	65*	0.4*	1.7*	5*	125*
7–12 months	1666	50*	400*	5*	2.5	0.3*	0.4*	4*	0.3*	80*	0.5*	1.8*	6*	150*
CHILDREN														
1–3 years	1000	15	600*	6	30	0.5	0.5	6	0.5	150	0.9	2*	8*	200*
4–8 years	1333	25	600*	7	55	0.6	0.6	8	0.6	200	1.2	3*	12*	25*
MALES														
9–13 years	2000	45	600*	11	60	0.9	0.9	12	1.0	300	1.8	4*	20*	375*
14–18 years	3000	75	600*	15	75	1.2	1.3	16	1.3	400	2.4	5*	25*	550*
19–30 years	3000	90	600*	15	120	1.2	1.3	16	1.3	400	2.4	5*	30*	550*
FEMALES														
9–13 years	2000	45	600*	11	60	0.9	0.9	12	1.0	300	1.8	4*	20*	375*
14–18 years	2333	65	600*	15	75	1.0	1.0	14	1.2	400	2.4	5*	25*	400*
19–30 years	2333	75	600*	15	90	1.1	1.1	14	1.3	400	2.4	5*	30*	425*

Continued

21

TABLE 21.5

DIETARY REFERENCE INTAKES: RECOMMENDED INTAKES FOR INDIVIDUALS—VITAMINS—CONT'D

Life Stage	Vit. A[a] (IU)	Vit. C (mg/day)	Vit. D[b,c] (IU)	Vit. E[d] (IU)	Vit. K (mCg/day)	Thiamin (mg/day)	Riboflavin (mg/day)	Niacin[e] (mg/day)	Vit. B6 (mg/day)	Folate[f] (mCg/day)	Vit. B12 (mCg/day)	Pantothenic Acid (mg/day)	Biotin (mCg/day)	Choline[g] (mg/day)
PREGNANCY														
≤18 years	2500	80	600*	15	75*	1.4	1.4	18	1.9	600	2.6	6*	30*	450*
19–30 years	2567	85	600*	15	90*	1.4	1.4	18	1.9	600	2.6	6*	30*	450*
LACTATION														
≤18 years	4000	115	600*	19	75*	1.4	1.6	17	2.0	500	2.8	7*	35*	550*
19–30 years	4333	120	600*	19	90*	1.4	1.6	17	2.0	500	2.8	7*	35*	550*

[a]One international unit (IU) = 0.3 mCg retinol equivalent.

[b]One mCg cholecalciferol = 40 IU vitamin D.

[c]In the absence of adequate exposure to sunlight.

[d]One IU = 1 mg vitamin E.

[e]As niacin equivalents (NE). 1 mg of niacin = 60 mg of tryptophan; 0 to 6 months = preformed niacin (not NE).

[f]As dietary folate equivalents (DFE). 1 DFE = 1 mCg food folate = 0.6 mCg of folic acid from fortified food or as a supplement consumed with food = 0.5 mCg of a supplement taken on an empty stomach.

[g]Although AIs have been set for choline, there are few data to assess whether a dietary supply of choline is required at all life stages, and it may be that the choline requirement can be met by endogenous synthesis at some of these stages.

NOTE: This table presents recommended dietary allowances (RDAs) in **bold type** and adequate intakes (AIs) in regular type followed by an asterisk (*). RDAs and AIs may both be used as goals for individual intake. RDAs are set to meet the needs of almost all (97% to 98%) individuals in a group. For healthy breastfed infants, the AI is the mean intake. The AI for other life stage and gender groups is believed to cover needs of all individuals in the group, but lack of data or uncertainty in the data prevents specifying with confidence the percentage of individuals covered by this intake.

Modified from Otten JJ, Hellwig JP, Meyers LD, eds. *Dietary Reference Intakes: The Essential Guide to Nutrient Requirements.* National Academies Press; 2006. http://www.nap.edu

TABLE 21.6

VITAMIN D LABORATORY INTERPRETATION

25-Hydroxy Vitamin D	Value (ng/mL)
Severe deficiency	<10
Deficiency	<10–20
Insufficiency	>20–<30
Optimal level	≥30[a]

[a]Cutoff values are not yet well defined. Controversy exists regarding the optimal 25-hydroxy vitamin D level. Some experts recommend a level of 20 to 30 ng/mL as being sufficient. These are the Johns Hopkins Hospital Pediatrics guidelines used for dosing.

NOTE: 1,25-dihydroxy vitamin D is the physiologically active form, but 25-hydroxy vitamin D is the value to monitor for vitamin D deficiency as it approximates body stores of vitamin D.

a. Breastfed term infants should receive 1 mg/kg/day of an oral iron supplement beginning at 4 months of age, preferably from iron-fortified cereal or, alternatively, elemental iron.

b. Breastfed preterm infants should receive 2 mg/kg/day by 1 month of age, which should continue until the infant is weaned to iron-fortified formula or begins eating complementary foods.

c. Formula-fed term infants receive adequate iron from fortified formula.

d. Formula-fed preterm infants need 2 mg/kg/day, which is the amount supplied by iron-fortified formulas.

2. Fluoride[30]

a. Consider fluoride supplementation for those patients who use bottled water or home filtration systems. Some home water treatment systems can reduce fluoride levels.

b. For infants and children at high risk for the development of caries, fluoride supplementation ranging from 0.25 to 1 mg/day is recommended, according to the American Dental Association's schedule.

c. Fluoridated toothpaste is recommended for all children starting at tooth eruption, using a smear (grain-of-rice-sized) until age 3 and then a pea-sized amount after that time.

E. Fiber Requirements (Table 21.8)

VI. BREASTFEEDING AND THE USE OF HUMAN MILK

A. Benefits of Breast Milk[31]

1. Decreased risk of infections (e.g., otitis media, respiratory), necrotizing enterocolitis, inflammatory bowel, sudden infant death syndrome (SIDS)

2. Decreased incidence of atopic conditions, obesity, and diabetes

B. Contraindications to Breastfeeding[31] (Box 21.2)

1. Tobacco smoking is not contraindicated but is strongly discouraged because of an association with increased risks of SIDS, respiratory disease, and infections in exposed infants.

TABLE 21.7

DIETARY REFERENCE INTAKES: RECOMMENDED INTAKES—ELEMENTS

Life Stage	Calcium (mg/day)	Chromium (mcg/day)	Copper (mcg/day)	Fluoride (mg/day)	Iodine (mcg/day)	Iron (mg/day)	Magnesium (mg/day)	Manganese (mg/day)	Molybdenum (mcg/day)	Phosphorus (mg/day)	Selenium (mcg/day)	Zinc (mg/day)
INFANTS												
0–6 months	200*	0.2*	200*	0.01*	110*	0.27*	30*	0.003*	2*	100*	15*	2*
7–12 months	260*	5.5*	220*	0.5*	130*	11	75*	0.6*	3*	275*	20*	3
CHILDREN												
1–3 years	700	11*	340	0.7*	90	7	80	1.2*	17	460	20	3
4–8 years	1000	15*	440	1.0*	90	10	130	1.5*	22	500	30	5
MALES												
9–13 years	1300	25*	700	2*	120	8	240	1.9*	34	1250	40	8
14–18 years	1300	35*	890	3*	150	11	410	2.2*	43	1250	55	11
19–30 years	1000	35*	900	4*	150	8	400	2.3*	45	700	55	11
FEMALES												
9–13 years	1300	21*	700	2*	120	8	240	1.6*	34	1250	40	8
14–18 years	1300	24*	890	3*	150	15	360	1.6*	43	1250	55	9
19–30 years	1000	25*	900	3*	150	18	310	1.8*	45	700	55	8
PREGNANCY												
≤18 years	1300	29*	1000	3*	220	27	400	2.0*	50	1250	60	13
19–30 years	1000	30*	1000	3*	220	27	350	2.0*	50	700	60	11
LACTATION												
≤18 years	1300	44*	1300	3*	290	10	360	2.6*	50	1250	70	14
19–30 years	1000	45*	1300	3*	290	9	310	2.6*	50	700	70	12

NOTE: This table presents recommended dietary allowances (RDAs) in **bold type** and adequate intakes (AIs) in regular type followed by an asterisk (*). RDAs and AIs may both be used as goals for individual intake. RDAs are set to meet the needs of almost all (97% to 98%) individuals in a group. For healthy breastfed infants, the AI is the mean intake. The AI for other life stage and gender groups is believed to cover needs of all individuals in the group, but lack of data or uncertainty in the data prevents specifying with confidence the percentage of individuals covered by this intake.

Modified from Otten JJ, Hellwig JP, Meyers LD, eds. *Dietary Reference Intakes: The Essential Guide to Nutrient Requirements.* National Academies Press; 2006. Includes updates from Ross AC, Taylor CL, Yaktine AL, Del Valle HB,

TABLE 21.8

FIBER REQUIREMENTS: ADEQUATE INTAKE[a]

Age	Total Fiber (g/day)
0–12 months	Not determined
1–3 years	19
4–8 years	25
9–13 years, boys	31
9–13 years, girls	26
14–18 years, boys	38
14–18 years, girls	26
Pregnancy	28
Lactation	29

[a]Adequate intake (AI). If sufficient scientific evidence unavailable to establish recommended dietary allowance (RDA), an AI is usually developed. For healthy breastfed infants, the AI is the mean intake. AI for other life-stage and gender groups is believed to cover the needs of all healthy individuals in the group, but a lack of data or uncertainty in the data prevents specifying with confidence the percentage of individuals covered by this intake.

g, Grams.

Modified from Otten JJ, Hellwig JP, Meyers LD, eds. *Dietary Reference Intakes: The Essential Guide to Nutrient Requirements.* National Academies Press; 2006.

BOX 21.2

CONTRAINDICATIONS TO BREASTFEEDING

Infant galactosemia

Maternal human T-cell lymphotropic virus I/II infection

Maternal untreated brucellosis

Maternal HIV (developed countries)

Maternal active, untreated tuberculosis (may give expressed BM)

Maternal active HSV lesions on breast (may give expressed BM)

Maternal varicella infection 5 days before through 2 days after delivery (may give expressed BM)

Maternal use of diagnostic or therapeutic radioactive isotopes, antimetabolites, or chemotherapeutic agents

Illicit street drugs such as cannabis, cocaine, phencyclidine, etc.

BM, Breast milk; *HIV,* human immunodeficiency virus; *HSV,* herpes simplex virus.
Modified from American Academy of Pediatrics, Section on Breastfeeding. Policy Statement—Breastfeeding and the Use of Human Milk. *Pediatrics.* 2012;129:e827–e841.

2. Alcohol should be limited to the occasional intake of 2 oz of liquor, 8 oz of wine, or two beers for the average 60 kg woman >2 hours prior to the onset of nursing.
3. Methadone and buprenorphine are not contraindications, if the mother is in a stable maintenance program and not using street drugs.

C. Use of Milk Bank Donor Human Milk[32]

1. Most commonly used in low-birth-weight infants (<1.5 kg)
2. Can be considered in infants with intestinal disease with documented intolerance to specialized infant formulas

D. Safe Handling of Breast Milk[33]

1. Freshly expressed or pumped milk can be stored at room temperature for up to 4 hours, in the refrigerator for up to 4 days, in the freezer for approximately 6 months (up to 12 months), and in an insulated cooler bag with frozen packs up to 24 hours while traveling.
2. Once breast milk is thawed to room temperature or warmed, it should be used within 2 hours.

E. Breastfeeding Resources

See Section IX.C.

VII. ENTERAL NUTRITION

A. Feeding the Healthy Infant

1. Recommended formula amount by age[34]
   a. 1st days of life: 1 to 2 ounces every 2 to 3 hours
   b. 1st month: 2 to 4 ounces every 3 to 4 hours
   c. 2nd month: 5 to 6 ounces every 4 to 5 hours
   d. 3rd to 5th month: 6 to 7 ounces every 4 to 5 hours
   e. 6th to 8th month: 24 to 32 ounces in 24 hours
   f. 8th to 10th month: 16 to 32 ounces in 24 hours
   g. 10th to 12th month: 12 to 24 ounces in 24 hours
2. Properties of formula options for healthy infants and toddlers (Table 21.9)
3. Appropriate preparation and fortification of formulas (Table 21.10)
4. Methods to further increase calories, protein, carbohydrate, fat, or a combination (Table 21.11)

B. Available Formulas for Patients With Specific Clinical Conditions or for Those Requiring Special Diets (Tables 21.12 and 21.13)

C. Use of Enteral Tube Feeds[35]

1. Insufficient oral intake (e.g., anorexia nervosa, food aversion, malabsorption, increased needs)
2. As a primary therapy (e.g., metabolic or inflammatory bowel disease, fasting intolerance)
3. Oral motor dysfunction (e.g., prematurity, neuromuscular and neurologic disease)
4. Abnormal gastrointestinal tract (e.g., congenital malformations, esophageal stenosis, intestinal pseudo-obstruction)
5. Injury/critical illness (e.g., burn, trauma, surgery, sepsis, malignancy)

D. Features of the Most Common Oral Rehydration Solutions (Table 21.14)

VIII. PARENTERAL NUTRITION

A. Indications for the Use of Parenteral Nutrition[36-38]

1. Inability to feed enterally or when alimentation via gastrointestinal tract is restricted >3 to 5 days (or earlier for premature infants and neonates)
2. Chronic gastrointestinal dysfunction and/or malabsorption
3. Increased gastrointestinal losses or requirements

TABLE 21.9
PROPERTIES OF FEEDING OPTIONS FOR HEALTHY INFANTS AND CHILDREN

	Examples	Calories (kcal/oz)	Carbohydrate Source	Protein Source	Unique Properties	Indications
Human milk		20	Lactose	Human milk	See Section VI.A	Preferred for most infants
Cow's milk–based formulas	Enfamil Infant, Similac Advance, Similac Sensitive, Gerber Good Start Gentle	20	Lactose	Cow's milk		Typical term infant
Toddler/child	Boost Kids Essential, Carnation Instant Breakfast Essential, Compleat Pediatric, Nutren Junior, Pediasure Enteral, Pediasure	20–45	Lactose	Cow's milk	Milk-based Contain added iron, vitamin C, E, and zinc, DHA/AA, calcium	Age 1 year to 10–13 years

AA, Amino acids; *DHA*, docosahexaenoic acid; *kcal*, kilocalorie; *oz*, ounce.
Data from O'Connor N. Infant formula. *Am Fam Phys.* 2009;79(7):565–570, Table 21.9; and Comparison of breast milk and available infant formulas: https://www.aafp.org/afp/2009/0401/p565.html, Table 1.

TABLE 21.10

PREPARATION OF INFANT FORMULAS FOR MOST FULL-TERM STANDARD AND SOY FORMULAS[a]

Formula Type	Desired Caloric Concentration (kcal/oz)	Amount of Formula 13 oz = 1 can	Water (oz)	Approximate Final Volume (oz)
Liquid concentrates (40 kcal/oz)	20	13 oz	13 oz	26 oz
	22	13 oz	11 oz	24 oz
	24	13 oz	9 oz	22 oz
	26	13 oz	7 oz	20 oz
	27	13 oz	6 oz (3/4 cup)	19 oz
	30	13 oz	4.3 oz	17.3 oz
Powder (approx 44 kcal/scoop)[b]	20	1 scoop	2 oz	2 oz
	22	3 scoop	5.5 oz	6 oz
	24	3 scoops	5 oz	5.5 oz
	26	6 scoops	9 oz	10 oz
	27	6 scoops	8.5 oz	10 oz
	30	6 scoops	7.5 oz	9 oz

[a]Does not apply to Enfacare, Neocate Infant, Alfamino Infant, or NeoSure. Of note, Enfamil A.R. and Similac for Spit-Up is not recommended to be concentrated greater than 24 kcal/oz. Use a packed measure for Nutramigen and Pregestimil; all others unpacked powder.

[b]Slight variations in brands, range 40 to 45 kcal/scoop.

kcal, Kilocalorie; *oz*, ounce.

Modified from University of Michigan Hospitals & Health Centers. Powdered and liquid concentrate recipe chart. https://www.med.umich.edu/1libr/pa/FormulaAdjustmentstandard.pdf

TABLE 21.11

COMMON CALORIC MODULARS[a]

Component	Calories
PROTEIN	
Beneprotein (powder)	25 kcal/scoop (6 g protein)
ProSource protein powder	30 kcal/scoop (6 g protein)
Complete Amino Acid Mix (powder)	3.28 kcal/g (0.82 g protein)
	2.9 g/teaspoon (9.5 kcal, 2.38 g protein)
Abbott Liquid Protein Fortifier	0.67 kcal/mL (0.167 g protein/mL)
CARBOHYDRATE	
SolCarb	3.75 kcal/g; 23 kcal/tbsp
Polycal	3.84 kcal/g; 28 kcal/tbsp; 20 kcal/scoop
FAT	
MCT oil[b]	7.7 kcal/mL
Vegetable oil	8.3 kcal/mL
Microlipid (emulsified LCT)	4.5 kcal/mL
Liquigen (emulsified MCT)[b]	4.5 kcal/mL
FAT AND CARBOHYDRATE	
Duocal (powder)	42 kcal/tbsp; 25 kcal/scoop (59% carb, 41% fat, 35% fat as MCT)

[a]Use these caloric supplements when you want to increase protein, carbohydrate, or fat; or when you have reached the maximum concentration tolerated and wish to further increase caloric density.

[b]Medium-chain triglyceride (MCT) oil is unnecessary unless there is fat malabsorption.

Carb, Carbohydrate; *g*, grams; *kcal*, kilocalorie; *LCT*, long chain–triglyceride; *MCT*, medium chain–triglyceride; *mL*, milliliter; *tbsp*, tablespoon.

TABLE 21.12

FORMULA PROPERTIES AND INDICATIONS FOR SPECIFIC CONDITIONS

	Examples	Calories (kcal/oz)	Carbohydrate Source	Protein Source	Unique Properties	Indications
Human milk fortifiers					Contain protein, carbohydrates, fat, vitamins, and minerals	Preterm infants, especially <1500 g who are receiving human milk
Preterm formulas	Enfamil Premature, Similac Special Care Advance	24	Lactose	Cow's milk	Higher protein, calcium, magnesium, phosphorous, and vitamin A and D Contain taurine	Generally use until infant weighs 1800–2000 g or until 34 weeks corrected gestational age
Enriched or transitional formula	Enfamil Enfacare, Similac Neosure	22	Lactose	Cow's milk	Higher protein, calcium, magnesium, and phosphorous	Transition from preterm to enriched as described above until age 6–12 months
Cow's milk–based formulas	Enfamil Infant, Similac Advance, Similac Sensitive	20	Lactose	Cow's milk		Typical term infant
Soy formulas	America's Store Brand Soy, Enfamil ProSobee, Gerber Good Start Soy, Similac Soy Isomil, Similac for Diarrhea	20	Corn-based	Soy	Contain higher protein concentration and supplemental amino acids	Galactosemia, congenital lactase deficiency, strict vegan families Should NOT be used for preterm infants (increased risk of poor growth, osteopenia of prematurity)

Continued

21

TABLE 21.12

FORMULA PROPERTIES AND INDICATIONS FOR SPECIFIC CONDITIONS—CONT'D

	Examples	Calories (kcal/oz)	Carbohydrate Source	Protein Source	Unique Properties	Indications
						Avoided in infants with milk protein intolerance given association with soy allergy
Hydrolyzed casein	Alimentum, Nutramigen, Pregestimil	20	Corn or sucrose	Casein	Easier to digest Hypoallergenic	IgE-mediated milk protein allergy Fat malabsorption
Partially hydrolyzed whey	Gerber Good Start Gentle, Gerber Good Start Soothe, Similac Pro-Total Comfort	20	Corn or sucrose	Hydrolyzed whey + casein or 100% whey	Reduced lactose content	May reduce risk of developing allergic diseases (especially eczema), improve gastric emptying, decrease colic, but data limited and may differ between products
Amino acid	Neocate Infant and Junior, Elecare Infant and Junior, Alfamino Infant and Junior, PurAmino Infant and Junior	20	Corn or sucrose	Amino acids	Easier to digest Nonallergenic	Milk protein allergy Severe malabsorption

g, Grams; *kcal,* kilocalorie; *oz,* ounce.

Data from O'Connor N. Infant formula. *Am Fam Phys.* 2009;79(7):565–570; Comparison of breast milk and available infant formulas: https://www.aafp.org/afp/2009/0401/p565.html. Additional sources listed in references.

TABLE 21.13

ADDITIONAL FORMULAS FOR SPECIAL CLINICAL CIRCUMSTANCES

INFANTS	
Severe carbohydrate intolerance	MJ3232A
	Ross Carbohydrate Free (RCF)
Requiring lower calcium and phosphorus	Similac PM 60/40

TODDLERS AND YOUNG CHILDREN AGED 1–10 YEARS	
Vegetarian, lactose intolerance, or milk protein intolerance	Bright Beginnings Soy Pediatric Drink
Protein allergy/intolerance and/or fat malabsorption	PediaSure Peptide (and Peptide 1.5)
	Pepdite Junior
	Peptamen Junior (with and without Prebio)
	Vivonex Pediatric
	EleCare Junior
	Neocate Junior
	Neocate Splash
	Alfamino Junior
	PurAmino Junior
Fat malabsorption, intestinal lymphatic obstruction, chylothorax	Monogen
	Enfaport
Increased caloric needs	Boost Kids Essentials
	Carnation Instant Breakfast Essentials
	Nutren Junior (also with fiber)
	PediaSure (also with fiber)
Requiring clear liquid diet	Resource Breeze
	Ensure Clear
Intractable epilepsy	KetoCal (3:1 and 4:1)
Blended formulas (using real foods)[a]	Pediasure Harvest
	Compleat Pediatric
	Compleat Organic Blends
	Compleat Pediatric Organic Blends
	Nourish
	Liquid Hope
	Kate Farms (Standard 1.0, Pediatric Standard 1.2, Peptide 1.5 and Pediatric Peptide 1.5)

OLDER CHILDREN AND ADULTS	
Enteral Nutrition (Tube Feeding)	
For malabsorption of protein and/or fat	Peptamen, Peptamen w/Prebio, Peptamen 1.0 and 1.5
	Pediasure Peptide 1.0 and 1.5
	Vital Peptide 1.5
	Perative
	Tolerex
	Vital High Protein
	Vital 1.0 Cal and AF 1.2 Cal, 1.5 Cal
	Vivonex Plus and Vivonex T.E.N.
For critically ill and/or malabsorption	Pulmocare
	Pivot 1.5 Cal
	Perative
For impaired glucose tolerance	Glucerna
	Glytrol
	Store-brand diabetic nutritional drink

Continued

TABLE 21.13

ADDITIONAL FORMULAS FOR SPECIAL CLINICAL CIRCUMSTANCES—CONT'D

For dialysis patients	Magnacal Renal
	Nepro
	NutriRenal
For patients with acute renal failure not on dialysis	Renalcal
	Suplena
Increased Caloric Needs (Oral)	
With a normal gastrointestinal (GI) tract	Boost, Boost with fiber
	Boost Plus, Boost High Protein
	Carnation Instant Breakfast Essentials with whole milk
	Ensure Original
	NUTRA Shake
For clear liquid diet	Resource Breeze
	Ensure Clear
For patients with cystic fibrosis (CF)	Scandishake with whole milk

[a]Some blended formulas can also be used for older children and adults. Tube bore size (French) and gravity versus bolus feeding recommendations vary; review each formula company's recommendations. Calories and nutrient information vary among formulas. Gradually changing from a nonblended formula may allow for optimal tolerance.

TABLE 21.14

ORAL REHYDRATION SOLUTIONS

Solution	Kcal/mL (kcal/oz)	Carbohydrate (g/L)	Na (mEq/L)	K (mEq/L)	Osmolality (mOsm/kg H$_2$0)
CeraLyte-50	0.16 (4.9)	Rice digest (40)	50	20	N/A
CeraLyte-70	0.16 (4.9)	Rice digest (40)	70	20	N/A
CeraLyte-90	0.16 (4.9)	Rice digest (40)	90	20	N/A
Enfalyte	0.12 (3.7)	Rice syrup solids (30)	50	25	160
Oral Rehydration Salts (WHO)	0.06 (2)	Dextrose (20)	90	20	330
Pedialyte (unflavored)	0.1 (3)	Dextrose (25)	45	20	250

g, Gram; *kcal,* kilocalorie; *kg,* kilogram; *L,* liter; *mL,* milliliter; *mOsm,* milliosmole; *oz,* ounce.

B. Starting and Advancing Parenteral Nutrition (Table 21.15)

C. Frequency of Monitoring Growth Parameters and Laboratory Studies in Patients on Parenteral Nutrition (Table 21.16)

D. Recommended Formulations of Parenteral Nutrition (Table 21.17)

TABLE 21.15

INITIATION AND ADVANCEMENT OF PARENTERAL NUTRITION FOR INFANTS THROUGH ADOLESCENTS[a,b]

Nutrient	Initial Dose	Advancement	Goals
Glucose	3.5%–10%	1%–5%/day	5–12 (max 14–18) mg/kg/min (rate of infusion)
Protein	0.8–3 g/kg/day	1 g/kg/day	0.8–4 g/kg/day
			10%–16% of calories
Fat[c]	1–2 g/kg/day	0.5–1 g/kg/day	1–3.5 g/kg/day[d]
			0.17 g/kg/hr (maximum rate of infusion)

[a]Acceptable osmolarity of parenteral nutrition through a peripheral line varies between 900 and 1050 osm/L by institution. An estimate of the osmolarity of parenteral nutrition can be obtained with the following formula: Estimated osmolarity = (dextrose concentration × 50) + (amino acid concentration × 100) + (mEq of electrolytes × 2). Consult individual pharmacy for hospital limitations.

[b]In general, infants require the higher concentration and/or rate of glucose, protein, and fat compared to older children and adolescents.

[c]Essential fatty acid deficiency may occur in fat-free parenteral nutrition within 2 to 4 weeks in infants and children and as early as 2 to 14 days in neonates. A minimum of 2% to 4% of total caloric intake as linoleic acid and 0.25% to 0.5% as linolenic acid is necessary to meet essential fatty acid requirements.

[d]If parenteral nutrition–associated cholestasis occurs, lipid minimization and/or use of fish oil or composite lipids should be considered.

g, Gram; *hr*, hour; *kg*, kilogram; *L*, liter; *mg*, milligram; *min*, minute; *osm*, osmole.

Modified from Corkins M, Balint J, Plogested S, eds. *The A.S.P.E.N. Pediatric Nutrition Support Core Curriculum.* American Society for Parenteral and Enteral Nutrition; 2010; Table 34.4.

TABLE 21.16

MONITORING SCHEDULE FOR PATIENTS RECEIVING PARENTERAL NUTRITION[a]

Variable	Initial Period[b]	Later Period[c]
GROWTH		
Weight	Daily	2 times/week
Height	Weekly (infants)	
	Monthly (children)	Monthly
Head circumference (infants)	Weekly	Monthly[d]
LABORATORY STUDIES		
Electrolytes and glucose	Daily ×3 or until stable	1–2× weekly
BUN/creatinine	Daily ×3 or until stable	1–2× weekly
Albumin or prealbumin	Weekly	Weekly
Ca^{2+}, Mg^{2+}, P	Daily ×3 or until stable	Weekly
ALT, AST, ALP	Weekly	Weekly
Total and direct bilirubin	Weekly	Weekly
CBC with differential	Daily ×3 or until stable	1–2× weekly
Triglycerides	Daily until stable	Weekly
Vitamins	—	As indicated
Trace minerals	—	As indicated

[a]For patients on long-term parenteral nutrition, monitoring every 24 weeks is adequate in most cases.

[b]The period before nutritional goals are reached or during any period of instability.

[c]When stability is reached, no changes in nutrient composition.

[d]Weekly in preterm infants.

ALP, Alkaline phosphatase; *ALT*, alanine transaminase; *AST*, aspartate transaminase; *BUN*, blood urea nitrogen; *CBC*, complete blood cell count; *Ca*, calcium; *Mg*, magnesium; *P*, phosphorous.

Modified from Worthington P, Balint J, Bechtold M, et al. When is parental nutrition appropriate? *J Parent Enter Nutr.* 2017;41(3); Table 13.2.

TABLE 21.17

PARENTERAL NUTRITION FORMULATION RECOMMENDATIONS

Electrolyte	Preterm	Term Infants/Children	Adolescents and Children >50 mg
Sodium (mEq/kg)	2–5	2–5	1–2
Potassium (mEq/kg)	2–4	2–4	1–2
Calcium	2–4 mEq/kg	0.5–4 mEq/kg	10–20 mEq/day
Phosphorus	1–2 mmol/kg	0.5–2 mmol/kg	10–40 mmol/day
Magnesium	0.3–0.5 mEq/kg	0.3–0.5 mEq/kg	10–30 mEq/day
Acetate and chloride	As needed for acid base balance		

Trace Element	Preterm Neonates <3 kg (mCg/kg/day)	Term Neonates 3–10 kg (mCg/kg/day)	Children 10–40 kg (mCg/kg/day)	Adolescents >40 kg (per day)
Zinc	400	50–250	50–125	2–5 mg
Copper[a]	20	20	5–20	200–500 mg
Manganese[a]	1	1	1	40–100 mCg
Chromium	0.05–0.2	0.2	0.14–0.2	5–15 mCg
Selenium	1.5–2	2	1–2	40–60 mCg

[a]Copper and manganese needs may be lowered in cholestasis.

From Mirtallo J, Canada T, Johnson D, et al. Safe practices for parenteral nutrition. *J Parenter Enteral Nutr.* 2004;28(6):S29–S70; and Corkins M, Balint J, Plogested S, eds. *The A.S.P.E.N. Pediatric Nutrition Support Core Curriculum.* American Society for Parenteral and Enteral Nutrition; 2010, Tables 34.5 and 34.7.

IX. WEB RESOURCES

A. Professional and Government Organizations

- Growth charts and nutrition information: https://www.cdc.gov/growthcharts/cdc_charts.htm
- American Academy of Pediatrics (AAP) children's health topics: http://www.healthychildren.org
- Academy of Nutrition and Dietetics: http://www.eatright.org
- American Society for Parenteral and Enteral Nutrition: http://www.nutritioncare.org
- U.S. Department of Agriculture Healthy Eating Guidelines: http://www.choosemyplate.gov
- Bright Futures: Nutrition and Pocket Guide: https://downloads.aap.org/AAP/PDF/Bright%20Futures/BFNutrition3rdEdPocketGuide.pdf
- AAP Committee on Nutrition: https://www.aap.org/en/community/aap-committees/committee-on-nutrition/

B. Infant and Pediatric Formula Company Websites

- Enfamil, Enfacare, Nutramigen, and Pregestimil: http://www.meadjohnson.com
- Carnation, Good Start, Nutren, Peptamen, Vivonex, Boost, Alfamino, and Resource: https://www.nestlehealthscience.us/ and http://medical.gerber.com/

- Alimentum, EleCare, Ensure, NeoSure, PediaSure, Pedialyte, and Similac: https://www.abbottnutrition.com/content/dam/an/abbottnutrition/pdf/product-guides/Pediatric%20Nutrition%20Handbook%202022Q3.pdf
- Bright Beginnings: http://www.brightbeginnings.com
- America's Store Brand: http://www.storebrandformula.com
- KetoCal, Neocate, and Pepdite: http://www.nutricia-na.com
- Liquid Hope and Nourish: https://www.functionalformularies.com/
- Kate Farms: https://www.katefarms.com/

C. Breastfeeding Resources

- LactMed is an online resource from the National Library of Medicine/National Institutes of Health (N/IH) that provides information on the safety of maternal medications and breastfeeding: https://www.ncbi.nlm.nih.gov/books/NBK501922/
- Video instruction on breastfeeding techniques from Stanford Newborn Nursery: http://newborns.stanford.edu/Breastfeeding/FifteenMinuteHelper.html
- Academy of Breastfeeding Medicine Protocols for the Care of Breastfeeding Mothers and Infants. Management of common breastfeeding-related challenges discussed: https://www.bfmed.org/protocols
- National Institute of Child Health and Human Development—Breastfeeding: https://www.nichd.nih.gov/health/topics/breastfeeding/Pages/default.aspx
- La Leche League is an international organization that provides mother-to-mother support, encouragement, information, and education. This organization hosts free lactation consultant-led support groups to connect mothers locally. While there are some excellent articles and the support groups can provide access to a lactation consultant, this group does support co-sleeping, and anticipatory guidance regarding the danger of co-sleeping and SIDS is necessary when providing parents with this resource: https://www.llli.org/

REFERENCES

A complete list of references can be found online.

Chapter 22

Oncology

Lawrence Gersz, MD, MBA and Rebecca Xi, MD

⊗ See additional content online.

🔊 **Audio Case File 22.1** Initial presentation and workup of acute lymphoblastic leukemia

I. NONSPECIFIC SYMPTOMS IN THE PRIMARY CARE SETTING (TABLE 22.1)[1,2]

TABLE 22.1

RED FLAGS FOR MALIGNANCY[1,2]

Finding	Red Flags
Lymphadenopathy	• Nontender • Rubbery or hard • Increase in size over 2–4 weeks or persisting >6 weeks • >2 cm or >1 cm in supraclavicular fossa • Associated fever, night sweats, weight loss, orthopnea
Joint/bone pain	• Pain causing awakening from sleep • Pain worse at night • Back pain causing neurologic deficits • Persisting >2 weeks • Associated with swelling • Palpable mass • Limping or refusal to walk • Lack of improvement with NSAIDs • Pathologic fracture
Headache	• New onset • Pain causing awakening from sleep • Pain worse with lying down • Persistent morning headaches • Associated emesis • Occipital region • Vision changes with or without papilledema • Cranial nerve palsies • Associated personality changes • Altered gait or frequent falls
Hepatosplenomegaly or palpable abdominal mass	• Always investigate • Associated with pain, anorexia, fever, vomiting

NSAIDs, Nonsteroidal antiinflammatory drugs.

II. PEDIATRIC HEMATOLOGIC MALIGNANCIES (TABLE 22.2)[3-4]

TABLE 22.2

COMMON PEDIATRIC HEMATOLOGIC MALIGNANCIES[1,2]

Malignancy	Clinical Presentation	Initial Workup	Epidemiology, Prognosis
ALL, AML	Fever, pallor, petechiae/ecchymoses, lethargy, malaise, anorexia, bone/joint pain **Exam:** Lymphadenopathy, hepatosplenomegaly, abnormal neurologic exam, testicular enlargement **AML** may include subcutaneous nodules, gingival hyperplasia, chloromas (solid collection of leukemic cells) **T-cell ALL** commonly presents with anterior mediastinal mass	CBC with differential, peripheral smear; CMP with phosphate, uric acid, LDH important to assess for tumor lysis CXR to assess for mediastinal mass Blood and urine cultures if febrile Definitive diagnosis requires lumbar puncture (evaluate for CNS involvement), bone marrow biopsy, flow cytometry	**ALL:** Most common pediatric cancer (approximately 25% in <15 years). Peaks at age 2–5 years. Overall 5-year survival rate exceeds 90%. **AML:** Peaks in first year of life, risk increases again after adolescence. Survival rate ~60%–70%; acute promyelocytic leukemia best prognosis
Lymphoma HD, NHL	Painless, firm lymphadenopathy (often supraclavicular or cervical nodes) Cough, shortness of breath, "B symptoms" (fevers, night sweats, weight loss)	CBC with differential, peripheral smear, electrolytes, include CRP, UA, LDH CXR to assess for mediastinal mass Diagnosis made through lymph node biopsy and/or in some cases, fluid sampling. Full staging with PET/CT	15% of childhood malignancies HD peak incidence occurs in bimodal distribution (15–34 years old and >55 years) NHL incidence increases with age, more common in second decade of life Prognosis: HD highly curable (95% survival with stage I disease and 75% for stage IV); NHL prognosis varies with histology and stage
Histiocytic Disease Nonmalignant proliferation of monocytes, macrophages, or dendritic cells	Scaly rash, long bone pain, fever, weight loss, diarrhea, dyspnea, painless lymphadenopathy, polydipsia, polyuria	Triglycerides, fibrinogen, ferritin, urine osmolality Imaging to detect lytic lesions: Skeletal survey, followed by CT/MRI, bone scan/PET	**Langerhans Cell Histiocytosis:** Median age at presentation 30 months **Rosai Dorfman:** Higher incidence among African Americans in first 2 decades of life

NOTE: Laboratory testing and imaging suggestions are meant as a guide for evaluation of a potential malignancy. Patients warranting definitive testing should be referred to an oncologist.

ALL, Acute lymphocytic leukemia; *AML,* acute myeloid leukemia; *CBC,* complete blood count; *CMP,* complete metabolic panel; *CNS,* central nervous system; *CRP,* c-reactive protein; *CT,* computed tomography; *CXR,* chest x-ray; *HD,* Hodgkin disease; *IV,* intravenous; *LDH,* lactate dehydrogenase; *MRI,* magnetic resonance imaging; *NHL,* non-Hodgkin lymphoma; *PET,* positron emission tomography; *UA,* urinalysis.

III. PEDIATRIC SOLID TUMOR MALIGNANCIES (TABLE 22.3)[3-4]

TABLE 22.3
PEDIATRIC SOLID TUMOR MALIGNANCIES[1,2]

Malignancy	Clinical Presentation	Initial Workup	Epidemiology, Prognosis
Neuroblastoma: Malignant tumor of neural crest cell origin	Abdominal pain and/or mass (hard, nontender), periorbital ecchymosis, spinal cord compression, Horner syndrome, Paraneoplastic syndromes (secretory diarrhea, diaphoresis, opsoclonus-myoclonus)	Abdominal ultrasound Definitive diagnosis requires CT chest/abdomen/pelvis, urine catecholamines (HVA/VMA), MIBG scan, biopsy	Most common malignancy in infancy; median age of diagnosis 17 months 8% childhood malignancies, 15% of deaths caused by childhood malignancy **Prognosis:** Favorable prognosis if age of diagnosis <1 year, Stage I, II, IV-S, absence of N-myc amplification
Wilms tumor (Nephroblastoma)	Abdominal mass with or without abdominal pain May see hypertension, hematuria, anemia (bleeding within the tumor)	Liver and renal function tests, urinalysis Abdominal ultrasound, chest/abdominal CT or MRI Diagnosis requires biopsy	Peaks at age 3–4 years Survival rate 90% (poorer prognosis with diffuse anaplasia)
Bone tumors: Osteosarcoma, Ewing sarcoma	**Osteosarcoma:** Bone pain or mass (typically in epiphysis/metaphysis of long bones) not relieved with conservative treatment **Ewing sarcoma:** Bone pain and swelling, most commonly in femur or pelvis	X-ray of primary site, followed by MRI Metastasis evaluation: CT of chest, PET scan	**Osteosarcoma:** Peaks in adolescence during maximum growth velocity **Ewing:** Peaks between 10 and 20 years **Prognosis:** Cure rate for localized disease: 60%–70% Poor prognosis with metastatic disease, primary tumor of axial skeleton, poor necrosis at time of resection (osteosarcoma)
Rhabdomyosarcoma: Soft tissue malignant tumor of skeletal muscle origin	Rapidly growing mass, may be painful Symptoms based on location **HEENT:** Periorbital swelling, proptosis, chronic otitis	CT or MRI of primary site Diagnosis requires tissue biopsy, immunohistochemical staining	Peak at 2–6 years and in adolescence **Prognosis:** Based on stage, extent of surgical resection, and histopathology (alveolar histopathology poorer prognosis than

Malignancy	Clinical Presentation	Initial Workup	Epidemiology, Prognosis
	media, dysphagia, neck mass **GU tract:** Paratesticular swelling, hematuria, urinary frequency/retention		embryonal); favorable prognostic factors include localized disease, >90% tumor necrosis at resection, age between 1 and 10 years at presentation
Retinoblastoma (Rb)	Leukocoria (retrolental mass), strabismus, hyphema, irregular pupil(s)	Ophthalmology referral MRI brain to evaluate pineal gland if bilateral	Peaks at age 2 years Survival at 5 years >90% 66%–75% tumors are unilateral *Rb1* mutations carry risk for second malignancies (osteosarcoma, soft tissue sarcoma, malignant melanoma)
Hepatic tumors: Hepatoblastoma, Hepatocellular carcinoma (HCC)	Painless abdominal mass, anorexia, emesis, abdominal pain, fever Hepatoblastoma may be associated with anemia, thrombocytosis	CBC, LFTs, AFP, hepatitis B and C titers Abdominal ultrasound	Hepatoblastoma peaks at age <3 years HCC peaks after 10 years of age (associated with hepatitis B and C) **Prognosis:** Hepatoblastoma favorable prognosis pending tumor resection at diagnosis; HCC carries poor prognosis
Gonadal/germ cell tumors	**Testicular tumors:** Nontender scrotal mass, hydrocele **Ovarian tumors:** Typically asymptomatic until quite large **Hormone-producing tumors:** Amenorrhea, precocious puberty, hirsutism	AFP, β-hCG, CXR, abdominal ultrasound, followed by CT or MRI	Peaks <4 years, then again in adolescence Overall cure rate >80% Favorable prognostic factors include <12 years of age, lack of thoracic involvement

NOTE: Laboratory testing and imaging suggestions are meant as a guide for evaluation of a potential malignancy. Patients warranting definitive testing should be referred to an oncologist.

AFP, α-Fetoprotein; *β-hCG*, beta human chorionic gonadotropin; *CBC*, complete blood cell count; *CT*, computed tomography; *CXR*, chest x-ray; *GU*, genitourinary; *HEENT*, head eyes ears nose throat; *HVA/VMA*, homovanillic acid/vanillylmandelic acid (urine catecholamines); *LFTs*, liver function tests; *MIBG*, metaiodobenzylguanidine; *MRI*, magnetic resonance imaging; *PET*, positron emission tomography.

IV. PEDIATRIC CENTRAL NERVOUS SYSTEM (CNS) TUMORS[3-4,7-10] (TABLE 22.4)

A. Epidemiology

1. Most common solid tumors in children
2. Leading cause of childhood cancer deaths
3. Highest incidence in infants and children under 5 years old

B. Clinical Presentation

1. Early/generalized symptoms: Headache, lethargy/fatigue, nausea/emesis, gait abnormalities; increased head circumference in infants
2. Later symptoms related to tumor location: Seizures, altered language, encephalopathy, hemiplegia/hemi-sensory deficit, facial weakness, neuroendocrine effects (precocious/delayed puberty, diabetes insipidus), visual changes, abnormal movements, back pain, sphincter disturbance

C. Initial Workup

1. Thorough neurologic exam, including fundoscopic exam
2. Neurosurgery/neurooncology consultation
3. Labs: Presurgical tests (complete blood count [CBC], electrolytes, blood type, coagulation factors, crossmatching); endocrine tests for suprasellar tumors; α fetoprotein (AFP) and β human chorionic gonadotropin (β-hCG) if germinoma suspected
4. Imaging: Magnetic resonance imaging (MRI) of brain (sometimes spine) with and without intravenous (IV) contrast

D. Management Principles

1. High-dose dexamethasone: Often administered to reduce tumor-associated edema
2. Consider seizure prophylaxis for those at high risk of seizures or seizure history.

V. ONCOLOGIC EMERGENCIES[4,11-18,19]

A. Fever and Neutropenia (Fig. 22.1)

1. **Etiology:** Fever with temperature ≥38.0°C (some centers and medical associations also use 38.0°C sustained over an hour to define fever) in the setting of neutropenia (absolute neutrophil count [ANC] <500 cells/μL or <1000 cells/μL but expected to drop to <500 cells/μL in the next 48 hours). Presumed serious infection in a neutropenic host. While fevers may be caused by other etiologies including medications, presume infection until proven otherwise.
2. **Presentation:** May appear ill with fatigue, lethargy, or localized pain. Can also appear well yet have subtle signs of compensated shock, including chills, rigors, tachypnea, or tachycardia. May deteriorate after initial doses of antibiotics
3. **Management:** Broad-spectrum antibiotics with anti-pseudomonal coverage should be administered within 60 minutes of presentation to medical facility. NOTE: Antibiotic administration may lead to clinical

TABLE 22.4

PEDIATRIC CENTRAL NERVOUS SYSTEM TUMORS[1-2,5-7]

Tumor (Incidence)	Epidemiology	Location	Prognosis
Glioma (40%)	**Low-grade:** Average age of diagnosis: 6.5–9 years; male predominance **High-grade:** 9–10 years; 1:1 male-female ratio	Occur throughout the CNS Low-grade astrocytomas commonly occur in cerebellum, hypothalamic, third ventricular region, optic nerve	Low-grade: 50%–100% depending on ability to resect
Embryonal tumor: Most commonly medulloblastoma (20%)	Most common group of malignant CNS tumors Bimodal distribution, peaking at 3–4 years, then again between 8–10 years	Commonly located in the midline cerebellar vermis Older patients can present in cerebellar hemisphere	5-year survival 50%–80% Poorer outcome if presents under 4 years of age given general avoidance of radiation if possible
Ependymoma: Derived from ependymal lining of ventricular system (10%)	Median age 6 years	~70% occur in the posterior fossa Can occur in supratentorial region, spinal cord Usually noninvasive, can extend into ventricular lumen	Long-term survival ~40% after undergoing gross total resection
Craniopharyngioma: Arise from embryonic remnant of Rathke pouch (5%–10%)	In childhood, peaks between 8–10 years of age Rarely occurs in infancy	Occur in suprasellar region adjacent to optic chiasm Minimally invasive	5 year survival 70%–90% Associated with significant morbidity (panhypopituitarism, growth failure, visual loss)
Germ cell tumor (3%–5%)	Peak incidence 10–12 years of age	Commonly arise in midline locations (pineal and suprasellar region)	5-year survival 40%–70%

CNS, Central nervous system.

sepsis secondary to release of endotoxin from Gram-negative bacteria. May consider early discharge (prior to ANC recovery) at 48 to 72 hours in certain low-risk populations

B. Hyperleukocytosis/Leukostasis

1. **Etiology:** Elevated white blood cell (WBC) count (usually >100,000/μL) in patients with newly diagnosed leukemia, which leads to leukostasis in the microcirculation and diminished tissue perfusion (notably in CNS,

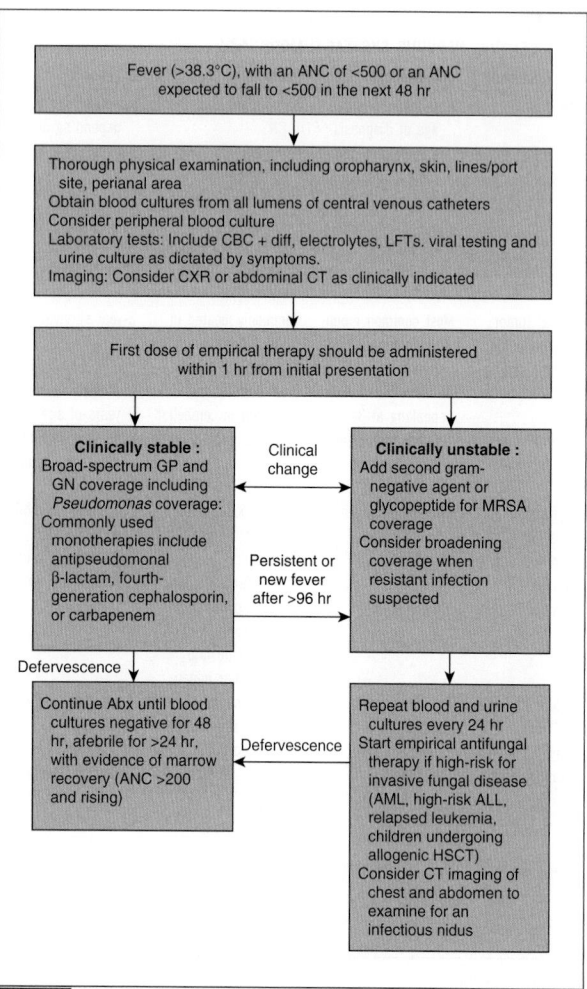

FIGURE 22.1

Algorithm for the management of fever and neutropenia in children with cancer and/or undergoing hematopoietic stem cell transplantation. NOTE: Some centers and medical associations also use 38.0°C sustained over an hour to define fever. *Abx*, Antibiotics; *ALL*, acute lymphocytic leukemia; *AML*, acute myeloid leukemia; *ANC*, absolute neutrophil count; *CBC*, complete blood cell count; *CT*, computed tomography; *CXR*, chest x-ray; *diff*, differential; *GN*, Gram-negative; *GP*, Gram-positive; *HSCT*, hematopoietic stem cell transplantation; *LFTs*, liver function tests; *MRSA*, methicillin-resistant *Staphylococcus aureus*. (Data from Lehrnbecher T, Robinson P, Fisher B, et al. Guideline for the management of fever and neutropenia in children with cancer and hematopoietic stem-cell transplantation recipients: 2017 update. *J Clin Oncol.* 2017;35:2082–2094.)

kidneys, and lungs). Leukostasis occurs more commonly and at lower WBC counts in acute myeloid leukemia (AML) than in acute lymphocytic leukemia (ALL).

2. **Presentation:** Hypoxia, tachypnea, dyspnea, and pulmonary hemorrhage from pulmonary leukostasis. Mental status changes, headaches, seizures, and papilledema from cerebral leukostasis. May also see gastrointestinal bleeding, abdominal pain, renal insufficiency, priapism, and/or intracranial hemorrhage. Hyperleukocytosis may be asymptomatic.

3. **Management:**
   a. Prompt initiation of chemotherapy is the most effective approach.
   b. Consider leukapheresis or exchange transfusion only if evidence of symptomatic leukostasis (although any improvement will be short term).
   c. Transfuse platelets to keep count above at least 20,000/μL to prevent hemorrhage.[3]
   d. Avoid red blood cell (RBC) transfusions if possible, which increase viscosity. If required, consider partial exchange transfusion.
   e. Hydration and allopurinol should be initiated, as hyperleukocytosis increases the risk of tumor lysis syndrome.
   f. Treat coagulopathy aggressively.

C. Tumor Lysis Syndrome

1. **Etiology:** Rapid lysis of tumor cells releases intracellular contents into the bloodstream spontaneously before treatment or during early stages of chemotherapy (especially Burkitt lymphoma, T-cell leukemia/lymphoma, acute leukemias with hyperleukocytosis).

2. **Presentation:** Hyperuricemia, hyperkalemia, hyperphosphatemia (with secondary hypocalcemia). Can lead to acute kidney injury. Usually asymptomatic, but may present with nausea, anorexia, diarrhea, dark and/or decreased urine output, muscle cramps, heart palpitations

3. **Diagnosis:** CBC, basic metabolic panel (BMP), phosphorus, uric acid, lactate dehydrogenase (LDH), electrocardiogram (ECG)

4. **Prevention and management:**
   a. Hydration: IV fluids (without potassium, calcium, phosphate or bicarbonate) at twice maintenance rate. Keep urine-specific gravity <1.010 and urine output >100 mL/m^2/hr. Alkalinization is no longer recommended, given increased risk of calcium phosphate precipitation.
   b. Hyperuricemia: Allopurinol inhibits formation of uric acid and should only be given PO (see Formulary for dosing). Rasburicase converts uric acid to the more soluble allantoin and should be used if *two* of the following criteria are met: uric acid ≥8 mg/dL, WBC >50,000/μL, LDH >2× ULN (upper limit of normal), creatinine >1.5× ULN, CHF/pulmonary edema **OR** if uric acid ≥8 mg/dL despite 48 hours of allopurinol. Do not use rasburicase with patients with known G6PD deficiency, as it may result in methemoglobinemia.

    c. Monitor potassium, calcium, phosphorus, uric acid, and urinalysis closely (up to Q2 hr for high-risk patients). There is an increased risk of calcium phosphate precipitation when Ca × Phos >60. Consider early use of sevelamer.

    d. See Chapter 11 for management of abnormal electrolytes and Chapter 19 for dialysis indications.

D. Spinal Cord Compression

1. **Etiology:** Intrinsic or extrinsic compression of spinal cord. Occurs most commonly with metastases from brain tumors, spinal tumors, soft tissue sarcomas, neuroblastoma, lymphoma

2. **Presentation:** Back pain (localized or radicular), weakness, sensory loss, bowel or bladder dysfunction, gait abnormalities. Prognosis for recovery based on duration and level of disability at presentation

3. **Diagnosis:** MRI (preferred) or computed tomography (CT) scan of spine. Spine radiography is less sensitive.

4. **Management:**

    a. In the presence of neurologic abnormalities, strong history, and/or rapid progression of symptoms, consider immediate dexamethasone. NOTE: Steroids may prevent accurate diagnosis/staging of leukemia/lymphoma; plan diagnostic procedure and LP as soon as possible.

    b. If tumor type is known and chemosensitive, emergent chemotherapy is indicated.

    c. If tumor type is unknown or debulking may remove most/all of tumor, emergent neurosurgery consultation may be indicated to decompress the spine in select cases. Emergent radiotherapy (RT) may also be considered.

E. Increased Intracranial Pressure (ICP)

1. **Etiology:** Ventricular obstruction or impaired cerebral spinal fluid (CSF) flow. Most commonly seen with brain tumors but also with intracranial hemorrhage, thrombosis, meningeal involvement by tumor, or infection.

2. **Presentation:** Headaches, altered mental status, irritability, lethargy, nuchal rigidity, emesis, abnormal vision; Cushing triad and pupillary changes are late and ominous findings

3. **Diagnosis:**

    a. Evaluate for vital sign changes (i.e., Cushing triad [↓ heart rate, ↑ systolic blood pressure, irregular respirations]).

    b. Funduscopic evaluation for papilledema

    c. Obtain CT/ultrafast MRI or MRI of the head (MRI preferred for diagnosis of posterior fossa tumors).

4. **Management:**

    a. See Chapter 1 for management principles.

    b. Obtain emergent neurosurgical consultation.

    c. If tumor is the cause, start IV dexamethasone (see Formulary for dosing).

F. Other Neurologic Emergencies: Cerebrovascular Accident (CVA), Seizures

1. **CVA etiology:** Hyperleukocytosis, coagulopathy, thrombocytopenia, radiation (fibrosis) or chemotherapy-related (e.g., l-asparaginase–induced hemorrhage or thrombosis, methotrexate). Most common in patients with AML or any form of leukemia with hyperleukocytosis
2. **Seizure etiology:** Most common in primary CNS tumors with supratentorial location, tumors metastatic to CNS, meningeal leukemia, or chemotherapy-related (intrathecal [IT] cytarabine, IT/IV methotrexate)
3. See Chapters 1 and 20 for diagnosis and management.

G. Superior Vena Cava Syndrome/Superior Mediastinal Syndrome

1. **Etiology:** Compression of venous drainage and trachea, most commonly caused by mediastinal mass. Usually seen with T-lymphoblastic lymphoma, Hodgkin lymphoma, mature B-cell lymphoma, and germ cell tumors
2. **Presentation:** Dyspnea, cough, wheeze, stridor, orthopnea, headaches, facial swelling or plethora, dizziness
3. **Diagnosis:** Two-view chest radiograph. If mediastinal mass present, obtain CT or MRI to further assess. Avoid sedation, high risk for airway obstruction
4. **Management:**
   a. Control airway (mass usually too distal for intubation), place in upright position, and administer supplemental oxygen.
   b. Diagnosis through least invasive means necessary, including peripheral blood flow cytometry, percutaneous node biopsy, and/or effusion drainage
   c. Empiric therapy: Radiotherapy, steroids, chemotherapy.
      NOTE: Steroids can confound diagnosis and/or staging.

H. Typhlitis (Neutropenic Enterocolitis)

1. **Etiology:** Inflammation of bowel wall, typically localized to cecum. Associated with bacterial or fungal invasion. Associated with prolonged neutropenia
2. **Presentation:** Right lower quadrant abdominal pain, nausea/emesis, diarrhea, fever (may be absent early in course). Risk for perforation
3. **Diagnosis:**
   a. Careful serial abdominal examinations
   b. Abdominal ultrasound may be considered (may show pneumatosis intestinalis, bowel wall edema), although CT abdomen with IV and PO contrast is most sensitive form of imaging.
4. **Management:**
   a. Bowel rest: NPO on IV fluids; consider nasogastric decompression
   b. Broad anaerobic and Gram-negative antibiotic coverage
   c. Surgical consultation

I. Cytokine Release Syndrome (CRS)

1. **Etiology:** Newer immunologic agents (e.g., chimeric antigen receptor T [CAR-T] therapy and specific antibodies) can provoke release of cytokines causing systemic inflammation and hemodynamic instability.
2. **Presentation:** Early symptoms include fever, headache, myalgia, or mild evidence of hemodynamic instability (tachycardia) that can progress quickly to cardiovascular collapse and multiorgan dysfunction.
3. **Diagnosis:** Based on clinical features. Consider obtaining CRP and ferritin, although nondiagnostic.
4. **Management:**
   a. Place on continuous monitor, closely watch for hypotension, institute supportive care measures (acetaminophen, cold packs), obtain blood cultures, and administer appropriate antibiotics based on ANC and clinical status.
   b. Treat hypotension with IV fluids (although use cautiously since patients are at risk of capillary leak). If refractory, may require vasopressors and intensive care unit-level care
   c. Administer tocilizumab: Recombinant humanized monoclonal antibody targeting the IL-6 receptor
   d. Closely monitor neurologic status. Patient should be on seizure prophylaxis.
   e. For mild/moderate CRS, avoid use of glucocorticoids as they can deplete or eradicate CAR-T cell therapy. Severe CRS may require the use of tocilizumab in combination with glucocorticoids.

VI. COMMONLY USED CHEMOTHERAPEUTIC DRUGS, ASSOCIATED ACUTE AND LONG-TERM TOXICITIES (TABLE 22.5)

TABLE 22.5

COMMONLY USED CHEMOTHERAPEUTIC DRUGS AND ASSOCIATED ACUTE TOXICITIES

Drug Name (By Class)	Toxicity[a]	Acute Monitoring and Care	Long-Term Toxicity
ALKYLATORS	**Significant myelosuppression, severe nausea, impaired fertility**	**Myelosuppression supportive care, aggressive antiemetics, pretreatment fertility consult**	**Gonadal dysfunction, delayed/arrested puberty, infertility, secondary AML/ myelodysplasia**
Busulfan	Seizures, SOS/VOD, acute/chronic lung injury	Monitor weight, abdominal girth, bilirubin; seizure prophylaxis	Pulmonary fibrosis, cataracts
Carmustine	Hypotension, chronic lung injury	Slow infusion, PFTs	Pulmonary fibrosis
Cyclophosphamide		Hyperhydration and **mesna** to prevent	Urinary tract toxicity, bladder malignancy

Drug Name (By Class)	Toxicity[a]	Acute Monitoring and Care	Long-Term Toxicity
	Myocardial necrosis, hemorrhagic cystitis, SIADH	hemorrhagic cystitis; ECG	
Ifosfamide	Mental status changes, encephalopathy (rarely progressing to death), renal tubular damage, hemorrhagic cystitis, Fanconi syndrome	Monitor creatinine, magnesium, phosphate, potassium; hyperhydration and **mesna** to prevent hemorrhagic cystitis; methylene blue for neurotoxicity	Renal toxicity, hypertension
Lomustine	Disorientation, fatigue		Pulmonary fibrosis
Melphalan	Severe mucositis, pulmonary fibrosis	Aggressive oral hygiene, ophthalmologic examination	
Procarbazine	Encephalopathy; adverse effects with tyramine-rich foods, ethanol, MAOIs, meperidine, and many other drugs	Avoid serotonergic agents/modulators, diet low in tyramine (avoid aged cheese/meats, beer, pickled food, soy sauce)	
Temozolomide	Headache, seizures, thrombocytopenia		
Thiotepa	Encephalopathy, rash, burns, desquamation of skin, lower extremity weakness	Frequent bathing	
NUCLEOTIDE ANALOGS	**Myelosuppression, mucositis, transaminitis**	**Supportive care, monitor LFTs**	
Clofarabine	Capillary leak syndrome, SOS/VOD, nephrotoxicity, hyperbilirubinemia	Monitor creatinine; monitor weight, abdominal girth, bilirubin	
Cytarabine (Ara-C)	Ara-C syndrome (maculopapular rash, fever), conjunctivitis, severe mucositis, ataxia, respiratory distress rapidly progressing to pulmonary edema	Corticosteroid eye drops; coverage for viridans streptococci with fever, systemic steroids for Ara-C syndrome	High dose: Neurocognitive deficits (executive function, attention, memory, fine motor dexterity), clinical leukoencephalopathy (spasticity, ataxia, dysarthria, seizure)

Continued

TABLE 22.5

COMMONLY USED CHEMOTHERAPEUTIC DRUGS AND ASSOCIATED ACUTE TOXICITIES—CONT'D

Drug Name (By Class)	Toxicity[a]	Acute Monitoring and Care	Long-Term Toxicity
Fludarabine	Transaminitis, neurotoxicity, immunosuppression (nonmyelosuppressive)	Monitor creatinine (decreased clearance results in increased risk of neurotoxicity)	
Mercaptopurine (6-MP)	Hepatotoxicity (increased risk in TPMT deficiency), pancreatitis	LFTs, hepatic dysfunction, VOD	
Thioguanine	Hepatotoxicity (increased risk in TPMT deficiency), SOS	LFTs, hepatic dysfunction, VOD	
DNA MODIFYING AGENTS			
Bleomycin (DNA strand breaker)	Anaphylaxis, pneumonitis, pulmonary fibrosis	PFTs	Interstitial pneumonitis, pulmonary fibrosis
Carboplatin (DNA cross-linker)	Nephrotoxicity, ototoxicity, peripheral neuropathy	Monitor creatinine, adjust dose based on creatinine clearance, audiology evaluation	Sensorineural hearing loss, tinnitus, vertigo, peripheral sensory neuropathy, renal toxicity, hypertension
Cisplatin (DNA cross-linker)	Nephrotoxicity (related to cumulative dose), severe emesis, hypomagnesemia, hypophosphatemia, ototoxicity	Monitor creatinine, magnesium, phosphorous; audiology evaluation; aggressive antiemetic regimen	Peripheral sensory neuropathy, renal toxicity, hypertension
Etoposide (topoisomerase inhibitor)	Anaphylaxis (rare), hypotension, hyperbilirubinemia, transaminitis, secondary malignancy (AML)	Slow infusion if hypotension; change formulation to etoposide phosphate if anaphylaxis; monitor bilirubin and LFTs	AML
OTHER CHEMOTHERAPEUTIC AGENTS			
Asparaginase (Enzyme)	Pancreatitis, hypersensitivity reaction (acute and delayed), coagulopathy (thrombosis and bleeding), hyperammonemia	Monitor serum asparaginase activity levels, high index of suspicion for clots/bleeds, consider amylase/lipase with abdominal pain	No known long-term effects

Drug Name (By Class)	Toxicity[a]	Acute Monitoring and Care	Long-Term Toxicity
Dactinomycin (antibiotic)	Rash, hypocalcemia, radiation recall (rash), SOS	Monitor calcium; monitor weight, abdominal girth, bilirubin	No known long-term effects
Daunorubicin and doxorubicin, mitoxantrone (adriamycin) (anthracyclines)	Arrhythmia, cardiomyopathy/heart failure (related to cumulative dose), severe mucositis, severe emesis, red urine and bodily fluids (dauno/doxo), blue-green urine (mitoxantrone), radiation recall	Limit cumulative dose; echocardiogram; consider **dexrazoxane** for cardioprotection	AML, cardiomyopathy, arrhythmias, subclinical left ventricular dysfunction
Methotrexate (MTX) (folate antagonist)	Mucositis, diarrhea, renal dysfunction, encephalopathy, chemical arachnoiditis (intrathecal), photosensitivity, leukoencephalopathy, osteoporosis	**Leucovorin** to reduce mucositis with high-dose therapy; oral hygiene; monitor neurologic exam and developmental milestones	Reduced bone mineral density, renal toxicity, hypertension, hepatic dysfunction High dose: Neurocognitive deficits (executive function, attention, memory, fine motor dexterity), clinical leukoencephalopathy (spasticity, ataxia, dysarthria, seizure)
Vinblastine, vincristine, and vinorelbine (Microtubule inhibitors)	Constipation, bone and jaw pain, peripheral and autonomic sensory and motor neuropathy, foot drop, SIADH (rare), hyperbilirubinemia, transaminitis	Bowel regimen; monitor for neuropathy; fatal if given intrathecally; bilirubin, and LFTs	Peripheral sensory or motor neuropathy (areflexia, weakness, paresthesias, foot drop), vasospastic attacks (Raynaud phenomenon)
MOLECULARLY TARGETED AGENTS			
Alemtuzumab (Campath) (monoclonal Ab binds CD52 on mature lymphocytes)	Severe infusion reactions (hypotension, bronchospasm, ARDS, anaphylaxis), infections	Antimicrobial prophylaxis	
Blinatumomab (bi-specific T-cell engager)	CRS, neurotoxicity	Dexamethasone	
Brentuximab (chimeric monoclonal Ab binds CD30)	Peripheral neuropathy, diarrhea		

Continued

TABLE 22.5

COMMONLY USED CHEMOTHERAPEUTIC DRUGS AND ASSOCIATED ACUTE TOXICITIES—CONT'D

Drug Name (By Class)	Toxicity[a]	Acute Monitoring and Care	Long-Term Toxicity
CAR-T cells (immune cells genetically modified to bind tumor-specific antigens)	CRS, neurotoxicity (headache, confusion, encephalopathy, seizure), HLH	**Tocilizumab** (anti-IL-6R), steroids if severe/refractory	
Dinutuximab (monoclonal Ab binds GD-2; for use in neuroblastoma)	Rash/hives, rigors, severe pain, neuropathy, hyponatremia, hepatotoxicity, hypocalcemia, capillary leak syndrome, ocular neurologic disorders	Monitor sodium, calcium, LFTs; aggressive pain management	
Imatinib (Gleevec), dasatinib, nilotinib (tyrosine kinase inhibitors)	Congestive heart failure, edema, pleural effusions, rash, night sweats, myelosuppression	ECG, serial echocardiograms	
Nivolumab (PD-1 checkpoint inhibitor) and pembrolizumab (CTLA-4 checkpoint inhibitor)	Autoimmune manifestations (colitis, dermatitis, hepatitis, nephritis, pneumonitis, etc.)		
Rituximab (Rituxan) (chimeric monoclonal Ab binds CD20 on B cells)	Infusion reaction, urticaria	Hep B testing before use, slow infusion for first dose, immune reconstitution may be very delayed post therapy	

[a]All chemotherapeutic medications may cause nausea, vomiting, fever, immunosuppression, mucositis, gastrointestinal upset.

AML, Acute myeloid leukemia; *ARDS*, acute respiratory distress syndrome; *CAR-T cell therapy*, chimeric antigen receptor T-cell; *CRS*, cytokine release syndrome; *ECG*, electrocardiogram; *LFTs*, liver function tests; *MAOIs*, monoamine oxidase inhibitors; *PFTs*, pulmonary function tests; *SIADH*, syndrome of inappropriate antidiuretic hormone; *SOS*, sinusoidal obstruction syndrome; *TPMT*, thiopurine S-methyltransferase; *VOD*, venoocclusive disease.

Data from *Physician's Desk Reference*. 71st ed. Medical Economics; 2017; and Taketomo CK, Hodding JH, Kraus DM. *American Pharmaceutical Association Pediatric Dosage Handbook*. 16th ed. Lexi-Comp, *Pediatric & Neonatal Dosage Handbook*, 25th ed.; and Micromedex 2.0 (2018).

VII. COMMON CHEMOTHERAPY COMPLICATIONS AND SUPPORTIVE CARE[3,13]

A. Cytopenias: Anemia, Thrombocytopenia, Neutropenia

1. **Etiology:** Chemotherapy, medication, radiation, marrow infiltration, blood loss, hemolysis, consumptive coagulopathy
2. **Management:**
   a. See Chapter 14 for details on transfusion.
   b. Anemia: Hemoglobin thresholds for pRBC transfusions in cancer patients are based on clinical status and symptoms (often ≤8 g/dL).
   c. Thrombocytopenia: In general, maintain platelet count above 10,000/μL. Patients with active bleeding, fever, or before selected procedures (e.g., lumbar puncture, intramuscular injection) may require higher thresholds. Consider maintaining at higher levels for patients who have brain tumors, recent brain surgery, or history of stroke.
   d. Neutropenia:
      (1) Broad-spectrum antibiotics with concomitant fever (see Fig. 22.1).
      (2) Granulocyte colony-stimulating factor (GCSF) to assist in recovery of neutrophils may be considered in some patient populations and regimens.
3. Transfuse only irradiated and leukoreduced packed red blood cells (pRBCs) and single-donor platelets; cytomegalovirus (CMV)-negative or leukofiltered pRBCs/platelets for CMV-negative patients. Use leukofiltered pRBCs/platelets for those who may undergo transplant in the future to prevent alloimmunization or for those who have had nonhemolytic febrile transfusion reactions. Many oncology patients have nonhemolytic reactions (fever, rash, hypotension, respiratory distress) to pRBCs and/or platelet transfusion and should subsequently be premedicated with diphenhydramine and/or acetaminophen.

B. Mucositis

1. **Etiology:** Damage to endothelial cells of the GI tract from chemotherapy, leading to breakdown of the mucosa. Typically peaks in the first 1 to 2 weeks after chemotherapy
2. **Presentation:** Oropharyngeal pain, abdominal pain, nausea, vomiting, diarrhea, intolerance of oral intake
3. **Prevention and management:** Supportive care aimed at pain control and nutrition. Local pain control with lidocaine-containing mouthwashes and bicarbonate rinses. Systemic pain control often requires patient-controlled analgesia (PCA) infusion. Total parenteral nutrition (TPN) is commonly required. Low threshold to evaluate for contributing viral infection (e.g., herpes simplex virus)

C. Nausea and Emesis

1. **Etiology:** Chemotherapy side effect. Also suspect opiate therapy, GI and CNS radiotherapy, obstructive abdominal process, elevated ICP, certain antibiotics, or hypercalcemia.

2. **Presentation:** Can be acute (within 24 hours of chemotherapy initiation), delayed (beyond 24 hours), or anticipatory in subsequent cycles
3. **Therapy:** Hydration plus one or more antiemetic medications (Table 22.6; see Formulary for dosing)

TABLE 22.6

ANTIEMETIC THERAPIES[3]

Antiemetic Classes	Common Agents	Common Adverse Effects
Serotonin (5-HT3) antagonists	Ondansetron, granisetron	QT prolongation, QRS widening, constipation
Histamine-1 antagonist	Diphenhydramine, scopolamine	Sedation, urinary retention, blurred vision
Benzodiazepines	Lorazepam	Sedation
Dopamine antagonists	Metoclopramide, prochlorperazine, promethazine	Sedation, extrapyramidal effects, QT prolongation; rarely, seizures or neuroleptic malignant syndrome Consider diphenhydramine to reduce risk of extrapyramidal symptoms.
Substance P receptor antagonists	Aprepitant, fosaprepitant	Exercise caution with agents metabolized by CYP3A4.
Steroids (helpful in patients with brain tumors and prophylaxis for delayed nausea/vomiting)	Dexamethasone	Hypertension, hyperglycemia, bradycardia, osteoporosis/osteonecrosis
Cannabinoids (also an appetite stimulant)	Dronabinol	Hallucinations, dizziness
Antipsychotics (useful in patients with refractory vomiting, can help comorbid depression)	Olanzapine	Weight gain, sedation, insulin resistance, QT prolongation; extrapyramidal side effects (rare)

VIII. ANTIMICROBIAL PROPHYLAXIS IN ONCOLOGY PATIENTS[20-22] (TABLE 22.7)

NOTE: Treatment length and dosage may vary per protocol.

TABLE 22.7

ANTIMICROBIAL PROPHYLAXIS IN ONCOLOGY PATIENTS[3,20-22]

Organism	Medication	Indication
Pneumocystis jirovecii	TMP-SMX: 2–3 consecutive days per week Alternatives: atovaquone, dapsone, or pentamidine	Patients receiving chemotherapy and/or HSCT; and usually at least 3–6 months after therapy completion
HSV, CMV, VZV	Acyclovir or valacyclovir (dosing is different for zoster, varicella, and mucocutaneous HSV)	At risk for prolonged neutropenia (HSCT, AML, induction chemotherapy for high-risk leukemia, or reinduction therapy for relapsed leukemia)

Organism	Medication	Indication
Candida albicans	Fluconazole Alternatives: voriconazole or micafungin	Patients with leukemia or after HSCT (usually at least 28 days)
Gram-positive and Gram-negative organisms	Levofloxacin	HSCT or leukemias with prolonged severe neutropenia until counts normalize

AML, Acute myeloid leukemia; *CMV,* cytomegalovirus; *HSCT,* hematopoietic stem cell transplantation; *HSV,* herpes simplex virus; *TMP-SMX,* trimethoprim–sulfamethoxazole; *VZV,* varicella zoster virus.

IX. HEMATOPOIETIC STEM CELL TRANSPLANTATION (HSCT) (ALSO CALLED BONE MARROW OR STEM CELL TRANSPLANTATION)[3,4,23]

A. Goal
Administer healthy functioning hematopoietic stem cells from the bone marrow, peripheral blood, or umbilical cord blood to a patient whose bone marrow is diseased (e.g., hematologic malignancy) or depleted (after treatment with intense myeloablative chemotherapy). HSCT is also used for some congenital and acquired hematologic, immunologic, and metabolic disorders.

B. Preparative Regimens
1. **Myeloablative:** Elimination of recipient's diseased marrow with high-dose chemotherapy or chemotherapy plus total body irradiation (TBI) before stem cell infusion. Generally, provides greater anticancer activity but carries a higher risk of treatment-related organ injury
2. **Nonmyeloablative:** Reduced-intensity conditioning regimen in which marrow is not fully ablated, allowing recovery of autologous hematopoiesis if patient fails to engraft. Associated with decreased treatment-related morbidity and mortality but higher incidence of graft rejection

C. Types of HSCT
1. Allogeneic
   a. Recipient receives donor stem cells from a genetically similar but nonidentical donor, following a preparative regimen that includes chemotherapy ± radiation ± serotherapy. Donors undergo human leukocyte antigen (HLA) typing to determine if they are an adequate "match" to the recipient. Possible donors include HLA-matched siblings, fully or partially HLA-matched unrelated donors, umbilical cord blood units, and HLA-haploidentical (half-matched) related donors.
   b. Increased level of mismatch between donor and recipient increases the risk for graft-versus-host disease (GVHD) but may offer greater graft-versus-leukemia (GVL) immunologic treatment effect.

c. Used commonly for leukemias, myelodysplastic syndrome, hemophagocytic lymphohistiocytosis, and a number of nonmalignant hematologic, immunologic, and metabolic disorders

2. Autologous
   a. Donor is recipient. Stem cells are harvested from the patient, stored, and given back after the patient has received myeloablative doses of chemotherapy.
   b. Generally, lacks GVHD or GVL effect
   c. Used for high-risk neuroblastoma, lymphoma, and various high-risk solid tumors, which have demonstrated improved disease control after higher intensity chemotherapy that would otherwise be limited by excessive marrow suppression

D. Engraftment

1. Recipient's bone marrow is repopulated with donor stem cells that proliferate and mature.
2. Usually starts within 2 to 4 weeks from graft infusion and may present with an inflammatory response but can be significantly delayed with certain conditions such as drug toxicity or infection
3. Defined as an ANC more than 500/μL for 3 consecutive days

X. COMPLICATIONS OF HSCT[3,4,23-26]

A. Graft-Versus-Host Disease (GVHD)

1. **Etiology:** Donor T-cell–mediated reaction to unique host antigens. Risk factors include HLA disparity, source of stem cells (peripheral blood > bone marrow > umbilical cord blood), magnitude of conditioning-related tissue injury, and posttransplant infections.
2. **Presentation:** Acute GVHD most commonly occurs within 6 weeks of transplantation, typically within 100 days of transplantation; rarely, it may occur or persist beyond this time. Chronic GVHD traditionally presents >100 days after transplant but may occur earlier and persist.
   a. Maculopapular skin rash. Can progress to bullous lesions resembling toxic epidermal necrolysis
   b. GI symptoms: Anorexia, dyspepsia, nausea, vomiting, abdominal cramping, secretory diarrhea
   c. Liver: Direct hyperbilirubinemia ± transaminitis
   d. Chronic GVHD can involve nearly any organ. Can include sclerodermatous or lichenoid skin changes, cholestasis/hepatitis, lung involvement (restrictive or obstructive), and/or dry eyes and mouth
3. **Diagnosis:** Triad of rash, abdominal cramping with diarrhea, hyperbilirubinemia. Tissue biopsy of skin or mucosa can provide histologic confirmation, demonstrating lymphocytic infiltration and apoptosis. See Section XIII (EC Table 22.1) for clinical staging.
4. **Prevention and management:**

a. Prophylaxis: Immunosuppression with posttransplant cyclophosphamide, cyclosporine, mycophenolate mofetil, tacrolimus, and/or sirolimus; adjuvants include methotrexate and prednisone

b. First-line treatment: Grade 1 and 2 acute GVHD may be treated locally with topical steroids (skin) or nonabsorbable enteral steroids (gut). First-line systemic treatment of acute and chronic GVHD is corticosteroids, often with an additional immunosuppressant

c. NOTE: Patients with chronic cGVHD are functionally asplenic and significantly immunosuppressed, requiring antimicrobial prophylaxis.

B. Sinusoidal Obstructive Syndrome (SOS); Previously Known as Venoocclusive Disease (VOD)

1. **Etiology:** Injury to endothelial cells leads to activation of the clotting cascade in liver sinusoids, causing erythrocyte congestion and occlusive fibrosis of terminal intrahepatic venules and sinusoids. Occurs as a consequence of hematopoietic cell transplantation, hepatotoxic chemotherapy, and/or high-dose liver radiation. Typically occurs within 3 weeks of the insult, most common at the end of the first week after transplant

2. **Presentation:** Tender hepatomegaly, hyperbilirubinemia, edema, ascites, unexplained weight gain, thrombocytopenia refractory to transfusions

3. **Diagnosis:** Based upon the Cairo/Cooke revised criteria[26] with any two of the following:
   a. Elevated bilirubin (>2 mg/dL)
   b. Unexpected weight gain (>5% compared to baseline weight pre-HSCT)
   c. Excessive platelet transfusions consistent with refractory thrombocytopenia post-HSCT
   d. Hepatomegaly for age or increased size over pre-HSCT
   e. Right upper quadrant pain
   f. Ascites confirmed by physical exam and/or imaging studies
   g. Reversal of portal venous flow (hepatofugal flow) by Doppler ultrasound

      OR

   h. Any one of the following criteria following HSCT:
      (1) Hepatic biopsy consistent with SOS/VOD
      (2) Unexplained elevated portal venous wedge pressure

4. **Prevention and treatment:**
   a. Prevention: Ursodeoxycholic acid from conditioning through 90 days posttransplant
   b. Treatment: Mild/moderate SOS can be managed with supportive care, including fluid and sodium restriction and diuretics. Defibrotide is the only approved pharmacologic treatment modality, with improved outcomes with earlier initiation and a 50% response rate. Criteria for defibrotide use include renal or pulmonary dysfunction and severe SOS/VOD. Maintain coagulation factors, platelets, and RBCs in a stable range secondary to consumption.

XI. CANCER SURVIVORSHIP[5,27-29]

A. Understand the Diagnosis

Obtain comprehensive treatment summary from oncologist summarizing diagnosis, chemotherapeutic agents, radiation, surgeries, history of HSCT, and adverse drug reactions.

B. Monitoring

1. Determine any potential toxicities by organ system based upon treatments received and devise a plan for routine evaluation.
2. See Table 22.5 and https://www.survivorshipguidelines.org for common late effects of therapy.
3. Multidisciplinary follow-up with clinician, social work, physical therapist, occupational therapist, neuropsychology/neuropsychiatry, nutritionist, and dentist.

A. VACCINATIONS IN ONCOLOGY AND HSCT PATIENTS: SEE CHAPTER 16

XII. FERTILITY PRESERVATION[30]

All newly diagnosed patients should be evaluated and counseled early on after treatment plans are made for the risk of infertility. It is important to identify which, if any, gonadotoxic therapies will be used for oncologic treatment. Different fertility preservation options are available depending on a patient's risk category (low, intermediate, high).

The choice of fertility preservation methodology is dependent on age and location of cancer. Among the chemotherapeutic drugs, alkylating agents have been shown to be associated with ovarian damage. Other risk factors for infertility include radiation to the abdomen and pelvis and surgery removing part or all reproductive organs.

For females, options include oocyte or ovarian cryopreservation, ovarian suppression, and ovarian transposition. For males, the primary option is sperm cryopreservation, though an experimental option of testicular tissue cryopreservation is available for prepubertal males.

A. Resources for Patients and Families

1. Fertility Hope (Livestrong): http://www.fertilehope.org
2. ASCO Survivorship Guidelines for Fertility Preservation: https://ascopubs.org/doi/abs/10.1200/JOP.18.00160
3. NCCN Adolescent & Young Adult Guidelines: https://www.nccn.org/guidelines

XIII. WEB RESOURCES

- National Cancer Institute (NCI): https://www.cancer.gov/cancertopics/pdq/pediatrictreatment
- NCI Clinical Trial Database: https://www.cancer.gov/clinicaltrials

- Surveillance, Epidemiology, and End Results (SEER) from NCI: http://seer.cancer.gov/
- Children's Oncology Group: https://www.childrensoncologygroup.org
- Long-term follow-up guidelines for survivors of pediatric cancer: http://www.survivorshipguidelines.org/
- Children's Oncology Camping Association, International: https://www.cocai.org/

REFERENCES

A complete list of references can be found online.

Chapter 23

Palliative Care

Sapna Desai, MD

See additional content online.

Audio Case File 23.1 End of life decision making in the adolescent palliative care patient

I. INTRODUCTION TO HOSPICE AND PALLIATIVE MEDICINE

A. Definition of Palliative Care[1,2]

1. Palliative care is the active total care of the child's body, mind, and spirit with the intent to prevent and relieve suffering, with a special focus on symptom control.
2. Palliative medicine supports the best quality of life for the child and family. It can be provided along with disease-directed treatment from the time of diagnosis of serious illness.
3. See Fig. 23.1 for the current accepted model for palliative care.

B. Definition of Hospice

1. Hospice care is an insurance benefit that may be initiated for patients who have a terminal illness with a life expectancy estimated to be 6 months or less.
2. It specializes in care at the end of life to promote a child's comfort and to support loved ones in their bereavement.

C. Concurrent Care for Children[3]

1. Prior to the Affordable Care Act, Medicaid would only provide either curative treatment or hospice services to those who qualified.
2. Now, children living with life-limiting or life-threatening conditions who are enrolled in Medicaid (and some other insurance providers) can receive both curative/life-prolonging treatments and hospice services.

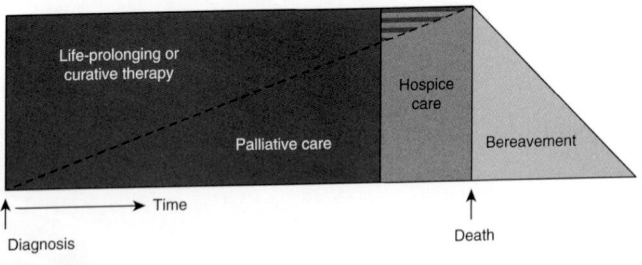

FIGURE 23.1

Current accepted model for palliative care.

D. Team Composition

1. Hospice and palliative care teams are robust and interdisciplinary.
2. They may include physicians, nurses, nurse practitioners, physician assistants, psychologists, counselors, social workers, child life specialists, pastoral care, patient care coordinators, and bereavement coordinators.

E. Timing of Palliative Care Consults

1. Palliative care teams can become involved at any point during a child's life, but it is best to involve them as early as possible.
2. Prenatal consults may be done with parents to help them with planning, decision making, and development of a birth plan.

II. COMMUNICATION AND DECISION-MAKING

A. Decision-Making Tools[4]

1. Provide framework for discussion with families regarding medical issues, quality of life, family goals, preferences, and other contextual preferences, such as spirituality and culture.
2. **Advance directives:**
   a. Adolescents 18 years and older can name another adult to make healthcare decisions if they cannot speak for themselves.
   b. Children younger than 18 years can participate in decision-making with tools such as "Five Wishes" and "Voicing My Choices."

B. Structuring Family Meetings[5]

1. Make sure all necessary individuals are present and understand the meeting's purpose.
2. A pre-meeting with the healthcare team is helpful to make sure all clinicians agree about the patient's condition and recommendations.
3. Identify who will facilitate the meeting.
4. **Choose a private location with minimal distraction.**
5. Always have water and tissues available.
6. Begin by introducing all participants and the meeting's purpose.
7. Assess what the family knows and expects regarding the patient's condition.
8. Describe the clinical situation, providing the big picture and then asking family members if they would like or are ready for more details.
9. Encourage each family member to express concerns and questions.
10. Explore the patient's and family's values and how they influence decision making.
11. Propose goals for the patient's care that reflect the stated values.
12. Provide a concrete follow-up plan.

C. Breaking Bad News[6]

1. Prepare yourself: Know the medical information, know what you will say, ask the patient/family if they want someone specific present with them for the discussion.
2. Prepare the family/patient: Give a brief, calm statement that leads into the news.

3. State the news: Do this clearly, concisely, and as definitively as possible.
4. Wait for the patient/family's reaction: Resist the urge to say more, allowing others to speak first.
5. Reflect the response back: "This news is clearly very upsetting to you."
6. Legitimize the reaction: "It is understandable that you would be upset."
7. Explore: "What upsets you most about this news?"
8. Provide realistic hope.
9. Discuss next steps (if appropriate at this time): "May I address your concerns now and talk about the next steps for treatment, or would you like more time?"

D. Other Tools for Difficult Conversations

1. Assess spirituality according to the "FICA" tool[7]:
   a. **F**aith and belief: "Do you consider yourself spiritual or religious?"
   b. **I**mportance in life: "What importance does your faith or belief system have in your life?"
   c. **C**ommunity: "Are you a part of a spiritual or religious community?"
   d. **A**ddress in care: "How would you like me, your healthcare provider, to address these issues in your healthcare?"
2. "Ask-tell-ask"[8]
   a. **Ask** the patient/family to describe their understanding of the situation or issue.
   b. **Tell** them what you need to communicate in a straightforward manner.
   c. **Ask** them questions to assess their understanding.
3. "Hope together" with the patient/family while also preparing for all possible outcomes.

III. CARE OF THE DYING CHILD

A. Limiting Interventions

The following options should be considered.

1. Do not attempt resuscitation (DNAR)/allow natural death (AND): Foregoing cardiopulmonary resuscitation (CPR) and other resuscitative interventions as part of a care plan that emphasizes comfort and quality of living
2. Do not intubate (DNI): Although, if clinically appropriate, may still allow the initiation of continuous positive-pressure ventilation or may help in managing symptoms
3. Do not escalate treatment: The choice to forego changes in treatment, even as a patient's condition worsens, because death is expected Examples include the following:
   a. Do not increase the dose of current medications (e.g., vasopressors).
   b. Do not add new medications (e.g., antibiotics).
   c. Do not initiate new interventions (e.g., dialysis, mechanical ventilation).
   d. However, one may still initiate and increase interventions to treat pain and reduce suffering.

4. Discontinuing current interventions: The option of discontinuing interventions that prolong the dying process must also be discussed.
5. Medical orders for life-sustaining treatment (MOLST) and physician orders for life-sustaining treatment (POLST) forms:
   a. These are portable and enduring medical order forms completed by patients or their authorized decision-makers and are signed by a physician.
   b. They contain orders regarding CPR and other life-sustaining treatments.
   c. If a state offers one of these forms, the orders are valid for emergency medical service providers as well as healthcare providers and facilities within that state.
   d. A copy must be provided to the patient or authorized decision maker within 48 hours of completion or sooner if the patient is to be transferred.
   e. Refer to your state's laws prior to completing any documentation.
   f. Additional information for US providers can be found at https://www.polst.org.

B. Involving the Child in Conversations About Death[9-12]

1. See Table 23.1 for the development of death concepts in children.[13]
2. A minor child has the capacity to meaningfully participate in medical decision making if he or she demonstrates the ability to do all of the following:
   a. Communicate understanding of the medical information
   b. State his or her preference
   c. Communicate understanding of the consequences of decisions

TABLE 23.1

CONCEPTUALIZATION OF DEATH IN CHILDREN

Age Range	Characteristics	Concepts of Death	Interventions
0–2 years	Achieve object permanence May sense something is wrong	None	Provide maximal comfort with familiar persons and favorite toys.
2–6 years	Magical thoughts	Believe death is temporary Do not personalize death Believe death can be caused by thoughts	Minimize separation from parents, correct perceptions that the illness is punishment.
6–12 years	Concrete thoughts	Understand death can be personal Interested in details of death	Be truthful, evaluate fears, provide concrete details if requested, allow participation in decision making.
12–18 years	Reality becomes objective Capable of self-reflection	Search for meaning, hope, purpose, and value of life	Be truthful, allow expression of strong feelings, allow participation in decision making.

3. Helpful documents are available for purchase from the nonprofit Aging with Dignity (see Section IV.B).
   a. Five Wishes: This is a legal advance directive with versions tailored for adolescents.
   b. Voicing My Choices: A workbook for adolescents intended to complement Five Wishes
   c. My Wishes: A simple booklet for younger children to help them share their preferences

C. Outpatient Care

1. Provide continuity of care and advanced symptom management.
2. Focus on both patient and caregiver stress and support.

D. Supporting Patients Throughout the Dying Process[13-16, 22]

1. See Table 23.2 for normal changes that occur as death approaches and their recommended management.
2. See Table 23.3 for appropriate dosing of recommended medications. (NOTE: Doses may be different for other indications.)
3. Integrative therapies can be utilized. For example, aromatherapy can be used for comfort and symptoms such as nausea, vomiting, pain, and anxiety.

TABLE 23.2

SYMPTOMATIC MANAGEMENT OF THE DYING PATIENT

System	Changes as Death Approaches	Interventions
Neurologic	Pain Overactive senses (hearing last to diminish) Increased need for sleep with occasional surge of energy to play or socialize	Morphine as needed Dim lights and reduce noise, provide soft background music
Cardiovascular	Heart rate increases, blood pressure decreases, pulse weakens, and skin becomes cooler	Inform family that death is near
Respiratory	Increased secretions Air hunger	Turn every few hours, elevate head of bed, frequent mouth care (avoid deep suctioning) Hyoscyamine Positive pressure through handheld fan Supplemental room air or oxygen as needed Morphine
Gastrointestinal	Nausea and vomiting Decreased appetite, preference for liquids Natural dehydration, fevers	Ondansetron or prochlorperazine Ice chips, moist mouth swabs Antipyretics per rectum
Dermatologic	Pruritus	Diphenhydramine
Psychiatric	Decreased interactions with outside world as thoughts and emotions are increasingly directed inward Agitation or delirium	Provide reassurance to family Frequently orient child to surroundings, surround with family and speak calmly Lorazepam and haloperidol if needed

TABLE 23.3

DOSING FOR MEDICATIONS USED IN PALLIATIVE CARE[13,20, 22-24]

Indication	Medication	Initial Regimen
Pain	Morphine	0.2–0.4 mg/kg/dose PO, SC, SL, PR Q2–4 hr[a]
		0.1–0.2 mg/kg/dose IV Q2–4 hr[a]
		NOTE: Morphine should be titrated to symptomatic relief.
	Hydromorphone[b]	0.03–0.08 mg/kg/dose PO Q2–4 hr
		0.015–0.02 mg/kg/dose IV, SC Q2–4 hr
	Oxycodone	0.1 mg/kg/dose PO 4hr (adult dose 5-10 mg)
Neuropathic pain	Gabapentin[b]	3–5 mg/kg/dose QHS day 1, BID day 2, then TID day 3
		(titrate to effect, max dose per day 3600 mg)
Dyspnea	Morphine	0.1–0.25 mg/kg/dose PO, SC, SL, PR Q2–4 hr
		0.05–0.1 mg/kg/dose IV Q2–4 hr
Agitation	Lorazepam	0.02–0.05 mg/kg/dose PO, IV, SL, PR Q4–8 hr
	Haloperidol	0.01–0.02 mg/kg/dose PO, IM, SC, IV Q8–12 hr
Pruritus	Diphenhydramine	0.5–1 mg/kg/dose PO, IV Q6–8 hr
Nausea/Vomiting	Prochlorperazine	0.1–0.15 mg/kg/dose PO, PR Q6–8 hr
	Ondansetron	0.15 mg/kg/dose PO, IV Q6–8 hr (max dose 8 mg)
	Granisetron	0.01 mg/kg IV/PO Q12hr (max 1 mg/dose)
	Olanzapine	0.1 mg/kg PO once daily (max 10 mg, titrate down in cases
		of oversedation)
Seizures	Diazepam	0.3–0.5 mg/kg/dose PR Q2–4 hr
	Lorazepam	0.05–0.1 mg/kg/dose SC, SL, IV Q2–4 hr
Secretions	Glycopyrrolate	0.04–0.1 mg/kg PO (max 8 mg/day)
		0.004–0.01 mg/kg (4–10 mCg/kg) IV, SC

NOTE: For *adult*-sized patients, see Formulary for adult dosing recommendations.

[a]Infants <6 months should receive one-third to one-half the dose. For adolescents, consider starting adult dosing of 10 to 30 mg/dose PO, 2 to 15 mg/dose IV.

[b]Medication has not been studied in neonates.

BID, Twice daily; *IV,* intravenous; *PO,* oral; *PR,* rectal; *QHS,* nightly; *SC,* subcutaneous; *SL,* sublingual; *TID,* three times daily.

4. Management of refractory distress
   a. Palliative sedation therapy is rarely required in pediatrics.
   b. The intent of palliative sedation therapy is relief of intolerable suffering from refractory symptoms by decreasing level of consciousness through sedation.
   c. Medications are titrated to symptom relief.
   d. Ensure that all appropriate symptom management strategies have been attempted, including expert consultation and nonpharmacologic approaches. Expert advice from palliative medicine experts is strongly recommended.

E. Pronouncing Death[17]

1. Preparation
   a. Know the child's name and gender.
   b. Be prepared to answer simple, pertinent questions from family and friends.
   c. Consult with nursing staff for relevant information, such as recent events and family dynamics.

    d. Determine the need and call for interdisciplinary support, such as social work, child life, pastoral care, and/or a bereavement coordinator.

2. Entering the room
   a. Enter quietly and respectfully along with the primary nurse.
   b. **Introduce yourself and identify your role.**
   c. Determine the relationship of those in the room.
   d. Inform the family of the purpose of your visit ("I am here to examine your child") and invite them to remain in the room.

3. Procedure for pronouncement
   a. Check ID bracelet and pulse.
   b. Respectfully check response to tactile stimuli.
   c. Check for spontaneous respirations for a minimum of 1 minute.
   d. Check for heart sounds for a minimum of 1 minute.
   e. Record the time of death.
   f. Inform the family of death ("[Child's name] has died").
   g. Remember to convey sympathy ("I'm so sorry for your loss").
   h. Offer to contact other family members.

4. Documentation of death in the chart
   a. Write date, time of death, and the provider pronouncing the death.
   b. Document absence of pulse, respirations, and heart sounds.
   c. Identify family members who were present and informed of death.
   d. Document notification of the attending physician.

F. Explaining Autopsies[18]

1. Definitions
   a. **Autopsy:** Definitive examination of a deceased patient to determine the cause of death
   b. **Forensic autopsy:** Legally mandated examination to determine cause of death in a criminal investigation
   c. **Rapid autopsy:** Urgent removal of tissues for research uses

2. Answers to frequently asked questions
   a. A voluntary autopsy can look at all parts of a patient's body or only some.
   b. An autopsy will not affect the patient's body cosmetically and should not affect funeral or viewing arrangements.
   c. An autopsy takes 2 to 4 hours to perform and should not delay funeral/burial arrangements.

3. Benefits of autopsy
   a. For families:
      (1) May provide closure regarding diagnosis
      (2) May help identify possible genetic or other etiologies for unexplained death
   b. For providers: Clarifies potential diagnostic errors and uncertainties

G. Organ Donation

1. Most hospitals have a special third-party team that coordinates organ donations.

2. Inform family members, if they are interested, that this team may be visiting soon to explain the process.

H. Completing Death Certificates[17]

1. Locate a copy of a sample death certificate for reference.
2. Cardiopulmonary arrest or respiratory arrest is NOT an acceptable primary cause of death.
3. For specific instructions for your state and/or institution, contact the Office of Decedent Affairs at your institution.
4. If you are completing a handwritten death certificate:
   a. Use BLACK INK ONLY and complete *Physician sections.*
   b. DO NOT use abbreviations (e.g., May 1 not 5/1).
   c. DO NOT cross out or use correction fluid; you must begin again if mistakes are made.

I. Interacting with Loved Ones After a Child's Death

1. It is appropriate to send condolence cards, contact families, or attend funerals after a child has died. These are all appropriate physician activities that are deeply valued by bereaved families. Families want to know that their children are not forgotten.
2. Numerous services are available for families, including pastoral care, social work, bereavement coordinators, community support groups, counseling services, and bereavement follow-up programs.

IV. WEB RESOURCES

- Center to Advance Palliative Care: https://www.capc.org
- Aging With Dignity: https://agingwithdignity.org/
- The American Academy of Hospice and Palliative Medicine: https://www.aahpm.org
- The National Hospice and Palliative Care Organization: https://www.nhpco.org

REFERENCES

A complete list of references can be found online.

Chapter 24

Psychiatry

Jelina Marie V. Castillo, MD, MPH

⊗ See additional content online.

I. OVERVIEW

A. General Approach

1. Screening:
   a. Surveillance for mental health issues should occur at all well child visits from early childhood through adolescence.
   b. The Pediatric Symptom Checklist (PSC) is a general mental health checklist that screens for a broad array of disorders (Table 24.1).[1]
2. See the *Diagnostic and Statistical Manual of Mental Disorders*, fifth edition (DSM-5), for a full list of psychiatric diagnoses.[2]
3. Pharmacotherapy for many disorders may be managed or monitored by the pediatrician.[3]

B. Mental Status Exam

1. General appearance: Dress, self-care, demeanor, attitude, behavior, developmental milestones
2. Motor activity: Activity level (restless, fidgety, stereotyped, or ritualized movements)
3. Speech and language: Fluency, comprehension, rate, rhythm, volume, expressive and receptive skills
4. Mood and affect: Stated by patient and observed by clinician
5. Thought form: Goal directed nature of thoughts, coherence, organization
6. Thought content:
   a. What patient is thinking about
   b. Mood, suicidal ideation, homicidal ideation, delusions
7. Abnormal perceptual phenomena: Illusions, hallucinations
8. Insight, judgment, cognition developmentally appropriate

C. Behavioral Interventions

1. Brief behavioral interventions can be done based on primary presenting problem or symptoms prior to escalation of care (Table 24.4).

II. POSTPARTUM DEPRESSION

A. Diagnosis

1. Depression occurring in the 12-month period after birth
2. Maternal depression is important to identify and treat given the substantial impact on the health of the developing infant. Impaired

TABLE 24.1

MENTAL HEALTH SCREENING TOOLS BY DIAGNOSIS

Suspected Diagnosis	Screening Test	Age Group	Administration Time	Completed By
General psychosocial screening	Pediatric Symptom Checklist (PSC)	Ages 4–16 >11 years for child/adolescent self-report[a]	5 min	Different versions can be completed by parent or child/adolescent.
Postpartum depression	Edinburgh Postnatal Depression Scale	All postpartum mothers until child is 12 months of age	5 min	Mother
Attention-deficit/hyperactivity disorder (ADHD)	Vanderbilt Diagnostic Rating Scales	6–12 years[a]	10 min	Parent and teacher
Anxiety	Generalized Anxiety Disorder-7 (GAD-7)	>12 years[a]	5 min	Parent or child/adolescent
Depression	Patient Health Questionnaire-2 (PHQ-2) and Patient Health Questionnaire-9 (PHQ-9)	>12 years[b]	10 min	Child/adolescent
Eating disorders	Eating Disorder Screen for Primary Care (ESP)	Any age	1 min	Child/adolescent

[a]Recommendation based on validated age for screening tool, however can screen at any age if clinical suspicion

[b]Recommendation based on US Preventative Services Task Force (USPTF), however can screen at any age of clinical suspicion

Listed are the most common screening tools; however, more are available via The American Academy of Pediatrics. Mental health tools for pediatrics. In: *Addressing Mental Health Concerns in Pediatrics: A Practical Resource Toolkit for Clinicians.* 2nd ed. 2021.[1]

24

TABLE 24.2

BRIEF INTERVENTIONS FOR COMMON PEDIATRIC PRIMARY CARE PROBLEMS

Presenting Problem Area	Most Common Elements of Related Evidence-Based Practices
Anxiety	Graded exposure, modeling
ADHD and oppositional problems	Tangible rewards, praise for child and parent, help with monitoring, time-out, effective commands and limit setting, response cost
Low mood	Cognitive and/or coping methods, problem-solving strategies, activity scheduling, behavioral rehearsal, social skills building

Modified from Wissow LS, et al. Integrating children's mental health into primary care.[4]

maternal attachment may compromise the social, cognitive, and behavioral development of the infant.[5]
3. Differential diagnosis: Postpartum blues, other postpartum mood disorders such as bipolar mood disorder, postpartum psychosis

B. Epidemiology

1. According to CDC analysis of Pregnancy Risk Assessment Monitoring System, 13.2% of women self-reported depressive symptoms postpartum in 2018.[6]

C. Evaluation

1. Universal screening is recommended for all postpartum women.
2. A history of depression doubles the risk of postpartum depression and should prompt careful assessment for postpartum symptoms.[7]
3. Screening can be done using The Edinburgh Postnatal Depression Scale.

D. Management

1. Referral to mother's primary care physician or a mental health expert is preferred.[8]

III. COMMON PSYCHIATRIC CONDITIONS OF CHILDREN AND ADOLESCENTS

A. Attention-Deficit/Hyperactivity Disorder (ADHD)

1. Diagnosis:
   a. DSM-5 diagnostic criteria:
      (1) Inattention, impulsivity/hyperactivity that are more frequent and severe than typically observed in children of the same developmental age
      (2) Symptoms must persist for 6 months or more, occur before the age of 12 years, and should be evident in two or more settings (e.g., home and school).[2]
      (3) Persistent pattern of inattention and/or hyperactivity-impulsivity that interferes with functioning or development
      (4) Subtypes: Combined, predominantly inattentive, or predominantly hyperactive/impulsive

b. If the medical history is unremarkable, no further laboratory or testing is required. Psychological and neuropsychological testing is not required for diagnosis but is recommended if other academic or developmental concerns are present.

c. Differential diagnosis: Conduct disorder, oppositional defiant disorder, anxiety, depression, or learning disorder. Vanderbilt Diagnostic Rating Scale scoring can help differentiate between these diagnoses.

d. Adverse childhood events (ACE) or trauma exposure can also contribute to an ADHD-like presentation, so referral for therapy can also be useful in this context. See Chapter 9 for more information on ACE and trauma.

2. Epidemiology:

a. According to the National Survey of Children's Health, prevalence of ADHD for 2- to 17- year-olds was 9.4%, with boys being more likely and earlier to be diagnosed than girls.[9]

b. Most affected children continue to meet the diagnostic criteria for ADHD through adolescence.

3. Evaluation:

a. Evaluate all children who have academic and/or behavioral concerns for ADHD using Vanderbilt Diagnostic Rating Scales for parent and teacher. Vanderbilt can also be used to monitor changes in behavior and efficacy of interventions[10] (see Table 24.1).

4. Management:

a. Pharmacologic treatment works best with behavioral therapy as an adjunct.[10]

b. Refer to Table 24.2 for brief behavioral interventions.

c. Referral for behavioral therapy may be tried alone in preschool-age children (4 to 5 years old).

d. Before starting stimulant medication, take a history to exclude cardiac symptoms, Wolff-Parkinson-White syndrome, a family history of sudden death, hypertrophic cardiomyopathy, and long QT syndrome. If there is a cardiac history, referral for further testing to a cardiologist is recommended prior to initiating treatment. Screening electrocardiography is not required if there is no personal or family history of cardiac disease.[11]

e. See Table 24.3 for pharmacologic treatment. The ADHD Medication guide (https://www.adhdmedicationguide.com) provides visual information.

f. Titrate medications to maximal symptom control with minimal side effects. Symptom control is expected within 1 week of medication initiation.

g. Common side effects of stimulants include appetite suppression, abdominal pain, headaches, palpitations, and sleep disturbance.[10]

h. If the first stimulant is ineffective, consider an alternative class of stimulant. Second-line options as alternative therapy or as an

TABLE 24.3

COMMONLY USED PSYCHOTROPIC MEDICATIONS

Class	Drug Name	FDA Approved Ages	Starting Dose	Titration	Maximum Dose
Antidepressant/ Anxiolytics	Fluoxetine (Prozac)	7+ years (OCD) 8+ years (MDD)	10 mg	10 mg weekly	20 mg/24 hr
	Sertraline (Zoloft)	6+ years (OCD)	≤12 yo 12.5 ≥13 yo 25 mg	≤12 yo 25 mg weekly ≥13 yo 50 mg weekly	200 mg/24 hr
	Escitalopram (Lexapro)	12+ years (MDD)	10 mg	10 mg after 3 weeks	20 mg/24 hr
Methylphenidate Preparations	Methylphenidate (Ritalin)	6+ years	0.3 mg/kg/dose (or 2.5–5mg)	0.1 mg/kg (or 5–10 mg) weekly	2 mg/kg/24 hr or 60 mg/24 hr for <50 kg or 100 mg/24 hr for >50 kg
	Methylphenidate (Concerta)	6+ years	18 mg	18 mg weekly	6–12 yo: 54 mg/24 hr 13–17 yo: 72 mg/24 hr
	Dexmethylphenidate (Focalin)	6+ years	6–17 yo Immediate: 2.5 mg ER: 5 mg ≥18 yo Immediate: 2.5 mg ER: 20 mg/24 hr	6–17 yo Immediate: 2.5–5 mg ER: 5 mg weekly ≥18 yo Immediate: 2.5–5 mg ER: 10 mg weekly	6–17yo Immediate: 20 mg/24 hr ER: 30 mg/24 hr ≥18 yo Immediate: 20 mg/24 hr ER: 40 mg/24 hr
Amphetamine Preparations	Lisdexamfetamine (Vyvanse)	6+ years	<18 yo 20 mg ≥18 yo 30 mg	10–20 mg weekly	70 mg/24 hr
	Dextroamphetamine + amphetamine (Adderall)	3+ years (IR) 6+ years (ER)	3–5 yo 2.5 mg ≥6 yo 5 mg	3–5 yo 2.5 mg weekly ≥6 yo 5 mg weekly	40 mg/24 hr Or >50 kg 60 mg/24 hr

Non-stimulant options				
Clonidine extended release (Kapvay)	6+ years	≤45 kg 0.05 mg >45 kg 0.1 mg	≤45 kg 0.05 mg every 3–7 days >45 kg 0.1 mg every 3–7 days	27–40.5 kg 0.2 mg/24 hr 40.5–45 kg 0.3 mg/24 hr >45 kg 0.4 mg/24 hr
Guanfacine immediate-release (Tenex)	12+ years	≤45 kg 0.5 mg >45 kg 1 mg	≤45 kg 0.5 mg every 3–4 days >45 kg 1 mg every 3–4 days	27–40.5 kg 2 mg/24 hr 40.5–45 kg 3 mg/24 hr >45 kg 4 mg/24 hr
Guanfacine extended release (Intuniv)	6+ years	1 mg	1 mg weekly	6–12 yo 4 mg/24 hr >12 yo 7 mg/24 hr
Atomoxetine (Strattera)	6+ years	≤70 kg 0.5 mg/kg/24 hr >70 kg 40 mg	≤70 kg 1.2 mg/kg/24 hr After 3 days >70 kg 80 mg After 3 days	≤70 kg 1.4 mg/kg/24 hr or 100 mg >70 kg 100 mg
Antipsychotic for Acute Agitation				
Haloperidol (Haldol IM)	Not established	6–12 yo 1–3 mg >12 yo 2–5 mg	6–12 yo Q4–8 hr PRN >12 yo Q1 hr PRN	0.15 mg/kg/24 hr

IR, Immediate Release; *ER*, Extended Release; ASD, Autism spectrum disorder; GAD, generalized anxiety disorder; MDD, major depressive disorder; OCD, obsessive-compulsive disorder.

Modified from the Centers for Medicare and Medicaid Services factsheets (https://www.CMS.gov) and the U.S. Food and Drug Administration.

24

augmenting agent to stimulant therapy include guanfacine, clonidine, and atomoxetine.[3,10] If multiple medication trials prove ineffective, consultation with a psychiatrist is suggested.

B. Oppositional Defiant Disorder (ODD)

1. Diagnosis:
   a. DSM-5 diagnostic criteria: Angry/irritable mood with argumentative/defiant behavior and vindictiveness for 6 or more months
   b. Behavior must be present with at least one non-sibling.
2. Epidemiology:
   a. According to the National Survey of Children's Health, prevalence of ODD for 3- to 17-year-olds was 4.6% in 2007. Prevalence of these disorders was twice as high among boys as among girls. Age of onset approximately 6 years of age, frequently comorbid with ADHD.[12]
3. Evaluation:
   a. Many screening tools are available, including the Vanderbilt Assessment Scale (see Table 24.1).[13]
4. Management:
   a. No evidence for pharmacologic intervention as first-line therapy for ODD
   b. Refer to Table 24.2 brief behavioral interventions.
   c. Combination of cognitive behavioral therapy (CBT) and parent management training (PMT) may be most effective as first-line intervention.[14]

C. Anxiety Disorders

1. Diagnosis:
   a. A group of disorders characterized by excessive fear, anxiety, and related behavioral disturbances. May present with fear or worry and without recognizing that their fear or anxiety is unreasonable
   b. Commonly presents as somatic complaints of headache and abdominal pain. Patients with many primary care visits for such complaints may benefit from formal anxiety screening.
   c. Fear/anxiety may affect school performance or manifest as school avoidance.
   d. Crying, irritability, angry outbursts, and disruptive behavior are expressions of fear and an effort to avoid anxiety-provoking stimuli.
   e. Consider screening for adverse childhood experiences (ACE) or trauma exposure (see Chapter 9 for more information).
   f. DSM-5 diagnostic criteria vary based on the specific disorder[2]: (1) generalized anxiety disorder, (2) separation anxiety disorder, (3) social anxiety disorder, (4) selective mutism, (5) specific phobia, (6) panic disorder, (7) agoraphobia
   g. Differential diagnosis: Obsessive-compulsive disorder, posttraumatic stress disorder

2. Epidemiology:
   a. According to the National Survey of Children's Health, prevalence of anxiety diagnosis for 6- to 17-year-olds per parent report was 6.4% in 2011–2012, increased from 5.5% in 2007.[15]
   b. There are ongoing studies on the effect of the COVID-19 pandemic on prevalence of anxiety in youth related to the social isolation and increase in social stressors. Meta-analysis of global data suggests increase of clinically elevated anxiety symptoms by 20.5%.[16]
3. Evaluation:
   a. Multiple tools, such as the Generalized Anxiety Disorder-7 (GAD-7) and Self-Report for Childhood Anxiety Related Emotional Disorders (SCARED), are available (see Table 24.1).
4. Management (Fig. 24.1):
   a. CBT with or without pharmacotherapy (Table 24.3) based on the disorder and its severity[17]
   b. Refer to Table 24.2 for brief behavioral interventions.[4]

D. Depressive and Mood Disorders

1. Diagnosis:
   a. A group of disorders characterized by mood changes as well as somatic and cognitive symptoms that disrupt functioning
   b. DSM-5 major depressive disorder diagnostic criteria:
      (1) Five or more of the following symptoms for 2 or more weeks: Must include either depressed mood/irritability OR anhedonia; changes in appetite/weight, sleep, or activity; fatigue or loss of energy; guilt/worthlessness; decreased concentration; suicidality
      (2) Symptoms cause significant impairment in functioning.
      (3) Symptoms not due to substance use or a medical condition
      (4) No history of manic episodes[19]
   c. Other depressive disorders are defined by their own diagnostic criteria[2]:
      (1) Disruptive mood dysregulation disorder
      (2) Persistent depressive disorder (dysthymia)
      (3) Premenstrual dysphoric disorder
   d. Differential diagnosis: Bipolar disorder, adjustment disorder, demoralization
2. Epidemiology:
   a. According to the National Survey of Children's Health, prevalence of depression diagnosis for 6- to 17-year-olds per parent report was 4.9% in 2011–2012.[15]
   b. There are ongoing studies on the effect of the COVID-19 pandemic on the prevalence of depression in youth related to the social isolation and increase in social stressors. Meta-analysis of global data suggests increase of clinically elevated depressive symptoms by 25.2%.[16]
   c. Common comorbid conditions: Anxiety disorders, disruptive behavior disorders, ADHD, substance use

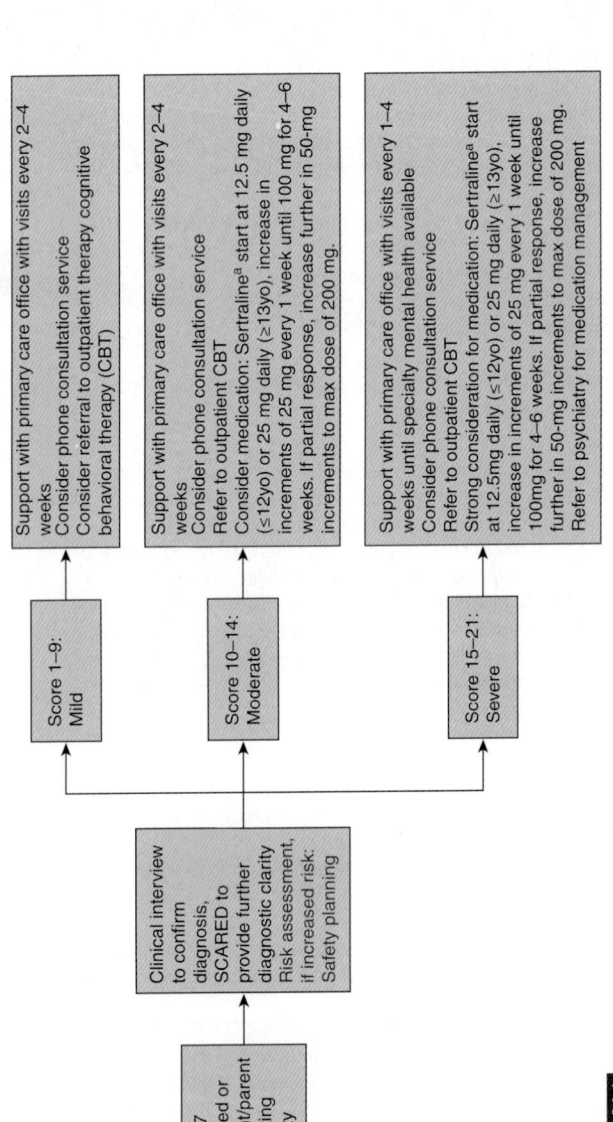

FIGURE 24.1

Management of anxiety.

[a]There is no reason to believe sertraline is superior to other SSRIs such as fluoxetine or escitalopram. Sertraline recommendation based on Child/Adolescent Anxiety Multimodal Study (CAMS) 2010.[18]

3. Evaluation:
   a. Routine screening is recommended for patients 12 years of age or older according to United States Preventative Services Taskforce (USPSTF); however, may consider younger if clinical concern
   b. Multiple screening tools are available (see Table 24.1). The Patient Health Questionnaire (PHQ-2) is a brief but effective tool for use in adolescents.[20]
   c. All patients with suspected depressive symptoms should be screened for suicidal ideation and referred for emergency evaluation if serious thoughts and/or action plans are endorsed (see Section IV.A).
4. Management (Fig. 24.2)
   a. Refer to Table 24.2 for brief behavioral interventions.[4]
   b. Selective serotonin reuptake inhibitors (SSRIs) may be initiated in the primary care setting.
   c. Referral to subspecialist may be required depending on severity or in the case of treatment failure (see Fig. 24.2).
   d. Antidepressant medications (Table 24.3) and CBT combined are recommended as studies show these will have benefit earlier than medication or CBT alone. [21]
   e. Counsel patients that SSRIs may take up to 4 to 6 weeks for peak effect.
   f. SSRIs have a black box warning from the US Food and Drug Administration (FDA) concerning a possible increase in suicidal thoughts or behaviors after initiation of medication.
      (1) The basis of this warning was a large meta-analysis that found no increase in completed suicides but a small increase in suicidal ideation.[22]
      (2) Professional mental health groups support the continued use of SSRIs in treating depression in children and adolescents because the benefits outweigh potential risks.[22]

E. Eating Disorders

1. Diagnosis[2]:
   a. Anorexia nervosa
      (1) Restricted energy intake and low weight (body mass index [BMI] <18.5 kg/m^2; severity stratified by BMI)
      (2) Fear of gaining weight
      (3) Disturbance in perception of body weight or shape
   b. Bulimia nervosa
      (1) Recurrent episodes of binge eating that occur at least once a week for 3 months
      (2) Recurrent inappropriate compensatory mechanisms to prevent weight gain (e.g., diuretic or laxative use, exercise) or purging (self-induced vomiting)
      (3) Self-evaluation excessively influenced by body shape or weight

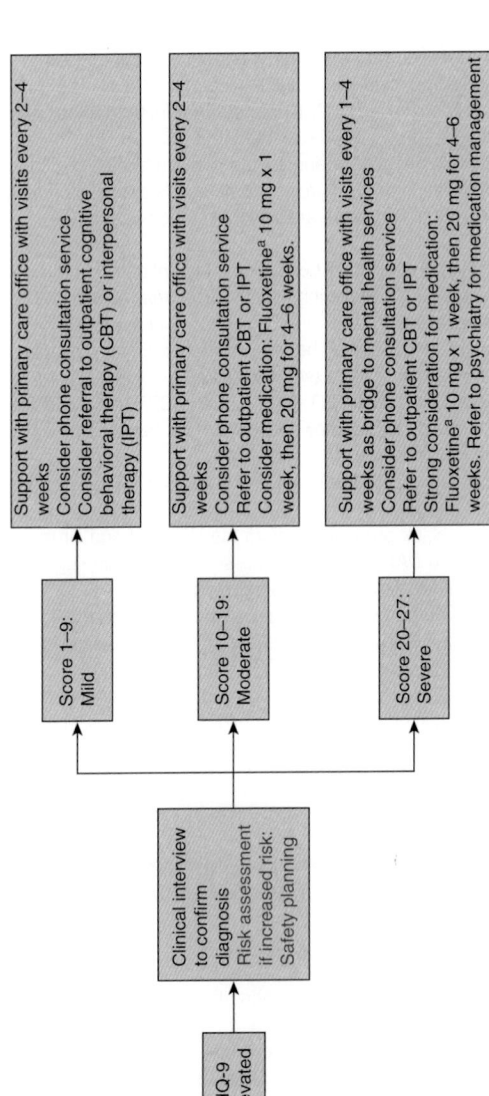

FIGURE 24.2

Management of depressive disorders.

[a]There is no reason to believe fluoxetine is superior to other SSRIs such as sertraline or escitalopram. Fluoxetine recommendation based on The Treatment for Adolescents with Depression Study (TADS) Study 2008.[21]

2. Epidemiology:
    a. According to the National Comorbidity Survey Adolescent Supplement, in the United States the lifetime prevalence of eating disorders was 2.7%; twice as prevalent among females (3.8%) than males (1.5%).[23]
    b. Common comorbidities: Mood and anxiety disorders
3. Evaluation:
    a. Many screening tools available, including the Eating Disorder Screen for Primary Care (ESP), the SCOFF (Sick, Control, One, Fat, Food) Questionnaire, and the Eating Attitudes Test (EAT-26) (see Table 24.1)[1]
4. Management:
    a. Aimed at nutritional rehabilitation, therapy (family-based or as a component of day treatment programs) and treatment of comorbid psychiatric illness. Hospitalization may be needed in cases of medical instability. See Chapter 21 for management of refeeding syndrome.
    b. SSRIs indicated in the treatment of bulimia nervosa (see Table 24.3). No medications have been approved for use in anorexia nervosa.[24]

F. Substance Use Disorders

1. Epidemiology:
    a. According to the National Survey on Drug Use and Health, 4.7% of adolescents ages 12 to 17 reported illicit drug use in the past year. Interviews from 2001 to 2004 for the National Comorbidity Survey Replication Adolescent Supplement estimated 8.3% prevalence of substance use disorder.[12]
    b. Common comorbid conditions: ADHD, disruptive behavior disorders, mood disorders, anxiety disorders
2. For more information on diagnosis, evaluation, and management, please see Chapter 5.

IV. PSYCHIATRIC EMERGENCIES

A. Suicide

1. Diagnosis:
    a. Thoughts or plans to end one's life or not wanting to live anymore. Screening must be done to ensure safety of patient.
2. Epidemiology:
    a. In 2019 suicide was the second leading cause of death among 10- to 34-year-olds.[25]
3. Evaluation:
    a. Inpatient, outpatient, and emergency department settings: Use the Ask Suicide-Screening Questions (ASQ) (Table 24.4). This tool is validated for identifying pediatric patients at risk for suicide.
4. Management: (see Table 24.4)

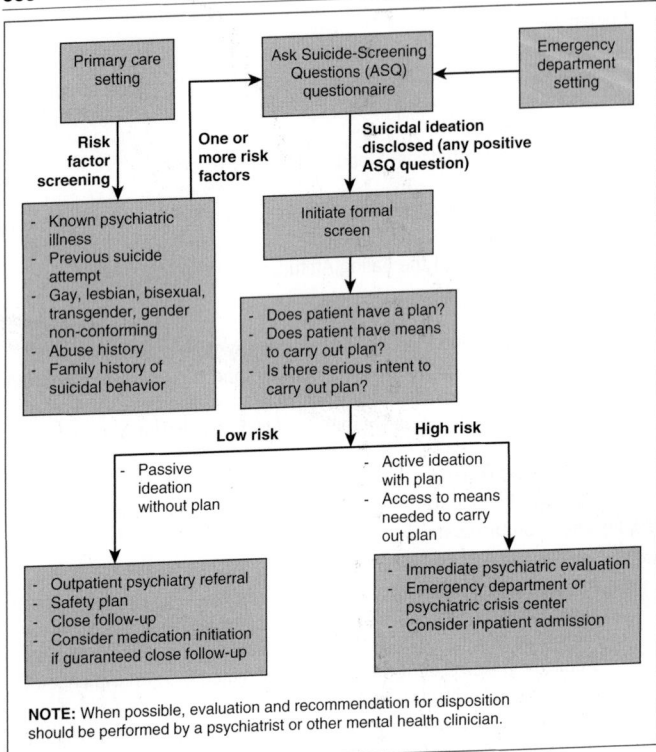

FIGURE 24.3

Suicide screening and assessment.

a. Goal is to determine disposition (inpatient versus outpatient) and develop a safety plan with caregivers (see Table 24.4).

b. Any positive reply to a screening question warrants further evaluation by the pediatrician and consideration of referral to a psychiatrist or other mental health professional.

B. Aggression or Impulsivity[26,27]

1. Diagnosis:

a. Agitation can be defined as disruptive behavior occurring during periods of emotional distress.

b. Manifestations include:

(1) Excessive motor activity: Pacing, fidgeting

(2) Verbal aggression: Yelling, shouting, rapid pressured speech, threats

(3) Physical aggression: Hitting, throwing things

TABLE 24.4

SUICIDE SAFETY PLAN AND SCREENING

Validated for identifying pediatric patients at risk for suicide.

1. In the past few weeks, have you wished you were dead?
2. In the past few weeks, have you felt that you or your family would be better off if you were dead?
3. In the past week, have you been having thoughts about killing yourself?
4. Have you ever tried to kill yourself?

Any affirmative response constitutes a positive screen.

COMPONENTS OF SAFETY PLAN

1. Understanding warning signs that crisis may be developing
2. Coping strategies
3. People or social settings that can provide distraction
4. People who can be reached for help
5. Referral to professional agencies or Suicide and Crisis Lifeline 988 during crisis, or saving these numbers into personal phone
6. Making the environment safe, ensuring means of suicide such as weapons or medications are not readily available

Data from the Ask Suicide-Screen Questions (ASQ) Toolkit. National Institute of Mental Health, National Institutes of Health. Available from: http://www.nimh.nih.gov/labs-at-nimh/asq-toolkit-materials/index.shtml; and the Stanley-Brown Safety Plan https://suicidesafetyplan.com/forms/

   c. Acute aggression and impulsivity can occur as a manifestation of psychiatric illness, substance intoxication or withdrawal, grief, or organic disease.

2. Management:
   a. Determine the etiology by reviewing vital signs, presenting history, past diagnoses, past episodes of aggression (Fig. 24.4). Attempt to rule out underlying medical cause (e.g., ingestion, traumatic brain injury).
   b. Nonpharmacologic
     (1) Low-stimulation environment (e.g., dim lights, move child away from busy areas, avoid unnecessary interventions)
     (2) Communicate in a calm, neutral, empathetic tone at eye level using simple language.
     (3) Utilize distraction techniques and Child Life Services if available.
   c. Pharmacologic: Therapy choice should target the etiology of agitation (see Fig. 24.4).
   d. Restraints and seclusion: Reserved for cases where both nonpharmacologic and pharmacologic interventions fail. Regulations and requirements for use vary by state.
     (1) Close monitoring required
     (2) Frequent reassessment of necessity of restraints

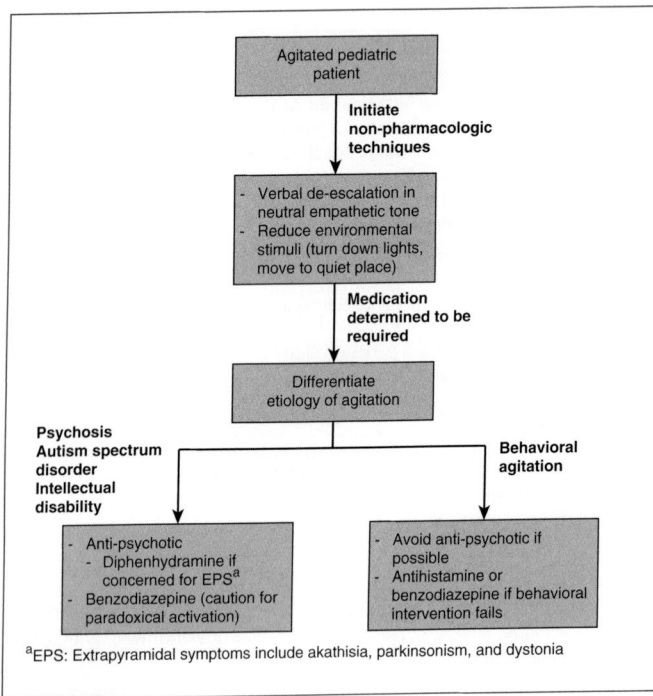

FIGURE 24.4

Agitation management algorithm.

V. WEB RESOURCES

- ADHD Medication Guide: https://www.adhdmedicationguide.com
- AAP Mental Health Toolkit: https://publications.aap.org/toolkits/pages/mental-health-toolkit
- Template for Creating a Safety Plan: https://suicidesafetyplan.com/forms/

REFERENCES

A complete list of references can be found online.

Chapter 25

Pulmonology and Sleep Medicine

Saskia Groenewald, MD

⊗ See additional content online.

I. EVALUATION OF PULMONARY GAS EXCHANGE

A. Pulse Oximetry[1-3]

1. Noninvasive and indirect measurement of arterial O_2 saturation (SaO_2) estimated by light absorption characteristics of oxygenated and deoxygenated hemoglobin in peripheral blood.
2. Limitations:
   a. Measures oxygen saturation, not O_2 delivery to tissues
   b. Insensitive to hyperoxia. See eFig. 25.1 for oxyhemoglobin dissociation curve.
   c. Artificially increased by: Carboxyhemoglobin levels >1% to 2%
   d. Artificially decreased by: Intravenous dyes, opaque nail polish, and methemoglobin levels >1%
   e. Unreliable when pulse signal is poor: Hypothermia, hypovolemia, shock, edema, movement artifact

B. Capnography[4,5]

1. Measures CO_2 concentration of expired gas by infrared or mass spectroscopy
2. End-tidal CO_2 ($ETCO_2$) correlates with $PaCO_2$ (usually within 5 mmHg in healthy subjects).
3. Used to evaluate proper placement of an endotracheal tube, to monitor ventilation in mechanically ventilated patients, to assess effectiveness of CPR, and during polysomnography

C. Blood Gases[6-8]

1. Arterial blood gas (ABG): Most accurate way to assess oxygenation (PaO_2), ventilation ($PaCO_2$), and acid–base status (pH and HCO_3^-). See Chapter 28 for normal mean values.
2. Venous blood gas (VBG): $PvCO_2$ averages 6 to 8 mmHg higher than $PaCO_2$; venous pH is slightly lower than arterial pH.
3. Capillary blood gas (CBG): Correlation with ABG is generally best for pH, moderate for PCO_2, and worst for PO_2.

D. Analysis of Acid–Base Disturbances[9-11]

Determine primary disturbance (metabolic versus respiratory), then assess for mixed disorder by calculating expected compensatory response. See Chapter 11 for details.

II. PULMONARY FUNCTION TESTS (PFT)

Provide objective and reproducible measurements of airway function and lung volumes. Used to characterize disease, assess severity, and follow response to therapy

A. Peak Expiratory Flow Rate (PEFR)[12,13]

Maximal flow rate generated during a forced expiratory maneuver.

1. Used to follow the course of asthma and response to therapy by comparing current PEFR with the previous "personal best" and the normal predicted value
2. Limitations: Measurement is effort dependent and can be difficult to determine normal values based on patient factors. Cannot be done reliably by many young children
3. Normal predicted PEFR values for children (Table 25.1)

B. Maximal Inspiratory and Expiratory Pressures[14,15]

Maximal pressure generated during inhalation and exhalation against a fixed obstruction. Used as a measure of respiratory muscle strength

1. Maximal inspiratory pressure (MIP) is in the range of 80 to 120 cm H_2O at all ages. A low MIP may be an indication for ventilatory support.
2. Maximum expiratory pressure (MEP) increases with age and is greater in males. A low MEP correlates with decreased effectiveness of coughing.

C. Spirometry (for Children ≥6 Years)[16,17]

Plot of airflow versus time during rapid, forceful, and complete expiration from total lung capacity (TLC) to residual volume (RV) is useful to characterize different patterns of airway obstruction (Fig. 25.1). Usually performed before and after bronchodilation to assess response to therapy or after bronchial challenge to assess airway hyperreactivity.

TABLE 25.1
PREDICTED AVERAGE PEAK EXPIRATORY FLOW RATES FOR NORMAL CHILDREN

Height in Inches (cm)	PEFR (L/min)	Height in Inches (cm)	PEFR (L/min)
43 (109)	147	56 (142)	320
44 (112)	160	57 (145)	334
45 (114)	173	58 (147)	347
46 (117)	187	59 (150)	360
47 (119)	200	60 (152)	373
48 (122)	214	61 (155)	387
49 (124)	227	62 (157)	400
50 (127)	240	63 (160)	413
51 (130)	254	64 (163)	427
52 (132)	267	65 (165)	440
53 (135)	280	66 (168)	454
54 (137)	293	67 (170)	467
55 (140)	307		

PEFR, Peak expiratory flow rate.
Data from Voter KZ. Diagnostic tests of lung function. *Pediatr Rev.* 1996;17:53–63.

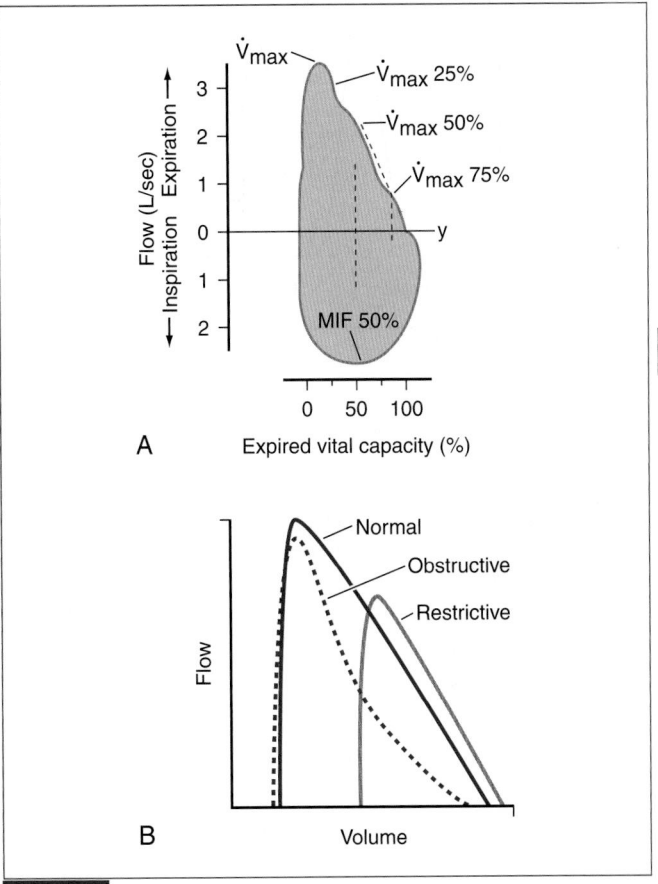

FIGURE 25.1

(A) Normal flow–volume curve. Maximal inspiratory flow (MIF). (B) Obstructive pattern seen in asthma or cystic fibrosis; restrictive pattern seen in interstitial lung disease. (B, Data from Baum GL, Wolinsky E. *Textbook of Pulmonary Diseases*. 5th ed. Little, Brown; 1994.)

1. Important definitions (Fig. 25.2)
   a. Forced vital capacity (FVC): Maximum volume of air exhaled from the lungs after a maximum inspiration
   b. Forced expiratory volume in 1 second (FEV_1): Volume exhaled during the first second of the FVC maneuver
2. Interpretation of spirometry and lung volume readings[18] (Table 25.2).

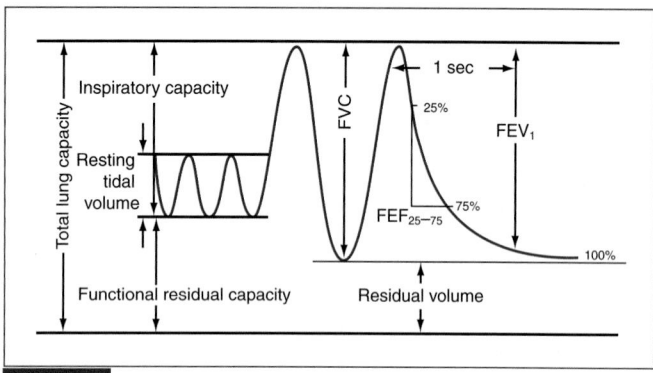

Lung volumes. *FEF$_{25-75}$*, Forced expiratory flow between 25% and 75% of FVC; *FEV$_1$*, forced expiratory volume in 1 second; *FVC*, forced vital capacity.

TABLE 25.2

INTERPRETATION OF SPIROMETRY AND LUNG VOLUME READINGS

	Obstructive Disease (Asthma, Cystic Fibrosis)	Restrictive Disease (Interstitial Fibrosis, Scoliosis, Neuromuscular Disease)
SPIROMETRY		
FVC[a]	Normal or reduced	Reduced
FEV$_1$[a]	Reduced	Reduced[d]
FEV$_1$/FVC[b]	Reduced	Normal
FEF$_{25-75}$	Reduced	Normal or reduced[d]
PEFR[a]	Normal or reduced	Normal or reduced[d]
LUNG VOLUMES		
TLC[a]	Normal or increased	Reduced
RV[a]	Increased	Reduced
RV/TLC[c]	Increased	Unchanged
FRC	Increased	Reduced

[a]Normal range: ±20% of predicted.
[b]Normal range: >85%.
[c]Normal range: 20 ± 10%.
[d]Reduced proportional to FVC.

FEF$_{25-75}$, forced expiratory flow between 25% and 75% of FVC; *FEV$_1$*, forced expiratory volume in 1 second; *FRC*, functional residual capacity; *FVC*, forced vital capacity; *PEFR*, peak expiratory flow rate; *RV*, residual volume; *TLC*, total lung capacity.

III. ASTHMA[12-13,19]

A. Definition

A chronic inflammatory disease with reversible constriction of airway smooth muscles, mucus production, and edema that lead to obstruction and air trapping. Commonly manifests as recurrent episodes of wheezing, breathlessness, chest tightness, and cough. The inflammation causes increased airway hyperreactivity to a variety of stimuli: viral infections, cold air, exercise, emotions, environmental allergens, and pollutants.

B. Clinical Presentation

1. Cough, increased work of breathing (tachypnea, retractions, accessory muscle use), wheezing, hypoxemia, and variable expiratory airflow limitation. Crackles may also be present with asthma exacerbations.
2. No audible wheezing may indicate very poor air movement and severe bronchospasm.
3. Radiographic findings: Peri-bronchial thickening, hyperinflation, patchy atelectasis

C. Treatment

1. See Chapter 1 for acute management of status asthmaticus.
2. The National Asthma Education and Prevention Program Coordinating Committee Expert Panel Working Group of the National Heart, Lung, and Blood Institute recently published its 2020 Focused Updates to the Asthma Management Guidelines:
    a. Stepwise management recommendations summarized in Figs. 25.3 to 25.8
    b. In children ages 0 to 4 years with intermittent asthma (recurrent wheezing triggered only by URIs), recommend short course inhaled corticosteroids (ICS) along with short-acting beta-agonist (SABA) at onset of infection.
    c. The preferred treatment for ages 5 to 11 and 12+ with moderate to severe persistent asthma (steps 3 and 4) already taking low- or medium-dose ICS is a single inhaler with ICS-formoterol (referred to as single maintenance and reliever therapy, or "SMART") used both daily and as needed.
    d. For ages 12+: Addition of a long-acting muscarinic antagonist (LAMA) as an add-on therapy (preferred step 5, option in step 3+).
    e. A biologic (omalizumab for ages ≥5, additional options for ages 12+) should be considered for steps 5 and 6.
    f. In children ≥5 years with mild/moderate asthma and allergen sensitization, the use of subcutaneous immunotherapy as an adjunct treatment to standard pharmacotherapy is recommended in steps 2 through 4.
    g. Fractional exhaled nitric oxide (FeNO) is a biomarker that can be measured and used used to predict the level of inflammation in the lungs.
    h. Using FeNO measurement as an adjunct to the evaluation process in individuals ≥5 years is recommended if further diagnostic clarification is needed but should not be used to predict risk of future exacerbations or severity.
    i. In children with asthma who do not have sensitization to specific indoor allergens, the allergen-mitigation interventions is NOT recommended as part of routine asthma management.[13]
3. Initial classification and initiation of treatment for ages 0 to 4, 5 to 11, and ≥12 years (Figs. 25.3, 25.4, and 25.5).

Classifying asthma severity and initiating treatment in children 0–4 years of age

Classifying severity in children who are not currently taking long-term control medication.

Components of severity		Classification of asthma severity (0–4 years of age)			
		Intermittent	Persistent		
			Mild	Moderate	Severe
Impairment	Symptoms	≤2 days/week	>2 days/week but not daily	Daily	Throughout the day
	Nighttime awakenings	0	1–2×/month	3–4×/month	>1×/week
	Short-acting β₂-agonist use for symptom control (not prevention of EIB)	≤2 days/week	>2 days/week but not daily	Daily	Several times per day
	Interference with normal activity	None	Minor limitation	Some limitation	Extremely limited
Risk	Exacerbations requiring oral systemic corticosteroids	0–1/year	≥2 exacerbations in 6 months requiring oral systemic corticosteroids, or ≥4 wheezing episodes/1 year lasting >1 day AND risk factors for persistent asthma		
		← Consider severity and interval since last exacerbation. Frequency and severity may fluctuate over time. → Exacerbations of any severity may occur in patients in any severity category.			

- Level of severity is determined by both impairment and risk. Assess impairment domain by caregiver's recall of previous 2–4 weeks. Assign severity to the most severe category in which any feature occurs.
- At present, there are inadequate data to correspond frequencies of exacerbations with different levels of asthma severity. For treatment purposes, patients who had ≥2 exacerbations requiring oral corticosteroids in the past 6 months, or ≥4 wheezing episodes in the past year, and who have risk factors for persistent asthma may be considered the same as patients who have persistent asthma, even in the absence of impairment levels consistent with persistent asthma.

FIGURE 25.3

Guidelines for classifying asthma severity and initiating treatment in infants and young children (aged 0–4 years). (Modified from National Asthma Education and Prevention Program [NAEPP]—Expert Panel Report 3. Guidelines for the Diagnosis and Management of Asthma. August 2007.)

4. Stepwise approach to continued management for ages 0 to 4, 5 to 11, and ≥12 years (Figs. 25.6, 25.7, and 25.8)
5. Additional management guidelines available from the Global Initiative for Asthma[19]

D. Prevention of Exacerbations[19]

1. Ensure up-to-date immunizations, including influenza and COVID-19.
2. Create an asthma action plan.
3. Identify and minimize asthma triggers and environmental exposures.
4. Assess symptom control, inhaler technique, and medication adherence with regular clinical evaluations.

CLASSIFYING ASTHMA SEVERITY AND INITIATING TREATMENT IN CHILDREN 5–11 YEARS OF AGE

Assessing severity and initiating therapy in children who are not currently taking long-term control medication

Components of severity		Classification of asthma severity (5–11 years of age)			
		Intermittent	Persistent		
			Mild	Moderate	Severe
Impairment	Symptoms	≤2 days/week	>2 days/week but not daily	Daily	Throughout the day
	Nighttime awakenings	≤2×/month	3–4×/month	>1×/week but not nightly	Often 7×/week
	Short-acting β₂-agonist use for symptom control (not prevention of EIB)	≤2 days/week	>2 days/week but not daily	Daily	Several times per day
	Interference with normal activity	None	Minor limitation	Some limitation	Extremely limited
	Lung function	• Normal FEV₁ between exacerbations • FEV₁ >80% predicted • FEV₁/FVC >85%	• FEV₁ >80% predicted • FEV₁/FVC >80%	• FEV₁ = 60%–80% predicted • FEV₁/FVC = 75%–80%	• FEV₁ <60% predicted • FEV₁/FVC <75%
Risk	Exacerbations requiring oral systemic corticosteroids	0–1/year (see note)	≥2/year (see note)		
		Consider severity and interval since last exacerbation. Frequency and severity may fluctuate over time for patients in any severity category.			
		Relative annual risk of exacerbations may be related to FEV₁.			

Key: EIB, exercise-induced bronchospasm; FEV₁, forced expiratory volume in 1 second; FVC, forced vital capacity; ICS, inhaled corticosteroids

Notes
- The stepwise approach is meant to assist, not replace, the clinical decision making required to meet individual patient needs.
- Level of severity is determined by both impairment and risk. Assess impairment domain by patient's/caregiver's recall of previous 2–4 weeks and spirometry. Assign severity to the most severe category in which any feature occurs.
- At present, there are inadequate data to correspond frequencies of exacerbations with different levels of asthma severity. In general, more frequent and intense exacerbations (e.g., requiring urgent, unscheduled care, hospitalization, or ICU admission) indicate greater underlying disease severity. For treatment purposes, patients who had ≥2 exacerbations requiring oral systemic corticosteroids in the past year may be considered the same as patients who have persistent asthma, even in the absence of impairment levels consistent with persistent asthma.

FIGURE 25.4

Guidelines for classifying asthma severity and initiating treatment in children 5 to 11 years of age. (Modified from National Asthma Education and Prevention Program [NAEPP]—Expert Panel Report 3. Guidelines for the Diagnosis and Management of Asthma. August 2007.)

**CLASSIFYING ASTHMA SEVERITY AND INITIATING
TREATMENT IN YOUTHS ≥12 YEARS OF AGE**

Assessing severity and initiating treatment for patients who are not currently taking long-term control medications

Components of severity		Classification of asthma severity ≥12 years of age			
			Persistent		
		Intermittent	Mild	Moderate	Severe
Impairment **Normal** FEV_1/FVC: 8–19 yr 85% 20–39 yr 80% 40–59 yr 75% 60–80 yr 70%	Symptoms	≤2 days/week	>2 days/week but not daily	Daily	Throughout the day
	Nighttime awakenings	≤2×/month	3–4×/month	>1×/week but not nightly	Often 7×/week
	Short-acting β_2-agonist use for symptom control (not prevention of EIB)	≤2 days/week	>2 days/week but not daily, and not more than 1 time on any day	Daily	Several times per day
	Interference with normal activity	None	Minor limitation	Some limitation	Extremely limited
	Lung function	• Normal FEV_1 between exacerbations • FEV_1 >80% predicted • FEV_1/FVC normal	• FEV_1 >80% predicted • FEV_1/FVC normal	• FEV_1 >60% but <80% predicted • FEV_1/FVC reduced 5%	• FEV_1 <60% predicted • FEV_1/FVC reduced >5%
Risk	Exacerbations requiring oral systemic corticosteroids	0–1/year (see note)	≥2/year (see note) →→→		
		Consider severity and interval since last exacerbation. ← Frequency and severity may fluctuate over time → for patients in any severity category.			
		Relative annual risk of exacerbations may be related to FEV_1.			

Key: FEV_1, forced expiratory volume in 1 second; FVC, forced vital capacity; ICU, intensive care unit

Notes
- The stepwise approach is meant to assist, not replace, the clinical decision making required to meet individual patient needs.
- Level of severity is determined by both impairment and risk. Assess impairment domain by patient's/caregiver's recall of previous 2–4 weeks and spirometry. Assign severity to the most severe category in which any feature occurs.
- At present, there are inadequate data to correspond frequencies of exacerbations with different levels of asthma severity. In general, more frequent and intense exacerbations (e.g., requiring urgent, unscheduled care, hospitalization, or ICU admission) indicate greater underlying disease severity. For treatment purposes, patients who had ≥2 exacerbations requiring oral systemic corticosteroids in the past year may be considered the same as patients who have persistent asthma, even in the absence of impairment levels consistent with persistent asthma.

FIGURE 25.5

Guidelines for classifying asthma severity and initiating treatment in youths 12 years and older. (Modified from National Asthma Education and Prevention Program [NAEPP]—Expert Panel Report 3. Guidelines for the Diagnosis and Management of Asthma. August 2007.)

Stepwise approach for management of asthma in individuals ages 0–4 years

Treatment	Intermittent asthma	Management of persistent asthma in individuals ages 0–4 years				
	Step 1	Step 2	Step 3	Step 4	Step 5	Step 6
Preferred	PRN SABA and At the start of RTI: Add short course daily ICS^	Daily low-dose ICS and PRN SABA	Daily medium-dose ICS and PRN SABA	Daily medium-dose ICS-LABA and PRN SABA	Daily high-dose ICS-LABA and PRN SABA	Daily high-dose ICS-LABA + oral systemic corticosteroid and PRN SABA
Alternative		Daily montelukast* or Cromolyn,* and PRN SABA		Daily medium-dose ICS + montelukast* and PRN SABA	Daily high-dose ICS + montelukast* and PRN SABA	Daily high-dose ICS + montelukast* + oral systemic corticosteroid and PRN SABA

For children age 4 years only, see step 3 and step 4 on management of persistent asthma in individuals ages 5–11 years diagram.

Assess control

- First check adherence, inhaler technique, environmental factors,^ and comorbid conditions.
- **Step up** if needed; reassess in 4–6 weeks
- **Step down** if possible (if asthma is well controlled for at least 3 consecutive months)

Consult with asthma specialist if step 3 or higher is required. Consider consultation at step 2.
Control assessment is a key element of asthma care. This involves both impairment and risk. Use of objective measures, self-reported control, and health care utilization are complementary and should be employed on an ongoing basis, depending on the individual's clinical situation.

Abbreviations: ICS, inhaled corticosteroid; LABA, long-acting beta₂-agonist; SABA, inhaled short-acting beta₂-agonist; RTI, respiratory tract infection; PRN; as needed

^ Updated based on the 2020 guidelines.

* Cromolyn and montelukast were not considered for this update and/or have limited availability for use in the United States. The FDA issued a boxed warning for montelukast in March 2020.

FIGURE 25.6

Stepwise approach for managing asthma in infants and young children (aged 0–4 years). (Modified from National Asthma Education and Prevention Program [NAEPP]—2020 Focused Updates to the Asthma Management Guidelines. December 2020.)

Ages 5–11 years: Stepwise approach for management of asthma

	Management of persistent asthma in individuals ages 5–11 years					
	Intermittent asthma					
Treatment	Step 1	Step 2	Step 3	Step 4	Step 5	Step 6
Preferred	PRN SABA	Daily low-dose ICS and PRN SABA	Daily and PRN combination low-dose ICS-formoterol ▲	Daily and PRN combination medium-dose ICS-formoterol ▲	Daily high dose ICS-LABA and PRN SABA	Daily high-dose ICS-LABA + oral systemic corticosteroids and PRN SABA
Alternative		Daily LTRA,* or Cromolyn,* or Nedocromil,* or Theophylline,* and PRN SABA	Daily medium-dose ICS and PRN SABA or Daily low-dose ICS-LABA, or daily low-dose ICS + LTRA,* or daily low-dose ICS +Theophylline,* and PRN SABA	Daily medium-dose ICS-LABA and PRN SABA or Daily medium-dose ICS + LTRA,* or daily medium-dose ICS + Theophylline,* and PRN SABA	Daily high-dose ICS + LTRA* or daily high-dose ICS + Theophylline,* and PRN SABA	Daily high-dose ICS + LTRA* + oral systemic corticosteroid or daily high-dose ICS + Theophylline* + oral systemic corticosteroid, and PRN SABA
			Steps 2–4: Conditionally recommend the use of subcutaneous immunotherapy as an adjunct treatment to standard pharmacotherapy in individuals ≥ 5 years of age whose asthma is controlled at the initiation, buildup, and maintenance phases of immunotherapy ▲		Consider omalizumab**▲	

Assess control

- First check adherence, inhaler technique, environmental factors, ▲ and comorbid conditions.
- **Step up** if needed; reassess in 2–6 weeks
- **Step down** if possible (if asthma is well controlled for at least 3 consecutive months)

Consult with asthma specialist if step 4 or higher is required. Consider consultation at step 3.

Control assessment is a key element of asthma care. This involves both impairment and risk. Use of objective measures, self-reported control, and health care utilization are complementary and should be employed on an ongoing basis, depending on the individual's clinical situation.

FIGURE 25.7

Stepwise approach for managing asthma in children 5 to 11 years. Abbreviations: ICS, inhaled corticosteroid; LABA, long-acting beta2-agonist; LTRA, leukotriene receptor antagonist; SABA, inhaled short-acting beta2-agonist ▲ Updated based on the 2020 guidelines. * Cromolyn, Nedocromil, LTRAs including montelukast, and Theophylline were not considered in this update and/or have limited availability for use in the United States, and/or have an increased risk of adverse consequences and need for monitoring that make their use less desirable. The FDA issued a Boxed Warning for montelukast in March 2020. ** Omalizumab is the only asthma biologic currently FDA-approved for this age range. (Modified from National Asthma Education and Prevention Program [NAEPP]— 2020

Quick-relief medications	• Use SABA as needed for symptoms. The intensity of treatment depends on severity of symptoms: Up to 3 treatments at 20-minute intervals as needed.
	• In steps 3 and 4, the preferred option includes the use of ICS-formoterol 1 to 2 puffs as needed up to a maximum total daily maintenance and rescue dose of 8 puffs (36 mcg).▲
	• **Caution:** Increasing use of SABA or use >2 days a week for symptom relief (not prevention of EIB) generally indicates inadequate control and may require a step up in treatment.
Each step: Assess environmental factors, provide patient education, and manage comorbidities▲	• In individuals with sensitization (or symptoms) related to exposure to pests‡: Conditionally recommend integrated pest management as a single or multicomponent allergen-specific mitigation intervention.▲
	• In individuals with sensitization (or symptoms) related to exposure to identified indoor allergens, conditionally recommend a multi-component allergen-specific mitigation strategy.▲
	• In individuals with sensitization (or symptoms) related to exposure to dust mites, conditionally recommend impermeable pillow/mattress covers only as part of a multicomponent allergen-specific mitigation intervention, but not as a single component intervention.▲
Notes	• The terms ICS-LABA and ICS-formoterol indicate combination therapy with both an ICS and a LABA, usually and preferably in a single inhaler.
	• Where formoterol is specified in the steps, it is because the evidence is based on studies specific to formoterol.
	• In individuals ages 5–11 years with persistent allergic asthma in which there is uncertainty in choosing, monitoring, or adjusting anti-inflammatory therapies based on history, clinical findings, and spirometry, FeNO measurement is conditionally recommended as part of anongoing asthma monitoring and management strategy that includes frequent assessment.

FIGURE 25.7 CONT'D

Stepwise approach for management of asthma in individuals ages 12 years and older

Treatment		Intermittent asthma	Management of persistent asthma in individuals ages 12+ years				
		Step 1	Step 2	Step 3	Step 4	Step 5	Step 6■
Preferred		PRN SABA	Daily low-dose ICS and PRN SABA or PRN concomitant ICS and SABA▲	Daily and PRN combination low-dose ICS-formoterol▲	Daily and PRN combination medium-dose ICS-formoterol▲	Daily medium-high dose ICS-LABA + LAMA and PRN SABA▲	Daily high-dose ICS-LABA + oral systemic corticosteroids + PRN SABA
Alternative			Daily LTRA* and PRN SABA or Cromolyn,* or Nedocromil,* or Zileuton,* or Theophylline,* and PRN SABA	Daily medium-dose ICS and PRN SABA or Daily low-dose ICS-LABA, or daily low-dose ICS + LAMA, or daily low-dose ICS + LTRA,▲ and PRN SABA or Daily low-dose ICS + Theophylline,* or Zileuton,* and PRN SABA	Daily medium-dose ICS-LABA or daily medium-dose ICS + LAMA, and PRN SABA▲ or Daily medium-dose ICS + LTRA,* or daily medium-dose ICS + Theophylline,* or daily medium-dose ICS + Zileuton,* and PRN SABA	Daily medium-high dose ICS-LABA or daily high-dose ICS + LTRA,* and PRN SABA	

Steps 2–4: Conditionally recommend the use of subcutaneous immunotherapy as an adjunct treatment to standard pharmacotherapy in individuals ≥ 5 years of age whose asthma is controlled at the initiation, buildup, and maintenance phases of immunotherapy▲

Consider adding asthma biologics (e.g., anti-IgE, anti-IL5, anti-IL5R, anti-IL4/IL13)**

Assess control

- First check adherence, inhaler technique, environmental factors,▲ and comorbid conditions.
- **Step up** if needed; reassess in 2–6 weeks
- **Step down** if possible (if asthma is well controlled for at least 3 consecutive months)

Consult with asthma specialist if step 4 or higher is required. Consider consultation at step 3.
Control assessment is a key element of asthma care. This involves both impairment and risk. Use of objective measures, self-reported control, and health care utilization are complementary and should be employed on an ongoing basis, depending on the individual's clinical situation.

FIGURE 25.8
Stepwise approach for managing asthma in youths 12 years and older. (Modified from National Asthma Education and Prevention Program [NAEPP]— 2020 Focused Updates to the Asthma Management Guidelines. December 2020.)

Abbreviations: ICS, inhaled corticosteroid; LABA, long-acting beta₂-agonist; LAMA, long-acting muscarinic antagonist; LTRA, leukotriene receptor antagonist; SABA, inhaled short-acting beta₂-agonist

▲ Updated based on the 2020 guidelines.

˟ Cromolyn, Nedocromil, LTRAs including Zileuton and montelukast, and Theophylline were not considered for this update, and/or have limited availability for use in the United States, and/or have an increased risk of adverse consequences and need for monitoring that make their use less desirable. The FDA issued a boxed warning for montelukast in March 2020.

˟˟ The AHRQ systematic reviews that informed this report did not include studies that examined the role of asthma biologics (e.g. anti-IgE, anti-IL5, anti-IL5R, anti-IL4/IL13). Thus, this report does not contain specific recommendations for the use of biologics in asthma in steps 5 and 6.

▪ Data on the use of LAMA therapy in individuals with severe persistent asthma (step 6) were not included in the AHRQ systematic review and thus no recommendation is made.

Notes for individuals ages 12+ years diagram

Quick-relief medications	• Use SABA as needed for symptoms. The intensity of treatment depends on the severity of symptoms: Up to 3 treatments at 20-minute intervals as needed. • In steps 3 and 4, the preferred option includes the use of ICS-formoterol 1 to 2 puffs as needed up to a maximum total daily maintenance and rescue dose of 12 puffs (54 mcg).▲ • **Caution:** Increasing use of SABA or use >2 days a week for symptom relief (not prevention of EIB) generally indicates inadequate control and may require a step up in treatment.
Each step: Assess environmental factors, provide patient education, and manage comorbidities ▲	• In individuals with sensitization (or symptoms) related to exposure to pests‡: Conditionally recommend integrated pest management as a single or multicomponent allergen-specific mitigation intervention.▲ • In individuals with sensitization (or symptoms) related to exposure to identified indoor allergens, conditionally recommend a multi-component allergen-specific mitigation strategy.▲ • In individuals with sensitization (or symptoms) related to exposure to dust mites, conditionally recommend impermeable pillow/mattress covers only as part of a multicomponent allergen-specific mitigation intervention, but not as a single component intervention.▲
Notes	• The terms ICS-LABA and ICS-formoterol indicate combination therapy with both an ICS and a LABA, usually and preferably in a single inhaler. • Where formoterol is specified in the steps, it is because the evidence is based on studies specific to formoterol. • In individuals ages 12 years and older with persistent allergic asthma in which there is uncertainty in choosing, monitoring, or adjusting antiinflammatory therapies based on history, clinical findings, and spirometry, FeNO measurement is conditionally recommended as part of an ongoing asthma monitoring and management strategy that includes frequent assessment. • Bronchial thermoplasty was evaluated in step 6. The outcome was a conditional recommendation against the therapy.

FIGURE 25.8 CONT'D

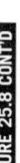

5. Consider specialist referral for formal PFT's, monitoring, and indoor allergen-mitigation strategies for sensitized children.

IV. BRONCHIOLITIS[20-27]

A. Definition

1. Lower respiratory tract infection common in infants and children aged 2 years and younger
2. Characterized by acute inflammation, edema, and necrosis of airway epithelium, leading to increased mucus production and bronchospasm
3. Most commonly caused by respiratory syncytial virus (RSV) but can also be seen with other viruses, including human rhinovirus, parainfluenza, adenovirus, mycoplasma, and human metapneumovirus

B. Clinical Presentation

1. Rhinitis and cough, which may progress to tachypnea, wheezing, rales, use of accessory muscles, and/or nasal flaring. Transient apnea may also be seen.
2. Radiographic findings: Hyperinflation and atelectasis
3. Radiographs and viral testing should NOT be routinely obtained.

C. Treatment

Mainstay is supportive care.

1. Assess risk factors for severe disease, such as age less than 12 weeks, a history of prematurity, underlying cardiopulmonary disease, or immunodeficiency.
2. Clinicians should NOT administer albuterol, epinephrine, systemic corticosteroids, or chest physiotherapy to previously healthy infants and children with a first-time diagnosis of bronchiolitis. Antibiotics should be administered only for concomitant bacterial infection.
3. Nebulized hypertonic saline may be considered for hospitalized patients but should not be administered as a therapy in emergency department settings.
4. Clinicians may choose to not give supplemental oxygen therapy if saturations are greater than 90% or use continuous pulse oximetry for monitoring if not requiring oxygen therapy.
5. Nasogastric or intravenous fluid is necessary when infant is unable to maintain oral hydration.
6. There is insufficient evidence to recommend or go against nasal suctioning as a way to clear upper airway obstruction resulting from mucus production. Deep suctioning can cause airway trauma and is not recommended because of the potential to lengthen hospitalization.[23]
7. Heated humidified high-flow nasal cannula oxygen may decrease work of breathing and need for escalation of care in children at risk for progression to respiratory failure, but conflicting data exist.[22,27]
8. RSV immunoprophylaxis with palivizumab is recommended for high-risk infants (see Chapter 16).

V. BRONCHOPULMONARY DYSPLASIA (BPD)[28-33]

A. Definition

1. Also known as chronic lung disease of prematurity or neonatal chronic lung disease and is due to disruption of pulmonary development
2. Chronic pulmonary condition that usually evolves after premature birth, characterized by the need for oxygen supplementation >21% for at least 28 days after birth
3. Thought to be a result of airway inflammation, damage from hyperoxia, hypoxia, or mechanical ventilation; results in interference with normal lung alveolar, airway, and vascular development
4. Risk factors: Prematurity, IUGR, maternal smoking, perinatal infection, mechanical ventilation, supplemental oxygen requirement

B. Clinical Presentation

Children with BPD may have persistent respiratory symptoms, airway hyperreactivity, and supplemental oxygen requirements, especially during intercurrent illness. Respiratory disease may persist into adulthood for a subset of individuals.

C. Diagnosis

Severity based on oxygen requirement at time of assessment and characterized as mild if on room air, moderate if requiring <30% oxygen, or severe if requiring >30% oxygen and/or positive pressure.

1. If gestational age at birth <32 weeks: Assess infant at 36 weeks' postmenstrual age or at discharge to home, whichever comes first.
2. If gestational age at birth >32 weeks: Assess infant at 28 to 56 days postnatal age or at discharge to home, whichever comes first.

D. Treatment

1. Children with BPD often require some combination of the following for their lung disease: Bronchodilators, antiinflammatory agents (corticosteroids), supplemental oxygen therapy, diuretics, tracheostomy and prolonged mechanical ventilation for severe cases, RSV prophylaxis (see Chapter 16 for indications).
2. Minimize further lung damage and promote healing by ensuring adequate nutrition given increased caloric needs, carefully monitor fluid status, use low tidal volumes with mechanical ventilation, set oxygen goals per gestational age, and prioritize weaning respiratory support.
3. Children with BPD need close monitoring for complications, which can affect additional organ systems: Pulmonary or systemic hypertension, electrolyte abnormalities, nephrocalcinosis (from chronic diuretics), neurodevelopmental or growth delay, sleep-disordered breathing, aspiration from dysphagia and/or GER, more severe infections with RSV or influenza.

A. Definition
Autosomal recessive disorder in which mutations of the cystic fibrosis transmembrane conductance regulator (*CFTR*) gene reduce the function of a chloride channel that usually resides on the surface of epithelial cells in the airways, pancreatic ducts, biliary tree, intestine, vas deferens, and sweat glands, resulting in progressive obstructive pulmonary disease and pancreatic exocrine insufficiency

B. Clinical Manifestations (Fig. 25.9)

C. Diagnosis (Fig. 25.10)
Diagnosing CF is a multistep process; a complete evaluation involves the following:

1. Newborn screening (NBS): Utilizes blood immunoreactive trypsinogen (IRT) level and/or *CFTR* gene mutation analysis
2. Quantitative pilocarpine iontophoresis (sweat chloride) test: Gold standard for diagnosis. False-positive results can be seen in untreated adrenal insufficiency, glycogen storage disease type 1, fucosidosis, hypothyroidism, nephrogenic diabetes insipidus, ectodermal dysplasia, malnutrition, mucopolysaccharidosis, and panhypopituitarism.
3. Genetic analysis: Over 2500 *CFTR* gene mutations have been described. CFTR gene sequencing can be performed if a variant is not identified on the CFTR mutation screening pane.
4. Comprehensive medical history, family history, and physical exam.

D. Treatment
Patients with CF should be managed within a CF Foundation–accredited care center. Current annual care recommendations are four office visits, four respiratory cultures, and two PFTs.

1. **Pulmonary**
   a. Airway clearance therapy to mobilize airway secretions and facilitate expectoration: Often manual/mechanical percussion and postural drainage. Older children may use high-frequency chest wall oscillation, mechanical chest percussors, or oscillatory positive expiratory pressure (PEP) handheld devices.
   b. Aerosolized medications to enhance mucociliary clearance: Recombinant human DNAase (dornase alfa) and aerosolized hypertonic saline to hydrate airway mucus and stimulate cough.
   c. Chronic antibiotics: If *Pseudomonas aeruginosa* is persistently present in airway cultures, consider chronic aerosolized antibiotic. Chronic azithromycin therapy has been shown to decrease exacerbations.
   d. CFTR modulator therapy: Effective for patients with specific mutations that produce CFTR protein. Can be used in combination. See Table 25.3 and Formulary for dosing.

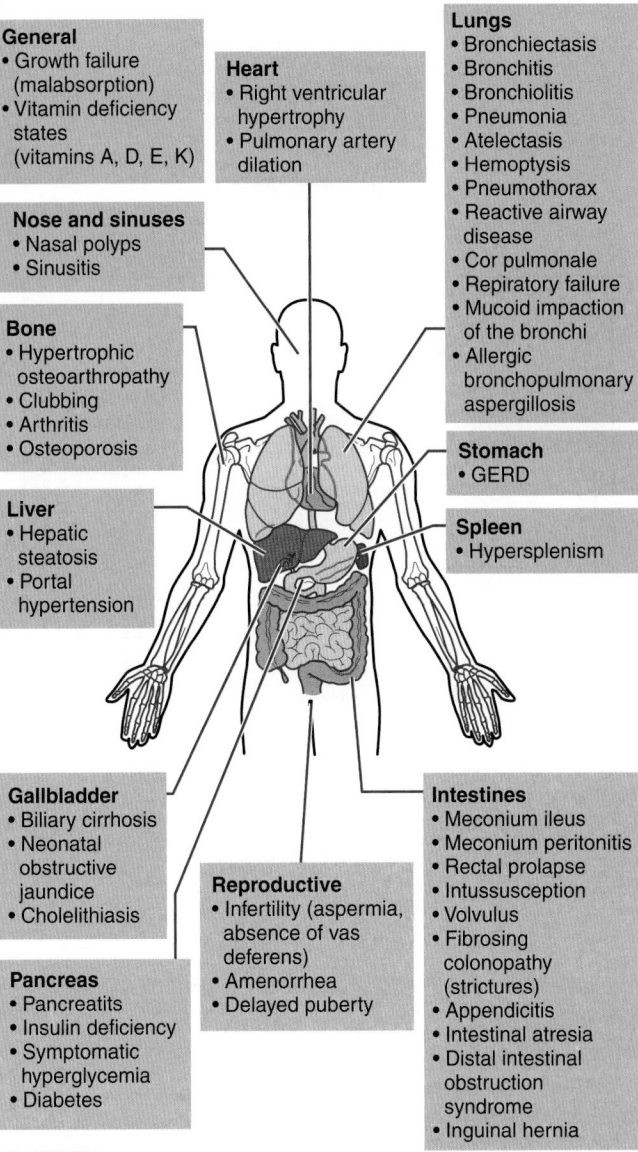

General
- Growth failure (malabsorption)
- Vitamin deficiency states (vitamins A, D, E, K)

Nose and sinuses
- Nasal polyps
- Sinusitis

Bone
- Hypertrophic osteoarthropathy
- Clubbing
- Arthritis
- Osteoporosis

Liver
- Hepatic steatosis
- Portal hypertension

Gallbladder
- Biliary cirrhosis
- Neonatal obstructive jaundice
- Cholelithiasis

Pancreas
- Pancreatits
- Insulin deficiency
- Symptomatic hyperglycemia
- Diabetes

Heart
- Right ventricular hypertrophy
- Pulmonary artery dilation

Lungs
- Bronchiectasis
- Bronchitis
- Bronchiolitis
- Pneumonia
- Atelectasis
- Hemoptysis
- Pneumothorax
- Reactive airway disease
- Cor pulmonale
- Repiratory failure
- Mucoid impaction of the bronchi
- Allergic bronchopulmonary aspergillosis

Stomach
- GERD

Spleen
- Hypersplenism

Reproductive
- Infertility (aspermia, absence of vas deferens)
- Amenorrhea
- Delayed puberty

Intestines
- Meconium ileus
- Meconium peritonitis
- Rectal prolapse
- Intussusception
- Volvulus
- Fibrosing colonopathy (strictures)
- Appendicitis
- Intestinal atresia
- Distal intestinal obstruction syndrome
- Inguinal hernia

FIGURE 25.9

Clinical manifestations of cystic fibrosis. (Modified from Kliegman R. *Nelson Essentials of Pediatrics.* Elsevier Saunders; 2019.)

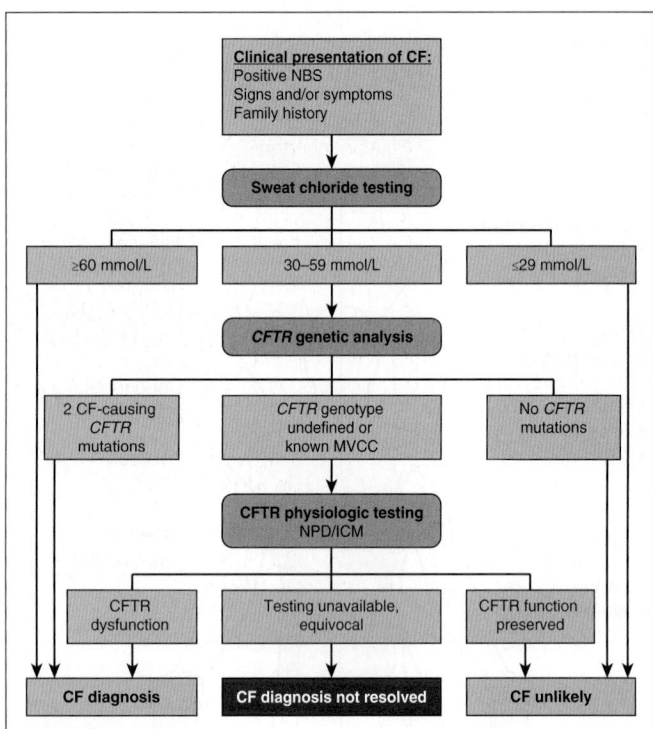

FIGURE 25.10

Diagnosis of cystic fibrosis. *CF*, Cystic fibrosis; *CFTR*, cystic fibrosis transmembrane conductance regulator; *ICM*, intestinal current measurement; *MVCC*, mutation of varying clinical consequence; *NBS*, newborn screen; *NPD*, nasal potential difference. (Modified from Farrell DW, White TB, Ren CL, et al. Diagnosis of cystic fibrosis: consensus guidelines from the cystic fibrosis foundation. *J Pediatr.* 2017;181S:S4-S15.e1. https://doi.org/10.1016/j.jpeds.2016.09.064)

    e. Intermittent use of IV antibiotics when hospitalized for exacerbations. Common bacteria that cause exacerbations include *P. aeruginosa* and *Staphylococcus aureus*. No current consensus regarding antibiotic choice, dosing, or duration

    f. Allergic bronchopulmonary aspergillosis (ABPA) treatment: Oral corticosteroids, antifungal therapy can be a helpful adjunct therapy

    g. Lung transplantation

TABLE 25.3

CFTR MODULATORS

CFTR Modulator	Indications	Therapeutic Approach
Kalydeco (ivacaftor tablets and oral granules)	Patients at least 4 months or older Must have one mutation in the *CFTR* gene or one of 97 specified mutations, as noted in the prescribing information	CFTR Potentiator
Orkambi (lumacaftor/ivacaftor tablets)	Patients at least 2 years of age or older Must be homozygous for F508del mutation in the *CFTR* gene	Corrector + Potentiator
Symdeko (tezacaftor/ivacaftor and ivacaftor tablets)	Patients at least age 6 years or older Must be homozygous for the F508del mutation or have one of 154 specified mutations as noted in the prescribing information	Corrector + Potentiator
Trikafta (elexacaftor/tezacaftor/ ivacaftor and ivacaftor tablets)	Patients aged 6 years and older Must have at least one copy of the F508del mutation or one of 177 specified mutations as noted in the prescribing information	Potentiator + Corrector + Corrector

CFTR, Cystic fibrosis transmembrane conductance regulator.
Data from prescriber information from Trikafda, Kalydeco, Orkambi, Symdeko ([44,45,46]).

2. **Extrapulmonary**
   a. Pancreatic and liver disease
      (1) Pancreatic enzyme replacement therapy prior to meals to improve digestion and intestinal absorption of dietary protein and fat
      (2) Fat-soluble vitamin A, D, E, and K supplementation
      (3) Nutritional supplementation to maintain body mass index (BMI) ≥50th percentile
      (4) Monitoring for CF-related diabetes or liver disease
   b. Infertility
      (1) Men have absence of the vas deferens; however, assisted fertilization is possible using aspiration of viable sperm from testes.
      (2) Women who are healthy have relatively normal fertility.
   c. Decreased life expectancy. Survival continues to improve, and median predicted survival age is more than 48 years.

VII. OBSTRUCTIVE SLEEP APNEA SYNDROME (OSAS)[47-53]

A. Definition

Disorder of breathing during sleep characterized by prolonged partial upper airway obstruction and/or intermittent complete obstruction that disrupts normal ventilation during sleep and normal sleep patterns

B. Clinical Presentation

1. Nighttime symptoms: Habitual snoring ± intermittent pauses in breathing, increased respiratory effort, sleepwalking, enuresis, and/or sweating
2. Daytime symptoms: Inattention, learning problems, and behavioral issues. Young children rarely present with daytime sleepiness.
3. Long-term complications: Neurocognitive impairment, behavioral problems, poor growth, cardiac dysfunction, systemic and pulmonary hypertension
4. Risk factors: Adenotonsillar hypertrophy, obesity, family history of OSAS, craniofacial or laryngeal anomalies, prematurity, nasal/pharyngeal inflammation, cerebral palsy, neuromuscular disease

C. Diagnosis

1. All children and adolescents should be routinely screened for snoring.
2. If a child snores on a regular basis and has any of the complaints or findings shown in Box 25.1, clinicians should obtain a polysomnogram or, if polysomnography is not available, refer the patient to a sleep specialist or otolaryngologist for more extensive evaluation.
3. Polysomnography criteria for OSAS diagnosis (one of the following):
   a. One or more obstructive or mixed apnea or hypopnea events per hour (AHI ≥1).

BOX 25.1
SYMPTOMS AND SIGNS OF OBSTRUCTIVE SLEEP APNEA SYNDROME

I. History

Frequent snoring (≥3 nights/week)
Labored breathing during sleep
Gasping/snorting noises or observed episodes of apnea
Mouth breathing
Sleep enuresis (especially secondary enuresis)
Sleeping in a seated position or with the neck hyperextended
Cyanosis
Headache on awakening
Daytime sleepiness
Attention-deficit/hyperactivity disorder
Learning problems

II. Physical Examination

Underweight or overweight
Tonsillar hypertrophy
Adenoidal facies
Micrognathia/retrognathia
High-arched palate
Failure to thrive
Hypertension

Modified from Marcus CL, Brooks LJ, Draper KA, et al. Diagnosis and management of childhood obstructive sleep apnea syndrome. *Pediatrics.* 2012;130:575–584.

b. Obstructive hypoventilation ($PaCO_2$ >50 mmHg) for >25% of sleep time coupled with snoring, paradoxical thoracoabdominal movement, or flattening of nasal airway pressure waveform
4. No standard severity classifications but commonly classified as mild, moderate, or severe based on number of AHI events

D. Treatment

1. Adenotonsillectomy is recommended as first-line treatment of patients with OSAS documented with an overnight polysomnogram, especially adenotonsillar hypertrophy present. Patients should be reevaluated postoperatively to determine whether further treatment is required.
   a. High-risk children warrant a more comprehensive evaluation and postoperative admission for monitoring.
2. Watchful waiting for up to 6 months can be considered for otherwise healthy children with mild/moderate OSAS along with supportive care (sleep hygiene practices, nasal saline spray, treatment for allergies)
3. Continuous positive airway pressure is recommended as treatment if adenotonsillectomy is not performed or if OSAS persists postoperatively.
4. Weight loss for patients who are overweight or obese
5. Intranasal corticosteroids may be considered for children with mild OSAS. Follow-up is needed to assess symptoms and monitor possible adverse effects of long-term intranasal steroids. Oral leukotriene inhibitor (e.g., montelukast) can also be considered.
6. Rapid maxillary expansion (RME) and use of a mandibular advancement device can be used to increase upper airway patency in children with certain orofacial features.
7. Craniofacial surgery and tracheostomy are reserved for severe cases in children with syndromic craniofacial abnormalities.

VIII. INFANT AND CHILD SLEEP[53-54]

A. Sleep Duration

1. Recommended average sleep duration varies by age (Table 25.4).
2. Sleep concerns are common in childhood. Inadequate or poor-quality sleep can have negative impacts on health, behavior, and learning.
   a. Chronic sleep insufficiency is associated with increased risk of obesity, depression, hypertension, diabetes, and poor academic performance.
3. See online content for a discussion of common childhood sleep disorders.

B. Sleep-Related Infant Death[55-58]

1. **Definition**
   a. Sleep-related infant death: Sudden unexplained infant death (SUID) that occurs during an observed or unobserved sleep period
   b. Sudden infant death syndrome (SIDS): Cause assigned to infant death that cannot be explained after thorough case investigation
2. **Epidemiology**
   a. In 2020, the SUID rate was 92.9 deaths per 100,000 live births. Disproportionately affects African-American and Native American populations[57]

TABLE 25.4	

RECOMMENDED AVERAGE SLEEP DURATION

Age Group	Duration of Sleep (Per 24 Hours)
Infants (4–12 months)	12–16 hours[a]
Toddlers (1–2 years)	11–14 hours[a]
Preschool-aged children (3–5 years)	10–13 hours[a]
School-aged children (6–12 years)	9–12 hours
Teenagers (13–18 years)	8–10 hours

[a]Recommended sleep duration in 24-hour period includes naps.

Modified from Paruthi S, Brooks LJ, D'Ambrosio C, et al. Recommended amount of sleep for pediatric populations: a consensus statement of the American Academy of Sleep Medicine. *J Clin Sleep Med.* 2016;12(6):785–786.

    b. Peak incidence at 1 to 4 months, with 90% occurring before 6 months

3. Safe infant sleep

Most recent evidence-based safe infant sleep recommendations to reduce the risk of sleep-related infant death from the 2016 AAP guidelines include[56]:

    a. Back to sleep during every episode of sleep until age 1 year

    b. Using a firm sleep surface without soft objects or loose bedding

    c. Room-sharing with the infant on a separate surface, ideally for the first year of life, but at least for the first 6 months

    d. Avoidance of overheating and head covering

    e. Avoidance of alcohol, illicit drugs, and smoke exposure during pregnancy and after birth

    f. Protective factors that should be recommended: Regular prenatal care, breastfeeding, routine immunizations, offering pacifier at sleep times

    g. Modeling of safe sleep by healthcare providers/staff, daycare provides, and in advertising

    h. Home cardiorespiratory monitors should not be used as a strategy to reduce the risk of SIDS

IX. BRIEF RESOLVED UNEXPLAINED EVENT (BRUE)[58-59]

A. Definition

Formerly termed an *apparent life-threatening event (ALTE)*, a BRUE is defined as an event occurring in an infant younger than 1 year when the observer reports a sudden, brief (<1 minute), and now-resolved episode of at least one of the following:

1. Cyanosis or pallor
2. Absent, decreased, or irregular breathing
3. Marked change in tone (hyper- or hypotonia)
4. Altered level of responsiveness

B. Differential Diagnosis

Differential diagnoses that should be evaluated for during the history and physical exam include gastroesophageal reflux (GER), seizure, nonaccidental

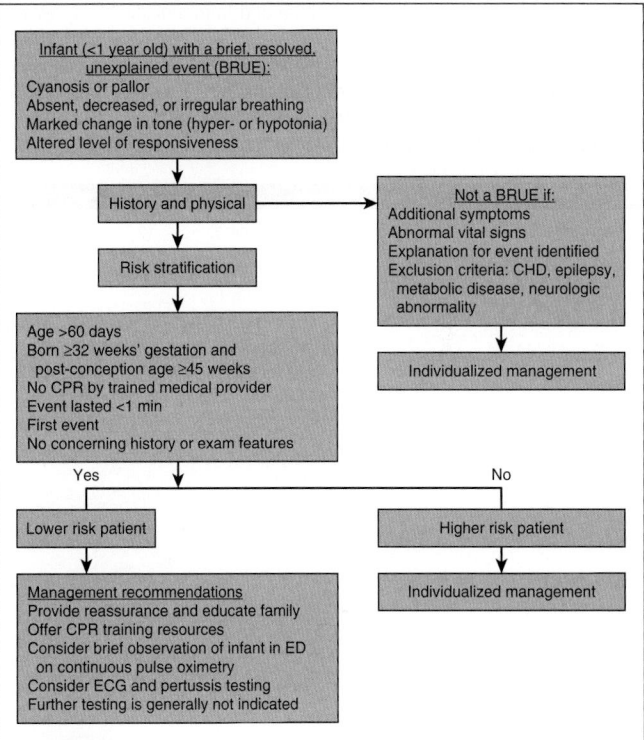

FIGURE 25.11

Algorithm for diagnosis, risk stratification, and management of BRUE. *CHD*, Congenital heart disease; *CPR*, cardiopulmonary resuscitation; *ECG*, electrocardiogram; *ED*, emergency department. (Modified from Tieder JS, Bonkowsky JL, Etzel RA, et al. AAP Clinical Practice Guideline: brief resolved unexplained events [formerly apparent life-threatening events] and evaluation of lower-risk infants. May 2016.)

trauma, cardiac arrhythmia, inborn errors of metabolism, and lower respiratory tract infection. If an explanation for the event is identified, then it is not a BRUE.

C. Management

Algorithm for diagnosis, risk stratification, and management of patients with BRUE (Fig. 25.11)

X. WEB RESOURCES

- American Lung Association: https://www.lung.org
- Cystic Fibrosis Foundation: https://www.cff.org

- American Academy of Allergy, Asthma and Immunology: https://www.aaaai.org
- National Heart Lung and Blood Institute: National Asthma Education and Prevention Program: https://www.nhlbi.nih.gov
- American Thoracic Society: https://www.thoracic.org
- American Academy of Sleep Medicine: https://www.aasm.org

REFERENCES

A complete list of references can be found online.

Chapter 26

Radiology

Urveel Mukesh Shah, MD

🔗 See additional content online.

I. GENERAL PEDIATRIC PRINCIPLES

A. Use Imaging Judiciously

1. Ionizing radiation is a carcinogen. Children are at increased risk of its effects given their potentially greater lifetime exposure, small size leading to greater penetration, and higher rates of cell division.[1]
2. Use evidence-based guidelines to inform appropriate imaging choice.[1]
3. See Table 26.1 for relative radiation by imaging study.
4. Choose appropriate modality to obtain a diagnostic image while reducing unnecessary patient exposure to ionizing radiation.
5. Limit imaging to indicated areas to improve resolution and minimize unnecessary radiation exposure.
6. Provide adequate clinical background when ordering imaging studies to assist radiologist.

B. Terminology

1. Radiographs and computed tomography (CT): Fewer x-rays penetrate dense structures than structures that are less dense. In terms of density, air/gas < fat < fluid < soft tissue < bone < metal. Structures that are less dense than surrounding tissue appear darker on the radiograph (more

TABLE 26.1

COMPARATIVE RADIATION EXPOSURE

Radiation Source	mSv	Equivalent Chest X-Rays	Equivalent Flight Hours	Equivalent Background Radiation
CXR (single view)	0.01	1	3	1 day
Abdominal XR (2 views)	0.05	5	17	5 days
Chest CT	3	300	1000	12 months
Head CT	4	400	1300	16 months
Abdominal CT	5	500	1670	20 months

CT, Computed tomography; *CXR*, chest x-ray;

Data from Zitelli BJ, McIntire SC, Nowalk AJ, Garrison J. *Zitelli and Davis' Atlas of Pediatric Physical Diagnosis.* 8th ed. Elsevier; 2023; Image Gently. *What Parents Should Know About CT Scans for Children.* 2016; Flight Radiation Calculator. (n.d.). Updated January 10, 2023. https://www.omnicalculator.com/other/flight-radiation

x-rays pass through them). Structures that are denser than surrounding tissues appear whiter. More dense structures are referred to as higher in attenuation.

2. Ultrasound: Described with ability to reflect sound waves (echogenicity) compared to the tissue around them. The more echoes a structure demonstrates, the more sound waves are reflected. Anechoic(without echoes) structures are darker than hypoechoic structures, which are darker than hyperechoic structures. Fluid transmits sound well, so a bladder filled with urine can appear anechoic because the fluid transmits soundwaves better than the soft tissues that surround the bladder. Air and gas have characteristically bright echoes because the air reflects sound waves.

II. CHOOSING THE RIGHT STUDY

1. See Table 26.2 for descriptions of imaging modalities.
2. CT versus magnetic resonance imaging (MRI): CT is often more readily available, can be performed quickly, and in most cases does not require sedation; however, CT raises safety concerns regarding radiation exposure. MRI uses nonionizing radiation and may require sedation due to longer imaging time.[1]
3. Contrast: Helps distinguish selected body areas from surrounding tissue. Oral and rectal contrast is used for bowel opacification. Intravenous contrast is used to opacify vessels and solid organs and can be helpful in cases of suspected infection/inflammation, malignancy, and trauma.

III. HEAD

Head ultrasound (HUS) can be used for infants with open anterior fontanelles (up until about 6 months of age). **CT** is preferred for acute situations (e.g., trauma, hemorrhage) and for evaluating bone structure or calcifications. **MRI** offers better soft-tissue contrast and visualization of brain anatomy and is, therefore, preferred for most nontraumatic intracranial pathology. **MRI fast sequences** (such as ultrafast [UF] MRI) uses shorter sequences targeted for anatomic assessment of ventricular size and shunt position without requiring sedation. Does not allow for adequate delineation and diagnosis of other brain pathology[1]

A. Head Trauma

1. **Preferred imaging:** Noncontrast head CT. Use the Pediatric Emergency Care Applied Research Network (PECARN) rules to decide whether imaging is indicated (see Chapter 2).[2,3]

B. CSF Shunt Malfunction

1. **Preferred imaging:** Ultrafast brain MRI (UF MRI) and shunt series (radiographs evaluating shunt tubing course)
2. **Other imaging:** CT if UF MRI is not available or contraindicated

TABLE 26.2

OVERVIEW OF IMAGING MODALITIES

Modality/Description	Ionizing Radiation	Advantages	Disadvantages/ Limitations	Relative Cost
Conventional radiographs (CR) Uses x-rays to create 2D images based on density	Yes	Fast, portable, readily available	2D only, limited soft-tissue contrast	+
Ultrasound (US) Uses high-frequency sound waves to produce image, can evaluate blood flow with Doppler or contrast	No	Portable, real-time imaging, multiplanar	Operator dependent, limited in obese patients, poor penetration of air-filled viscera and bone, may require preparation (e.g., fasting or full bladder)	++
Computed tomography (CT) Uses multiple x-rays to produce cross-sectional image, delineates bones, soft tissue, calcifications	Yes	Fast, cross sectional, more detailed than CR, multiplanar capabilities	Uses ionizing radiation, rare potential side effects from intravenous contrast if used (anaphylaxis, nephrotoxicity)	+++
Magnetic resonance imaging (MRI) Uses motion of protons in magnetic fields, field gradients, and radio waves to produce detailed cross-sectional images	No	High resolution of soft tissue, multiplanar capabilities, dynamic applications	Lengthy, image quality may be degraded by motion, may require sedation in some patients, contraindicated for certain implantable devices	++++
Fluoroscopy Uses x-rays and contrast to evaluate dynamic processes	Yes	Real-time imaging	Requires contrast, high radiation dose	++
Nuclear medicine (commonly PET, Meckel scan, SPECT) Uses radioactive tracer to delineate patterns of concentration or elimination of tracer, can be superimposed with MRI or CT	Yes	Functional, dynamic capabilities, various studies may be paired with CT or MRI for improved spatial resolution	Uses ionizing radiation, may require sedation	++++

2D, Two dimensional; *PET,* positron emission tomography; *SPECT,* single photon emission computed tomography.
Modified from Zitelli BJ, McIntire SC, Nowalk AJ, Garrison J. *Zitelli and Davis' Atlas of Pediatric Physical Diagnosis.* 8th ed. Elsevier; 2023.

26

C. Orbital Cellulitis

1. **Preferred imaging:** Orbital contrast-enhanced CT (eFig. 26.1)[4]

IV. NECK AND AIRWAY

Conventional radiography (CR) (anteroposterior (AP) and lateral neck views) are preferred initial imaging.[5,6]

A. Normal Anatomy

1. Normal anatomy (Figs. 26.1 and 26.2)
2. Reading lateral C-spine radiographs
   a. Must visualize skull base, C1 to C7, top of T1
   b. Assess alignment on lateral radiograph by evaluating four curvilinear contour lines: anterior vertebral, posterior vertebral, spinolaminar, tips of spinous process (Fig. 26.3).
   c. Evaluate vertebral bodies for fractures, displacement, subluxation, dislocations. Vertebral bodies should be similar/slightly increasing in height when descending below C2 (eFig. 26.2).
   d. Evaluate prevertebral soft tissues.

B. Cervical Spine Trauma

1. **Initial imaging:** CR, lateral and AP
2. **Other imaging:** MRI if high clinical suspicion of C-spine injury without CR findings

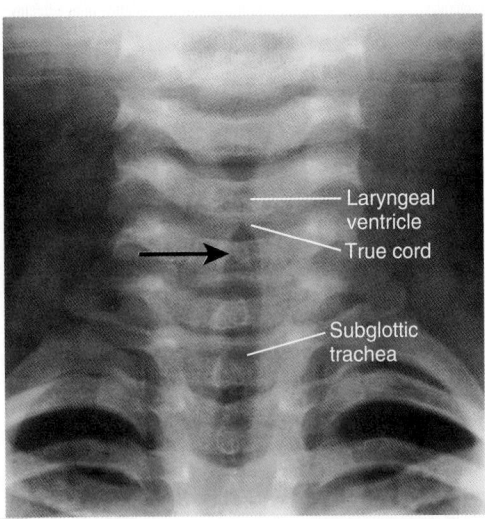

FIGURE 26.1

Anteroposterior neck radiograph with normal anatomy. Note, the vocal cords have a normal convex impression upon the subglottic airway resulting in rounded shoulders *(arrow)*. (Modified from Blickman JG, Van Die L. *Pediatric Radiology: The Requisites.* 3rd ed. Elsevier; 2009, Fig. 2.17B.)

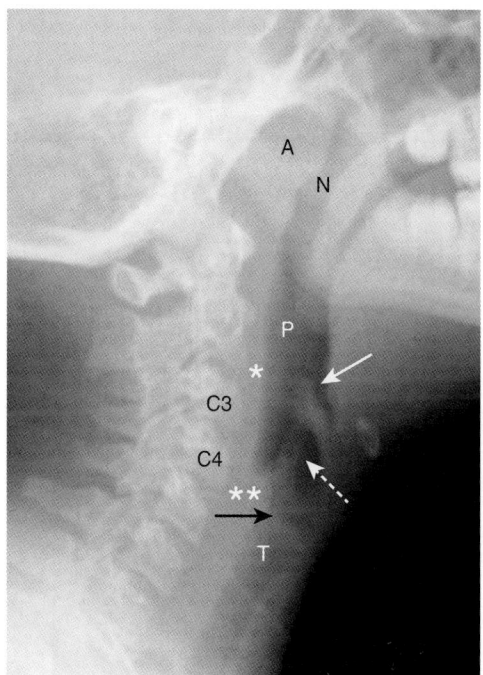

FIGURE 26.2

Normal soft tissue lateral neck radiograph. The adenoids *(A)* are seen at the base of the skull and are adjacent to the nasopharyngeal airway *(N)*. More distally is the pharynx *(P)*. The epiglottis *(solid white arrow)* is bounded superiorly by air in the vallecula. The aryepiglottic folds are paired structures extending posteriorly from the epiglottis *(dotted white arrow)*. The laryngeal ventricle *(black arrow)* separates the false vocal cords above from the true cords elow. The trachea *(T)* starts below the true cords. The normal prevertebral soft tissue thickness is less than one-half the width of the adjacent vertebral body above *C3/C4 ** and less than the width of the adjacent vertebral body below C3/C4 *(**)*. (Modified from Herring W. *Learning Radiology: Recognizing the Basics.* 3rd ed. Elsevier; 2016, Fig. 28.12.)

C. Classic Findings of Upper Airway Conditions on Conventional Radiographs

1. Croup: AP and lateral radiographs with subglottic airway narrowing *(steeple sign)* and dilation of hypopharynx. Evaluate for possible foreign bodies or subglottic airway masses (eFig. 26.3).
2. Epiglottitis: Enlarged, indistinct epiglottis on lateral radiograph *(thumbprint sign)* (eFig. 26.4)
3. Retropharyngeal abscess or pharyngeal mass: Soft tissue air or enlargement of prevertebral soft tissues not explained by neck flexion (eFig. 26.5)

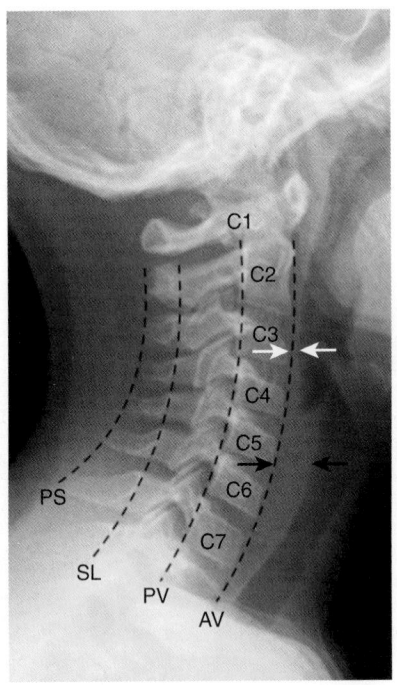

Normal lateral cervical spine radiograph. Four curvilinear lines drawn along normal landmarks can be used to help evaluate alignment: anterior vertebral line *(AV)*, posterior vertebral line *(PV)*, spinolaminar line *(SL)*, posterior spinous line *(PS)*.

D. Foreign Body

1. **Preferred imaging:** CR, AP and lateral of neck and chest. With suspicion of foreign body in airways, obtain both expiratory and inspiratory radiographs. Bilateral decubitus for younger children who cannot hold breath on command[7]
2. **Findings:** Radiopaque foreign bodies visualized. *Indirect signs*: Persistent hyperinflation of affected lung on expiratory and decubitus radiographs, atelectasis/consolidation distal to obstruction[7]

E. Tracheoesophageal Fistula and Esophageal Atresia

1. **Initial imaging:** CR; upper GI (UGI) rarely needed
2. **Findings:** Distended air-filled pharyngeal pouch and failure to pass esophagogastric tube indicates esophageal atresia (EA). Presence of distal bowel gas indicates concurrent distal TEF.[8]

F. Vascular Rings, Aortic Arch Variants, and Pulmonary Sling

1. **Preferred imaging:** Contrast-enhanced CT angiography (CTA) or MR angiography (MRA) for diagnosis
2. **Other imaging:** Echocardiography (ECHO) in neonates and infants may be able to directly visualize vascular ring.[9] Radiographs and fluoroscopic studies may suggest need for cross-sectional imaging. Neck and chest CR may show displacement or compression of tracheal air column. Fluoroscopic esophagram may show extrinsic compression of esophagus.[7]

V. CHEST

CR used for initial imaging. **CT** useful for evaluating lung parenchyma, pleura, and osseous thorax; important for identifying oncologic disease.[1,6] **US** can evaluate pleura, lung parenchyma, and diaphragmatic motion.[6]

A. Normal Anatomy (Fig. 26.4 and eFig. 26.6)
B. Pulmonary Infections

1. **Preferred imaging:** CR, PA and lateral when possible
2. **Other imaging:** CT with IV contrast for suspected complications, including pulmonary abscess, empyema, bronchopleural fistula, lung necrosis, or recurrent infection. US for parapneumonic effusions, empyema, and evaluating feasibility of percutaneous drainage[6,9]
3. **Lower airway inflammation:** Examples include asthma and bronchiolitis. Chest radiographs in asthma and bronchiolitis are most often normal. They can demonstrate nonspecific findings that often overlap with other infections such as bilateral pulmonary opacities, peribronchial thickening (cuffing), hyperinflation, subsegmental atelectasis (eFig. 26.7).[9]
4. **Pneumonia:** Difficult to distinguish between bacterial and nonbacterial with imaging alone (both can be present)
   a. **CXR findings:** Pneumonia can demonstrate alveolar consolidation and air bronchograms (eFig. 26.8).[9,10] Viral pneumonia may be accompanied by hyperinflation, air trapping, and atelectasis. Bacterial pneumonia may have lobar or segmental airway opacification and expansion.

   b. Localizing pneumonia on CXR:
      (1) *Silhouette sign*: Loss of normal borders between thoracic structures of same density; used to localize lung pathology (Table 26.3).[10]
      (2) *Spine sign*: Vertebral bodies of thoracic spine normally become more radiolucent upon visual inspection inferiorly from the thoracic inlet to the diaphragm. Soft tissue or fluid density involving posterior lower lobe adds density, causing spine to become more radiopaque, which can suggest a consolidation.[1,10]

26

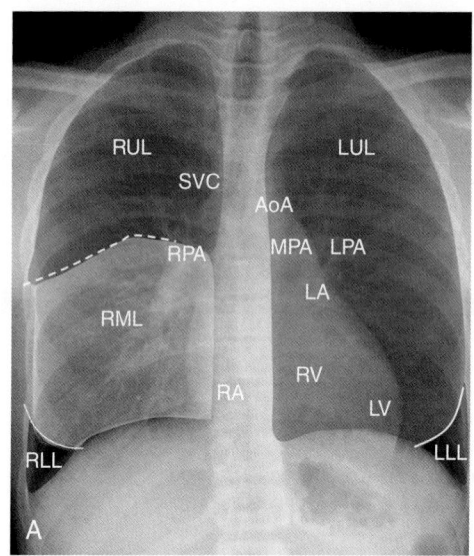

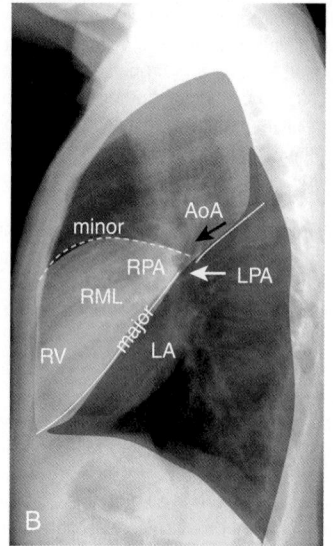

FIGURE 26.4

Normal lung and cardiac anatomy as seen on anteroposterior (A) and lateral (B) chest radiograph. *AoA,* Aortic arch; *RPA,* right pulmonary artery; *LPA,* left pulmonary artery; *RA,* right atrium; *RV,* right ventricle; *LA,* left atrium; *LV,* left ventricle; *black arrow,* posterior wall of bronchus intermedius; *white arrow,* left upper lobe airway; *RUL,* right upper lobe, *RML,* right middle lobe; *RLL,* right lower lobe; *LUL,* left upper lobe; *LLL,* left lower lobe.

TABLE 26.3

USING THE SILHOUETTE SIGN TO HELP LOCALIZE PNEUMONIA

Silhouetted Structure	Lobe
Ascending aorta	Right upper lobe
Right heart border	Right middle lobe
Right diaphragm	Right lower lobe
Descending aorta	Left upper or lower lobe
Left heart border	Lingula of left upper lobe
Left diaphragm	Left lower lobe

from Herring W. *Learning Radiology: Recognizing the Basics.* 4th ed. Elsevier; 2020, Table 9.4.

C. Neonatal Lung Disease

1. Respiratory distress syndrome (RDS, or hyaline membrane disease): Most common in preterm newborns. Hypoinflation, symmetrical hazy or granular pulmonary opacities, prominent air bronchograms, poor definition of pulmonary vessels[6-8] (Fig. 26.5)

2. Transient tachypnea of the newborn (TTN): Most common in term newborns. Interstitial edema, small pleural effusions, increased vascular markings, mildly enlarged cardiothymic silhouette, hyperinflation[6,7]

3. Meconium aspiration syndrome: Most common in term and postterm newborns, often with history of meconium. Bilateral, coarsened, and asymmetric opacities often described as "rope-like" and extending from the bilateral hila. Also with asymmetric areas of hyperinflation and atelectasis. Can be associated with pneumothorax, pneumomediastinum, or pleural effusions[7,8]

4. Neonatal pneumonia: Can occur in preterm and term newborns. Appear as symmetric, bilateral, diffuse pulmonary opacities with hyperinflation.[7] Can appear similar to RDS. Often associated with pleural effusions (whereas RDS are less likely to be associated with pleural effusions)

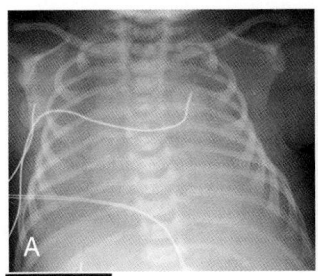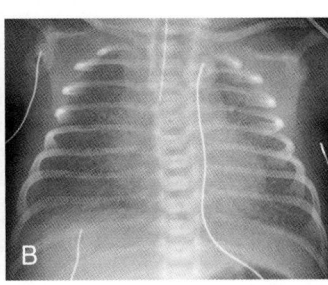

FIGURE 26.5

Infant respiratory distress syndrome. (A) Initial chest radiograph in a premature newborn with respiratory distress; demonstrates hypoinflated lungs and diffuse hazy granular opacities. (B) After intubation and surfactant administration, aeration in lungs has improved. (From Walters MM, Robertson RL. *Pediatric Radiology: The Requisites.* 4th ed. Elsevier; 2017. Fig 2.67.)

D. Mediastinal Masses
1. **Differential diagnosis** (Table 26.4)[1]
2. **Preferred imaging:** CR followed by contrast-enhanced CT
3. **Findings:** Middle mediastinal masses silhouetting the heart border and aorta[1]

VI. HEART

See Chapter 7. **ECHO** is the first-line imaging modality. Dynamic **cardiac MR (CMR)** evaluates cardiac and extracardiac anatomy; gold standard for quantifying ventricular volume, mass, and ejection fraction; creates a three-dimensional reconstruction of complex congenital heart disease (CHD) without ionizing radiation. **Cardiac CT** is alternative if CMR is contraindicated (see Fig. 26.4 for normal cardiac findings on CXR).[1,8]

VII. ABDOMEN

CR used for initial workup for most suspected abdominal pathologies; two-view studies (supine and upright) may be necessary to further evaluate in some clinical situations (e.g., intestinal obstruction or free air). Decubitus and cross-table lateral views can help localize free air, foreign bodies, and enteric tubes.[7] **US** is the initial modality of choice for suspected abdominal masses, ascites, appendicitis, abscesses, and biliary pathology.[1] **CT** is preferred for trauma and intestinal obstruction.[1] **MRI** is becoming more frequently utilized, including magnetic resonance cholangiopancreatography **(MRCP)** for evaluating pancreaticobiliary obstructions not directly visualized on ultrasound, abnormal pancreaticobiliary anatomy, and trauma. Magnetic resonance enterography **(MRE)** in known or suspected inflammatory bowel disease can be used to assess disease activity, extent of bowel involvement, and extra-intestinal complications.[1] **Cross-sectional imaging** (US, CT, or MR) may be necessary for suspected inflammation, infection, tumors, and lymphadenopathy, especially if large and/or invasive. **Upper GI (UGI) series** can assess

---

TABLE 26.4

MEDIASTINAL MASS DIFFERENTIAL DIAGNOSIS

Anterior compartment	Thymus (normal, hyperplasia, cyst, thymoma, carcinoma), teratoma, dermoid, lymphoma, ectopic thyroid, lymphatic malformation, lipoma
Middle compartment	Lymph nodes, lymphoma, foregut abnormalities (bronchopulmonary malformations, cysts), prominent vessels/dilations/aneurysms, pericardial abnormalities
Posterior compartment	Neurogenic tumors (ganglioneuroma, neuroblastoma, ganglioneuroblastoma), nerve sheath tumors (schwannoma, neurofibroma, malignant peripheral nerve sheath tumor), congenital lesions (bronchogenic or neurenteric cysts, sequestration)
Superior compartment	Lymphatic malformation, cystic hygroma, bronchogenic cyst, neurogenic tumors

Modified from Walters MM, Robertson RL. *Pediatric Radiology: The Requisites.* 4th ed. Elsevier; 2017, Box 2.1 and Ranganath SH, Lee EY, Restrepo R, Eisenberg RL. Mediastinal masses in children. *AJR Am J Roentgenol.* 2012 Mar;198(3):W197-216. doi: 10.2214/AJR.11.7027.

for proximal (esophagus to duodenojejunal junction) obstruction in neonates, malrotation, anatomic malformations, and motility problems.[7]

A. Normal Abdominal X-Ray and Bowel Gas Pattern

1. Neonatal bowel gas pattern: Gas should be present in stomach immediately after birth and in colon by 24 hours (eFig. 26.9).[6,11] Bowel loops resemble polygons or honeycombs, and there should be uniform distribution and spacing between them.[5]
2. After infancy, pockets of gas should be visualized in small bowel, colon, and rectum.
3. Small bowel seen if contains gas, located centrally, has valvulae (extends across bowel) (Fig. 26.6)
4. Large bowel contains gas and stool, located peripherally, has haustra (extends partially across bowel) (see Fig. 26.6).

B. Pneumoperitoneum (Free Intraperitoneal Air)

1. **Preferred imaging:** CR including upright imaging (cross-table or lateral decubitus if patient unable to stand or sit)
2. **Other imaging:** CT can confirm diagnosis and may be used to identify source of abnormal bowel or perforation, detects small amounts of air not seen on CR.[10]

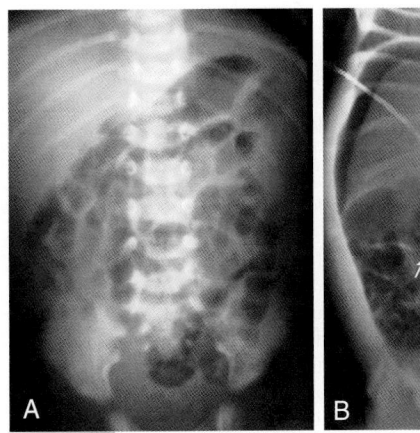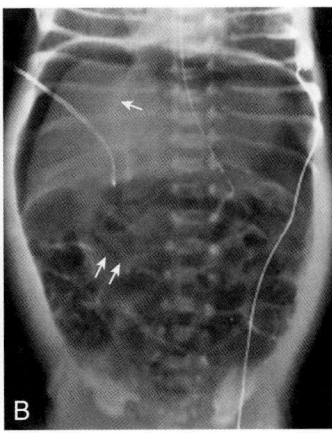

FIGURE 26.6

Normal abdominal x-ray and free intraperitoneal air. A normal abdominal radiograph (A) with evenly distributed gas throughout nondilated loops of small and large bowel. An anteroposterior supine abdominal radiograph (B) in a baby with necrotizing enterocolitis and free air demonstrated generalized lucency throughout the abdomen. Note that free air outlines the falciform ligament ("football sign") *(arrow)*, and air is seen on both sides of the bowel wall ("Rigler sign") *(double arrows)*. (From Walters MM, Robertson RL. *Pediatric Radiology: The Requisites.* 4th ed. Elsevier; 2017, p. 93, Fig 4.1 image A only and Fig 4.4, labeled as B.)

3. **Findings:**
   a. *Continuous diaphragm sign:* Air outlines inferior aspect of diaphragm, including underneath heart silhouette.
   b. *Falciform ligament sign*: Ability to visualize the typically indistinct falciform ligament as free air surrounds it (and displaces surrounding soft tissue) (see Fig. 26.6)
   c. *Football sign*: Oval appearance of abdominal cavity outlined by gas with visualization of falciform ligament, seen in massive pneumoperitoneum (see Fig. 26.6)[10]

C. Neonatal Enterocolitis (NEC, see Chapter 18)

1. **Initial imaging:** CR, include cross-table lateral or left decubitus views to evaluate for free air[7]
2. **CR findings:** *Nonspecific signs*: Diffuse gaseous distention, a nonspecific, but common finding, or persistence of focally/asymmetrically dilated bowel loop (fixed loop sign) may indicate an ileus, which is often the earliest radiographic sign. *Pathognomonic signs*: In the setting of clinically suspected necrotizing enterocolitis, radiographic signs of pneumatosis and portal venous gas are DIAGNOSTIC. (Fig. 26.7).[7]
3. **Other imaging:** Intestinal US if high clinical suspicion for NEC and CR nonspecific or inconclusive, as can depict changes in bowel motion, bowel distension, free abdominal fluid, organized fluid collections, bowel wall thickness, pneumatosis, pneumoperitoneum and bowel wall perfusion[12]

D. Neonatal Intestinal Obstruction

1. Difficult to distinguish small from large bowel in neonates on radiographs[5]
2. **Initial imaging:** CR to decipher high obstruction (stomach to proximal ileum) from low obstruction (distal ileum to colon)
3. **Further imaging:** UGI series (obstruction proximal to ligament of Treitz), UGI series with small bowel follow-through (ligament of Treitz to ileocecal junction), contrast enema (distal colon to ileocecal junction)[5,7,9]
4. High intestinal obstruction
   a. **CR findings:** Few dilated loops of bowel may indicate a proximal obstruction.
   b. Duodenal obstruction: Double bubble on CR (eFig. 26.10), reflecting gas in dilated stomach and proximal duodenum with absence of gas distally. Obstruction may be partial or complete, due to duodenal atresia, stenosis, web, malrotation with midgut volvulus, or annular pancreas. If partial obstruction, UGI series may help with further differentiation.[7]
   c. Malrotation with midgut volvulus: Abnormal rotation of the duodenojejunal loop resulting in a short mesenteric root and malposition of the duodenojejunal junction (normally located at or more superior to the level of the duodenal bulb and to the left of the spine). UGI series is the gold standard and can evaluate for duodenal

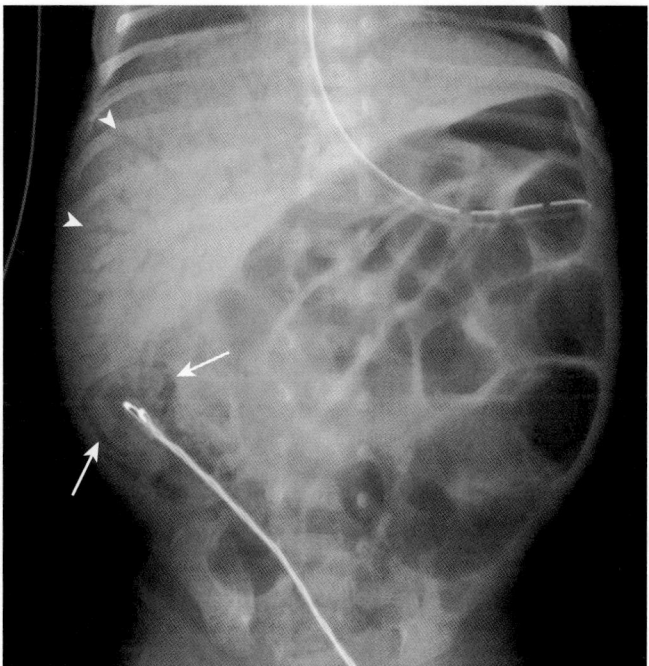

FIGURE 26.7

Necrotizing enterocolitis (NEC) in a premature infant. Radiography shows multiple dilatated bowel loops with multiple areas of circumferential lucency *(arrows)* along the bowel wall, consistent with pneumatosis. Note portal venous gas *(arrowheads)* as branching, tubular lucencies overlying the liver. (From Donnelly LF. *Fundamentals of Pediatric Imaging.* 2nd ed. Elsevier; 2017, p. 92, Fig. 5.1.)

   obstruction (either from Ladd bands or from volvulus).[5,7] CT may be
   performed for identification in older children (eFig. 26.11).
5. Low intestinal obstruction (Table 26.5)
   a. **CR findings:** Multiple dilated loops of bowel can indicate a distal
      obstruction; assess further with contrast enema.
   b. Ileal atresia: Contrast enema opacifies microcolon (diffusely small
      caliber large bowel). Rectum is normally distensible. Contrast refluxes
      into distal ileum at point of atresia as it is unable to reflux further.
      Bowel proximal to the obstruction in the distal ileum is gas filled and
      dilated.
   c. Hirschsprung disease: Contrast enema shows "transition zone"
      between nondilated aganglionic distal colon and distended, proximal
      colon with normal ganglion cells.[7]

TABLE 26.5

LOW INTESTINAL OBSTRUCTION

	Dilated Segment	Nondilated Segment
Ileal atresia	Proximal to point of atresia (no opacification on contrast enema because it cannot pass point of atresia)	Distal to point of atresia (microcolon)
Hirschsprung disease	Proximal, dilated, normal bowel with ganglion cells (will opacify with contrast enema)	Distal aganglionic bowel
Meconium ileus	Proximal to terminal ileum (will opacify with contrast enema)	Terminal ileum (microcolon) with filling defects (meconium pellets)

    d. Meconium ileus: Contrast enema opacifies a microcolon. Contrast refluxes into nondilated terminal ileum, which contains impacted meconium pellets. Bowel proximal to terminal ileum is dilated[5,7] (eFig. 26.12). Meconium ileus is seen almost exclusively in children with cystic fibrosis.

E. Pyloric Stenosis

1. Commonly presents with forceful, nonbilious "projectile" emesis between 2 to 6 weeks old, rare after 3 months of age unless preterm child
2. **Preferred imaging:** Pylorus US
3. **Findings:** Abnormal wall thickness of pyloric muscularis (≥ 3 mm) and elongation of pyloric channel (>15 to 17 mm)[10]

F. Intussusception

1. **Preferred imaging:** Abdominal US[1]
2. **Findings:** Donut or target sign, indicating a mass with bowel-in-bowel configuration[1]
3. **Treatment:** Pneumatic or water soluble contrast enema reduction under fluoroscopic guidance[1]

G. Ileus

1. **Preferred imaging:** CR
2. **Findings:** Small and large bowel distention.[1,10] May not be able to identify transition point on radiographs

H. Bowel Obstruction

1. **Initial imaging:** CR. Supine view for identifying gas pattern or paucity of bowel gas. Upright/erect, cross-table lateral, or lateral decubitus can identify free air and air-fluid levels in the appropriate clinical scenario (eFig. 26.13).
2. **Other imaging:** CT with IV and, ideally oral contrast helps determine obstruction site and detect complications such as ischemia.[10] *NOTE: CR has limited sensitivity for localizing bowel obstruction; therefore, CT should be obtained if obstruction clinically suspected.*
3. **Findings:** Dilated loops of bowel proximal to obstruction, little to no air in rectum[1]

I. Appendicitis

1. **Preferred imaging:** Abdominal US
2. **Other imaging:** MRI if high suspicion for appendicitis and US unable to visualize appendix. CT if benefits of obtaining diagnostic image outweigh the risks of exposure to ionizing radiation, patient unstable, or MRI unavailable/patient cannot tolerate MRI[1,7]
3. **US findings:** Fluid-filled, noncompressible, blind-ending tubular structure greater than 6 mm in diameter with wall thickening/hyperemia, and surrounding inflammatory changes.[1,7] May also see appendicolith and sonographic evidence for perforation (disrupted appendix and/or fluid collections). If US able to visualize a normal appendix in its entirety with no signs of inflammation in abdomen, likely no further imaging is indicated.

J. Esophageal Foreign Bodies

1. **Preferred imaging:** CR (for a radiodense foreign body), evaluate entire GI tract (neck, chest, abdomen)
2. **Other imaging:** Esophagram with water-soluble contrast if suspicion high but CR negative and suspected radiolucent foreign body[7]
3. **Findings:** Most commonly lodged at thoracic inlet. May see mass effect on adjacent structures from swelling caused by foreign body
   a. Coins (most common): Flat object on frontal view with radiodense edge visualized on lateral
   b. Disk batteries (or button batteries): Metallic disk with peripheral lucent rim and step-off, best seen along its short axis. Must identify as may cause serious electrical burn or chemical injury[7]

K. Abdominal Trauma

1. **Preferred imaging:** CT with IV contrast
2. **Other imaging:** If hemodynamically unstable, rapid bedside US using focused assessment with sonography for trauma (FAST) protocol to evaluate for free fluid.[7] FAST evaluates bilateral upper quadrants, bilateral pericolic gutters, pelvis, and pericardium[1] (eFig. 26.14).

L. Gallbladder Disease

1. **Preferred imaging:** RUQ US. Patients should fast for 6 hours prior to allow for gallbladder filling.[1]
2. **Findings:** Mobile, echogenic structures with posterior acoustic shadowing in cholelithiasis. Sludge may appear mobile or adherent. Gallbladder wall thickening (>3 mm), positive sonographic Murphy sign (localized tenderness with transducer palpation over gallbladder), sludge, and pericholecystic fluid with cholelithiasis in acute cholecystitis.[1] Biliary tree dilation may indicate inflammation and/or obstruction (including choledochal cysts/congenital abnormalities in young patients) in appropriate clinical setting.

M. Pancreatitis

1. **Initial imaging:** US
2. **Other imaging:** CT with IV contrast to evaluate for potential complications. MRCP for detecting choledocholithiasis and biliary/pancreatic duct anomalies[13]

3. **US findings:** Abnormal pancreatic echogenicity, peripancreatic fluid, or fluid collection.[1,7] Pancreatic ductal dilation can indicate chronicity.

VIII. GENITOURINARY TRACT

Renal and bladder ultrasound (RBUS): Generally acceptable first-line imaging modality; evaluates kidneys, ureters, and bladder; can assess calculi, urinary tract dilation. **Fluoroscopic voiding cystourethrogram (VCUG), radionuclide cystourethrography (RNC),** and **contrast-enhanced voiding urosonography (ceVUS)** assess for vesicoureteral reflux. **Nuclear renal scintigraphy (Mag-3 scan)** assesses renal perfusion, function, and excretion. **Cross-sectional imaging** (CT, MR, MR urography) assesses genitourinary (GU) tract anatomy, tumors, or obstruction. Additionally, MR urography can evaluate renal perfusion and excretion. Unenhanced CT can assess collecting system calculi.[7] See Chapter 19 for additional detail.

A. Urinary Tract Infection
See Chapter 19.

B. Nephrolithiasis/Urolithiasis

1. **Preferred imaging:** US or noncontrast CT[1,7]
2. **US findings:** Usually echogenic, shadowing foci[7]
3. **CT findings:** Radiodense stones, dilated ureteral or collection system, ureteral wall thickening, asymmetric enlargement, or edema of kidney[1]

C. Testicular Pathology

1. **Preferred imaging:** US scrotum and testicles[1]
2. **Testicular torsion findings:** Affected testicle is frequently enlarged with heterogeneous echogenicty, and with diminished/absent blood flow. Torsed spermatic cord may be visualized.[1]
3. **Acute epididymo-orchitis findings:** Enlarged epididymis with increased blood flow in epididymis and testicle, scrotal thickening, reactive hydrocele[1]

D. Ovarian Pathology

1. **Preferred imaging:** Pelvic US
2. **Ovarian cyst findings:** Well-circumscribed anechoic structures arising from ovary measuring more than 3 cm in diameter. Hyperechoic material or thin, lace-like septations within cyst indicate possible hemorrhage.[9]
3. **Ovarian torsion findings:** Variable appearance, usually asymmetrically enlarged solid ovary with multiple peripheral follicles[9] and edematous ovarian parenchyma. Absence or presence of flow on duplex not a reliable indicator of torsion[7]

E. Congenital Hydronephrosis

1. Normally first detected on fetal US, defined as AP renal pelvis diameter greater than 4 mm in second trimester and greater than 7 mm in third trimester
2. **Preferred imaging:** US to confirm postnatally, as can resolve spontaneously. Do not perform until at least 48 hours after delivery given

risk of false negatives or underestimation of severity due to relative dehydration and low glomerular filtration rate.[1]

3. **Findings:** Dilation of the renal pelvis (>10 mm), calyces, and/or ureters especially with with abnormal sonographic appearance of the kidneys, clinical suspicion for obstruction or reflux, or family history may warrant further evaluation with VCUG and followup US between 1 and 6 months to confirm resolution.[1,14]

IX. MUSCULOSKELETAL

CR is the primary initial imaging modality for assessment in trauma, infection, and suspected bone lesions.[7] **MRI** provides superior contrast resolution of soft tissue and bone marrow; preferred for internal derangement, infection, and tumors of bone and soft tissue. Use IV contrast to delineate inflammation, ischemia, suspected vascular anomalies, and masses.[1] **US** used for superficial soft-tissue masses, vascular anomalies, and suspected joint effusions.

A. Fractures and Trauma

1. **Preferred imaging:** CR. For long bones, obtain at least two projections. For joints, obtain at least three projections and evaluate proximal and distal joint. Fractures may not be seen on initial CR; consider repeat CRs in 7 to 10 days, which may show evidence of healing.[1,7]
2. **Findings:** Abrupt disruption of the cortex or acute angulation of smooth contour of normal bone.[10] *Indirect signs:* Soft-tissue swelling, joint effusion, periosteal reaction (if subacute or healing)
3. Describing fractures[10]:
   a. **Location:** Laterality, location on bone, relation to joint (intra-articular, extra-articular), involvement of growth plate (Table 26.6)
   b. **Type:** Complete (through whole cortex), incomplete (retains some continuity [e.g., plastic, bowing, torus, greenstick]),

TABLE 26.6

SALTER-HARRIS CLASSIFICATION OF GROWTH PLATE INJURY

Class I	Class II	Class III	Class IV	Class V
Fracture along growth plate	Fracture along growth plate with metaphyseal extension	Fracture along growth plate with epiphyseal extension	Fracture across growth plate, including metaphysis and epiphysis	Crush injury to growth plate without obvious fracture

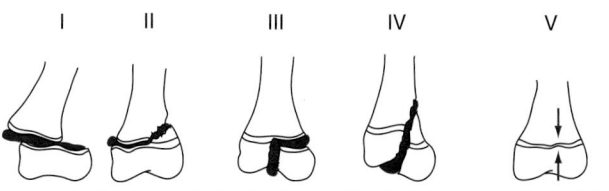

I II III IV V

   c. **Number of fragments:** Simple (two fragments) or comminuted (>2)
   d. **Orientation of fracture lines:** Transverse (perpendicular to long axis), oblique (diagonal in orientation relative to long axis), spiral
   e. **Relationship** between fracture fragments: Displacement (amount distal fragment is offset relative to proximal fragment), angulation (angle between fragments), apposition (amount of contact between fragments), shortening (amount of overlap between fragments, change in bone length), distraction (distance fragments are separated in longitudinal axis), rotation (orientation of joint at one end of fracture relative to joint at other end)
   f. **Open versus closed:** Open or compound (communication between fracture and outside atmosphere), closed or simple
   g. **Common pediatric fracture patterns:** See Chapter 2.
  4. Elbow XRs
   a. **Anterior humeral line:** Line drawn tangential to anterior humeral cortex should bisect middle third of capitellum. If line more anterior, supracondylar fracture should be suspected (Figs. 26.8 and 26.9).[10] Of note, children under 4 years old can normally have tangential line cross the anterior one-third of capitellum.
   b. **Radiocapitellar line:** Line drawn through the center and parallel to long axis of radius should pass through the center of capitellum. If it does not, dislocation should be suspected (see Figs. 26.8 and 26.9).[14]
   c. **Ossification centers:** Mnemonic CRITOE commonly used to remember sequential order of appearance (eTable 26.1 and eFig. 26.15)[15]
   d. **Fat pad:** Normal lateral view of flexed elbow shows only anterior fat pad (lucency). Elevated anterior fat pad and visible posterior fat pad indicate intra-articular injury and possible radial neck or supracondylar humerus fracture (*positive fat-pad sign*) (Fig. 26.10).[12]
   e. **Hourglass sign** ("figure-of-eight"): On a true lateral view, an hourglass or figure-of-eight configuration can be visualized on the distal humerus (see Fig. 26.10).

B. Osteomyelitis

1. **Initial imaging:** CR. Findings often lag 7 to 14 days after symptom onset; however, may identify alternative diagnosis such as fractures or tumors.[1]
2. **Preferred imaging:** MRI. Findings can be seen as early as 24 to 48 hours after symptom onset.[1,16]
3. **Findings:** Metaphysis of long bones most frequently affected. CR: Soft tissue swelling, bony destruction or demineralization, cortical loss, periosteal reaction[16]

C. Hip Disorders

1. Developmental dysplasia of the hip
   a. **Preferred imaging:** US, typically around 6 weeks of age
   b. **Other imaging:** Once femoral heads ossify (within 3 to 6 months), CR more helpful[7]

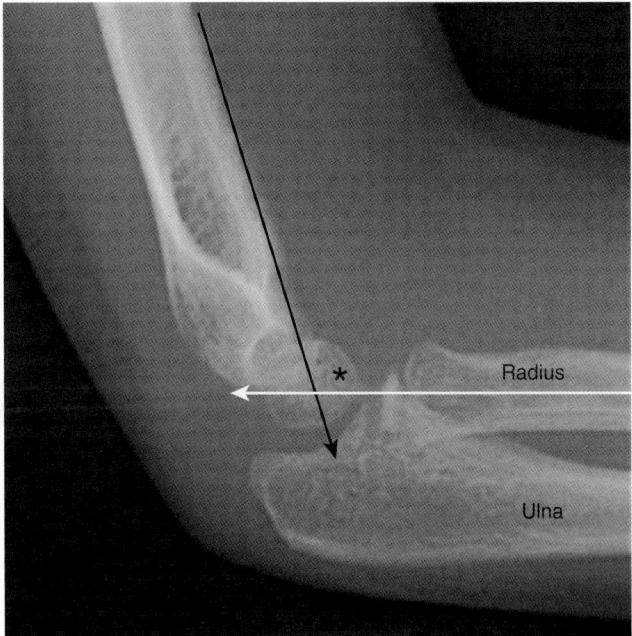

FIGURE 26.8

Normal elbow alignment on lateral radiograph. The anterior humeral line *(black arrow)* is drawn along the anterior cortex of the humerus and should intersect the middle third of the capitellum *(asterisk)*. The radiocapitellar line *(white arrow)* is drawn along the axis of the radius. (Modified from Coley BD. *Caffey's Pediatric Diagnostic Imaging.* 13th ed. Elsevier; 2019, p. 1439, Fig. 142.19.)

2. Idiopathic avascular necrosis of femoral head (Legg-Calvé-Perthes disease)
   a. **Initial imaging:** CR, AP pelvis, and frog-leg lateral hip
   b. **Other imaging:** MRI, more sensitive for early disease (especially cartilaginous changes), useful if CR is nondiagnostic[7]
   c. **Findings:** Sclerotic femoral head, widened joint space, curvilinear subchondral lucency from subchondral fracture *(crescent sign)*[7]
3. Slipped capital femoral epiphysis (SCFE)
   a. **Initial imaging:** CR, AP and frog-leg lateral views of pelvis
   b. **Other imaging:** MRI is helpful in evaluation for early changes of SCFE and of contralateral hip.
   c. **Findings:** Asymmetric widening, irregularity, and/or lucency of proximal femoral physis, posterior and inferomedial displacement of femoral head relative to femoral neck (ice cream falling off cone). SCFE can lead to femoral head avascular necrosis. Can assess femoral head position by drawing line along lateral aspect of the femoral neck (Klein's line), which should intersect the capital femoral epiphysis in normal anatomy (eFig. 26.16)[7]

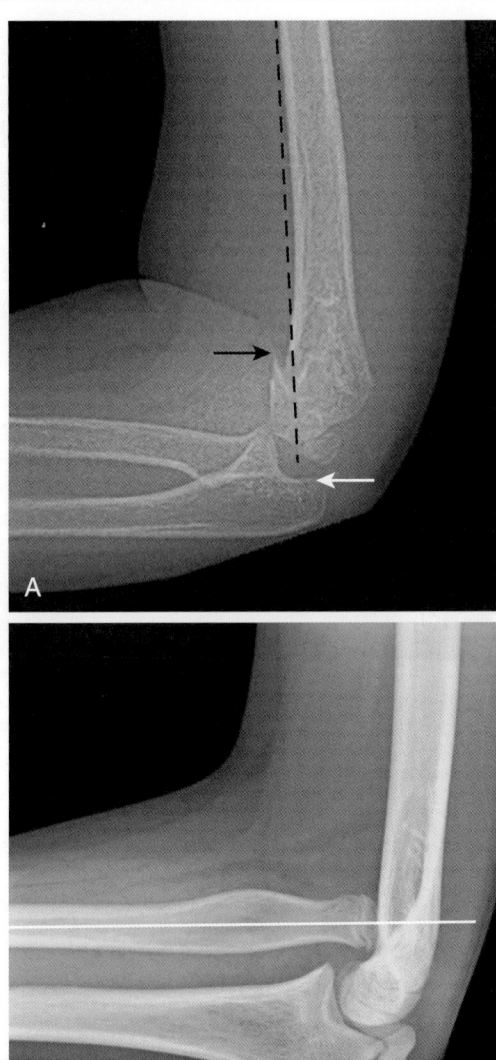

FIGURE 26.9

(A) Abnormal anterior humeral line seen in a supracondylar humeral fracture. The anterior humeral line *(dashed line)* courses anterior to the capitellum *(white arrow)* in a minimally displaced fracture of the supracondylar humerus *(black arrow)*. (B) Abnormal radiocapitellar line in a radial head dislocation. Radiocapitellar line *(white line)* drawn along the axis of the radius courses superior to the capitellum instead of intersecting the capitellum.

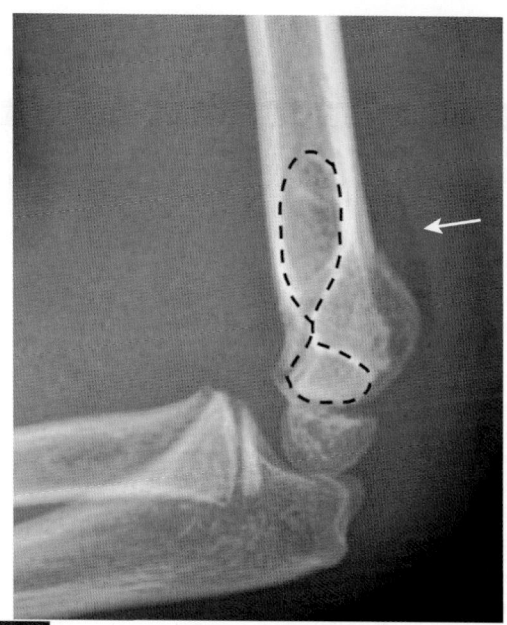

FIGURE 26.10

Lateral radiograph of elbow demonstrates visible posterior fat pad *(white arrow)*, "positive fat-pad sign." Note the "hourglass sign" *(dashed line)*.

D. Scoliosis

1. **Initial imaging:** CR, upright PA view. Sitting or supine reserved for nonambulatory patients. Lateral view not necessary for initial screening; include if known scoliosis[9]

2. **Findings:** Lateral spinal curvature greater than 10 degrees as measured by Cobb method[9]

E. Bone Lesions

1. **Initial imaging:** CR, usually diagnostic[1]

2. **Other imaging:** MRI defines extent of lesion and staging of malignant lesions[1]

3. **Findings:** *Benign lesions:* Well-demarcated from normal bone, sclerotic margin around lesion, nonaggressive growth pattern. *Pathologic lesions:* Not well demarcated from surrounding normal bone, possible accompanying soft tissue mass, periosteal reaction, destructive bone changes (eFig. 26.17 to eFig. 26.21)[1]

F. Skeletal Survey in Suspected Nonaccidental Trauma

1. **Imaging:** CR at presentation and 2 weeks after presentation. Follow-up surveys may identify new or healing fractures (eFig. 26.22).[5]

2. Evaluate for fractures inconsistent with history or developmental stage or other findings suspicious for nonaccidental trauma (NAT) (see Chapter 2).

X. CONFIRMING TUBE PLACEMENT AND LINE INSERTION

A. Central Venous Catheter

1. *Upper extremity*: Tip in superior vena cava (SVC) at cavoatrial junction or proximal atrium (Fig. 26.11)
2. *Lower extremity*: Tip in inferior vena cava (IVC) within 1 cm of diaphragm

B. Umbilical Lines (Fig. 26.12)

1. Umbilical artery catheter (UAC): *High-lying (preferred)*: Tip above diaphragm between T6 and T9. *Low-lying*: Tip just above bifurcation of aorta between L3 and L4
2. Umbilical venous catheter (UVC): Tip near inferior cavoatrial junction
3. UACs distinguished from UVCs by initial downward course from umbilicus into internal iliac artery and subsequent ascent into the common iliac artery and aorta. UVCs extend immediately superior from umbilicus. UVC is more anteriorly located than UAC on lateral view radiographs.

C. Nasogastric Tube

1. Tip below diaphragm in stomach, overlying gastric bubble

D. Nasoduodenal Tube

1. Tube should pass through stomach, cross midline to the right abdomen into duodenal bulb, and end into the duodenum.

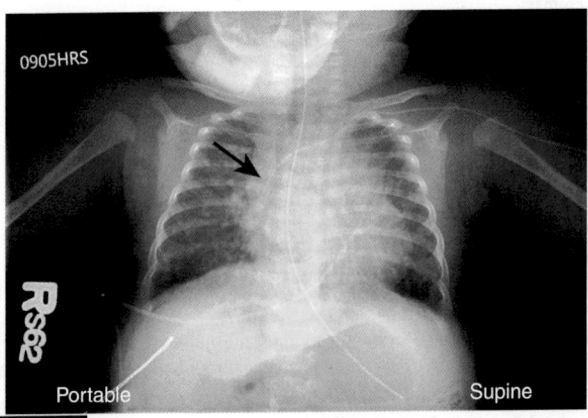

FIGURE 26.11

Central line placement on anteroposterior chest radiograph for line inserted in arm or neck. *Arrow* indicates termination of catheter at junction of superior vena cava and right atrium.

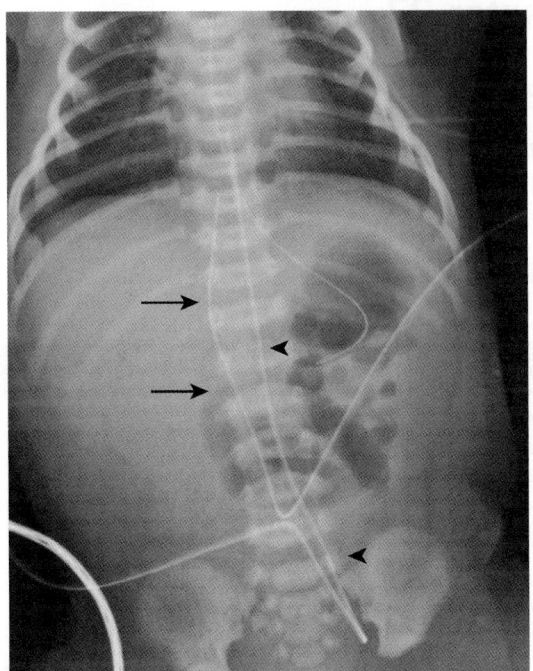

FIGURE 26.12

Umbilical catheters. Umbilical venous catheter (UVC) terminates at inferior cavoatrial junction *(arrows)*. The umbilical arterial catheter (UAC) first descends the iliac artery before it ascends the aorta and terminates in a typical "high" position, at T7 *(arrowheads)*.

E. Endotracheal Tube

1. Tip between T1 and the carina.

XI. WEB RESOURCES

- American College of Radiology Appropriateness Criteria: http://www.acr. org/Clinical-Resources/ACR-Appropriateness-Criteria
- Image Gently Alliance: http://www.imagegently.org
- Society for Pediatric Radiology: http://www.pedrad.org

REFERENCES

A complete list of references can be found online.

Chapter 27

Rheumatology

Emma Vaimberg, MD

See additional content online.

🔊 **Audio Case File 27.1** A systematic approach to differentiating the various childhood arthritic conditions

I. BRIEF OVERVIEW OF CLINICAL CHARACTERISTICS OF RHEUMATOLOGIC DISEASES

A. Juvenile Idiopathic Arthritis (JIA)[1-4]

1. Most common rheumatologic condition in children
2. Classification criteria
   a. Arthritis of one or more joints defined as: joint swelling, limitation in range of motion, and/or tenderness
   b. Symptoms lasting at least 6 weeks
   c. Symptom onset less than 16 years of age
3. See Table 27.1 for information by JIA subtypes.[5]
4. Treatment varies based on JIA subtype, but can include:
   a. Nonspecific therapies: Non-Steroidal Anti-Inflammatory Drugs (NSAIDs), corticosteroids
   b. Disease-modifying antirheumatic drugs (DMARDs), such as methotrexate, leflunomide, azathioprine
   c. Biologic agents, such as antitumor necrosis factor (anti-TNF), anti-interleukin 1 (IL-1), anti-interleukin 6 (IL-6), abatacept, and ustekinumab
5. Macrophage activation syndrome (MAS)[6]
   a. A severe disorder that develops in 7% to 17% of patients with systemic JIA
   b. Clinical features: Persistent fever, mental status changes, lymphadenopathy, hepatosplenomegaly
   c. Associated lab findings include severe and precipitous cytopenias with associated coagulopathies and hepatic dysfunction, marked hyperferritinemia with precipitous or paradoxical drop in erythrocyte sedimentation rate (ESR) and fibrinogen, elevated lactate dehydrogenase (LDH), and triglycerides, evidence of hemophagocytic macrophages in bone marrow or other tissue.
   d. MAS can also complicate other diseases, such as systemic lupus erythematosus and Kawasaki disease.
   e. First-line therapy includes pulse dose IV corticosteroids, IL-1 and IL-6 blockade. Cyclosporine A and Janus kinase (JAK) inhibitors can also be used in refractory disease.

TABLE 27.1

CLASSIFICATION OF JUVENILE IDIOPATHIC ARTHRITIS (JIA)[1,5]

ILAR JIA Subtype (% of Total Patients)	Demographics	Arthritis Characteristics	Definition	Other Features
Oligoarticular (40%–50%)	• F > M predominance • Peak age of onset: 2–4 years	Typically lower extremity large joints: knees and ankles	1–4 joint involvement within the first 6 months of disease Two subtypes: • Persistent: Affects ≤4 joints for entire clinical course • Extended: Involves >4 joints after first 6 months of disease	60%–70% ANA positive Uveitis is common with an overall prevalence of 30%. Prevalence of uveitis in persistent oligoarticular JIA and extended oligoarticular JIA is 16% and 25%, respectively.
Polyarticular-rheumatoid factor negative (20%–35%)	• F > M predominance • Peak age of onset: 2–4 years and 10–14 years	Involves small and large joints, can be symmetric or asymmetric	≥5 joints involved within the first 6 months of disease	50% ANA positive 10% HLA-B27 positive Uveitis prevalence: 4%
Polyarticular-rheumatoid factor positive (<10%)	• F > M predominance • Peak age of onset: 9–12 years	Symmetric polyarthritis	≥5 joints involved within the first 6 months of disease	40% ANA positive 10%–15% HLA-B27 positive Rheumatoid nodules: Nontender subcutaneous nodules found on bony prominences, extensor surfaces, or adjacent to joints Uveitis prevalence: 2%
Systemic (5%–15%)	• M = F predominance • Peak age of onset: 1–5 years	Oligo- or polyarticular, usually involves knees, wrists, and ankles.	Arthritis with daily (quotidian) fevers for ≥2 weeks with 1 or more associated features.	20% ANA positive 5%–10% HLA-B27 positive Uveitis prevalence: 1%

27

Continued

TABLE 27.1

CLASSIFICATION OF JUVENILE IDIOPATHIC ARTHRITIS (JIA)[1,5]—CONT'D

ILAR JIA Subtype (% of Total Patients)	Demographics	Arthritis Characteristics	Definition	Other Features
		The cervical spine can also be involved.	• Evanescent erythematous rash • Generalized lymphadenopathy • Hepatomegaly and/or splenomegaly • Serositis Macrophage activation syndrome (MAS) most commonly associated with systemic JIA	
Enthesitis-related arthritis (10%–15%)	• M > F predominance • Peak age of onset: 9–12 years	Mostly lower extremity small and large joints. Can involve axial skeleton	Both arthritis and enthesitis OR Arthritis or enthesitis with at least 2 additional features: • Axial spine involvement (including sacroiliitis) • HLA-B27 positive • Arthritis onset in males older than 6 years old • Symptomatic Anterior uveitis • First-degree relative with HLA-B27 associated disease	20% ANA positive 60%–80% HLA-B27 positive Uveitis prevalence: 7% Uveitis is typically acute symptomatic type
Psoriatic arthritis (5%–10%)	• F > M predominance • Peak age of onset: 2–4 years and 9–11 years	Involves wrists and small joints of the hands and feet initially but can progress to larger joints without effective treatment	Both arthritis and psoriasis OR Arthritis with at least 2 additional features: • Dactylitis • Nail pitting or onycholysis • Psoriasis in first-degree relative	40% ANA positive 20% HLA-B27 positive Uveitis prevalence: 10%

Undifferentiated (5%)	Arthritis that does not meet criteria for the above subtypes, or fulfills criteria for 2 or more subtypes	30% ANA positive 25% HLA-B27 positive Uveitis prevalence: 11%

ANA, Antinuclear antibodies; *F,* female; *HLA,* human leukocyte antigen; *ILAR,* International League of Associations for Rheumatology; *M,* male; *RF,* rheumatoid factor; *TMJ,* temporomandibular joint.

B. Systemic Lupus Erythematosus (SLE)[1,2,7-10]

1. Epidemiology
   a. 90% female, typically during reproductive years. However, F:M ratio closer to 5:1 for childhood onset disease
   b. Childhood onset accounts for up to 20% of cases
   c. Average age of onset: 12 years
   d. Higher prevalence in non-Caucasian individuals
2. Heterogeneous clinical manifestations. Patients with SLE may not fit all of the classification criteria. However, these classification criteria can be used to support a clinical diagnosis.
   a. American College of Rheumatology (ACR) criteria: Positive diagnosis **requires at least four** of the following:
      (1) Malar rash, discoid rash, photosensitivity, oral ulcers, arthritis, serositis (pleuritis or pericarditis), renal disorder (persistent proteinuria or cellular casts), neurologic disorder (seizures, psychosis), hematologic disorder (hemolytic anemia, leukopenia, lymphopenia, thrombocytopenia), positive antinuclear antibody (ANA), other immunologic disorder (positive anti–double-stranded DNA [dsDNA], anti-Smith or antiphospholipid antibodies)
   b. Systemic Lupus International Collaborating Clinics (SLICC) criteria: Positive diagnosis requires four items (at least one clinical and one immunologic) OR biopsy-proven lupus nephritis with positive ANA or anti-dsDNA.
      (1) Clinical: Acute cutaneous, chronic cutaneous, oral ulcers, alopecia, synovitis, serositis, renal disorder, neurologic disorder, hemolytic anemia, leukopenia, thrombocytopenia
      (2) Positive immunologic testing: ANA, anti-dsDNA, anti-Smith, antiphospholipid, low C3/C4 complements or CH50, direct Coombs test in the absence of hemolytic anemia
   3. Other clinical symptoms: Unexplained recurrent fever, weight loss, fatigue, anorexia, myalgia, arthralgia

4. Common autoantibodies
   a. ANAs are present in >99% of children with SLE.
   b. anti-dsDNA and anti-Smith are highly specific for SLE.
   c. anti-Ro (SSA) and anti-La (SSB) can be seen in SLE and can be associated with Sjögren syndrome and neonatal lupus (see Neonatal SLE).
5. Renal involvement
   a. 20% to 75% of children under 18 years will have renal involvement.
   b. 18% to 50% progress to end-stage kidney disease.
   c. Kidney biopsy can be helpful for both disease management and prognostication.
6. Treatment varies depending on disease severity and end-organ system involvement.
   a. NSAIDs
   b. Corticosteroids
   c. Hydroxychloroquine
   d. Methotrexate
   e. Azathioprine
   f. Leflunomide
   g. Cyclophosphamide
   h. Mycophenolate mofetil
   i. Biologics such as rituximab and belimumab
   j. Adjunctive therapy with antihypertensives and renoprotective agents

C. Drug-Induced SLE[11]

1. Some inciting drugs include: hydralazine, minocycline, procainamide, quinidine, isoniazid, interferon-alfa, chlorpromazine, ethosuximide, carbamazepine, anti-TNF therapy.
2. Usually with milder disease than idiopathic SLE
3. Presenting symptoms: Arthralgias, myalgias, fever, weight loss, serositis, polyarthritis
4. Rarely involves renal disorders and neuropsychiatric symptoms
5. More common lab findings: Positive ANA, anti-histone, anti-dsDNA
6. Treatment involves removal of the offending agent and, for severe disease, can include short-term immunosuppressive therapies.

D. Neonatal SLE[12-14]

1. Neonates born to mothers with positive anti-Ro (anti-SSA) or anti-La (anti-SSB) can develop a transient lupus-like syndrome due to transplacental passage of these autoantibodies.
2. Frequently, the mothers are healthy and do not have known autoimmune disease. The mothers may have isolated positive anti-Ro or anti-La, primary Sjögren syndrome, or SLE.
3. Clinical features in the neonate include: rash (annular erythema on eyelids and scalp, papular or plaque-like lesions), hepatomegaly, thrombocytopenia, hemolytic anemia, congenital atrioventricular heart block (1st, 2nd, or 3rd degree), and hydrops fetalis.
4. Neonates with heart block may require permanent pacemaker and are at continued risk for cardiac dysfunction later in life.

5. Other inflammatory features in the neonate resolve as maternal autoantibodies are cleared. Often within 6 months
6. Treatment for neonatal lupus is dependent on presenting symptoms and cardiac involvement.
7. Treatment may include steroids, cardiac pacing, and IVIG.

E. Vasculitis[1,2,15,16]

1. Refer to Table 27.2.
2. Treatment
   a. Note that treatment recommendations are largely based on adult studies because of limited clinical trials in pediatric patients.
   b. Single Hub and Access point for pediatric Rheumatology in Europe (SHARE) initiative first-line treatment recommendations for most severe vasculitis may include corticosteroids, cyclophosphamide, and/or plasma exchange. Rituximab may also be used.
      (1) In Table 27.2, this is referred to as "first-line vasculitis therapy."

F. Sarcoidosis[2,26,27]

1. Epidemiology
   a. Prepubertal: Very rare
   b. During puberty and postpuberty: Peak onset at 13 to 15 years; males and females are equally affected
2. Multisystem, infiltrative, noncaseating granulomatous disease of unknown etiology; lung is the most commonly involved organ
   a. Pulmonary: Bilateral hilar adenopathy, restrictive and obstructive disease
   b. Ocular: Anterior uveitis, conjunctival granulomas
   c. Cutaneous: Erythema nodosum, plaques, alopecia
   d. CNS: Bilateral or unilateral Bell palsy (more common in postpubertal children, seizures (more common in prepubertal children), aseptic meningitis
3. Definitive diagnosis with lymph node biopsy; elevated angiotensin-converting enzyme (ACE) levels can be helpful but not diagnostic
4. Blau syndrome and early-onset sarcoidosis are two monogenic forms of sarcoidosis characterized by polyarthritis, uveitis, and dermatitis; symptom onset <4 years
5. Systemic immune suppression is often needed for treatment.

G. Scleroderma[2,28]

1. Both juvenile localized scleroderma and juvenile systemic sclerosis typically present in mid-childhood between 6 and 11 years of age, with a female predominance
2. In children, localized scleroderma is more common than systemic sclerosis and involves skin, muscle, and bone.
3. Treatment of localized scleroderma includes topical and systemic therapies such as corticosteroids, methotrexate, tacrolimus, imiquimod, and phototherapy.
4. Systemic sclerosis: Diffuse and limited disease; diffuse disease characterized by severe Raynaud syndrome, resulting in digital ulcers,

TABLE 27.2

CHILDHOOD VASCULITIS SYNDROMES[1,2,15,16]

Vasculitis	Involved Vessels	Epidemiology	Clinical Manifestations	Treatment
Takayasu arteritis[17]	Large arteries	Predominantly young adult women. If childhood onset; more likely in adolescence but can be seen in all age groups	Aneurysms, thrombosis, and stenosis of large arteries, hypertension is common	• First-line vasculitis therapy • Therapy will also likely include hypertension management, which may be medically managed or require revascularization procedures • Maintenance therapy may include: methotrexate, azathioprine, or mycophenolate mofetil or other biologics
Kawasaki disease	Medium-sized arteries	Children <5 years old	Fever, rash, lymphadenopathy, conjunctival injection, peripheral edema. See Chapter 7 for diagnostic criteria.	• First-line: IVIG, aspirin • Treatment refractory options: corticosteroids, infliximab
Polyarteritis nodosa[17,18]	Medium-sized arteries Histopathology with inflammatory infiltrates of vessel walls and fibrinoid necrosis	Slight female predominance, most cases presenting at 9–10 years of age, but there is wide age spectrum	• Typical presentation with fever and weight loss • Commonly associated symptoms include: skin involvement (livedo reticularis, tendon nodules, infarcts, purpura), myalgia, kidney involvement (hypertension), and peripheral neuropathy.	• For mild disease: corticosteroids ± NSAIDs • For severe disease: first-line vasculitis therapy • For treatment of refractory disease, can consider: TNF blockade, B-cell depleting therapy, or IL-6 blockade

Immunoglobulin A (IgA) vasculitis (Henoch-Schönlein purpura)[17,19]	Arterioles and venules, IgA-containing immune deposits seen on biopsy	Most common pediatric vasculitis, typically presents between 3 and 12 years old, Chronic renal disease develops in 1%–2% of children	Palpable purpura involving buttocks and lower extremities, colicky abdominal pain, subcutaneous or scrotal edema, migratory arthralgias/arthritis, renal disease, glomerulonephritis, intussusception (frequently ileoileal)	• First-line: Supportive care • Corticosteroids can be used in the setting of severe GI disease. • Chronic corticosteroids, azathioprine, or mycophenolate mofetil may be used in refractory disease.
Microscopic polyangiitis (MPA)[20-22]	Necrotizing vasculitis of arterioles, venules, and capillaries	Very rare in pediatrics	Necrotizing glomerulonephritis and pulmonary capillaritis leading to alveolar hemorrhage and hemoptysis	• First-line vasculitis therapy • Refractory disease: Consider B cell-depleting biologic therapies.
Granulomatosis with polyangiitis (GPA)[20,22]	Necrotizing small and medium-size vessel vasculitis with granulomatous inflammation	Most common ANCA-associated vasculitis in pediatrics	Diagnosis with at least 3 of the following: • Histopathology with granulomatous inflammation • Upper airway involvement: epistaxis, sinusitis, otitis media, and hearing loss	• First-line vasculitis therapy • Refractory disease: Consider B cell-depleting biologic therapies.

Continued

27

TABLE 27.2

CHILDHOOD VASCULITIS SYNDROMES[1,2,15,16]—CONT'D

Vasculitis	Involved Vessels	Epidemiology	Clinical Manifestations	Treatment
			Pulmonary involvement: nodules, infiltrates, hemorrhage ANCA positive Renal Involvement: glomerulonephritis Laryngotracheobronchial stenoses	
Eosinophilic granulomatosis with polyangiitis (Churg-Strauss syndrome)[22]	Necrotizing vasculitis of small arteries and veins	Very rare in pediatrics	Associated with asthma, nasal polyps, and allergic rhinitis	• First-line vasculitis therapy • Mepolizumab (anti IL-5 monoclonal antibody) may also be used.
Behcet disease[23]	Occlusive vasculitis in arterioles and veins	M = F prevalence in childhood. Males more frequently with severe vasculitis and uveitis. Females more frequently with genital ulcers and erythema nodosum, peak age of onset 8–12 years, often associated with HLA-B51	Defined by the presence of oral ulcers (at least 3 in a year), along with two of the following: recurrent genital ulcers, ocular disease, skin lesions, and a positive pathergy test (traumatic injury to skin results in development of a sterile pustule in 24–48 hours)	• For oral/genital ulcers and anterior uveitis: Topical corticosteroids • For disease refractory to topical steroids OR as a first-line agent for posterior uveitis and retinal vasculitis: Systemic corticosteroids • Colchicine can be used for prevention of recurrent ulcers. • Alternative options for severe disease: Anti-TNF agents, azathioprine, cyclophosphamide, cyclosporine A

| Raynaud phenomenon[24,25] | Exaggerated vasoconstriction dictated by vascular, neural, and intravascular abnormalities | More common in women Can be idiopathic or associated with disorders such as SLE, mixed connective tissue disease, scleroderma, antiphospholipid antibody syndrome | Response to cold or emotional stress: Sudden onset color change in digits with demarcated skin pallor due to constricted blood flow, followed by cyanotic skin, and finally erythema with reperfusion; similar findings can be seen at sites other than digits; ischemic disease more likely to be seen in patients with a secondary cause | • First line for primary Raynaud syndrome: supportive care and education
• Pharmacologic management: calcium-channel blockers
• Management of critical digital ulcers: hospitalization with intensive vasodilator therapy and anti-platelet therapy (aspirin). If no improvement with initial management in a few hours, escalation to heparin and more intensive vasodilation is recommended. |

27

GI, Gastrointestinal; *URI*, upper respiratory infection. *NSAID*, Non-Steroidal Anti-Inflammatory Drug; *TNF*, Tumor Necrosis Factor; *IVIG*, Intravenous Immunoglobulin; *IL*, Interleukin; *ANCA*, Anti-Neutrophil Cytoplasmic Antibodies; *SLE*, Systemic Lupus Erythematosus

pulmonary arterial hypertension (PAH), pulmonary fibrosis, esophageal dysmotility, renal disease
5. Treatment of systemic sclerosis involves management of the symptoms and underlying systemic inflammation.
   a. Raynaud syndrome: Nifedipine or PDE-5 inhibitors
   b. PAH: Endothelin receptor antagonist, PDE-5 inhibitors, riociguat, epoprostenol
   c. Skin and lung disease: Methotrexate, cyclophosphamide, and biologic therapy
   d. GI disease: Proton pump inhibitors, prokinetic medications
   e. Renal disease: ACE inhibitors

H. Sjögren Syndrome[2,29]

1. Female-to-male ratio 5:1 in children, age of onset 7 to 14 years old
2. Widespread lymphocytic infiltration of salivary and lacrimal glands with secondary atrophy and obliteration of secretory acini
3. Keratoconjunctivitis sicca: Dry eyes secondary to decreased tear production by lacrimal glands
4. Xerostomia: Dry mouth from decreased salivary gland production
5. May present as parotid gland swelling in children
6. Other possible system involvement: MSK, pulmonary, neurologic, renal
7. Treatment focuses mostly on symptomatic relief and management of chronic glandular changes.
   a. Keratoconjunctivitis sicca: Artificial tears
   b. Xerostomia: Sugar-free hard candies or chewing gum
   c. Systemic immune modulation and suppressing medications such as hydroxychloroquine, corticosteroids, methotrexate, and biologic therapy

I. Juvenile Dermatomyositis (JDM)[2,30]

1. More common in females (up to 2.5:1 female:male)
2. Median age of onset: 7 years old
3. Typically symmetric muscle weakness, involves more central musculature
4. Cutaneous findings: Gottron papules overlying knuckles and knees (91%), heliotrope rash (83%), malar rash (42%)
5. Treatment options depend on disease severity and prognosis and include the use of systemic immune modulation and suppressing medications such as intravenous immunoglobulins (IVIG), hydroxychloroquine, corticosteroids, methotrexate, mycophenolate mofetil, and biologic agents.

J. Other Rheumatologic Disorders[2,31,32]

1. **Reactive arthritis**
   a. Sterile inflammatory arthritis in response to a preceding (<4 weeks) bacterial infection, particularly of the gastrointestinal or genitourinary tracts
   b. Common triggers: *Salmonella, Yersinia, Campylobacter, Shigella, Chlamydia trachomatis*

    c. Involves acute asymmetrical oligoarticular arthritis of larger joints, often the lower extremities

    d. Can be associated with fever, weight loss, fatigue, tendinitis, bursitis, anterior uveitis, conjunctivitis, erythema nodosum, urethritis, and cervicitis

    e. Therapies include treatment of the precipitating infection, if needed, and supportive care for arthritis symptoms with NSAIDs. Can consider intraarticular or systemic steroids for NSAID-refractory arthritis

2. **Reactive arthritis after a streptococcal infection**

    a. Acute rheumatic fever (ARF)

      (1) Clinical features: Arthritis, carditis, erythema marginatum, nodules, Sydenham chorea

      (2) Pathogenesis: M protein from Group A *Streptococcus* induces production of autoimmune antibodies that are cross-reactive.

      (3) Typically occurs 2 to 3 weeks after tonsillopharyngitis infection

      (4) Treatment: Arthritis is responsive to NSAIDs, transient, and migratory.

        (a) Poststreptococcal reactive arthritis

          (i) Does not meet diagnostic criteria for ARF

          (ii) Typically occurs sooner after streptococcal infection (7–10 days)

          (iii) Can involve large and small joints and axial skeleton

          (iv) Arthritis is less responsive to NSAIDs, persistent, and additive.

          (v) Cardiac involvement is less common but can occur.

K. Multisystem Inflammatory Syndrome in Children (MIS-C)[33-35]

1. Emergence of MIS-C co-occurred with the 2019 SARS-CoV-2 pandemic. MIS-C is a postinfectious inflammatory syndrome after symptomatic or asymptomatic infection with the SARS-CoV-2 virus.

2. It is a rare complication of SAR-CoV-2 virus infection.

3. Case Definition for MIS-C was derived by the Centers for Disease Control and Prevention (CDC):

    An individual aged <21 years who presents with fever (>38.0° C for >24 hours, or subjective fever lasting >24 hours), laboratory evidence of inflammation, and evidence of clinically severe illness requiring hospitalization affecting multiple organ systems (>2) **AND** without other plausible diagnosis **AND** positive for current or recent SARS-CoV-2 infection by reverse transcription polymerase chain reaction, serology, or antigen test or confirmed COVID-19 case within 4 weeks of onset of symptoms

4. Common clinical features include: fever, mucocutaneous lesions, conjunctivitis, mucositis, peripheral edema, lymphadenopathy, diarrhea, vomiting, abdominal pain, coronary artery aneurysm, myocarditis and cardiac dysfunction, altered mental status, seizures, focal neurologic deficits, respiratory failure, hypotension, and shock. Some develop acute renal failure and pancreatitis.

5. Common laboratory findings: Evidence of systemic inflammation including cytopenia, elevated ESR, C-reactive protein (CRP), elevated ferritin, coagulopathy with prolonged PTT/PT, and elevated d-dimer. Evidence of cardiac involvement with elevated pro-BNP and troponin

6. MIS-C can be complicated by macrophage activation syndrome (see section on Juvenile Idiopathic Arthritis).

7. The American College of Rheumatology provides continued guidance on evaluation and management of MIS-C.
   a. Suggested workup includes: complete blood count (CBC), comprehensive metabolic panel (CMP), PTT, PT, INR, CRP, ESR, ferritin, fibrinogen, d-dimer, troponin, Pro-BNP, EKG, echocardiogram.
   b. Evaluation for infectious and noninfectious causes during workup for MIS-C is recommended.
   c. Treatment includes: IVIG, systemic steroids, biologic therapy with agents such as anakinra (IL-1 blockade), or TNF inhibition with infliximab.
   d. Adjunctive therapies include: antiplatelet and anticoagulation with aspirin, enoxaparin, or warfarin for coronary artery involvement. Anticoagulation in patient with MIS-C and coronary artery aneurysms may be guided by the American Heart Association recommendations for Kawasaki disease (see Chapter 7 for a full discussion of cardiac involvement in MIS-C and Kawasaki disease). MIS-C patients with thrombosis should be on anticoagulation (low-dose aspirin and therapeutic) for 3 months or depending on resolution of thrombi on imaging at 4 to 6 weeks postdiagnosis.

8. Treatment teams should include input from Rheumatology, Cardiology, Infectious Disease, and Hematology, and if other organ systems involved, may also include: Nephrology, Neurology, Gastroenterology/Hepatology.

II. INTERPRETATION OF LAB STUDIES USED IN THE DIAGNOSIS AND MONITORING OF RHEUMATOLOGIC DISORDERS[1]

Most laboratory studies used to diagnose rheumatic diseases are nonspecific, and results must be interpreted within the context of the full clinical picture. Once a diagnosis is established, however, some studies may be used to follow the clinical course, indicating flares or remission of the disease.

A. Acute Phase Reactants: Indicate presence of inflammation when elevated. Elevation is nonspecific and can result from trauma, infection, rheumatologic disorder or malignancy

1. Erythrocyte sedimentation rate (ESR)[36,37]
   a. Measure of the rate of fall of red blood cells in the first 1 hour after collection in anticoagulated blood within a vertical tube; reflects level of rouleaux formation caused by acute-phase reactants
   b. Can be falsely lowered in afibrinogenemia, polycythemia, and hemoglobinopathies

    c. Increased levels can be seen in pregnancy, obesity, increasing age, and anemia

2. C-reactive protein (CRP)[38,39]
   a. It is a nonspecific marker of inflammation; however:
      (1) In most active-phase rheumatologic diseases CRP will increase to 1–10 mg/dL.
      (2) CRP >10 mg/dL raises concern for bacterial infection or systemic vasculitis.
         (a) Increases and decreases rapidly owing to short half-life (~19 hours)
         (b) Not a useful marker of inflammation in SLE

B. Autoantibodies (See Table 27.3 for Association With Rheumatologic Diseases)[36,39-43]

1. Antinuclear autoantibodies (ANA)
   a. Can be useful in the diagnosis of SLE
   b. Can be positive in other autoimmune diseases such as scleroderma (systemic and local), JIA, and JDM
   c. Can be used to stratify risk of uveitis in patients with JIA
   d. Can be positive in up to 33% of asymptomatic individuals, depending on cut-off titers used
2. Anti-dsDNA (double-stranded DNA)
   a. Highly specific for SLE
   b. Associated with lupus nephritis
3. Anti-centromere antibodies
   a. Highly specific for systemic sclerosis (>99%)
   b. Is not a sensitive test for the diagnosis of systemic sclerosis (19%)
4. Anti-Scl 70
   a. Antibodies against topoisomerase I
   b. In adulthood it is not very sensitive (43%) but highly specific (90%) for systemic sclerosis
   c. Can predict increased risk for pulmonary involvement in systemic sclerosis
5. Anti-Neutrophil Cytoplasmic Antibodies (ANCA)
   a. cANCA/PR3-ANCA: Mostly associated with GPA
   b. pANCA/MPO-ANCA: Mostly associated with MPA, polyarteritis nodosa, SLE
6. Rheumatoid factor (RF)
   a. IgM to the Fc portion of IgG
   b. Can be used in the classification of specific subtypes of JIA
   c. Can also be seen in Sjögren syndrome, SLE, sarcoidosis, systemic sclerosis
7. Anticyclic citrullinated peptide antibodies (anti-CCP)
   a. Highly specific for rheumatoid arthritis in adults
   b. In the pediatric population, primarily seen in polyarticular RF+ JIA
   c. Associated with more aggressive disease

TABLE 27.3

COMMON RHEUMATOLOGIC DISEASES AND AUTOANTIBODIES

Disease	Associated Antibody	Interpretation of Results	Clinical Considerations
SLE	ANA Anti-double-stranded DNA Anti-Smith Antiphospholipids	ANA sensitivity >95% Anti-dsDNA specificity is 97% Anti-Smith specificity 55%–100%	Most patients with positive ANA do not have SLE, but almost all patients with SLE have a positive ANA. Measure anti-dsDNA when ANA positive. Anti-phospholipids present in up to 50% of SLE patients; associated with thrombosis and fetal loss
Juvenile idiopathic arthritis	ANA	ANA positive in 80% of those with oligoarticular type	Typically RF and CCP negative; when positive, may indicate erosive disease
Vasculitis	ANCA-cytoplasmic/PR3 (proteinase-3) ANCA-perinuclear/MPO (myeloperoxidase)	90% of patients with active GPA and MPA are ANCA positive	c-ANCA associated with GPA p-ANCA associated with MPA and Churg-Strauss
Dermatomyositis/ polymyositis	ANA Anti-Jo-1	Specificity of Anti-Jo-1 99% ANA may be normal	Anti-Jo-1 associated with polymyositis with interstitial lung disease and JDM
Mixed connective tissue disease	Anti-RNP	The presence of antibodies to RNP is required for diagnosis	Also present in SLE, systemic sclerosis
Scleroderma	ANA Anticentromere Anti-Scl-70	ANA sensitivity >85% Anticentromere specificity >98%	Anti-Scl-70 associated with diffuse systemic sclerosis, while anticentromere with limited disease
Sjögren syndrome	Anti-Ro/SS-A Anti-La/SS-B	Anti-Ro sensitivity 75%	Associated with neonatal cutaneous lupus Incidence of congenital heart block increased for infants born to mothers with high titers of anti-Ro and anti-La
Drug-induced SLE	Antihistone	Sensitivity >95%	Antihistone antibodies do not distinguish drug-induced lupus from SLE.

ANA, Antinuclear antibody; *ANCA,* antineutrophil cytoplasmic antibodies; *CCP,* cyclic citrullinated peptide; *GPA,* granulomatosis with polyangiitis; *JDM,* juvenile dermatomyositis; *MPA,* microscopic polyangiitis; *SLE,* systemic lupus erythematosus.

Data from Stone JH. *Current Diagnosis & Treatment in Rheumatology.* 4th ed. McGraw-Hill Medical; 2021.

C. Complement: The complement system is composed of a series of plasma proteins and cellular receptors that function together to mediate host defense and inflammation. Inflammatory processes may increase the synthesis or consumption of these proteins.

1. Total hemolytic complement level (CH_{50})
   a. Assay that assesses the complement pathway as a whole
   b. Low levels indicate reduced function or low levels of complement proteins.
   c. Typically low values are seen in SLE, acute poststreptococcal glomerulonephritis, and subacute bacterial endocarditis.
2. C3/C4
   a. Commonly measured in the diagnosis and clinical monitoring of SLE
   b. Low levels indicate high levels of immune complex deposition.

III. MEDICATIONS: MECHANISMS OF ACTION, TOXICITIES, AND RECOMMENDED SURVEILLANCE[2] (SEE TABLE 27.4)

IV. Primary Care Management of Rheumatologic Diseases[54-57]
A. Vaccination (See Chapter 16)

1. Patients on immunosuppressive therapies cannot receive live vaccines but can receive killed/inactivated vaccines.
2. Special considerations should be made for immunocompromised patients on biologics and other immunosuppressive therapy.
3. Patients who have received IVIG should not have live vaccines for up to 11 months following the IVIG administration.

B. Weight Management

1. As a result of chronic inflammation, malnutrition can be a common comorbidity in children with rheumatologic conditions.
2. Obesity is a common concern given the frequent use of corticosteroids.

C. Bone and Skin Health

1. Chronic steroid use, presence of arthritis, and many medications used in the maintenance therapy of rheumatologic diseases increase the risk for osteopenia. Ensure adequate calcium and vitamin D intake and weight-bearing activities.
2. Patients with SLE and dermatomyositis are particularly vulnerable to ultraviolet radiation. It is recommended that patients use broad-spectrum sunscreen with a high sun-protection factor (SPF) and not use tanning booths.

D. Reproductive Health

1. Many medications used in the treatment of rheumatologic diseases are teratogenic.
2. The American College of Rheumatology provides recommendations for the use of contraceptives and reproductive assistance (see Chapter 5 for more information regarding contraception).

TABLE 27.4

COMMON MEDICATIONS USED IN PEDIATRIC RHEUMATOLOGY[2,44-53]

Medication	Mechanism of Action	Side Effects	Recommended Surveillance
NONSPECIFIC THERAPIES			
Nonsteroidal antiinflammatory drugs (NSAIDs): naproxen, ibuprofen, celecoxib, meloxicam, acetylsalicylic acid	Cyclooxygenase (COX) inhibitor	Nephrotoxic, GI bleed	No specific surveillance recommendations. However, periodic evaluation for medication side effects is advised.
Corticosteroids: prednisone, prednisolone, methylprednisolone	Antiinflammatory and immunosuppressive, predominant effects on T-cells	Growth suppression, osteoporosis, avascular necrosis, Cushing syndrome, CNS: mood and behavioral disturbance, cataracts, glaucoma, hypertension	No specific surveillance recommendations. However, periodic evaluation for medication side effects is advised.
Intravenous immunoglobulins (IVIG)	Multiple proposed mechanisms of action	Infusion reaction, anaphylactoid reactions, aseptic meningitis	Labs: Immunoglobulin levels prior to initiation
DISEASE-MODIFYING ANTIRHEUMATIC DRUGS (DMARDS)			
Methotrexate	Folic acid analogue, targets dihydrofolate reductase (DHFR) and thymidylate synthetase (TYMS) to decrease de novo purine synthesis	GI upset, hepatotoxicity, hematologic toxicity (macrocytic anemia, leukopenia, thrombocytopenia, pancytopenia), teratogenicity	• Labs: CBC, liver enzymes, creatinine • Timing: At initiation, 4–8 weeks after initiation, then every 12 weeks once stable
Hydroxychloroquine	Exact mechanism of action is unknown. A number of proposed mechanisms exist: inhibit self-antigen binding, inhibit neutrophil function, decrease effect of prostaglandins on end-	Retinal toxicity, GI upset, headache, anxiety	Obtain baseline ophthalmology exam within first month of therapy and then annually.

Drug	Mechanism	Adverse Effects	Monitoring
	targets, decrease production of inflammatory molecules (TNF, IL-6, IFN-γ).		
Sulfasalazine	Exact mechanism of action is unknown. A number of proposed mechanisms exist: Decrease enzyme activity involved in the formation of leukotrienes and prostaglandins, impacts gut bacterial growth, which may have an impact in spondyloarthropathies.	Photosensitivity, oral ulcer, Steven-Johnson syndrome	• Labs: CBC with differential, liver enzymes, creatinine, urine analysis • Timing: At initiation, every 1–2 weeks with dose adjustments, then every 3 months while on stable dose • Consider testing for G6PD deficiency on initiation. • Obtain immunoglobulins every 6 months.
Leflunomide	Inhibits de novo pyrimidine synthesis	GI upset, hepatotoxicity, alopecia, teratogenicity	• Labs: CBC with differential, liver enzymes, creatinine • Timing: At initiation, every 2–4 weeks with dose adjustments, then every 3 months while on stable dose
CYTOTOXIC AGENTS			
Azathioprine	Purine analog that inhibits de novo purine synthesis	Common: GI upset Rare: hepatotoxicity, interstitial pneumonitis, maculopapular rash, cytopenias	• CBC with differential at initiation, every 1–2 weeks with dose adjustments, then every 4–12 weeks while on stable dose • Liver enzymes, BUN, creatinine at initiation, every 4 weeks with dose adjustments, then every 12 weeks while on stable dose • TPMT genotype and/or activity at initiation
Mycophenolate	Inhibits monophosphate dehydrogenase to inhibit de novo guanine synthesis	GI upset, cytopenias, opportunistic infections, teratogenic	• Labs: CBC with differential every 4–12 weeks

Continued

27

TABLE 27.4

COMMON MEDICATIONS USED IN PEDIATRIC RHEUMATOLOGY[2,44-53]—CONT'D

Medication	Mechanism of Action	Side Effects	Recommended Surveillance
Cyclophosphamide	Alkylating agent	Hemorrhagic cystitis, GI upset, alopecia, leukopenia, thrombocytopenia, infertility	• Vitals when administering IV formulation (ensure pretreatment with Mesna and intravenous fluids) • Close urine output and urine specific gravity monitoring • Labs: CBC with differential on day 7–10 postinfusion
Cyclosporine	Calcineurin inhibitor	Hypertension, hepatotoxicity, nephrotoxicity	• Labs: CBC with differential, liver enzymes, BUN, creatinine, urine analysis • Timing: At initiation, continued until desired cyclosporine trough level is reached, and then monthly • Blood pressure monitoring
BIOLOGIC AGENTS			
Antitumor necrosis factor-alpha agents (anti-TNF-α)[44]	• Etanercept: Small protein with anti-TNF ligand bound to Fc portion of human IgG • Adalimumab: Binds soluble and membrane-bound TNF • Infliximab: Binds soluble and membrane-bound TNF	Common: Infection, infusion-related reaction, GI upset, headache Rare: Hepatotoxic, hematologic malignancy	• Labs: CBC with differential, liver enzymes • Timing: At initiation, then every 12 weeks • Screen for viral hepatitis and tuberculosis prior to initiation
Rituximab[45]	Anti-CD20 monoclonal antibody	Common: Infection, GI upset, anemia, peripheral edema, headache, muscle spasms Rare: Infusion-related reaction, HBV reactivation, progressive multifocal leukoencephalopathy	• Labs: CBC, liver enzymes, GGT • Timing: At initiation, then every 4–12 weeks • Screen for viral hepatitis and tuberculosis prior to initiation • Assess Immunoglobulin levels every 3 months • Assess B-cell CD19/20 depletion 1 month before and after infusion

Tocilizumab[46]	IL-6 receptor monoclonal antibody	Infection, headache, hypertension, hepatotoxic, injection site reactions	• Labs: CBC with differential, liver enzymes, lipid panel • Timing: At initiation, time of second infusion, then every 2–4 weeks, lipid screening 4–8 weeks after initiation, then every 6 months • Screen for viral hepatitis and tuberculosis prior to initiation.
Canakinumab[47]	Binds to IL-1β	GI upset, headache, infection, vertigo	• Labs: CBC with differential, liver enzymes, lipid panel • Timing: At initiation, then every 12 weeks, lipid panel after 2–3 months of therapy • Screen for latent tuberculosis prior to initiation: Tuberculosis testing.
Anakinra	IL-1 receptor antagonist	Injection-site reactions	• Labs: CBC with differential, liver enzymes, lipid panel • Timing: At initiation, then every 12 weeks, lipid panel 2–3 months after starting therapy • Screen for viral hepatitis and tuberculosis prior to initiation and intermittently during use.
Janus kinase (JAK) inhibitors: Tofacitinib[48], baricitinib[49], ruxolitinib	Numerous subtypes of JAK proteins exist; small molecule drugs inhibit the dimerization of JAK proteins to prevent further downstream signaling.	Risk of serious bacterial, mycobacterial, and fungal infections, anemia, thrombocytopenia, neutropenia, hepatotoxicity, thrombosis	• Labs: CBC with differential, liver enzymes, lipid panel • Timing: At initiation, every 4–8 weeks with dose adjustments, then every 3 months once at stable dose • Close monitoring of heart rate and blood pressure • Screen for viral hepatitis and latent tuberculosis prior to initiation.

27

Continued

TABLE 27.4

COMMON MEDICATIONS USED IN PEDIATRIC RHEUMATOLOGY[2,44-53] —CONT'D

Medication	Mechanism of Action	Side Effects	Recommended Surveillance
Abatacept[50]	Fusion protein that inhibits T-cell activation	GI upset, fever, teratogenicity, infusion reaction	• Labs: CBC with differential, liver enzymes • Timing: At initiation, then every 12 weeks • Screen for viral hepatitis and tuberculosis prior to initiation. • Close monitoring of vital signs during infusion (every 30 minutes)
Ustekinumab[51-53]	IgG antibody that inhibits downstream effects of inflammatory molecules, such as IL-12 and IL-23	Nasopharyngitis, upper respiratory tract infections, headache, cardiovascular events seen in adult studies (myocardial infarction, stroke)	• Screen for hepatitis and tuberculosis prior to initiation. • Labs: CBC with differential, complete metabolic panel • Timing: At initiation, every 3–6 months • Measure trough concentrations in between infusions • Monitor for signs of posterior reversible encephalopathy syndrome (PRES)

BUN, Blood urea nitrogen; *CBC,* complete blood count; *CMP,* comprehensive metabolic panel; *DMARD,* disease-modifying antirheumatic drug; *GI,* gastrointestinal; *IV,* intravenous; *LFT,* liver function test; *SIADH,* syndrome of inappropriate antidiuretic hormone; *s/p,* status post; *TB,* tuberculosis; *TNF,* tumor necrosis factor.

E. Ophthalmologic

1. Individuals with JIA should have regular ophthalmology screenings.
   a. Screening intervals are dependent on uveitis risk, presence of disease, and current therapy.

F. Laboratory Monitoring

1. As a primary care provider, be aware that multiple medications require frequent monitoring. Ensure the patient has adequate follow-up with their primary rheumatologist.

REFERENCES

A complete list of references can be found online.

PART III

REFERENCE

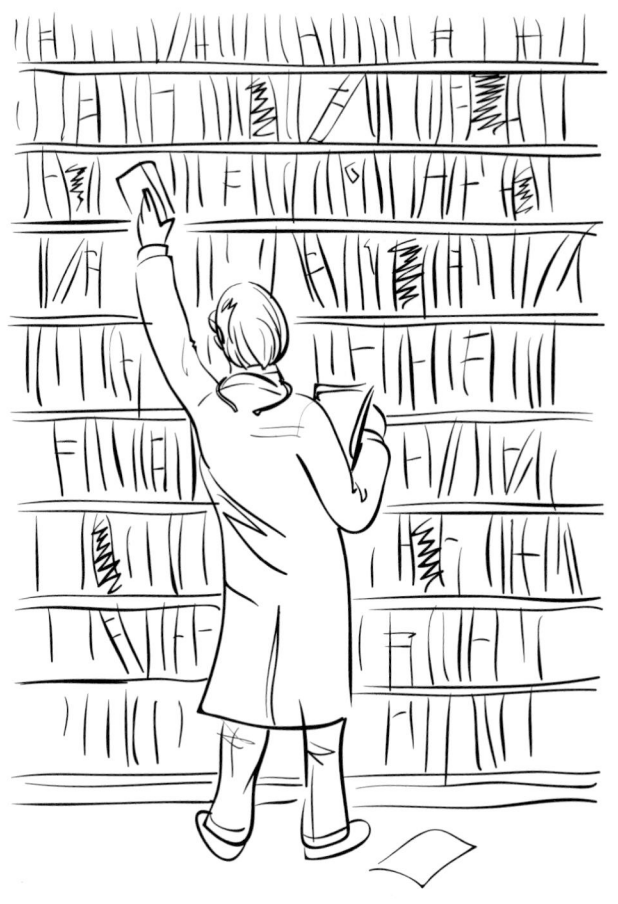

Chapter 28

Blood Chemistry and Body Fluids

Camille C. Anderson, MD

See additional content online.

Determining normal reference ranges of laboratory studies in pediatric patients poses some major challenges. Available literature is often limited due to small sample sizes of patients used to derive these suggested reference ranges.

The following values have been compiled from both published literature and the Johns Hopkins Hospital Department of Pathology. Reference range values vary with the analytic method used. Consult your laboratory for its analytic method and range of reference values, and for less commonly used parameters that are beyond the scope of this text. **Additional reference laboratory values may be found in Chapter 10 (Endocrinology), Chapter 14 (Hematology), and Chapter 15 (Immunology and Allergy).**

Special thanks to Lori Sokoll, PhD, and Nadia Ayala-Lopez, PhD, for their guidance in preparing this chapter.

I. REFERENCE VALUES

(Table 28.1)

II. EVALUATION OF BODY FLUIDS

A. **Evaluation of Cerebrospinal Fluid: See Table 28.2.**
B. **Evaluation of Urine: See Table 28.3.**
C. **Evaluation of Transudate/Exudate: See eTable 28.1.**
D. **Evaluation of Synovial Fluid: See eTable 28.2.**

III. CONVERSION FORMULAS

A. **Temperature**
1. **To convert degrees Celsius to degrees Fahrenheit:**

$$[(9/5) \times \text{Celsius}] + 32$$

2. **To convert degrees Fahrenheit to degrees Celsius:**

$$(\text{Fahrenheit} - 32) \times (5/9)$$

B. **Length and Weight**
1. **Length:** To convert inches to centimeters, multiply by 2.54.
2. **Weight:** To convert pounds to kilograms, divide by 2.2.

TABLE 28.1

REFERENCE VALUES

	Conventional Units	SI Units
ALANINE AMINOTRANSFERASE (ALT)[1]		
0 to <1 year	5–33 U/L	5–33 U/L
1 to <13 years	9–25 U/L	9–25 U/L
13–19 years (male)	9–24 U/L	9–24 U/L
13 to <19 years (female)	8–22 U/L	8–22 U/L
ALBUMIN[a,1]		
0–14 days	3.3–4.5 g/dL	33–45 g/L
15 days to <1 year	2.8–4.7 g/dL	28–47 g/L
1 to <8 years	3.8–4.7 g/dL	38–47 g/L
8 to <15 years	4.1–4.8 g/dL	41–48 g/L
15 to <19 years (male)	4.1–5.1 g/dL	41–51 g/L
15 to <19 years (female)	4.0–4.9 g/dL	40–49 g/L
ALKALINE PHOSPHATASE[1]		
0–14 days	90–273 U/L	90–273 U/L
15 days to <1 year	134–518 U/L	134–518 U/L
1 to <10 years	156–369 U/L	156–369 U/L
10 to <13 years	141–460 U/L	141–460 U/L
13 to <15 years (male)	127–517 U/L	127–517 U/L
13 to <15 years (female)	62–280 U/L	62–280 U/L
15 to <17 years (male)	89–365 U/L	89–365 U/L
15 to <17 years (female)	54–128 U/L	54–128 U/L
17 to <19 years (male)	59–164 U/L	59–164 U/L
17 to <19 years (female)	48–95 U/L	48–95 U/L
AMMONIA[2]		
0–14 days	0–161.8 mCg/dL	0–95 mcmol/L
15 days to 6 years	0–115.8 mCg/dL	0–68 mcmol/L
>6 years	0–122.6 mCg/dL	0–72 mcmol/L
AMYLASE[1]		
0–14 days	3–10 U/L	3–10 U/L
15 days to <13 weeks	2–22 U/L	2–22 U/L
13 weeks to <1 year	3–50 U/L	3–50 U/L
1 year to <19 years	25–101 U/L	25–101 U/L
ANTISTREPTOLYSIN-O TITER[1]		
0 to <6 months	0 IU/mL	0 IU/mL
6 months to <1 year	0–30 IU/mL	0–30 IU/mL
1 to <6 years	0–104 IU/mL	0–104 IU/mL
6 to <19 years	0–331 IU/mL	0–331 IU/mL
ASPARTATE AMINOTRANSFERASE (AST)[1]		
0–14 days	32–162 U/L	32–162 U/L
15 days to <1 year	20–67 U/L	20–67 U/L
1 to <7 years	21–44 U/L	21–44 U/L
7 to <12 years	18–36 U/L	18–36 U/L
12 to <19 years (male)	14–35 U/L	14–35 U/L
12 to <19 years (female)	13–26 U/L	13–26 U/L

BICARBONATE[1]

0–14 days	5–20 mEq/L	5–20 mmol/L
15 days to <1 year	10–24 mEq/L	10–24 mmol/L
1 to <5 years	14–24 mEq/L	14–24 mmol/L
5 to <15 years	17–26 mEq/L	17–26 mmol/L
Male 15 to <19 years	18–28 mEq/L	18–28 mmol/L
Female 15 to <19 years	17–26 mEq/L	17–26 mmol/L

BILIRUBIN (TOTAL)[1]

See Chapter 18 for more complete information about neonatal hyperbilirubinemia.

0–14 days	0.19–16.60 mg/dL	3.3–283.8 mcmol/L
15 days to <1 year	0.05–0.68 mg/dL	0.8–11.7 mcmol/L
1 to <9 years	0.05–0.40 mg/dL	0.8–6.8 mcmol/L
9 to <12 years	0.05–0.55 mg/dL	0.8–9.4 mcmol/L
12 to <15 years	0.10–0.70 mg/dL	1.7–11.9 mcmol/L
15 to <19 years	0.10–0.84 mg/dL	1.7–14.4 mcmol/L

BILIRUBIN (DIRECT)[1]

0–14 days	0.33–0.71 mg/dL	5.7–12.1 mcmol/L
15 days to <1 year	0.05–0.30 mg/dL	0.8–5.2 mcmol/L
1 to <9 years	0.05–0.20 mg/dL	0.8–3.4 mcmol/L
9 to <13 years	0.05–0.29 mg/dL	0.8–5.0 mcmol/L
13 to <19 years (female)	0.10–0.39 mg/dL	1.7–6.7 mcmol/L
13 to <19 years (male)	0.11–0.42 mg/dL	1.9–7.1 mcmol/L

BLOOD GAS, ARTERIAL (BREATHING ROOM AIR)[3]

	pH	PaO$_2$ (mmHg)	PaCO$_2$ (mmHg)
Cord blood (umbilical artery)	7.18–7.38	5.7–30.5	42–74[4]
Newborn (birth)	7.11–7.36	8–24	27–40
5–10 min	7.09–7.30	33–75	27–40
30 min	7.21–7.38	31–85	27–40
60 min	7.26–7.49	55–80	27–40
1 day	7.29–7.45	54–95	27–40
Child/adult	7.35–7.45	83–108	32–48

NOTE: Venous blood gases can be used to assess acid-base status, not oxygenation. PvCO$_2$ is 2–8 mmHg higher than PaCO$_2$, and pH is slightly lower. Peripheral venous samples are strongly affected by the local circulatory and metabolic environment. Arterialized capillary blood gases correlate better than venous samples with arterial pH and PaCO$_2$.[3]

C-REACTIVE PROTEIN (HIGH SENSITIVITY)[1]

0–14 days	0.3–6.1 mg/L	0.3–6.1 mg/L
15 days to <15 years	0.1–1.0 mg/L	0.1–1.0 mg/L
15 to <19 years	0.1–1.7 mg/L	0.1–1.7 mg/L

CALCIUM (IONIZED)[2]

0 to <1 month	4.4–5.4 mg/dL	1.10–1.35 mmol/L
1 month to adult	4.44–5.2 mg/dL	1.11–1.30 mmol/L

CALCIUM (TOTAL)[1]

0 to <1 year	8.5–11.0 mg/dL	2.1–2.7 mmol/L
1 year to <19 years	9.2–10.5 mg/dL	2.3–2.6 mmol/L

Continued

28

TABLE 28.1

REFERENCE VALUES—CONT'D

CARBON MONOXIDE (CARBOXYHEMOGLOBIN)[5]

Nonsmoker	<2% of total hemoglobin
Smoker	<10% of total hemoglobin

CHLORIDE (SERUM)[6]

3–5 years	100–107 mEq/L	100–107 mmol/L
6–11 year	101–107 mEq/L	101–107 mmol/L
12–29 years (male)	101–106 mEq/L	101–106 mmol/L
12–29 years (female)	100–107 mEq/L	100–107 mmol/L

CHOLESTEROL

(See LIPIDS, further on)

COPPER[7]

6 months to 2 years	72–178 mCg/dL	11.3–28.0 mcmol/L
3–4 years	80–160 mCg/dL	12.6–25.2 mcmol/L
5–6 years	76–167 mCg/dL	12.0–26.3 mcmol/L
7–8 years	79–147 mCg/dL	12.4–23.1 mcmol/L
9–10 years	84–154 mCg/dL	13.2–24.2 mcmol/L
11–12 years	73–149 mCg/dL	11.5–23.4 mcmol/L
13–14 years	66–137 mCg/dL	10.4–21.6 mcmol/L
15–16 years	60–132 mCg/dL	9.4–20.8 mcmol/L
17–18 years	59–146 mCg/dL	9.3–23.0 mcmol/L

CREATINE KINASE[8]

6 months to 2 years (male)	50–272 U/L	50–272 U/L
6 months to 2 years (female)	38–260 U/L	38–260 U/L
3–5 years (male)	59–296 U/L	59–296 U/L
3–5 years (female)	42–227 U/L	42–227 U/L
6–8 years (male)	54–275 U/L	54–275 U/L
6–8 years (female)	50–231 U/L	50–231 U/L
9–11 years (male)	55–324 U/L	55–324 U/L
9–11 years (female)	52–256 U/L	52–256 U/L
12–14 years (male)	63–407 U/L	63–407 U/L
12–14 years (female)	45–257 U/L	45–257 U/L
15–17 years (male)	68–914 U/L	68–914 U/L
15–17 years (female)	45–458 U/L	45–458 U/L

CREATININE (SERUM) (ENZYMATIC)[1]

0–14 days	0.32–0.92 mg/dL	29–82 mcmol/L
15 days to <2 years	0.10–0.36 mg/dL	9–32 mcmol/L
2 to <5 years	0.20–0.43 mg/dL	18–38 mcmol/L
5 to <12 years	0.31–0.61 mg/dL	27–54 mcmol/L
12 to <15 years	0.45–0.81 mg/dL	40–72 mcmol/L
15 to <19 years (male)	0.62–1.08 mg/dL	55–96 mcmol/L
15 to <19 years (female)	0.49–0.84 mg/dL	43–74 mcmol/L

ERYTHROCYTE SEDIMENTATION RATE (ESR)[9]

0 to <1 month	≤2 mm/hr
1 month–12 years	≤20 mm/hr

| >12 years (male) | ≤15 mm/hr | |
| >12 years (female) | ≤20 mm/hr | |

FERRITIN[1]

4 to <15 days	100–717 ng/mL	224–1611 pmol/L
15 days to <6 months	14–647 ng/mL	31–1454 pmol/L
6 months to <1 year	8–182 ng/mL	19–409 pmol/L
1 to <5 years	5–100 ng/mL	12–224 pmol/L
5 to <14 years	14–79 ng/mL	31–177 pmol/L
14 to <19 years (female)	6–67 ng/mL	12–152 pmol/L
14 to <16 years (male)	13–83 ng/mL	28–186 pmol/L
16 to <19 years (male)	11–172 ng/mL	25–386 pmol/L

FOLATE (RBC)[2]

| | ≥366 ng/mL | ≥829 nmol/L |

FOLATE (SERUM)[2]

Deficient	≤3.9 ng/mL	≤8.8 nmol/L
Indeterminate	4.0–5.8 ng/mL	9.1–13.1 nmol/L
Normal	≥5.9 ng/mL	≥13.4 nmol/L

GAMMA-GLUTAMYL TRANSFERASE (GGT)[1]

0–14 days	23–219 U/L	23–219 U/L
15 days to <1 year	8–127 U/L	8–127 U/L
1 to <11 years	6–16 U/L	6–16 U/L
11 to <19 years	7–21 U/L	7–21 U/L

GLUCOSE

See Chapter 10.

HAPTOGLOBIN[1]

0–14 days	0–10 mg/dL	0–0.10 g/L
15 days to <1 year	7–221 mg/dL	0.07–2.21 g/L
1 to <12 years	7–163 mg/dL	0.07–1.63 g/L
12 to <19 years	7–179 mg/dL	0.07–1.79 g/L

HEMOGLOBIN A1c

See Chapter 10.

HEMOGLOBIN F, % TOTAL HEMOGLOBIN[2]

0–1 month	45.8–91.7	
2 months	32.7–85.2	
3 months	14.5–73.7	
4 months	4.2–56.9	
5 months	1.0–38.1	
6–8 months	0.9–19.4	
9–12 months	0.6–11.6	
13–23 months	0.0–8.5	
2 years and older	0.0–2.1	

IRON[1]

0 to <14 years	16–128 mCg/dL	2.8–22.9 mcmol/L
14–19 years (male)	31–168 mCg/dL	5.5–30.0 mcmol/L
14–19 years (female)	20–162 mCg/dL	3.5–29.0 mcmol/L

Continued

28

TABLE 28.1

REFERENCE VALUES—CONT'D

LACTATE[10]

0–90 days	9–32 mg/dL	1.0–3.5 mmol/L
3–24 months	9–30 mg/dL	1.0–3.3 mmol/L
2–18 years	9–22 mg/dL	1.0–2.4 mmol/L

LACTATE DEHYDROGENASE[1]

0–14 days	309–1222 U/L	309–1222 U/L
15 days to <1 year	163–452 U/L	163–452 U/L
1 to <10 years	192–321 U/L	192–321 U/L
10 to <15 years (male)	170–283 U/L	170–283 U/L
10 to <15 years (female)	157–272 U/L	157–272 U/L
15 to <19 years	130–250 U/L	130–250 U/L

LEAD

See Chapter 3.

LIPASE[1]

0 to <19 years	4–39 U/L	4–39 U/L

LIPIDS[11]

	Desirable	Borderline	High[b]
Total cholesterol	<170 mg/dL (4.4 mmol/L)	170–199 mg/dL (4.4–5.1 mmol/L)	≥200 mg/dL (5.2 mmol/L)
LDL	<110 mg/dL (2.8 mmol/L)	110–129 mg/dL (2.8–3.3 mmol/L)	≥130 mg/dL (3.4 mmol/L)
Non-HDL	<120 mg/dL (3.1 mmol/L)	120–144 mg/dL (3.1–3.7 mmol/L)	≥145 mg/dL (3.8 mmol/L)
HDL	>45 mg/dL (1.2 mmol/L)	40–45 mg/dL (1.0–1.2 mmol/L)	<40 mg/dL (1.0 mmol/L)
Triglycerides (0–9 years)	<75 mg/dL (0.8 mmol/L)	75–99 mg/dL (0.8–1.1 mmol/L)	≥100 mg/dL (1.1 mmol/L)
Triglycerides (10–19 years)	<90 mg/dL (1.0 mmol/L)	90–129 mg/dL (1.0–1.5 mmol/L)	≥130 mg/dL (1.5 mmol/L)

	Conventional Units	SI Units

MAGNESIUM[1]

0–14 days	1.99–3.94 mg/dL	0.82–1.62 mmol/L
15 days to <1 year	1.97–3.09 mg/dL	0.81–1.27 mmol/L
1 to <19 years	2.09–2.84 mg/dL	0.86–1.17 mmol/L

OSMOLALITY[2]

0–16 years	271–296 mOsm/kg	271–296 mmol/kg
17 years and older	280–303 mOsm/kg	280–303 mmol/kg

PHOSPHORUS[1]

0–14 days	5.6–10.5 mg/dL	1.8–3.4 mmol/L
15 days to <1 year	4.8–8.4 mg/dL	1.5–2.7 mmol/L
1 to <5 years	4.3–6.8 mg/dL	1.4–2.2 mmol/L
5 to <13 years	4.1–5.9 mg/dL	1.3–1.9 mmol/L

13 to <16 years (male)	3.5–6.2 mg/dL	1.1–2.0 mmol/L
13 to <16 years (female)	3.2–5.5 mg/dL	1.0–1.8 mmol/L
16 to <19 years	2.9–5.0 mg/dL	0.9–1.6 mmol/L

PORCELAIN[12]

0 to <1 year	10.11–20.22 mg/dL	6.20–19.56 mmol/L
1 to <19 years	6.30–20.21 mg/dL	11.09–20.22 mmol/L

POTASSIUM[3]

Preterm	3.0–6.0 mEq/L	3.0–6.0 mmol/L
Newborn	3.7–5.9 mEq/L	3.7–5.9 mmol/L
Infant	4.1–5.3 mEq/L	4.1–5.3 mmol/L
3–5 years	3.9–4.6 mEq/L	3.9–4.6 mmol/L
6 years and older	3.8–4.9 mEq/L	3.8–4.9 mmol/L

PREALBUMIN[1]

0–14 days	2–12 mg/dL	0.02–0.12 g/L
15 days to <1 year	5–24 mg/dL	0.05–0.24 g/L
1 to <5 years	12–23 mg/dL	0.12–0.23 g/L
5 to <13 years	14–26 mg/dL	0.14–0.26 g/L
13 to <16 years	18–31 mg/dL	0.18–0.31 g/L
16 to <19 years (male)	20–35 mg/dL	0.20–0.35 g/L
16 to <19 years (female)	17–33 mg/dL	0.17–0.33 g/L

RHEUMATOID FACTOR[1]

0–14 days	9.0–17.1 IU/mL	9.0–17.1 IU/mL
15 days to <19 years	0–9.0 IU/mL	0–9.0 IU/mL

SODIUM[6]

3–5 years	135–142 mEq/L	135–142 mmol/L
6–15 years	136–143 mEq/L	136–143 mmol/L
16–49 years (male)	137–143 mEq/L	137–143 mmol/L
16–49 years (female)	137–142 mEq/L	137–142 mmol/L

TOTAL IRON-BINDING CAPACITY (TIBC)[2]

0–2 months	59–175 mCg/dL	11–31 mcmol/L
3 months to 17 years	250–400 mCg/dL	45–72 mcmol/L
18 years and older	240–450 mCg/dL	43–81 mcmol/L

TOTAL PROTEIN[1]

0–14 days	5.3–8.3 g/dL	53–83 g/L
15 days to <1 year	4.4–7.1 g/dL	44–71 g/L
1 to <6 years	6.1–7.5 g/dL	61–75 g/L
6 to <9 years	6.4–7.7 g/dL	64–77 g/L
9 to <19 years	6.5–8.1 g/dL	65–81 g/L

TRANSFERRIN[1]

0 to <9 weeks	104–224 mg/dL	1.04–2.24 g/L
9 weeks <1 year	107–324 mg/dL	1.07–3.24 g/L
1 to <19 years	220–337 mg/dL	2.2–3.37 g/L

Continued

TABLE 28.1		
REFERENCE VALUES—CONT'D		

TRIGLYCERIDES		
(See LIPIDS, earlier)		

UREA NITROGEN[1]		
0–14 days	2.8–23.0 mg/dL	1.0–8.2 nmol/L
15 days to <1 year	3.4–16.8 mg/dL	1.2–6.0 nmol/L
1 to <10 years	9.0–22.1 mg/dL	3.2–7.9 nmol/L
10 to <19 years (male)	7.3–21 mg/dL	2.6–7.5 nmol/L
10 to <19 years (female)	7.3–19 mg/dL	2.6–6.8 nmol/L

URIC ACID[1]		
0–14 days	2.8–12.7 mg/dL	164–757 mcmol/L
15 days to <1 year	1.6–6.3 mg/dL	94–377 mcmol/L
1 to <12 years	1.8–4.9 mg/dL	106–289 mcmol/L
12 to <19 years (male)	2.6–7.6 mg/dL	156–454 mcmol/L
12 to <19 years (female)	2.6–5.9 mg/dL	153–349 mcmol/L

VITAMIN A (RETINOL)[1]		
0 to <1 year	8.0–53.6 mg/dL	0–2 mcmol/L
1 to <11 years	27.5–44.4 mg/dL	1–2 mcmol/L
11 to <16 years	24.9–55.0 mg/dL	1–2 mcmol/L
16 to <19 years	28.7–75.1 mg/dL	1–3 mcmol/L

VITAMIN B$_1$ (THIAMINE), WHOLE BLOOD[3]		
	90–140 nmol/L	90–140 nmol/L

VITAMIN B$_2$ (RIBOFLAVIN)[3]		
	4–24 mCg/dL	106–638 nmol/L

VITAMIN B$_{12}$ (COBALAMIN)[1]		
5 days to <1 year	259–1576 pg/mL	191–1163 pmol/L
1 to <9 years	283–1613 pg/mL	209–1190 pmol/L
9 to <14 years	252–1125 pg/mL	186–830 pmol/L
14 to <17 years	244–888 pg/mL	180–655 pmol/L
17 to <19 years	203–811 pg/mL	150–599 pmol/L

VITAMIN C (ASCORBIC ACID)[3]		
	0.4–1.5 mg/dL	23–85 mcmol/L

VITAMIN D (1,25-DIHYDROXY-VITAMIN D)[13]		
0 to <1 year	32–196 pg/mL	77–471 pmol/L
1 to <3 years	47–151 pg/mL	113–363 pmol/L
3 to <19 years	45–102 pg/mL	108–246 pmol/L

VITAMIN D (25-HYDROXY-VITAMIN D)[14,15]		
Deficient	<12 ng/mL	<30 nmol/L
Insufficient	12–20 ng/mL	30–50 nmol/L
Sufficient[c]	>20 ng/mL	>50 nmol/L
Excess	>50–60 ng/mL	>125–150 nmol/L

VITAMIN E (α-TOCOPHEROL)[1]		
0 to <1 year	0.2–2.1 mg/dL	5.0–50.0 mcmol/L
1 to <19 years	0.6–1.4 mg/dL	14.5–33.0 mcmol/L

ZINC[7]		
6 months to 2 years	56–125 mCg/dL	8.6–19.1 mcmol/L
3–4 years	60–120 mCg/dL	9.2–18.4 mcmol/L
5–6 years	64–117 mCg/dL	9.8–17.9 mcmol/L
7–8 years	65–125 mCg/dL	9.9–19.1 mcmol/L
9–10 years	66–125 mcg/dL	10.1–19.1 mcmol/L
11–12 years	66–127 mCg/dL	10.1–19.4 mcmol/L
13–14 years	69–124 mCg/dL	10.6–19.0 mcmol/L
15–16 years	62–123 mCg/dL	9.5–18.8 mcmol/L
17–18 years	62–133 mCg/dL	9.5–20.3 mcmol/L

[a]Assay with bromocresol green.
[b]It is important to note that these values have not been validated to demonstrate increased risk of atherosclerosis or cardiovascular events.
[c]Controversy exists regarding optimal 25-hydroxyvitamin D level. Some experts recommend a level ≥30 ng/mL as sufficient.[16]

TABLE 28.2

EVALUATION OF CEREBROSPINAL FLUID

WBC		
Age	**Count/mcL (median)**	**95th Percentile**
0–28 days[17]	0–12[a] (4)	16
29–60 days[17]	0–8[a] (2)	11
Child[19]	0–7	

GLUCOSE		
Age	**Median**	**5th Percentile**
0–28 days[17]	45 mg/dL	35 mg/dL
29–60 days[17]	47 mg/dL	37 mg/dL
	Conventional Units	**SI Units**
Infant, child[3]	60–80 mg/dL	3.3–4.4 mmol/L
Adult[3]	40–70 mg/dL	2.2–3.9 mmol/L

PROTEIN		
Age	**Median**	**95th Percentile**
0–28 days[17]	66 mg/dL	118 mg/dL
29–60 days[17]	49 mg/dL	91 mg/dL
	Conventional Units	**SI Units**
6 months to 2 years[18]	6–25 mg/dL	60–250 mg/L
2–6 years[18]	5–25 mg/dL	50–250 mg/L
6–12 years[18]	5–28 mg/dL	50–280 mg/L
12–18 years[18]	6–34 mg/dL	60–340 mg/L

OPENING PRESSURE (LATERAL RECUMBENT POSITION[19,20])	
1–18 years	11.5–28 cm H_2O[a]
Respiratory variations	0.5–1 cm H_2O

[a]10th to 90th percentiles.
WBC, White blood cell.

TABLE 28.3

EVALUATION OF URINE

Urine Analyte	Reference Range
ALBUMIN[3,19]	
Random (first morning urine)	
Male	<22 mg urine albumin/g creatinine
Female	<30 mg urine albumin/g creatinine
24-hr collection	
4–16 years (male)	3.35–13.15 mg/1.73 m²/day
4–16 years (female)	3.75–18.34 mg/1.73 m²/day
CALCIUM[10]	
Random	
1 month–1 year	0.03–0.81 mg/mg creatinine
1–2 years	0.03–0.56 mg/mg creatinine
2–3 years	0.02–0.5 mg/mg creatinine
3–5 years	0.02–0.41 mg/mg creatinine
5–7 years	0.01–0.3 mg/mg creatinine
7–10 years	0.01–0.25 mg/mg creatinine
10–14 years	0.01–0.24 mg/mg creatinine
14–17 years	0.01–0.24 mg/mg creatinine
24-hr collection	
2–18 years (male)	0.75–3.79 mg/kg/day
2–18 years (female)	0.73–3.41 mg/kg/day
CHLORIDE[3,21]	
Random	
Male	25–253 mmol/g creatinine
Female	39–348 mmol/g creatinine
24-hr collection	
Infant	2–10 mmol/day
Child <6 years	15–40 mmol/day
6–10 years (male)	36–110 mmol/day
6–10 years (female)	18–74 mmol/day
10–14 years (male)	64–176 mmol/day
10–14 years (female)	36–173 mmol/day
Adult	110–250 mmol/day
CREATININE[3]	
Random	
3–5 years	15–152 mg/dL
6–11 years	14–196 mg/dL
12–13 years	21–215 mg/dL
14–29 years	19–305 mg/dL
24-hr collection	
Infant	8–20 mg/kg/day
Child	8–22 mg/kg/day
Adolescent	8–30 mg/kg/day
Adult (male)	14–26 mg/kg/day
Adult (female)	11–20 mg/kg/day

POTASSIUM[3,21]

Random	
Male	13–116 mmol/g creatinine
Female	8–129 mmol/g creatinine
24-hr collection	
6–10 years (male)	17–54 mmol/day
6–10 years (female)	8–37 mmol/day
10–14 years (male)	22–57 mmol/day
10–14 years (female)	18–58 mmol/day
Adult	25–125 mmol/day

PROTEIN[5,19]

Random	
6 months to 24 months	<0.5 mg protein/mg creatinine
>2 years	<0.2 mg protein/mg creatinine
24-hr collection	
At rest	50–80 mg/day
After intense exercise	<250 mg/day

SODIUM[3,21]

Random	
Male	23–229 mmol/g creatinine
Female	26–297 mmol/g creatinine
24-hr collection	
6–10 years (male)	41–115 mmol/day
6–10 years (female)	20–69 mmol/day
10–14 years (male)	63–177 mmol/day
10–14 years (female)	48–168 mmol/day
Adult (male)	40–220 mmol/day
Adult (female)	27–287 mmol/day

UREA NITROGEN[3,21]

Random	
Male	102–352 mmol/g creatinine
Female	112–416 mmol/g creatinine
24-hr collection	10–20 g/day

URINE OSMOLALITY[21]

Random	50–1,200 mOsm/kg H_2O, depending on fluid intake
On average fluid intake	300–900 mOsm/kg H_2O
After 12-hr fluid restriction	>850 mOsm/kg H_2O
24-hr collection	~300–900 mOsm/kg H_2O

28

REFERENCES

A complete list of references can be found online.

Chapter 29

Biostatistics and Evidence-Based Medicine

Michael R. Rose, MD, MPH

See additional content online.

Audio Case File 29.1 Evidence based medicine: a discussion on race based in clinical practice guideline

I. BIOSTATISTICS AND EVIDENCE-BASED MEDICINE (EBM)[1-3]

Evidence-based medicine is perhaps best encapsulated by Sackett's classic definition (and the accompanying Venn diagram, see Fig. 29.1): "the conscientious, explicit, and judicious use of current best evidence in making decisions about the care of individual patients. The practice of evidence-based medicine means integrating individual clinical expertise with the best available external clinical evidence from systematic research."[1]

1. **Formulate the clinical question (PICO process):** e.g., "Should I choose D5 0.9% saline or D5 0.45% saline for maintenance fluids for this 6-month-old with bronchiolitis and poor oral intake?"
   a. **Patient, population, and/or problem:** Decide what question you seek to answer and for whom (i.e., infants requiring maintenance IV fluids).
   b. **Intervention:** Describe the intervention under investigation (i.e., D5 0.9% saline)
   c. **Compare:** Compare the intervention with alternative or current standard of care (i.e., D5 0.45% saline).
   d. **Outcomes:** Formulate outcome(s) of interest for your question. (i.e., rates of electrolyte derangements, acute kidney injury, length of stay).
2. Search for evidence to answer the question.
   a. **Define search terms** that fit the clinical questions (i.e., isotonic vs. hypotonic fluids in pediatrics).
   b. **Develop search strategy** using primary sources such as PubMed or secondary sources such as Cochrane, UpToDate, ClinicalKey, or society guidelines. These strategies are not mutually exclusive and often used best in conjunction.
3. Critical appraisal of the evidence It is important to assess studies for both internal validity (study was conducted in an unbiased fashion) and external validity (study results are applicable in the "real world").
   a. Studies investigating an intervention are almost always best answered with randomized controlled trials (RCTs) given their ability to eliminate residual confounding (i.e., confounding we cannot anticipate, identify, and control for in nonrandomized studies). Key questions to ask:

What is evidence-based medicine?

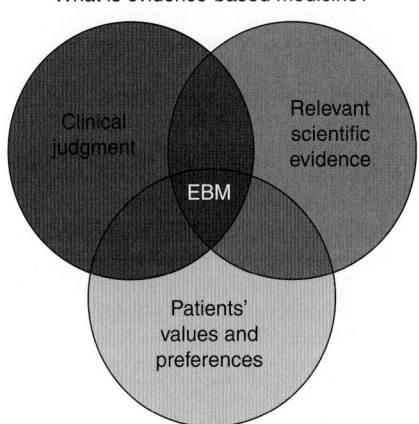

FIGURE 29.1

Venn diagram of evidence-based medicine. (Modified from Sackett DL, Rosenberg WMC, Gray JAM, et al. Evidence based medicine: what it is and what it isn't. *BMJ*. 1996;312:71. https://doi.org/10.1136/bmj.312.7023.71)

(1) Were participants (truly) randomized?
(2) Was the control/comparator group appropriate? (Beware of "straw man" comparators, e.g., new chemotherapeutic trialed against out-of-date standard of care.)
(3) Were the participants/investigators blinded? (When not feasible, think how this may affect the outcome.)
   (a) **Placebo effect:** Treatment benefit due to perception of treatment
   (b) **Nocebo effect:** Adverse effects due to perception of treatment
   (c) **Hawthorne effect:** Participant change of behavior from being studied
   (d) **Observer-expectancy bias:** Researcher's belief in efficacy of a treatment affects their actions
(4) Was the analysis appropriate?
   (a) **Intention to treat (ITT):** Analyzing outcomes based on initial group assignment regardless of receipt of intervention (almost always the proper analysis to minimize bias)
   (b) **As-treated analysis:** Analyzing outcomes based on receipt of intervention, not initial assignment (almost always incorrect due to participant crossover not being random)
(5) Were the outcomes clinically important (or a reasonable proxy to infer clinical relevance)?
(6) Was the study properly powered? Were power calculations performed prospectively?

    (a) **Underpowered study:** May statistically miss clinically meaningful benefits and harms. Smaller studies can miss important but uncommon harms

    (b) **Overpowered study:** May find statistically significant outcomes that are clinically insignificant

    (c) Beware of the use of composite outcomes to increase statistical power, which may come at the consequence of clinical relevance if power increase is driven by a nonclinically important outcome.

b. Studies investigating diagnosis (i.e., JAMA rational clinical exam, lab test characteristics, imaging modality comparisons)

    (1) Was the test compared with the appropriate reference standard? (Ideally this should be the "gold standard" test.)

    (2) Was the test assessed in the appropriate population? (This is an especially important in extrapolating results from adults to pediatric patients.)

c. Studies investigating prognosis

    (1) Where were patients in their course at the start of the study?

    (2) Were they followed up over sufficient time to detect the outcomes of interest?

    (3) Beyond the point estimate, how precise is the prognosis?

d. Factors that increase the likelihood of causality between variable and outcome

    (1) The relationship is temporal.

    (2) The association is strong.

    (3) The relationship is dose dependent.

    (4) The findings were replicated.

    (5) The findings have bio-plausibility.

    (6) The association fades with cessation of intervention.

    (7) The findings are consistent with prior knowledge.

e. **Bias:** Consider the many known types of bias and how they may affect the results.

    (1) **Selection biases:** Caused by a nonrandom or dissimilar sample (between cases/controls or exposed/unexposed) from a population. This is mitigated by randomization and selection of participants who are representative of the target population.

        (a) **Sampling bias:** The sample studied is not representative of population results that are extrapolated to (e.g., RCT performed in healthy volunteers but results inform treatment of sicker patients).

        (b) **Loss to follow-up bias:** The patients who are lost to follow-up are not randomly distributed (i.e., patients experiencing severe side effects were more likely to drop out of study, leaving only those who tolerated treatment).

        (c) **Exclusion bias:** Certain populations (e.g., children) were excluded from a study limiting external validity of results.

    (2) **Information bias:** Caused by flawed collection of information about exposures and outcomes. Mitigated by blinding

researchers and participants (see above) and standardizing data collection

   (a) **Recall bias:** Awareness of disorder alters recall by subjects.
   (b) **Lead-time bias:** Early detection is confused with increased survival.

(3) Other important biases

   (a) **Confounding:** A variable associated with both the disease and the exposure (risk factor), leading to detection of a false relationship between the disease and exposure if the researchers do not control for the confounder. Can be controlled for by adjustment, matching, and/or blinding, but best controlled for by randomization (e.g., ice cream sales increase violence is confounded by hot weather)
   (b) **Effect modifier (interaction):** A variable that modifies the observed effect of an exposure on disease (e.g., a new drug is effective in female children but not male children, then sex is an effect modifier). Can be controlled for by stratification
   (c) Directed acyclic graphs (DAGs) can be drawn to help assessment for confounders, effect modifiers, colliders, and other biases.
   (d) A more complete list of common biases can be found at https://catalogofbias.org/biases/

f. Assess value: Value is broadly defined as outcomes per cost. Ask whether the intervention is likely to be of high value, low value, or no value.[4]

   (1) **High-value care:** The intervention either improves outcomes, decreases cost, or both.
      (a) Expensive interventions can be high value if they have large benefit.
      (b) Low-cost interventions can be low value if they have negligible or no benefit.
      (c) High-value interventions may still increase the overall cost of care.
      (d) The cutoff between high and low value care is subjective and decided based on a society's values and resources.
   (2) **Low-value care:** There is some benefit, but it is not worth the cost (or its savings are not worth how much it worsens outcomes).
   (3) **No-value care:** The intervention adds no clinical benefit. Also known as a "Things We Do For No Reason"

g. Apply evidence: If the evidence is scientifically valid and clinically important, integrate it with your clinical expertise and the patient's values and preferences.

II. BIOSTATISTICS AND EPIDEMIOLOGY

A. Statistical Tests

The following statistical tests are used to determine whether observed differences are statistically significant (Table 29.1).[5-7]

1. **Parametric tests** are used when data follow a particular distribution (e.g., a normal distribution—a bell-shaped distribution where the median, mean, and mode are all equal). These tests are generally more powerful.

TABLE 29.1

COMMONLY USED STATISTICAL TESTS

Purpose of Test	Parametric Test	Nonparametric Test	Example
Compares two independent samples	Two-sample (unpaired) t test	Mann-Whitney U test	To compare girls' heights with boys' heights
Compares two sets of observations on a single sample	One-sample (paired) t test	Wilcoxon matched pairs test	To compare weight of infants before and after a feeding
Compares three or more sets of observations made on a single sample	One-way analysis of variance (F test) using total sum of squares	Kruskal-Wallis analysis of variance by ranks	To determine whether plasma glucose level is higher 1 hr, 2 hr, or 3 hr after a meal
As above, but tests the influence (and interaction) of two different variables	Two-way analysis of variance (ANOVA)	Two-way analysis of variance by ranks	In the above example, to determine whether the results differ in male and female subjects
Tests the null hypothesis that the distribution of a categorical variable is the same in two (or more) independent samples	χ^2 (chi square) test	Fisher exact test	To assess whether acceptance into medical school is more likely if the applicant was born in Britain
Assesses the strength of the straight-line association between two continuous variables	Product moment correlation coefficient (Pearson r)	Spearman rank correlation coefficient ($r\sigma$)	To assess whether and to what extent plasma HbA1C concentration is related to plasma triglyceride concentration in patients with diabetes
Describes the numeric relation between two quantitative variables, allowing one value to be predicted from the other	Regression by least squares method	Nonparametric regression (various tests)	To see how peak expiratory flow rate varies with height
Describes the numerical relationship between a dependent variable and several predictor variables (covariates)	Multiple regression by least squares method	Nonparametric regression (various tests)	To determine whether and to what extent a person's age, body fat, and sodium intake determine his or her blood pressure

Modified from Greenhalgh T. How to read a paper: Statistics for the non-statistician. I: Different types of data need different statistical tests. *BMJ.* 1997;315(7104):364–366.

2. **Nonparametric tests** are used when a particular distribution cannot be assumed. They rank data rather than taking absolute differences into account.
3. **Unpaired tests** compare values from independent samples.
4. *Paired tests* are performed on paired data. For example, where the same parameter is measured on each patient before and after an intervention.
5. **Two-tailed tests** should be used when an intervention could potentially lead to either an increase or decrease of the outcome.
6. **One-tailed tests** should be used when an intervention can have only one plausible effect on the outcome.

B. Statistical Terminology

1. **α (Alpha): Significance level of a statistical test**[5,8]
   a. **α:** Probability of making a **type I error**; the probability of rejecting the null hypothesis (i.e., no effect exists) when the null hypothesis is true (i.e., a difference is seen by chance alone).
   b. **α**, the preset level of significance, is typically set at less than 0.05 in medical research, which allows interpretation with 95% certainty that a detected association is true.
   c. The **P value** is the probability of obtaining the observed values if the null hypothesis is true. For example, if $P = 0.01$, there is a 1 in 100 chance of the values being from chance alone. The P value is judged against **α**, the preset level of significance. If P is less than the significance level **α**, the detected association is considered significant. Even if a P value is significant, it can still turn out to not be true. A P value can also be statistically significant but not clinically significant (e.g., a trial of a new antiviral shortens viral URI symptoms by one hour compared to placebo).

2. **β (Beta): Power of a statistical test**
   a. **β:** Probability of making a **type II error**; the probability of accepting the null hypothesis when the alternative hypothesis is true (i.e., no difference is seen even though there is one). Power is influenced by sample size, effect size, and variance.
   b. **Power = 1 − β:** Probability of correctly rejecting the null hypothesis (i.e., finding a difference when there truly is one)
   c. **Power** is typically set at a minimum of 0.80, which allows interpretation with 80% certainty that a detected lack of association is true.

3. **Sample size:** The number of subjects required in a study to detect an effect with a predetermined power and **α**.

4. **95% confidence interval:** Describes the values between which there is a 95% chance that the true population value falls. When confidence intervals for groups overlap, they have no statistically significant difference.

C. Types of Study Designs[9] (see Table 29.2)

D. Measurement of Disease Occurrence and Treatment Effects[5]

See Table 29.3 for equations in this section.

TABLE 29.2
STUDY DESIGN COMPARISON

Design Type	Cross-Sectional	Case-Control (Retrospective)	Cohort (Usually Prospective, Occasional Retrospective)	Clinical Trial (Experimental)	Systematic Reviews/ Meta-Analysis
Definition	In study population, concurrently measure outcome (disease) and risk factor Compare proportion of diseased group with risk factor to proportion of nondiseased group with risk factor	Define cases (with outcome of interest) and controls (without outcome) Compare proportion of cases with exposure (risk factor) to proportion of controls with exposure (risk factor)	In study population, define exposed group (with risk factor) and nonexposed group (without risk factor) Over time, compare proportion of exposed group with outcome (disease) to proportion of nonexposed group with outcome (disease)	In study population, randomly assign subjects to receive intervention or receive no intervention Compare rate of outcomes between intervention and control groups	Combine data from multiple independent studies to maximize precision and power in testing for statistical significance
Advantages	Defines prevalence Short time to complete Inexpensive	Good for rare diseases/outcomes Small sample size Shorter study times Less expensive Can study association of multiple exposures with outcome	Defines incidence Stronger evidence for causality Decreases biases (sampling, measurement, reporting) Can study association of exposure with multiple outcomes	Randomized controlled trial is gold standard Randomization reduces confounding Best evidence for causality	Higher statistical power Can control for interstudy variation
Disadvantages	Selection bias Weak evidence for causality	Highest potential for biases Weak evidence for causality Unable to determine prevalence, incidence	Expensive Long study times May not be feasible for rare diseases/outcomes Factors related to exposure and outcome may falsely alter effect of exposure on outcome (confounding)	Expensive Risks of experimental treatments in humans Longer study time Not suitable for rare diseases/ outcomes	Publication bias. Only as good as the studies included in the analysis.

Modified from Hulley SB, Cummings SR, Browner WS, et al. *Designing Clinical Research.* 4th ed. Lippincott Williams & Wilkins; 2013:84–207.

TABLE 29.3

GRID FOR CALCULATIONS IN CLINICAL STUDIES

	Disease or Outcome	
Exposure or Risk Factor or Treatment	**Positive**	**Negative**
Positive	A	B
Negative	C	D

Also known as a contingency table.

1. **Prevalence:** Proportion of population who has a disease at a point in time. Obtained in cross-sectional studies

$$\text{Prevalence} = \frac{\text{Number of total cases}}{\text{Population size}}$$

2. **Incidence:** Rate of people developing a disease in the population during a defined time period. Obtained in cohort studies and clinical trials

$$\text{Incidence} = \frac{\text{Number of new cases}}{\text{Population size}} \text{ per unit of time}$$

3. **Relative risk (RR):** The ratio of incidence of disease among people with an exposure to incidence of disease among people without the exposure. Obtained in cohort studies and clinical trials. RR cannot be obtained in case-control studies

$$RR = \frac{\dfrac{A}{A+B}}{\dfrac{C}{(C+D)}}$$

   a. RR = 1: No effect of exposure or treatment on outcome
   b. RR <1: Exposure or treatment protective against outcome
   c. RR >1: Exposure or treatment increases the outcome
   d. The **relative risk reduction (RRR)**, which measures the strength of the impact of an exposure or treatment, is equal to $1 - RR$.

4. **Odds ratios (ORs):** The ratio of the odds of an exposed person developing a disease to the odds of a nonexposed person developing the disease. OR are obtained in case-control studies, cohort studies, and clinical trials.

$$OR = \frac{\dfrac{A}{B}}{\dfrac{C}{D}} = \frac{A \times D}{B \times C}$$

a. OR approximates RR when the disease is rare (incidence <0.10).
b. OR =1: No association between risk factor and disease
c. OR <1: Suggests that risk factor is protective against disease
d. OR >1: Suggests positive association between risk factor and disease

5. **Risk difference:** The difference between the risk of the outcome in control and the risk of the outcome in treatment group. If the risk of the outcome is decreased by the treatment, **absolute risk reduction (ARR)** is used. If the risk of the outcome is increased by the treatment, **absolute risk increase (ARI)** is used.

$$ARR = \frac{C}{(C+D)} - \frac{A}{(A+B)}$$
$$ARI = \frac{A}{(A+B)} - \frac{C}{(C+D)}$$

6. **Number needed to treat (NNT):** Number of patients who need to be treated to prevent one undesired outcome, expressed as the inverse of ARR.

$$NNT = \frac{1}{ARR}$$

7. **Number needed to harm (NNH):** Number of patients who need to be treated to cause one additional patient harm, expressed as the inverse of ARI.

$$NNH = \frac{1}{ARI}$$

E. Measurements of Test Performance[5]
See Table 29.4 for equations in this section.

1. **Validity:** The ability of a test to indicate which patients have or do not have disease. Intrinsic to the test—not affected by disease prevalence
   a. **Sensitivity:** Proportion of all patients with disease who have a positive test. Measures the ability of the test to correctly identify those who have the disease. Use a highly sensitive test to help rule out a disease.

$$Sensitivity = \frac{TP}{TP + FN}$$

   b. **Specificity:** Proportion of all patients without disease who have a negative test. Measures the ability of the test to correctly identify those who do not have the disease. Use a highly specific test to help confirm a disease.

$$Specificity = \frac{TN}{TN + FP}$$

TABLE 29.4

GRID FOR EVALUATING A CLINICAL TEST

	Disease Status	
Test Result	**Has Disease**	**Does Not Have Disease**
Positive	TP (true positive)	FP (false positive)
Negative	FN (false negative)	TN (true negative)

2. **Predictive value**
   a. **Positive predictive value (PPV):** Proportion of those with positive tests who truly have disease. PPV is increased with higher disease prevalence.

$$PPV = \frac{TP}{TP + FP}$$

3. **Negative predictive value (NPV):** Proportion of those with negative tests who truly do not have disease. NPV is increased with lower disease prevalence.

$$NPV = \frac{TN}{TN + FN}$$

4. **Likelihood ratio (LR):** Incorporates the validity of a test (sensitivity and specificity) to determine the magnitude of the effect of a test result on changing the pretest probability. Used with Bayes nomogram (Fig. 29.2) to estimate posttest probability of a disease based on a given test result. Tests that provide the greatest impetus to changing clinical management are those with an LR ≥10 (for positive tests) or LR ≤0.1 (for negative tests). LR is unaffected by disease prevalence.

$$LR \text{ for positive test} = \frac{\text{Sensitivity}}{1 - \text{Specificity}}$$

$$LR \text{ for negative test} = \frac{1 - \text{Sensitivity}}{\text{Specificity}}$$

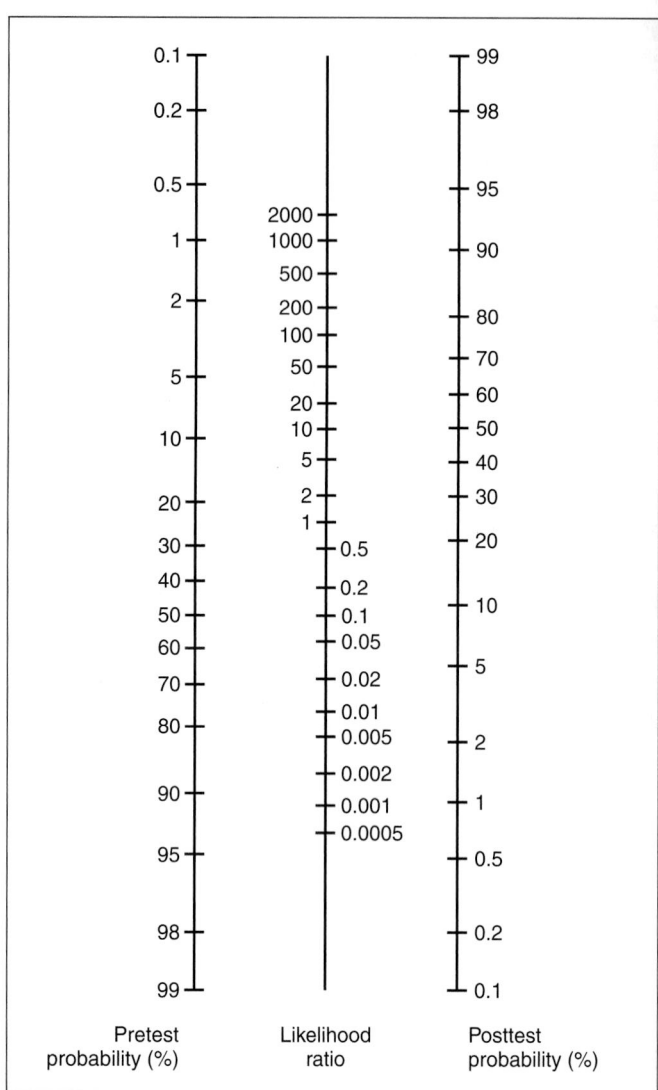

FIGURE 29.2

Bayes nomogram: draw a line connecting the baseline probability (pretest probability) with the value for the likelihood ratio for the test used. Extend this line to the right to find the posttest probability. (Modified from Fagan TJ. Nomogram for Bayes Theorem. *N Engl J Med.* 1975;293[5]:257.)

III. WEB RESOURCES

A. Evidence-Based Resources

- Agency for Healthcare Research and Quality: https://www.ahrq.gov/research/findings/evidence-based-reports/index.html
- Centre for Evidence Based Medicine: https://www.cebm.net
- Cochrane Reviews: https://www.cochranelibrary.com
- JAMA evidence: https://jamaevidence.mhmedical.com/
- JAMA The Rational Clinical Examination: https://jamanetwork.com/collections/6257/the-rational-clinical-examination
- NICE Guidance: https://www.nice.org.uk/guidance
- PubMed: https://www.ncbi.nlm.nih.gov/pubmed
- U.S. Preventive Services Task Force: https://www.uspreventiveservicestaskforce.org/uspstf/

B. Biostatistics and Epidemiology Resources

- BMJ Statistics at Square One: https://www.bmj.com/collections/statsbk/index.dtl
- Centers for Disease Control and Prevention Epi Info: https://www.cdc.gov/epiinfo/
- JAMA Users' Guide to the Medical Literature: https://jamanetwork.com/collections/44069/users-guide-to-the-medical-literature

REFERENCES

A complete list of references can be found online.

PART IV

FORMULARY

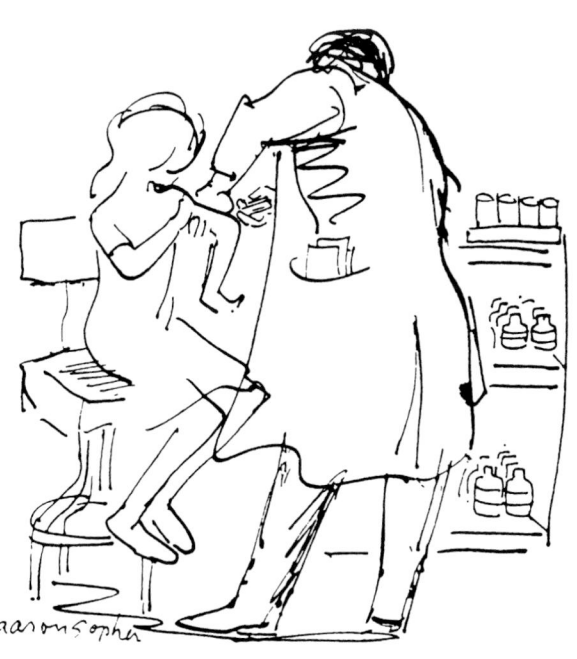

Chapter 30

Drug Dosages

Carlton K.K. Lee, PharmD, MPH

I. NOTE TO READER

The author has made every attempt to check dosages and medical content for accuracy. Because of the incomplete data on pediatric dosing, many drug dosages will be modified after the publication of this text. We recommend that the readers check product information and published literature for changes in dosing, especially for newer medicines. The US Food and Drug Administration (FDA) provides the following pediatric drug information data sources:

- New Pediatric Labeling Information: https://www.fda.gov/science-research/pediatrics/pediatric-labeling-changes
- Drug Safety Report Updates: https://www.fda.gov/advisory-committees/pediatric-advisory-committee/pediatric-advisory-recommendations-and-updates
- Ongoing and completed clinical research study information of pediatric medicines in development is located in https://www.clinicaltrials.gov/

To prevent prescribing errors, the use of abbreviations has been greatly discouraged. The following is a list of abbreviations that The Joint Commission considers prohibited for use.

THE JOINT COMMISSION

Official "Do Not Use" List[a]

Do Not Use	Potential Problem	Use Instead
U (unit)	Mistaken for "0" (zero), the number "4" (four) or "cc"	Write "unit"
IU (International Unit)	Mistaken for IV (intravenous) or the number 10 (ten)	Write "International Unit"
Q.D., QD, q.d., qd (daily)	Mistaken for each other	Write "daily"
Q.O.D., QOD, q.o.d, qod (every other day)	Period after the Q mistaken for "I" and the "O" mistaken for "I"	Write "every other day"
Trailing zero (X.0 mg)[b]	Decimal point is missed	Write X mg
Lack of leading zero (.X mg)	Decimal point is missed	Write 0.X mg
MS	Can mean morphine sulfate or magnesium sulfate	Write "morphine sulfate"
MSO_4 and $MgSO_4$	Confused for one another	Write "magnesium sulfate"

[a]Applies to all orders and all medication-related documentation that is handwritten (including free-text computer entry) or on preprinted forms.

[b]Exception: A "trailing zero" may be used only where required to demonstrate the level of precision of the value being reported, such as for laboratory results, imaging studies that report size of lesions, or catheter/tube sizes. It may not be used in medication orders or other medication-related documentation.

ADDITIONAL ABBREVIATIONS, ACRONYMS, AND SYMBOLS (FOR POSSIBLE FUTURE INCLUSION IN THE OFFICIAL "DO NOT USE" LIST)

Do Not Use	Potential Problem	Use Instead
> (greater than) < (less than)	Misinterpreted as the number "7" (seven) or the letter "L" Confused for one another	Write "greater than" Write "less than"
Abbreviations for drug names	Misinterpreted due to similar abbreviations for multiple drugs	Write drug names in full
Apothecary units	Unfamiliar to many practitioners Confused with metric units	Use metric units
@	Mistaken for the number "2" (two)	Write "at"
cc	Mistaken for U (units) when poorly written	Write "mL" or "ml" or "milliliters" ("mL" is preferred)
μg	Mistaken for mg (milligrams), resulting in one thousand-fold overdose	Write "mCg" or "micrograms"

II. SAMPLE ENTRY

Pharmacogenomics: Indicates need for assessing patient genotype or genetic polymorphism affecting dosing, drug selection, or anticipated pharmacological effects. ─────────────

Liver: Indicates need for caution or need for dose adjustment in hepatic impairment. ─────────────

Kidney: Indicates need for caution or need for dose adjustment in renal impairment (see also Chapter 31). ─────────────

Breast: Refer to explanation of breast-feeding categories (see p. 764). ─────────────

Pregnancy: Refer to explanation of pregnancy categories (see p. 764). ─────────────

How Supplied

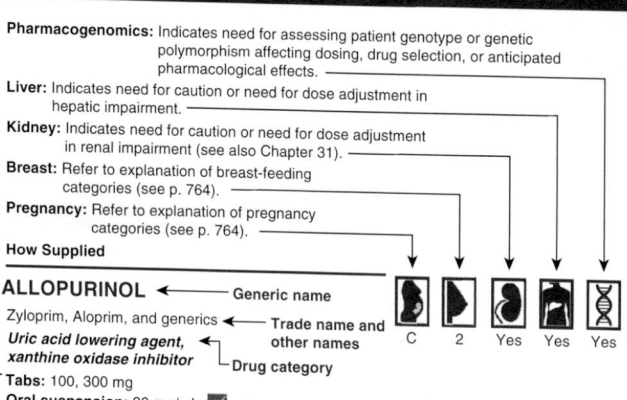

ALLOPURINOL ◄──── Generic name

Zyloprim, Aloprim, and generics ◄──── Trade name and other names

Uric acid lowering agent, ◄──── *xanthine oxidase inhibitor* └── Drug category

C   2   Yes   Yes   Yes

Tabs: 100, 300 mg
Oral suspension: 20 mg/mL
Injection (Aloprim and generics): 500 mg
Contains ~ 1.45 mEq Na/500 mg drug
For use in tumor lysis syndrome, see Chapter 22 for additional information.

Mortar and pestle: Indicates need for extemporaneous compounding by a pharmacist

Child:

    Oral: 10 mg/kg/24 hr PO ÷ BID–QID; **max. dose:** 800 mg/24 hr
    Injectable: 200 mg/m^2/24 hr IV ÷ Q6–12 hr; **max. dose:** 600 mg/24 hr

Adult:

    Oral: 200–800 mg/24 hr PO ÷ BID–TID

    Injectable: 200–400 mg/m^2/24 hr IV ÷ Q6–12 hr; **max. dose:** 600 mg/24 hr

Drug dosing

Discontinue use at the first appearance of skin rash or other signs of an allergic reaction. **Avoid** use in individuals with HLA-B*58:01 allele as they are at significant risk for developing severe cutaneous adverse reactions (e.g., Stevens-Johnson syndrome and TEN).

Side effects include rash, neuritis, hepatotoxicity, renal function impairment, GI disturbance, bone marrow suppression, and drowsiness.

Adjust dose in renal insufficiency (see Chapter 31). Must maintain adequate urine output and alkaline urine.

Drug interactions: increases serum theophylline level; may increase the incidence of rash with ampicillin and amoxicillin; increased risk of toxicity with azathioprine, didanosine, and mercaptopurine; and increased risk of hypersensitivity reactions with ACE inhibitors and thiazide diuretics. Use with didanosine is **contraindicated** due to increased risk for didanosine toxicity. Rhabdomyolysis has been reported with clarithromycin use.

IV dosage form is very alkaline and must be **diluted to a minimum concentration** of 6 mg/mL and infused over 30 min.

The manufacturer advises not to breastfeed during treatment with allopurinol for one week after the last dose as limited data indicate a maternal dose of 300 mg daily can provide near-therapeutic dose and plasma levels in an exclusively breastfed infant.

Brief remarks about side effects, drug interactions, precautions, therapeutic monitoring, and other relevant information

III. EXPLANATION OF BREASTFEEDING CATEGORIES

See sample entry on previous page.

1 Compatible

2 Use with caution

3 Unknown with concerns

X Contraindicated

? Safety not established

IV. EXPLANATION OF PREGNANCY CATEGORIES

A Adequate studies in pregnant women have not demonstrated a risk to the fetus in the first trimester of pregnancy, and there is no evidence of risk in later trimesters.

B Animal studies have not demonstrated a risk to the fetus, but there are no adequate studies in pregnant women; or animal studies have shown an adverse effect, but adequate studies in pregnant women have not demonstrated a risk to the fetus during the first trimester of pregnancy, and there is no evidence of risk in later trimesters.

C Animal studies have shown an adverse effect on the fetus, but there are no adequate studies in humans; or there are no animal reproduction studies and no adequate studies in humans.

D There is evidence of human fetal risk, but the potential benefits from the use of the drug in pregnant women may be acceptable despite its potential risks.

X Studies in animals or humans demonstrate fetal abnormalities or adverse reaction; reports indicate evidence of fetal risk. The risk of use in pregnant women clearly outweighs any possible benefit.

? Pregnancy category not established

V. NOMOGRAM AND EQUATION FOR BODY SURFACE AREA

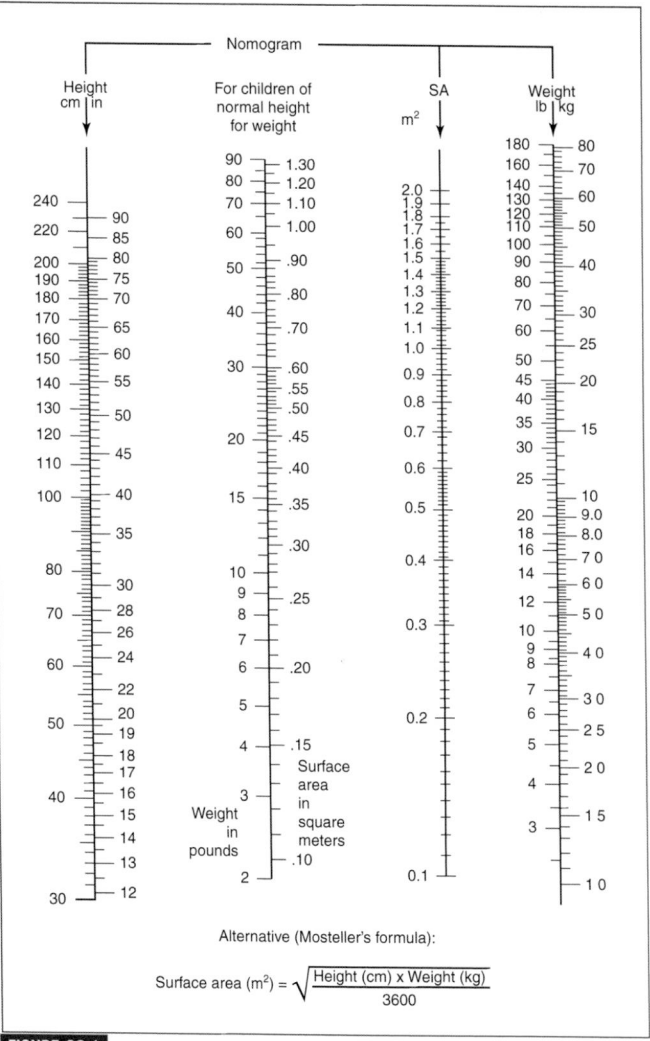

Nomogram

| Height cm | in | For children of normal height for weight | SA m² | Weight lb | kg |

Alternative (Mosteller's formula):

$$\text{Surface area (m}^2) = \sqrt{\frac{\text{Height (cm)} \times \text{Weight (kg)}}{3600}}$$

FIGURE 30.1

Nomogram and equation for body surface area. (From Kliegman RM, Stanton BF, Schor NF, et al., eds. *Nelson Textbook of Pediatrics.* 20th ed. Elsevier; 2016.)

VI. DRUG INDEX

Trade Name(s)	Generic Name
1,25-dihydroxycholecalciferol	Calcitriol
2-PAM[a]	Pralidoxime Chloride
3TC[a]	Lamivudine
5-aminosalicylic acid	Mesalamine
5-ASA	Mesalamine
5-FC[a]	Flucytosine
5-Fluorocytosine[a]	Flucytosine
8-Arginine Vasopressin[a]	Vasopressin
9-Fluorohydrocortisone[a]	Fludrocortisone Acetate
27% Elemental Ca	Calcium Chloride
A-200	Pyrethrins
Abelcet	Amphotericin B Lipid Complex
Absorica	Isotretinoin
Abstra	Fentanyl
Accolate	Zafirlukast
AccuNeb (prediluted nebulized solution)	Albuterol
Accutane	Isotretinoin
Acetadote	Acetylcysteine
Acticin	Permethrin
Actigall	Ursodiol
Actiq	Fentanyl
Activase	Alteplase
Acular, Acular LS	Ketorolac
Acuvail	Ketorolac
Aczone	Dapsone
Adalat CC	Nifedipine
Adderall, Adderall XR	Dextroamphetamine + Amphetamine
Adenocard	Adenosine
Adoxa	Doxycycline
Adrenaline	Epinephrine HCl
Advair Diskus, Advair HFA	Fluticasone Propionate and Salmeterol
Advil, Children's Advil	Ibuprofen
Aerospan	Flunisolide
Afrin	Oxymetazoline
AK-Poly-Bac Ophthalmic	Bacitracin + Polymyxin B
AK-Sulf	Sulfacetamide Sodium Ophthalmic
AKTob	Tobramycin
AK-Tracin Ophthalmic	Bacitracin
Albuminar	Albumin, Human
Albutein	Albumin, Human
Aldactone	Spironolactone
Aleve [OTC]	Naproxen/Naproxen Sodium
Allegra, Allegra ODT	Fexofenadine
Allegra-D 12 Hour, Allegra-D 24 Hour	Fexofenadine + Pseudoephedrine
Allergen Ear Drops	Antipyrine and Benzocaine
Aloprim	Allopurinol
Almacone, Almacone II Double Strength	Aluminum Hydroxide with Magnesium Hydroxide

Trade Name(s)	Generic Name
Alsuma	Sumatriptan Succinate
AlternaGEL	Aluminum Hydroxide
Alu-Cap	Aluminum Hydroxide
Alvesco	Ciclesonide
AmBisome	Amphotericin B, Liposomal
Amicar	Aminocaproic Acid
Amikin	Amikacin Sulfate
Amnesteem	Isotretinoin
Amoclan	Amoxicillin-Clavulanic Acid
Amoxil	Amoxicillin
Amphadase	Hyaluronidase
Amphocin	Amphotericin B
Amphojel	Aluminum Hydroxide
Anacin	Aspirin
Anaprox	Naproxen/Naproxen Sodium
Ancef	Cefazolin
Ancobon	Flucytosine
Anectine	Succinylcholine
Antilirium	Physostigmine Salicylate
Antipyrine and Benzocaine Otic	Antipyrine and Benzocaine
Antizol	Fomepizole
Anzemet	Dolasetron
Apresoline	Hydralazine Hydrochloride
Apriso	Mesalamine
Aquachloral Supprettes	Chloral Hydrate
Aquasol A	Vitamin A
Aquasol E	Vitamin E
Aquavit-E	Vitamin E
Aralen	Chloroquine HCl/Phosphate
Aranesp	Darbepoetin Alfa
Arbinoxa	Carbinoxamine
Arestin	Minocycline
Aridol	Mannitol
Aristospan	Triamcinolone
ASA[a]	Aspirin
Asacol, Asacol HD	Mesalamine
Asmanex Twisthaler	Mometasone Furoate
Aspirin Free Anacin	Acetaminophen
Astelin	Azelastine
Astepro	Azelastine
Astragraf XL	Tacrolimus
Ativan	Lorazepam
AtroPen	Atropine Sulfate
Atrovent	Ipratropium Bromide
Augmentin, Augmentin ES-600, Augmentin XR	Amoxicillin-Clavulanic Acid
Auralgan (available in Canada)	Antipyrine and Benzocaine
Auro Ear Drops	Carbamide Peroxide
Avinza	Morphine Sulfate
Avita	Tretinoin
Ayr Saline	Sodium Chloride—Inhaled Preparations

Trade Name(s)	Generic Name
Azactam	Aztreonam
Azasan	Azathioprine
Azasite	Azithromycin
Azo-Standard [OTC]	Phenazopyridine HCl
Azulfidine, Azulfidine EN-Tabs	Sulfasalazine
Baciguent Topical	Bacitracin
Bactrim	Sulfamethoxazole and Trimethoprim
Bactroban, Bactroban Nasal	Mupirocin
BAL[a]	Dimercaprol
Beconase AQ	Beclomethasone Dipropionate
Benadryl	Diphenhydramine
Benzac AC Wash 2½, 5, 10; Benzac 5, 10	Benzoyl Peroxide
Beta-Val	Betamethasone
Bethkis	Tobramycin
Biaxin, Biaxin XL	Clarithromycin
Bicillin C-R, Bicillin C-R 900/300	Penicillin G Preparations—Penicillin G Benzathine and Penicillin G Procaine
Bicillin L-A	Penicillin G Preparations—Benzathine
Bio-Statin	Nystatin
Bloxiverz	Neostigmine
Bleph-10	Sulfacetamide Sodium Ophthalmic
Brevibloc	Esmolol HCl
Brevoxyl Creamy Wash	Benzoyl Peroxide
Brisdelle	Paroxetine
British anti-Lewisite	Dimercaprol
Bufferin	Aspirin
Bumex	Bumetanide
Buminate	Albumin, Human
Cafcit	Caffeine Citrate
Cafergot	Ergotamine Tartrate + Caffeine
Calcidol	Ergocalciferol
Caldolor	Ibuprofen
Calan, Calan SR	Verapamil
Calciferol	Ergocalciferol
Calcijex	Calcitriol
Calcionate	Calcium Glubionate
Calciquid	Calcium Glubionate
Cal-Citrate	Calcium Citrate
Calcium disodium versenate	Edetate (EDTA) Calcium Disodium
Cal-Glu	Calcium Gluconate
Cal-Lac	Calcium Lactate
Calphron	Calcium Acetate
Camphorated opium tincture	Paregoric
Canasa	Mesalamine
Cancidas	Caspofungin
Cankaid	Carbamide Peroxide
Capoten	Captopril
Carafate	Sucralfate
Carbatrol	Carbamazepine
Cardene, Cardene SR	Nicardipine

Trade Name(s)	Generic Name
Cardizem, Cardizem SR, Cardizem CD, Cardizem LA	Diltiazem
Carnitor	Carnitine
Catapres, Catapres TTS	Clonidine
Cathflo Activase	Alteplase
Cayston	Aztreonam
Ceclor, Ceclor CD	Cefaclor
Cecon	Ascorbic Acid
Cefotan	Cefotetan
Ceftin	Cefuroxime Axetil
Cefzil	Cefprozil
Celestone	Betamethasone
CellCept	Mycophenolate Mofetil
Cephulac	Lactulose
Ceptaz	Ceftazidime
Cerebyx	Fosphenytoin
Chemet	Succimer
Chloromycetin	Chloramphenicol
Chlor-Trimeton	Chlorpheniramine Maleate
Cholestyramine Light	Cholestyramine
Chronulac	Lactulose
Ciloxan ophthalmic	Ciprofloxacin
Cipro, Cipro XR, Ciprodex, Cipro HC Otic	Ciprofloxacin
Citracal	Calcium Citrate
Claforan	Cefotaxime
Claravis	Isotretinoin
Claritin, Claritin Children's Allergy, Claritin RediTabs	Loratadine
Claritin-D 12 Hour, Claritin-D 24 Hour	Loratadine + Pseudoephedrine
Cleocin-T, Cleocin	Clindamycin
Cogentin	Benztropine Mesylate
Colace	Docusate
Colocort	Hydrocortisone
CoLyte	Polyethylene Glycol—Electrolyte Solution
Compazine	Prochlorperazine
Concerta	Methylphenidate HCl
Copegus	Ribavirin
Cordarone	Amiodarone HCl
Cordron-D NR, Cordron-D	Carbinoxamine + Pseudoephedrine
Coreg, Coreg CR	Carvedilol
Cortef	Hydrocortisone
Cortenema	Hydrocortisone
Cortifoam	Hydrocortisone
Cortisporin Otic	Polymyxin B Sulfate, Neomycin Sulfate, Hydrocortisone
Co-Trimoxazole	Sulfamethoxazole and Trimethoprim
Coumadin	Warfarin
Covera-HS	Verapamil
Cozaar	Losartan
Crolom	Cromolyn
Cruex	Clotrimazole
Cuprimine	Penicillamine

Trade Name(s)	Generic Name
Curosurf	Surfactant, Pulmonary/Poractant Alfa
Cutivate	Fluticasone Propionate
Cuvposa	Glycopyrrolate
Cyanoject	Cyanocobalamin/Vitamin B_{12}
Cyclogyl	Cyclopentolate
Cyclomydril	Cyclopentolate with Phenylephrine
Cyomin	Cyanocobalamin/Vitamin B_{12}
Cytovene	Ganciclovir
D-3, D3-5, D3-50	Cholecalciferol
Dantrium	Dantrolene
Daraprim	Pyrimethamine
Daytrana	Methylphenidate HCl
DDAVP[a]	Desmopressin Acetate
DDS[a]	Dapsone
D Drops	Cholecalciferol
Debrox	Carbamide Peroxide
Decadron	Dexamethasone
Deltasone	Prednisone
Delzicol	Mesalamine
Deodorized tincture of opium	Opium Tincture
Depacon	Valproic Acid
Depakene	Valproic Acid
Depakote, Depakote ER	Divalproex Sodium
Depen	Penicillamine
Depo-Medrol	Methylprednisolone
Depo-Provera	Medroxyprogesterone
Depo-Sub Q Provera 104	Medroxyprogesterone
Desquam-E 5, Desquam-E 10	Benzoyl Peroxide
Desyrel (previously available as)	Trazodone
Dexedrine Spansules	Dextroamphetamine
DexFerrum	Iron—Injectable Preparations (iron dextran)
Dexpak Taperpak	Dexamethasone
DextroStat	Dextroamphetamine ± Amphetamine
Di-5-ASA[a]	Olsalazine
Dialume	Aluminum Hydroxide
Diaminodiphenyl sulfone	Dapsone
Diamox	Acetazolamide
Diastat, Diastat AcuDial	Diazepam
Dificid	Fidaxomicin
Diflucan and others	Fluconazole
Digibind, DigiFab	Digoxin Immune Fab (Ovine)
Digitek	Digoxin
Dilacor XR	Diltiazem
Dilantin, Dilantin Infatab	Phenytoin
Dilaudid, Dilaudid-HP	Hydromorphone HCl
Di-mesalazine	Olsalazine
Dimetapp Children's Cold and Allergy	Brompheniramine with Phenylephrine
Diovan	Valsartan
Dipentum	Olsalazine

Trade Name(s)	Generic Name
Diprolene, Diprolene AF	Betamethasone
Diprosone	Betamethasone
DisperMox	Amoxicillin
Ditropan, Ditropan XL	Oxybutynin Chloride
Diuril	Chlorothiazide
DMSA [dimercaptosuccinic acid][a]	Succimer
Dobutrex (previously available as)	Dobutamine
Dolophine	Methadone HCl
Doryx	Doxycycline
Doxidan	Bisacodyl
Dramamine, Children's Dramamine	Dimenhydrinate
Drisdol	Ergocalciferol
Dulcolax	Bisacodyl
Dulera	Mometasone Furoate + Formoterol Fumarate
Duraclon	Clonidine
Duragesic	Fentanyl
Duramist 12-Hr Nasal	Oxymetazoline
Duricef	Cefadroxil
Dycill	Dicloxacillin Sodium
Dymista	Azelastine and Fluticasone
Dynacin	Minocycline
Dyrenium	Triamterene
EC-Naprosyn	Naproxen
Efidac/24-Pseudoephedrine	Pseudoephedrine
Elavil	Amitriptyline
Elidel	Pimecrolimus
Elimite	Permethrin
Eliphos	Calcium Acetate
Elitek	Rasburicase
Elixophyllin	Theophylline
Elocon	Mometasone Furoate
Enfamil D-Vi-Sol	Cholecalciferol
EMLA, Eutectic mixture of lidocaine and prilocaine	Lidocaine and Prilocaine
E-Mycin	Erythromycin Preparations
Enbrel	Etanercept
Endocet	Oxycodone and Acetaminophen
Endodan	Oxycodone and Aspirin
Enemeez	Docusate
Enlon	Edrophonium Chloride
Entocort EC	Budesonide
Enulose	Lactulose
Epaned	Enalapril Maleate
EpiPen	Epinephrine HCl
Epitol	Carbamazepine
Epivir, Epivir-HBV	Lamivudine
Epogen	Epoetin Alfa
Epsom salts	Magnesium Sulfate
Ergomar	Ergotamine Tartrate
Ery-Ped	Erythromycin

Trade Name(s)	Generic Name
Erythrocin, Pediamycin, E-Mycin, Ery-Ped	Erythromycin
Erythropoietin	Epoetin Alfa
Eryzole	Erythromycin Ethylsuccinate and Acetylsulfisoxazole
Exalgo	Hydromorphone HCl
Extina	Ketoconazole
Famvir	Famciclovir
Fansidar	Pyrimethamine + Sulfadoxine
Felbatol	Felbamate
Fentora	Fentanyl
Feosol	Iron—Oral Preparations (Ferrous sulfate)
Fergon	Iron—Oral Preparations (Ferrous sulfate)
Fer-In-Sol	Iron—Oral Preparations (Ferrous gluconate)
Ferrlecit	Iron—Injectable Preparations (Ferric gluconate)
Fetroja	Cefiderocol
Feverall	Acetaminophen
Fiberall	Psyllium
First-Lansoprazole	Lansoprazole
First-Omeprazole	Omeprazole
FK506	Tacrolimus
Flagyl, Flagyl ER	Metronidazole
Flebogamma DIF	Immune Globulin
Fleet Babylax	Glycerin
Fleet Laxative, Fleet Bisacodyl	Bisacodyl
Fleet Mineral Oil	Mineral Oil
Fleet, Fleet Phospho-Soda	Sodium Phosphate
Fletcher's Castoria	Senna/Sennosides
Flonase HFA	Fluticasone Propionate
Florinef Acetate	Fludrocortisone Acetate
Flovent Diskus	Fluticasone Propionate
Floxin, Floxin Otic	Ofloxacin
Flumadine	Rimantadine
Fluohydrisone	Fludrocortisone Acetate
Fluoritab	Fluoride
Focalin, Focalin XR	Dexmethylphenidate
Folvite	Folic Acid
Foradil Aerolizer	Formoterol
Fortamet	Metformin
Fortaz	Ceftazidime
Fortical Nasal Spray	Calcitonin—Salmon
Foscavir	Foscarnet
Fulvicin U/F, Fulvicin P/G	Griseofulvin
Fungizone	Amphotericin B
Furadantin	Nitrofurantoin
Gabitril	Tiagabine
Gablofen	Baclofen
Galzin	Zinc Salts, Systemic
Gammaplex	Immune Globulin

Trade Name(s)	Generic Name
Gamma benzene hexachloride[a]	Lindane
Gammaked	Immune Globulin
Garamycin	Gentamicin
Gastrocrom	Cromolyn
Gas-X	Simethicone
Gengraf	Cyclosporine Modified
GlucaGen, Glucagon Emergency Kit	Glucagon HCl
Glucophage, Glucophage XR	Metformin
Gly-Oxide	Carbamide Peroxide
Glycate	Glycopyrrolate
GoLYTELY	Polyethylene Glycol—Electrolyte Solution
Gralise	Gabapentin
Granisol	Granisetron
Grifulvin V	Griseofulvin
Grisactin	Griseofulvin
Gris-PEG	Griseofulvin
Gyne-Lotrimin 3, Gyne-Lotrimin	Clotrimazole
H.P. Acthar Gel	Corticotropin
Haldol, Haldol Decanoate 50, Haldol Decanoate 100	Haloperidol
Hecoria	Tacrolimus
Hexadrol	Dexamethasone
Horizant	Gabapentin
Humatin	Paromomycin Sulfate
Hydro-Tussin CBX	Carbinoxamine + Pseudoephedrine
Hylenex	Hyaluronidase
Hypersal	Sodium Chloride—Inhaled Preparations
Imitrex	Sumatriptan Succinate
Imodium, Imodium AD	Loperamide
Imuran	Azathioprine
Inapsine	Droperidol
Inderal, Inderal LA	Propranolol
Indocin, Indocin SR, Indocin IV	Indomethacin
Infasurf	Surfactant, Pulmonary/Calfactant
INFeD	Iron—Injectable Preparations (iron dextran)
INH[a]	Isoniazid
Intal (previously available as)	Cromolyn
Intropin (previously available as)	Dopamine
Intuniv	Guanfacine
Invanz	Ertapenem
Iosat	Potassium Iodide
Iquix	Levofloxacin
Isentress, Isentress HD	Raltegravir
IsonaRif	Isoniazid
Isoptin SR	Verapamil
Isopto Carpine	Pilocarpine HCl
Isopto Hyoscine	Scopolamine Hydrobromide
Isuprel	Isoproterenol
Jantoven	Warfarin
Kadian	Morphine Sulfate

Trade Name(s)	Generic Name
Kantrex	Kanamycin
Kaopectate	Bismuth Subsalicylate
Kao-Tin	Bismuth Subsalicylate
Kapvay	Clonidine
Kayexalate	Sodium Polystyrene Sulfonate
Keflex	Cephalexin
Kemstro	Baclofen
Kenalog	Triamcinolone
Keppra, Keppra XR	Levetiracetam
Ketalar	Ketamine
Kionex	Sodium Polystyrene Sulfonate
Klonopin	Clonazepam
Klout	Pyrethrins with Piperonyl Butoxide
Kondremul	Mineral Oil
Konsyl	Psyllium
K-PHOS Neutral	Phosphorus Supplements
Kristalose	Lactulose
Kytril	Granisetron
Lamictal, Lamictal ODT, Lamictal XR	Lamotrigine
Laniazid	Isoniazid
Lanoxin	Digoxin
Lariam	Mefloquine HCl
Lasix	Furosemide
Lax-Pills	Senna/Sennosides
Lazanda	Fentanyl
L-Carnitine	Carnitine
Levaquin, Quixin, Iquix	Levofloxacin
Levocarnitine	Carnitine
Levophed and others	Norepinephrine Bitartrate
Lialda	Mesalamine
Licide	Pyrethrins with Piperonyl Butoxide
Lidoderm	Lidocaine
Lioresal	Baclofen
Liquid Pred	Prednisone
Lithobid	Lithium
L-M-X	Lidocaine
Loniten (previously available as)	Minoxidil
Lopressor, Toprol-XL	Metoprolol
Lotrimin AF	Clotrimazole
Lotrimin AF	Miconazole
Lovenox	Enoxaparin
Luminal	Phenobarbital
Luride	Fluoride
Luvox CR	Fluvoxamine
Maalox, Maalox Maximum Strength Liquid	Aluminum Hydroxide with Magnesium Hydroxide
Macrobid	Nitrofurantoin
Macrodantin	Nitrofurantoin
Mag-200, Mag-Ox 400, Uro-Mag	Magnesium Oxide
Marinol	Dronabinol

Trade Name(s)	Generic Name
Maxidex	Dexamethasone
Maxipime	Cefepime
Maxivate	Betamethasone
Maxolon	Metoclopramide
Medrol, Medrol Dosepack	Methylprednisolone
Mefoxin	Cefoxitin
Mephyton	Phytonadione/Vitamin K_1
Mepron	Atovaquone
Merrem	Meropenem
Mestinon	Pyridostigmine Bromide
Metadate ER	Methylphenidate HCl
Metamucil	Psyllium
Methadose	Methadone HCl
Methylin, Methylin ER	Methylphenidate HCl
Metozolv	Metoclopramide
MetroCream	Metronidazole
MetroGel, MetroGel-Vaginal	Metronidazole
MetroLotion	Metronidazole
Miacalcin, Miacalcin Nasal Spray	Calcitonin—Salmon
Micatin	Miconazole
Microzide	Hydrochlorothiazide
Milk of Magnesia	Magnesium Hydroxide
Millipred	Prednisolone
Minocin	Minocycline
Mintezol	Thiabendazole
Mintox	Aluminum Hydroxide with Magnesium Hydroxide
MiraLax	Polyethylene Glycol—Electrolyte Solution
Monistat	Miconazole
Motrin, Children's Motrin	Ibuprofen
MS Contin	Morphine Sulfate
Mucomyst	Acetylcysteine
Mucosol	Acetylcysteine
Murine Ear	Carbamide Peroxide
Myambutol	Ethambutol HCl
Mycamine	Micafungin Sodium
Mycelex, Mycelex-7	Clotrimazole
Mycobutin	Rifabutin
Mycostatin	Nystatin
Myfortic	Mycophenolate Sodium
Mylanta Gas	Simethicone
Mylanta, Mylanta Extra Strength	Aluminum Hydroxide with Magnesium Hydroxide
Mylicon	Simethicone
Myorisan	Isotretinoin
Mysoline	Primidone
Nallpen	Nafcillin
Naprelan	Naproxen/Naproxen Sodium
Narcan	Naloxone
Nasacort AQ	Triamcinolone

Trade Name(s)	Generic Name
Nasalcrom	Cromolyn
Nasarel	Flunisolide
Nascobal	Cyanocobalamin/Vitamin B_{12}
Nasonex	Mometasone Furoate
Nebcin	Tobramycin
NebuPent	Pentamidine Isethionate
Nembutal	Pentobarbital
NeoBenz Micro	Benzoyl Peroxide
Neo-fradin	Neomycin Sulfate
Neo-Polycin	Neomycin/Polymyxin B/Bacitracin
NeoProfen (IV)	Ibuprofen
Neoral	Cyclosporine
Neosporin, Neosporin Ophthalmic, Neo To Go	Neomycin/Polymyxin B/Bacitracin
Neosporin GU Irrigant	Neomycin/Polymyxin B
Neo-Synephrine	Phenylephrine HCl
Neo-Synephrine 12-Hr Nasal	Oxymetazoline
Nephron	Epinephrine, Racemic
Neupogen, G-CSF	Filgrastim
Neurontin	Gabapentin
Neut	Sodium Bicarbonate
Nexiclon XR	Clonidine
Nexium	Esomeprazole
Nexterone	Amiodarone HCl
Niacor	Niacin (Vitamin B_3)
Niaspan	Niacin (Vitamin B_3)
Nicotinic acid	Niacin (Vitamin B_3)
Nifediac CC	Nifedipine
Niferex	Iron—Oral Preparations
Nilstat	Nystatin
Nipride (previously available as)	Nitroprusside
Nitro-Bid	Nitroglycerin
Nitro-Dur	Nitroglycerin
Nitro-Mist	Nitroglycerin
Nitropress	Nitroprusside
Nitrostat	Nitroglycerin
Nitro-Time	Nitroglycerin
Nix	Permethrin
Nizoral, Nizoral A-D	Ketoconazole
Noritate	Metronidazole
Normal Serum Albumin (Human)	Albumin, Human
Normodyne	Labetalol
Noroxin	Norfloxacin
Norvasc	Amlodipine
Nostrilla	Oxymetazoline
NuCort	Hydrocortisone
NuLYTELY	Polyethylene Glycol—Electrolyte Solution
Nutr-E-Sol	Vitamin E/α-Tocopherol
NVP[a]	Nevirapine
Nydrazid	Isoniazid
OCL[a]	Polyethylene Glycol—Electrolyte Solution

Trade Name(s)	Generic Name
Ocean	Sodium Chloride—Inhaled Preparations
Ocuflox	Ofloxacin
Ocusulf-10	Sulfacetamide Sodium Ophthalmic
Omnaris	Ciclesonide
Ofirmev	Acetaminophen
Omeprazole and Syrspend SF Alka	Omeprazole
Omnicef	Cefdinir
Omnipaque 140, Omnipaque 180, Omnipaque 240, Omnipaque 300, and Omnipaque 350	Iohexol
Omnipen	Ampicillin
Onfi	Clobazam
Onmel	Itraconazole
Opticrom	Cromolyn
Optivar	Azelastine
Oralone	Corticosteroid
Oramorph SR	Morphine Sulfate
Orapred, Orapred ODT	Prednisolone
Oraqix	Lidocaine and Prilocaine
Orasone	Prednisone
OraVerse	Phentolamine Mesylate
Orazinc	Zinc Salts, Systemic
Os-Cal	Calcium Carbonate
Osmitrol	Mannitol
OsmoPrep	Sodium Phosphate
Oxtellar	Oxcarbazepine
Oxy-5, Oxy-10	Benzoyl Peroxide
OxyContin	Oxycodone
Oxytrol	Oxybutynin Chloride
Pacerone	Amiodarone HCl
Palgic	Carbinoxamine
Pamelor	Nortriptyline Hydrochloride
Pamix	Pyrantel Pamoate
Panadol	Acetaminophen
Paracetamol	Acetaminophen
Pataday	Olopatadine
Patanase	Olopatadine
Patanol	Olopatadine
Pathocil	Dicloxacillin Sodium
Paxil, Paxil CR	Paroxetine
Pediaflor	Fluoride
Pedia-Lax	Glycerin
Pediamycin	Erythromycin Preparations
Pediapred	Prednisolone
Pediazole	Erythromycin Ethylsuccinate and Acetylsulfisoxazole
PediOtic	Polymyxin B Sulfate, Neomycin Sulfate, Hydrocortisone
Pentam 300	Pentamidine Isethionate
Pentasa	Mesalamine

Trade Name(s)	Generic Name
Pepcid, Pepcid AC [OTC], Maximum Strength Pepcid AC [OTC], Pepcid Complete [OTC], Pepcid RPD	Famotidine
Pepto-Bismol	Bismuth Subsalicylate
Percocet	Oxycodone and Acetaminophen
Percodan	Oxycodone and Aspirin
Perforomist	Formoterol
Periactin (previously available as)	Cyproheptadine
Periostat	Doxycycline
Pexeva	Paroxetine
Pfizerpen	Penicillin G Preparations—Aqueous Potassium and Sodium
PGE_1[a]	Alprostadil
Phazyme	Simethicone
Phenergan	Promethazine
Phenytek	Phenytoin
PhosLo	Calcium Acetate
Phoslyra	Calcium Acetate
Pilopine HS	Pilocarpine HCl
Pima	Potassium Iodide
Pin-Rid	Pyrantel Pamoate
Pin-X	Pyrantel Pamoate
Pipracil	Piperacillin
Pitressin	Vasopressin
Plaquenil	Hydroxychloroquine
Plasbumin	Albumin, Human
Polymox	Amoxicillin
Polysporin Ophthalmic	Bacitracin + Polymyxin B
Polysporin Topical	Bacitracin + Polymyxin B
Polytrim Ophthalmic Solution	Polymyxin B Sulfate and Trimethoprim Sulfate
Posture-D	Calcium Phosphate, Tribasic
Potassium Phosphate	Phosphorus Supplements
Pradaxa	Dabigatran etexilate mesylate
Precedex	Dexmedetomidine
Prelone	Prednisolone
Prevacid, Prevacid SoluTab	Lansoprazole
Prevalite	Cholestyramine
Prilosec, Prilosec OTC	Omeprazole
Primacor	Milrinone
Primaxin IV	Imipenem and Cilastatin
Principen	Ampicillin
Prinivil	Lisinopril
Privigen	Immune Globulin
ProAir HFA	Albuterol
Procardia, Procardia XL	Nifedipine
ProCentra	Dextroamphetamine Sulfate
Procrit	Epoetin Alfa
Proglycem	Diazoxide
Prograf	Tacrolimus
Pronestyl	Procainamide

Trade Name(s)	Generic Name
Pronto	Pyrethrins
Prostaglandin E₁	Alprostadil
Prostigmin	Neostigmine
Prostin VR Pediatric	Alprostadil
Protonix	Pantoprazole
Protopam	Pralidoxime Chloride
Protopic	Tacrolimus
Protostat	Metronidazole
Proventil, Proventil HFA (aerosol inhaler)	Albuterol
Provera	Medroxyprogesterone
Prozac, Prozac Weekly	Fluoxetine Hydrochloride
Pseudo Carb Pediatric	Carbinoxamine + Pseudoephedrine
PTU[a]	Propylthiouracil
Pulmicort Respules, Pulmicort Flexhaler	Budesonide
Pulmozyme	Dornase Alfa/DNase
Pyrazinoic acid amide	Pyrazinamide
Pyridium	Phenazopyridine HCl
Pyrinyl	Pyrethrins
Qnasl	Beclomethasone Dipropionate
Quelicin, Quelicin-1000	Succinylcholine
Questran, Questran Light	Cholestyramine
Quinidex	Quinidine
Quixin	Levofloxacin
QVAR[a]	Beclomethasone Dipropionate
Raniclor	Cefaclor
Rapamune	Sirolimus
Rayos	Prednisone
Rebetol	Ribavirin
Reese's Pinworm	Pyrantel Pamoate
Regitine	Phentolamine Mesylate
Reglan	Metoclopramide
Regonal	Pyridostigmine Bromide
Renova	Tretinoin
Resectisol	Mannitol
Restasis	Cyclosporine, Cyclosporine Microemulsion, Cyclosporine Modified
Retin-A, Retin-A Micro	Tretinoin
Retrovir, AZT	Zidovudine
Revatio	Sildenafil
Reversol	Edrophonium Chloride
Revonto	Dantrolene
R-Gene 10	Arginine Chloride
Rhinaris	Sodium Chloride—Inhaled Preparations
Rhinocort Aqua Nasal Spray	Budesonide
Ribasphere	Ribavirin
RID	Pyrethrins
Rifadin	Rifampin
Rifamate	Isoniazid + Rifampin
Rifater	Pyrazinamide + Isoniazid + Rifampin
Rimactane	Rifampin

Trade Name(s)	Generic Name
Riomet	Metformin
Risperdal, Risperdal M-Tab, Risperdal Consta	Risperidone
Ritalin, Ritalin SR, Ritalin LA	Methylphenidate HCl
Robinul	Glycopyrrolate
Rocaltrol	Calcitriol
Rocephin	Ceftriaxone
Rogaine, Men's Rogaine Extra Strength	Minoxidil
Romazicon	Flumazenil
Rowasa, SfRowasa	Mesalamine
Roxanol	Morphine Sulfate
Roxicet	Oxycodone and Acetaminophen
Roxicodone	Oxycodone
Roxilox	Oxycodone and Acetaminophen
RuLox Plus	Aluminum Hydroxide with Magnesium Hydroxide
S-2 Inhalant	Epinephrine, Racemic
Sabril	Vigabatrin
Salagen	Pilocarpine HCl
Salicylazosulfapyridine	Sulfasalazine
Sal-Tropine	Atropine Sulfate
Sancuso	Granisetron
Sandimmune	Cyclosporine
Sandostatin, Sandostatin LAR Depot	Octreotide Acetate
Sani-Supp	Glycerin
Sarafem	Fluoxetine Hydrochloride
SAS[a]	Sulfasalazine
Saxenda	Liraglutide
Scopace	Scopolamine Hydrobromide
Selsun and others	Selenium Sulfide
Senna-Gen	Senna/Sennosides
Senokot	Senna/Sennosides
Septra	Sulfamethoxazole and Trimethoprim
Serevent Diskus	Salmeterol
Sildec	Carbinoxamine + Pseudoephedrine
Silvadene	Silver Sulfadiazine
Simply Saline	Sodium Chloride—Inhaled Preparations
Singulair	Montelukast
Slo-Niacin	Niacin (Vitamin B_3)
Slow FE	Iron—Oral Preparations
Sodium Phosphate	Phosphorus Supplements
Solodyn	Minocycline
Solu-cortef	Hydrocortisone
Solu-Medrol	Methylprednisolone
Soluspan	Betamethasone
Sporanox	Itraconazole
SPS[a]	Sodium Polystyrene Sulfonate
SSD Cream, SSD AF Cream	Silver Sulfadiazine
SSKI[a]	Potassium Iodide
Stadol	Butorphanol
Stavzor	Valproic Acid
Stimate	Desmopressin Acetate

Trade Name(s)	Generic Name
Stomach Relief, Stomach Relief Max St, Stomach Relief Plus	Bismuth Subsalicylate
Strattera	Atomoxetine
Streptase	Streptokinase
Sublimaze	Fentanyl
Sudafed	Pseudoephedrine
Sulfatrim	Sulfamethoxazole and Trimethoprim
Sulfazine, Sulfazine EC	Sulfasalazine
Sunkist Vitamin C	Ascorbic Acid
Suprax	Cefixime
Surfak	Docusate
Surfaxin	Surfactant, Pulmonary/Lucinactant
Survanta	Surfactant, Pulmonary/Beractant
Symbicort	Budesonide and Formoterol
Symmetrel	Amantadine Hydrochloride
Synagis	Palivizumab
Synercid	Quinupristin and Dalfopristin
Synthroid	Levothyroxine T_4
Tambocor	Flecainide Acetate
Tamiflu	Oseltamivir Phosphate
Tapazole	Methimazole
Tazicef	Ceftazidime
Tazidime	Ceftazidime
Tegretol, Tegretol-XR	Carbamazepine
Tempra	Acetaminophen
Tenex	Guanfacine
Tenormin	Atenolol
Tensilon	Edrophonium Chloride
Tetrahydrocannabinol	Dronabinol
THC[a]	Dronabinol
Theo-24	Theophylline
Theochron	Theophylline
Thera-Ear	Carbamide Peroxide
Thermazene	Silver Sulfadiazine
Thorazine	Chlorpromazine
ThyroSafe	Potassium Iodide
ThyroShield	Potassium Iodide
Tiazac	Diltiazem
Tigan	Trimethobenzamide HCl
Timentin	Ticarcillin and Clavulanate
Tinactin	Tolnaftate
Tirosint	Levothyroxine
Tisit	Pyrethrins
TMP-SMX[a]	Sulfamethoxazole and Trimethoprim
TOBI, TOBI Podhaler	Tobramycin
Tobrex	Tobramycin
Tofranil, Tofranil-PM	Imipramine
Topamax	Topiramate
Topiragen	Topiramate
Toprol-XL	Metoprolol
Totacillin	Ampicillin

Trade Name(s)	Generic Name
tPA[a]	Alteplase
Trandate	Labetalol
Transderm Scop	Scopolamine Hydrobromide
Trianex	Corticosteroid
Triaz	Benzoyl Peroxide
Triderm	Corticosteroid
Trileptal	Oxcarbazepine
Trilisate and others	Choline Magnesium Trisalicylate
TriLyte	Polyethylene Glycol—Electrolyte Solution
Trimethoprim-Sulfamethoxazole	Sulfamethoxazole and Trimethoprim
Trimox	Amoxicillin
Trokendi XR	Topiramate
Tums	Calcium Carbonate
Tylenol	Acetaminophen
Tylenol #1, #2, #3, #4	Codeine and Acetaminophen
Tylox	Oxycodone and Acetaminophen
Uceris	Budesonide
Unasyn	Ampicillin/Sulbactam
Unithroid, Unithroid Direct	Levothyroxine
Urecholine	Bethanechol Chloride
Uro-KP-Neutral	Phosphorus Supplements
Urolene Blue	Methylene Blue
Urso 250, Urso Forte	Ursodiol
Vagistat-3	Miconazole
Valcyte	Valganciclovir
Valium	Diazepam
Valtrex	Valacyclovir
Vancocin	Vancomycin
Vantin	Cefpodoxime Proxetil
VariZig	Varicella-Zoster Immune Globulin (Human)
Vasotec	Enalapril Maleate
Vasotec IV	Enalaprilat
Veetids	Penicillin V Potassium
Venofer	Iron—Injectable Preparations (iron sucrose)
Ventolin HFA	Albuterol
Veramyst	Fluticasone Propionate
Verelan, Verelan PM	Verapamil
Veripred	Prednisolone
Vermox	Mebendazole
Versed (previously available as)	Midazolam
VFEND	Voriconazole
Viagra	Sildenafil
Vibramycin	Doxycycline
Victoza	Liraglutide
Vimpat	Lacosamide
Viramune, Viramune XR	Nevirapine
Virazole	Ribavirin
Visicol	Sodium Phosphate
Visine LR	Oxymetazoline
Vistaril	Hydroxyzine

Trade Name(s)	Generic Name
Vistide	Cidofovir
Vitamin B$_1$	Thiamine
Vitamin B$_2$	Riboflavin
Vitamin B$_{12}$	Cyanocobalamin/Vitamin B$_{12}$
Vitamin B$_3$	Niacin/Vitamin B$_3$
Vitamin B$_6$	Pyridoxine
Vitamin C	Ascorbic Acid
Vitrase	Hyaluronidase
Vitrasert	Ganciclovir
VoSpire ER	Albuterol
Vyvanse	Lisdexamfetamine
VZIG	Varicella-Zoster Immune Globulin (Human)
WinRho-SDF	Rh$_0$ (D) Immune Globulin Intravenous (Human)
Wycillin	Penicillin G Preparations—Procaine
Wymox	Amoxicillin
Xarelto, Xarelto Starter Pack	Rivaroxaban
Xolegel	Ketoconazole
Xopenex, Xopenex HFA	Levalbuterol
Xylocaine	Lidocaine
Zarontin	Ethosuximide
Zaroxolyn	Metolazone
Zegerid	Omeprazole
Zemuron	Rocuronium
Zenatane	Isotretinoin
Zenzedi	Dextroamphetamine Sulfate
Zerbaxa	Ceftolozane with Tazobactam
Zestril	Lisinopril
Zetonna	Ciclesonide
Zinacef	Cefuroxime
Zirgan	Ganciclovir
Zithromax, Zithromax TRI-PAK, Zithromax Z-PAK, Zmax	Azithromycin
Zoderm	Benzoyl Peroxide
Zofran	Ondansetron
Zolicef	Cefazolin
Zoloft	Sertraline HCl
Zonegran	Zonisamide
ZORprin	Aspirin
Zosyn	Piperacillin with Tazobactam
Zovirax	Acyclovir
Zyloprim	Allopurinol
Zyrtec, Children's Zyrtec	Cetirizine
Zyrtec-D 12 Hour	Cetirizine + Pseudoephedrine
Zyvox	Linezolid

[a]Common abbreviation or other name (not recommended for use when writing a prescription).

TABLE 30.1

EXAMPLES OF INDUCERS AND INHIBITORS OF CYTOCHROME P450 SYSTEM

Isoenzyme	Substrates (Drugs Metabolized by Isoenzyme)	Inhibitors[a]	Inducers
CYP1A2	Caffeine, theophylline, estradiol, propranolol	Cimetidine, quinolones, fluvoxamine, ketoconazole, lidocaine	Carbamazepine, smoking, phenobarbital, rifampin
CYP2B6	Cyclophosphamide, efavirenz, propofol	Paroxetine, sertraline	Carbamazepine, (fos)phenytoin, phenobarbital, rifampin
CYP2C9/10	Warfarin, phenytoin, tolbutamide, fluoxetine, sulfamethoxazole, fosphenytoin	Amiodarone, fluconazole, ibuprofen, indomethacin, nicardipine	Carbamazepine, (fos)phenytoin, rifampin, phenobarbital
CYP2C19	Diazepam, PPIs, phenytoin, desogestrel, ifosfamide, phenobarbital, sertraline, voriconazole	Cimetidine fluvoxamine, fluconazole, isoniazid, PPIs, sertraline	Carbamazepine, (fos)phenytoin, rifampin
CYP2D6	Captopril, codeine, haloperidol, dextromethorphan, tricyclic antidepressants, hydrocodone, oxycodone, phenothiazines, metoprolol, propranolol, paroxetine, venlafaxine, risperidone, flecainide, sertraline, aripiprazole, fluoxetine, lidocaine, fosphenytoin, ritonavir	Chlorpromazine, cinacalcet, dexmedetomidine, cocaine, cimetidine, quinidine, ritonavir, fluoxetine, sertraline, amiodarone	None known
CYP2E1	Acetaminophen, alcohol, isoniazid, theophylline, isoflurane	Disulfiram	Alcohol
CYP3A4	Amlodipine, aripiprazole, budesonide, cocaine, clonazepam, diltiazem, efavirenz, erythromycin, estradiol, fentanyl, fluticasone, nifedipine, verapamil, cyclosporine, carbamazepine, cisapride, tacrolimus, midazolam, alfentanil, diazepam, ifosfamide, imatinib, itraconazole, ketoconazole, cyclophosphamide, PPIs, haloperidol, lidocaine, medroxyprogesterone, methadone, methylprednisolone, salmeterol, theophylline, quetiapine, ritonavir, indinavir, sildenafil, ivacaftor	Erythromycin, cimetidine, clarithromycin, isoniazid, ketoconazole, itraconazole, metronidazole, sertraline, ritonavir, indinavir, imatinib, nicardipine, propofol, quinidine	Rifampin, (fos)phenytoin, phenobarbital, carbamazepine, dexamethasone, lumacaftor

NOTE: The cytochrome P450 enzyme system is composed of different isoenzymes. Each isoenzyme metabolizes a unique group of drugs or substrates. When an inhibitor of a particular isoenzyme is introduced, the serum concentration of any drug or substrate metabolized by that particular isoenzyme will increase. When an inducer of a particular isoenzyme is introduced, the serum concentration of drugs or substrates metabolized by that particular isoenzyme will decrease.

PPI, Proton pump inhibitor.

[a]Only strong and some moderate inhibitors are listed here. Weak inhibitors also exist.

Data from Taketomo CK, Hodding JH, Kraus DM. *American Pharmaceutical Association Pediatric Dosage Handbook.* 16th ed. Lexi-Comp; 2009; Zevin S, Benowitz NL. Drug interactions with tobacco smoking. An update. *Clin Pharmacokinet.* 1999;36:425–438; Cupp MJ, Tracy TS. Cytochrome P450: new nomenclature and clinical implications. *Am Fam Physician.* 1998;57:107–116.

A

ACETAMINOPHEN
Tylenol, Tempra, Panadol, FeverAll, Anacin Asprin
Free, Mapap, Paracetamol, Ofirmev, and many
others
Analgesic, antipyretic

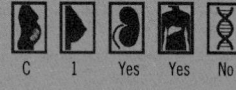

C 1 Yes Yes No

Tabs [OTC]: 325, 500 mg
Chewable tabs [OTC]: 80, 160 mg; some may contain phenylalanine
Child suspension/syrup [OTC]: 160 mg/5 mL; may contain sodium benzoate and propylene glycol
Oral liquid [OTC]: 160 mg/5 mL; may contain sodium benzoate and propylene glycol
Elixir [OTC]: 160 mg/5 mL; may contain sodium benzoate and propylene glycol
Extended release tabs [OTC]: 650 mg
Capsules [OTC]: 325, 500 mg
Dispersible tabs (Tylenol Children's Meltaways) [OTC]: 80, 160 mg; contain sucralose
Suppositories (FeverAll and generics) [OTC]: 80, 120, 325, 650 mg; contain polysorbate 80
Injection:
    Ofirmev and generics: 10 mg/mL (100 mL); preservative free

**PO/PR (maximum daily doses include all routes of acetaminophen administration and
DO NOT exceed 5 doses in 24 hours):**
    Term neonate: 10—15 mg/kg/dose PO/PR Q4—6 hr; **max. dose:** 75 mg/kg/24 hr. Some
    advocate loading doses of 20—25 mg/kg/dose for PO dosing or 30 mg/kg/dose for PR dosing.
    Pediatric: 10—15 mg/kg/dose PO/PR Q4—6 hr; **max. dose:** 75 mg/kg/24 hr or 4 g/24 hr. For rectal
    dosing, some may advocate a 40—45 mg/kg/dose loading dose.
Dosing by weight (preferred) or age (PO/PR Q4—6 hr; DO NOT exceed 5 doses in 24 hours):

Weight (lbs)	Weight (kg)	Age	Dosage (mg)
6—11	2.7—5	0—3 mo	40
12—17	5.1—7.7	4—11 mo	80
18—23	7.8—10.5	1—2 yr	120
24—35	10.6—15.9	2—3 yr	160
36—47	16—21.4	4—5 yr	240
48—59	21.5—26.8	6—8 yr	320 to 325
60—71	26.9—32.3	9—10 yr	325 to 400
72—95	32.4—43.2	11 yr	480 to 500

Adult: 325—650 mg/dose
Max. dose: 4 g/24 hr, 5 doses/24 hr
IV (maximum daily doses include all routes of acetaminophen administration):
    Neonate (≥32 weeks' gestation) and infant:
        ≤28 days old: 12.5 mg/kg/dose Q6 hr IV up to a **maximum** of 50 mg/kg/24 hr
        ≥29 days old to <2 yr: 15 mg/kg/dose Q6 hr IV up to a **maximum** of 60 mg/kg/24 hr
    Child (≥2—12 yr) and adolescent (≥13 yr)/adult: 15 mg/kg/dose Q6 hr, *OR* 12.5 mg/kg/dose Q4 hr IV
    up to the following **maximum** dose by patient weight:
        <50 kg: 75 mg/kg/24 hr up to 3750 mg/24 hr with a **maximum** single dose of 15 mg/kg/dose up to
        750 mg
        ≥50 kg: 75 mg/kg/24 hr up to 4000 mg/24 hr with a **maximum** single dose of 15 mg/kg/dose up to
        1000 mg

Continued

ACETAMINOPHEN *continued*

Adolescent (≥13 yr) and adult (≥50 kg): 1000 mg Q6 hr, *OR* 650 mg Q4 hr up to a **maximum** of 4000 mg/24 hr with a **maximum** single dose of 1000 mg/dose

Does not possess antiinflammatory activity. Safety and efficacy for acute pain and fever in children ≥2 years old are supported by controlled clinical trials. **Use with caution** in patients with known G6PD deficiency.

$T_{1/2}$: 1—3 hr, 2—5 hr in neonates; metabolized in the liver; see Chapter 3 and acetylcysteine for management of drug overdose.

Some preparations contain alcohol (7%—10%) and/or phenylalanine; all suspensions should be shaken before use.

May be used for the treatment of patent ductus arteriosus when standard NSAID is contraindicated or has failed. Most commonly reported dosage is 15 mg/kg dose Q6 hr IV/PO for 3 days (may be given up to 7 days or with a repeated 3-day course).

May decrease the activity of lamotrigine and increase the activity/toxicity of busulfan, warfarin, and zidovudine. Barbiturates, phenytoin, rifampin, and anticholinergic agents (e.g., scopolamine) may decrease the effect of acetaminophen. Increased risk for hepatotoxicity may occur with barbiturates, carbamazepine, phenytoin, carmustine (with high acetaminophen doses), chronic alcohol use, and inducers of CYP 450 2E1 (e.g., isoniazid). **Adjust dose in renal failure (see Chapter 31).**

FOR IV USE: Administer dose undiluted over 15 min. Most common side effects with IV use include nausea, vomiting, constipation, pruritus, agitation, and atelectasis in children; and nausea, vomiting, headache, and insomnia in adults. Rare risk of serious skin reactions (e.g., SJS, TEN) has been reported.

ACETAZOLAMIDE
Various generics; previously available as Diamox
Carbonic anhydrase inhibitor, diuretic

C   1   Yes   Yes   No

Tabs: 125, 250 mg
Oral suspension: 25 mg/mL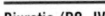
Capsules (extended release): 500 mg
Injection (sodium): 500 mg
Contains 2.05 mEq Na/500 mg drug

Diuretic (PO, IV)

   Child: 5 mg/kg/dose once daily or every other day
   Adult: 250—375 mg/dose once daily or every other day

Glaucoma
   Child:
      PO: 8—30 mg/kg/24 hr ÷ Q6—8 hr; **max. dose:** 1000 mg/24 hr
      IM/IV: 20—40 mg/kg/24 hr ÷ Q6 hr; **max. dose:** 1000 mg/24 hr
   Adult:
      PO (Simple chronic; open angle): 1000 mg/24 hr ÷ Q6 hr
      IV (Acute secondary; closed angle): For rapid decrease in intraocular pressure, administer 500 mg/ dose IV.

Seizures (extended release product not recommended):
   Child and adult: 8—30 mg/kg/24 hr ÷ Q6—12 hr PO; **max. dose:** 1 g/24 hr

Urine alkalization:
   Adult: 5 mg/kg/dose PO repeated BID-TID over 24 hr

ACETAZOLAMIDE *continued*

Management of hydrocephalus (see remarks): Start with 20 mg/kg/24 hr ÷ Q8 hr PO/IV; may increase to 100 mg/kg/24 hr up to a **max. dose** of 2 g/24 hr.

Pseudotumor cerebri (PO; see remarks):

Child: Start with 25 mg/kg/24 hr ÷ once daily-QID; increase by 25 mg/kg/24 hr until clinical response or as tolerated up to a **maximum** of 100 mg/kg/24 hr.

Adolescent: Start with 1 g/24 hr ÷ once daily-QID; increase by 250 mg/24 hr until clinical response or as tolerated up to a **maximum** of 4 g/24 hr.

Contraindicated in hepatic failure, severe renal failure (GFR <10 mL/min), and hypersensitivity to sulfonamides.

$T_{1/2}$: 2–6 hr; **do not use** sustained release capsules in seizures; **IM** injection may be painful; bicarbonate replacement therapy may be required during long-term use (see Citrate Mixtures or Sodium Bicarbonate). For use in pseudotumor cerebri, doses of 60 mg/kg/24 hr may be required.

Possible side effects (more likely with long-term therapy) include GI irritation, paresthesias, sedation, hypokalemia, acidosis, reduced urate secretion, aplastic anemia, polyuria, and development of renal calculi.

May increase toxicity of carbamazepine and cyclosporine. Aspirin may increase toxicity of acetazolamide. May decrease the effects of salicylates, lithium, and phenobarbital. False-positive urinary protein may occur with several assays. **Adjust dose in renal failure (see Chapter 31).**

ACETYLCYSTEINE
Various generics, Acetadote; previously available as Mucomyst
Mucolytic, antidote for acetaminophen toxicity

    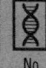

| B | ? | No | Yes | No |

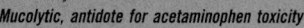

Solution for inhalation or oral use: 100 mg/mL (10%) (4, 10, 30 mL) or 200 mg/mL (20%) (4, 10, 30 mL); may contain EDTA

Injectable (Acetadote and generics): 200 mg/mL (20%) (30 mL); may contain EDTA 0.5 mg/mL
Preservative-free versions of the inhalation and oral solutions and injectable forms exist.

Acetaminophen poisoning (see Chapter 3 for additional information):

PO: 140 mg/kg (**max.** 15 g/dose) × 1, followed by 70 mg/kg/dose (**max.** 7.5 g/dose) Q4 hr for a total of 17 doses. Repeat dose if vomiting occurs with 1 hr of administration.

IV (see remarks): 150 mg/kg (**max.** 15 g/dose) × 1 diluted in D_5W or D_5W $^1/_2$ NS administered over 60 min, followed by 50 mg/kg (**max.** 5 g/dose) diluted in D_5W administered over 4 hr, then 100 mg/kg (**max.** 10 g/dose) diluted in D_5W administered over 16 hr. Recommended weight-based drug dilution volumes:

Weight (kg)	Volume of D_5W or D_5W $^1/_2$ NS for 150 mg/kg Loading Dose Administered Over 60 min	Volume of D_5W for 50 mg/kg Second Dose Administered Over 4 hr	Volume of D_5W for 100 mg/kg Third Dose Administered Over 16 hr
≤20	3 mL/kg	7 mL/kg	14 mL/kg
>20 to ≤40	100 mL	250 mL	500 mL
>40	200 mL	500 mL	1000 mL

Nebulizer:

Infant: 1–2 mL of 20% solution (diluted with equal volume of H_2O, or sterile saline to equal 10%), or 2–4 mL of 10% solution; administer TID-QID

Continued

ACETYLCYSTEINE *continued*

Child: 3—5 mL of 20% solution (diluted with equal volume of H_2O, or sterile saline to equal 10%), or 6—10 mL of 10% solution; administer TID-QID

Adolescent: 5—10 mL of 10% or 20% solution; administer TID-QID

Distal intestinal obstruction syndrome in cystic fibrosis:

Adolescent and adult: 10 mL of 20% solution (diluted in a sweet drink) PO QID with 100 mL of 10% solution PR as an enema once daily-QID

Use with caution in asthma. For nebulized use, give inhaled bronchodilator 10—15 min before use and follow with postural drainage and/or suctioning after acetylcysteine administration. Prior hydration is essential for distal intestinal obstruction syndrome treatment.

May induce bronchospasm, stomatitis, drowsiness, rhinorrhea, nausea, vomiting, and hemoptysis. Serious hypersensitivity reactions have been reported with IV use in children. Be aware of potential fluid overload resulting in hyponatremia with IV volume dilution; reduce diluent volume if needed.

For IV use, elimination $T_{1/2}$ is longer in newborns (11 hr) than in adults (5.6 hr). $T_{1/2}$ is increased by 80% in patients with severe liver damage (Child-Pugh score of 7—13) and biliary cirrhosis (Child-Pugh score of 5—7). A 2-bag IV administration method for acetaminophen poisoning has been associated with less cutaneous and systemic nonallergic anaphylactic reactions with similar efficacy (≥12 yr: 200 mg/kg infused IV over 4 hr followed by 100 mg/kg infused over 16 hr; **max. total dose:** 30 g).

For oral administration, chilling the solution and mixing with carbonated beverages, orange juice, or sweet drinks may enhance palatability.

ACTH

See Corticotropin.

ACYCLOVIR
Zovirax, Avaclyr, and generics
Antiviral

 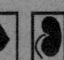 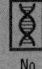

B   2   Yes   No   No

Capsules: 200 mg
Tabs: 400, 800 mg
Oral suspension: 200 mg/5 mL (473 mL); may contain parabens
Ointment: 5% (5, 15, 30 g)
Cream: 5% (5 g); may contain propylene glycol
Ophthalmic ointment (Avaclyr): 3% (3.5 g)
Injection in solution (with sodium): 50 mg/mL (10, 20 mL)
Contains 4.2 mEq Na/1 g drug

IMMUNOCOMPETENT:

Neonatal (HSV and HSV encephalitis; birth—3 mo):

Initial IV therapy (duration of therapy: 14 days for cutaneous/mucous membrane infection or 21 days for CNS/disseminated infection):

<34 wk postmenstrual age: 40 mg/kg/24 hr ÷ Q12 hr IV

≥34 wk postmenstrual age: 60 mg/kg/24 hr ÷ Q8 hr IV

Oral therapy for HSV suppression and neurodevelopment following treatment with IV acyclovir for 14—21 days: 300 mg/m^2/dose Q8 hr PO × 6 mo

HSV encephalitis (duration of therapy: 14—21 days):

Birth—3 mo: Use aforementioned IV dosage.

3 mo—12 yr: 60 mg/kg/24 hr ÷ Q8 hr IV

≥12 yr: 30 mg/kg/24 hr ÷ Q8 hr IV

ACYCLOVIR *continued*

Mucocutaneous HSV (including genital, ≥12 yr):

  Initial infection:

  IV: 15 mg/kg/24 hr or 750 mg/m²/24 hr ÷ Q8 hr × 5—7 days

  PO: 1000—1200 mg/24 hr ÷ 3—5 doses per 24 hr × 7—10 days. For pediatric dosing, use 40—80 mg/kg/24 hr ÷ Q6—8 hr × 5—10 days (**max. pediatric dose:** 1000 mg/24 hr)

  Recurrence (≥12 yr):

  PO: 1000 mg/24 hr ÷ 5 doses per 24 hr × 5 days, or 1600 mg/24 hr ÷ Q12 hr × 5 days, or 2400 mg/24 hr ÷ Q8 hr × 2 days

  Chronic suppressive therapy (≥12 yr):

  PO: 800 mg/24 hr ÷ Q12 hr for up to 1 yr

Zoster:

  IV (all ages): 30 mg/kg/24 hr or 1500 mg/m²/24 hr ÷ Q8 hr × 7—10 days

  PO (≥12 yr): 4000 mg/24 hr ÷ 5×/24 hr × 5—7 days

Varicella:

  IV (≥2 yr): 30 mg/kg/24 hr or 1500 mg/m²/24 hr ÷ Q8 hr × 7—10 days

  PO (≥2 yr): 80 mg/kg/24 hr ÷ QID × 5 days (begin treatment at earliest signs/symptoms); **max. dose:** 3200 mg/24 hr

Max. dose of oral acyclovir in children = 80 mg/kg/24 hr

IMMUNOCOMPROMISED:

HSV:

  IV (all ages): 750—1500 mg/m²/24 hr ÷ Q8 hr × 7—14 days

  PO (≥2 yr): 1000 mg/24 hr ÷ 3—5 times/24 hr × 7—14 days; **max. dose** for child: 80 mg/kg/24 hr

HSV prophylaxis:

  IV (all ages): 750 mg/m²/24 hr ÷ Q8 hr during risk period

  PO (≥2 yr): 600—1000 mg/24 hr ÷ 3—5 times/24 hr during risk period; **max. dose** for child: 80 mg/kg/24 hr

Varicella or zoster:

  IV (all ages): 1500 mg/m²/24 hr ÷ Q8 hr × 7—10 days

  PO (consider using valacyclovir or famciclovir for better absorption):

  Infant and child: 20 mg/kg/dose (**max.** 800 mg) Q6 hr × 7—10 days

  Adolescent and adult: 20 mg/kg/dose (**max.** 800 mg) 5 times daily × 7—10 days

Max. dose of oral acyclovir in children = 80 mg/kg/24 hr

TOPICAL:

Cream (see remarks):

  Herpes labialis (≥12 and adult): Apply to affected areas 5 times a day × 4 days.

Ointment:

  Immunocompromised genital or mucocutaneous HSV: Apply ½-inch ribbon of 5% ointment for 4-inch square surface area 6 times a day × 7 days.

OPHTHALMIC:

Herpes simplex keratitis (≥2 yr and adolescent): Apply 1 cm (½-inch) ribbon onto the lower eyelid of affected eye(s) 5 times a day while awake (∼Q3 hr) until corneal ulcer heals, then reduce dosage to TID for 7 days.

See most recent edition of the AAP Red Book for further details. Use with **caution** in patients with preexisting neurologic or **renal impairment (adjust dose; see Chapter 31)** or dehydration. Adequate hydration and slow (1 hr) IV administration are essential to prevent crystallization in renal tubules. **Do not use** topical product on the eye or for the prevention of recurrent HSV infections. Oral absorption is unpredictable (15%—30%); consider using valacyclovir or famciclovir for better absorption. Use ideal body weight for obese patients when calculating dosages. Resistant strains of HSV and VZV have been reported in immunocompromised patients (e.g., advanced HIV infection).

Continued

ACYCLOVIR *continued*

Inflammation or phlebitis at the injection site and transient elevations of sCr and BUN are the most frequent IV use side effects. Can cause renal impairment and has been associated with headache, vertigo, insomnia, encephalopathy, GI tract irritation, elevated liver function tests, rash, urticaria, arthralgia, fever, and adverse hematologic effects. Probenecid decreases acyclovir renal clearance. Acyclovir may increase the concentration of tenofovir, and meperidine and its metabolite (normeperidine).

Topical cream acyclovir 5% in combination with hydrocortisone 1% (Xerese) is indicated for herpes labialis (≥6 yr and adults) at a dosage of 5 applications per day for 5 days. Use a finger cot or rubber glove when applying topical cream or ointment.

Ophthalmic ointment: Patient should close their eyes for 1–2 min after each application and wipe away any excess ointment. Most common side effects include stinging, punctuate keratitis, and follicular conjunctivitis. Blepharitis and hypersensitivity reactions have been reported. Do not use contact lenses during therapy.

ADAPALENE ± BENZOYL PEROXIDE
Differin and generics
In combination with benzoyl peroxide: Epiduo, Epiduo Forte
Synthetic retinoic acid derivative; topical acne product

C   ?   No   No   No

Topical cream: 0.1% (45 g)
Topical gel: 0.1% [OTC] (15, 45 g), 0.3% (45 g); some preparations may contain parabens and propylene glycol
Topical lotion: 0.1% (59 mL); some preparations may contain parabens and propylene glycol
Topical solution as a swab: 0.1% (1.2 g per swab; 14 swabs per box)
In combination with benzoyl peroxide:
  Topical gel:
    Epiduo and generics: 0.1% adapalene + 2.5% benzoyl peroxide (45 g)
    Epiduo Forte: 0.3% adapalene + 2.5% benzoyl peroxide (45, 60 g)
  Topical gel as a swab: 0.1% adapalene + 2.5% benzoyl peroxide (1.2 g per swab; 14 swabs per box)

Adapalene (≥12 yr and adult; see remarks): Apply a thin film of cream, gel, or lotion to affected areas of cleansed and dried skin QHS. Limited data in children 7 to ≤12 yr
Adapalene and benzoyl peroxide (see remarks): Apply a thin film to affected areas of cleansed and dried skin once daily.
  Epiduo: Indicated for children ≥9 yr and adults with limited data in children 7 to <9 yr
  Epiduo Forte: Indicated for children ≥12 yr and adults

Avoid contact with eyes, mucous membranes, abraded skin, and open wounds; excessive sun exposure; and use of other irritating topical products. A mild, transitory warm or stinging sensation of the skin may occur during the first 4 wk of use. Clean and dry the skin before each use.
ADAPALENE: Onset of therapeutic benefits seen in 8–12 wk. Common side effects include dry skin, erythema, and scaly skin. When compared with tretinoin in clinical trials for acne vulgaris, adapalene was as effective and had a more rapid onset of clinical effects with less skin irritation.
ADAPALENE + BENZOYL PEROXIDE: Contraindicated in patients with a history of benzoyl peroxide hypersensitivity reactions. **Avoid** or minimize exposure to artificial (e.g., tanning beds) or natural light to prevent photosensitivity reactions; sunscreen products and protective apparel use are recommended. Onset of therapeutic benefits seen in 4–8 wk. Side effects reported in placebo-controlled studies include dry skin, erythema, skin irritation, and contact dermatitis. When

ADAPALENE ± BENZOYL PEROXIDE *continued*

compared with isotretinoin in a clinical trial for nodulocystic acne, adapalene + benzoyl peroxide plus doxycycline was not inferior to isotretinoin and was less effective in reducing the number of total lesions (nodules, papules/pustules, and comedones).

ADDERALL

See Dextroamphetamine ± Amphetamine.

ADENOSINE
Generics; previously available as Adenocard
Antiarrhythmic

    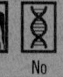

C   ?   No   No   No

Injection: 3 mg/mL (2, 4 mL); preservative free

Supraventricular tachycardia (follow each dose with NS flush; see remarks):
  Neonate: 0.05—0.1 mg/kg by rapid IV push over 1—2 sec; may increase dose by
    0.05—0.1 mg/kg increments every 2 min to a **max. single dose** of 0.3 mg/kg or until
    termination of SVT
  Child: 0.1 mg/kg **(initial max. dose:** 6 mg) by rapid IV/IO push over 1—2 sec; may repeat in 2 min at
    0.2 mg/kg IV/IO, then 0.3 mg/kg IV/IO after 2 min **(all subsequent max. single doses:** 12 mg), or
    until termination of SVT
  Adolescent and adult ≥50 kg: 6 mg rapid IV push over 1—2 sec; if no response after 1—2 min, give 12
    mg rapid IV push. May repeat a second 12 mg dose after 1—2 min if required. **Max. single dose:**
    12 mg

Contraindicated in 2nd and 3rd degree AV block or sick-sinus syndrome unless pacemaker
  placed. **Use with caution** in combination with digoxin (enhanced depressant effects on
  SA and AV nodes). If necessary, doses may be administered IO. $T_{1/2}$: <10 sec.
May precipitate bronchoconstriction, especially in asthmatics. Side effects include transient asystole,
  facial flushing, headache, shortness of breath, dyspnea, nausea, chest pain, and lightheadedness.
Carbamazepine and dipyridamole may increase the effects/toxicity of adenosine. Methylxanthines (e.g.,
  caffeine and theophylline) may decrease the effects of adenosine.

ALBUMIN, HUMAN
Albuked, Albumin-ZLB, Albutein, Kedbumin,
Plasbumin, and many others
*Blood product derivative, plasma volume
expander*

C   ?   No   No   No

Injection: 5% (50 mg/mL) (50, 100, 250, 500 mL); 25% (250 mg/mL) (20, 50, 100 mL); both
  concentrations contain 130—160 mEq Na/L

Hypoalbuminemia:
  Child: 0.5—1 g/kg/dose **(max. dose:** 25 g/dose) IV over 30—120 min; repeat Q1—2 days
    PRN
  Adult: 25 g/dose IV over 30—120 min; repeat Q1—2 days PRN
  Max. dose: 2 g/kg/24 hr
Hypovolemia:
  Child: 0.5—1 g/kg/dose IV rapid infusion; after 15-30 min, may repeat PRN

Continued

ALBUMIN, HUMAN *continued*

Adult: 12.5—25 g/dose IV rapid infusion; after 15—30 min, may repeat PRN

Contraindicated in cases of CHF or severe anemia; rapid infusion may cause fluid overload; hypersensitivity reactions may occur; may cause rapid increase in serum sodium levels. Recommended maximum infusion rates:

Product Concentration	Patients With Normal Plasma Volume	Patients With Hypoproteinemia
5%	2—4 mL/min	5—10 mL/min
25%	1 mL/min	2—3 mL/min

Caution: 25% concentration is considered **contraindicated** in preterm infants due to risk of IVH. Use product-specific recommended in-line filter size. Both 5% and 25% products are isotonic but differ in oncotic effects. Dilutions of the 25% product should be made with D_5W or NS; **avoid sterile water as a diluent.**

ALBUTEROL
ProAir HFA, Proventil HFA, Ventolin HFA (aerosol inhaler); ProAir RespiClick, ProAir Digihaler (breath activated aerosol powder inhaler); AccuNeb (prediluted nebulized solution); and many generics
β₂ adrenergic agonist

    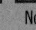

C   1   No   No   No

Tabs: 2, 4 mg
Oral solution: 2 mg/5 mL (473 mL)
Aerosol inhaler (HFA): 90 mCg/actuation
    ProAir HFA: (200 actuations/inhaler) (8.5 g)
    Proventil HFA: (200 actuations/inhaler) (6.7 g)
    Ventolin HFA: (60 actuations/inhaler) (8 g), (200 actuations/inhaler) (18 g)
    Generic: (6.7, 8.5, 18 g)
Breath-activated aerosol powder inhaler:
    ProAir RespiClick and ProAir Digihaler: 90 mCg/actuation (200 actuations/inhaler) (0.65 g); contains milk proteins and small amounts of lactose. ProAir Digihaler contains an electronic event monitor that detects, records, and stores data on inhaler use events, including peak inspiratory flow rate.
Nebulization solution (dilution required): 0.5% (5 mg/mL) (0.5, 20 mL); some preparations may be preservative free (see remarks)
Prediluted nebulized solution: 0.63 mg in 3 mL NS, 1.25 mg in 3 mL NS, and 2.5 mg in 3 mL NS (0.083%); some preparations may be preservative free (see remarks)

Inhalations (nonacute use; see remarks):
    Aerosol (HFA): 2 puffs (90 mCg/puff) Q4—6 hr PRN
    Breath-activated aerosol (see remarks):
      >4 yr: 2 inhalations (90 mCg/inhalation) Q4—6 hr PRN
    Nebulization:
      <1 yr: 0.05—0.15 mg/kg/dose Q4—6 hr
      1—5 yr: 1.25—2.5 mg/dose Q4—6 hr
      5—12 yr: 2.5 mg/dose Q4—6 hr
      >12 yr: 2.5—5 mg/dose Q4—8 hr
For use in acute exacerbations, more aggressive dosing may be used.

ALBUTEROL *continued*

Exercise-induced bronchospasm (administered 15–30 min before exercise):
Aerosol (HFA): 2 puffs (90 mCg/puff)
Breath-activated aerosol (see remarks): 2 inhalations (90 mCg/inhalation)
Oral (highly discouraged—see remarks):
2–6 yr: 0.3 mg/kg/24 hr PO ÷ TID; **max. dose:** 12 mg/24 hr
6–12 yr: 6 mg/24 hr PO ÷ TID; **max. dose:** 24 mg/24 hr
>12 yr and adult: 2–4 mg/dose PO TID-QID; **max. dose:** 32 mg/24 hr

Inhaled doses may be given more frequently than indicated. In such cases, consider cardiac monitoring and monitoring of serum potassium (hypokalemia). Systemic effects are dose related. Verify the concentration of the nebulization solution used. Continuous nebulization treatment with an albuterol product containing the benzalkonium chloride preservative has been reported to have a longer duration of treatment and need for additional respiratory support when compared to a preservative-free albuterol product.

Safety and efficacy for the treatment of symptoms or bronchospasms associated with obstructive airway disease have not been demonstrated for children <4 yr of age (either dose studied was not optimal in this age or drug is not effective in this age group).

Use of oral dosage form is discouraged due to increased side effects and decreased efficacy compared with inhaled formulations.

Possible side effects include tachycardia, palpitations, tremor, insomnia, nervousness, nausea, and headache.

The use of tube spacers or chambers may enhance efficacy of the HFA metered dose inhalers and have been proven to be just as effective and sometimes safer than nebulizers. **Do not** use a spacer device with any of the breath-activated inhaler dosage forms. Breath-activated dosage forms require patients to generate a minimum inspiratory flow rate of ≥30 L/min for proper dose activation. **Do not** wash or place any part of the ProAir RespiClick or ProAir Digihaler inhaler in water.

ALLOPURINOL
Zyloprim, Aloprim, and generics
Uric acid lowering agent, xanthine oxidase inhibitor

C   3   Yes   Yes   Yes

Tabs: 100, 300 mg
Oral suspension: 20 mg/mL
Injection (Aloprim and generics): 500 mg
Contains ∼1.45 mEq Na/500 mg drug

For use in tumor lysis syndrome, see Chapter 22 for additional information. See remarks for genomic considerations.
Child:
Oral: 10 mg/kg/24 hr PO ÷ BID-QID; **max. dose:** 800 mg/24 hr
Injectable: 200 mg/m^2/24 hr IV ÷ Q 6–12 hr; **max. dose:** 600 mg/24 hr
Adult:
Oral: 200–800 mg/24 hr PO ÷ BID-TID
Injectable: 200–400 mg/m^2/24 hr IV ÷ Q 6–12 hr; **max. dose:** 600 mg/24 hr

Discontinue use at the first appearance of skin rash or other signs of an allergic reaction. **Avoid** use in individuals with HLA-B*58:01 allele as they are at significant risk for developing severe cutaneous adverse reactions (e.g., Stevens-Johnson syndrome and TEN).

Side effects include rash, neuritis, hepatotoxicity, renal function impairment, GI disturbance, bone marrow suppression, and drowsiness.

Continued

ALLOPURINOL *continued*

Adjust dose in renal insufficiency (see Chapter 31). Must maintain adequate urine output and alkaline urine.

Drug interactions: Increases serum theophylline level; may increase the incidence of rash with ampicillin and amoxicillin; increased risk of toxicity with azathioprine, didanosine, and mercaptopurine; and increased risk of hypersensitivity reactions with ACE inhibitors and thiazide diuretics. Use with didanosine is **contraindicated** due to increased risk for didanosine toxicity. Rhabdomyolysis has been reported with clarithromycin use.

IV dosage form is very alkaline and must be **diluted to a minimum concentration** of 6 mg/mL and infused over 30 min.

The manufacturer advises not to breastfeed during treatment with allopurinol for 1 week after the last dose as limited data indicate a maternal dose of 300 mg daily can provide near-therapeutic dose and plasma levels in an exclusively breastfed infant.

ALMOTRIPTAN MALATE
Generics; previously available as Axert
Antimigraine agent, selective serotonin agonist

  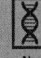

C   3   Yes   Yes   No

Tabs: 6.25, 12.5 mg

Treatment of acute migraines with or without aura:
  Oral (safety of an average of >4 headaches in a 30-day period has not been established; see remarks):
    Child ≥12 and adult: Start with 6.25—12.5 mg PO × 1. If needed in 2 hr, a second dose may be administered. **Max. daily dose:** 2 doses/24 hr and 25 mg/24 hr

Contraindicated in ischemic/vasospastic coronary artery disease, significant underlying cardiovascular disease, cerebrovascular syndromes, peripheral vascular disease, uncontrolled hypertension, or hemiplegic/basilar migraine. **Do not** administer with any ergotamine-containing medication or ergot-type medication, any other 5-HT₁ agonist (e.g., triptans), methylene blue, or with/within 2 wk of discontinuing an MAO inhibitor or linezolid.

FDA-labeled indication for adolescents is acute migraine treatment in patients with a history of migraine lasting ≥4 hr when left untreated. Efficacy for the treatment of migraine-associated symptoms of nausea, photophobia, and phonophobia was not established for adolescents.

Most common side effects include dizziness, somnolence, headache, paresthesia, nausea, and vomiting. Reported serious adverse effects include coronary artery spasm, ischemia (myocardial, gastrointestinal, peripheral vascular), cerebral/subarachnoid hemorrhage, cerebrovascular accident/disease, and vision loss.

Use with **caution** in renal impairment (CrCl ≤30 mL/min) or hepatic impairment; use initial dose of 6.25 mg dose with a **max. daily dose** of 12.5 mg/24 hr.

Almotriptan is a minor substrate for CYP 450 2D6 and 3A4. Use lower initial single dose of 6.25 mg with **maximum daily dose** of 12.5 mg if receiving a potent CYP 450 3A4 inhibitor (e.g., itraconazole, ritonavir). **Do not use** almotriptan in the presence of renal or hepatic impairment and receiving a potent CYP 3A4 inhibitor.

Doses may be administered with or without food.

ALPROSTADIL
Prostin VR Pediatric, and generics, prosta-
glandin E₁, PGE₁
Prostaglandin E₁, vasodilator

    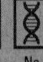

?   ?   No   No   No

ALPROSTADIL *continued*

Injection: 500 mCg/mL (1 mL); contains dehydrated alcohol

Neonate:
  Initial: 0.05—0.1 mCg/kg/min. Advance to 0.2 mCg/kg/min if necessary.
  Maintenance: When increase in PaO₂ is noted, decrease immediately to lowest effective dose. Usual
    dosage range: 0.01—0.4 mCg/kg/min; doses >0.4 mCg/kg/min not likely to produce additional
    benefit.
To prepare infusion: See p. iii.

For palliation only. Continuous vital sign monitoring essential. May cause apnea (10%—12%;
  especially in those weighing <2 kg at birth), fever, seizures, flushing, bradycardia,
  hypotension, diarrhea, gastric outlet obstruction, and reversible cortical proliferation of long bones
  (with prolonged use). May decrease platelet aggregation.

ALTEPLASE
Activase, Cathflo Activase, tPA
Thrombolytic agent, tissue plasminogen activator

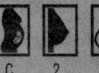   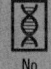

C   2   Yes   Yes   No

Injection:
  Cathflo Activase: 2 mg
  Activase: 50 mg (29 million unit), 100 mg (58 million unit)
All products contain: L-arginine and polysorbate 80

Occluded IV catheter:
  Aspiration method: Use 1 mg/1 mL concentration as follows:
    Central venous line (dosage per lumen, treating one lumen at a time):
      <30 kg: Instill a volume equal to 110% of internal lumen volume of the catheter **NOT exceeding**
        2 mg.
      ≥30 kg: 2 mg each lumen
    Subcutaneous port: Instill a volume equal to 110% of internal lumen and line volume of the port
      NOT exceeding 2 mg.
    Instill into catheter over 1—2 min and leave in place for 2 hr before attempting blood withdrawal.
      After 2 hr, attempts to withdraw blood may be made every 2 hr for 3 attempts. Dose may be
      repeated once in 24 hr using a longer catheter dwell time of 3—4 hr. After 3—4 hr (repeat dose),
      attempts to withdraw blood may be made every 2 hr for 3 attempts. **DO NOT** infuse into patient.
  **Systemic thrombolytic therapy (limited data, use in consultation with a hematologist; see
  remarks):**
    Low-dose initial infusion:
      <90 days old: 0.06 mg/kg/hr; **max. dose:** 2 mg/hr
      ≥90 days old—21 yr: 0.03 mg/kg/hr; **max. dose:** 2 mg/hr
    High-dose initial infusion: 0.1—0.5 mg/kg/hr; **max. dose:** 25 mg/hr
    Dosage regimens ranging from lower dosages (0.01 mg/kg/hr) to higher dosages (0.1—0.6 mg/kg/hr)
      have been reported (*Chest* 2008;133:887—968S). The length of continuous infusion is variable as
      patients may respond to longer or shorter courses of therapy.

Current use in the pediatric population is limited. May cause bleeding, rash, angioedema, and
  increased prothrombin time. Rare fatal hypersensitivity reaction has been reported.
THROMBOLYTIC USE: History of stroke, transient ischemic attacks, other neurologic disease,
  and hypertension are **contraindications for adults** but considered **relative contraindications for
  children**. Monitor fibrinogen, thrombin clotting time, PT, and aPTT when used as a thrombolytic. For
  systemic thrombosis therapy, efficacy has been reported at 40%—97% with the risk for bleeding at

Continued

ALTEPLASE *continued*

3%–27%. Poor efficacy in VTE in children has been recently reported. **Use with caution** in severe hepatic or renal dysfunction (systemic use only).

Newborns have reduced plasminogen levels (~50% of adult values), which decrease the thrombolytic effects of alteplase. Plasminogen supplementation may be necessary.

ALUMINUM HYDROXIDE
Various generics; previously available as Amphojel
Antacid, phosphate binder

 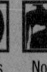 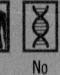

? ? Yes No No

Oral suspension [OTC]: 320 mg/5 mL (473 mL)
Each 5 mL suspension contains <0.13 mEq Na.

Antacid (see remarks):
  Child: 320–960 mg PO 1–3 hr PC and QHS PRN
  Adult: 640 mg PO 1–3 hr PC and QHS PRN; **max. dose:** 3840 mg/24 hr
Hyperphosphatemia (administer all doses with meals and titrate to normal serum phosphorus):
  Child: 50–150 mg/kg/24 hr ÷ Q4–6 hr PO
  Adult: 300–600 mg TID PO with meals
  Max. dose (all ages): 3000 mg/24 hr

AVOID long-term use. Chronic antacid use is not recommended for children with GERD.
  Use with caution in patients with renal failure and upper GI hemorrhage.
Interferes with the absorption of several orally administered medications, including digoxin, ethambutol, indomethacin, isoniazid, naproxen, mycophenolate, tetracyclines, fluoroquinolones (e.g., ciprofloxacin), and iron. In general, **do not** take oral medications within 1–2 hr of taking aluminum dose unless specified.

May cause constipation, decreased bowel motility, encephalopathy, and phosphorus depletion.

ALUMINUM HYDROXIDE WITH MAGNESIUM HYDROXIDE
Mylanta Maximum Strength, Almacone Antacid
Antigas, Almacone Double Strength, and many
other generics (see remarks); previously available as Maalox
Antacid

   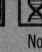

? ? Yes No No

Chewable tabs [OTC]: (Al [OH]$_3$: Mg [OH]$_2$)
  Almacone and generics: 200 mg AlOH, 200 mg MgOH, and 25 mg simethicone
Oral suspension [OTC] (see remarks):
  Almacone Antacid Antigas, and generics: each 5 mL contains 200 mg AlOH, 200 mg MgOH, and 20 mg simethicone (150, 360, 720 mL); some preparations may contain 0.2% alcohol, benzyl alcohol, or propylene glycol
  Mylanta Maximum Strength, Almacone Double Strength, and generics: each 5 mL contains 400 mg AlOH, 400 mg MgOH, and 40 mg simethicone (360, 480 mL); some preparations may contain benzyl alcohol
  Many other combinations exist.
  Contains 0.03–0.06 mEq Na/5 mL

Antacid (mL volume dosages are based on the 200 mg AlOH, 200 mg MgOH, and 20 mg simethicone per 5 mL oral suspension concentration):

ALUMINUM HYDROXIDE WITH MAGNESIUM HYDROXIDE *continued*

Child ≤12 yr: 0.5—1 mL/kg/dose (**max. dose:** 20 mL/dose) PO 1—3 hr PC and HS PRN
>12 yr and adult: 10—20 mL PO 1—3 hr PC and HS PRN; **max. dose:** 80 mL/24 hr

Chronic antacid use is not recommended for children with GERD. May have laxative effect.
May cause hypokalemia. **Use with caution** in patients with renal insufficiency (magnesium),
gastric outlet obstruction. **Do not use** for hyperphosphatemia.

Interferes with the absorption of the benzodiazepines, chloroquine, digoxin, naproxen, mycophenolate,
phenytoin, quinolones (e.g., ciprofloxacin), tetracyclines, and iron. In general, do not take oral
medications within 1—2 hr of taking antacid dose unless specified.

DO NOT use Maalox Total Relief (bismuth subsalicylate), Mylanta New Tonight Soothing Liquid
(calcium carbonate + magnesium hydroxide + simethicone), Maalox Regular Strength or Children's
Chewable Tablets and Children's Mylanta Chewable Tablets (calcium carbonate), Maalox Maximum
Strength Chewable (calcium carbonate and simethicone), and Mylanta Gas (simethicone), as these
products do not contain aluminum hydroxide and magnesium hydroxide.

AMANTADINE HYDROCHLORIDE
Immediate release dosage forms: generics;
previously available as Symmetrel
Extended release dosage forms: Gocovri, Osmo-
lex ER
Antiviral agent

C   3   Yes   Yes   No

Capsule: 100 mg
Tabs: 100 mg
Extended release capsule (Gocovri; see remarks): 68.5, 137 mg
Extended release tabs (Osmolex ER; see remarks): 129, 193 mg
Oral solution: 50 mg/5 mL (480 mL); may contain parabens

Influenza A prophylaxis and treatment (for treatment, it is best to initiate therapy
immediately after the onset of symptoms; within 2 days; use immediate release dosage
forms and see remarks):
1—9 yr: 5 mg/kg/24 hr PO ÷ BID; **max. dose:** 150 mg/24 hr
≥10 yr:
  <40 kg: 5 mg/kg/24 hr PO ÷ BID; **max. dose:** 200 mg/24 hr
  ≥40 kg: 200 mg/24 hr PO ÷ BID
Duration of therapy:
  Prophylaxis:
    Single exposure: At least 10 days
    Repeated/uncontrolled exposure: Up to 90 days
    Use with influenza A vaccine when possible.
  Symptomatic treatment:
    Continue for 24—48 hr after disappearance of symptoms.
Traumatic brain injury (limited data; use immediate release dosage forms):
  ≥6 yr to <16 yr: 4—6 mg/kg/24 hr PO ÷ BID with the suggested **maximum** dosage:
    <10 yr or <40 kg: 150 mg/24 hr
    ≥10 yr or ≥40 kg: 200 mg/24 hr
  ≥16 yr: 100 mg PO BID x 14 days, then increase to 150 mg PO BID. If needed, may increase dose to
    200 mg PO BID only after 3 weeks from the initiation of therapy.

The CDC has reported resistance to influenza A and does not recommend its use for treatment
and prophylaxis. Check with local microbiology laboratories and the CDC for seasonal

Continued

AMANTADINE HYDROCHLORIDE *continued*

susceptibility/resistance. Individuals immunized with live attenuated influenza vaccine should not receive amantadine prophylaxis for 14 days after the vaccine.

Preliminary studies in traumatic brain injury suggest improved cognition in children that were more recently injured (<2 years after injury).

Do not use in the first trimester of pregnancy. **Use with caution** in patients with liver disease, seizures, renal disease, congestive heart failure, peripheral edema, orthostatic hypotension, history of recurrent eczematoid rash, and in those receiving CNS stimulants. **Adjust dose in patients with renal insufficiency (see Chapter 31).**

Extended release capsule and tablet dosage forms are indicated for the treatment of dyskinesia in patients with Parkinson disease receiving levodopa-based therapy.

May cause dizziness, anxiety, depression, mental status change, rash (livedo reticularis), nausea, orthostatic hypotension, edema, CHF, and urinary retention. Impulse control disorder has been reported. Neuroleptic malignant syndrome has been reported with abrupt dose reduction or discontinuation (especially if patient is receiving neuroleptics).

AMIKACIN SULFATE
Various generics; previously available as Amikin
Antibiotic, aminoglycoside

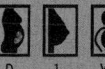   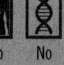

| D | 1 | Yes | No | No |

Injection: 250 mg/mL (2, 4 mL); may contain sodium bisulfite

Initial empirical dosage; patient-specific dosage defined by therapeutic drug monitoring (see remarks).
Neonate: See the following table.

Postconceptional Age (wk)	Postnatal Age (days)	Dose (mg/kg/dose)	Interval (hr)
≤29[a]	0—7	18	48
	8—28	15	36
	>28	15	24
30—34	0—7	18	36
	>7	15	24
≥35	ALL	15	24[b]

[a]Or significant asphyxia, PDA, indomethacin use, poor cardiac output, reduced renal function.
[b]Use Q36 hr interval for HIE patients receiving whole-body therapeutic cooling.

Infant and child: 15—22.5 mg/kg/24 hr ÷ Q8 hr IV/IM; infants and patients requiring higher doses (e.g., cystic fibrosis) may receive initial doses of 30 mg/kg/24 hr ÷ Q8 hr IV/IM
Cystic fibrosis (if available, use patient's previous therapeutic mg/kg dosage):
    Conventional Q8 hr dosing: 30 mg/kg/24 hr ÷ Q8 hr IV
    High-dose extended interval (once daily) dosing (limited data): 30—35 mg/kg/24 hr Q24 hr IV
Nontuberculous mycobacterium (part of a multiple drug regimen):
    Infant and child: 15—30 mg/kg/dose Q24 hr IV; **max. dose:** 1500 mg/24 hr
    Adolescent: 10—15 mg/kg/dose Q24 hr IV; **max. dose:** 1500 mg/24 hr
    Adult: 15 mg/kg/24 hr ÷ Q8—12 hr IV/IM
    Initial max. dose: 1.5 g/24 hr, then monitor levels

Use with **caution** in preexisting renal, vestibular, or auditory impairment; concomitant anesthesia or neuromuscular blockers, neurotoxic; concomitant neurotoxic, ototoxic, or nephrotoxic drugs; sulfite sensitivity; and dehydration. **Adjust dose in renal failure**

AMIKACIN SULFATE *continued*

(see Chapter 31). Longer dosing intervals may be necessary for neonates receiving indomethacin for PDAs and for all patients with poor cardiac output. Rapidly eliminated in patients with cystic fibrosis or burns, and in febrile neutropenic patients. CNS penetration is poor beyond early infancy.

Therapeutic Drug Monitoring Goals:

Dosing Method/ Indication	Peak Level	Trough Level	Recommended Serum Sampling Time
Conventional dosing	20—30 mg/L; 25—30 mg/L for CNS, pulmonary, bone, life-threatening, *Pseudomonas* infections and febrile neutropenia	5—10 mg/L	Trough within 30 min before the third consecutive dose and peak 30—60 min after the administration of the third consecutive dose (at steady state)
High-dose extended interval (Q24 hr) for cystic fibrosis	80—120 mg/L	<10 mg/L	Trough within 30 min before the 2nd dose and peak 30—60 min after administration of 2nd dose
Extended interval (Q24 hr) for nontuberculous mycobacterium	20—40 mg/L	<10 mg/L	Trough within 30 min before the 2nd dose and peak 30—60 min after administration of 2nd dose

For initial dosing in obese patients, use an adjusted body weight (ABW). ABW = ideal body weight + 0.4 (total body weight − ideal body weight).

May cause ototoxicity, nephrotoxicity, neuromuscular blockade, and rash. Loop diuretics may potentiate the ototoxicity of all aminoglycoside antibiotics.

A liposomal inhalation product, Arikayce, is currently approved in adults as part of a multi-drug treatment regimen for *Mycobacterium avium complex* (MAC) lung disease.

AMINOCAPROIC ACID
Amicar and generics
Hemostatic agent

| C | ? | Yes | No | No |

Tabs: 500, 1000 mg
Oral liquid/syrup: 250 mg/mL (240, 480 mL); may contain 0.2% methylparaben and 0.05% propylparaben
Injection: 250 mg/mL (20 mL); may contain 0.9% benzyl alcohol

Child (IV/PO):
    Loading dose: 100—200 mg/kg
    Maintenance: 50—100 mg/kg/dose Q4—6 hr; **max. dose:** 24—30 g/24 hr
Adult (IV/PO): 4—5 g during the first hour, followed by 1 g/hr × 8 hr or until bleeding is controlled.
    Max. dose: 30 g/24 hr

Continued

AMINOCAPROIC ACID *continued*

Contraindications: DIC, hematuria. **Use with caution** in patients with cardiac or renal disease. Should not be given with factor IX complex concentrates or antiinhibitor coagulant concentrates because of risk for thrombosis. Dose should be reduced by 75% in oliguria or end stage renal disease. Hypercoagulation may be produced when given in conjunction with oral contraceptives.

May cause nausea, diarrhea, malaise, weakness, headache, decreased platelet function, hypotension, and false increase in urine amino acids. Elevation of serum potassium may occur, especially in patients with renal impairment. Prolonged use may increase risk for skeletal muscle weakness and rhabdomyolysis.

AMINOPHYLLINE
Various generics
Bronchodilator, methylxanthine

    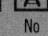

C   1   No   Yes   No

Injection: 25 mg/mL (79% theophylline) (10, 20 mL)
Note: Pharmacy may dilute IV dosage forms to enhance accuracy of neonatal dosing.

Neonatal apnea:
   Loading dose: 5—6 mg/kg IV
   Maintenance dose: 1—2 mg/kg/dose Q6—8 hr, IV
Asthma exacerbation and reactive airway disease:
   IV loading: 6 mg/kg IV over 20 min (each 1.2 mg/kg dose raises the serum theophylline concentration 2 mg/L)
   IV maintenance: Continuous IV drip:
     Neonate: 0.2 mg/kg/hr
     6 wk—6 mo: 0.5 mg/kg/hr
     6 mo—1 yr: 0.6—0.7 mg/kg/hr
     1—9 yr: 1—1.2 mg/kg/hr
     9—12 yr and young adult smoker: 0.9 mg/kg/hr
     >12 yr healthy nonsmoker: 0.7 mg/kg/hr
     The above total daily doses may also be administered IV ÷ Q4—6 hr.

Consider milligrams of theophylline available when dosing aminophylline. For oral route of administration, use theophylline.

Monitoring serum levels is essential, especially in infants and young children. Intermittent dosing for infants and children 1—5 yr may require Q4 hr dosing regimen due to enhanced metabolism/clearance. Side effects: restlessness, GI upset, headache, tachycardia, seizures (may occur in absence of other side effects with toxic levels)

Therapeutic level (as theophylline): for asthma, 10—20 mg/L; for neonatal apnea, 6—13 mg/L

Recommended guidelines for obtaining levels:
   IV bolus: 30 min after infusion
   IV continuous: 12—24 hr after initiation of infusion
   PO liquid, immediate release tab (theophylline product):
     Peak: 1 hr post dose
     Trough: just before dose
   PO sustained release (theophylline product):
     Peak: 4 hr post dose
     Trough: just before dose

Ideally, obtain levels after steady state has been achieved (after at least 1 day of therapy). Liver impairment, cardiac failure, and sustained high fever may increase theophylline levels. See Theophylline for drug interactions.

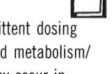

AMINOPHYLLINE *continued*

Use in breastfeeding may cause irritability to infant. It is recommended to avoid breastfeeding for 2 hr after IV or 4 hr after immediate release oral intermittent dose.

AMIODARONE HCL
Pacerone, Nexterone, and generics
Antiarrhythmic, Class III

    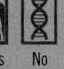

| D | 3 | Yes | Yes | No |

Tabs (Pacerone and generics): 100, 200, 400 mg
Oral suspension: 5 mg/mL
Injection: 50 mg/mL (3, 9, 18 mL) (contains 20.2 mg/mL benzyl alcohol and 100 mg/mL polysorbate 80 or Tween 80)
Premixed injection (Nexterone): 1.5 mg/mL (100 mL) (iso-osmotic solution, each 1 mL contains 15 mg sulfbutylether β-cyclodextrin [SBECD; see remarks], 0.362 mg citric acid, 0.183 mg sodium citrate, and 42.1 mg dextrose), 1.8 mg/mL (200 mL) (iso-osmotic solution, each 1 mL contains 18 mg SBECD, 0.362 mg citric acid, 0.183 mg sodium citrate, and 41.4 mg dextrose)
Contains 37.3% iodine by weight

See algorithms in front of book for arrest dosing.
Child PO for tachyarrhythmia:
   <1 yr: 600–800 mg/1.73 m²/24 hr ÷ Q12–24 hr × 4–14 days and/or until adequate control achieved, then reduce to 200–400 mg/1.73 m²/24 hr
   ≥1 yr: 10–15 mg/kg/24 hr ÷ Q12–24 hr × 4–14 days and/or until adequate control achieved, then reduce to 5 mg/kg/24 hr ÷ Q12–24 hr if effective
Child IV for tachyarrhythmia (limited data):
   5 mg/kg (**max. dose:** 300 mg) over 30–60 min followed by a continuous infusion starting at 5 micrograms (mCg)/kg/min; infusion may be increased up to a **max. dose** of 15 mCg/kg/min or 20 mg/kg/24 hr or 2200 mg/24 hr
Adult PO for ventricular arrhythmias:
   Loading dose: 800–1600 mg/24 hr ÷ Q8–12 hr for 1–3 wk
   Maintenance: 600–800 mg/24 hr ÷ Q12–24 hr × 1 mo, then 200 mg Q12–24 hr
   Use lowest effective dose to minimize adverse reactions.
Adult IV for ventricular arrhythmias:
   Loading dose: 150 mg over 10 min (15 mg/min) followed by 360 mg over 6 hr (1 mg/min); followed by a maintenance dose of 0.5 mg/min. Supplemental boluses of 150 mg over 10 min may be given for breakthrough VF or hemodynamically unstable VT, and the maintenance infusion may be increased to suppress the arrhythmia. **Max. dose:** 2.1 g/24 hr

---

Used in the resuscitation algorithm for ventricular fibrillation/pulseless ventricular tachycardia (**see front of book for arrest dosing and back cover for PALS algorithm**). Overall use of this drug may be limited due to its potentially life-threatening side effects and the difficulties associated with managing its use.

Contraindicated in severe sinus node dysfunction, marked sinus bradycardia, second- and third-degree AV block. **Use with caution** in hepatic impairment.

Long elimination half-life (IV single dose: 9–36 days, chronic oral dosing: 40–55 days). Major metabolite N-desethylamiodarone is active with a long half-life (IV single dose: 9–30 days; chronic oral dosing: 61 days). Use of premixed injection (Nexterone) is not recommended in renal insufficiency due to accumulation of cyclodextrin excipient.

Increases cyclosporine, digoxin, phenytoin, tacrolimus, warfarin, calcium channel blockers, theophylline, and quinidine levels. Amiodarone is a CYP P450 3A3/4 substrate and inhibits CYP 3A3/4, 2C9, and 2D6. Risk of rhabdomyolysis is increased when used with simvastatin at doses greater than 20 mg/24 hr and lovastatin at doses greater than 40 mg/24 hr. Serious symptomatic bradycardia has been reported when used with sofosbuvir.

Continued

AMIODARONE HCL *continued*

Proposed therapeutic level with chronic oral use: 1—2.5 mg/L

Asymptomatic corneal microdeposits should appear in all patients. Alters liver enzymes, thyroid function. Pulmonary fibrosis reported in adults. May cause worsening of preexisting arrhythmias with bradycardia and AV block. May also cause hypotension, anorexia, nausea, vomiting, dizziness, paresthesias, ataxia, tremor, SIADH, and hypothyroidism or hyperthyroidism. Drug rash with eosinophilia and systemic symptoms (DRESS), acute respiratory distress syndrome, and anaphylactic reactions have been reported. IV administration at much higher concentrations and rates of infusion has been reported to increase the risk for hepatic injury.

Correct hypokalemia, hypocalcemia, or hypomagnesemia whenever possible before use as these conditions may exaggerate QTc prolongation.

Intravenous continuous infusion concentration for peripheral administration **should not exceed** 2 mg/mL (minimizes the risk for phlebitis) and **must be** diluted with D_5W. The intravenous dosage form can leach out plasticizers such as DEHP. It is recommended to reduce the potential exposure to plasticizers in pregnant women and children at the toddler stages of development and younger by using alternative methods of IV drug administration.

Oral administration should be consistent with regard to meals because food increases the rate and extent of oral absorption.

AMITRIPTYLINE
Generics; previously available as Elavil
Antidepressant, tricyclic (TCA)

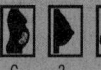 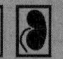 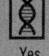

C   2   No   Yes   Yes

Tabs: 10, 25, 50, 75, 100, 150 mg
Oral suspension: 10 mg/mL, 20 mg/mL
Oral syrup: 1 mg/mL

See remarks for genomic considerations.

Antidepressant:

Child: Start with 1 mg/kg/24 hr ÷ TID PO for 3 days; then increase to 1.5 mg/kg/24 ÷ TID. Dose may be gradually increased to a **max. dose** of 5 mg/kg/24 hr if needed. Monitor ECG, BP, and heart rate (HR) for doses >3 mg/kg/24 hr.

Adolescent: 10 mg TID PO and 20 mg QHS; dose may be gradually increased up to a **max. dose** of 200 mg/24 hr if needed.

Adult: 40—100 mg/24 hr ÷ QHS-BID PO; dose may be gradually increased up to 300 mg/24 hr if needed; gradually decrease dose to lowest effective dose when symptoms are controlled.

Augment analgesia for chronic pain:

Child: Initial: 0.1 mg/kg/dose QHS PO; increase as needed and tolerated over 2—3 wk to 0.5—2 mg/kg/dose QHS.

Migraine prophylaxis (limited data):

Child: Initial 0.1—0.25 mg/kg/dose QHS PO; increase as needed and tolerated every 2 wk by 0.1—0.25 mg/kg/dose up to a **max. dose** of 2 mg/kg/24 hr or 75 mg/24 hr. For doses >1 mg/kg/24 hr, divide daily dose BID and monitor ECG.

Adult: Initial 10—25 mg/dose QHS PO; reported range of 10—400 mg/24 hr

---

Contraindicated in narrow-angle glaucoma, seizures, severe cardiac disorders, and patients who received MAO inhibitors within 14 days. See Chapter 3 for management of TCA toxic ingestion.

$T_{1/2}$ = 9—25 hr in adults. **Maximum** antidepressant effects may not occur for 2 wk or more after initiation of therapy. **Do not abruptly discontinue therapy in patients receiving high doses for prolonged periods.**

Therapeutic levels (sum of amitriptyline and nortriptyline): 100—250 ng/mL. Recommended serum sampling time: obtain a single level 8 hr or more after an oral dose (following 4—5 days of

AMITRIPTYLINE *continued*

continuous dosing). Amitriptyline is a substrate for CYP 450 1A2, 2C9, 2C19, 2D6, and 3A3/4 and inhibitor for CYP 450 1A2, 2C19, 2C9, 2D6, and 2E1. Rifampin can decrease amitriptyline levels. Amitriptyline may increase side effects of tramadol.

Pharmacogenomic dosing considerations for CYP 2D6 and 2C19 phenotype (*Clinical Pharmacology and Therapeutics.* 2016;102[1]:37—44):

Phenotype	CYP 2D6 Ultra-Rapid Metabolizer	CYP 2D6 Normal Metabolizer	CYP 2D6 Intermediate Metabolizer	CYP 2D6 Poor Metabolizer
CYP 2C19 Ultra-rapid or Rapid Metabolizer	Avoid use, use alternative therapy	Consider alternative therapy not metabolized by CYP 2C19	Consider alternative therapy not metabolized by CYP 2C19	Avoid use; use alternative therapy
CYP 2C19 Normal Metabolizer	Avoid use but if use necessary, titrate to higher target dose	Use recommended initial dose	Consider a 25% initial dose reduction	Avoid use but if use necessary, consider 50% initial dose reduction
CYP 2C19 Intermediate Metabolizer	Avoid use; use alternative therapy	Use recommended initial dose	Consider a 25% initial dose reduction	Avoid use but if use necessary, consider 50% initial dose reduction
CYP 2C19 Poor Metabolizer	Avoid use; use alternative therapy	Avoid use but if use necessary, consider 50% initial dose reduction	Avoid use; use alternative therapy	Avoid use; use alternative therapy

Side effects include sedation, urinary retention, constipation, dry mouth, dizziness, drowsiness, liver enzyme elevation, and arrhythmia. May discolor urine (blue/green). QHS dosing during first weeks of therapy will reduce sedation. Monitor ECG, BP, CBC at start of therapy and with dose changes. Decrease dose if PR interval reaches 0.22 sec, QRS reaches 130% of baseline, HR rises greater than 140/min, or if BP is >140/90. Tricyclics may cause mania. **For antidepressant use, monitor for clinical worsening of depression and suicidal ideation/behavior following the initiation of therapy or after dose changes.**

AMLODIPINE
Norvasc, Norliqva, Katerzia, and generics
Calcium channel blocker, antihypertensive

    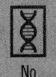

C   2   No   Yes   No

Continued

AMLODIPINE *continued*

Tabs: 2.5, 5, 10 mg
Oral solution (Norliqva): 1 mg/mL (150 mL); contains 4% v/v alcohol
Oral suspension: 1 mg/mL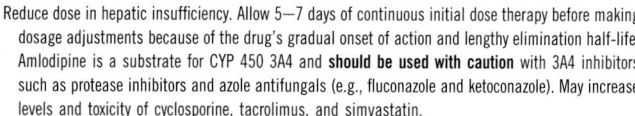
   Katerzia: 1 mg/mL (150 mL); contains polysorbate 80 and sodium benzoate

Hypertension:
   Child:
      <6 yr: Start with 0.1 mg/kg/dose (**max. dose:** 5 mg) PO once daily—BID; dosage may be gradually increased to a **max. dose** of 0.6 mg/kg/24 hr up to 5 mg/24 hr.
      ≥6–17 yr: Start with 2.5 mg PO once daily; dosage may be gradually increased to a **max. dose** of 10 mg/24 hr.
   Adult: 5–10 mg/dose once daily PO; use 2.5 mg/dose once daily PO in patients with hepatic insufficiency. **Max. dose:** 10 mg/24 hr

Use with caution in combination with other antihypertensive agents. Younger children (<6 yr) may require higher mg/kg doses than older children and adults. A BID dosing regimen may provide better efficacy in children.

Reduce dose in hepatic insufficiency. Allow 5–7 days of continuous initial dose therapy before making dosage adjustments because of the drug's gradual onset of action and lengthy elimination half-life. Amlodipine is a substrate of the CYP 450 3A4 and **should be used with caution** with 3A4 inhibitors such as protease inhibitors and azole antifungals (e.g., fluconazole and ketoconazole). May increase levels and toxicity of cyclosporine, tacrolimus, and simvastatin.

Dose-related side effects include edema, dizziness, flushing, fatigue, and palpitations. Other side effects include headache, nausea, abdominal pain, and somnolence.

Limited data report amlodipine present in breast milk at low levels, undetectable in infant plasma with no adverse effects to breastfed infants.

AMMONUL

See Sodium Phenylacetate + Sodium Benzoate.

AMOXICILLIN
Various generics; previously available as Amoxil
and Trimox
Antibiotic, aminopenicillin

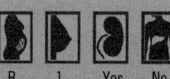

B   1   Yes   No   No

Oral suspension: 125, 250 mg/5 mL (80, 100, 150 mL); and 200, 400 mg/5 mL (50, 75, 100 mL)
Caps: 250, 500 mg
Tablets: 500, 875 mg
Chewable tabs: 125, 250 mg; may contain phenylalanine

Neonate — ≤3 mo: 20–30 mg/kg/24 hr ÷ Q12 hr PO
Child:
   Standard dose: 25–50 mg/kg/24 hr ÷ Q8–12 hr PO
   High dose (resistant *Streptococcus pneumoniae*; see remarks): 80–90 mg/kg/24 hr ÷ Q8–12 hr PO
   Max. dose: 2–3 g/24 hr; some experts recommend a **maximum** dosage up to 4 g/24 hr
Adult:
   Mild/moderate infections: 250 mg/dose Q8 hr PO OR 500 mg/dose Q12 hr PO
   Severe infections: 500 mg/dose Q8 hr PO OR 875 mg/dose Q12 hr PO
   Max. dose: 2–3 g/24 hr

AMOXICILLIN *continued*

Tonsillitis/pharyngitis (*S. pyogenes*): 50 mg/kg/24 hr ÷ Q12 hr PO × 10 days; **max. dose:** 1 g/24 hr
SBE prophylaxis: Administer dose 30—60 min before procedure.
   Child: 50 mg/kg PO × 1; **max.** 2 g/dose
   Adult: 2 g PO × 1
Early Lyme disease:
   Child: 50 mg/kg/24 hr ÷ Q8 hr PO × 14—21 days; **max. dose:** 1.5 g/24 hr
   Adult: 500 mg/dose Q8 hr PO × 14—21 days

Renal elimination. **Adjust dose in renal failure (see Chapter 31).** Serum levels about twice those achieved with equal dose of ampicillin. Fewer GI effects, but otherwise similar to ampicillin. Side effects: rash and diarrhea. Rash may develop with concurrent EBV infection. May increase warfarin's effect by increasing INR.

High-dose regimen is recommended in respiratory infections (e.g., CAP), acute otitis media, and sinusitis, owing to increasing incidence of penicillin-resistant pneumococci. **Chewable tablets may contain phenylalanine and should not be used by patients with phenylketonuria.**

AMOXICILLIN-CLAVULANIC ACID
Augmentin, Augmentin ES-600, and generics
Antibiotic, aminopenicillin with β-lactamase inhibitor

 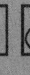   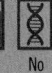

B   1   Yes   No   No

Tabs:
   For TID dosing: 250, 500 mg (with 125 mg clavulanate)
   For BID dosing: 875 mg amoxicillin (with 125 mg clavulanate)
Extended release tabs (previously available as Augmentin XR): 1 g amoxicillin (with 62.5 mg clavulanate)
Chewable tabs:
   For BID dosing (7:1 amoxicillin:clavulanate): 200, 400 mg amoxicillin (28.5 and 57 mg clavulanate, respectively); contains saccharin and aspartame
Oral suspension:
   For TID dosing (4:1 amoxicillin:clavulanate): 125, 250 mg amoxicillin/5 mL (31.25 and 62.5 mg clavulanate/5 mL, respectively) (75, 100, 150 mL); contains saccharin
   For BID dosing:
      7:1 amoxicillin:clavulanate: 200, 400 mg amoxicillin/5 mL (28.5 and 57 mg clavulanate/5 mL, respectively) (50, 75, 100 mL)
      14:1 amoxicillin:clavulanate (Augmentin ES-600 and generics): 600 mg amoxicillin/5 mL; contains 42.9 mg clavulanate/5 mL) (75, 125, 200 mL); contains saccharin and/or aspartame
   Contains 0.63 mEq K$^+$ per 125 mg clavulanate (Augmentin ES-600 contains 0.23 mEq K$^+$ per 42.9 mg clavulanate)

Dosage based on amoxicillin component (see remarks for resistant *S. pneumoniae*).
Infant 1—<3 mo: 30 mg/kg/24 hr ÷ Q12 hr PO (recommended dosage form is 125 mg/5 mL suspension)
Child ≥3 mo:
   Non—high-dose amoxicillin regimens:
      <40 kg:
         TID dosing (see remarks): 20—40 mg/kg/24 hr ÷ Q8 hr PO
         BID dosing (see remarks): 25—45 mg/kg/24 hr ÷ Q12 hr PO
      ≥40 kg: Use adult dosage.
   High-dose amoxicillin regimens:

Continued

AMOXICILLIN-CLAVULANIC ACID *continued*

>≥3 mo and <40 kg (use 14:1 amoxicillin:clavulanate dosage form, Augmentin ES-600, or generic
oral suspension): 90 mg/kg/24 hr ÷ Q8—12 hr PO; Q8 hr recommended for CAP, orbital
cellulitis, and severe infections
>>≥**40 kg:** Use adult dosage.

Adult: 250—500 mg/dose Q8 hr PO or 875 mg/dose Q12 hr PO for more severe and respiratory
infections

Extended release tablet:
>≥**16 yr and adult:** 2 g Q12 hr PO × 10 days for acute bacterial sinusitis, 7—10 days for community-
acquired pneumonia, or 5—10 days for acute otitis media

See Amoxicillin for additional comments. **Adjust dose in renal failure (see Chapter 31).**
Contraindicated in patients with a history of cholestatic jaundice/hepatic dysfunction
associated with amoxicillin-clavulanic acid. Extended release tablet dosage form is **contraindicated**
in patients with CrCl <30 mL/min.

Clavulanic acid extends the activity of amoxicillin to include β-lactamase—producing strains of
Haemophilus influenzae, Moraxella catarrhalis, Neisseria gonorrhoeae, and some *Staphylococcus
aureus* and may increase the risk for diarrhea.

The BID dosing schedule is associated with less diarrhea. For BID dosing, the 875 mg, 1 g tablets, the
200 mg, 400 mg chewable tablets or the 200 mg/5 mL, 400 mg/5 mL, 600 mg/5 mL suspensions
should be used. These BID dosage forms contain phenylalanine and **should not be used** by patients
with phenylketonuria. For TID dosing, the 250 mg, 500 mg tablets, the 125 mg, 250 mg chewable
tablets, or the 125 mg/5 mL, 250 mg/5 mL suspensions should be used.

Higher doses of 80—90 mg/kg/24 hr (amoxicillin component) have been recommended for resistant
strains of *S. pneumoniae* in acute otitis media and pneumonia (use BID formulations containing 7:1
or 14:1 ratio of amoxicillin to clavulanic acid or Augmentin ES-600, respectively).

The 250 or 500 mg tablets **cannot** be substituted for Augmentin XR tablets.

AMPHETAMINE
Evekeo, Evekeo ODT, Adzenys XR-ODT, Dyanavel
XR
CNS stimulant

   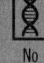

C   3   No   No   No

Tabs, immediate release:
>**Evekeo and generics:** 5, 10 mg; both tablets are scored

Immediate release dispersible tabs:
>**Evekeo ODT:** 5, 10, 15, 20 mg

Extended release dispersible tabs:
>**Adzenys XR-ODT:** 3.1, 6.3, 9.4, 12.5, 15.7, 18.8 mg

Extended release oral suspension:
>**Dyanavel XR:** 2.5 mg/mL (464 mL); contains parabens and polysorbate 80

DO NOT substitute extended release formulations for other amphetamine products on a milligram per
milligram basis due to differences in potency and pharmacokinetic profiles. If converting from other
amphetamine products, discontinue that treatment first and titrate new dosage form as indicated in
the drug dosage section.

Attention-deficit/hyperactivity disorder:
Immediate release tabs (Evekeo and generics) and dispersible tabs (Evekeo ODT) (PO):
>**3—5 yr:** 2.5 mg/24 hr QAM; increase by 2.5 mg/24 hr at weekly intervals until desired response.
Incremental dosages may be administered BID-TID with the first dose at awakening and
subsequent doses spaced at 4—6 hr intervals. Doses rarely exceed 40 mg/24 hr.

AMPHETAMINE *continued*

≥**6 yr and adolescent:** 5 mg once daily or BID; increase by 5 mg/24 hr at weekly intervals until desired response. Incremental dosages may be administered BID-TID with the first dose at awakening and subsequent doses spaced at 4–6 hr intervals. Doses rarely exceed 40 mg/24 hr.

Extended release suspension (Dyanavel XR; PO):

≥**6 yr and adolescent:** Start at 2.5 or 5 mg/24 hr QAM; increase by 2.5–10 mg/24 hr every 4–7 days until desired response up to a **maximum dose** of 20 mg/24 hr.

Extended release dispersible tabs (see how-supplied section, earlier; Adzenys XR-ODT; PO):

6–17 yr: 6.3 mg/24 hr QAM; increase by 3.1 or 6.3 mg/24 hr at weekly intervals until desired response. **Max. dose:** 6–12 yr: 18.8 mg/24 hr; 13–17 yr: 12.5 mg/24 hr

Adult: 12.5 mg/24 hr QAM

If converting from Adderall XR, see dosage equivalent information in Adzenys XR-ODT product information.

Narcolepsy:

Immediate release tabs (Evekeo and generics; PO):

6–12 yr: 5 mg QAM; increase by 5 mg/24 hr at weekly intervals until desired response. Incremental doses may be administered with the first dose at awakening and subsequent doses (5 or 10 mg) spaced at 4–6 hr intervals. Usual daily dosage range: 5–60 mg/24 hr in divided doses

≥**13 yr and adult:** 10 mg QAM; increase by 10 mg/24 hr at weekly intervals until desired response. Incremental doses may be administered with the first dose at awakening and subsequent doses (5 or 10 mg) spaced at 4–6 hr intervals. Usual daily dosage range: 5–60 mg/24 hr in divided doses

Use with caution in presence of hypertension or cardiovascular disease. **Avoid use** in known serious structural cardiac abnormalities, cardiomyopathy, serious heart rhythm abnormalities, coronary artery disease, or other serious cardiac problems that may increase risk of sympathomimetic effects of amphetamines (sudden death, stroke, and MI have been reported).

Contraindicated with MAO inhibitors, including linezolid and IV methylene blue, as a hypertensive crisis may occur if used within 14 days of discontinuance of MAO inhibitor. Serotonin syndrome may occur when used in combination with MAO inhibitors, SSRIs, serotonin norepinephrine reuptake inhibitors (SNRIs), triptans, TCAs, fentanyl, lithium, tramadol, tryptophan, buspirone, and St. John's wort.

Amphetamine is a minor substrate of CYP 450 2D6. Alkalinizing agents should be **avoided** as they can increase the effects/toxicity of amphetamine by decreasing its secretion.

Not recommended for patients <3 yr of age. Medication should generally not be used in children <5 yr, because diagnosis of ADHD in this age group is extremely difficult (use in consultation with a specialist). Interrupt administration occasionally to determine need for continued therapy.

Common side effects include headache, insomnia, anorexia (monitor growth), abdominal pain, anxiety, mood swings, and agitation. Psychotic disorder, peripheral vascular disease (including Raynaud phenomenon), intestinal ischemia, and cerebrovascular accident have been reported.

Evekeo has an additional labeled indication for the treatment of exogenous obesity in ≥12 yr and adults. Doses may be administered with or without food. **Do not** crush or chew the extended release dispersible tabs (Adzenys XR-ODT). Shake oral suspension bottle (Dyanavel XR) well before dispensing and administering each dose.

AMPHOTERICIN B DEOXYCHOLATE (CONVENTIONAL)
Various generics; previously available as
Fungizone
Antifungal, polyene

B   ?   Yes   Yes   No

Continued

AMPHOTERICIN B DEOXYCHOLATE (CONVENTIONAL) *continued*

Injection: 50 mg vials

IV: Mix with D₅W to concentration 0.1 mg/mL (peripheral administration) or 0.25 mg/mL (central line only). pH >4.2. Infuse over 2—6 hr.

Optional test dose: 0.1 mg/kg/dose IV up to **max. dose** of 1 mg (followed by remaining initial dose)

Initial dose: 0.5—1 mg/kg/24 hr; if test dose NOT used infuse first dose over 6 hr and monitor frequently during the first several hours.

Increment: Increase as tolerated by 0.25—0.5 mg/kg/24 hr once daily or every other day. Use larger dosage increment (0.5 mg once daily) for critically ill patients.

Usual maintenance:

Once daily dosing: 0.5—1 mg/kg/24 hr once daily

Every other day dosing: 1.5 mg/kg/dose every other day

Max. dose: 1.5 mg/kg/24 hr

Intrathecal (limited data): 25—100 mCg Q48—72 hr. Increase to 500 mCg as tolerated. Dosages as high as 1500 mCg have been recommended by the 2018 AAP Red Book.

Bladder irrigation for urinary tract mycosis (limited data): 5—15 mg in 100 mL sterile water for irrigation at 100—300 mL/24 hr. Instill solution into bladder, clamp catheter for 1—2 hr, then drain; repeat TID—QID for 2—5 days.

Monitor renal, hepatic, electrolyte, and hematologic status closely. Hypercalciuria, hypokalemia, hypomagnesemia, RTA, renal failure, acute hepatic failure, hypotension, and phlebitis may occur. **For dosing information in renal failure, see Chapter 31.**

Common infusion-related reactions include fever, chills, headache, hypotension, nausea, and vomiting; may premedicate with acetaminophen and diphenhydramine 30 min before and 4 hr after infusion. Meperidine useful for chills. Hydrocortisone, 1 mg/mg ampho (**max.:** 25 mg) added to bottle may help to prevent immediate adverse reactions. Use total body weight for obese patients when calculating dosages.

Salt loading with 10—15 mL/kg of NS infused prior to each dose may minimize the risk of nephrotoxicity. Maintaining sodium intake of >4 mEq/kg/24 hr in premature neonates may also reduce risk for nephrotoxicity. Nephrotoxic drugs such as aminoglycosides, chemotherapeutic agents, and cyclosporine may result in synergistic toxicity. Hypokalemia may increase the toxicity of neuromuscular blocking agents and cardiac glycosides.

Although there are no breastfeeding data for amphotericin, many experts believe it is compatible since the drug is highly protein bound, has a large molecular weight, and is not absorbed orally.

AMPHOTERICIN B LIPID COMPLEX
Abelcet, ABLC
Antifungal, polyene

    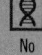

| B | ? | Yes | Yes | No |

Injection: 5 mg/mL (20 mL)
(Formulated as a 1:1 molar ratio of amphotericin B to lipid complex composed of dimyristoylphosphatidylcholine and dimyristoylphosphatidylglycerol)

IV: 5 mg/kg/24 hr once daily
Candidiasis:

IV: 3—5 mg/kg/24 hr once daily
Cryptococcal meningitis:

IV: 5 mg/kg/24 hr once daily; use in combination with flucytosine or fluconazole for HIV

Mix with D₅W to concentration 1 or 2 mg/mL for fluid-restricted patients.

AMPHOTERICIN B LIPID COMPLEX *continued*

Infusion rate: 2.5 mg/kg/hr; shake the infusion bag every 2 hr if total infusion time exceeds 2 hr. **Do not** use an in-line filter.

Monitor renal, hepatic, electrolyte, and hematologic status closely. Thrombocytopenia, anemia, leukopenia, hypokalemia, hypomagnesemia, diarrhea, respiratory failure, skin rash, nephrotoxicity, and increases in liver enzymes and bilirubin may occur. See Conventional Amphotericin B for drug interactions.

Highest concentrations achieved in spleen, lung, and liver from human autopsy data from one heart transplant patient. CNS/CSF levels are lower than amphotericin B, liposomal (AmBisome). In animal models, concentrations are higher in the liver, spleen, and lungs but the same in the kidneys when compared with conventional amphotericin B. Pharmacokinetics in renal and hepatic impairment have not been studied.

Common infusion-related reactions include fever, chills, rigors, nausea, vomiting, hypotension, and headache; may premedicate with acetaminophen, diphenhydramine, and meperidine (see Conventional Amphotericin B remarks).

AMPHOTERICIN B, LIPOSOMAL
AmBisome and generics
Antifungal, polyene

 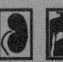 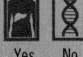

B   ?   Yes   Yes   No

Injection: 50 mg (vials); contains soy, 900 mg sucrose
(Formulated in liposomes composed of hydrogenated soy phosphatidylcholine, cholesterol, distearoylphosphatidylglycerol, and α-tocopherol)

Systemic fungal infections: 3–5 mg/kg/24 hr IV once daily; an upper dosage limit of 10 mg/kg/24 hr has been suggested based on pharmacokinetic endpoints and risk for hypokalemia. However, dosages as high as 15 mg/kg/24 hr have been used. Dosages as high as 10 mg/kg/24 hr have been used in patients with *Aspergillus*.
Empiric therapy for febrile neutropenia: 3 mg/kg/24 hr IV once daily
Cryptococcal meningitis in HIV: 6 mg/kg/24 hr IV once daily
Leishmaniasis (a repeat course may be necessary if infection does not clear):
  Immunocompetent: 3 mg/kg/24 hr IV on days 1 to 5, 14, and 21
  Immunocompromised: 4 mg/kg/24 hr IV on days 1 to 5, 10, 17, 24, 31, and 38
Mix with D₅W to concentration 1–2 mg/mL (0.2–0.5 mg/mL may be used for infants and small children).
Infusion rate: Administer dose over 2 hr; infusion may be reduced to 1 hr if well tolerated. A ≥1-micron inline filter may be used.

Closely monitor renal, hepatic, electrolyte, and hematologic status. Thrombocytopenia, anemia, leukopenia, tachycardia, hypokalemia, hypomagnesemia, hypocalcemia, hyperglycemia, diarrhea, dyspnea, skin rash, low back pain, nephrotoxicity, and increases in liver enzymes and bilirubin may occur. Rhabdomyolysis has been reported. Safety and effectiveness in neonates have not been established as lipid-based formulations may have reduced tissue penetration as compared with conventional formulations in neonates. See Conventional Amphotericin B for drug interactions.

Compared with conventional amphotericin B, higher concentrations are found in the liver and spleen; and similar concentrations found in the lungs and kidney. CNS/CSF concentrations are higher than other amphotericin B products. Pharmacokinetics in renal and hepatic impairment have not been studied.

Common infusion-related reactions include fever, chills, rigors, nausea, vomiting, hypotension, and headache; may premedicate with acetaminophen, diphenhydramine, and meperidine (see Conventional Amphotericin B remarks).

Continued

Mix with D₅W to concentration 1–2 mg/mL

AMPHOTERICIN B, LIPOSOMAL *continued*

False elevations of serum phosphate have been reported with the PHOSm assay (used in Beckman Coulter analyzers).

AMPICILLIN
Many generics
Antibiotic, aminopenicillin

B   1   Yes   No   No

Caps: 500 mg
Injection: 125, 250, 500 mg; 1, 2, 10 g
Contains 3 mEq Na/1 g IV drug

Neonate (IM/IV):
  ≤34 wk gestation:
    Postnatal age ≤7 days old: 100 mg/kg/24 hr ÷ Q12 hr
    Postnatal age 8–<28 days old: 150 mg/kg/24 hr ÷ Q12 hr
  >34 wk gestation:
    Postnatal age ≤28 days old: 150 mg/kg/24 hr ÷ Q8 hr
  Group B streptococcal meningitis (independent of gestational age):
    Postnatal age ≤7 days old: 300 mg/kg/24 hr ÷ Q8 hr
    Postnatal age 8–<28 days old: 300 mg/kg/24 hr ÷ Q6 hr
Infant/child (see remarks):
  Mild-moderate infections:
    IM/IV: 100–200 mg/kg/24 hr ÷ Q6 hr; **max dose:** 8 g/24 hr
    PO: 50–100 mg/kg/24 hr ÷ Q6 hr; **max. PO dose:** 2 g/24 hr
  Severe infections: 300–400 mg/kg/24 hr ÷ Q4–6 hr IM/IV; **max. dose:** 12 g/24 hr
  Community-acquired pneumonia in a fully immunized patient (IV/IM):
    ***S. pneumoniae* penicillin MIC ≤2.0 or *H. influenzae* (β-lactamase negative):** 150–200 mg/kg/24 hr ÷ Q6 hr
    ***S. pneumoniae* penicillin MIC ≥4.0:** 300–400 mg/kg/24 hr ÷ Q6 hr
    Max. IV/IM dose: 12 g/24 hr
Adult:
  IM/IV: 500–3000 mg Q4–6 hr; **max. dose:** 14 g/24 hr
  PO: 250–500 mg Q6 hr
SBE prophylaxis (when PO administration is not feasible):
  Moderate-risk patients:
    Child: 50 mg/kg/dose (**max. dose:** 2 g/dose) × 1 IV/IM 30 min before procedure
    Adult: 2 g/dose × 1 IV/IM 30 min before procedure
  High-risk patients with GU and GI procedures: Aforementioned doses PLUS gentamicin 1.5 mg/kg × 1 (**max. dose:** 120 mg) IV within 30 min of starting procedure. Followed by ampicillin 25 mg/kg/dose IV (or PO amoxicillin) × 1, 6 hr later.

Use higher doses with shorter dosing intervals to treat CNS disease and severe infection. CSF penetration occurs only with inflamed meninges. **Adjust dose in renal failure (see Chapter 31).**

Produces the same side effects as penicillin, with cross-reactivity. Rash commonly seen at 5–10 days and rash may occur with concurrent EBV infection or allopurinol use. May cause interstitial nephritis, diarrhea, and pseudomembranous enterocolitis. Chloroquine reduces ampicillin's oral absorption.

AMPICILLIN/SULBACTAM
Unasyn and generics
Antibiotic, aminopenicillin with β-lactamase inhibitor

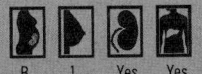

B   1   Yes   Yes   No

Injection:
  1.5 g = ampicillin 1 g + sulbactam 0.5 g
  3 g = ampicillin 2 g + sulbactam 1 g
  15 g = ampicillin 10 g + sulbactam 5 g
Contains 5 mEq Na per 1.5 g drug combination

Dosage based on ampicillin component:
  Neonate:
    Premature (based on pharmacokinetic data): 100 mg/kg/24 hr ÷ Q12 hr IM/IV
    Full term: 100 mg/kg/24 hr ÷ Q8 hr IM/IV
  Infant ≥1 mo and child (see remarks):
    Mild/moderate infections: 100—200 mg/kg/24 hr ÷ Q6 hr IM/IV; **max. dose:** 2 g ampicillin/dose
    Meningitis/severe infections: 200—400 mg/kg/24 hr ÷ Q4—6 hr IM/IV; **max. dose:** 2 g ampicillin/dose
  Adult: 1—2 g Q6—8 hr IM/IV; **max. dose:** 8 g ampicillin/24 hr

Similar spectrum of antibacterial activity to ampicillin with the added coverage of
  β-lactamase—producing organisms. Total sulbactam dose **should not exceed** 4 g/24 hr.
Use higher doses with shorter dosing intervals to treat CNS disease and severe infection. Hepatic
  dysfunction (e.g., hepatitis and cholestatic jaundice) and allergic reaction resulting in acute myocardial
  ischemia have been reported. Monitor hepatic function in patients with hepatic impairment.
Adjust dose in renal failure (see Chapter 31). Similar CSF distribution and side effects to ampicillin.
  Postmarking adverse reactions reported include abdominal pain, melena, gastritis, stomatitis,
  dyspepsia, black hairy tongue, dizziness, dyspnea, TEN, and urticaria.

ANTIPYRINE AND BENZOCAINE (OTIC)
Antipyrine and Benzocaine Otic and generics;
previously available as Auralgan
Otic analgesic, cerumenolytic

    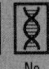

C   2   No   No   No

Otic solution: antipyrine 5.4%, benzocaine 1.4% (15 mL); may contain oxyquinoline sulfate

Otic analgesia: Fill external ear canal (2—4 drops) Q1—2 hr PRN. After instillation of the
  solution, a cotton pledget should be moistened with the solution and inserted into the meatus.
Cerumenolytic: Fill external ear canal (2—4 drops) TID for 2—3 days.

Benzocaine sensitivity may develop; not intended for prolonged use. **Contraindicated if**
  tympanic membrane perforated or PE tubes in place. Local reactions (e.g., burning, stinging)
  and hypersensitivity reactions may occur. Risk of benzocaine-induced methemoglobinemia
  may be increased in infants aged ≤3 mo.

ARGININE HYDROCHLORIDE—INJECTABLE PREPARATION
R-Gene 10
Metabolic alkalosis agent, urea cycle disorder treatment agent, growth hormone diagnostic agent

    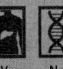

B   ?   Yes   Yes   No

Continued

ARGININE HYDROCHLORIDE—INJECTABLE PREPARATION *continued*

Injection: 10% (100 mg/mL) arginine hydrochloride, contains 47.5 mEq chloride per 100 mL (300 mL)
Osmolality: 950 mOsmol/L

Used as a secondary alternative agent for patients that are unresponsive or unable to receive sodium chloride and potassium chloride.

Correction of hypochloremia (IV): Arginine chloride dose in milliequivalents (mEq) = $0.2 \times$ patient's weight (kg) $\times$ (103 − patient's serum chloride in mEq/L). Administer $\frac{1}{2}$ to $\frac{2}{3}$ of the calculated dose and reassess.

Drug administration: Do not exceed an IV infusion rate of 1 g/kg/hr (4.75 mEq/kg/hr). Drug may be administered without further dilution but should be diluted to reduce risk of tissue irritation.

Hyperammonemia in metabolic disorders: See Chapter 13.

Contraindicated in renal or hepatic failure. Use with **extreme caution** as overdosages may result in hyperchloremic metabolic acidosis, cerebral edema, and death. Hypersensitivity reactions, including anaphylaxis, and hematuria have been reported.

Arginine hydrochloride is metabolized to nitrogen-containing products for renal excretion. Excess arginine increases the production of nitric oxide (NO) to cause vasodilation/hypotension. Closely monitor acid/base status. Hyperglycemia, hyperkalemia, GI disturbances, IV extravasation, headache, and flushing may occur.

In addition to its use for chloride supplementation, arginine is used in urea cycle disorder therapy (increase arginine levels and prevent breakdown of endogenous proteins) and as a diagnostic agent for growth hormone (stimulates pituitary release of growth hormone).

ARIPIPRAZOLE
Abilify, Abilify Maintena, Abilify MyCite (Starter or Maintenance Kit), and generics
Atypical antipsychotic (2nd generation)

C   3   No   No   Yes

Tabs: 2, 5, 10, 15, 20, 30 mg

Abilify MyCite: 2, 5, 10, 15, 20, 30 mg; contains an ingestible event marker sensor inside the tablet to monitor adherence

Starter Kit: Each respective strength starter kit comes with 30 tablets, one MYCITE pod device, and 7 MYCITE adhesive strips.

Maintenance Kit: Each respective strength maintenance kit comes with 30 tablets and 7 MYCITE adhesive strips.

Tabs, orally disintegrating (ODT): 10, 15 mg; contains phenylalanine
Oral solution: 1 mg/mL (150 mL); may contain parabens
Intramuscular suspension for injection (extended release):
Abilify Maintena: 300, 400 mg

Irritability Associated With Autistic Disorder:

6−17 yr: Start at 2 mg PO once daily × 7 days, then increase to 5 mg PO once daily. If needed, dose may be increased in 5 mg increments ≥7 days in duration up to a **maximum** dose of 15 mg/24 hr. Patients should be periodically evaluated to determine the continued need for maintenance treatment.

Schizophrenia:

13−17 yr: Start at 2 mg PO once daily × 2 days, followed by 5 mg PO once daily × 2 days, then to the recommended target dose of 10 mg PO once daily. If necessary, dose may be increased in 5 mg increments up to a **maximum** of 30 mg/24 hr (30 mg/24 hr was not shown to be more effective than 10 mg/24 hr in clinical trials). Patients should be periodically evaluated to determine the continued need for maintenance treatment.

ARIPIPRAZOLE *continued*

Bipolar 1 Disorder (monotherapy or adjunctive therapy):

  10—17 yr: Start at 2 mg PO once daily × 2 days, followed by 5 mg PO once daily × 2 days, then to the recommended target dose of 10 mg PO once daily. If necessary, dose may be increased in 5 mg increments up to a **maximum** of 30 mg/24 hr.

Tourette Disorder:

  6—18 yr (patients should be periodically evaluated to determine the continued need for maintenance treatment):

    <50 kg: Start at 2 mg PO once daily × 2 days, then increase to the target dose of 5 mg PO once daily. If necessary after 7 days, dose may be increased to 10 mg PO once daily.

    ≥50 kg: Start at 2 mg PO once daily × 2 days, followed by 5 mg PO once daily × 5 days, and then 10 mg PO once daily. If necessary after 7 days, dose may be increased in 5 mg increments of ≥7 days in duration **up to** a **maximum** of 20 mg/24 hr.

Monitor for clinical worsening of depression and suicidal ideation/behavior after initiation of therapy or after dose changes. **Avoid** use of extended-release IM injection with CYP 450 inducers, including carbamazepine, for >14 days. Higher cumulative doses and longer treatment duration may increase risk for irreversible tardive dyskinesia.

Weight gain, constipation, GI discomfort, akathisia, dizziness, extrapyramidal symptoms, headaches, insomnia, sedation, blurred vision, and fatigue are common. May cause leukopenia, neutropenia, agranulocytosis, hiccups, hyperthermia, neuroleptic malignant syndrome, hyperglycemia, orthostatic hypotension (risk for falls), and prolongation of the QT interval (use considered contraindicated with other medications prolonging the QT interval). Rare impulse-control problems (e.g., compulsive or uncontrollable urges to gamble, binge eat, shop, and to have sex), oculogyric crisis, and DRESS have been reported.

Primarily metabolized by the CYP 450 2D6 and 3A4 enzymes. Dosage reduction for using half of the usual dose has been recommended for those who are either known CYP 450 2D6 poor metabolizers; or nonpoor CYP 450 2D6 metabolizers taking strong CYP 450 2D6 (e.g., quinidine, fluoxetine, paroxetine) or 3A4 (e.g., itraconazole, clarithromycin) inhibitors. Use of $\frac{1}{4}$ the usual dose has been recommended for known CYP 2D6 poor metabolizers taking either a strong 2D6 or 3A4 inhibitor; or nonpoor CYP 450 2D6 metabolizers taking both strong 2D6 AND 3A4 inhibitors.

Consult with a pediatric psychiatrist for use in ADHD, conduct disorder, and PDD-NOS. Oral doses may be administered with or without meals. Do not split orally disintegrating tablet dosage form.

ARNUITY ELLIPTA

See Fluticasone Preparations.

ASCORBIC ACID
Vitamin C; many brands and generics
Water-soluble vitamin

A/C   1   No   No   No

Tabs [OTC]: 100, 250, 500 mg, 1 g
Chewable tabs [OTC]: 100, 250, 500 mg; some may contain aspartame
Tabs (timed release) [OTC]: 0.5, 1.5 g
Caps [OTC]: 500, 1000 mg
Extended release caps [OTC]: 500 mg
Injection: 500 mg/mL (50 mL); may contain sodium hydrosulfite or edetate disodium
Oral liquid [OTC]: 500 mg/5 mL (120, 236, 473 mL); may contain propylene glycol, saccharin, sodium benzoate

Continued

ASCORBIC ACID *continued*

Oral crystals or powder [OTC]: 1 g per 1/4 teaspoonful (120 g, 480 g)
Some products may contain approximately 5 mEq Na/1 g ascorbic acid.

Scurvy (PO/IM/IV/SC):
    Child: 100—300 mg/24 hr ÷ once daily-BID for at least 2 wk
    Adult: 100—250 mg once daily-BID for at least 2 wk
U.S. Recommended Daily Allowance (RDA):
    See Chapter 21.

Adverse reactions: nausea, vomiting, heartburn, flushing, headache, faintness, dizziness, and
hyperoxaluria. Use high doses with **caution** in G6PD patients. May cause false-negative and
false-positive urine glucose determinations with glucose oxidase and cupric sulfate tests, respectively.
May increase the enteral absorption of aluminum hydroxide and iron; and increase the adverse/toxic
effects of deferoxamine. 200 mg oral vitamin C per 30 mg iron has been recommended to enhance
enteral iron absorption. May reduce the effects of amphetamines.
Oral dosing is preferred with or without food. IM route is the preferred parenteral route. Protect the
injectable dosage form from light.
Pregnancy Category changes to "C" if used in doses greater than the RDA.

ASPIRIN
ASA, various trade names and generics
Nonsteroidal antiinflammatory agent, antiplatelet agent, analgesic

    D   2   Yes   Yes   No

Tabs/caplet [OTC]: 325, 500 mg
Tabs, enteric coated [OTC]: 81, 325, 650 mg
Tabs, time release [OTC]: 81, 325 mg
Tabs, buffered [OTC]: 325, 500 mg; may contain magnesium, aluminum, and/or calcium
Caplet, buffered [OTC]: 500 mg; may contain calcium
Tabs, chewable [OTC]: 81 mg
Suppository [OTC]: 300 mg (12s)

Analgesic/antipyretic: 10—15 mg/kg/dose PO/PR Q4—6 hr up to total of 60—80 mg/kg/24 hr
    Max. dose: 4 g/24 hr
Antiinflammatory: 60—100 mg/kg/24 hr PO ÷ Q6—8 hr
Kawasaki disease (see remarks): 80—100 mg/kg/24 hr PO ÷ QID for during febrile phase (up to
14 days) until defervesces for 48—72 hr, then decrease to 3—5 mg/kg/24 hr PO QAM. Continue for
at least 8 wk or until both platelet count and ESR are normal. Alternatively, a lower initial febrile
phase dosage of 30—50 mg/kg/24 hr PO ÷ QID is used in Japan and Western Europe because there
are no data to suggest this or the higher 80—100 mg/kg/24 hr dosage regimen is superior.

Do not use in children <16 yr for treatment of varicella or flu-like symptoms (risk for Reye
syndrome), in combination with other NSAIDs, or in severe renal failure. **Use with caution** in
bleeding disorders, renal dysfunction, gastritis, and gout. May cause GI upset, allergic reactions,
liver toxicity, and decreased platelet aggregation.
Drug interactions: May increase effects of methotrexate, valproic acid, and warfarin, which may lead to
toxicity (protein displacement). Buffered dosage forms may decrease absorption of ketoconazole and
tetracycline. GI bleeds have been reported with concurrent use of SSRIs (e.g., fluoxetine, paroxetine,
sertraline).
Therapeutic levels: antipyretic/analgesic: 30—50 mg/L, antiinflammatory: 150—300 mg/L. Tinnitus
may occur at levels of 200—400 mg/L. Recommended serum sampling time at steady state: Obtain

ASPIRIN *continued*

trough level just prior to dose following 1—2 days of continuous dosing. Peak levels obtained 2 hr (for nonsustained release dosage forms) after a dose may be useful for monitoring toxicity. **Adjust dose in renal failure (see Chapter 31).**

For breastfeeding considerations:

High-dose aspirin regimens: Use of an alternative drug is recommended.

Low-dose (75—162 mg/24 hr) aspirin regimens: Avoid breastfeeding for 1—2 hr after a dose.

For pregnancy considerations: Low-dose regimens are currently recommended for certain pregnancy-related conditions such as the prevention of preeclampsia. However, **DO NOT** use non-low-dose regimens at >20 weeks' gestation as it may cause problems to the unborn child or complications during delivery.

ATENOLOL
Tenormin and generics
β₁ selective adrenergic blocker

 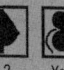 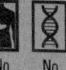

D 2 Yes No No

Tab: 25, 50, 100 mg
Oral suspension: 2 mg/mL

Hypertension:
    Child and adolescent: 0.5—1 mg/kg/dose PO once daily—BID; **max. dose:** 2 mg/kg/24 hr up to 100 mg/24 hr
    Adult: 25—100 mg/dose PO once daily—BID; **max. dose:** 100 mg/24 hr

Infantile hemangioma (limited data):
    Infant and child <2 yr: 1 mg/kg/dose PO once daily x 6 mo

Contraindicated in pulmonary edema and cardiogenic shock. May cause bradycardia, hypotension, second- or third-degree AV block, dizziness, fatigue, lethargy, and headache. **Use with caution** in diabetes and asthma. Wheezing and dyspnea have occurred when daily dosage exceeds 100 mg/24 hr. Postmarketing evaluation reports a temporal relationship for causing elevated LFTs and/or bilirubin, hallucinations, psoriatic rash, thrombocytopenia, visual disturbances, and dry mouth. **Avoid** abrupt withdrawal of the drug. Does not cross the blood-brain barrier; lower incidence of CNS side effects compared with propranolol. Neonates born to mothers receiving atenolol during labor or while breastfeeding may be at risk for hypoglycemia.

Use with disopyramide, amiodarone, or digoxin may enhance bradycardic effects. **Adjust dose in renal impairment (see Chapter 31).**

ATOMOXETINE
Strattera and generics
Norepinephrine reuptake inhibitor, ADHD agent

C 3 No Yes Yes

Capsules: 10, 18, 25, 40, 60, 80, 100 mg

Child ≥6 yr and adolescent ≤70 kg (see remarks):
    Start with 0.5 mg/kg/24 hr PO QAM and increase after a minimum of 3 days to approximately 1.2 mg/kg/24 hr PO ÷ QAM or BID (morning and late afternoon/early evening).
    Max. daily dose: 1.4 mg/kg/24 hr or 100 mg, whichever is less
    If used with a strong CYP 450 2D6 inhibitor (e.g., fluoxetine, paroxetine, quinidine) or in patients with reduced CYP 450 2D6 activity: Maintain aforementioned initial dose for 4 wk and increase to a max. of 1.2 mg/kg/24 hr only if symptoms **do not** improve and initial dose is tolerated.

Child ≥6 yr and adolescent >70 kg (see remarks):

Continued

ATOMOXETINE *continued*

Start with 40 mg PO QAM and increase after a minimum of 3 days to approximately 80 mg/24 hr PO ÷ QAM or BID (morning and late afternoon/early evening). After 2–4 wk, dose may be increased to a **max.** of 100 mg/24 hr if needed.

If used with a strong CYP 450 2D6 inhibitor (e.g., fluoxetine, paroxetine, quinidine) or in patients with reduced CYP 450 2D6 activity: Maintain aforementioned initial dose for 4 wk and increase to 80 mg/24 hr only if symptoms **do not** improve and initial dose is tolerated.

Contraindicated in patients with narrow-angle glaucoma, pheochromocytoma, and severe cardiac disorders. **Do not** administer with or within 2 wk after discontinuing an MAO inhibitor; fatal reactions have been reported. **Use with caution** in hypertension, tachycardia, cardiovascular or cerebrovascular diseases, or with concurrent albuterol therapy. Increased risk of suicidal thinking has been reported; closely monitor for clinical worsening, agitation, aggressive behavior, irritability, suicidal thinking or behaviors, and unusual changes in behavior when initiating (first few months) or at times of dose changes (increases or decreases). Patients with bipolar disorders may be at increased risk for developing mania or mixed episodes.

Atomoxetine is a CYP 450 2D6 substrate; poor 2D6 metabolizers compared with normal have been reported to have higher rates of adverse effects (insomnia, weight loss, constipation, depression, tremor, and excoriation), greater improvement of ADHD symptoms with lower final dose requirements.

Doses >1.2 mg/kg/24 hr in patients ≤70 kg have not been shown to be of additional benefit. Reduce dose (initial and target doses) by 50% and 75% for patients with moderate (Child-Pugh Class B) and severe (Child-Pugh Class C) hepatic insufficiency, respectively.

Major side effects include GI discomfort, vomiting, fatigue, anorexia, dizziness, and mood swings. Hypersensitivity reactions, aggression, irritability, psychotic or manic symptoms, priapism, allergic reactions, severe liver injury, alopecia, and hyperhidrosis have also been reported. Consider interrupting therapy in patients who are not growing or gaining weight satisfactorily.

Doses may be administered with or without food. Atomoxetine can be discontinued without tapering.

ATOVAQUONE
Mepron and generics
Antiprotozoal

C   3   Yes   Yes   No

Oral suspension: 750 mg/5 mL (210 mL); contains benzyl alcohol

Pneumocystis jiroveci (carinii) pneumonia (PCP):
Treatment (21-day course):
Child: 30–40 mg/kg/24 hr PO ÷ BID with fatty foods; **max. dose:** 1500 mg/24 hr. Infants 4–24 mo may require higher doses of 45 mg/kg/24 hr.
Adult: 750 mg/dose PO BID
Prophylaxis (1st episode and recurrence):
Child 1–3 mo or >24 mo: 30 mg/kg/24 hr PO once daily; **max. dose:** 1500 mg/24 hr
Child 4–24 mo: 45 mg/kg/24 hr PO once daily: **max. dose:** 1500 mg/24 hr
Adult: 1500 mg/dose PO once daily

Toxoplasma gondii:
Child:
First episode prophylaxis and recurrence prophylaxis: Use *P. jiroveci* prophylaxis dosages ± pyrimethamine 1 mg/kg/dose (**max.** 25 mg/dose) PO once daily PLUS leucovorin 5 mg PO Q3 days.
Adult:
Treatment: 1500 mg/dose PO BID ± (sulfadiazine 1000–1500 mg PO Q6 hr or pyrimethamine PLUS leucovorin) for a minimum of 6 weeks

ATOVAQUONE *continued*

First episode prophylaxis: 1500 mg/dose PO once daily ± pyrimethamine 25 mg PO once daily PLUS leucovorin 10 mg PO once daily

Recurrence prophylaxis: 750 mg/dose PO Q6–12 hr ± pyrimethamine 25 mg PO once daily PLUS leucovorin 10 mg PO once daily

Not recommended in the treatment of severe *P. jiroveci* (lack of clinical data). Patients with GI disorders or severe vomiting and who cannot tolerate oral therapy should consider alternative IV therapies. Rash, pruritus, sweating, GI symptoms, LFT elevation, dizziness, headache, insomnia, anxiety, cough, and fever are common. Anemia, Stevens-Johnson syndrome, hepatitis, renal/urinary disorders, and pancreatitis have been reported.

Metoclopramide, rifampin, rifabutin, and tetracycline may decrease atovaquone levels. Shake oral suspension well before dispensing all doses. Take all doses with high-fat foods to maximize absorption.

ATROPINE SULFATE
AtroPen, Isopto Atropine, and many generics
Anticholinergic agent

   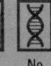

C   2   No   No   No

Injection (vials): 0.4, 1 mg/mL
Injection (prefilled syringe): 0.25 mg/5 mL, 0.5 mg/5 mL, 1 mg/10 mL
Injection (autoinjector for IM use):
 AtroPen 0.25 mg: Delivers a single 0.25 mg (0.3 mL) dose (yellow-colored pen)
 AtroPen 0.5 mg: Delivers a single 0.5 mg (0.7 mL) dose (blue-colored pen)
 AtroPen 1 mg: Delivers a single 1 mg (0.7 mL) dose (dark red-colored pen)
 AtroPen 2 mg: Delivers a single 2 mg (0.7 mL) dose (green-colored pen)
Ophthalmic Dosage Forms:
 Ointment: 1% (3.5 g)
 Solution:
  Isopto Atropine: 1% (5 mL); contains benzalkonium chloride
  Generics: 1% (2, 5, 15 mL)

Preintubation dose (use 1 mg/mL concentration for IM route; see remarks):

 Neonate: 0.01–0.02 mg/kg/dose IV (over 1 min)/IM prior to other premedications
 Child: 0.02 mg/kg/dose IV/IO/IM; **max. dose:** 0.5 mg/dose
 Adult: 0.5 mg/dose IV/IM
Cardiopulmonary resuscitation/bradycardia (see remarks):
 Child: 0.02 mg/kg/dose IV/IO/IM (use 1 mg/mL for IM) Q5 min × 2–3 doses PRN; **max. single dose:** 0.5 mg in children, 1 mg in adolescents; **max total dose:** 1 mg children, 2 mg adolescents
  ET tube administration: 0.04–0.06 mg/kg (dilute with NS to volume of 1–2 mL and follow dose with 1 mL NS); may repeat once if needed
 Adult: 0.5–1 mg/dose IV Q5 min; **max. total dose:** 3 mg
Bronchospasm: 0.025–0.05 mg/kg/dose (**max. dose:** 2.5 mg/dose) in 2.5 mL NS Q6–8 hr via nebulizer
Nerve agent and insecticide poisoning for muscarinic symptoms (organophosphate or carbamate poisoning) (IV/IO/IM/ET; dilute in 1–2 mL NS for ET administration):
 Child: 0.05–0.1 mg/kg Q 5–10 min until bronchial or oral secretions terminate
 Adolescent: 1–3 mg/dose Q 3–5 min until bronchial or oral secretions terminate
 Adult: 2–5 mg/dose Q3–5 min until bronchial or oral secretions terminate

Continued

ATROPINE SULFATE *continued*

AtroPen device (IM route): Inject as soon as exposure is known or suspected. Give one dose for mild symptoms and two additional doses (total three doses) in rapid succession 10 min after the first dose for severe symptoms as follows:

Child <6 mo (<7 kg): 0.25 mg
Child 6 mo—4 yr (7—18 kg): 0.5 mg
Child 4—10 yr (18—41 kg): 1 mg
Child >10 yr and adult (>41 kg): 2 mg

Ophthalmic (uveitis; see remarks):
Child: (0.5% solution; prepared by diluting equal volume of the 1% atropine ophthalmic solution with artificial tears) 1—2 drops in each eye once daily—TID
Adult: (1% solution) 1—2 drops in each eye once daily—BID

Contraindicated in glaucoma, obstructive uropathy, tachycardia, and thyrotoxicosis, except for severe or life-threatening muscarinic symptoms. Use with **caution** in patients sensitive to sulfites.

Use in neonatal bradycardia is no longer recommended. Data suggest the use of a minimum 0.1 mg dose may not be warranted for the preintubation indication. Use of the minimum 0.1 mg dose could result in an overdose in younger patients.

Side effects include: dry mouth, blurred vision, fever, tachycardia, constipation, urinary retention, CNS signs (dizziness, hallucinations, restlessness, fatigue, headache).

Use injectable solution for nebulized use; can be mixed with albuterol for simultaneous administration. AtroPen dosage form is designed for IM administration to the outer thigh.

Ophthalmic use is not recommended for children less than 3 mo of age due to risk for systemic absorption.

AURALGAN

See Antipyrine and Benzocaine.

AZATHIOPRINE
Imuran, Azasan, and generics
Immunosuppressant

D   2   Yes   Yes   Yes

Oral suspension: 50 mg/mL
Tabs:
Imuran and generics: 50 mg (scored)
Azasan and generics: 75, 100 mg (scored)
Injection: 100 mg

Immunosuppression (see remarks for genomic considerations):
Child and adult:
Initial: 3—5 mg/kg/24 hr IV/PO once daily
Maintenance: 1—3 mg/kg/24 hr IV/PO once daily

Increased risk for hepatosplenic T-cell lymphoma has been reported in adolescents and young adults. Toxicity: Bone marrow suppression, rash, stomatitis, hepatotoxicity, alopecia, arthralgias, and GI disturbances.

Use $\frac{1}{4}$—$\frac{1}{3}$ dose when given with xanthine oxidase inhibitors (e.g., allopurinol). Patients with low or absent thiopurine methyl transferase (TPMT) or nucleotide diphosphatase (NUDT15) may be at increased risk for severe and life-threatening myelotoxicity. Consider alternative therapy in patients

AZATHIOPRINE *continued*

with homozygous TPMT or NUDT15 deficiency and reduced dosages in patients with heterozygous deficiency. Individuals with the low-functioning alleles for NUDT15 are common among Asian ancestry and Hispanic ethnicity.

Severe anemia has been reported when used in combination with captopril or enalapril. Monitor CBC, platelets, total bilirubin, alkaline phosphatase, BUN, and creatinine. Pancytopenia and bone marrow suppression have been reported with concomitant use of pegylated interferon and ribavirin in patients with hepatitis C. Progressive multifocal leukoencephalopathy (PML) has been reported. **Adjust dose in renal failure (see Chapter 31).**

Administer oral doses with food to minimize GI discomfort. To minimize infant exposure via breastmilk, avoid breastfeeding for 4—6 hr after administering a maternal dose.

AZELASTINE
Generics; previously available as Astepro and Opitvar
Antihistamine

  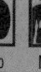 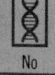

C ? No No No

Nasal spray (generics; previously available as Astepro):
 0.1% (delivers 137 mCg/spray) (200 actuations per 30 mL); contains benzalkonium chloride and EDTA
 0.15% (delivers 205.5 mCg/spray) (200 actuations per 30 mL); contains benzalkonium chloride and EDTA
Ophthalmic drops (generics; previously available as Opitvar): 0.05% (0.5 mg/mL) (6 mL); contains benzalkonium chloride

Seasonal allergic rhinitis:
 0.1% strength:
  Child 2—11 yr: 1 spray each nostril BID
  ≥12 yr and adult: 1—2 sprays each nostril BID
 0.15% strength:
  Child 6—12 yr: 1 spray each nostril BID
  ≥12 yr and adult: 1—2 sprays each nostril BID or 2 sprays each nostril once daily
Perennial allergic rhinitis:
 0.1% strength:
  ≥6 mo—<12 yr: 1 spray each nostril BID
 0.15% strength:
  6—<12 yr: 1 spray each nostril BID
  ≥12 yr and adult: 2 sprays each nostril BID
Ophthalmic:
 ≥3 yr and adult: Instill 1 drop into each affected eye BID.

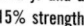

NASAL USE: Drowsiness may occur despite nasal route of administration (**avoid** concurrent use of alcohol or CNS depressants). Bitter taste, nausea, nasal burning, pharyngitis, weight gain, fatigue, nasal sores, and epistaxis may also occur. Also available in combination with fluticasone as Dymista with labeled dosing information of 1 spray each nostril BID for seasonal allergic rhinitis (≥6 yr and adult).

OPHTHALMIC USE: Eye burning and stinging have been reported in about 30% of patients receiving the ophthalmic dosage form. **Should not be used** to treat contact lens—related irritation. Soft contact lens users should wait at least 10 min after dose instillation before they insert their lenses.

AZELASTINE AND FLUTICASONE
Dymista and generics
Intranasal antihistamine and corticosteroid combination

    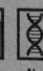

C ? No No No

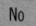

Continued

AZELASTINE AND FLUTICASONE *continued*

Nasal spray: 137 mcg azelastine and 50 mcg fluticasone per spray (23 g delivers 120 doses); contains benzalkonium chloride, EDTA, and polysorbate 80

Seasonal allergic rhinitis:
   Child >6 yr, adolescent, and adult: 1 spray each nostril BID

May cause drowsiness. **Avoid use** with recent nasal ulcers, nasal surgery, or nasal trauma. Use with ketoconazole, ritonavir, or other strong CYP 450 3A4 inhibitors may increase fluticasone levels and result in systemic corticosteroid effects, including Cushing syndrome and adrenal suppression. Monitor growth velocity in children with prolonged use. See azelastine and fluticasone preparations for remarks on intranasal route of administration for additional information.

AZITHROMYCIN					
Zithromax, Zithromax TRI-PAK, Zithromax Z-PAK, AzaSite, and generics					
Antibiotic, macrolide	B	2	Yes	Yes	No

Tablets: 250, 500, 600 mg
   TRI-PAK and generics: 500 mg (3s as unit dose pack)
   Z-PAK and generics: 250 mg (6s as unit dose pack)
Oral suspension: 100 mg/5 mL (15 mL), 200 mg/5 mL (15, 22.5, 30 mL)
Oral powder (sachet): 1 g (3s, 10s)
Injection: 500 mg; contains 9.92 mEq Na/1 g drug
Ophthalmic solution (AzaSite): 1% (2.5 mL); contains benzalkonium chloride

Infant and child (see remarks):
   Community acquired pneumonia (≥3 mo):
      Tablet or oral suspension (mild infection or step-down therapy): 10 mg/kg (**max. dose:** 500 mg) PO on day 1, followed by 5 mg/kg/24 hr (**max. dose:** 250 mg/24 hr) PO once daily on days 2–5
      IV and PO regimen (severe infection): 10 mg/kg/dose (**max. dose:** 500 mg/dose) IV once daily for at least 2 days followed by 5 mg/kg/dose (**max. dose:** 250 mg/dose) PO once daily to complete a 5-day course
   Pharyngitis/tonsillitis (Group A streptococcal; 2–15 yr): 12 mg/kg/24 hr PO once daily × 5 days (**max. dose:** 500 mg/24 hr)
   Acute sinusitis (≥6 mo): 10 mg/kg/dose (**max. dose:** 500 mg) PO once daily × 3 days
   Pertussis:
      1–<6 mo: 10 mg/kg/dose PO once daily × 5 days
      ≥6 mo: 10 mg/kg/dose (**max. dose:** 500 mg) PO × 1, followed by 5 mg/kg/dose (**max. dose:** 250 mg) PO once daily on days 2–5
   ***Mycobacterium avium* complex in HIV (see www.aidsinfo.nih.gov/guidelines for most current recommendations):**
      Prophylaxis for first episode: 20 mg/kg/dose PO Q7 days (**max. dose:** 1200 mg/dose); alternatively, 5 mg/kg/24 hr PO once daily (**max. dose:** 250 mg/dose) with or without rifabutin
      Prophylaxis for recurrence: 5 mg/kg/24 hr PO once daily (**max. dose:** 250 mg/dose), plus ethambutol 15 mg/kg/24 hr (**max. dose:** 900 mg/24 hr) PO once daily with or without rifabutin 5 mg/kg/24 hr (**max. dose:** 300 mg/24 hr)
      Treatment: 10–12 mg/kg/24 hr PO once daily (**max. dose:** 500 mg/24 hr) × 1 mo or longer, plus ethambutol 15–25 mg/kg/24 hr (**max. dose:** 1 g/24 hr) PO once daily with or without rifabutin 10–20 mg/kg/24 hr (**max. dose:** 300 mg/24 hr)
   Endocarditis prophylaxis: 15 mg/kg/dose (**max. dose:** 500 mg) PO × 1, 30–60 min before procedure

AZITHROMYCIN *continued*

Antiinflammatory agent in cystic fibrosis:

<18 kg: 10 mg/kg/dose PO every Mondays, Wednesdays, and Fridays

18–<36 kg: 250 mg PO every Mondays, Wednesdays, and Fridays

≥36 kg: 500 mg PO every Mondays, Wednesdays, and Fridays

Adolescent and adult:

Pharyngitis, tonsillitis, skin, and soft tissue infection: 500 mg PO day 1, then 250 mg/24 hr PO on days 2–5

Mild/moderate bacterial COPD exacerbation: Aforementioned 5-day dosing regimen OR 500 mg PO once daily × 3 days

Community acquired pneumonia:

Tablets (outpatient regimen): 500 mg PO day 1, then 250 mg/24 hr PO on days 2–5

IV and tablet regimen (inpatient regimen): 500 mg IV once daily × 3 days followed by 500 mg PO once daily to complete a 7- to 10-day regimen (IV and PO)

Sinusitis:

Tablets: 500 mg PO once daily × 3 days

Uncomplicated chlamydial cervicitis or urethritis: Single 1 g dose PO

Gonococcal cervicitis or urethritis: Single 2 g dose PO

Acute PID (chlamydia): 500 mg IV once daily × 1–2 days followed by 250 mg PO once daily to complete a 7-day regimen (IV and PO)

***Mycobacterium avium* complex in HIV (see www.aidsinfo.nih.gov/guidelines for most recent recommendations):**

Prophylaxis for first episode: 1200 mg PO Q7 days with or without rifabutin 300 mg PO once daily

Prophylaxis for recurrence: 500 mg PO once daily, plus ethambutol 15 mg/kg/dose PO once daily, with or without rifabutin 300 mg PO once daily

Treatment: 500–600 mg PO once daily with ethambutol 15 mg/kg/dose PO once daily with or without rifabutin 300 mg PO once daily

Endocarditis prophylaxis: 500 mg PO × 1, 30–60 min before procedure

Antiinflammatory agent in cystic fibrosis: Use same dosing in children.

Ophthalmic:

≥1 yr and adult: Instill one drop into the affected eye(s) BID, 8–12 hr apart, × 2 days, followed by one drop once daily for the next 5 days

No longer recommended for otitis media due to increased resistant pathogens.
Contraindicated in hypersensitivity to macrolides and history of cholestatic jaundice/ hepatic dysfunction associated with prior use. **Use with caution** in impaired hepatic function, GFR <10 mL/min (limited data), hypokalemia, hypomagnesemia, bradycardia, arrhythmias, prolonged QT intervals, and receiving medications that can cause the aforementioned conditions of caution. May cause increase in hepatic enzymes, cholestatic jaundice, GI discomfort, and pain at injection site (IV use). Compared with other macrolides, less risk for drug interactions. Nelfinavir may increase azithromycin levels; monitor for liver enzyme abnormalities and hearing impairment. Vomiting, diarrhea, and nausea have been reported at higher frequency in otitis media with 1-day dosing regimen. Exacerbations of myasthenia gravis/syndrome, serious skin reactions (e.g., SJS and TEN), infantile hypertrophic pyloric stenosis, decreased lymphocytes, and elevated bilirubin, BUN, and creatinine have been reported. CNS penetration is poor.

Aluminum- and magnesium-containing antacids decrease absorption. Tablet and oral suspension dosage forms may be administered with or without food. Extended release oral suspension should be taken on an empty stomach (at least 1 hr before or 2 hr following a meal). Intravenous administration is over 1–3 hr; **do not** give as a bolus or IM injection.

Ophthalmic Use: Do not wear contact lenses. Eye irritation is the most common side effect.

AZTREONAM
Azactam, Cayston, and generic intravenous products
Antibiotic, monobactam

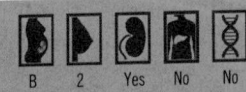

B   2   Yes   No   No

Injection: 1, 2 g; each 1 g drug contains approximately 780 mg L-arginine
Nebulizer solution (Cayston): 75 mg powder to be reconstituted with the supplied diluent of 1 mL
0.17% sodium chloride (28-day course kit contains 84 sterile vials of Cayston and 88 ampules of
sterile diluent)

Neonate:
   30 mg/kg/dose IV/IM (higher doses may be necessary for meningitis):
      Gestational age <34 wk:
         ≤7 days old: Q12 hr
         >7 days old: Q8 hr
      Gestational age ≥34 wk:
         ≤7 days old: Q8 hr
         >7 days old: Q6 hr
Child: 90–120 mg/kg/24 hr ÷ Q6–8 hr IV/IM; **max. dose:** 2 g/dose and 8 g/24 hr
Cystic fibrosis: 150–200 mg/kg/24 hr ÷ Q6–8 hr IV/IM (**max. dose:** 8 g/24 hr). Alternatively, higher
   doses have been used at 200–300 mg/kg/24 hr ÷ Q6 hr IV/IM (**max. dose:** 12 g/24 hr)
Adult: Moderate infections: 1–2 g/dose Q8–12 hr IV/IM
   Severe infections: 2 g/dose Q6–8 hr IV/IM
   Max. dose: 8 g/24 hr
Inhalation:
   Cystic fibrosis prophylaxis therapy:
      ≥7 yr and adult: 75 mg TID (minimum 4 hr between doses) administered in repeated cycles of 28
      days on drug followed by 28 days off drug. Administer each dose with the Altera Nebulizer System.

Typically indicated in multidrug resistant aerobic gram-negative infections when β-lactam
therapy is contraindicated. Well-absorbed IM. **Use with caution** in arginase deficiency.
Low cross-allergenicity between aztreonam and other β-lactams. Adverse reactions:
thrombophlebitis, eosinophilia, leukopenia, neutropenia, thrombocytopenia, elevation
of liver enzymes, hypotension, seizures, and confusion. Good CNS penetration. Probenecid
and furosemide increase aztreonam levels. **Adjust dose in renal failure (see Chapter 31).**
INHALATIONAL USE: Cough, nasal congestion, wheezing, pharyngolaryngeal pain, pyrexia, chest
discomfort, abdominal pain, and vomiting may occur. Bronchospasm has been reported. Use the
following order of administration: bronchodilator first, chest physiotherapy, other inhaled
medications (if indicated), and aztreonam last. Cayston vials and diluent ampules should be stored
in the refrigerator (2-8° C), but once they are removed from the refrigerator, they can be stored at
room temperature for up to 28 days. Cayston vials should be protected from light.

B

BACITRACIN ± POLYMYXIN B
Various ophthalmic and topical generic products
In combination with polymyxin B: AK-Poly-Bac
Ophthalmic, Polycin, Double Antibiotic Topical,
Polysporin Topical and others
Antibiotic, topical

C   ?   No   No   No

BACITRACIN:
Ophthalmic ointment: 500 units/g (3.5 g)
Topical ointment (OTC): 500 units/g (1, 14, 15, 28, 30, 454 g)

BACITRACIN ± POLYMYXIN B *continued*

BACITRACIN IN COMBINATION WITH POLYMYXIN B:

Ophthalmic ointment (AK-Poly-Bac Ophthalmic, Polycin, and generics): 500 units bacitracin +10,000 units polymyxin B/g (3.5 g)

Topical ointment (OTC): 500 units bacitracin +10,000 units polymyxin B/g (15, 30 g)

BACITRACIN:
Child and adult:

Topical: Apply to affected area once daily–TID.

Ophthalmic: Apply 0.25- to 0.5-inch ribbon into the conjunctival sac of the infected eye(s) Q3–12 hr; frequency depends on severity of infection. Administer Q3–4 hr × 7–10 days for mild/moderate infections.

BACITRACIN + POLYMYXIN B:
Child and adult:

Topical: Apply ointment to affected area once daily–TID.

Ophthalmic: Apply 0.25- to 0.5-inch ribbon into the conjunctival sac of the infected eye(s) Q3–12 hr; frequency depends on severity of infection. Administer Q3–4 hr × 7–10 days for mild/moderate infections.

Hypersensitivity reactions to bacitracin and/or polymyxin B can occur. **Do not use** topical ointment for the eyes or for a duration of >7 days. Side effects may include rash, itching, burning, and edema.

Ophthalmic dosage form may cause temporary blurred vision and retard corneal healing. For ophthalmic use, wash hands before use and **avoid contact** of tube tip with skin or eye.

For neomycin-containing products, see Neomycin/Polymyxin B/± Bacitracin.

BACLOFEN
Lioresal, Gablofen, Lyvispah, Ozobax, Fleqsuvy, and generics
Centrally acting skeletal muscle relaxant

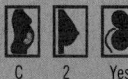

| C | 2 | Yes | No | No |

Tabs: 5, 10, 20 mg

Oral granules (Lyvispah): 5, 10, 20 mg (90 packets); contains saccharin

Oral suspension: 5, 10 mg/mL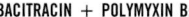

Fleqsuvy: 5 mg/mL (120, 300 mL); contains propylene glycol and sodium benzoate

Oral solution (Ozobax and generics): 1 mg/mL (473 mL); may contain parabens

Injection:

Gablofen: 50 mCg/mL (1 mL), 0.5 mg/mL (20 mL), 1 mg/mL (20 mL), 2 mg/mL (20 mL); preservative free

Lioresal: 50 mCg/mL (1 mL), 0.5 mg/mL (20 mL), 2 mg/mL (5, 20 mL); preservative free

Generics: 0.5 mg/mL (20 mL), 1 mg/mL (20 mL), 2 mg/mL (20 mL); preservative free

Oral: Dosage increments, if tolerated, are made at 3-day intervals until desired effect or max. dose is achieved. Initiate first dosage level at QHS, followed by Q12 hr and then Q8 hr. Dosage increments are made by first increasing the QHS dosage, followed by the morning dosage and then the remaining mid-day dosage.

Child (PO, see remarks):

<20 kg: Start at 2.5 mg QHS, increase in 2.5 mg increments, if needed, up to the recommended **max. dose**, below.

≥20–50 kg: Start at 5 mg QHS, increase in 5 mg increments, if needed, up to the recommended **max. dose**, below.

>50 kg: Start at 10 mg QHS, increase in 10 mg increments, if needed, up to the recommended **max. dose**, below.

Continued

BACLOFEN *continued*

Recommended max. PO dose:
2 yr–<8 yr: 60 mg/24 hr
8–16 yr: 80 mg/24 hr
>16 yr: 120 mg/24 hr
Adult (PO):
Start at 5 mg TID, increase in 5 mg increments, if needed, up to a **maximum** of 80 mg/24 hr.
Intrathecal continuous infusion maintenance therapy (not well established):
<12 yr: Average dose of 274 mCg/24 hr (range: 24–1199 mCg/24 hr) has been reported.
≥12 yr and adult: Most required 300–800 mCg/24 hr (range: 12–2003 mCg/24 hr with limited experience at doses >1000 mCg/24 hr).

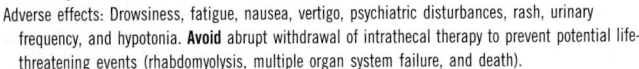

Avoid abrupt withdrawal of drug. **Use with caution** in patients with seizure disorder or impaired renal function. Approximately 70%–80% of the drug is excreted in the urine unchanged. Administer oral doses with food or milk.

Adverse effects: Drowsiness, fatigue, nausea, vertigo, psychiatric disturbances, rash, urinary frequency, and hypotonia. **Avoid** abrupt withdrawal of intrathecal therapy to prevent potential life-threatening events (rhabdomyolysis, multiple organ system failure, and death).

Cases of intrathecal mass at the tip of the implanted catheter leading to withdrawal symptoms have been reported. Inadvertent subcutaneous injection may occur with improper access of the reservoir refill septum and may result in an overdose. Sterile techniques must be used with intrathecal use, accounting for all nonsterile external surfaces.

Usual maintenance oral dosage range observed from a collection of smaller prospective and retrospective studies suggests the following (see dosage section for initial dose titration):
<2 yr: 10–20 mg/24 hr ÷ Q8 hr to a **maximum** of 40 mg/24 hr
2–7 yr: 20–40 mg/24 hr ÷ Q8 hr to a **maximum** of 60 mg/24 hr
≥8 yr: 30–40 mg/24 hr ÷ Q8 hr to a **maximum** of 200 mg/24 hr

Caution: Multiple concentrations of the oral liquid dosage form exist (e.g., 1, 5, 10 mg/mL). This is important to consider when completing the medication reconciliation process for needing to determine the dosage in milligrams and NOT the dosage volume that may result in an under- or overdose when using the incorrect medication concentration.

Oral granules dosage form may be administered directly into the mouth or mixed into liquids or soft foods (e.g., applesauce, yogurt, or pudding). Recommended enteral feeding tube size for administering granules: nasogastric (>8 FR), gastrostomy (>12 FR), percutaneous endoscopic gastrostomy (>14 FR), and gastrojejunostomy (>16 FR); see product information for additional details with feeding tube administration.

BALOXAVIR MARBOXIL
Xofluza
Antiviral, endonuclease inhibitor

   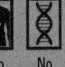

C   ?   No   No   No

Tabs: 40, 80 mg (1 tablet blister card)
Oral suspension: 2 mg/mL (20 mL)

Treatment of influenza (initiate therapy within 48 hr of onset of symptoms):
Child 1–<12 yr (limited data):
<20 kg: 2 mg/kg/dose PO once
≥20 kg: 40 mg PO once
≥12 yr and adult:
<80 kg: 40 mg PO once
≥80 kg: 80 mg PO once

BALOXAVIR MARBOXIL *continued*

Pediatric phase 3 comparison trial with oseltamivir (MINISONE-2) showed comparable efficacy and baloxavir was well tolerated. May be used for influenza postexposure prophylaxis for children ≥12 yr and adults using the same treatment dosage; data are limited for <12 yr old for this indication. Human pregnancy information currently not available.

Adverse effects reported in clinical trials include diarrhea, bronchitis, nasopharyngitis, headache, and nausea.

Baloxavir marboxil is a prodrug that is rapidly converted to the active baloxavir following oral administration. No clinically meaningful pharmacokinetics differences with moderate hepatic impairment (Child-Pugh class B) or with creatinine clearances ≥50 mL/min. Pharmacokinetics have not been evaluated in severe hepatic and/or severe renal impairment.

Primarily metabolized by UGT1A3 with minor contribution from CYP3A4. May reduce the efficacy of intranasal live attenuated influenza vaccine.

Dose may be administered with or without food. **Avoid** coadministration with dairy products, calcium, aluminum, magnesium, multivitamins with minerals, iron, selenium, or zinc, because decreased absorption of baloxavir may occur. Oral suspension dosage form must be administered within 10 hours after reconstitution.

BECLOMETHASONE DIPROPIONATE
QVAR Redihaler, Beconase AQ, Qnasl Children's, Qnasl
Corticosteroid

C   2   No   Yes   No

Breath-activated inhalation aerosol, oral:
    QVAR Redihaler: 40 mCg/inhalation (10.6 g provides 120 inhalations), 80 mCg/inhalation (10.6 g provides 120 inhalations)
Inhalation aerosol, nasal:
    Qnasl Children's: 40 mCg/inhalation (6.8 g provides 60 metered doses)
    Qnasl: 80 mCg/inhalation (10.6 g provides 120 metered doses)
Inhalation suspension, nasal:
    Beconase AQ: 42 mCg/inhalation (25 g provides 180 metered doses); contains benzalkonium chloride

---

Oral inhalation (QVAR Redihaler) (patient requires an inspiratory flow rate of approximately 30 L/min for optimal drug delivery; see remarks):
Asthma maintenance therapy:
    4–11 yr: Start at 40 mCg BID. If response is inadequate after 2 wk, may increase dose to the recommended **maximum dose** of 80 mCg BID.
    ≥12 yr and adult:
        Corticosteroid naïve: Start at 40–80 mCg BID; **max. dose:** 320 mCg BID
        Previous corticosteroid use: Start at 40–160 mCg BID; **max. dose:** 320 mCg BID
Nasal inhalation for allergic rhinitis:
    Beconase AQ:
        6–12 yr: Start with 1 spray (42 mCg) each nostril BID, may increase to the **maximum dose** of 2 sprays each nostril BID if needed. Once symptoms are controlled, decrease dose to 1 spray each nostril BID.
        >12 yr and adult: 1–2 spray(s) (42–84 mCg) each nostril BID
        Maximum dose (>6 yr and adult): 2 sprays each nostril BID or 336 mCg/24 hr
    Qnasl Children's:
        4–11 yr: 1 spray (40 mCg) each nostril once daily; **max. dose:** 2 sprays total (80 mCg)/24 hr

Continued

BECLOMETHASONE DIPROPIONATE *continued*

Qnasl:
 12 yr and adult: 2 sprays (160 mCg) each nostril once daily; **max. dose:** 4 sprays (320 mCg)/24 hr

Not recommended for children <4 yr with oral inhalation and <6 yr (Beconase AQ) or <4 yr (Qnasl Children's) with the nasal administration because of unknown safety and efficacy. Dose should be titrated to lowest effective dose. **Avoid** using higher-than-recommended doses. **Avoid** use of nasal dosage form in recent nasal ulcers, nasal surgery, or nasal trauma. Nasal septal perforation has been reported with nasal product. Psychiatric and behavioral changes have been reported in children with the oral inhalation product. Routinely monitor growth of pediatric patients with chronic use of all dosage forms.

For mild asthma exacerbation in patients with mild/moderate disease, no history of life-threatening exacerbations, and a good asthma self-management plan, limited data in adolescents and adults suggest a temporary quadrupling of the maintenance dosage when asthma control starts to deteriorate. Revert back to baseline maintenance dose after symptoms stabilize or up to a **maximum** of 14 days of the quadrupled dose; whichever comes first. **DO NOT** use this management strategy for children <12 years of age due to the lack of efficacy and increased risk for decreasing linear growth.

When converting from fluticasone to beclomethasone for oral inhalation use, consider the following:

Fluticasone MDI (Flovent HFA)	Fluticasone DPI (Flovent Diskus)	Beclomethasone BAI (QVAR Redihaler)
44 mCg: 2 puffs BID	50 mCg: 2 inhalations BID	40 mCg: 1 puff BID
110 mCg: 2 puffs BID	100 mCg: 2 inhalations BID	40 mCg: 2 puffs BID
220 mCg: 2 puffs BID	250 mCg: 2 inhalations BID	80 mCg: 2 puffs BID

BAI, Breath-activated inhaler; *DPI,* dry powder inhaler; *MDI,* metered dose inhaler.

CYP 450 3A4 inhibitors (e.g., ketoconazole, erythromycin, and protease inhibitors) or significant hepatic impairment may increase systemic exposure of beclomethasone.

Monitor for hypothalamic, pituitary, adrenal, or growth suppression, and hypercorticism. Rinse mouth and gargle with water after oral inhalation; may cause thrush.

QVAR Redihaler is a breath-activated inhaler device and requires the patient to have a minimum inspiratory flow rate of 30 L/min for proper dose activation and does not require priming. **Do not** shake the Redihaler device with the cap open, and **do not use** it with a tube spacer or volume holding chamber.

BENZOYL PEROXIDE
BP Gel, BP Wash, Oxy-5, Oxy-10, PanOxyl, and
many other products
Topical acne product

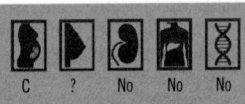

C   ?   No   No   No

Liquid wash [OTC]: 2.5% (240 mL), 5% (120, 150, 240 mL), 7% (480 mL), 10% (120, 150, 240 mL)
Liquid cream wash [OTC]: 4% (170 g), 7% (180 g)
Bar [OTC]: 10% (113 g)
Lotion [OTC]: 5% (30, 120 mL), 8% (297 g), 10% (30, 120 mL)
Cream [OTC]: 5% (3, 30 g), 10% (30 g)
Gel [OTC]: 2.5% (60 g), 5% (42.5, 60, 90 g), 6.5% (113 g), 8% (113 g), 10% (42.5, 60, 90 g)
NOTE: Some preparations may contain alcohol and come in combination packs of cleansers and creams at various strengths.

BENZOYL PEROXIDE *continued*

Combination product with erythromycin (Benzamycin and generics):
 Gel: 30 mg erythromycin and 50 mg benzoyl peroxide per g (23.3, 46 g); some preparations may contain 20% alcohol.
Combination product with clindamycin:
 Gel: 10 mg clindamycin and 50 mg benzoyl peroxide per g (25, 35, 50 g), 12 mg clindamycin and 25 mg benzoyl peroxide per g (50 g), 12 mg clindamycin and 50 mg benzoyl peroxide per g (45 g); some preparations may contain methylparaben.
  Acanya: 12 mg clindamycin and 25 mg benzoyl peroxide per g (50 g); contains propylene glycol
  Neuac: 12 mg clindamycin and 50 mg benzoyl peroxide per g (45 g); contains parabens
  Onexton: 12 mg clindamycin and 37.5 mg benzoyl peroxide per g (3.5, 50 g); contains propylene glycol
Combination product with adapalene: See Adapalene ± Benzoyl Peroxide.

Acne (child ≥12 yr and adult, see remarks):
 Cleansers (liquid wash, or bar): Wet affected area prior to application. Apply and wash once daily—BID; rinse thoroughly, and pat dry. Modify dose frequency or concentration to control the amount of drying or peeling.
 Lotion, cream, or gel: Cleanse skin, and apply small amounts over affected areas once daily initially; increase frequency to BID—TID, if needed. Modify dose frequency or concentration to control drying or peeling.
 Combination products (these products have not been evaluated beyond 12 weeks of use):
  Generics: Apply once daily to affected areas after washing and drying skin. The 10 mg clindamycin and 50 mg benzoyl peroxide per g product may be administered BID (morning and evening).
  Acanya and Onexton: Apply pea-sized amount to affected areas once daily after washing and drying skin.
  Neuac: Apply a thin layer QHS to affected areas after washing and drying skin.

Contraindicated in known history of hypersensitivity to product's components (benzoyl peroxide, clindamycin, or erythromycin). **Avoid** contact with mucous membranes and eyes. May cause skin irritation, stinging, dryness, peeling, erythema, edema, and contact dermatitis. Anaphylaxis has been reported with products containing clindamycin and benzoyl peroxide.
Concomitant topical acne therapy should be used with caution due to possible cumulative irritancy effect. Concurrent use with tretinoin (Retin-A) will increase risk of skin irritation. Products containing clindamycin and erythromycin should not be used in combination.
Any single application resulting in excessive stinging or burning may be removed with mild soap and water. Lotion, cream, and gel dosage forms should be applied to dry skin.
Data are limited for use <12 yr of age.

BENZTROPINE MESYLATE
Generics; previously available as Cogentin
Anticholinergic agent, drug-induced dystonic reaction antidote, anti-Parkinson agent

   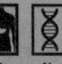

? ? No No No

Injection: 1 mg/mL (2 mL)
Tabs: 0.5, 1, 2 mg

Drug-induced extrapyramidal symptoms (PO/IM/IV; see remarks):
 >3 yr: 0.02—0.05 mg/kg/dose once daily—BID
 Adult: 1—4 mg/dose once daily—BID

Continued

BENZTROPINE MESYLATE *continued*

Acute dystonic reactions (IM/IV; see remarks):
   Child: 0.02 mg/kg/dose (**max. dose:** 1 mg) × 1
   Adult: 1—2 mg/dose × 1

Contraindicated in myasthenia gravis, GI/GU obstruction, untreated narrow-angle glaucoma, and peptic ulcer. Use IV route **only** when PO and IM routes are not feasible. May cause anticholinergic side effects, especially constipation and dry mouth. Drug interactions include: potentiate CNS depressant effects when used with CNS depressants; enhance CNS side effects of amantadine; and inhibit the response of neuroleptics. This medication has not been formally assigned a pregnancy category by the FDA. The Australian pregnancy ratings have deemed use in pregnancy to a limited number of women without an increase in frequency of malformation or other direct/indirect harmful effects.
Onset of action: 15 min for IV/IM and 1 hr for PO.
Oral doses should be administered with food to decrease GI upset.

BERACTANT

See Surfactant, pulmonary.

BETAMETHASONE
Injection: Celestone Soluspan and generics
Topical: Diprolene, Luxiq, Sernivo, and generics
Corticosteroid

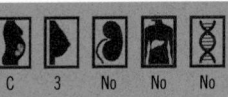

C   3   No   No   No

Na Phosphate and Acetate:
   Injection suspension (Celestone Soluspan and generics): 6 mg/mL (3 mg/mL Na phosphate +3 mg/mL betamethasone acetate) (5 mL); may contain benzalkonium chloride and EDTA
Dipropionate:
   Topical cream: 0.05% (15, 45 g)
   Topical emulsion (Sernivo): 0.05% (120 mL); contains parabens
   Topical lotion: 0.05% (60 mL); may contain 46.8% alcohol and propylene glycol
   Topical ointment: 0.05% (15, 45 g)
Valerate:
   Topical cream: 0.1% (15, 45 g)
   Topical foam (Luxiq and generics): 1.2 mg/g (50, 100 g); may contain 60.4% ethanol, cetyl alcohol, stearyl alcohol, and propylene glycol
   Topical lotion: 0.1% (60 mL); may contain 47.5% isopropyl alcohol
   Topical ointment: 0.1% (15, 45 g)
Dipropionate augmented:
   Topical cream: 0.05% (15, 50 g); contains propylene glycol
   Topical gel: 0.05% (15, 50 g); contains propylene glycol
   Topical lotion: 0.05% (60 mL); contains 30% isopropyl alcohol
   Topical ointment (Diprolene and generics): 0.05% (15, 45, 50 g); contains propylene glycol

All dosages should be adjusted based on patient response and severity of condition
   (see remarks).
Antiinflammatory:
   Child:
      IM: 0.0175—0.125 mg/kg/24 hr or 0.5—7.5 mg/m²/24 hr Q6—12 hr

BETAMETHASONE *continued*

Adolescent and adult:
IM: 0.6—9 mg/24 hr ÷ Q12—24 hr

Topical (use smallest amount for shortest period of time to avoid adrenal suppression, and reassess diagnosis if no improvement is achieved after 2 wk; see remarks):

Valerate and dipropionate forms:
Child and adult: Apply to affected areas once daily—BID.

Dipropionate augmented forms (see remarks):
≥13 yr—adult: Apply to affected areas once daily—BID.

Max. dose: 14 days and the following specific dosage form maximum amount
Cream, ointment, and gel: 50 g/wk
Lotion: 50 mL/wk

Use with caution in hypothyroidism, cirrhosis, ulcerative colitis, and history of allergic reactions to corticosteroids. See Chapter 8 for relative steroid potencies and doses based on body surface area. Betamethasone is inadequate when used alone for adrenocortical insufficiency because of its minimal mineralocorticoid properties. Like all steroids, may cause hypertension, pseudotumor cerebri, acne, Cushing syndrome, adrenal axis suppression, GI bleeding, hyperglycemia, and osteoporosis.

Betamethasone is a substrate for CYP 450 3A4, and use with a strong inhibitor (e.g., ketoconazole and itraconazole) may lead to increased exposure and side effects of betamethasone.

Na phosphate and acetate injectable suspension recommended for IM, intra-articular, intrasynovial intralesional, soft tissue use only; but **not** for IV use. Topical betamethasone dipropionate augmented (Diprolene and Diprolene AF) is **not recommended** in children ≤12 yr owing to the higher risk for adrenal suppression.

Injectable IM dosage form is used in premature labor to stimulate fetal lung maturation.

BICITRA

See Citrate Mixtures.

BISACODYL
Dulcolax, Ducodyl, Bisacodyl EC, Fleet Bisacodyl, and various other names
Laxative, stimulant

B   1   No   No   No

Tabs (enteric coated) [OTC]: 5 mg
Suppository [OTC]: 10 mg
Enema (Fleet Bisacodyl) [OTC]: 10 mg/30 mL (37.5 mL)
Delayed release tabs [OTC]: 5 mg

Oral (administered 6 hr before desired effect):
Child (3—10 yr): 5 mg once daily
>10 yr and adolescent: 5—10 mg once daily
Adult: 5—15 mg once daily

Rectal suppository (see remarks):
2—10 yr: 5 mg once daily
>10 yr and adolescent: 5—10 mg once daily
Adult: 10 mg once daily

Continued

BISACODYL *continued*

Rectal enema (as a single dose):
    2—10 yr: 5 mg (15 mL) × 1
    >10—18 yr: 5—10 mg (15—30 mL) × 1
    Adult: 10 mg (30 mL) × 1

Do not use in newborn period. Instruct patient/parent that tablets should be swallowed whole, **not** chewed or crushed; **not** to be given within 1 hr of antacids or milk. May cause abdominal cramps, nausea, vomiting, and rectal irritation. Oral usually effective within 6—10 hr; rectal usually effective within 15—60 min.

Antacids may decrease the effect of bisacodyl and may cause the premature release of the delayed release formulation prior to reaching the large intestine. Use of suppository should be retained in the rectum for 15—20 min.

BISMUTH SUBSALICYLATE
Pepto-Bismol, Bismatrol, Pink Bismuth, Stomach
Relief, Stomach Relief Extra Strength, and
many others (see remarks)
Antidiarrheal, gastrointestinal ulcer agent

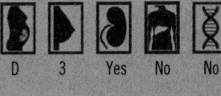

D   3   Yes   No   No

Liquid [OTC]:
    Pepto-Bismol, Bismatrol, Pink Bismuth, Stomach Relief, and others: 262 mg/15 mL (240, 360, 480 mL)
    Stomach Relief Extra Strength: 525 mg/15 mL (237 mL)
Chewable tabs [OTC]: 262 mg; may contain aspartame
Contains 102 mg salicylate per 262 mg tablet; or 129 mg salicylate per 15 mL of the 262 mg/15 mL liquid

Diarrhea:
    Child: 100 mg/kg/24 hr ÷ 5 equal doses for 5 days; **max. dose:** 4.19 g/24 hr
    Dosage by age: *Give following dose Q30 min to 1 hr PRN up to a **max. dose** of 8 doses/24 hr:*
        3—5 yr: 87.3 mg (1/3 tablet or 5 mL of 262 mg/15 mL)
        6—8 yr: 174.7 mg (2/3 tablet or 10 mL of 262 mg/15 mL)
        9—11 yr: 262 mg (1 tablet or 15 mL of 262 mg/15 mL)
        ≥12 yr—adult: 524 mg (2 tablets or 30 mL of 262 mg/15 mL)
Helicobacter pylori **gastric infection** (as part of a 3 or 4 drug combination therapy; doses not well established for children):
    Child: 8 mg/kg/24 hr PO ÷ BID × 10—14 days, or 262 mg PO QID × 7—14 days has been reported.
    Adult: 300 mg PO QID × 10—14 days

Generally not recommended in children <16 yr with chicken pox or flu-like symptoms (risk for Reye syndrome), in combination with other nonsteroidal antiinflammatory drugs, anticoagulants, or oral antidiabetic agents, or in severe renal failure. **Use with caution** in bleeding disorders, renal dysfunction, gastritis, and gout. May cause darkening of tongue and/or black stools, GI upset, impaction, and decreased platelet aggregation.

Drug combination appears to have antisecretory and antimicrobial effects with some antiinflammatory effects. Absorption of bismuth is negligible, whereas approximately 80% of the salicylate is absorbed. Decreases absorption of tetracycline. The salicylate component may increase the effects/toxicity of antiplatelet, anticoagulant, and blood glucose—lowering medications and increase nephrotoxicity risk when used with ACE inhibitors.

DO NOT use Children's Pepto (calcium carbonate) because it does not contain bismuth subsalicylate. **Avoid use in renal failure (see Chapter 31).**

BOSENTAN
Tracleer and generics
Endothelin receptor antagonist

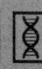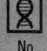

X   3   No   Yes   No

Tabs: 62.5, 125 mg
Dispersible tabs (to be dissolved in water to make an oral suspension):
  Tracleer: 32 mg (scored); contains aspartame
Oral suspension: 6.25 mg/mL

Pulmonary arterial hypertension (see remarks):
  2015 AHA/ATS Pediatric Pulmonary Hypertension Guidelines:
    <10 kg: Start at 1 mg/kg/dose PO BID, then increase to 2 mg/kg/dose PO BID.
    10–20 kg: Start at 15.625 mg PO BID, then increase to 31.25 mg PO BID.
    >20–40 kg: Start at 31.25 mg PO BID, then increase to 62.5 mg PO BID.
    >40 kg: Start at 62.5 mg PO BID, then increase to 125 mg PO BID.
  Alternative FDA-labeled dosing by age and weight (PO):

Age	Weight (kg)	Dosage (PO)
≤12 yr	4–8	16 mg BID
	>8–16	32 mg BID
	>16–24	48 mg BID
	>24–40	64 mg BID
>12 yr	≤40	62.5 mg BID
	>40	62.5 mg BID × 4 wk, then 125 mg BID

Dosage Modification for Transaminase Elevation:

ALT/AST Levels	Dosage Adjustment
>3 to ≤5× ULN	Reconfirm by another aminotransferase test; if confirmed, modify dosage regimen (always reassess aminotransferase levels within 3 days and Q2 wk thereafter to any dosage reintroduction or reduction): ≤12 yr, and >12 yr and ≤40 kg: Interrupt therapy. If aminotransferase returns to pretreatment levels, reintroduce with dosage prior to interruption. >12 yr and >40 kg, and adult: Reduce dosage to 62.5 mg PO BID; or interrupt therapy and monitor aminotransferase levels Q2 wk (if aminotransferase levels return to pretreatment levels, continue with most recent dosage or 62.5 mg PO BID).
>5 to ≤8× ULN	Reconfirm by another aminotransferase test; if confirmed, stop treatment and monitor aminotransferase at least Q2 wk. Once aminotransferase returns to pretreatment levels, consider reintroduction of bosentan and reassess aminotransferase within 3 days and Q2 wk thereafter to any dosage reintroduction or reduction: ≤12 yr, and >12 yr and ≤40 kg: Dosage prior to discontinuing >12 yr and >40 kg, and adult: 62.5 mg PO BID
>8× ULN	All ages: Discontinue treatment permanently

ULN, Upper limit of normal.

Continued

BOSENTAN *continued*

Contraindicated in women who are or may become pregnant and with concurrent use of cyclosporine (increases bosentan concentrations) or glyburide (increases risk for hepatotoxicity). Due to these risks, bosentan is available only through the Tracleer REMS program, where prescribers and pharmacies need to be certified. See www.BosentanREMSProgram.com or call 1-866-359-2612 for more information.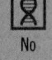

Baseline and monthly monitoring of serum aminotransferases and bilirubin; and pregnancy tests for females of reproductive potential (two forms of birth control required) are required. Use should be **avoided** in patients with preexisting hepatic impairment (baseline aminotransferases >3 times the usual normal limit).

May cause respiratory tract infections, anemia (dose related), edema, increased liver aminotransferases (see dosage modification; higher incidence in adults), and pyrexia. Decreased sperm counts, liver cirrhosis, liver failure, DRESS, thrombocytopenia, and sinusitis have been reported.

Bosentan is substrate for the CYP2C9 and 3A4 enzymes, and OATP1B1/SLCO1B1 transporter. It also induces CYP2C9 and 3A4; may decrease sildenafil levels. Reduces the effectiveness of hormonal contraceptives.

Doses may be administered orally with or without food.

BREO ELLIPTA

See Fluticasone Furoate + Vilanterol.

BROMPHENIRAMINE WITH PHENYLEPHRINE
Children's Dimetapp Cold and Allergy, Rynex PE,
Ru-Hist D, and many other products
Antihistamine + decongestant

C   3   No   No   No

Oral liquid/syrup (Children's Dimetapp Cold and Allergy, Rynex PE, and others) [OTC]:
Brompheniramine 1 mg + phenylephrine 2.5 mg/5 mL (118, 237 mL); contains propylene glycol and sodium benzoate

Tabs (Ru-Hist D) [OTC]: Brompheniramine 4 mg + phenylephrine 10 mg

NOTE: Other combination products exist, using the Dimetapp name; always check the specific ingredients and their concentration (amount) with each specific product.

All doses based on brompheniramine component (see remarks).
  2 to <6 yr: 1 mg Q4 hr PRN PO up to a **max. dose** of 6 mg/24 hr
  6–12 yr: 2 mg Q4 hr PRN PO up to a **max. dose** of 12 mg/24 hr
  ≥12 yr and adult: 4 mg Q4 hr PRN PO up to a **max. dose** of 24 mg/24 hr
Alternatively, dosing based on specific dosage forms/products. CAUTION: These products may be available in different concentrations (see remarks).
  Oral, liquid/syrup (Children's Dimetapp Cold and Allergy and Rynex PE):
    6 to <12 yr: 10 mL Q4 hr PRN PO up to a **max. dose** of 60 mL/24 hr
    ≥12 yr and adult: 20 mL Q4 hr PRN PO up to a **max. dose** of 120 mL/24 hr
  Oral, tab (Ru-Hist D):
    6 to <12 yr: 0.5 tab Q4 hr PRN PO **not to exceed** 3 tablets/24 hr
    ≥12 yr and adult: 1 tab Q4 hr PRN PO **not to exceed** 6 tablets/24 hr

Generally not recommended for treating URIs for infants. No proven benefit for infants and young children with URIs. Over-the-counter (OTC or nonprescription) use of this product is **not recommended** for children <6 yr old due to reports of serious adverse effects (cardiac and respiratory distress, convulsions, and hallucinations) and fatalities (from unintentional overdosages, including combined use of other OTC products containing the same active ingredients).

BROMPHENIRAMINE WITH PHENYLEPHRINE *continued*

Contraindicated with use of MAO inhibitors (concurrent use and within 14 days after discontinuing MAO inhibitor). **Use with caution** in narrow-angle glaucoma, bladder neck obstruction, asthma, pyloroduodenal obstruction, symptomatic prostatic hypertrophy, hypertension, coronary artery disease, diabetes mellitus, and thyroid disease. Discontinue use 48 hr prior to allergy skin testing. May cause drowsiness, fatigue, CNS excitation, xerostomia, blurred vision, and wheezing.

BUDESONIDE
Pulmicort Respules, Pulmicort Flexhaler, Ortikos, Tarpeyo, Uceris, and generics; previously available as Rhinocort Allergy Nasal Spray and Entocort EC
Corticosteroid

    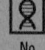
B/C   2/?   No   Yes   No

Nasal spray (generics; previously available as Rhinocort Allergy) [OTC]: 32 mCg/actuation (8.43 mL delivers 120 sprays); may contain disodium EDTA and polysorbate 80
Nebulized inhalation suspension (Pulmicort Respules and generics): 0.25 mg/2 mL, 0.5 mg/2 mL, 1 mg/2 mL (30s); may contain disodium EDTA and polysorbate 80
Oral breath-activated inhalation powder (Pulmicort Flexhaler): 90 mCg/metered dose (165 mg, delivers 60 doses), 180 mCg/metered dose (225 mg, delivers 120 doses); contains lactose
Delayed or extended release capsule:
  Tarpeyo: 4 mg
  Ortikos: 6, 9 mg
Enteric coated granules in a capsule (generics; previously available as Entocort EC): 3 mg
Extended release tablet (Uceris and generics): 9 mg
Rectal foam (Uceris): 2 mg per metered dose (33.4 g, delivers 14 doses; 2 canisters per kit)

Nebulized inhalation suspension (see remarks):
  Child 1—8 yr:
    No prior steroid use: 0.5 mg/24 hr ÷ once daily—BID; **max. dose:** 0.5 mg/24 hr
    Prior inhaled steroid use: 0.5 mg/24 hr ÷ once daily—BID; **max. dose:** 1 mg/24 hr
    Prior oral steroid use: 1 mg/24 hr ÷ once daily—BID; **max. dose:** 1 mg/24 hr
  NIH Asthma Guideline 2007 recommendations (divide daily doses once daily—BID):
    Child 0—4 yr:
      Low dose: 0.25—0.5 mg/24 hr
      Medium dose: >0.5—1 mg/24 hr
      High dose: >1 mg/24 hr
    Child 5—11 yr:
      Low dose: 0.5 mg/24 hr
      Medium dose: 1 mg/24 hr
      High dose: 2 mg/24 hr
Oral inhalation (see remarks):
  Pulmicort Flexhaler (patient requires an inspiratory flow rate of approximately 60 L/min for optimal drug delivery):
    Child ≥6—17 yr: Start at 180 mCg BID; **max. dose:** 720 mCg/24 hr.
    ≥18 yr and adult: Start at 180—360 mCg BID; **max. dose:** 1440 mCg/24 hr.
    NIH Asthma Guideline 2007 recommendations (divide daily doses BID):
      Child 5—11 yr:
        Low dose: 180—400 mCg/24 hr
        Medium dose: >400—800 mCg/24 hr
        High dose: >800 mCg/24 hr

Continued

BUDESONIDE *continued*

Child ≥12 and adolescent:
Low dose: 180—600 mCg/24 hr
Medium dose: >600—1200 mCg/24 hr
High dose: >1200 mCg/24 hr

Nasal inhalation:

≥6 to <12 yr: Start at 1 spray (32 mCg) in each nostril once daily. If needed, increase to 2 sprays (64 mCg) each nostril once daily. Then reduce dose back to initial dose when symptoms improve. Max. nasal dose: 128 mCg/24 hr (4 sprays/24 hr).

≥12 yr to adult: Start at 2 sprays (64 mCg) in each nostril once daily. When symptoms improve, reduce dose to 1 spray (32 mCg) each nostril once daily. Usual max. dose is 128 mCg/24 hr (4 sprays/24 hr) but some may require 256 mCg/24 hr (8 sprays/24 hr) initially with a subsequent reduced dosage to improve symptoms.

Crohn disease:

Child ≥6 yr (see remarks): Data are limited; only the following dosages have been reported. Additional studies are needed.

Active disease: 9 mg/24 hr PO once daily or ÷ Q8 hr × 7—8 wk

Maintenance of remission: 6 mg PO once daily × 3—4 wk

In addition, a report in 10—19 yr old children demonstrated higher remission rates with an induction dose of 12 mg PO once daily × 4 wk, followed by 9 mg PO once daily × 3 wk, followed by 6 mg PO once daily × 3 wk.

Adult:

Active disease: 9 mg PO QAM × 8 wk; if remission is not achieved, a second 8-wk course may be given.

Maintenance of remission: 6 mg PO once daily for up to 3 mo. If symptom control is maintained at 3 mo, taper dosage to compete cessation. Remission therapy beyond 3 mo has not shown to provide substantial clinical benefit.

Ulcerative colitis, induction of remission (Uceris and generics):

Adult:

Extended release oral tablet: 9 mg PO QAM for up to 8 wk

Rectal foam: 2 mg PR BID × 2 wk followed by 2 mg PR once daily × 4 wk

Reduce maintenance dose to as low as possible to control symptoms. May cause pharyngitis, cough, epistaxis, nasal irritation, and HPA-axis suppression. Rinse mouth after each use via the oral inhalation route. Nebulized budesonide has been shown effective in mild to moderate croup at doses of 2 mg × 1. Ref: *N Engl J Med.* 331(5):285.

For mild asthma exacerbation in patients with mild/moderate disease, no history of life-threatening exacerbations, and a good asthma self-management plan, limited data in adolescents and adults suggest a temporary quadrupling of the maintenance dosage when asthma control starts to deteriorate. Revert back to baseline maintenance dose after symptoms stabilize or up to a **maximum** of 14 days of the quadrupled dose, whichever comes first. **DO NOT** use this management strategy for children <12 years of age due to the lack of efficacy and increased risk for decreasing linear growth.

Hypersensitivity reactions, including anaphylaxis, have been reported with the inhaled route. Anaphylactic reactions, rectal bleeding, peripheral edema, mood swings, increased blood pressure, rash, and benign intracranial hypertension have been reported with oral route of administration.

Safety and effectiveness for mild/moderate Crohn disease have been established for children 8—17 yr old weighing ≥25 kg. Safety and efficacy have NOT been established in pediatric patients for the maintenance of clinical remission of mild/moderate Crohn disease. Although the reported safety profile in pediatric Crohn disease is consistent with adults, there may be increased risk for decreased growth velocity due to higher systemic absorption of corticosteroids in children with Crohn disease.

BUDESONIDE *continued*

CYP 450 3A4 inhibitors (e.g., ketoconazole, erythromycin, protease inhibitors) or significant
hepatic impairment may increase systemic exposure of budesonide (inhalation and PO routes).

Onset of action for oral inhalation and nebulized suspension is within 1 day and 2—8 days,
respectively, with peak effects at 1—2 wk and 4—6 wk, respectively.

For nasal use, onset of action is seen after 1 day with peak effects after 3—7 days of therapy.
Discontinue therapy if no improvement in nasal symptoms after 3 wk of continuous therapy.

Pulmicort Flexhaler is a breath-activated device that requires the patient to have an inspiratory flow
rate of approximately 60 L/min for optimal drug delivery.

Pregnancy category is "B" for inhalation routes of administration and "C" for the oral and rectal routes.

Breastfeeding category is "2" for inhalation routes and "?" for the rectal route. Breastfeeding with the
oral route of administration may result in budesonide exposure to the infant up to 10 times higher than
that by the inhalation route. **Do not** crush or chew the oral capsule dosage form.

BUDESONIDE AND FORMOTEROL
Symbicort and generics
*Corticosteroid and long-acting β₂ adrenergic
agonist*

   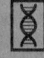

C   2   No   Yes   No

Aerosol inhaler:
>   80 mCg budesonide + 4.5 mCg formoterol fumarate dihydrate (6.9 g delivers 60 inhalations, 10.2 g
>   delivers approximately 120 inhalations)
>   160 mCg budesonide + 4.5 mCg formoterol fumarate dihydrate (6 g delivers 60 inhalations, 10.2 g
>   delivers approximately 120 inhalations)

Asthma maintenance therapy:
>   **5—11 yr (NIH Asthma Guideline 2007 recommendations) and 6 to <12 yr (FDA labeling);
>   see remarks:** Two inhalations BID of 80 mCg budesonide + 4.5 mCg formoterol; **max. dose:** 4
>   inhalations/24 hr
>
>   **≥12 yr and adult (see remarks):**
>>   **No prior inhaled steroid use:** Start with two inhalations BID of 80 mCg budesonide + 4.5 mCg
>>   formoterol **OR** 160 mCg budesonide + 4.5 mCg formoterol, depending on severity.
>>   **Prior low to medium doses of inhaled steroid use:** Start with two inhalations BID of 80 mCg
>>   budesonide + 4.5 mCg formoterol.
>>   **Prior medium to high doses of inhaled steroid use:** Start with two inhalations BID of 160 mCg
>>   budesonide + 4.5 mCg formoterol.
>>   **Max. dose:** 2 inhalations of 160 mCg budesonide + 4.5 mCg formoterol BID

See Budesonide and Formoterol for remarks. Should only be used for patients not adequately
controlled on other asthma-controller medications (e.g., low- to medium-dose inhaled
corticosteroids) or whose disease severity requires the use of two maintenance therapies. Titrate to
the lowest effective strength after asthma is adequately controlled.

Reported side effects at ≥3% and more frequently compared with budesonide alone include URI,
pharyngitis, headache, and rhinitis.

As-needed rescue combination low-dose inhaled corticosteroid (ICS) and formoterol is preferred over
short-acting beta-agonists (SABA) for adolescent and adult patients with asthma for all asthma severity
levels (2022 GINA guidelines; see www.ginasthma.org/gina-reports for the latest updates). Significant
reduction in ED visits/hospitalizations with PRN ICS-formoterol compared to daily ICS and PRN SABA; and
greater reduction in severe asthma exacerbations in adults and adolescents previously taking SABA
alone with PRN ICS-formoterol compared with daily ICS and PRN SABA were also reported. **DO NOT**
substitute formoterol with a slower onset, long-acting beta-agonist (LABA) such as salmeterol.

Continued

BUDESONIDE AND FORMOTEROL *continued*

Proper patient education including dosage administration technique is essential; see patient package insert for detailed instructions. Rinse mouth after each use.

BUMETANIDE Bumex and generics *Loop diuretic*	 C ? No Yes No

Tabs: 0.5, 1, 2 mg
Injection: 0.25 mg/mL (4, 10 mL); some preparations may contain 1% benzyl alcohol

Edema:
Neonate and infant (see remarks): PO/IM/IV
  ≤6 mo: 0.01–0.05 mg/kg/dose once daily or every other day
Infant and child: PO/IM/IV
  >6 mo: 0.015–0.1 mg/kg/dose once daily–QID; **max. dose:** 10 mg/24 hr
Adult:
  PO: 0.5–2 mg/dose as a single dose. If needed, repeat dose(s) in 4–5 hour intervals up to two additional doses.
  IM/IV: 0.5–1 mg (over 1–2 min for IV). May give additional doses Q2–3 hr PRN
  Max. dose (PO/IM/IV): 10 mg/24 hr

Cross-allergenicity may occur in patients allergic to sulfonamides. Dosage reduction may be necessary in patients with hepatic dysfunction. Administer oral doses with food.
Side effects include cramps, dizziness, hypotension, headache, electrolyte losses (hypokalemia, hypocalcemia, hyponatremia, hypochloremia), and encephalopathy. May also lead to metabolic alkalosis. Serious skin reactions (e.g., Stevens-Johnson, TEN) have been reported.
Drug elimination has been reported to be slower in neonates with respiratory disorders compared with neonates without. May displace bilirubin in critically ill neonates. **Maximal** diuretic effect for infants ≤6 mo has been reported at 0.04 mg/kg/dose with greater efficacy seen at lower dosages.

BUTORPHANOL Generics; previously available as Stadol *Narcotic, analgesic*	 C 3 Yes Yes No

Injection: 1 mg/mL (1 mL), 2 mg/mL (1, 2 mL)
Nasal solution: 10 mg/mL (2.5 mL); 1 mg per spray

Child (limited data): 0.01–0.02 mg/kg/dose (**max. dose:** 2 mg/dose) IV Q3–4 hr PRN. Use of  a single dose of 0.03 mg/kg IV has been reported in postoperative patients.
Adult:
  IV: 1 mg/dose Q3–4 hr PRN; usual dosage range: 0.5–2 mg Q3–4 hr PRN
  IM: 2 mg/dose Q3–4 hr PRN; usual dosage range: 1–4 mg Q3–4 hr PRN
  Intranasal: 1 spray (1 mg) in one nostril × 1; an additional 1 mg dose may be given at 1–1.5 hr if needed. This 2-dose sequence may be repeated in 3–4 hr if needed. Alternatively, the patient may receive 2 mg initially (1 mg in each nostril) only if they remain recumbent if drowsiness or dizziness occurs; an additional dose may be given 3–4 hr later.

BUTORPHANOL *continued*

A synthetic mixed agonist/antagonist opioid analgesic used when alternative treatment options are ineffective or not tolerated. **Contraindicated** in patients hypersensitive to benzethonium chloride. **Use with caution** in hypotension, thyroid dysfunction, renal or hepatic impairment, and concomitant CNS depressants. **Suggested dosage reduction** in renal impairment (IV/IM): 75% of usual dose for GFR 10–50 mL/min and 50% of usual dose for GFR <10 mL/min with an increase in dosage interval based on duration of clinical effects. A 50% IV/IM dosage reduction with increased dosage interval has been recommended in hepatic dysfunction. Reduced dosage for intranasal administration for both renal and hepatic impairment: initial dose should not exceed 1 mg.

Butorphanol is a P450 3A4 substrate. Cytochrome P450 3A4 inhibitors may increase butophanol's effects and toxicity (fatal respiratory depression).

Common side effects include drowsiness, dizziness, insomnia (nasal spray), nausea, vomiting, nasal congestion (nasal spray). Severe respiratory depression has been reported with use of nasal solutions.

Onset of action: 5–10 min (IV); 0.5–1 hr (IM); and within 15 min (intranasal). **Duration:** 3–4 hr (IV/IM) and 4–5 hr (intranasal).

C

CAFFEINE CITRATE
Cafcit and generics
Methylxanthine, respiratory stimulant

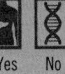

C 2 Yes Yes No

Injection: 20 mg/mL (3 mL)
Oral liquid: 20 mg/mL (3 mL), also available as powder for compounding 10 or 20 mg/mL
20 mg/mL caffeine citrate salt = 10 mg/mL caffeine base

Doses expressed in mg of caffeine citrate.
Apnea of prematurity:
    Loading dose: 20–25 mg/kg IV/PO × 1
    Maintenance dose: 5–10 mg/kg/dose PO/IV Q24 hr, to begin 24 hr after loading dose

Avoid use in symptomatic cardiac arrhythmias. **Do not use** caffeine benzoate formulations in neonates; it has been associated with kernicterus. **Use with caution** in impaired renal or hepatic function; monitor serum concentration to prevent toxicity.

Therapeutic levels: 5–25 mg/L. Cardiovascular, neurologic, or GI toxicity reported at serum levels >50 mg/L. Recommended serum sampling time: obtain trough level within 30 min prior to a dose. Steady state is typically achieved 3 wk after initiation of therapy. Levels obtained prior to steady state are useful for preventing toxicity.

For IV administration, give loading dose over 30 min and maintenance dose over 10 min.

CALCITONIN—SALMON
Miacalcin and generics; previously available as
Fortical and Miacalcin as nasal sprays
Hypercalcemia antidote, antiosteoporotic

    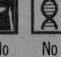

C ? No No No

Injection (Miacalcin and generics): 200 U/mL (2 mL); contains phenol

Continued

CALCITONIN—SALMON *continued*

Nasal spray: 200 U/metered dose (3.7 mL provides at least 30 doses); may contain benzalkonium chloride or chlorobutanol

Osteogenesis imperfecta:
>6 mo—adolescent: 2 U/kg/dose IM/SC 3 times per week

Hypercalcemia (see remarks):
Adult: Start with 4 U/kg/dose IM/SC Q12 hr; if response is unsatisfactory after 1 or 2 days, may increase dose to 8 U/kg/dose Q12 hr. If response remains unsatisfactory after 2 more days, increase to a **max. dose** of 8 U/kg/dose Q6 hr.

Paget disease (see remarks):
Adult: Start with 100 U IM/SC once daily initially, followed by lower maintenance dose of 50 U 3 times per week if sufficient.

Contraindicated in patients sensitive to salmon protein or gelatin. Because of hypersensitivity risk (e.g., bronchospasm, airway swelling, anaphylaxis), skin test is recommended before initiating IM/SC therapy. For skin test, prepare a 10-U/mL dilution with normal saline (NS), administer 0.1 mL intradermally, and observe for 15 min for wheal or significant erythema. Tachyphylaxis has been reported after 2–3 days of use for the treatment of hypercalcemia of malignancy.

Nausea, abdominal pain, diarrhea, flushing, and inflammation/urticaria at the injection site have been reported with IM/SC route of administration. May decrease lithium levels via enhanced urinary clearance. Hypocalcemia and increased risk for malignancies have been reported in a meta-analysis.

Intranasal use currently indicated for postmenopausal osteoporosis in adults. Nasal irritation (alternate nostrils to reduce risk), rhinitis, and epistaxis may occur with the intranasal product.

Tremors have been reported with both intranasal and injectable routes of administration.

If the injection volume exceeds 2 mL, use IM route and multiple sites of injection.

CALCITRIOL
1,25-dihydroxycholecalciferol, Rocaltrol, and generics
Active form vitamin D, fat soluble

   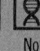

C   2   No   No   No

Caps (Rocaltrol and generics): 0.25, 0.5 mCg; may contain parabens
Oral solution (Rocaltrol and generics): 1 mCg/mL (15 mL)
Injection (generics; previously available as Calcijex): 1 mCg/mL (1 mL); contains EDTA

Neonatal hypocalcemia: 0.25—1 mCg/dose PO once daily
Hypoparathyroidism (evaluate dosage at 2- to 4-wk intervals and note the different mCg/dose vs. mCg/kg/dose per respective age group below):
Child >1 yr and adult: Initial dose of 0.25 mCg/dose PO once daily. May increase daily dosage by 0.25 mCg at 2- to 4-wk intervals. Usual maintenance dosage as follows:
<1 yr (limited data): 0.02—0.06 mCg/kg/dose PO once daily
1—5 yr: 0.25—0.75 mCg/dose PO once daily
>6 yr and adult: 0.5—2 mCg/dose PO once daily

Renal failure: See the National Kidney Foundation guidelines at https://kdigo.org/guidelines/ckd-mbd/

Most potent vitamin D metabolite available. Should not be used to treat 25-OH vitamin D deficiency; use cholecalciferol or ergocalciferol. Monitor serum calcium and phosphorus, and parathyroid hormone (PTH) in dialysis patients. **Avoid** concomitant use of Mg^{2+}-containing antacids. IV dosing applies if patient is undergoing hemodialysis.

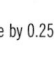

CALCITRIOL *continued*

Contraindicated in patients with hypercalcemia or vitamin D toxicity. Side effects include: weakness, headache, vomiting, constipation, hypotonia, polydipsia, polyuria, myalgia, metastatic calcification, etc. Allergic reactions, including anaphylaxis, have been reported. May increase serum creatinine in predialysis patients.

CALCIUM ACETATE
Calphron, Phoslyra, and generics; previously
available as PhosLo; 25% elemental Ca
Calcium supplement, phosphorus-lowering agent

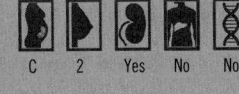

C   2   Yes   No   No

Tabs (Calphron [OTC] and generics): 667 mg (169 mg elemental Ca)
Capsules (Generics; previously available as PhosLo): 667 mg (169 mg elemental Ca)
Oral solution (Phoslyra): 667 mg/5 mL (473 mL) (169 mg elemental Ca per 5 mL); contains
  methylparabens and propylene glycol
Each 1 g of salt contains 12.7 mEq or 6.34 mmol (250 mg) elemental Ca.

Doses expressed in mg of calcium acetate.
Hyperphosphatemia (see remarks):
  Child and adolescent: Start with 667—1000 mg PO with each meal. If needed, dosage may be titrated
    every 2—4 wk up to the recommended limits from the KDOQI guidelines:
    Calcium intake as phosphate binders: 1500 mg elemental calcium/24 hr
    Total calcium intake from all sources: 2000 mg elemental calcium/24 hr
  Adult: Start with 1334 mg PO with each meal. Dosage may be increased gradually every 2—3 wk to
    bring serum phosphorus levels below 6 mg/dL, as long as hypercalcemia does not occur. Most
    patients require 2001—2668 mg PO with each meal.

Contraindicated in ventricular fibrillation. **Use with caution** in renal impairment, as
hypercalcemia may develop in end-stage renal failure. Nausea and hypercalcemia may occur.
Approximately 40% of dose is systemically absorbed under fasting conditions and up to 30% in
nonfasting conditions. May reduce absorption of fluoroquinolones, tetracyclines, and iron and
effectiveness of polystyrene sulfonate. May potentiate effects of digoxin.
1 g calcium acetate binds to 45 mg phosphorus.
Administer with meals and plenty of fluids for use as a phosphorus-lowering agent. Calcium is
excreted in breast milk and is not expected to harm the infant, provided maternal serum calcium is
appropriately monitored.

CALCIUM CARBONATE
Tums, Children's Pepto, Maalox Children's, and
many others including generics; 40% elemental Ca
Calcium supplement, antacid

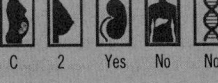

C   2   Yes   No   No

Tab, chewable [OTC]: 500, 750, 1000, 1250 mg; may contain aspartame
  Children's Pepto, Maalox Children's [OTC]: 400 mg
Tab [OTC]: 648, 1250, 1500 mg
Oral suspension [OTC]: 1250 mg/5 mL (473 mL); may contain parabens
Powder [OTC]: 800 mg/2 g (480 g)
Each 1 g of salt contains 20 mEq or 10 mmol (400 mg) elemental Ca.
Some products may be combined with vitamin D; check package labeling.

Continued

CALCIUM CARBONATE *continued*

Hypocalcemia: (Doses expressed in mg of elemental calcium. To convert to mg of salt, divide elemental dose by 0.4.)
  Neonate: 50—150 mg/kg/24 hr ÷ Q4—6 hr PO; **max. dose:** 1 g/24 hr
  Child: 45—65 mg/kg/24 hr PO ÷ QID
  Adult: 1—2 g/24 hr PO ÷ TID—QID
Antacid: (Doses expressed in mg of calcium carbonate; chronic use NOT recommended in GERD.)
  2—5 yr and ≥10.9 kg: 375—400 mg PO as symptoms occur; **max. dose:** 1500 mg/24 hr
  >6—11 yr: 750—800 mg PO as symptoms occur; **max. dose:** 3000 mg/24 hr
  >11 yr and adult: 500—3000 mg PO as symptoms occur; **max. dose:** 7500 mg/24 hr

See Calcium Acetate for **contraindications, precautions,** and drug interactions. Side effects: constipation, hypercalcemia, hypophosphatemia, hypomagnesemia, nausea, vomiting, headache, and confusion. Some products may contain trace amounts of sodium. Administer with plenty of fluids. For use as a phosphorus-lowering agent, administer with meals. Calcium is excreted in breast milk and is not expected to harm the infant, provided maternal serum calcium is appropriately monitored.

CALCIUM CHLORIDE
Various generics; 27% elemental Ca
Calcium supplement

    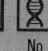

C   2   Yes   No   No

Injection: 100 mg/mL (10%) (1.36 mEq Ca/mL) (10 mL)
Prefilled syringe for injection: 100 mg/mL (10%) (1.36 mEq Ca/mL) (10 mL)
Each 1 g of salt contains 13.6 mEq or 6.8 mmol (273 mg) elemental Ca.

Doses expressed in mg of calcium chloride.
Cardiac arrest or calcium channel blocker toxicity (see remarks):
  Neonate, infant, and child: 20 mg/kg/dose (**max. dose:** 1000 mg/dose) IV/IO Q10 min PRN; if effective, an infusion of 20—50 mg/kg/hr may be used
  Adult: 500—1000 mg/dose IV Q10 min PRN
MAXIMUM IV ADMINISTRATION RATES (in mg of calcium chloride):
  IV push: Do not exceed 100 mg/min (over 10—20 sec in cardiac arrest).
  IV infusion: Do not exceed 45—90 mg/kg/hr with a **max. concentration** of 20 mg/mL.

Contraindicated in ventricular fibrillation. **Not recommended** for asystole and electromechanical dissociation. **Use with caution** in renal impairment, as hypercalcemia may develop in end-stage renal failure. May potentiate effects of digoxin. Routine use in cardiac arrest is NOT recommended due to the lack of improved survival.
Use IV with extreme caution. Extravasation may lead to necrosis. Hyaluronidase may be helpful for extravasation. Central line administration is preferred IV route of administration. **Do not use** scalp veins. **Do not administer IM or SC routes.**
Rapid IV infusion associated with bradycardia, hypotension, and peripheral vasodilation. May cause hyperchloremic acidosis.
Calcium is excreted in breast milk and is not expected to harm the infant, provided maternal serum calcium is appropriately monitored.

CALCIUM CITRATE
Calcitrate, Citracal Petites, Citracal Maximum Plus, Citracal Gummies, Viactiv Calcium and Bone Strengthening, and generics; 21% elemental Ca
Calcium supplement

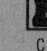   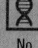

C   2   Yes   No   No

CALCIUM CITRATE *continued*

Tabs:
Calcitrate and generics [OTC]: 950 mg (200 mg elemental Ca)
Generics [OTC]: 1040 mg (218 mg elemental Ca)
Caplets:
Citracal Petites [OTC]: 200 mg elemental Ca and 250 IU vitamin D_3 with 2.5 mg sodium
Citracal Maximum Plus [OTC]: 325 mg elemental Ca and 500 IU vitamin D_3 with 2.75 mg zinc, 0.225 mg copper, 0.575 mg manganese, and 2.5 mg sodium
Some products may be combined with vitamin D; check package labeling.
Chewable tabs:
Citracal Gummies [OTC]: 250 mg elemental Ca and 500 IU vitamin D3 with 105 mg phosphorus and 12.5 mg sodium
Viactiv Calcium and Bone Strengthening [OTC]: 650 mg elemental Ca and 500 IU vitamin D3 with 40 mCg vitamin K, and 10 mg sodium
Each 1 g of salt contains 10.5 mEq or 5.25 mmol (211 mg) elemental Ca.

Doses expressed as mg of elemental calcium. To convert to mg of salt, divide elemental dose by 0.21.
Hypocalcemia:
Neonate: 50—150 mg/kg/24 hr ÷ Q4—6 hr PO; **max. dose:** 1 g/24 hr
Child: 45—65 mg/kg/24 hr PO ÷ QID
Adult: 1—2 g/24 hr PO ÷ BID—TID

See Calcium Acetate for **contraindications, precautions,** and drug interactions. Side effects: constipation, hypercalcemia, hypophosphatemia, hypomagnesemia, nausea, vomiting, headache, and confusion.

Administer with meals for use as a phosphorus-lowering agent. For hypocalcemia, do not administer with or before meals/food and take plenty of fluids.

Calcium is excreted in breast milk and is not expected to harm the infant, provided maternal serum calcium is appropriately monitored.

CALCIUM GLUCONATE
Cal-Glu and generics, 9.3% elemental Ca
Calcium supplement

   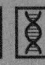 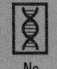

| C | 2 | Yes | No | No |

Tabs [OTC]: 50 mg
Caps (Cal-Glu) [OTC]: 500 mg
Injection: 100 mg/mL (10%) (0.465 mEq Ca/mL) (10, 50, 100 mL); may contain up to 512 mCg aluminum per 1000 mL (0.512 mCg per 100 mg calcium gluconate); see remarks
Ready to use injection in sodium chloride: 20 mg/mL (0.093 mEq Ca/mL) (50, 100 mL); contains 0.675% NaCl and may contain up to 100 mCg aluminum per 1000 mL (0.5 mCg per 100 mg calcium gluconate); see remarks
Each 1 g of salt contains 4.65 mEq or 2.33 mmol (93 mg) elemental Ca.

Doses expressed in mg calcium gluconate.
Maintenance/hypocalcemia:
Neonate: IV: 200—800 mg/kg/24 hr ÷ Q6 hr
Infant:
IV: 200—500 mg/kg/24 hr ÷ Q6 hr
PO: 400—800 mg/kg/24 hr ÷ Q6 hr
Child: 200—500 mg/kg/24 hr IV or PO ÷ Q6 hr
Adult: 0.5—8 g/24 hr IV or PO ÷ Q6 hr

Continued

CALCIUM GLUCONATE *continued*

For cardiac arrest (see remarks):
    Infant and child: 60 mg/kg/dose (**max.** 3000 mg/dose) IV Q10—20 min PRN
    Adult: 1.5—3 g/dose IV Q10 min PRN
    Max. dose: 3 g/dose
For tetany:
    Neonate, infant, child: 100—200 mg/kg dose IV over 5—10 min; repeat dose 6 hr later if needed; **max. dose:** 500 mg/kg/24 hr
    Adult: 0.5—2 g IV over 10—30 min; repeat dose 6 hr later if needed.
MAXIMUM IV ADMINISTRATION RATES:
    IV push: Do not exceed 100 mg/min (over 10—20 sec in cardiac arrest).
    IV infusion: Do not exceed 200 mg/min with a **maximum** concentration of 50 mg/mL.

Contraindicated in ventricular fibrillation. **Use with caution** in renal impairment, as hypercalcemia may develop in end-stage renal failure. **Avoid** peripheral infusion because extravasation may cause tissue necrosis. IV infusion associated with hypotension and bradycardia. Also associated with arrhythmias in digitalized patients. May reduce absorption of fluoroquinolones, tetracyclines, iron, and effectiveness of polystyrene sulfonate with oral route of administration. Routine use in cardiac arrest is not recommended due to lack of improved survival. Use of calcium chloride IV may be preferred due to its more rapid increase of ionized calcium in critically ill children.

Do not administer IV dosage form via scalp veins and the IM or SC routes. IV dosage form may precipitate when mixed with bicarbonate or ceftriaxone. IV dosage form may also contain aluminum (see how-supplied section), and for patients with renal impairment (including premature infants), receipt of >4—5 mCg/kg/24 hr aluminum has been associated with CNS and bone toxicities.

Calcium is excreted in breast milk and is not expected to harm the infant, provided maternal serum calcium is appropriately monitored.

CALCIUM LACTATE
Cal-Lac and various generics; 13% elemental Ca
Calcium supplement

C   2   Yes   No   No

Tabs [OTC]: 100, 654 mg
Caps (Cal-Lac and generics) [OTC]: 500 mg
Each 1 g salt contains 6.48 mEq or 3.24 mmol (130 mg) elemental Ca.

Doses expressed in mg of calcium lactate.
Hypocalcemia:
    Neonate/Infant: 400—500 mg/kg/24 hr PO ÷ Q4—6 hr
    Child: 500 mg/kg/24 hr PO ÷ Q6—8 hr
    Adult: 1.5—3 g PO Q8 hr
    Max. dose: 9 g/24 hr

See Calcium Acetate for **contraindications, precautions,** and drug interactions. May cause constipation, headache, and hypercalcemia.

Administer with or following meals and with plenty of fluids. **Do not** dissolve tablets in milk.

Calcium is excreted in breast milk and is not expected to harm the infant, provided maternal serum calcium is appropriately monitored.

CALFACTANT

See Surfactant, pulmonary.

CANNABIDIOL
Epidiolex
Anticonvulsant

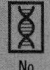

C 3 No Yes No

Oral solution: 100 mg/mL (60, 100 mL); contains ethanol and sesame oil

Lennox-Gastaut syndrome or Dravet syndrome (see remarks for therapy discontinuation):
  Child ≥2 yr and adult: Start at 2.5 mg/kg/dose PO BID × 1 wk, dosage may be increased
    to a maintenance dose of 5 mg/kg/dose PO BID. Dose may be further increased after 1 wk if needed
    and tolerated at weekly increments of 2.5 mg/kg/dose BID (5 mg/kg/24 hr) up to the **maximum** of
    20 mg/kg/24 hr. Those requiring a more rapid titration from 10 mg/kg/24 hr to 20 mg/kg/24 hr may
    be titrated no more frequently than Q48 hr.
  **Dosage reduction in moderate and severe hepatic impairment prior to initiation of therapy (slower
  dose titration has been suggested):**

Child-Pugh Category for Hepatic Impairment	Initial PO Dose (mg/kg/dose BID)	Maintenance PO Dose (mg/kg/dose BID)	Maximum PO Dose (mg/kg/dose BID)
B (moderate)	1.25	2.5	5
C (severe)	0.5	1	2

Cannabidiol is no longer a controlled substance (FDA: April 6, 2020). Common side effects
  include somnolence, decreased appetite, diarrhea, elevated transaminase (dose related or
  with concomitant valproic acid and clobazam use), fatigue, malaise and asthenia, rash,
  insomnia, and sleep disorder. Suicidal behavior and ideation, hypersensitivity reactions, elevated
  serum creatinine, respiratory failure, and increase risk for pneumonia with concomitant clobazam
  have been reported.
Monitor ALT, AST, and total bilirubin at baseline and 1, 3, 6 mo initially and periodically thereafter.
  More frequent monitoring is recommended with concurrent valproic acid or clobazam. Reduce dose
  or discontinue use in the presence of hepatic impairment.
Cannabidiol is a substrate for CYP 450 2C19 and 3A4; other moderate/strong inducers or inhibitors for
  these enzymes may affect its overall exposure. May increase the effects/toxicity of clobazam and
  diazepam because it may inhibit CYP 450 1A2, 2B6, 2C8, 2C9, and 2C19 and UGT 1A9 and 2B7
  transporters. May also inhibit P-glycoprotein transporters to increase effects/toxicity of sirolimus,
  tacrolimus, digoxin, and other P-glycoprotein substrates.
Teratogen data limited only to animal studies with evidence of developmental toxicities at similar
  exposure concentrations in humans receiving therapeutic doses. Patients exposed to cannabidiol
  during pregnancy are encouraged to register with the North American Antiepileptic Drug Pregnancy
  Registry at www.aedpregnancyregistry.org.
Administration with high-fat or high-calorie meals may increase absorption. Gradually taper when
  discontinuing medication; **avoid** abrupt discontinuation to reduce risk for increased seizures.
Use the supplied oral dosing syringe and bottle adapter and store the bottle of oral solution in the
  original bottle in the upright position at 59–86°F. Discard the unused portion of each bottle 12 wk
  after first opening.

CAPTOPRIL
Various generics; previously available as Capoten
Angiotensin-converting enzyme inhibitor,
antihypertensive

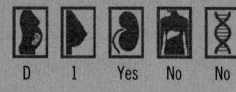

D   1   Yes   No   No

Tabs: 12.5, 25, 50, 100 mg
Oral suspension: 1 mg/mL

Hypertension:

Neonate: 0.01–0.05 mg/kg/dose PO Q8–12 hr

Infant: Initially 0.05–0.3 mg/kg/dose PO BID–TID; titrate upward if needed; **max. dose:** 6 mg/kg/24 hr

Child: Initially, 0.3–0.5 mg/kg/dose PO BID–TID; titrate upward if needed; **max. dose:** 6 mg/kg/24 hr up to 450 mg/24 hr

Adolescent and adult: Initially, 12.5–25 mg/dose PO BID–TID; increase weekly if necessary by 25 mg/dose to **max. dose:** 450 mg/24 hr. Usual dosage range: 25–100 mg/24 hr ÷ BID

Onset within 15–30 min of administration. Peak effect within 1–2 hr. **Adjust dose with renal failure (see Chapter 31).** Should be administered on an empty stomach 1 hr before or 2 hr after meals. Titrate to minimal effective dose. Lower doses should be used in patients with sodium and water depletion because of diuretic therapy.

Use with caution in collagen vascular disease and concomitant potassium-sparing diuretics. **Avoid use** with dialysis with high-flux membranes as anaphylactoid reactions have been reported. May cause rash, proteinuria, neutropenia, cough, angioedema (head, neck, and intestine), hyperkalemia, hypotension, or diminution of taste perception (with long-term use). Known to decrease aldosterone and increase renin production. **Do not** coadminister with angiotensin receptor blockers or aliskiren as use has been associated with increased risks for hypotension, hyperkalemia, and acute renal failure. Captopril is a CYP 450 2D6 substrate. Use with sirolimus, everolimus, temsirolimus, or sacubitril may increase risk for angioedema.

Captopril should be discontinued as soon as possible when pregnancy is detected.

CARBAMAZEPINE
Epitol, Tegretol, Tegretol-XR, Carbatrol, Equetro,
and various generics
Anticonvulsant

D   2   Yes   Yes   Yes

Tabs: 200 mg
Chewable tabs: 100 mg
Extended release tabs (Tegretol-XR and generics): 100, 200, 400 mg
Extended release caps (Carbatrol, Equetro, and generics): 100, 200, 300 mg
Oral suspension: 100 mg/5 mL (450 mL); may contain propylene glycol

Seizures (see remarks regarding specific dosage form dosing interval and pharmacogenomic considerations):

<6 yr:

Initial: 10–20 mg/kg/24 hr PO ÷ BID–TID (QID for oral suspension)
Increment: Q5–7 days up to **max. dose** of 35 mg/kg/24 hr PO

6–12 yr:

Initial: 10 mg/kg/24 hr PO ÷ BID (QID for oral suspension) up to **max. dose:** 100 mg/dose BID (50 mg/dose QID for oral suspension)

CARBAMAZEPINE *continued*

  Increment: 100 mg/24 hr at 1-wk intervals (÷ TID–QID) until desired response is obtained
  Maintenance: 20–30 mg/kg/24 hr PO ÷ BID-QID; usual maintenance dose is 400–800 mg/24 hr;
   max. dose: 1000 mg/24 hr
 >12 yr and adult:
  Initial: 200 mg PO BID (100 mg/dose QID for oral suspension)
  Increment: 200 mg/24 hr at 1-wk intervals (÷ BID-QID) until desired response is obtained
  Maintenance: 800–1200 mg/24 hr PO ÷ BID–QID
  Max. dose:
   Child 12–15 yr: 1000 mg/24 hr
   Child >15 yr: 1200 mg/24 hr
   Adult: 1.6–2.4 g/24 hr

Contraindicated for patients taking monoamine oxidase (MAO) inhibitors or who are sensitive
 to tricyclic antidepressants. Should not be used in combination with clozapine, owing to
 increased risk for bone marrow suppression and agranulocytosis. Increased risk for severe
 dermatologic reactions (e.g., Stevens-Johnson syndrome [SJS] and toxic epidermal necrolysis
 [TEN]) has been associated with the HLA-B*1502 (prevalent among Asian descent) and
 HLA-A*3101 (prevalent among Japanese, Native American, Southern Indian, and some Arabic
 ancestry) alleles.
Erythromycin, diltiazem, verapamil, cefixime, cimetidine, itraconazole, aprepitant, and INH may
 increase serum levels. Carbamazepine may decrease activity of warfarin, direct-acting oral
 anticoagulants (e.g., rivaroxaban, apixaban), doxycycline, oral contraceptives, cyclosporine,
 theophylline, phenytoin, benzodiazepines, ethosuximide, and valproic acid. Carbamazepine is a CYP
 450 3A3/4 substrate and inducer of CYP 450 1A2, 2C, and 3A3/4. The enzyme-inducing effects may
 increase effects/toxicity of cyclophosphamide. CYP 450 3A4 inhibitors may increase carbamazepine
 levels/toxicity.
Suggested dosing intervals for specific dosage forms: extended release tabs or caps (BID); chewable
 and immediate release tabs (BID–TID); oral suspension (TID–QID).
Doses may be administered with food. **Do not** crush or chew extended release dosage forms. Shake
 bottle well prior to dispensing oral suspension dosage form, and **do not** administer simultaneously
 with other liquid medicines or diluents.
Drug metabolism typically increases after the first month of therapy initiation due to hepatic
 autoinduction.
Therapeutic blood levels for seizures: 4–12 mg/L. Recommended serum sampling time: obtain trough
 level within 30 min prior to an oral dose. Steady state is typically achieved 1 mo following the
 initiation of therapy (following enzymatic autoinduction). Levels obtained prior to steady state are
 useful for preventing toxicity. Blood trough levels of 7–10 mg/L have been recommended for bipolar
 disorders.
Side effects include sedation, dizziness, diplopia, aplastic anemia, neutropenia, urinary retention,
 nausea, SIADH, and SJS. Suicidal behavior or ideation, hypogammaglobulinemia, and
 onychomadesis have been reported. Approximately one-third of patients who had hypersensitivity
 reactions will also experience the hypersensitivity to oxcarbazepine. Pretreatment complete blood
 counts (CBCs) and liver function tests (LFTs) are suggested. Patient should be monitored for
 hematologic and hepatic toxicity. Most common side effects with the IV route: dizziness,
 somnolence, blurred vision, diplopia, headache, infusion-related reaction, infusion site pain, and
 anemia.
Adjust dose in renal impairment (see Chapter 31).

CARBAMIDE PEROXIDE
Otic solution: Debrox, Auraphene-B, Clearcanal
Earwax Softener, GoodSense Ear Wax Removal,
and many generic products
Oral liquid: Gly-Oxide
Cerumenolytic, topical oral analgesic

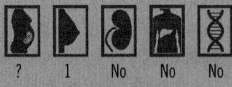

?   1   No   No   No

Otic solution (OTC): 6.5% (15 mL); may contain propylene glycol or alcohol
Oral liquid (OTC): 10% (Gly-Oxide) (15 mL)

Cerumenolytic:
  <12 yr: Tilt head sideways and instill 1—5 drops (according to patient size) into affected
    ear; retain drops in ear for several minutes. Remove wax by gently flushing the ear
    with warm water, using a soft rubber bulb ear syringe. Dose may be repeated BID PRN for
    up to 4 days.
  ≥12 yr: Following the same instructions as aforementioned, instill 5—10 drops into affected ear BID
    PRN for up to 4 days.
Oral analgesic (see remarks):
  ≥2 yr (able to follow instructions): Instill several drops of the oral liquid to affected area and
    expectorate after 2—3 min, *OR* place 10 drops on tongue and mix with saliva, swish for several
    minutes, and expectorate. Administer up to QID, after meals and QHS, for **up to 7 days.**

Otic solution: Contraindicated if tympanic membrane perforated; following otic surgery; ear
discharge, drainage, pain, irritation, or rash; or PE tubes in place. Tip of applicator should
not enter ear canal when used as a cerumenolytic.
Oral liquid: Prolonged use may result in fungal overgrowth. **Do not** rinse the mouth or drink for at least
5 min when using oral preparation.
Pregnancy category has not been formally assigned by the FDA.

CARBINOXAMINE
Karbinal ER, RyVent, and many generics
Antihistamine

C   3   No   No   No

Oral liquid: 4 mg/5 mL (118 mL); may contain propylene glycol
Extended release oral suspension (Karbinal ER): 4 mg/5 mL (480 mL); contains parabens and
  metasulfite
Tabs: 4, 6 mg
RyVent: 6 mg

Child (PO; see remarks):
  Immediate release dosage forms: 0.2—0.4 mg/kg/24 hr PO ÷ TID—QID; alternative
    dosing by age (**do not exceed** 0.4 mg/kg/24 hr):
      2—5 yr: 1—2 mg TID—QID
      6—11 yr: 2—4 mg TID—QID
      ≥12 yr: 4—8 mg TID—QID
  Extended release oral suspension (Karbinal ER; approximately 0.2—0.4 mg/kg/24 hr):
      2—3 yr: 3—4 mg Q12 hr
      4—5 yr: 3—8 mg Q12 hr
      6—11 yr: 6—12 mg Q12 hr
      ≥12 yr: 6—16 mg Q12 hr

CARBINOXAMINE *continued*

Adult (PO):
  Immediate release dosage forms: 4—8 mg TID—QID
  Extended release oral suspension (Karbinal ER): 6—16 mg Q12 hr

Generally not recommended for treating upper respiratory tract infections (URIs) for infants.
  No proven benefit for infants and young children with URIs. **The FDA does not recommend use for URIs in children <2 yr because of reports of increased fatalities.** Karbinal ER use is **contraindicated** in children <2 yr and in nursing mothers.
Contraindicated in acute asthma, hypersensitivity with other ethanolamine antihistamines, MAO inhibitors (prolongs and intensifies anticholinergic effects), severe hypertension, narrow-angle glaucoma, severe coronary artery disease, and urinary retention. Be aware that combination products containing a decongestant may exist.
May cause drowsiness, vertigo, dry mucus membranes, and headache. Paradoxical excitation reactions more likely in younger children. Contact dermatitis and CNS excitation have been reported.

CARNITINE
Levocarnitine, Carnitor, Carnitor SF, L-Carnitine, and generics
Nutritional supplement, amino acid

   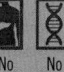

B   ?   Yes   No   No

Tabs (Carnitor and generics): 330 mg
Caps: 250 mg
Oral solution: 100 mg/mL (118 mL); contains methylparabens and propylparabens; Carnitor SF is a sugar-free product
Injection: 200 mg/mL (5 mL); preservative free

Primary carnitine deficiency:
  Oral:
    Child: 50—100 mg/kg/24 hr PO ÷ Q8—12 hr; increase slowly as needed and tolerated to **max. dose** of 3 g/24 hr
    Adult: 330 mg to 1 g/dose BID—TID PO; **max. dose:** 3 g/24 hr
Secondary carnitine deficiency:
  IV:
    Child and adult: 50 mg/kg as loading dose; may follow with 50 mg/kg/24 hr IV infusion (for severe cases); maintenance: 50 mg/kg/24 hr ÷ Q4—6 hr; increase to **max. dose** of 300 mg/kg/24 hr if needed

May cause nausea, vomiting, abdominal cramps, diarrhea, and body odor. Seizures have been reported in patients with or without a history of seizures.
Safety in end-stage renal disease (ESRD) has not been established. High doses to severely compromised renal function or ESRD on dialysis may result in accumulation of potentially toxic metabolites (trimethylamine and trimethylamine-*N*-oxide). Serious hypersensitivity reactions, including anaphylaxis, have been reported with IV use mostly in ESRD patients undergoing dialysis. Give bolus IV infusion over 2—3 min.

CARVEDILOL
Coreg, Coreg CR, and generics
Adrenergic antagonist (α and β), antihypertensive

C   ?   Yes   Yes   No

Continued

CARVEDILOL continued

Tabs: 3.125, 6.25, 12.5, 25 mg
Extended release caps (Coreg CR and generics): 10, 20, 40, 80 mg
Oral suspension: 0.1, 1.25, 1.67 mg/mL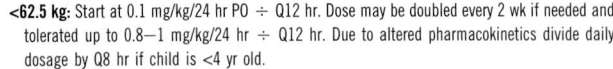

Heart failure:
Immediate release dosage forms (tablets and oral suspension; see remarks):
Infant, child, adolescent (2013 Canadian Cardiovascular Society Guidelines):

<62.5 kg: Start at 0.1 mg/kg/24 hr PO ÷ Q12 hr. Dose may be doubled every 2 wk if needed and tolerated up to 0.8—1 mg/kg/24 hr ÷ Q12 hr. Due to altered pharmacokinetics divide daily dosage by Q8 hr if child is <4 yr old.

≥62.5 kg: Start at 3.125 mg PO BID. Dose may be doubled every 2 wk if needed and tolerated up to 25 mg BID. 25 mg PO TID may be needed for patients weighing >75 kg.

Adult: Start at 3.125 mg PO BID × 2 wk; if needed and tolerated, may increase to 6.25 mg BID. Dose may be doubled every 2 wk if needed to the following **max. doses:**

<85 kg: 25 mg BID
≥85 kg: 50 mg BID

Extended release capsules:
Adult: Start at 10 mg PO once daily × 2 wk; if needed and tolerated, double the dose every 2 wk up to the **maximum** of 80 mg once daily.

Hypertension:
Adult:

Immediate release dosage forms: Start at 6.25 mg PO BID; dose may be doubled every 1—2 wk up to a **maximum** of 25 mg PO BID.

Extended release capsules: Start at 20 mg PO once daily × 1—2 wk; if needed and tolerated, increase to 40 mg PO once daily. If needed, dose may be further increased in 2-wk intervals up to a **maximum** of 80 mg/24 hr.

Immediate release and extended release products are NOT interchangeable on a mg-to-mg basis. **Contraindicated** in asthma or related bronchospastic disease, sick sinus syndrome, 2nd- or 3rd-degree heart block, severe bradycardia, cardiogenic shock, decompensated cardiac failure requiring IV inotropic therapy, and severe hepatic impairment (Child-Pugh class C).

Use with caution mild/moderate hepatic impairment (Child-Pugh class A or B), renal insufficiency, thyrotoxicosis, ischemic heart disease, diabetes, and cataract surgery. **Avoid abrupt withdrawal** of medication.

Children <3½ yr old may have faster carvedilol clearance and may require higher dosages or TID dosing. Carvedilol is a CYP 450 2D6 substrate. Digoxin, disopyramide, and dipyridamole may increase bradycardic effects.

Bradycardia, postural hypotension, peripheral edema, weight gain, hyperglycemia, diarrhea, dizziness, and fatigue are common. Hypersensitivity reactions have been reported. Chest pain, headache, vomiting, edema, and dyspnea have also been reported in children. Administering doses with food can reduce risk for orthostatic hypotension.

CASPOFUNGIN
Cancidas and generics
Antifungal, echinocandin

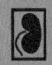 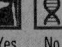

C   ?   No   Yes   No

Injection: 50, 70 mg; contains sucrose (39 mg in 50 mg vial and 54 mg in 70 mg vial) and mannitol (26 mg in 50 mg vial and 36 mg in 70 mg vial)

CASPOFUNGIN *continued*

Preterm neonate to <3 mo infant: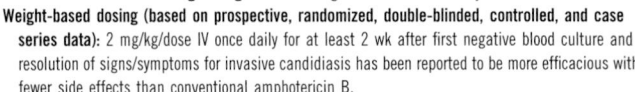
  BSA dosing (based on a small pharmacokinetic study, achieving similar plasma exposure as seen in adults receiving 50 mg/24 hr): 25 mg/m²/dose IV once daily
  Weight-based dosing (based on prospective, randomized, double-blinded, controlled, and case series data): 2 mg/kg/dose IV once daily for at least 2 wk after first negative blood culture and resolution of signs/symptoms for invasive candidiasis has been reported to be more efficacious with fewer side effects than conventional amphotericin B.
3 mo infant—17 yr (see remarks): 70 mg/m²/dose IV loading dose on day 1 followed by 50 mg/m²/dose IV once-daily maintenance dose. Increase the maintenance dose to 70 mg/m²/dose if response is inadequate or if the patient is receiving an enzyme-inducing medication (see remarks).
  Maximum loading and maintenance dose: 70 mg/dose
Adult (see remarks):
  Loading dose: 70 mg IV × 1
  Maintenance dose:
    Usual: 50 mg IV once daily. If tolerated and response is inadequate or if patient is receiving an enzyme-inducing medication (see remarks), increase to 70 mg IV once daily.
    Moderate hepatic insufficiency (Child-Pugh score 7—9): 35 mg IV once daily is recommended in the FDA label. However, several pharmacokinetic evaluations suggest the reduced dosage may result in subtherapeutic levels for these patients.

Use with caution in hepatic impairment and concomitant enzyme-inducing drugs. Higher maintenance doses (70 mg/m²/dose [not to exceed 70 mg] in children and 70 mg in adults) are recommended for concomitant use of enzyme inducers such as carbamazepine, dexamethasone, phenytoin, nevirapine, efavirenz, or rifampin. Use Mosteller formula for calculating body surface area (BSA).

Most common adverse effects (>10%) in children include fever, diarrhea, rash, elevated aspartate transaminase/alanine transaminase (ALT/AST), hypokalemia, hypotension, and chills. May also cause facial swelling, nausea/vomiting, headache, infusion site phlebitis, and LFT elevation. Anaphylaxis, TEN, SJS, and possible histamine-related reactions (angioedema, bronchospasm, and warmth sensation) have been reported. Hepatobiliary adverse effects have been reported in pediatric patients with serious underlying medical conditions.

Despite the FDA labeling recommendation for reducing the daily maintenance dose by 30% in moderate hepatic impairment (Child-Pugh score 7—9), several pharmacokinetic evaluations suggest this dose reduction may result in subtherapeutic levels.

Use with cyclosporine may cause transient increase in LFTs and caspofungin level elevations. May decrease tacrolimus levels.

Administer doses by slow IV infusion over 1 hr. **Do not** mix or co-infuse with other medications, and **avoid** using dextrose-containing diluents (e.g., D₅W).

CEFACLOR
Generics; previously available as Ceclor
Antibiotic, cephalosporin (second generation)
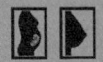   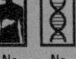
B   1   Yes   No   No

Caps: 250, 500 mg
Extended release tabs: 500 mg
Oral suspension: 125 mg/5 mL (150 mL); 250 mg/5 mL (150 mL); 375 mg/5 mL (100 mL)

Child >1 mo old (use regular release dosage forms): 20—40 mg/kg/24 hr PO ÷ Q8 hr;
  max. dose: 1 g/24 hr
  Q12 hr dosage interval option for pharyngitis (use oral suspension dosage form): 20 mg/kg/24 hr PO ÷ Q12 hr; **max. dose:** 1 g/24 hr

Continued

CEFACLOR *continued*

Adult: 250–500 mg/dose PO Q8 hr
 Extended release tablets: 500 mg/dose PO Q12 hr

Not recommended for otitis media or pharyngitis/tonsillitis. **Use with caution** in patients with penicillin allergy or renal impairment. Side effects include elevated LFTs, bone marrow suppression, and moniliasis. Probenecid may increase cefaclor concentrations. May cause positive Coombs test or false-positive test for urinary glucose (e.g., Clinitest, Benedict's solution, or Fehling's solution). Enzymatic glucose oxidase urinary glucose tests (e.g., Clinistix or Tes-Tape) are recommended. Serum sickness reactions have been reported in patients receiving multiple courses of cefaclor.

Do not crush, cut, or chew extended release tablets. Doses should be given on an empty stomach. **Extended release tablets not recommended for children. Adjust dose in renal failure (see Chapter 31).**

CEFADROXIL
Generics; previously available as Duricef
Antibiotic, cephalosporin (first generation)

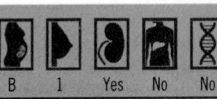

B   1   Yes   No   No

Oral suspension: 250 mg/5 mL (100 mL), 500 mg/5 mL (75, 100 mL)
Tabs: 1 g
Caps: 500 mg

Infant and child: 30 mg/kg/24 hr PO ÷ Q12 hr; **max. dose:** 2 g/24 hr
 Group A β-hemolytic streptococci pharyngitis/tonsillitis: 30 mg/kg/24 hr PO ÷ Q12–24 hr; **max. dose:** 1 g/24 hr
Adolescent and adult: 1–2 g/24 hr PO ÷ Q12–24 hr (administer Q12 hr for complicated UTIs); **max. dose:** 2 g/24 hr
 Group A β-hemolytic streptococci pharyngitis/tonsillitis: 1 g /24 hr PO ÷ Q12–24 hr; **max. dose:** 1 g/24 hr

See Cephalexin for **precautions** and interactions. Rash, nausea, vomiting, and diarrhea are common. Transient neutropenia and vaginitis have been reported. **Adjust dose in renal failure (see Chapter 31).**

CEFAZOLIN
Generics; previously available as Ancef
Antibiotic, cephalosporin (first generation)

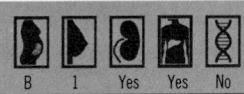

B   1   Yes   Yes   No

Injection: 0.5, 1, 10, 100 g
Frozen injection: 1 g/50 mL (contains 2 g dextrose to make an iso-osmotic solution), 2 g/100 mL (contains 4 g dextrose to make an iso-osmotic solution)
Contains 2.1 mEq Na/g drug

Neonate (IM/IV):
 Postnatal age ≤7 days:
  ≤2000 g: 50 mg/kg/24 hr ÷ Q12 hr
  >2000 g: 100 mg/kg/24 hr ÷ Q12 hr
 Postnatal age >7–28 days:
  ≤2000 g: 75 mg/kg/24 hr ÷ Q8 hr
  >2000 g: 150 mg/kg/24 hr ÷ Q8 hr
Infant >1 mo and child (IM/IV):
 Mild/moderate infection: 25–100 mg/kg/24 hr ÷ Q6–8 hr; **max. dose:** 6 g/24 hr

CEFAZOLIN *continued*

Severe infection: 100—150 mg/kg/24 hr ÷ Q6—8 hr (**max. dose:** 12 g/24 hr); 150 mg/kg/24 hr ÷ Q6—8 hr has been recommended for bone/joint infections
Adult: 1—2 g/dose Q8 hr IV/IM; **max. dose:** 12 g/24 hr
Bacterial endocarditis prophylaxis for dental and upper respiratory procedures:
Infant and child: 50 mg/kg IV/IM (**max. dose:** 1 g) 30—60 min before procedure
Adult: 1 g IV/IM 30—60 min before procedure

Use with caution in renal impairment or in penicillin-allergic patients. Does not penetrate well into cerebrospinal fluid (CSF). May cause phlebitis, leukopenia, thrombocytopenia, transient liver enzyme elevation, and false-positive urine-reducing substance (e.g., Clinitest, Benedict's solution, or Fehling's solution) and Coombs test. Enzymatic glucose oxidase urinary glucose tests (e.g., Clinistix or Tes-Tape) are recommended.

For dosing in obese patients, use higher end of the dosing recommendation. **Adjust dose in renal failure (see Chapter 31).**

CEFDINIR
Generics; previously available as Omnicef
Antibiotic, cephalosporin (third generation)

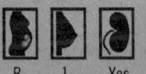 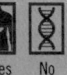

B   1   Yes   Yes   No

Caps: 300 mg
Oral suspension: 125 mg/5 mL (60, 100 mL), 250 mg/5 mL (60, 100 mL)

6 mo—12 yr:
Otitis media, sinusitis (not recommended as empiric monotherapy), pharyngitis/tonsillitis: 14 mg/kg/24 hr PO ÷ Q12—24 hr; **max. dose:** 600 mg/24 hr
Uncomplicated skin infections (see remarks): 14 mg/kg/24 hr PO ÷ Q12 hr; **max. dose:** 600 mg/24 hr
≥13 yr and adult:
Bronchitis, sinusitis, pharyngitis/tonsillitis: 600 mg/24 hr PO ÷ Q12—24 hr
Community-acquired pneumonia, UTI, uncomplicated skin infections (see remarks): 600 mg/24 hr PO ÷ Q12 hr

Use with caution in penicillin-allergic patients or in presence of renal impairment. Good Gram-positive cocci activity but may be inadequate for penicillin-resistant pneumococci. May cause diarrhea (especially in children <2 yr), headache, vaginitis, and false-positive urine-reducing substance (e.g., Clinitest, Benedict's solution, or Fehling's solution) and Coombs test. Enzymatic glucose oxidase urinary glucose tests (e.g., Clinistix or Tes-Tape) are recommended. Eosinophilia and abnormal LFTs have been reported with higher-than-usual doses.

Once-daily dosing has not been evaluated in pneumonia and skin infections. Probenecid increases serum cefdinir levels. **Avoid** concomitant administration with iron and iron-containing vitamins and antacids containing aluminum or magnesium (space 2 hr apart) to reduce the risk for decreasing antibiotic's absorption. May cause red stools when administered with iron and iron-containing products. Doses may be taken without regard to food. **Adjust dose in renal failure (see Chapter 31).**

CEFEPIME
Generics; previously available as Maxipime
Antibiotic, cephalosporin (fourth generation)

B   1   Yes   Yes   No

Injection: 0.5, 1, 2, 100 g
Premixed injection: 1 g/50 mL, 2 g/100 mL (iso-osmotic dextrose solutions)
Each 1 g drug contains 725 mg L-arginine.

Continued

CEFEPIME *continued*

Neonate (IV/IM):

  <14 days old: 60 mg/kg/24 hr ÷ Q12 hr
  ≥14 days old: 100 mg/kg/24 hr ÷ Q12 hr
  Meningitis or *Pseudomonas* infections:
    <1 kg and 0–14 days old, or 1–2 kg and <0–7 days old: 100 mg/kg/24 hr ÷ Q12 hr
    <1 kg and >14 days old, or 1–2 kg and >7 days old, or >2 kg and 0–30 days old: 150 mg/kg/24 hr ÷ Q8 hr
Child ≥2 mo (IV/IM): 100 mg/kg/24 hr ÷ Q12 hr; **max. dose:** 4 g/24 hr
  Meningitis, fever, and neutropenia, or serious infections: 150 mg/kg/24 hr ÷ Q8 hr; **max. dose:** 2 g/single dose or 6 g/24 hr
Cystic fibrosis: 150 mg/kg/24 hr ÷ Q8 hr IV/IM, up to a **max. dose** of 6 g/24 hr. Higher dose of 200 mg/kg/24 hr ÷ Q6 hr (**max. dose:** 8 g/24 hr) has been recommended for resistant *Pseudomonas* isolates.
Adult: 1–4 g/24 hr ÷ Q12 hr IV/IM
  Severe infections: 6 g/24 hr ÷ Q8 hr IV/IM
  Max. dose: 6 g/24 hr

Use with caution in patients with penicillin allergy or renal impairment. Good activity against *Pseudomonas aeruginosa* and other Gram-negative bacteria plus most Gram-positives (methicillin-sensitive *Staphylococcus aureus*). Extended/continuous infusion administration is an option for treating resistant isolates.

May cause thrombophlebitis, GI discomfort, transient increases in liver enzymes, and false-positive urine-reducing substance (e.g., Clinitest, Benedict's solution, or Fehling's solution) and Coombs test. Enzymatic glucose oxidase urinary glucose tests (e.g., Clinistix or Tes-Tape) are recommended. Probenecid increases serum cefepime levels. Encephalopathy, myoclonus, seizures (including nonconvulsive status epilepticus), aphasia, transient leukopenia, neutropenia, agranulocytosis, and thrombocytopenia have been reported. Reported neurotoxicity (e.g., encephalopathy, aphasia, myoclonus, and seizures) may be attributed to cefepime's concentration-dependent GABA inhibitory effects. **Adjust dose in renal failure (see Chapter 31).**

CEFIDEROCOL
Fetroja
Antibiotic, cephalosporin (siderophore type)

? · 1 · Yes · Yes · No

Injection: 1 g; contains sucrose
Contains 3.7 mEq Na/g drug

Infant <3 mo (limited data based on pharmacokinetic allometric scaling techniques to replicate similar adult exposure levels; infuse doses IV over 1 hr):

  <2 mo:
    <32 wk gestation: 30 mg/kg/dose IV Q8 hr
    ≥32 wk gestation: 40 mg/kg/dose IV Q8 hr
  2–<3 mo:
    <32 wk gestation: 40 mg/kg/dose IV Q8 hr
    ≥32 wk gestation: 60 mg/kg/dose IV Q8 hr
Child 3 mo–<18 yr (current dosage being evaluated in clinical trials for suspected or confirmed Gram-negative bacterial infections; infuse doses IV over 3 hr):
  <34 kg: 60 mg/kg/dose IV Q8 hr
  ≥34 kg: 2 g IV Q8 hr

CEFIDEROCOL *continued*

Adult:

Hospital-acquired pneumonia, ventilator-associated pneumonia, and UTI (infuse doses IV over 3 hr): 2 g IV Q8 hr

Possesses a unique mechanism of action for having a catechol side chain that chelates with iron to enable iron transport systems to deliver cefiderocol to the outer membrane of Gram-negative aerobic bacteria. Its cephalosporin moiety then exerts its bactericidal properties by binding to penicillin-binding proteins.

Use with caution in penicillin, cephalosporin, or beta-lactam allergic patients or in the presence of renal impairment **(adjust dose in renal failure; see Chapter 31).** Common side effects include injection site reaction, rash, increased LFTs, hypokalemia, diarrhea, constipation, GI disturbance, and headache. Hypomagnesemia, hypersensitivity reactions, atrial fibrillation, seizures, and increase in mortality in patients with carbapenem-resistant Gram-negative bacterial infections have been reported in adults. May cause false-positive results for urine dipstick tests (urine protein, ketones, or occult blood) and Coombs test.

CEFIXIME
Suprax and generics
Antibiotic, cephalosporin (third generation)

   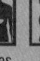 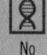

B   1   Yes   Yes   No

Oral suspension: 100 mg/5 mL (50 mL), 200 mg/5 mL (50, 75 mL), 500 mg/5 mL (10, 20 mL); may contain sodium benzoate
Chewable tabs: 100, 200 mg; contain aspartame
Caps: 400 mg

Infant (>6 mo) and child: 8 mg/kg/24 hr ÷ Q12–24 hr PO; **max. dose:** 400 mg/24 hr
  Alternative dosing for acute UTI: 16 mg/kg/24 hr ÷ Q12 hr on day 1, followed by 8 mg/kg/24 hr Q24 hr PO × 13 days. **Max. dose:** 400 mg/24 hr
Adolescent and adult: 400 mg/24 hr ÷ Q12–24 hr PO
  Uncomplicated cervical, urethral, or rectal infections due to *Neisseria gonorrhoeae* (not recommended as first-line cephalosporin by the CDC; ceftriaxone is preferred, use only when ceftriaxone is not available): 800 mg × 1 PO plus doxycycline 100 mg PO BID × 7 days

Use with caution in patients with penicillin allergy or renal failure. Adverse reactions include diarrhea (16% incidence reported in clinical trials), abdominal pain, nausea, and headaches. Transient increase in AST/ALT has been reported. Activity is inadequate against penicillin-resistant pneumococci.

Because of reduced bioavailability, do not use tablets for the treatment of otitis media. Probenecid increases serum cefixime levels. Unlike most cephalosporins, drug is excreted unchanged in the bile (5%–10%) and urine (50%). May increase carbamazepine serum concentrations. May cause false-positive urine-reducing substance (e.g., Clinitest, Benedict's solution, or Fehling's solution), Coombs test, and nitroprusside test for ketones. Enzymatic glucose oxidase urinary glucose tests (e.g., Clinistix or Tes-Tape) are recommended. **Adjust dose in renal failure (see Chapter 31).**

CEFOTAXIME
Generics; previously available as Claforan
Antibiotic, cephalosporin (third generation)

    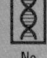

B   1   Yes   Yes   No

Injection: 1, 2 g
Contains 2.2 mEq Na/g drug

Continued

CEFOTAXIME *continued*

Neonate, IV/IM:
  Postnatal age ≤7 days (all weights): 100 mg/kg/24 hr ÷ Q12 hr
  Postnatal age 8—28 days:
    <1000 g:
      8—14 days postnatal: 100 mg/kg/24 hr ÷ Q12 hr
      15—28 days postnatal: 150 mg/kg/24 hr ÷ Q8 hr
    ≥1000 g: 150 mg/kg/24 hr ÷ Q8 hr
  Meningitis (minimum 21 days of therapy):
    Postnatal age ≤7 days and ≥2 kg: 100—150 mg/kg/24 hr ÷ Q8—12 hr
    Postnatal age >7 days and ≥2 kg: 150—200 mg/kg/24 hr ÷ Q6—8 hr
Infant and child (1 mo—12 yr and <50 kg): 150—200 mg/kg/24 hr ÷ Q6—8 hr IV/IM. Higher doses
  of 150—225 mg/kg/24 hr ÷ Q6—8 hr have been recommended for infections outside the CSF due
  to penicillin-resistant pneumococci.
  Meningitis: 200 mg/kg/24 hr ÷ Q6 hr IV/IM. Higher doses of 225—300 mg/kg/24 hr ÷ Q6—8 hr
    (some recommend 300 mg/kg/24 hr ÷ Q4—6 hr), in combination with vancomycin (dosed at CNS
    target levels), have been recommended for meningitis due to penicillin-resistant pneumococci.
  Max. dose: 12 g/24 hr
Child (>12 yr or ≥50 kg) and adult: 1—2 g/dose Q6—8 hr IV/IM
  Severe infection: 2 g/dose Q4—6 hr IV/IM
  Max. dose: 12 g/24 hr

Use with caution in penicillin allergy and renal impairment (reduce dosage). Toxicities similar
  to other cephalosporins: allergy, neutropenia, thrombocytopenia, eosinophilia, false-positive
  urine-reducing substance (e.g., Clinitest, Benedict's solution, or Fehling's solution) and Coombs
  test, elevated BUN, creatinine, and liver enzymes. Enzymatic glucose oxidase urinary glucose tests
  (e.g., Clinistix or Tes-Tape) are recommended. Probenecid increases serum cefotaxime levels.
Good CNS penetration. **Adjust dose in renal failure (see Chapter 31).**

CEFOTETAN
Generics; previously available as Cefotan
Antibiotic, cephalosporin (second generation)
B   1   Yes   Yes   No

Injection: 1, 2 g
Contains 3.5 mEq Na/g drug

Infant and child (IV/IM, limited data):
  Mild/moderate infection: 60 mg/kg/24 hr ÷ Q12 hr; **max. single dose:** 2 g/dose
  Severe infection: 100 mg/kg/24 hr ÷ Q12 hr; **max. single dose:** 2—3 g/dose
  Intra-abdominal infection: 40—80 mg/kg/24 hr ÷ Q12 hr; **max. dose:** 6 g/24 hr
Adolescent and adult: 2—4 g/24 hr ÷ Q12 hr IV/IM; **max. dose:** 6 g/24 hr
  PID: 2 g Q12 hr IV × 24—48 hr after clinical improvement. Doxycycline 100 mg Q12 hr PO/IV × 14
    days is also initiated at the same time.
Max. dose (all ages): 6 g/24 hr
**Preoperative prophylaxis (30—60 min before procedure; may repeat dose in 6 hr if lengthy
  procedure or excessive blood loss):**
  Child: 40 mg/kg/dose (**max. dose:** 2 g/dose) IV
  Adult: 1—2 g IV

Use with caution in penicillin-allergic patients or in presence of renal impairment. May cause
  disulfiram-like reaction with ethanol and increase effects/toxicities of anticoagulants,

CEFOTETAN *continued*

false-positive urine-reducing substance (e.g., Clinitest, Benedict's solution, or Fehling's solution), and false elevations of serum and urine creatinine (Jaffe method). Enzymatic glucose oxidase urinary glucose tests (e.g., Clinistix or Tes-Tape) are recommended. Hemolytic anemia and liver enzyme elevations have been reported. Good anaerobic activity but poor CSF penetration. **Adjust dose in renal failure (see Chapter 31).**

CEFOXITIN
Generics; previously available as Mefoxin
Antibiotic, cephalosporin (second generation)

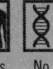

B　1　Yes　Yes　No

Injection: 1, 2, 10 g
Frozen injection: 1 g/50 mL 4% dextrose, 2 g/50 mL 2.2% dextrose (iso-osmotic solutions)
Contains 2.3 mEq Na/g drug

Neonate:
 <32 wk gestation:
  ≤7 days old: 70 mg/kg/24 hr ÷ Q12 hr IM/IV
  >7 days old: 105 mg/kg/24 hr ÷ Q8 hr IM/IV
 ≥32 wk gestation: 105 mg/kg/24 hr ÷ Q8 hr IM/IV
Infant and child:
 Mild/moderate infections: 80–100 mg/kg/24 hr ÷ Q6–8 hr IM/IV
 Severe infections: 100–160 mg/kg/24 hr ÷ Q4–6 hr IM/IV
Adult: 1–2 g/dose Q6–8 hr IM/IV
 Mild/moderate acute PID: 2 g IM x 1 and probenecid 1 g PO x 1, plus doxycycline 100 mg Q12 hr PO and metronidazole 500 mg Q12 hr PO × 14 days
 Severe acute PID: 2 g IV Q6 hr × 24–48 hr after clinical improvement. Doxycycline 100 mg Q12 hr PO/IV × 14 days is also initiated at the same time.
Max. dose (all ages): 12 g/24 hr
Preoperative prophylaxis (30–60 min before procedure; may repeat dose in 2 hr for lengthy procedure or excessive blood loss):
 Child: 40 mg/kg/dose (**max. dose:** 2 g/dose) IV
 Adult: 2 g IV

Use with caution in penicillin-allergic patients or in presence of renal impairment. Has good anaerobic activity but poor CSF penetration. May cause injection site reaction and thrombophlebitis. Transient increases in LFTs have been reported.
Probenecid increases serum cefoxitin levels. May cause false-positive urine-reducing substance (e.g., Clinitest, Benedict's solution, or Fehling's solution) and false elevations of serum and urine creatinine (Jaffe and KDA methods). Enzymatic glucose oxidase urinary glucose tests (e.g., Clinistix or Tes-Tape) are recommended.
Adjust dose in renal failure (see Chapter 31).

CEFPODOXIME PROXETIL
Generics; previously available as Vantin
Antibiotic, cephalosporin (third generation)

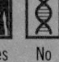

B　1　Yes　Yes　No

Tabs: 100, 200 mg
Oral suspension: 50, 100 mg/5 mL (50, 100 mL)

Continued

CEFPODOXIME PROXETIL *continued*

2 mo—11 yr: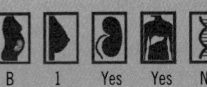
Otitis media: 10 mg/kg/24 hr PO ÷ Q12 hr × 5—10 days; **max. dose:** 400 mg/24 hr
Pharyngitis/tonsillitis: 10 mg/kg/24 hr PO ÷ Q12 hr × 5—10 days; **max. dose:** 200 mg/24 hr
Acute maxillary sinusitis: 10 mg/kg/24 hr PO ÷ Q12 hr × 10 days; **max. dose:** 400 mg/24 hr
≥12 yr—adult:
Exacerbation of chronic bronchitis, community-acquired pneumonia, and sinusitis: 400 mg/24 hr
   PO ÷ Q12 hr × 10 days (14 days for pneumonia)
Pharyngitis/tonsillitis: 200 mg/24 hr PO ÷ Q12 hr × 5—10 days
Skin/skin structure infection: 800 mg/24 hr PO ÷ Q12 hr × 7—14 days
Uncomplicated UTI: 200 mg/24 hr PO ÷ Q12 hr × 5—7 days

Use with caution in penicillin-allergic patients or in presence of renal impairment. May cause
diarrhea, nausea, vomiting, vaginal candidiasis, and false-positive urine-reducing substance
(e.g., Clinitest, Benedict's solution, or Fehling's solution) and Coombs test. Enzymatic glucose
oxidase urinary glucose tests (e.g., Clinistix or Tes-Tape) are recommended. Transient elevation of
ALT/SGPT has been reported in clinical trials.

Tablets should be administered with food to enhance absorption. Suspension may be administered
without regard to food. High doses of antacids or H_2 blockers may reduce absorption. Probenecid
increases serum cefpodoxime levels.

Cefpodoxime proxetil is a prodrug that is deesterified in the GI tract to the active cefpodoxime. **Adjust
dose in renal failure (see Chapter 31).**

CEFPROZIL
Generics; previously available as Cefzil
Antibiotic, cephalosporin (second generation)

B   1   Yes   Yes   No

Tabs: 250, 500 mg
Oral suspension: 125 mg/5 mL, 250 mg/5 mL (50, 75, 100 mL); contains aspartame and
phenylalanine

Otitis media:
   6 mo—12 yr: 30 mg/kg/24 hr PO ÷ Q12 hr; **max. dose:** 1 g/24 hr
Pharyngitis/tonsillitis:
   2—12 yr: 15 mg/kg/24 hr PO ÷ Q12 hr; **max. dose:** 1 g/24 hr
   ≥13 yr: 500 mg PO Q24 hr
Acute sinusitis:
   6 mo—12 yr: 15—30 mg/kg/24 hr PO ÷ Q12 hr; **max. dose:** 1 g/24 hr
   >12 yr: 250 or 500 mg PO Q12 hr
Uncomplicated skin infections:
   2—12 yr: 20 mg/kg/24 hr PO Q24 hr; **max. dose:** 500 mg/dose
   >12 yr: 250 mg PO Q12 hr or 500 mg PO Q12—24 hr
UTI:
   2—24 mo: 30 mg/kg/24 hr PO ÷ Q12 hr

Use with caution in penicillin-allergic patients or in presence of renal impairment. Oral
suspension contains aspartame and phenylalanine and should not be used by
phenylketonurics. May cause nausea, vomiting, diarrhea, liver enzyme elevations, and false-positive
urine-reducing substance (e.g., Clinitest, Benedict's solution, or Fehling's solution) and Coombs
test. Enzymatic glucose oxidase urinary glucose tests (e.g., Clinistix or Tes-Tape) are recommended.
Probenecid increases serum cefprozil levels. Absorption is not affected by food. **Adjust dose in renal
failure (see Chapter 31).**

CEFTAROLINE FOSAMIL
Teflaro
Antibiotic, cephalosporin (fifth generation)

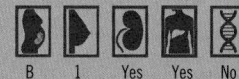

B   1   Yes   Yes   No

Injection: 400, 600 mg; contains L-arginine

Child (2 mo—<18 yr):

Acute bacterial skin and skin structure infection (ABSSSI) and community-acquired bacterial pneumonia (CABP):
  Infant <2 mo (ABSSSI indication only): 6 mg/kg/dose IV Q8 hr
  2 mo—<2 yr: 8 mg/kg/dose IV Q8 hr
  ≥2 yr—<18 yr:
    ≤33 kg: 12 mg/kg/dose IV Q8 hr
    >33 kg: 400 mg IV Q8 hr or 600 mg IV Q12 hr
Adult: 600 mg IV Q12 hr
Cystic fibrosis (limited data):
  Child ≥6 yr and adolescent: 15 mg/kg/dose IV Q8 hr (**max. dose:** 600 mg/dose) infused over 2 hr in 7 patients (mean age: 20.3 ± 8.0) achieved the targeted serum concentration time greater than the MIC of 60%.
  Adult: Pharmacokinetic simulations in 8 patients revealed dosages of 600 mg IV Q8 hr infused over 1 hr or 600 mg IV Q12 hr infused over 3 hr would achieve the targeted serum concentration time greater than the MIC of 60%.

Use with caution in penicillin allergy and renal impairment. Common side effects from pediatric trials include diarrhea, rash, vomiting, pyrexia, and nausea. Leukopenia and liver enzyme elevations have been reported.
Probenecid increases serum ceftaroline levels. Direct Coombs test seroconversion has been reported with use.
Adjust dose in renal failure (see Chapter 31).

CEFTAZIDIME
Tazicef and generics; previously available as Fortaz
Antibiotic, cephalosporin (third generation)

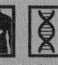

B   1   Yes   Yes   No

Injection: 1, 2, 6 g
Frozen injection: 1 g/50 mL 4.4% dextrose, 2 g/50 mL 3.2% dextrose (iso-osmotic solutions)
Contains 2.3 mEq Na/g drug

Neonate (IV/IM):

Postnatal age ≤7 days: 50 mg/kg/dose Q12 hr
Postnatal age >7—28 days:
  <1000 g:
    Postnatal age 8—14 days: 50 mg/kg/dose Q12 hr
    Postnatal age 15—28 days: 50 mg/kg/dose Q8 hr
  ≥1000 g: 50 mg/kg/dose Q8 hr
Meningitis:
  Postnatal age ≤7 days: 50 mg/kg/dose Q8—12 hr
  Postnatal age >7 days: 50 mg/kg/dose Q8 hr
Infant (>1 mo), child and adolescent (IV/IM):
  Mild/moderate infection: 100—150 mg/kg/24 hr ÷ Q8 hr; **max. dose:** 6 g/24 hr
  Meningitis: 150—200 mg/kg/24 hr ÷ Q8 hr (**max. dose:** 6 g/24 hr)

Continued

CEFTAZIDIME *continued*

Serious *Pseudomonas* infections: 200–300 mg/kg/24 hr ÷ Q8 hr (**max. dose:** 12 g/24 hr)
Cystic fibrosis: 200–400 mg/kg/24 hr ÷ Q6–8 hr (**max. dose:** 12 g/24 hr)
Adult (IV/IM): 1–2 g/dose Q8–12 hr; **max. dose:** 6 g/24 hr

Use with caution in penicillin-allergic patients or in presence of renal impairment. Good *Pseudomonas* coverage and CSF penetration. May cause rash, liver enzyme elevations, and false-positive urine-reducing substance (e.g., Clinitest, Benedict's solution, or Fehling's solution) and Coombs test. Enzymatic glucose oxidase urinary glucose tests (e.g., Clinistix or Tes-Tape) are recommended. Probenecid increases serum ceftazidime levels. **Adjust dose in renal failure (see Chapter 31).** Nonconvulsive status epilepticus, neuromuscular excitability, and myoclonia may occur with elevated levels of ceftazidime.

CEFTAZIDIME WITH AVIBACTAM
Avycaz
Antibiotic, cephalosporin (third generation with β-lactamase inhibitor)

?   1   Yes   Yes   No

Injection: 2 g ceftazidime and 0.5 g avibactam
Contains 3.2 mEq Na/g ceftazidime

All doses based on ceftazidime component and are infused over 2 hr.
Complicated UTI (including pyelonephritis; treat for 7–14 days):
≥3 mo–<6 mo: 40 mg/kg/dose IV Q8 hr
≥6 mo, child, and adolescent: 50 mg/kg/dose (**max.** 2 g/dose) IV Q8 hr
Adult: 2 g IV Q8 hr
Complicated intra-abdominal infections: Use same dosage for complicated UT in combination with metronidazole and treat for 5–14 days.
Nosocomial pneumonia (including VAP):
Adult: 2 g IV Q8 hr × 7–14 days

See Ceftazidime for additional remarks. Avibactam is a novel β-lactamase inhibitor of serine β-lactamases to improve ceftazidime's susceptibility to Enterobacteriaceae.
Clinical trial safety profiles in children and adults are similar, which include common side effects of vomiting, diarrhea, rash, and infusion site reactions. May cause false-positive urine-reducing substance (e.g., Clinitest, Benedict's solution, or Fehling's solution) and Coombs test. Enzymatic glucose oxidase urinary glucose tests (e.g., Clinistix or Tes-Tape) are recommended.
Adjust dose in renal failure (see Chapter 31). Australian Therapeutic Goods Administration reports animal reproductive toxicity without evidence of teratogenic effects with avibactam. Human studies of ceftazidime/avibactam are incomplete.

CEFTOLOZANE WITH TAZOBACTAM
Zerbaxa
Antibiotic, cephalosporin with β-lactamase inhibitor

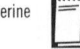

?   1   Yes   Yes   No

Injection: 1 g ceftolozane and 0.5 g tazobactam; contains 600 mg L-arginine
Contains 8.3 mEq Na/g ceftolozane

All doses based on ceftolozane component and are infused over 1 hr.
Neonate (limited data based on a single-dose pharmacokinetic [PK] evaluation where PK profiles in 13 neonates and infants <3 mo were comparable to older children receiving a single

CEFTOLOZANE WITH TAZOBACTAM *continued*

IV dose; <32 wk gestation and >7 days old [N=6] and >32 wk gestation and >7 days old [N=7]):
UTI: 20 mg/kg/dose IV Q8 hr
Severe infections: 40 mg/kg/dose IV Q8 hr
Infant, child, and adolescent:
  Complicated intra-abdominal infection and complicated UTI (including pyelonephritis): 20 mg/kg/dose (**max. dose:** 1 g/dose) IV Q8 hr for 5—14 days for intra-abdominal infection and 7—14 days for UTI
  Severe infections: 40 mg/kg/dose (**max. dose:** 2 g/dose) IV Q8 hr
Adult:
  Complicated intra-abdominal infection and UTI (including pyelonephritis): 1 g IV Q8 hr for 4—14 days for intra-abdominal infection and 7 days for UTI
  Hospital-acquired pneumonia and ventilator-associated pneumonia: 2 g IV Q8 hr for 8—14 days

Use is reserved for multi-drug-resistant Gram-negative bacterial infections, including *Pseudomonas aeruginosa* and *E. coli*. Tazobactam irreversibly inhibits certain β-lactamases, penicillinases, and cephalosporinases to extend ceftolozane's spectrum of activity. Safety and efficacy in children with hospital-acquired and ventilator-associated pneumonia are currently being evaluated.

Use with caution in penicillin, cephalosporin, or β-lactam allergic patients or in the presence of renal impairment **(adjust dose in renal failure; see Chapter 31).** Decreased efficacy has been reported in adults with baseline eGFR of 30—50 mL/min/1.73 m² in both intra-abdominal and UTI trials (monitor for changing renal function and adjust dosage accordingly). The manufacturer does not recommend use in children with an eGFR <50 mL/min/1.73 m² due to insufficient clinical data.

Common side effects in pediatric trials include thrombocytopenia, diarrhea, pyrexia, leukopenia, abdominal pain, vomiting, increased AST, and anemia. Common side effects in adult UTI trials include nausea, diarrhea, headache, and pyrexia. Increased hepatic transaminases, renal impairment, and diarrhea were observed in adult pneumonia trials.

CEFTRIAXONE				
Generics; previously available as Rocephin				
Antibiotic, cephalosporin (third generation)	B	1	Yes	Yes No

Injection: 0.25, 0.5, 1, 2, 10 g
Frozen injection: 1 g/50 mL 3.8% dextrose, 2 g/50 mL 2.4% dextrose (iso-osmotic solutions)
Contains 3.6 mEq Na/g drug

Neonate:
  Gonococcal ophthalmia or prophylaxis: 25—50 mg/kg/dose IM/IV × 1; **max. dose:** 250 mg/dose
Infant (>1 mo) and child:
  Mild/moderate infections: 50—75 mg/kg/24 hr ÷ Q12—24 hr IM/IV; **max. dose:** 2 g/24 hr
  Severe infections/meningitis (including penicillin-resistant pneumococci): 100 mg/kg/24 hr IM/IV ÷ Q12 hr; **max. dose:** 2 g/dose and 4 g/24 hr
  Penicillin-resistant pneumococci outside of the CSF: 80—100 mg/kg/24 hr ÷ Q12—24 hr (**max. dose:** 2 g/dose and 4 g/24 hr)
  Lyme disease: 50—75 mg/kg/dose (**max. dose:** 2 g/dose) IV once daily
  Acute otitis media: 50 mg/kg IM/IV (**max. dose:** 1 g) × 1; for persistent or relapse cases use 50 mg/kg IM/IV (**max. dose:** 1 g) Q24 hr × 3 doses
Adult: 1—2 g/dose Q12—24 hr IV/IM; **max. dose:** 2 g/dose and 4 g/24 hr

Continued

CEFTRIAXONE *continued*

Uncomplicated gonorrhea:
    <150 kg: 500 mg IM × 1
    ≥150 kg: 1 g IM x 1
PID (see latest CDC Sexually Transmitted Infections Treatment Guidelines):
    Mild/moderate acute: 0.5—1 g IM x 1 (following the above uncomplicated gonorrhea dosage), plus
    doxycycline 100 mg Q12 hr PO and metronidazole 500 mg Q12 hr PO × 14 days
    Severe acute: 1 g IV once daily, plus doxycycline 100 mg Q12 hr IV/PO and metronidazole 500 mg
    Q12 hr IV/PO to complete a 14-day course; convert to oral therapy after clinical improvement with
    IV therapy.
Bacterial endocarditis prophylaxis for dental and upper respiratory procedures:
    Infant and child: 50 mg/kg IV/IM (**max. dose:** 1 g) 30—60 min before procedure
    Adult: 1 g IV/IM 30—60 min before procedure

Contraindicated in neonates with hyperbilirubinemia. **Do not** administer with IV
calcium-containing solutions or products (mixed or administered simultaneously via different
lines) in neonates (<28 days old) because of risk of precipitation of ceftriaxone-calcium salt. Cases
of fatal reactions with calcium-ceftriaxone precipitates in lung and kidneys in preterm and full-term
neonates have been reported. **Do not** administer simultaneously with IV calcium-containing solutions
via a Y-site for any age group. IV calcium-containing products may be administered sequentially only
when the infusion lines are thoroughly flushed between infusions with a compatible fluid.
Use with caution in penicillin allergy; patients with gallbladder, biliary tract, liver, or pancreatic disease;
presence of renal impairment; or in neonates with continuous dosing (risk for hyperbilirubinemia). In
neonates, consider using an alternative third-generation cephalosporin with similar activity. Unlike
other cephalosporins, ceftriaxone is significantly cleared by the biliary route (35%—45%).
Rash, injection site pain, diarrhea, and transient increase in liver enzymes are common. May cause
reversible cholelithiasis, sludging in gallbladder, and jaundice. Reversible neurologic reactions
(e.g., encephalopathy, seizures, myoclonus) have been reported in post-marketing reports. May
interfere with serum and urine creatinine assays (Jaffe method) and cause false-positive urinary
protein and urinary reducing substances (e.g., Clinitest, Benedict's solution, or Fehling's solution).
Enzymatic glucose oxidase urinary glucose tests (e.g., Clinistix or Tes-Tape) are recommended.
For IM injections, dilute drug with either sterile water for injection or 1% lidocaine to a concentration
of 250 or 350 mg/mL (250 mg/mL has lower incidence of injection site reactions). Assess the
potential risk/benefit for using lidocaine as a diluent; see Lidocaine for additional remarks,
especially risk for methemoglobinemia.

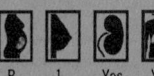

CEFUROXIME (IV, IM)/CEFUROXIME AXETIL (PO)
IV: Generics; previously available as Zinacef
PO: Generics; previously available as Ceftin
Antibiotic, cephalosporin (second generation)

    B   1   Yes   Yes   No

Injection: 0.75, 1.5 g
Injectable dosage forms contain 2.4 mEq Na/g drug.
Tabs: 250, 500 mg

IM/IV:
    Neonate:
        Postnatal age ≤7 days: 100 mg/kg/24 hr ÷ Q12 hr
        Postnatal age >7 days:
            <1 kg:
                8 to ≤14 days old: 100 mg/kg/24 hr ÷ Q12 hr

CEFUROXIME (IV, IM)/CEFUROXIME AXETIL (PO) *continued*

 ≥15 days old: 150 mg/kg/24 hr ÷ Q8 hr
 ≥1 kg: 150 mg/kg/24 hr ÷ Q8 hr
Infant (>3 mo)/child:
Mild/moderate infection: 75–100 mg/kg/24 hr ÷ Q8 hr; **max. dose:** 1500 mg/dose
Severe infection: 100–200 mg/kg/24 hr ÷ Q6–8 hr; **max. dose:** 1500 mg/dose
Adult: 750–1500 mg/dose Q8 hr; **max. dose:** 9 g/24 hr
PO (see remarks):
Child (3 mo–12 yr):
 Pharyngitis and tonsillitis (oral suspension): 20 mg/kg/24 hr ÷ Q12 hr; **max. dose:** 500 mg/24 hr
 Impetigo (oral suspension): 30 mg/kg/24 hr ÷ Q12 hr; **max. dose:** 1 g/24 hr
 Otitis media and sinusitis:
  Oral suspension: 30 mg/kg/24 hr ÷ Q12 hr; **max. dose:** 1 g/24 hr
  Oral tablet: 250 mg BID
 Lyme disease (alternative to doxycycline or amoxicillin):
  Oral suspension: 30 mg/kg/24 hr (**max. dose:** 1 g/24 hr) ÷ Q12 hr × 14–28 days
Child (≥13 yr):
 Sinusitis, otitis media, pharyngitis, and tonsillitis:
  Tab: 250 mg Q12 hr
Adult: 250–500 mg BID; **max. dose:** 1 g/24 hr

Use with caution in penicillin-allergic patients or in presence of renal impairment. May cause GI discomfort; thrombophlebitis at the infusion site; false-positive urine-reducing substance (e.g., Clinitest, Benedict's solution, or Fehling's solution) and Coombs test; and may interfere with serum and urine creatinine determinations by the alkaline picrate method. Enzymatic glucose oxidase urinary glucose tests (e.g., Clinistix or Tes-Tape) are recommended. Transient increases in liver enzymes have been reported. Not recommended for meningitis.

Oral suspension dosage form currently not available. Tablets and oral suspension are NOT bioequivalent and CANNOT be substituted on a mg/mg basis. Concurrent use of antacids, H$_2$ blockers, and proton pump inhibitors may decrease oral absorption. **Adjust dose in renal failure (see Chapter 31).**

CELECOXIB
Celebrex, Elyxyb, and generics
Nonsteroidal antiinflammatory agent (COX-2 selective)

 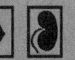

C/X   2   Yes   Yes   Yes

Capsules (Celebrex and generics): 50, 100, 200, 400 mg
Oral solution (Elyxyb): 120 mg/4.8 mL (4.8 mL); contains alcohol, cremophor, and levomenthol

Juvenile rheumatoid arthritis (JRA; ≥2 yr and adolescent; see remarks for dosage adjustment considerations):
 10–25 kg: 50 mg PO BID
 >25 kg: 100 mg PO BID
Adult (see remarks for dosage adjustment considerations):
 Analgesia: 100–200 mg PO BID
 Acute migraine with or without aura (Elyxyb): 120 mg PO × 1; **max. dose:** 120 mg/24 hr

Contraindicated for perioperative pain with coronary artery bypass graft (CABG) surgery. **Use with caution** in patients with systemic-onset JRA due to risk for serious adverse reactions

Continued

CELECOXIB *continued*

(e.g., disseminated intravascular coagulation). In adults, serious cardiovascular and GI
risks reported include thrombosis, myocardial infarction (MI), stroke, GI bleed, GI ulceration, and
GI perforation. Common adverse effects include headache, diarrhea, nausea, and hypertension.
DRESS, TEN, SJS, acute kidney injury, and hyperkalemia have also been reported.

Celecoxib is a substrate of CYP 450 2C9. Poor metabolizers of 2C9 should start with half the lowest
recommended dose and use with caution, or consider alternative therapy. Angiotensin-converting
enzyme (ACE) inhibitors, loop diuretics, and sodium phosphates may increase risk for renal
dysfunction. Oral corticosteroids, antiplatelet drugs (e.g., aspirin), anticoagulants, SSRIs, smoking,
alcohol use, older age, and poor health status may increase risk for GI bleeds with prolonged
treatment courses. Celecoxib may reduce the antihypertensive effects of ACE inhibitors and increase
the levels/toxicity of lithium, metoprolol, and methotrexate.

Not recommended for use in severe renal dysfunction and severe hepatic impairment (Child-Pugh
Class C). Reduce dose by 50% and monitor patient closely in moderate hepatic impairment (Child-
Pugh Class B).

Pregnancy category is "C" for prior to 30 weeks' gestation and "X" for 30 weeks and greater. **Avoid use**
at ≥30 weeks' gestation due to increased risk for premature closure of the fetal ductus arteriosus.
Limit dose and duration of use at 20–30 weeks' gestation for concerns of fetal renal dysfunction.

If patient is unable to swallow capsules whole, contents of the capsule may be added to applesauce
(stable for up to 6 hr refrigerated) and ingested with water.

CEPHALEXIN
Generics; previously available as Keflex
Antibiotic, cephalosporin (first generation)

B | 1 | Yes | Yes | No

Caps: 250, 500, 750 mg
Tabs: 250, 500 mg
Oral suspension: 125 mg/5 mL, 250 mg/5 mL (100, 200 mL)

Infant and child:
    Mild/moderate infection: 25–50 mg/kg/24 hr PO ÷ Q6 hr; **max. dose:** 2 g/24 hr. Less
    frequent dosing (Q8–12 hr) may be used for uncomplicated infections.
    Severe infection: 75–100 mg/kg/24 hr PO ÷ Q6 hr; **max. dose:** 4 g/24 hr
    Streptococcal pharyngitis and skin infections: 25–50 mg/kg/24 hr PO ÷ Q6–12 hr. Total daily
    dose may be divided Q12 hr for streptococcal pharyngitis (>1 yr).
    UTI: 25 mg/kg/dose PO Q6–8 hr; **max. dose:** 1 g/dose
Adult: 1–4 g/24 hr PO ÷ Q6 hr
Max. dose (all ages): 4 g/24 hr
Bacterial endocarditis prophylaxis for dental and upper respiratory procedures:
    Infant and child: 50 mg/kg PO (**max. dose:** 2 g) 30–60 min before procedure
    Adult: 2 g PO 30–60 min before procedure

Some cross-reactivity with penicillins. **Use with caution** in renal insufficiency. May cause GI
discomfort, false-positive urine-reducing substance (e.g., Clinitest, Benedict's solution, or
Fehling's solution) and Coombs test; false elevation of serum theophylline levels (HPLC method);
and false urinary protein test. Enzymatic glucose oxidase urinary glucose tests (e.g., Clinistix or Tes-
Tape) are recommended. Hemolytic anemia and slight increases in AST and ALT have been reported.

Probenecid increases serum cephalexin levels, and concomitant administration with cholestyramine
may reduce cephalexin absorption. May increase the effects of metformin.

Administer doses on an empty stomach; 2 hr prior to or 1 hr after meals. **Adjust dose in renal failure
(see Chapter 31).**

CETIRIZINE ± PSEUDOEPHEDRINE
Zyrtec, Zyrtec Allergy, Zyrtec Children's Allergy,
Zerviate, and many generics
In combination with pseudoephedrine:
Zyrtec-D 12 hr and generics
Antihistamine, less-sedating

    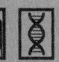

B/C 2 Yes Yes No

Oral solution or syrup (OTC): 5 mg/5 mL (120, 473 mL); contains parabens
Tabs (OTC): 5, 10 mg
Chewable tabs (OTC): 2.5, 5, 10 mg
Capsule (liquid filled; OTC): 10 mg
Dispersible/disintegrating tabs (OTC): 10 mg
Ophthalmic solution (Zerviate): 2.4 mg/1 mL (0.2 mL; 5 or 30 single-use vials per box; and 5, 7.5 mL multidose bottles); contains benzalkonium chloride and polyethylene glycol
In combination with pseudoephedrine (PE):
    Extended release tabs (OTC): 5 mg cetirizine + 120 mg PE

Cetirizine (see remarks for dosing in hepatic impairment):
    6 mo and <2 yr: 2.5 mg PO once daily; dose may be increased for children 12−23 mo to a
    max. dose of 2.5 mg PO Q12 hr
    2−5 yr: Initial dose: 2.5 mg PO once daily; if needed, may increase dose to a **max. dose** of 5 mg/24 hr
    once daily or divided BID
    ≥6 yr−adult: 5−10 mg PO once daily
    Ophthalmic use:
        ≥2 yr and adult: Instill 1 drop to affected eye(s) BID (approximately 8 hr apart).
**Cetirizine in combination with pseudoephedrine (PE) (see remarks for dosing in hepatic
impairment):**
    ≥12 yr and adult:
        Zyrtec-D 12 hr: 1 tablet PO BID

Generally not recommended for treating URIs for infants. No proven benefit for infants and
young children with URIs. The FDA does not recommend use for URIs in children <2 yr
because of reports of increased fatalities.
May cause headache, pharyngitis, GI symptoms, dry mouth, and sedation. Aggressive reactions and
convulsions have been reported. Has NOT been implicated in causing cardiac arrhythmias when
used with other drugs that are metabolized by hepatic microsomal enzymes (e.g., ketoconazole,
erythromycin).
In hepatic impairment, the following doses have been recommended:
    Cetirizine:
        <6 yr: Use not recommended
        6−11 yr: <2.5 mg PO once daily
        ≥12 yr−adult: 5 mg PO once daily
    Cetirizine in combination with pseudoephedrine (Zyrtec-D 12 and generics):
        ≥12 yr−adult: 1 tablet PO once daily
Doses may be administered without regard to food. For Zyrtec-D 12 Hr, see Pseudoephedrine for
additional remarks. Pregnancy category is "B" for cetirizine and "C" when combined with
pseudoephedrine. **Dosage adjustment is recommended in renal impairment (see Chapter 31).**
OPHTHALMIC USE: Common side effects include application site pain, ocular hyperemia, and reduced
visual acuity. Oculogyric crisis has been reported. Do not touch dropper tip to anything, and remove
contact lenses prior to administration (wait 10 min before reinserting lenses).

CHARCOAL, ACTIVATED

See Chapter 3.

CHLORAMPHENICOL
Generics
Antibiotic

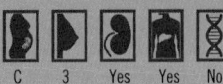

C 3 Yes Yes No

Injection: 1 g
Contains 2.25 mEq Na/g drug

Neonate IV (see remarks for therapeutic drug monitoring):
  Loading dose: 20 mg/kg
  Maintenance dose (first dose should be given 12 hr after loading dose):
    ≤7 days: 25 mg/kg/24 hr Q24 hr
    >7 days:
      ≤2 kg: 25 mg/kg/24 hr Q24 hr
      >2 kg: 50 mg/kg/24 hr ÷ Q12 hr
Infant/child/adult (see remarks for therapeutic drug monitoring): 50–75 mg/kg/24 hr IV ÷ Q6 hr
  Meningitis: 75–100 mg/kg/24 hr IV ÷ Q6 hr
Max. dose (all ages): 4 g/24 hr

Dose recommendations are just guidelines for therapy; monitoring of blood levels is essential.
  Follow hematologic status for dose-related or idiosyncratic marrow suppression. "Gray baby"
  syndrome may be seen with levels >50 mg/L. **Use with caution** in G6PD deficiency, renal or hepatic
  dysfunction, and neonates.
Concomitant use of phenobarbital and rifampin may lower chloramphenicol serum levels.
  Phenytoin may increase chloramphenicol serum levels. Chloramphenicol may increase the
  effects/toxicity of phenytoin, chlorpropamide, cyclosporine, tacrolimus, and oral
  anticoagulants and decrease absorption of vitamin B_{12}. Chloramphenicol is an inhibitor of
  CYP 450 2C9.
Therapeutic levels: Peak: 15–25 mg/L for meningitis and 10–20 mg/L for other infections. Trough:
  5–15 mg/L for meningitis and 5–10 mg/L for other infections. Recommended serum sampling
  time: trough within 30 min prior to next dose; peak 30 min after the end of infusion. Time to achieve
  steady state: 2–3 days for newborns; 12–24 hr for children and adults.

CHLOROQUINE PHOSPHATE
Generics; previously available as Aralen
Amebicide, antimalarial

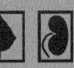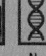

C 2 Yes Yes No

Tabs: 250, 500 mg as phosphate (150, 300 mg base, respectively)
Oral suspension: 16.67 mg/mL as phosphate (10 mg/mL base), 15 mg/mL as phosphate (9 mg/mL
  base)

Doses expressed in mg of chloroquine base:
  Malaria prophylaxis (start 1–2 wk prior to exposure and continue for 4 wk after leaving
    endemic area):
    Infant and child: 5 mg/kg/dose PO every week on the same day of the week; **max. dose:** 300 mg/
      dose
    Adult: 300 mg/dose PO every week on the same day of the week

CHLOROQUINE PHOSPHATE *continued*

Malaria treatment (chloroquine sensitive strains):
For treatment for malaria, consult with ID specialist or see the latest edition of the AAP Red Book.
Infant and child: 10 mg/kg/dose (**max. dose:** 600 mg/dose) PO × 1; followed by 5 mg/kg/dose
(**max. dose:** 300 mg/dose) 6, 24, and 48 hr after the initial dose
Adult: 600 mg/dose PO × 1; followed by 300 mg/dose 6, 24, and 48 hr after the initial dose

Contraindicated in the presence of retinal or visual field changes and known hypersensitivity
to 4-aminoquinoline compounds. **Use with caution** in liver disease, preexisting auditory
damage or seizures, G6PD deficiency, psoriasis, porphyria, or concomitant hepatotoxic drugs. May
cause nausea, vomiting, electrocardiogram (ECG) abnormalities, prolonged QT interval, blurred
vision, retinal and corneal changes (reversible corneal opacities), headaches, confusion, skeletal
muscle weakness, increased liver enzymes, and hair depigmentation. SJS, TEN, anaphylactic
reactions, and maculopathy and macular degeneration have been reported. False-positive test for
urine amphetamine screen may occur.

Antacids, ampicillin, and kaolin may decrease the absorption of chloroquine (allow 4-hr interval
between these drugs and chloroquine). Cimetidine may increase effects/toxicity of chloroquine. May
increase serum cyclosporine levels. Coadministration with mefloquine may increase risk of
convulsions. May reduce the antibody response to intradermal human diploid-cell rabies vaccine.
Monitor CBCs periodically with therapies of prolonged duration. **Adjust dose in renal failure (see
Chapter 31).**

CHLOROTHIAZIDE
Diuril and generics
Thiazide diuretic

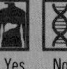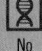

C/D	2	Yes	Yes	No

Oral suspension: 250 mg/5 mL (237 mL); contains 0.5% alcohol, 0.12% methylparaben, 0.02%
propylparaben, and 0.1% benzoic acid
Injection: 500 mg; contains 5 mEq Na/1 g drug

<6 mo:
PO: 20—40 mg/kg/24 hr ÷ Q12 hr
IV: Start at 5—10 mg/kg/24 hr ÷ Q12 hr; may increase to 20—40 mg/kg/24 hr ÷ Q12 hr if needed
≥6 mo:
PO: 10—40 mg/kg/24 hr ÷ Q12 hr; **maximum PO dose by age:**
   6 mo—<2 yr: 375 mg/24 hr
   2—12 yr: 1 g/24 hr
   >12 yr: 2 g/24 hr
IV: Start at 5—10 mg/kg/24 hr ÷ Q12—24 hr, may increase to 20 mg/kg/24 hr ÷ Q12 hr if needed
Adult: 500—2000 mg/24 hr ÷ Q12—24 hr IV; alternative IV dosing, some may respond to intermittent
dosing on alternate days or on 3—5 days each week
Adjunct therapy for neonatal hyperinsulinemia/hypoglycemia (limited data): 7—10 mg/kg/24 hr ÷
BID PO with diazoxide PO

Contraindicated in anuria. **Use with caution** in liver and severe renal disease and sulfonamide
hypersensitivity. May increase serum calcium, bilirubin, glucose, and uric acid. May cause
alkalosis, pancreatitis, dizziness, hypokalemia, and hypomagnesemia.
Avoid IM or subcutaneous administration.
Pregnancy category changes to "D" if used in pregnancy-induced hypertension.

CHLORPHENIRAMINE MALEATE
Chlor-Trimeton and generics
Antihistamine
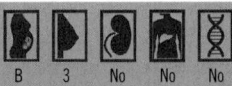
B 3 No No No

Tabs [OTC]: 4 mg
Sustained release tabs [OTC]: 12 mg
Syrup [OTC]: 2 mg/5 mL (120, 473 mL); may contain 5% alcohol and/or parabens

Doses may be administered as scheduled or PRN (see remarks).
Child <12 yr: 0.35 mg/kg/24 hr PO ÷ Q4—6 hr or dose based on age as follows:
 2—5 yr: 1 mg/dose PO Q4—6 hr; **max. dose:** 6 mg/24 hr
 6—11 yr: 2 mg/dose PO Q4—6 hr; **max. dose:** 12 mg/24 hr
≥12 yr—adult: 4 mg/dose Q4—6 hr PO; **max. dose:** 24 mg/24 hr
 Sustained release: 12 mg PO Q12 hr

Use with caution in asthma. May cause sedation, dry mouth, blurred vision, urinary retention,
 polyuria, and disturbed coordination. Young children may be paradoxically excited.
Found in many combinations, over-the-counter (OTC) cough and cold products are **not recommended**
 for children <6 yr old due to reports of serious adverse effects (cardiac and respiratory distress,
 convulsions, and hallucinations) and fatalities (from unintentional overdosages, including combined
 use of other OTC products containing the same active ingredients).
Administer doses with food. Sustained release forms are **NOT** recommended in children <6 yr and
 should **NOT** be crushed, chewed, or dissolved.

CHLORPROMAZINE
Generics; previously available as Thorazine
*Antiemetic, antipsychotic, phenothiazine
derivative*
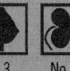
C 3 No No No

Tabs: 10, 25, 50, 100, 200 mg
Oral liquid concentrate: 30 mg/mL (120 mL), 100 mg/mL (240 mL)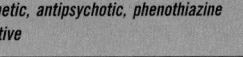
Injection: 25 mg/mL (1, 2 mL); may contain sodium metabisulfite and sodium sulfite

**Psychosis (gradually taper doses when discontinuing therapy to prevent withdrawal
 symptoms and minimize risk of relapse):**
Child >6 mo:
 PO: 2.5—6 mg/kg/24 hr ÷ Q4—6 hr; **max. PO dose:** 500 mg/24 hr
 IM/IV: 2.5—4 mg/kg/24 hr ÷ Q6—8 hr
 Max. IM/IV dose:
  <5 yr: 40 mg/24 hr
  5—12 yr: 75 mg/24 hr
Adult:
 PO: 10—25 mg/dose Q4—6 hr; **max. dose:** 1—2 g/24 hr
 IM/IV: Initial: 25 mg; repeat with 25—50 mg/dose; if needed, Q1—4 hr up to a **max. dose** of 400
  mg/dose Q4—6 hr
Antiemetic:
 Child (≥6 mo):
  IV/IM/PO: 0.5—1 mg/kg/dose Q6—8 hr PRN
  Max. IM/IV/PO dose:
   <5 yr or <22.7 kg: 40 mg/24 hr
   5—12 yr or 22.7—45.5 kg: 75 mg/24 hr

CHLORPROMAZINE *continued*

Adult:

IV/IM: 25—50 mg/dose Q4—6 hr PRN; **max. dose:** 300 mg/24 hr
PO: 10—25 mg/dose Q4—6 hr PRN; **max. dose:** 150 mg/24 hr

Adverse effects include drowsiness, jaundice, lowered seizure threshold, extrapyramidal/anticholinergic symptoms, hypotension (more with IV), arrhythmias, agranulocytosis, and neuroleptic malignant syndrome. May potentiate effect of narcotics, sedatives, and other drugs. Monitor BP closely. ECG changes include prolonged PR interval, flattened T waves, and ST depression; **do not use** in combination with fluoxetine, haloperidol, citalopram, and other drugs that can prolong the QT interval. **Do not administer oral liquid dosage form simultaneously with carbamazepine oral suspension;** an orange, rubbery precipitate may form.

CHOLECALCIFEROL
D—3, D3—5, D3—50, Decara, D Drops, Emfamil
D-Vi-Sol, Replesta, and many others
Vitamin D₃

    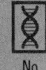

| A/D | 1 | No | No | No |

Tablet (OTC): 400; 1000; 2000; 3000; 5000; 50,000 IU
Caps (OTC): 1000; 2000; 5000; 10,000; 50,000 IU
  D3—5: 5000 IU
  Decara: 5,000, 25,000 IU
  D3—50: 50,000 IU
Chewable tablet (OTC): 400; 1000; 2000 IU
Chewable wafer (Replesta; OTC): 14,000 (8), 50,000 IU (4)
Oral drops (D Drops and others) [OTC]: 400 IU/drop (2.5, 10.3 mL), 600 IU/drop (2.8 mL), 1000 IU/drop (5, 10.3 mL), 2000 IU/drop (5, 10.3 mL), 4000 IU/drop (10.3 mL), 6000 IU/drop (10.3 mL)
Oral liquid (OTC): 400, 5000 IU/mL
  Emfamil D-Vi-Sol (OTC): 400 IU/mL (50 mL)
Conversion: 1000 IU is equivalent to 25 mCg of cholecalciferol

Dietary supplementation (see Chapter 21 for additional information):
  Preterm: 200—400 IU/24 hr PO
  Infant (<1 yr): 400 IU/24 hr PO
  Neonate and infant (breastfed and/or receiving <32 oz of formula): 400 IU/24 hr PO
  Child (≥1 yr) and adolescent: 400—600 IU/24 hr PO
  Cystic fibrosis: See specific cystic fibrosis specialty multivitamin product (e.g., DEKA Plus, MVW Complete, ADEK) for recommended dosages.
Vitamin D insufficiency and deficiency (PO):
  Patients without cystic fibrosis or malabsorptive conditions:

Vitamin D (25-OH) Level		
Age	**12—<20 ng/mL (Insufficiency)**	**<12 ng/mL (Deficiency)**
<1 yr	1000 IU once daily	2000—4000 IU once daily
≥1 yr	2000 IU once daily	5000—6000 IU once daily OR 50,000 IU once weekly

Continued

CHOLECALCIFEROL *continued*

Patients with non-cystic fibrosis malabsorptive conditions:

	Vitamin D (25-OH) Level	
Age	12—<20 ng/mL (Insufficiency)	<12 ng/mL (Deficiency)
<10 yr	2000 IU once daily	5000 IU once daily
≥10 yr	4000—6000 IU once daily	10,000 IU once daily OR 50,000 IU once weekly

Patients with cystic fibrosis:

	Vitamin D (25-OH) Level	
Age	20—<30 ng/mL (Insufficiency)	<20 ng/mL (Deficiency)
<1 yr	2000 IU once daily	5000 IU once daily
1—<10 yr	6000 IU once daily	50,000 IU once daily × 1 mo followed by either 10,000 IU once daily OR 50,000 IU once weekly
≥10 yr	10,000 IU once daily	50,000 IU once daily × 1 mo followed by either 10,000 IU once daily OR 50,000 IU once weekly

Rickets (with calcium supplementation; decrease to maintenance dosage when radiologically proven healing is achieved):
   Infant: 2000 IU PO once daily × ≥3 mo, followed by 400 IU once daily maintenance
   Child: 3000—6000 IU PO once daily × ≥3 mo, followed by 600 IU once daily maintenance
   Adolescent: 6000 IU PO once daily × ≥3 mo, followed by 600 IU once daily maintenance
Renal failure (CKD stages 2—5) and 25-OH vitamin D levels ≤30 ng/mL (monitor serum 25-OH vitamin D and corrected calcium/phosphorus 1 mo after initiation and Q3 mo thereafter):
   Child (PO):
      25-OH vitamin D <5 ng/mL: 8000 IU/24 hr × 4 wk, followed by 4000 IU/24 hr × 2 mo; OR 50,000 IU weekly × 4 wk, followed by 50,000 IU twice monthly × 3 mo
      25-OH vitamin D 5—15 ng/mL: 4000 IU/24 hr × 12 wk; OR 50,000 IU every other week × 12 wk
      25-OH vitamin D 16—30 ng/mL: 2000 IU/24 hr × 3 mo; OR 50,000 IU monthly × 3 mo
      Maintenance dose (after repletion): 200—1000 IU once daily

Biologic potency and oral absorption may be greater than ergocalciferol (vitamin D_2). Requires activation by the liver (25-hydroxylation) and kidney (1-hydroxylation) to the active form, calcitriol. Recommended time period to recheck serum 25-OH vitamin D is 3 mo after initiation or change in dosage.

Monitor serum Ca^{2+}, PO_4, 25-OH vitamin D (goal level for infant and child: ≥20 ng/mL) and alkaline phosphate. Serum Ca^{2+}, PO_4 product should be <70 mg/dL to avoid ectopic calcification. Serum 25-OH vitamin D level of ≥35 ng/mL has been used in cystic fibrosis patients to decrease the risk of hyperparathyroidism and bone loss.

Serum 25-OH vitamin D levels ≥100 ng/mL are considered toxic. Toxic effects in infants may result in nausea, vomiting, constipation, abdominal pain, loss of appetite, polydipsia, polyuria, muscle weakness, muscle/joint pain, confusion, and fatigue; renal damage may also occur.

Pregnancy category changes to "D" if used in doses above the U.S. RDA.

CHOLESTYRAMINE
Questran, Questran Light, Cholestyramine Light,
Prevalite, and generics
Antilipemic, binding resin

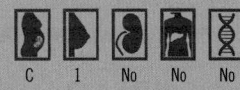

C   1   No   No   No

Powder for oral suspension:
    Questran and generics: 4 g anhydrous resin per 9 g powder (9 g—box of 60 packets, 378 g can)
    Questran Light: 4 g anhydrous resin per 5 g powder (5 g—box of 60 packets, 210 g can)
    Cholestyramine Light: 4 g anhydrous resin per 5.7 g powder with aspartame (5.7 g—box of 60
    packets, 239 g can)
    Prevalite: 4 g anhydrous resin per 5.5 g powder with aspartame (5.5 g—box of 42 or 60 packets,
    231 g can)

All doses based in terms of anhydrous resin. Titrate dose based on response and tolerance.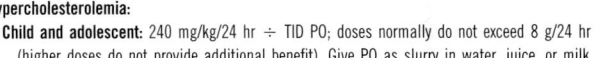
Hypercholesterolemia:
    Child and adolescent: 240 mg/kg/24 hr ÷ TID PO; doses normally do not exceed 8 g/24 hr
    (higher doses do not provide additional benefit). Give PO as slurry in water, juice, or milk
    before meals for better efficacy.
    Adult: 4 g once daily—BID PO; **max. dose:** 24 g/24 hr
Pruritus associated with cholestasis:
    Child: 240 mg/kg/24 hr ÷ BID—TID PO; suggested **max. dose:**
        ≤10 yr: 4—10 g/24 hr; higher doses may cause steatorrhea
        >10 yr and adolescent: 16 g/24 hr
    Adult: 4 g once daily or BID PO; may gradually increase dose to 16 g/24 hr. **Max. dose:** 24 g/24 hr

In addition to the use for managing hypercholesterolemia, drug may be used for itching
    associated with elevated bile acids, and diarrheal disorders associated with excess fecal
    bile acids or *Clostridium difficile* (pseudomembranous colitis). May also be applied topically for
    diaper dermatitis by preparing a 5% or 10% topical product with hydrophilic topical ointment
    (Aquaphor); other compounded topical formulations exist (e.g., Butt paste: Cholestyramine,
    sucralfate, zinc oxide, and Eucerin).
May cause constipation, abdominal distention, vomiting, vitamin deficiencies (A, D, E, K), and rash.
    Hyperchloremic acidosis may occur with prolonged use.
Give other oral medications 4—6 hr after cholestyramine or 1 hr before dose to avoid decreased
    absorption. High doses or long-term systemic therapy may decrease the absorption of folic acid,
    fat-soluble vitamins, and iron.

CICLESONIDE
Alvesco, Omnaris, Zetonna
Corticosteroid

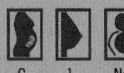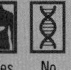

C   1   No   Yes   No

Aerosol inhaler (Alvesco): 80 mCg/actuation (6.1 g = 60 doses), 160 mCg/actuation (6.1 g = 60 doses)
Nasal spray:
    Omnaris (nasal suspension): 50 mCg/actuation (12.5 g = 120 doses); contains sodium EDTA
    Zetonna (nasal aerosol solution): 37 mCg/actuation (6.1 g = 60 doses)

Intranasal (allergic rhinitis):
    Omnaris:
        2—11 yr (limited data): 1 or 2 sprays (50 or 100 mCg) per nostril once daily. **Max. dose:** 200 mCg/
        24 hr

Continued

CICLESONIDE *continued*

FDA labeled seasonal allergic rhinitis for children ≥6 yr: 2 sprays (100 mCg) per nostril once daily

≥12 yr and adult: 2 sprays (100 mCg) per nostril once daily. **Max. dose:** 200 mCg/24 hr
Zetonna:
≥12 yr and adult: 1 spray (37 mCg) per nostril once daily. **Max. dose:** 74 mCg/24 hr
Oral inhalation (asthma; Alvesco):
Dosage recommended by the Global Initiative for Asthma (GINA) guidelines (current FDA labeled dosage information is for ≥12 yr and is listed below). All daily doses divided BID:

Age	Low Dose (mCg/24 hr)	Medium Dose (mCg/24 hr)	High Dose (mCg/24 hr)
6—11 yr	80	>80—160	>160 up to 640 mCg/24 hr
≥12 yr and adult	80—160	>160—320	>320 up to 640 mCg/24 hr

2—11 yr (limited data from randomized controlled studies in 4—11 and 2—6 yr of age, where efficacy could not be established): 40, 80, or 160 mCg/dose BID
≥12 yr and adult (FDA labeling):
Prior use with bronchodilator only: 80 mCg/dose BID; **max. dose:** 320 mCg/24 hr
Prior use with inhaled corticosteroid: 80 mCg/dose BID; **max. dose:** 640 mCg/24 hr
Prior use with oral corticosteroid: 320 mCg/dose BID; **max. dose:** 640 mCg/24 hr

Ciclesonide is a prodrug hydrolyzed to an active metabolite, des-ciclesonide via esterases in nasal mucosa and lungs; further metabolism via hepatic CYP3A4 and 2D6. Concurrent use with ketoconazole and other CYP 450 3A4 inhibitors may increase systemic des-ciclesonide levels. **Use with caution** and monitor in hepatic impairment.

Oral inhalation (asthma): Rinse mouth after each use. May cause headache, arthralgia, nasal congestion, nasopharyngitis, and URIs. Routinely monitor growth of pediatric patients. Maximum therapeutic benefit may not be achieved until 4 wk after initiation; consider dose increase if response is inadequate 4 wk after initial dosage.

Intranasal (allergic rhinitis): Clear nasal passages prior to use. May cause otalgia, epistaxis, nasopharyngitis, and headache. Nasal septal perforation has been reported. Patients should be free of nasal disease, except for allergic rhinitis, before starting therapy. Monitor linear growth of pediatric patients routinely. Onset of action: 24—48 hr; further improvement observed over 1—2 wk in seasonal allergic rhinitis or 5 wk in perennial allergic rhinitis. Discontinue use if nasal erosion, ulceration, or perforation occurs.

CIDOFOVIR
Generics; previously available as Vistide
Antiviral

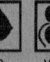

C   3   Yes   No   No

Injection: 75 mg/mL (5 mL); preservative free

Safety and efficacy have not been established in children.
CMV retinitis:
Adolescent and adult:
Induction: 5 mg/kg IV once weekly × 2 with probenecid and hydration

CIDOFOVIR *continued*

Maintenance: 5 mg/kg IV Q2 weeks with probenecid and hydration

Adenovirus infection in immunocompromised oncology patients (limited data and other regimens exist; see remarks):

Child:

Induction: 5 mg/kg/dose IV once weekly until PCR negative. Administer oral probenecid 1—1.25 g/m^2/dose (rounded to the nearest 250-mg interval) 3 hr before and 1 hr and 8 hr after each dose of cidofovir. Also give IV NS via IV at maintenance fluid concentration, 3 times, 1 hr before and 1 hr after cidofovir, followed by 2 times maintenance fluid for an additional 2 hr. For patients with renal dysfunction (see remarks), give 1 mg/kg/dose IV three times weekly until PCR negative.

Maintenance: 5 mg/kg/dose IV Q2 weeks with probenecid and hydration

Contraindicated in hypersensitivity to probenecid or sulfa-containing drugs; sCr >1.5 mg/dL, CrCl ≤55 mL/min, urine protein ≥100 mg/dL (2+ proteinuria), direct intraocular injection of cidofovir, and concomitant nephrotoxic drugs. **Renal impairment is the major dose-limiting toxicity.** IV NS prehydration and probenecid must be used (unless not indicated) to reduce risk of nephrotoxicity. May also cause nausea, vomiting, headache, rash, metabolic acidosis, uveitis, decreased intraocular pressure, and neutropenia.

Reported criteria for defining renal dysfunction in children include a sCr >1.5 mg/dL, GFR <90 mL/min/1.73 m^2, and >2+ proteinuria. For adults, reduce dose to 3 mg/kg if sCr increases 0.3—0.4 mg/dL from baseline. Discontinue therapy if sCr increases ≥0.5 mg/dL from baseline or development of ≥3+ proteinuria.

Administer doses via IV infusion over 1 hr at a concentration ≤8 mg/mL.

CIPROFLOXACIN
Cipro, Ciloxan ophthalmic, Cetraxal, Ciprodex,
Cipro HC Otic, Otovel Otic, and generics
Antibiotic, quinolone

    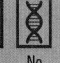

C   2   Yes   Yes   No

Tabs: 100, 250, 500, 750 mg
Oral suspension: 250 mg/5 mL (100 mL), 500 mg/5 mL (100 mL)
Premixed injection: 200 mg/100 mL 5% dextrose, 400 mg/200 mL 5% dextrose (iso-osmotic solutions)
Ophthalmic solution: 0.3% (2.5, 5, 10 mL); may contain benzalkonium chloride
Ophthalmic ointment (Ciloxan): 0.3% (3.5 g)
Otic solution (Cetraxal and generics): 0.5 mg/0.25 mL or 0.2% (14s)
Otic suspension:

With dexamethasone (Ciprodex and generics): 3 mg/mL (0.3%) ciprofloxacin + 1 mg/mL (0.1%) dexamethasone (7.5 mL); contains benzalkonium chloride
With hydrocortisone (Cipro HC Otic): 2 mg/mL (0.2%) ciprofloxacin + 10 mg/mL (1%) hydrocortisone (10 mL); contains benzyl alcohol
With fluocinolone (Otovel Otic and generics): 3 mg/mL (0.3%) ciprofloxacin + 0.25 mg/mL (0.025%) fluocinolone acetonide (0.25 mL; carton of 14s)

Neonate:
32—37 weeks' gestation: 10 mg/kg/dose IV Q12 hr
≥38 weeks' gestation: 15 mg/kg/dose IV Q12 hr

Child:

PO:
Mild/moderate infection: 20 mg/kg/24 hr ÷ Q12 hr; **max. dose:** 1 g/24 hr
Severe infection: 30—40 mg/kg/24 hr ÷ Q12 hr; **max. dose:** 1.5 g/24 hr

Continued

CIPROFLOXACIN *continued*

IV:

Severe infection: 10 mg/kg/dose Q8—12 hr; **max. dose:** 400 mg/dose

Complicated UTI or pyelonephritis (× 10—21 days):

PO: 20—40 mg/kg/24 hr ÷ Q12 hr; **max. dose:** 1.5 g/24 hr

IV: 18—30 mg/kg/24 hr ÷ Q8 hr; **max. dose:** 1.2 g/24 hr

Cystic fibrosis:

PO: 40 mg/kg/24 hr ÷ Q12 hr; **max. dose:** 2 g/24 hr

IV: 30 mg/kg/24 hr ÷ Q8 hr; **max. dose:** 1.2 g/24 hr

Anthrax (see remarks):

Inhalational/systemic/cutaneous: Start with 20—30 mg/kg/24 hr ÷ Q12 hr IV (**max. dose:** 800 mg/24 hr) and convert to oral dosing with clinical improvement at 20—30 mg/kg/24 hr ÷ Q12 hr PO (**max. dose:** 1 g/24 hr). Duration of therapy: 60 days (IV and PO combined)

Postexposure prophylaxis: 20—30 mg/kg/24 hr ÷ Q12 hr PO × 60 days; **max. dose:** 1 g/24 hr

Adult:

PO:

Immediate release: 250—750 mg/dose Q12 hr

Extended release tabs (Cipro XR and generics):

Uncomplicated UTI/cystitis: 500 mg/dose Q24 hr

Complicated UTI/uncomplicated pyelonephritis: 1000 mg/dose Q24 hr

IV: 400 mg/dose Q12 hr; 400 mg/dose Q8 hr for more severe/complicated infections

Anthrax (see remarks):

Inhalational/systemic/cutaneous: Start with 400 mg/dose Q12 hr IV and convert to oral dosing with clinical improvement at 500 mg/dose Q12 hr PO. Duration of therapy: 60 days (IV and PO combined)

Postexposure prophylaxis: 500 mg/dose Q12 hr PO × 60 days

Ophthalmic solution:

≥1 yr and adult: 1—2 drops Q2 hr while awake × 2 days, then 1—2 drops Q4 hr while awake × 5 days. Clinical efficacy for bacterial conjunctivitis has been demonstrated for neonates <31 days old in a randomized, double-blinded, multicenter, parallel-group clinical trial.

Ophthalmic ointment:

≥2 yr and adult: Apply 0.5-inch ribbon TID × 2 days, then BID × 5 days.

Otic:

Cetraxal and generics:

Acute otitis externa (≥1 yr and adult): 0.25 mL to affected ear(s) BID × 7 days

Ciprodex:

Acute otitis media with tympanostomy tubes or acute otitis externa (≥6 mo and adult): 4 drops to affected ear(s) BID × 7 days

Cipro HC Otic:

Otitis externa (>1 yr and adult): 3 drops to affected ear(s) BID × 7 days

Otovel Otic:

Acute otitis media with tympanostomy tubes (≥6 mo): 0.25 mL to affected ear(s) BID × 7 days

Systemic fluoroquinolones are associated with disabling and potentially permanent side effects of the tendons, muscles, joints, nerves, and central nervous system.

Can cause GI upset, renal failure, and seizures. GI symptoms, headache, restlessness, and rash are common side effects. Peripheral neuropathy, pseudotumor cerebri, severe hepatic necrosis, and psychiatric reactions have been reported. **Use with caution** in children <18 yr (like other quinolones, tendon rupture can occur during or after therapy, especially with concomitant corticosteroid use), alkalinized urine (crystalluria), seizures, excessive sunlight (photosensitivity), and renal dysfunction (**adjust systemic dose in renal failure; see Chapter 31**). Blood glucose

CIPROFLOXACIN *continued*

disturbances (hypoglycemia and hyperglycemia) have been reported in patients with diabetes who are receiving insulin or oral hypoglycemic agent.

Do not use otic suspension with perforated tympanic membranes and with viral infections of the external ear canal.

For dosing in obese patients, use an adjusted body weight (ABW). ABW = ideal body weight + 0.45 (total body weight − ideal body weight)

Combinational antimicrobial therapy is recommended for anthrax. For penicillin-susceptible strains, consider changing to high-dose amoxicillin (25—35 mg/kg/dose TID PO). See www.bt.cdc.gov for the latest information.

Inhibits CYP 450 1A2. Ciprofloxacin can increase effects and/or toxicity of caffeine, methotrexate, theophylline, warfarin, tizanidine (excessive sedation and dangerous hypotension), and cyclosporine. Probenecid increases ciprofloxacin levels.

Do not administer antacids or other divalent salts with or within 2—4 hr of oral ciprofloxacin dose.

Do not administer oral suspension through feeding tubes, because this dosage form adheres to the tube.

CITRATE MIXTURES *Alkalinizing agent, electrolyte supplement*		Yes	No	No
	? ?	Yes	No	No

Oral liquid:
Each mL of oral solution contains the following mEq of electrolyte:

	Na	K	Citrate or HCO₃
Tricitrates[a] or Sodium Citrate/Potassium Citrate and Citric Acid (473 mL)	1	1	2
Potassium Citrate and Citric Acid[a] (473 mL)	0	2	2
Sodium Citrate and Citric Acid[a] (30, 473 mL)	1	0	1
Oracit (15, 30, 500 mL)	1	0	1

[a]Sugar free.

Oral powder for oral solution:
  Cytra-K: Each packet of sugar-free powder contains 30 mEq each of potassium and citrate/HCO₃ (100 packets per box) and must be diluted in at least 6 ounces of cold water or juice.

Dilute dose in water or juice.
All mEq doses based on citrate.
Systemic alkalinization:
  Infant and child (PO): 2—3 mEq/kg/24 hr ÷ Q6—8 hr or 5—15 mL/dose Q6—8 hr (after meals and before bedtime) and adjust dose to desired serum bicarbonate level
  Adult (PO): 100—200 mEq/24 hr ÷ Q6—8 hr or 15—30 mL/dose Q6—8 hr (after meals and before bedtime)

Contraindicated in severe renal impairment and acute dehydration. **Use with caution** in patients already receiving potassium supplements or who are sodium restricted. May have laxative effect and cause hypocalcemia and metabolic alkalosis. Patients with active UTIs may attenuate the ability to increase urinary citrate by bacterial enzymatic degradation of citrate. Also, the rise in urinary pH may promote bacterial growth.

Continued

CITRATE MIXTURES *continued*

Adjust dose to maintain desired pH. 1 mEq of citrate is equivalent to 1 mEq HCO_3 in patients, as citrate is converted to CO_2 via the citric acid cycle in the mitochondria.

Potassium citrate has a pregnancy category of "C"; otherwise the pregnancy category is unknown for the other components to this medication.

CLARITHROMYCIN
Generics; previously available as Biaxin and
Biaxin XL
Antibiotic, macrolide

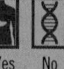

C   2   Yes   Yes   No

Film tablets: 250, 500 mg
Extended release tablets: 500 mg
Granules for oral suspension: 125, 250 mg/5 mL (50, 100 mL)

Infant and child:
  Acute otitis media, pharyngitis/tonsillitis, pneumonia, acute maxillary sinusitis, or uncomplicated skin infections: 15 mg/kg/24 hr PO ÷ Q12 hr; **max. dose:** 1 g/24 hr
  Pertussis (≥1 mo): 15 mg/kg/24 hr PO ÷ Q12 hr × 7 days; **max. dose:** 1 g/24 hr
  Bacterial endocarditis prophylaxis: 15 mg/kg (**max. dose:** 500 mg) PO 30–60 min before procedure
  Helicobacter pylori: 20 mg/kg/24 hr PO ÷ Q12 hr × 7–14 days; **max. dose:** 1 g/24 hr with amoxicillin and proton pump inhibitor with/without metronidazole
  ***Mycobacterium avium* complex (MAC):**
    Prophylaxis (1st episode and recurrence): 15 mg/kg/24 hr PO ÷ Q12 hr
    Treatment: 15 mg/kg/24 hr PO ÷ Q12 hr with other antimycobacterial drugs
    Max. dose (prophylaxis and treatment): 1 g/24 hr
Adolescent and adult:
  Pharyngitis/tonsillitis, acute maxillary sinusitis, bronchitis, pneumonia, or uncomplicated skin infections:
    Immediate release: 250–500 mg/dose Q12 hr PO
    Extended release tablet: 1000 mg Q24 hr PO (currently not indicated for pharyngitis/tonsillitis or uncomplicated skin infections)
Adult:
  Pertussis: 500 mg (immediate release)/dose Q12 hr PO × 7 days
  Bacterial endocarditis prophylaxis: 500 mg PO 30–60 min before procedure
  MAC:
    Prophylaxis (1st episode and recurrence): 500 mg/dose Q12 hr PO
    Treatment: 500 mg Q12 hr PO with other antimycobacterial drugs
  ***Helicobacter pylori* GI infection:** 500 mg Q12 hr PO × 7–14 days with proton pump inhibitor (lansoprazole or omeprazole) and amoxicillin

---

Contraindicated in patients allergic to erythromycin and history of cholestatic jaundice/hepatic dysfunction with prior use. As with other macrolides, clarithromycin has been associated with QT prolongation (**avoid use** with other drugs known to prolong QT interval) and ventricular arrhythmias, including ventricular tachycardia and torsades de pointes. May cause cardiac arrhythmias in patients also receiving cisapride. Side effects: diarrhea, nausea, abnormal taste, dyspepsia, abdominal discomfort (less than erythromycin but greater than azithromycin), and headache. Anaphylaxis, angioedema, hepatic dysfunction, rhabdomyolysis, SJS, and TEN have been reported.

CLARITHROMYCIN *continued*

May increase effects/toxicity of carbamazepine, theophylline, cyclosporine, digoxin, ergot alkaloids, fluconazole, midazolam, selected oral hypoglycemic agents, tacrolimus, triazolam, quetiapine, and warfarin. Substrate and inhibitor of CYP 450 3A4, and inhibits CYP 1A2.

Adjust dose in renal failure (see Chapter 31). Doses, regardless of dosage form, may be administered with food.

CLINDAMYCIN
Cleocin, Cleocin-T, Clindagel, Evoclin, Clindesse, Xaciato, and generics
Antibiotic, lincomycin derivative

 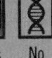

| B | 2 | Yes | Yes | No |

Caps: 75, 150, 300 mg
Oral solution: 75 mg/5 mL (100 mL); may contain ethyl parabens
Injection: 150 mg/mL (2, 4, 6, 60 mL); contains 9.45 mg/mL benzyl alcohol
Premixed injection in 5% dextrose or NS: 300 mg/50 mL, 600 mg/50 mL, 900 mg/50 mL; contains edetate disodium and may contain benzyl alcohol
Solution, topical: 1% (30, 60 mL); may contain 50% isopropyl alcohol and propylene glycol
Gel, topical (Cleocin-T, Clindagel, and generics): 1% (30, 60 g); may contain methylparaben and propylene glycol
Lotion, topical (Cleocin-T and generics): 1% (60 mL); may contain methylparaben
Foam, topical (Evoclin and generics): 1% (50, 100 g); contains 58% ethanol
See Benzoyl peroxide for combination topical product (clindamycin and benzoyl peroxide).
See Tretinoin for combination topical product (clindamycin and tretinoin).
Vaginal cream (Cleocin and generics): 2% (40 g); may contain benzyl alcohol or parabens
  Clindesse: 2% (5 g); contains parabens
Vaginal gel (Xaciato): 2% (25 g); contains benzyl alcohol
Vaginal suppository (Cleocin): 100 mg (3s)

Neonate (IV/IM):
≤**32 wk postmenstrual age:** 5 mg/kg/dose Q8 hr
33—40 wk postmenstrual age: 7 mg/kg/dose Q8 hr
>**40 wk postmenstrual age:** 9 mg/kg/dose Q8 hr

Child (>1 mo) and adolescent (see remarks for dosing in obesity):
  PO: 10—40 mg/kg/24 hr ÷ Q6—8 hr; **max. dose:** 1.8 g/24 hr
  IM/IV: 20—40 mg/kg/24 hr ÷ Q6—8 hr; **max. dose:** 2.7 g/24 hr

Adult:
  PO: 600—1800 mg/24 hr ÷ Q6—12 hr; **max. dose:** 2.4 g/24 hr
  IM/IV: 1200—2700 mg/24 hr ÷ Q6—12 hr; **max. IV dose:** 4.8 g/24 hr. **Max. IM dose:** 600 mg/dose

Topical for acne (≥12 yr and adult; administer after washing and fully drying the affected skin):
  Solution, lotion, or gel (Cleocin-T and generics): Apply to affected area BID.
  Clindagel or Evoclin (foam): Apply to affected area once daily.

Bacterial vaginosis (≥12 yr and adult):
  Suppositories: 100 mg/dose QHS × 3 days for nonpregnant patients
  Vaginal cream (2%): 1 applicator dose (5 g) QHS for 3 or 7 days in nonpregnant patients and for 7 days in pregnant patients in second and third trimesters.
    Clindesse (2%): 1 applicator dose (5 g) × 1 for nonpregnant patients
  Vaginal gel (2%; Xaciato): 1 applicator dose (5 g) × 1

Not indicated in meningitis; CSF penetration is poor. Clindamycin is no longer recommended for antibiotic prophylaxis for dental procedures.

Continued

CLINDAMYCIN *continued*

Pseudomembranous colitis may occur up to several weeks after cessation of therapy. May cause
diarrhea, rash, granulocytopenia, thrombocytopenia, or sterile abscess at injection site. Anaphylaxis,
DRESS, SJS, TEN, severe taste alterations including metallic taste (with high IV doses), and AKI have
been reported with systemic use. The intravenous product contains benzyl alcohol. Eye pain and
contact dermatitis have been reported with topical use.

Clindamycin may increase the neuromuscular blocking effects of tubocurarine and pancuronium. **Do
not exceed** IV infusion rate of 30 mg/min because hypotension and cardiac arrest have been
reported with rapid infusions. May diminish the effects of erythromycin when administered together.
In vitro studies indicate clindamycin is a substrate and inhibitor for CYP 450 3A4.

Dosage reduction may be required in severe renal or hepatic disease but not necessary in mild/
moderate conditions. Systemic clindamycin should be dosed based on total body weight regardless
of obesity. Oral liquid preparation may not be palatable; consider use of oral capsules as a sprinkle
onto applesauce or pudding.

CLOBAZAM
Onfi, Sympazan, and generics
Benzodiazepine, anticonvulsant

C   3   No   Yes   Yes

Tabs (Onfi and generics): 10, 20 mg
Oral film (Sympazan): 5, 10, 20 mg (60s)
Oral suspension (Onfi and generics): 2.5 mg/mL (120 mL); contains parabens, polysorbate 80, and
propylene glycol

Lennox-Gastaut (adjunctive therapy; see remarks):
  Child (≥2 yr) and adult (PO): Dosage increments (if needed) should not be more rapid than
  every 7 days.

Weight (kg)	Initial Dose	Dose at Day 8, if Needed	Dose at Day 15, if Needed
≤30 kg	5 mg once daily	5 mg BID	10 mg BID (**max. dose**)
>30 kg	5 mg BID	10 mg BID	20 mg BID (**max. dose**)

**Dosage adjustment for mild/moderate hepatic impairment (Child-Pugh score 5–9) and individuals
with poor CYP 450 2C19 activity (PO):**

Weight (kg)	Initial Dose	First Dose Increment, if Needed	Second Dose Increment, if Needed	Third Dose Increment, if Needed
≤30 kg	5 mg once daily × ≥14 days	5 mg BID × ≥7 days	10 mg BID (**max. dose**)	N/A
>30 kg	5 mg once daily × ≥7 days	5 mg BID × ≥7 days	10 mg BID × ≥7 days	20 mg BID (**max. dose**)

N/A, Not applicable.

CLOBAZAM *continued*

Seizures (generalized or partial, as monotherapy or adjunctive therapy; limited data and prescribing information from Canada and the United Kingdom):

Infant and child (<2 yr): Start at 0.5–1 mg/kg/24 hr (**max. dose:** 5 mg/24 hr) PO ÷ BID; if needed and tolerated, slowly increase dosage at 5- to 7-day intervals up to the **maximum** of 10 mg/24 hr.

2–16 yr: Start at 5 mg PO once daily; if needed and tolerated, slowly increase dosage at 5- to 7-day intervals up to the **maximum** of 40 mg/24 hr. Usual dosage range: 10–20 mg/24 hr or 0.3–1 mg/kg/24 hr ÷ BID

Use with caution in hepatic impairment (dose adjustment may be needed). **Do not** discontinue use abruptly, as seizures/withdrawal symptoms may occur. Common side effects include constipation, drooling, ataxia, drowsiness, insomnia, aggressive behavior, cough, and fever. SJS, TEN, urinary retention, hypothermia, leukopenia, and thrombocytopenia have been reported.

Do not use in combination with azelastine, olanzapine, sodium oxybate, and thioridazine; increases risk for adverse events. Proton pump inhibitors, azole antifungal agents (e.g., itraconazole and ketoconazole), St. John's wort, grapefruit juice, CNS depressants, cimetidine, calcium channel blockers, and strong/moderate CYP 2C19 inhibitors may increase the effects/toxicity of clobazam. Use with opioids may result in profound sedation, respiratory depression, coma, and mortality. Carbamazepine, rifamycin derivatives (e.g., rifampin), and theophylline may decrease the effects of clobazam. Clobazam is a major substrate for CYP 450 2C19 and P-glycoprotein, minor substrate for CYP 450 2B6 and 3A4, inhibitor of CYP 450 2D6, and inducer of CYP 3A4. Carefully review the patient's medication profile for other drug interactions each time clobazam is initiated or when a new drug is added to a regimen containing clobazam.

Doses may be taken with or without food. Tablets may be crushed and mixed with applesauce.

Oral film (Sympazan) uses same PO dosage with the following method for administration: Apply film on top of the tongue, allow it to dissolve, and swallow saliva in a normal manner. **Do not** chew, spit, or talk while film is dissolving. Doses may be taken with or without food but **do not** administer with liquids.

CLONAZEPAM
Klonopin and generics
Benzodiazepine, anticonvulsant

  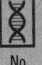

D   3   Yes   Yes   No

Tabs: 0.5, 1, 2 mg
Disintegrating oral tabs: 0.125, 0.25, 0.5, 1, 2 mg; contains phenylalanine
Oral suspension: 100 mCg/mL

Seizures:

Infant and child <10 yr or <30 kg:
Initial: 0.01–0.03 mg/kg/24 hr PO ÷ BID–TID; **maximum initial dose:** 0.05 mg/kg/24 hr
Increment: 0.25–0.5 mg/24 hr Q3 days, up to a **maximum maintenance dose** of 0.2 mg/kg/24 hr ÷ TID

Child ≥10 yr or ≥30 kg and adult:
Initial: 1.5 mg/24 hr PO ÷ TID
Increment: 0.5–1 mg/24 hr Q3–7 days up to a **maximum maintenance dose** of 20 mg/24 hr

Contraindicated in severe liver disease and acute narrow-angle glaucoma. Drowsiness, behavior changes, increased bronchial secretions, GI, CV, GU, and hematopoietic toxicity (thrombocytopenia, leukopenia) may occur. Monitor for depression, suicidal behavior/ideation, and unusual changes in behavior/mood. **Use with caution** in patients with compromised respiratory function, porphyria, and renal impairment. **Do not discontinue abruptly.**
$T_{1/2}$ = 24–36 hr.

Continued

CLONAZEPAM *continued*

Proposed therapeutic levels (not well established): 20–80 ng/mL. Recommended serum sampling time: Obtain trough level within 30 min prior to an oral dose. Steady state is typically achieved after 5–8 days continuous therapy using the same dose.

Carbamazepine, phenytoin, and phenobarbital may decrease clonazepam levels and effect. Drugs that inhibit CYP-450 3A4 isoenzymes (e.g., erythromycin) may increase clonazepam levels and effects/toxicity.

CLONIDINE
Kapvay, Catapres TTS, Duraclon, and generics;
previously available as Catapres
Central α adrenergic agonist, antihypertensive

   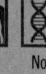

| C | 3 | Yes | No | No |

Tabs: 0.1, 0.2, 0.3 mg
Extended release oral tabs:
Kapvay and generics (12 hr dosing): 0.1 mg
Oral suspension: 20, 100 mCg/mL
Transdermal patch (Catapres TTS and generics): 0.1, 0.2, 0.3 mg/24 hr (7-day patch; 4 patches per box); contains metallic components (see remarks)
Injection, epidural (Duraclon and generics): 100, 500 mCg/mL (10 mL); preservative free

Neonatal abstinence syndrome, adjunctive therapy (use immediate release product; limited data): 0.5–1 mcg/kg/dose Q4–6 hr PO; use Q6 hr interval for preterm neonates

ADHD (Child ≥6 yr and adolescent):
Immediate release product (PO):
27–45 kg: Start with 0.05 mg QHS; if needed, increase by 0.05 mg/24 hr every 3–7 days as increments with BID, TID, and then QID dosing up to the following **max. dose:**
27–40.5 kg: 0.2 mg/24 hr
>40.5–45 kg: 0.3 mg/24 hr
>45 kg: Start with 0.1 mg QHS; if needed, increase by 0.1 mg/24 hr every 3–7 days as increments with BID, TID, and then QID dosing up to the **max. dose** of 0.4 mg/24 hr.
Extended release product (Kapvay and generics, PO): Start with 0.1 mg QHS; if needed, increase by 0.1 mg every 7 days by administering the dose BID up to a **maximum** of 0.4 mg/24 hr. Depending on dosage level, BID dosing should be either the same amount or with the higher dosage given at bedtime. If therapy is to be discontinued, slowly reduce dosage at ≤0.1 mg every 3 to 7 days to avoid withdrawal.

Hypertension (use immediate release products unless noted):
Child (PO): 2–5 mCg/kg/dose Q6–8 hr initially; if needed, increase at 5- to 7-day intervals up to 10 mCg/kg/dose Q6–8 hr; **max. dose:** 0.8 mg/24 hr
≥12 yr and adult (PO): 0.1 mg BID initially; increase in 0.1 mg/24 hr increments at weekly intervals until desired response is achieved (usual range: adolescent: 0.2–0.6 mg/24 hr ÷ BID; adult: 0.1–0.8 mg/24 hr ÷ BID); **max. dose:** 2.4 mg/24 hr
Transdermal patch (each patch lasts 7 days by rotating application sites, but more frequent patch change at every 5 days may be needed for children):
Child: Conversion to patch only after establishing an optimal oral dose first. Use a transdermal dosage closest to the established total oral daily dose.
Adult: Initial 0.1 mg/24 hr patch for first week. May increase dose by 0.1 mg/24 hr at 1–2 wk intervals PRN. Usual range: 0.1–0.3 mg/24 hr. Doses >0.6 mg/24 hr do not provide additional benefit.

Side effects: Dry mouth, dizziness, drowsiness, fatigue, constipation, anorexia, arrhythmias, and local skin reactions with patch. Somnolence, fatigue, URIs, irritability, throat pain, insomnia, nightmares, and emotional disorder were reported as common side effects in ADHD

CLONIDINE *continued*

clinical trials. May worsen sinus node dysfunction and AV block, especially for patients taking other sympatholytic drugs. **Do not abruptly discontinue;** signs of sympathetic overactivity may occur; taper gradually over >1 wk.

β-blockers may exacerbate rebound hypertension during and following the withdrawal of clonidine. If patient is receiving both clonidine and a β-blocker and clonidine is to be discontinued, the β-blocker should be withdrawn several days prior to tapering the clonidine. If converting from clonidine over to a β-blocker, introduce the β-blocker several days after discontinuing clonidine (after taper).

Monitor heart rate when used with digitalis, calcium channel blockers, and β-blockers. Use with diltiazem or verapamil may result in sinus bradycardia. Use with neuroleptics may induce/ exacerbate orthostatic hypotension, dizziness, and fatigue. Consider using lower dosages in renal impairment because the drug is primarily eliminated unchanged in the urine and signs of bradycardia, sedation, and hypotension may occur.

$T_{1/2}$: 44—72 hr (neonate), 6—20 hr (adult). Onset of action (antihypertensive): 0.5—1 hr for oral route, 2—3 days for transdermal route. **Do not** use transdermal route while patient is undergoing a magnetic resonance imaging (MRI) procedure; transdermal patches contain metals and may result in serious patient burns when undergoing MRI.

CLOTRIMAZOLE
Alevazol, Lotrimin AF, Gyne-Lotrimin 3, Gyne-
Lotrimin 7, and generics
Antifungal, imidazole

B/C	?	No	Yes	No

Oral troche: 10 mg
Cream, topical (Lotrimin AF and generics; OTC): 1% (15, 30, 45 g); may contain benzyl alcohol or parabens
Ointment, topical (Alevazol; OTC): 1% (56.7 g)
Solution, topical (OTC): 1% (10, 30 mL)
Vaginal cream (OTC):
  Gyne-Lotrimin 7 and generics: 1% (45 g)
  Gyne-Lotrimin 3 and generics: 2% (21 g)

Topical (cream, ointment, or solution):
  ≥2 yr—**adult:** Apply to affected skin areas BID; × 2 wk for cutaneous candidiasis, × 4—8 wk for tinea corporis/pedis.
Vaginal cream (>12 yr and adult; in addition to intravaginal use, may also apply to external vaginal area BID × 7 days PRN for itching and irritation):
  1 applicator dose (5 g) of 1% cream intravaginally QHS × 7—14 days, or
  1 applicator dose of 2% cream intravaginally QHS × 3 days
Oropharyngeal candidiasis:
  >3 yr—**adult:** Dissolve slowly (15—30 min) one troche in the mouth 5 times/24 hr × 14 days.

Systemic use: Do not use troches for systemic infections. Liver enzyme elevation, nausea, and
  vomiting may occur with troches.
Topical use: May cause erythema, blistering, or urticaria with topical use. **Avoid use** of tampons, douches, spermicides, other vaginal products, condoms, and diaphragms with vaginal cream. Vaginal cream can weaken latex.
Pregnancy code is a "B" for topical and vaginal dosage forms and "C" for troches.

CORTICOTROPIN
Acthar Gel, Cortrophin Gel; ACTH
Adrenocorticotropic hormone

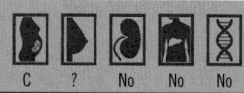

C   ?   No   No   No

Injection, repository gel: 80 U/mL (5 mL); contains phenol
1 unit = 1 mg

Infantile spasms (many regimens exist):
20–40 U/24 hr IM once daily × 6 wk or 150 U/m²/24 hr ÷ BID for 2 wk, followed by a
gradual 2 wk taper of 30 U/m²/dose QAM × 3 days, followed by 15 U/m²/dose QAM × 3 days,
followed by 10 U/m²/dose QAM × 3 days and 10 U/m²/dose every other morning × 6 days

Antiinflammatory:
≥2 yr and adolescent: 0.8 U/kg/24 hr ÷ Q12–24 hr IM

Contraindicated in infants <2 yr with suspected congenital infections, acute psychoses, CHF,
Cushing disease, primary adrenocortical insufficiency or adrenocortical hyperfunction,
TB, peptic ulcer, ocular herpes, fungal infections, recent surgery, and sensitivity to
porcine products. **Use with caution** in osteoporosis. Repository gel dosage form is only for
IM route.

Hypersensitivity reactions and injection site reactions may occur. Cases of anaphylaxis have been
reported. Similar adverse effects as corticosteroids. **Do not use** with live or live attenuated
vaccines.

CORTISONE ACETATE
Various generics
Corticosteroid

C/D   ?   No   No   No

Tabs: 25 mg

Antiinflammatory/immunosuppressive:
Child: 2.5–10 mg/kg/24 hr ÷ Q6–8 hr PO
Adult: 25–300 mg/24 hr ÷ Q12–24 hr PO

May produce glucose intolerance, Cushing syndrome, edema, hypertension, adrenal suppression,
cataracts, hypokalemia, skin atrophy, peptic ulcer, osteoporosis, and growth suppression.
Pregnancy category changes to "D" if used in the first trimester.

CO-TRIMOXAZOLE

See Sulfamethoxazole and Trimethoprim.

CROMOLYN
Nasalcrom, Gastrocrom, and generics; previously
available as Intal
Antiallergic agent, mast cell stabilizer

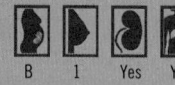

B   1   Yes   Yes   No

Nebulized solution: 10 mg/mL (2 mL)
Oral concentrate (Gastrocrom and generics): 100 mg/5 mL (5 mL)
Ophthalmic solution: 4% (10 mL)

CROMOLYN *continued*

Nasal spray (NasalCrom and generics) [OTC]: 4% (5.2 mg/spray) (100 sprays, 13 mL; 200 sprays, 26 mL); contains benzalkonium chloride and EDTA

Nebulization:

 Child ≥2 yr and adult: 20 mg Q6—8 hr

  Exercise-induced asthma: 20 mg × 1, 10—15 min prior to and no longer than 1 hr before exercise

Nasal:

 Child ≥2 yr and adult: 1 spray each nostril TID—QID; **max. dose:** 1 spray 6 times/24 hr

Ophthalmic:

 Child >4 yr and adult: 1—2 gtts 4—6 times/24 hr

Food allergy/inflammatory bowel disease (taper to lowest effective dose once desired effect is achieved):

 2—12 yr: 100 mg PO QID; give 15—20 min AC and QHS; **max. dose:** 40 mg/kg/24 hr

 >12 yr and adult: 200—400 mg PO QID; give 15—20 min AC and QHS

Systemic mastocytosis (taper to lowest effective maintenance dose once desired effect is achieved):

 Infant and child <2 yr: 20 mg/kg/24 hr ÷ QID PO; **max. dose:** <6 mo: 20 mg/kg/24 hr, ≥6 mo to <2 yr: 100 mg/dose or 40 mg/kg/24 hr

 2—12 yr: 100 mg PO QID; give 30 min AC and QHS; **max. dose:** 40 mg/kg/24 hr

 >12 yr and adult: 200 mg PO QID; give 30 min AC and QHS; **max. dose:** 40 mg/kg/24 hr

May cause rash, cough, bronchospasm, and nasal congestion. May cause headache, diarrhea with oral use. **Use with caution** in patients with renal or hepatic dysfunction because cromolyn is equally excreted unchanged in the urine and feces (bile).

Therapeutic response often occurs within 2 wk; however, a 4- to 6-wk trial may be needed to determine maximum benefit. Oral concentrate can only be diluted in water. Nebulized solution can be mixed with albuterol nebs.

CYANOCOBALAMIN/VITAMIN B₁₂
Dodex, Physicians EZ Use B-12, Vitamin Deficiency System B12, Nascobal, vitamin B₁₂, and generics
Vitamin (synthetic), water soluble

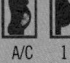 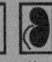

| A/C | 1 | Yes | No | No |

Tabs (OTC): 100, 250, 500, 1000 mCg
Extended release tabs: 1000 mCg
Sublingual tabs: 2500 mCg
Sublingual liquid: 3000 mCg/mL (52 mL)
Lozenges (OTC): 50, 100, 250, 500 mCg
Nasal spray (Nascobal): 500 mCg/spray (1.3 mL delivers 4 doses); contains benzalkonium chloride
Injection (Dodex and generics): 1000 mCg/mL (1, 10, 30); may contain benzyl alcohol
Injection kit (Physicians EZ Use B-12, Vitamin Deficiency System B12, and generics): 1000 mCg/mL (1 mL); may contain benzyl alcohol
Contains cobalt (4.35%), and some preparations may contain aluminum

U.S. RDA: See Chapter 21.
Vitamin B₁₂ deficiency, treatment:

 Child (IM or deep SC): 100 mCg/24 hr × 10—15 days followed by 100 mCg once or twice weekly for several months

  Maintenance: At least 60 mCg/mo

Continued

CYANOCOBALAMIN/VITAMIN B$_{12}$ *continued*

Adult (IM or deep SC): 100 mCg/24 hr × 6–7 days; if improvement, 100 mCg/dose every 3–4 days
× 2–3 wk. Use maintenance dose when hematologic values return to normal.

Maintenance: 100 mCg/mo

Pernicious anemia:

Child (IM or deep SC): 30–50 mCg/24 hr for at least 14 days to a total dose of 1000–5000 mCg

Maintenance: 100 mCg/mo

Adult (IM or deep SC): 100 mCg/24 hr × 6–7 days; if improvement, 100 mCg/dose every 3–4 days
× 2–3 wk. Use maintenance dose when hematologic values return to normal.

Maintenance:

IM/deep SC: 100 mCg/mo

Intranasal: 500 mCg in one nostril once weekly

Sublingual: 1000–2000 mCg/24 hr

Contraindicated in optic nerve atrophy. May cause hypokalemia, hypersensitivity (anaphylaxis
shock and death reported with parenteral use), pruritus, and vascular thrombosis. Vitamin
B$_{12}$ use may mask folate deficiency and unmask polycythemia vera.

Prolonged use of acid-suppressing medications may reduce cyanocobalamin oral absorption.

Pregnancy category changes to "C" if used in doses greater than the RDA or if administered by the
intranasal route.

Protect product from light. Some products may contain aluminum and may accumulate in renal
impairment. Oral route of administration is generally **not recommended** for pernicious anemia and
B$_{12}$ deficiency due to poor absorption. IV route of administration is **NOT recommended** because of a
more rapid elimination. See Chapter 21 for multivitamin preparations.

CYCLOPENTOLATE
Cyclogyl and generics
Anticholinergic, mydriatic agent

   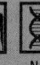

C   ?   No   No   No

Ophthalmic solution: 0.5% (15 mL), 1% (2, 5, 15 mL), 2% (2, 5, 15 mL); may contain benzalkonium
chloride

Administer dose approximately 40–50 min prior to examination/procedure.

Infant: Use of cyclopentolate/phenylephrine (Cyclomydril) due to lower cyclopentolate
concentration and reduced risk of systemic side effects

Child and adolescent: 1 drop of 0.5%–1% solution OU, followed by repeat drop, if necessary, in 5
min. Use 2% solution for heavily pigmented iris.

Adult: 1 drop of 1% solution OU, followed by another drop OU in 5 min. Use 2% solution for heavily
pigmented iris.

Do not use in narrow-angle glaucoma. May cause a burning sensation, behavioral disturbance,
tachycardia, and loss of visual accommodation. Psychotic reactions and behavioral
disturbances have been reported in children. To minimize absorption, apply pressure over
nasolacrimal sac for at least 2 min. CNS and cardiovascular side effects are common with the 2%
solution in children. **Avoid** feeding infants within 4 hr of dosing to prevent potential feeding
intolerance.

Onset of action: 15- to 60-min; duration of action: 6–24 hr; complete recovery of accommodation may
take several days for some patients. Observe patient closely for at least 30 min after dose.

CYCLOPENTOLATE WITH PHENYLEPHRINE
Cyclomydril
Anticholinergic/sympathomimetic, mydriatic agent

C ? No No No

Ophthalmic solution: 0.2% cyclopentolate and 1% phenylephrine (2, 5 mL); contains 0.1% benzalkonium chloride, EDTA, and boric acid

Neonate (administer dose approximately 40—50 min prior to examination/procedure; see remarks): 1 drop OU Q5—10 min; **max. dose:** 3 drops per eye
Infant, child, and adolescent (administer dose at least 15 min prior to examination; see remarks): 1 drop OU Q5—10 min PRN

Used to induce mydriasis. See Cyclopentolate for additional remarks.
Onset of action: 15—60 min. Duration of action: 4—12 hr.
Apply pressure over the nasolacrimal sac for 2—3 min after administration to minimize systemic absorption.

CYCLOSPORINE, CYCLOSPORINE MICROEMULSION, CYCLOSPORINE MODIFIED
Sandimmune, Gengraf, Neoral, Restasis, Verkazia, Cequa, and generics
Immunosuppressant

C 2 Yes Yes No

CYCLOSPORINE (Sandimmune and generics):
  Injection: 50 mg/mL (5 mL); contains 32.9% alcohol and 650 mg/mL polyoxyethylated castor oil (Cremophor EL)
  Oral solution: 100 mg/mL (50 mL); contains 12.5% alcohol
  Caps: 25, 50, 100 mg; contains 12.7% alcohol
CYCLOSPORINE MICROEMULSION (Neoral):
  Caps: 25, 100 mg
  Oral solution: 100 mg/mL (50 mL)
  All Neoral products contain 11.9% alcohol and propylene glycol.
CYCLOSPORINE MODIFIED (Gengraf):
  Caps: 25, 100 mg; contains 12.8% alcohol and propylene glycol
  Oral solution: 100 mg/mL (50 mL); contains propylene glycol
Ophthalmic emulsion:
  Restasis and generics: 0.05% (0.4 mL as 30 or 60 single-use vials/box); preservative free and contains polysorbate 80
  Verkazia: 0.1% (0.3 mL as 5 or 120 single-use vials/box); preservative free and contains poloxamer 188
Ophthalmic solution/drops (Cequa): 0.09% (0.25 mL in boxes of 60s); preservative free and contains Cremophor EL

Transplantation rejection prophylaxis: Neoral manufacturer recommends a 1:1 conversion ratio with Sandimmune. Because of its better absorption, lower doses of Neoral and Gengraf may be required. Exact dosing will vary depending on transplant type.
  Oral: 15 mg/kg/24 hr as a single dose given 4—12 hr pretransplantation; give same daily dose ÷ Q12—24 hr for 1—2 wk posttransplantation, then reduce by 5% per week to 3—10 mg/kg/24 hr ÷ Q12—24 hr

Continued

CYCLOSPORINE, CYCLOSPORINE MICROEMULSION, CYCLOSPORINE MODIFIED *continued*

IV: 5–6 mg/kg/24 hr as a single dose given 4–12 hr pretransplantation; administer over 2–6 hr; give same daily dose posttransplantation until patient able to tolerate oral form

Ophthalmic:

Keratoconjunctivitis sicca:

Ophthalmic emulsion (0.05%; Restasis and generics):

≥16 yr and adult: Instill one drop onto affected eye(s) Q12 hr.

Ophthalmic solution (0.09%; Cequa):

≥18 yr: Instill one drop onto affected eye(s) Q12 hr.

Severe vernal keratoconjunctivitis:

Ophthalmic emulsion:

Verkazia (0.1%):

≥4 yr and adult: Instill one drop onto affected eye(s) QID until resolution.

Restasis and generics (0.05%; limited data):

≥5 yr–14 yr: Instill one drop onto affected eye(s) QID.

May cause nephrotoxicity, hepatotoxicity, hypomagnesemia, hyperkalemia, hyperuricemia, hypertension, hirsutism, acne, GI symptoms, tremor, leukopenia, sinusitis, gingival hyperplasia, and headache. Encephalopathy, convulsions, lower extremity pain, vision and movement disturbances, and impaired consciousness have been reported, especially in liver transplant patients. Psoriasis patients previously treated with PUVA and, to a lesser extent, methotrexate or other immunosuppressive agents, UVB, coal tar, or radiation therapy are at increased risk for skin malignancies when taking Neoral or Gengraf.

Opportunistic infections and activation of latent viral infections have been reported.

BK virus—associated nephropathy has been observed in renal transplant patients.

Use caution with concomitant use of other nephrotoxic drugs (e.g., amphotericin B, aminoglycosides, nonsteroidal antiinflammatory drugs, and tacrolimus).

Plasma concentrations increased with the use of boceprevir, telaprevir, fluconazole, ketoconazole, itraconazole, erythromycin, clarithromycin, voriconazole, nefazodone, diltiazem, verapamil, nicardipine, carvedilol, and corticosteroids. Plasma concentrations decreased with the use of carbamazepine, nafcillin, rifampin, oxcarbazepine, bosentan, phenobarbital, octreotide, and phenytoin. May increase bosentan, dabigatran, methotrexate, repaglinide, and anthracycline antibiotics (e.g., doxorubicin, mitoxantrone, daunorubicin) levels/effects/toxicity. Use with nifedipine may result in gingival hyperplasia. Cyclosporine is a substrate and inhibitor for CYP 450 3A4 and P-glycoprotein.

Children may require dosages 2–3 times higher than adults. Plasma half-life 6–24 hr.

Monitor trough levels (just prior to a dose at steady state). Steady state is generally achieved after 3–5 days of continuous dosing. Interpretation will vary based on treatment protocol and assay methodology (RIA monoclonal vs. RIA polyclonal vs. HPLC), as well as whole blood vs. serum sample. Additional monitoring and dosage adjustments may be necessary in renal and hepatic impairment or when changing dosage forms.

For ophthalmic use: Ocular burning may occur. Remove contact lens prior to use; lens may be inserted 15 min after dose administration. May be used with artificial tears but need to be separated by 15 min from one another.

CYPROHEPTADINE
Various generics; previously available as Periactin
Antihistamine

    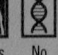

B   3   No   Yes   No

CYPROHEPTADINE *continued*

Tabs: 4 mg
Syrup: 2 mg/5 mL (473 mL); may contain alcohol 5%

Antihistaminic uses:
  Child: 0.25 mg/kg/24 hr or 8 mg/m²/24 hr ÷ Q8–12 hr PO or by age:
    2–6 yr: 2 mg Q8–12 hr PO; **max. dose:** 12 mg/24 hr
    7–14 yr: 4 mg Q8–12 hr PO; **max. dose:** 16 mg/24 hr
    ≥15 yr: 4 mg Q8 hr PO; usual range 12–16 mg/24 hr; **max. dose:** 0.5 mg/kg/24 hr
  Adult: Start with 12 mg/24 hr ÷ TID PO; dosage range: 12–32 mg/24 hr ÷ TID PO; **max. dose:** 0.5 mg/kg/24 hr
Migraine prophylaxis: 0.25–0.4 mg/kg/24 hr ÷ BID–TID PO up to the following **max. doses:**
  2–6 yr: 12 mg/24 hr
  7–14 yr: 16 mg/24 hr
  Adult: 0.5 mg/kg/24 hr or 32 mg/24 hr
Appetite stimulation (see remarks):
  ≥2 yr and adolescent: 0.25 mg/kg/24 hr ÷ Q12 hr PO up to the following **max. dose** by age: 2–6 yr: 12 mg/24 hr, 7–14 yr: 16 mg/24 hr, ≥15 yr: 32 mg/24 hr
  Alternative dosing by age:
    4–8 yr (limited data): 2 mg Q8 hr PO
    >13 yr and adult: Start with 2 mg Q6 hr PO; dose may be gradually increased to 8 mg Q6 hr over a 3-wk period.

Contraindicated in neonates, patients currently on MAO inhibitors, and patients suffering from asthma, glaucoma, or GI/GU obstruction. May produce anticholinergic side effects including sedation and appetite stimulation. Consider reducing dosage with hepatic insufficiency.
Allow 4 to 8 wk of continuous therapy for assessing efficacy in migraine prophylaxis. For use as an appetite stimulant, a dosing cycle of 3 wk on therapy followed by 1 wk off of therapy may enhance efficacy.

D

DABIGATRAN ETEXILATE MESYLATE
Pradaxa and generics
Anticoagulant, direct thrombin inhibitor

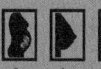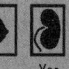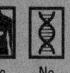
C   ?   Yes   No   No

Oral pellets (Pradaxa): 20, 30, 40, 50, 110, 150 mg (60 packets of pellets per carton)
Caps:
  Pradaxa: 75, 110, 150 mg; may contain carrageenan
  Generics: 75, 150 mg

Oral pellets and capsule dosage forms are NOT bioequivalent and are NOT interchangeable on a mg per mg basis.
Prevention and treatment of venous thromboembolic event (VTE; see remarks):
  Child 3 mo–<2 yr (using oral pellets):

Weight (kg)	Age (mo)	Dose (mg) PO BID
3–<4	3–<6	30
4–<5	3–<10	40
5–<7	3–<5	40

Continued

DABIGATRAN ETEXILATE MESYLATE *continued*

Weight (kg)	Age (mo)	Dose (mg) PO BID
	5—<24	50
7—<9	3—<4	50
	4—<9	60
	9—<24	70
9—<11	5—<6	60
	6—<11	80
	11—<24	90
11—<13	8—<18	100
	18—<24	110
13—<16	10—<11	100
	11—<24	140
16—<21	12—<24	140
21—<26	18—<24	180

Child 2—12 yr (PO BID; using oral pellets):
   7—<9 kg: 70 mg
   9—<11 kg: 90 mg
   11—<13 kg: 110 mg
   13—<16 kg:140 mg
   16—<21 kg: 170 mg
   21—<41 kg: 220 mg
   ≥41 kg: 260 mg
Child 8—<18 yr (PO BID; using oral capsules):
   11—<16 kg: 75 mg
   16—<26 kg: 110 mg
   26—<41 kg: 150 mg
   41—<61 kg: 185 mg
   61—<81 kg: 220 mg
   ≥81 kg: 260 mg
Adult (PO BID; using oral capsules): 150 mg

Contraindicated in mechanical prosthetic heart valves, active bleeding, and prior serious
   hypersensitivity reactions to dabigatran and any of its excipients. Use is **NOT** recommended
   in patients with triple-positive antiphospholipid syndrome due to the increase risk for recurrent
   thrombosis. Epidural or spinal hematomas may occur in patients receiving neuraxial anesthesia or
   undergoing spinal puncture and may result in paralysis.
Common side effects include esophagitis, gastritis, indigestion, GI hemorrhage, and hemorrhage.
   Alopecia, angioedema, neutropenia, and agranulocytosis have been reported. Idarucizumab is the
   reversal agent indicated for adults in situations of emergency surgery/urgent procedures and life-
   threatening/uncontrolled bleeding. Pediatric use of idarucizumab has not been established.
   Consider the use of an alternative anticoagulant to decrease the risk of thrombosis in situations
   where dabigatran is discontinued for reasons other than pathological bleeding or completion of a
   therapy course.
Safety and efficacy have been established in children 8—<18 years of age for the treatment
   and prophylaxis of venous thromboembolism. In a phase 3 pediatric treatment trial, site-specific
   bleeding rates were comparable to standard-of-care therapy (vitamin K antagonists, low molecular
   weight heparin, or fondaparinux) except for GI bleeds (5.7% vs. 1.8%). An open label study
   evaluating the safety of dabigatran prophylaxis following a treatment course of dabigatran noted

DABIGATRAN ETEXILATE MESYLATE *continued*

common side effects of dyspepsia, epistaxis, nausea, and menorrhagia. The adverse reaction profile for this pediatric trial was generally consistent with that of adult patients.

Adjust dose in renal impairment (see Chapter 31); pediatric renal impairment studies have not been completed. Dabigatran is a P-glycoprotein (P-gp)/ABCB1 substrate. **Avoid** use with rifampin (P-gp inducer). Use with a P-gp inhibitor in patients with renal impairment is likely to result in supratherapeutic/toxic effects.

BID dosing should be separated by Q12 hr when possible. **DO NOT** combine the capsule and pellet dosage forms as they are NOT bioequivalent. Capsules may be administered with or without food and **MUST NOT** be opened or chewed. Oral pellets are mixed with mashed carrot or banana, applesauce, or apple juice (see product information for specific instructions) for administration. **DO NOT** administer oral pellets via oral syringes or feeding tubes and **DO NOT** mix them with milk or any milk-containing products.

DANTROLENE
Dantrium, Revonto, Ryanodex, and generics
Skeletal muscle relaxant

   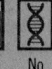

C   ?   No   Yes   No

Cap: 25, 50, 100 mg
Oral suspension: 5 mg/mL
Injection:
    Dantrium, Revonto, and generics: 20 mg; injectable solution containing 3 g mannitol per 20 mg drug
    Ryanodex : 250 mg; injectable suspension containing 125 mg mannitol, 25 mg polysorbate 80, 4 mg povidone K12 per 250 mg drug

Chronic spasticity:
  Child (≥5 yr):
    Initial: 0.5 mg/kg/dose (**max. dose:** 25 mg/dose) PO BID
    Increment: Increase frequency to TID—QID at 4- to 7-day intervals, then increase doses by 0.5 mg/kg/dose
    Max. dose: 3 mg/kg/dose PO BID—QID, up to 400 mg/24 hr
Malignant hyperthermia (infant, child, and adult):
  Prevention:
    PO: 4—8 mg/kg/24 hr ÷ Q6 hr × 1—2 days before surgery with last dose administered 3—4 hr prior to surgery
    IV (see remarks for specific dosage form administration rates): 2.5 mg/kg beginning 1.25 hr before anesthesia, additional doses PRN
  Treatment (see remarks for specific dosage form administration rates): 1 mg/kg IV, repeat PRN to **maximum cumulative dose** of 10 mg/kg, followed by a post-crisis regimen of 4—8 mg/kg/24 hr PO ÷ Q6 hr for 1—3 days

Contraindicated in active hepatic disease. Monitor transaminases for hepatotoxicity. **Use with caution** with cardiac or pulmonary impairment. May cause change in sensorium, drowsiness, weakness, diarrhea, constipation, incontinence, and enuresis. Rare cardiovascular collapse has been reported in patients receiving concomitant verapamil. May potentiate vecuronium-induced neuromuscular block.

Avoid unnecessary exposure of medication to sunlight. **Avoid** extravasation into tissues. A decrease in spasticity sufficient to allow daily function should be therapeutic goal. Discontinue if benefits are not evident in 45 days.

Continued

DANTROLENE *continued*

IV administration rates for malignant hyperthermia:

Dosage Form	Prevention Use	Treatment Use
Injectable solution	Over 1 hr	IV push
Injectable suspension	Over at least 1 min	IV push

DAPSONE
Aczone, Diaminodiphenyl sulfone, DDS, and generics
Antibiotic, sulfone derivative

C   2   Yes   Yes   No

Tabs: 25, 100 mg
Oral suspension: 2 mg/mL
Topical gel (Aczone and generics): 5%, 7.5% (60, 90 g); contains methylparaben

Pneumocystis jiroveci (formerly *carinii*) treatment:
  Child and adult: 2 mg/kg/24 hr PO once daily (**max. dose:** 100 mg/24 hr) with trimethoprim
    15 mg/kg/24 hr PO ÷ TID × 21 days
P. jiroveci (formerly *carinii*) prophylaxis (first episode and recurrence):
  Child ≥1 mo: 2 mg/kg/24 hr PO once daily; **max. dose:** 100 mg/24 hr. Alternative weekly dosing: 4 mg/
    kg/dose PO Q7 days; **max. dose:** 200 mg/dose
  Adult: 100 mg/24 hr PO ÷ once daily—BID as monotherapy; OR 50 mg PO once daily with
    pyrimethamine 50 mg PO Q7 days and leucovorin 25 mg PO Q7 days; other combination regimens
    with pyrimethamine and leucovorin may be used (see https://www.aidsinfo.gov)
Toxoplasma gondii prophylaxis (prevent first episode):
  Child ≥1 mo: 2 mg/kg/24 hr (**max. dose:** 25 mg/24 hr) PO once daily with pyrimethamine 1 mg/kg/24
    hr (**max.** 25 mg/dose) PO once daily and leucovorin 5 mg PO Q3 days
  Adolescent and adult: 50 mg PO once daily with pyrimethamine 50 mg PO Q7 days and leucovorin 25
    mg PO Q7 days; other combination regimens with pyrimethamine and leucovorin may be used (see
    https://www.aidsinfo.gov)
Leprosy (see http://www.who.int/en/ for the WHO latest recommendations, including combination
  regimens such as rifampin ± clofazimine):
  Child: 1–2 mg/kg/24 hr PO once daily; **max. dose:** 100 mg/24 hr
  Adult: 100 mg PO once daily
Acne vulgaris (topical gel; reevaluate patient if no improvement after 12 wk of therapy):
  5% gel (≥12 yr old): Apply small amount (pea size) of topical gel onto clean, acne-affected areas BID.
  7.5% gel (≥9 yr old): Apply small amount (pea size) of topical gel onto clean, acne-affected areas
    once daily.

Patients with HIV, glutathione deficiency, or G6PD deficiency may be at increased risk for
developing methemoglobinemia. Side effects include hemolytic anemia (dose related),
agranulocytosis, methemoglobinemia, aplastic anemia, nausea, vomiting, hyperbilirubinemia,
headache, nephrotic syndrome, and hypersensitivity reaction (sulfone syndrome). Cholestatic
jaundice, hepatitis, peripheral neuropathy, and suicidal intent have been reported with systemic
use.
Didanosine, rifabutin, and rifampin decrease dapsone levels. Trimethoprim increases dapsone levels.
Pyrimethamine, nitrofurantoin, primaquine, and zidovudine increase risk for hematological side
effects.
Oral suspension may not be absorbed as well as tablets.

DAPSONE *continued*

TOPICAL USE: Dry skin, erythema, and peeling of the skin may occur. Use of topical gel, followed by benzoyl peroxide for acne, has resulted in temporary local discoloration (yellow/orange) of the skin and facial hair. **Avoid use** of topical gel in G6PD deficiency or congenital/idiopathic methemoglobinemia.

DARBEPOETIN ALFA
Aranesp
Erythropoiesis stimulating protein

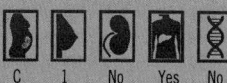

C   1   No   Yes   No

Injection: 25, 40, 60, 100, 200 mCg/1 mL (1 mL)
Single-dose prefilled injection syringe (27 gauge ¹/₂-inch needle): 10 mCg/0.4 mL (0.4 mL), 25 mCg/0.42 mL (0.42 mL), 40 mCg/0.4 mL (0.4 mL), 60 mCg/0.3 mL (0.3 mL), 100 mCg/0.5 mL (0.5 mL), 150 mCg/0.3 mL (0.3 mL), 200 mCg/0.4 mL (0.4 mL), 300 mCg/0.6 mL (0.6 mL), 500 mCg/1 mL (1 mL)

Both dosage forms contain polysorbate 80 (0.05 mg/mL) and mouse and/or hamster protein; albumin free and preservative free.

Anemia in chronic renal failure (see remarks):
  Receiving dialysis (initial dosage and adjust dose according to the table that follows; IV route is recommended for patients on hemodialysis):
    Infant, child, and adolescent: Start with 0.45 mCg/kg/dose IV/SC once weekly.
    Adult: Start with 0.45 mCg/kg/dose IV/SC once weekly, ***OR*** 0.75 mCg/kg/dose IV/SC once every 2 wk.
  Not receiving dialysis (initial dosage; adjust dose according to the table that follows):
    Infant, child, and adolescent: Start with 0.45 mCg/kg/dose IV/SC once weekly, ***OR*** 0.75 mCg/kg/dose IV/SC once every 2 wk.
    Adult: Start with 0.45 mCg/kg/dose IV/SC once every 4 wk.

DARBEPOETIN ALFA DOSE ADJUSTMENT IN ANEMIA ASSOCIATED WITH CHRONIC RENAL FAILURE

Response to Dose	Dose Adjustment
<1 g/dL increase in hemoglobin and below target range after 4 wk of therapy	Increase dose by 25% not more frequently than once monthly. Further increases, if needed, may be done at 4-wk intervals. Among those who do not adequately respond over a 12-wk escalation period, further dose increase is unlikely to improve response and may increase risks.
>1 g/dL increase in hemoglobin in any 2-wk period, or if hemoglobin exceeds and approaches 11 g/dL	Decrease dose by 25% or more
Hemoglobin continues to increase despite dosage reduction	Discontinue therapy; reinitiate therapy at a 25% lower dose of the previous dose after the hemoglobin starts to decrease

Anemia associated with chemotherapy (patients with nonmyeloid malignancies):
  Child (limited data) and adult (see remarks): Start with 2.25 mCg/kg/dose SC once weekly and adjust dose according to the table that follows:

Continued

DARBEPOETIN ALFA *continued*

DARBEPOETIN ALFA DOSE ADJUSTMENT IN ANEMIA ASSOCIATED WITH CHEMOTHERAPY

Response to Dose	Dose Adjustment
<1 g/dL increase in hemoglobin and remains below 10 g/dL after 6 wk of therapy	Increase dose to 4.5 mCg/kg/dose once weekly SC/IV
>1 g/dL increase in hemoglobin in any 2-wk period, or when hemoglobin reaches a level needed to avoid transfusion	Decrease dose by 40%
If hemoglobin exceeds a level needed to avoid transfusion	Hold therapy until hemoglobin approaches a level where transfusions may be required and restart at a reduced dose by 40%
Lack of response after 8 wk or completion of chemotherapy	Discontinue therapy

Conversion from epoetin alfa to darbepoetin alfa (see table below):

Previous Weekly Epoetin Alfa Dose (units/wk)[a]	Pediatric Weekly Darbepoetin Alfa Dose (mCg/wk) Administered SC/IV Once Weekly[b]	Adult Weekly Darbepoetin Alfa Dose (mCg/wk) Administered SC/IV Once Weekly[b]	Adult Once Every 2 wk Darbepoetin Alfa Dose (mCg Every 2 wk) Administered SC/IV Once Every 2 wk[c]
<1,500	Insufficient data	6.25	12.5
1,500–2,499	6.25	6.25	12.5
2,500–4,999	10	12.5	25
5,000–10,999	20	25	50
11,000–17,999	40	40	80
18,000–33,999	60	60	120
34,000–89,999	100	100	200
≥90,000	200	200	400

[a]200 units of epoetin alfa is equivalent to 1 mCg darbepoetin alfa.
[b]If patient was receiving epoetin alfa 2–3 times weekly, darbepoetin alfa should be administered once weekly.
[c]If patient was receiving epoetin alfa once weekly, darbepoetin alfa should be administered once every 2 wk.

Contraindicated in uncontrolled hypertension and patients hypersensitive to albumin/ polysorbate 80 or epoetin alfa. Darbepoetin alfa is not intended for patients requiring acute correction of anemia. **Use with caution** in seizures and liver disease. Erythema multiforme, SJS, and TEN have been reported. Evaluate serum iron, ferritin, and TIBC; concurrent iron supplementation may be necessary. Red cell aplasia and severe anemia associated with neutralizing antibodies to erythropoietin have been reported.

USE IN CHRONIC RENAL FAILURE: Higher doses may be needed for pediatric patients being switched from epoetin alfa than those for naïve patients. May cause edema, fatigue, GI disturbances, headache, blood pressure changes, fever, cardiac arrhythmia/arrest, infections, and myalgia. Higher risk for mortality and serious cardiovascular events have been reported with higher targeted hemoglobin levels (>11 g/dL). If hemoglobin levels do not increase or reach targeted levels despite appropriate dose titrations over a 12-wk period, (1) **do not** administer higher doses; use the lowest dose that will maintain hemoglobin levels to avoid the need for recurrent blood transfusions; (2) evaluate and treat other causes of anemia; (3) always follow the dose adjustment instructions; and (4) discontinue use if patient remains transfusion dependent.

DARBEPOETIN ALFA *continued*

USE IN CANCER: Use only for anemia due to myelosuppressive chemotherapy; not effective in reducing the need for transfusions in patients with anemia not due to chemotherapy. Shortened survival and time to tumor progression have been reported in patients with various cancers. May cause fatigue, fever, edema, dizziness, headache, GI disturbances, arthralgia/myalgia, and rash. Use lowest dose to avoid transfusions and **do not exceed hemoglobin levels >12 g/dL**; increased frequency of adverse events, including mortality and thrombotic vascular events, have been reported.

Prescribers and hospitals must enroll in and comply with the ESA APPRISE Oncology Program to prescribe and/or dispense this drug to cancer patients.

Monitor hemoglobin, BP, serum chemistries, and reticulocyte count. Increases in dose should not be made more frequently than once a month. For IV administration, infuse over 1—3 min.

DEFEROXAMINE MESYLATE Desferal and generics *Chelating agent*		
	C 2 Yes Yes No	

Injection: 500, 2000 mg

Acute iron poisoning (if using IV route, convert to IM as soon as the patient's clinical condition permits; see remarks):
  Child:
    IV: 15 mg/kg/hr
    IM: 50 mg/kg/dose Q6 hr
    Max. IV or IM dose: 6 g/24 hr
  Adult:
    IV: 15 mg/kg/hr
    IM: 1 g ×1, then 0.5 g Q4 hr ×2; may repeat 0.5 g Q4—12 hr
    Max. dose: 6 g/24 hr
Chronic iron overload (see remarks):
  Child and adolescent:
    IV: 20—40 mg/kg/dose over 8—12 hr once daily × 5—7 days per week; usual **max. dose:** 40 mg/kg/24 hr (child) or 60 mg/kg/24 hr (adolescent)
    SC: 20—40 mg/kg/dose once daily as infusion over 8—12 hr × 3—7 days per week; **max. dose:** 2 g/24 hr
  Adult:
    IV: 40—50 mg/kg/dose over 8—12 hr once daily × 5—7 days per week; **max. dose:** 60 mg/kg/24 hr
    IM: 0.5—1 g/dose once daily; **max. dose:** 1 g/24 hr
    SC: 1—2 g/dose once daily as infusion over 8—24 hr

Contraindicated in severe renal disease or anuria. **Not approved** for use in primary hemochromatosis. May cause flushing, erythema, urticaria, hypotension, tachycardia, diarrhea, leg cramps, fever, cataracts, hearing loss, nausea, and vomiting. Iron mobilization may be poor in children <3 yr. Serum creatinine elevation, acute renal failure, renal tubular disorders, and hepatic dysfunction have been reported.

Avoid use if glomerular filtration rate (GFR) <10 mL/min and administer 25%—50% of usual dose if GFR is 10—50 mL/min or patient is receiving continuous renal replacement therapy (CRRT).

High doses and concomitant low ferritin levels have also been associated with growth retardation. Growth velocity may resume to pretreatment levels by reducing the dosage. Acute respiratory distress syndrome (ARDS) has been reported following treatment with excessively high IV doses in patients with acute iron intoxication or thalassemia. Toxicity risk has been reported with infusions >8 mg/kg/hr for >4 days for thalassemia, and with infusions of 15 mg/kg/hr for >1 day for acute iron toxicity. Pulmonary toxicity was not seen in 193 courses.

Continued

DEFEROXAMINE MESYLATE *continued*

For IV infusion, **maximum rate:** 15 mg/kg/hr. Infuse IV infusion over 6—12 hr for mild/moderate iron intoxication and over 24 hr for severe cases, then reassess. SC route is via a portable controlled-infusion device and is **not recommended** in acute iron poisoning.

DESMOPRESSIN ACETATE
DDAVP, Stimate, and generics
Vasopressin analog, synthetic; hemostatic agent

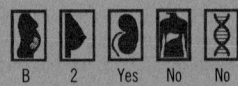

| B | 2 | Yes | No | No |

Tabs: 0.1, 0.2 mg
Injection: 4 mCg/mL (1, 10 mL); contains 9 mg NaCl/mL and may contain chlorobutanol
Nasal spray:
100 mCg/mL, 10 mCg/spray (50 sprays, 5 mL); contains 7.5 mg NaCl/mL and 0.2 mg benzalkonium chloride/mL
Stimate: 1500 mCg/mL, 150 mCg/spray (25 sprays, 2.5 mL); contains 7.5 mg NaCl/mL and 0.1 mg benzalkonium chloride/mL
Conversion: 100 mCg = 400 IU arginine vasopressin

Diabetes insipidus (see remarks):
Oral:
Child ≤12 yr: Start with 0.05 mg/dose BID; titrate to effect; usual dose range: 0.1—0.8 mg/24 hr.
Child >12 yr and adult: Start with 0.05 mg/dose BID; titrate dose to effect; usual dose range: 0.1—1.2 mg/24 hr ÷ BID—TID.
Nasal spray (titrate dose to achieve control of excessive thirst and urination. Morning and evening doses should be adjusted separately for diurnal rhythm of water turnover):
≥4—18 yr: Start at 10 mCg once daily, may titrate up to 30 mCg/24 hr ÷ once daily or BID (20 mCg AM and 10 mCg PM).
Adult: Start at 10 mCg once daily, may titrate up to 40 mCg/24 hr ÷ BID—TID.
Converting from IV dosage form: Give 10 times the IV dose intranasally, rounding down to the nearest 10 mCg.
Converting from PO dosage form: Intranasal dose is approximately 10- to 40-fold more potent than oral dose.
IV/SC:
<12 yr (limited data): 0.1—1 mCg/24 hr ÷ once daily—BID; start with lower dose and increase as needed.
≥12 yr and adult: 2—4 mCg/24 hr ÷ BID
Hemophilia A and von Willebrand disease:
Intranasal (≥11 mo, child and adolescent; using 150 mCg/spray product):
<50 kg: 150 mcg (1 spray) 2 hr before procedure
≥50 kg: 300 mcg (1 spray each nostril) 2 hr before procedure
IV (≥3 mo, child, adolescent): 0.3 mCg/kg/dose over 15—30 min, administered 30 min before procedure
Nocturnal enuresis (≥6 yr; see remarks):
Oral: 0.2 mg at bedtime; if needed, titrate to achieve desired effect by 0.2 mg Q3 days up to a **max. dose** of 0.6 mg/24 hr. Limit fluid intake to a minimum from 1 hr prior to desmopressin dosing until the next morning or at least 8 hr after dose administration.

Use with caution in hypertension, patients at risk for water intoxication with hyponatremia, and coronary artery disease. May cause headache, nausea, seizures, blood pressure changes, hyponatremia, nasal congestion, abdominal cramps, and hypertension.

DESMOPRESSIN ACETATE *continued*

Desmopressin is primarily excreted in the urine, and renal impairment may increase the elimination half-life (some consider use contraindicated when GFR is <50 mL/min).

NOCTURNAL ENURESIS: Intranasal formulations are no longer indicated by the FDA for primary **nocturnal enuresis** (children are susceptible for severe hyponatremia and seizures) or in patients with a history of hyponatremia. Patients using tablets should reduce their fluid intake to prevent potential water intoxication and hyponatremia, and have their therapy interrupted during acute illnesses that may lead to fluid and/or electrolyte imbalance.

Injection may be used SC or IV at approximately 10% of intranasal dose. Adjust fluid intake to decrease risk of water intoxication and monitor serum sodium.

If switching stabilized patient from intranasal route to IV/SC route, use 10% of intranasal dose. Peak effects: 1—5 hr with intranasal route; 1.5—3 hr with IV route; and 2—7 hr with PO route.

DEXAMETHASONE
Dexabliss, Dxevo, HiDex, TaperDex, ZCORT,
Maxidex, and various generics; previously
available as Decadron
Corticosteroid

C   3   No   No   No

Tabs: 0.5, 0.75, 1, 1.5, 2, 4, 6 mg
  Dexabliss, Dxevo: 1.5 mg [39 tabs (11 days)]
  HiDex: 1.5 mg [21 tabs (6 days)]
  TaperDex: 1.5 mg [21 tabs (6 days), 27 tabs (7 days), 49 tabs (12 days)]
  ZCORT: 1.5 mg [25 tabs (7 days)]
  Generic: 1.5 mg [21 tabs (6 days), 35 tabs (10 days), 51 tabs (13 days)]
Injection (sodium phosphate salt): 4 mg/mL (1, 5, 30 mL); 10 mg/mL (1, 10 mL); some preparations contain benzyl alcohol or methyl/propyl parabens
Oral elixir: 0.5 mg/5 mL (237 mL); some preparations contain 5% alcohol
Oral solution: 0.1, 1 mg/mL; some preparations contain 30% alcohol
Ophthalmic solution: 0.1% (5 mL)
Ophthalmic suspension (Maxidex): 0.1% (5 mL)

Airway edema/extubation:
  Infant, child, and adolescent: 0.5 mg/kg/dose (**max. dose:** 10 mg/dose) IV/IM/PO Q6 hr
  × 6 doses initiating therapy 6—12 hr prior to extubation

Asthma exacerbation:
  Infant, child, and adolescent: 0.6 mg/kg/dose (**max. dose:** 16 mg/dose) PO/IV/IM Q24 hr × 1 or 2 doses; use beyond 2 days increases risk for metabolic adverse effects
Croup:
  Infant and child: 0.6 mg/kg/dose PO/IV/IM ×1. **Usual max. dose:** 16 mg/dose
Antiemetic (chemotherapy induced):
  Initial: 10 mg/m^2/dose IV; **max. dose:** 20 mg
  Subsequent: 5 mg/m^2/dose Q6 hr IV
Antiinflammatory:
  Child: 0.08—0.3 mg/kg/24 hr PO, IV, IM ÷ Q6—12 hr
  Adult: 0.75—9 mg/24 hr PO, IV, IM ÷ Q6—12 hr
Cerebral edema (infant, child, and adolescent; limited data):
  Loading dose: 1—2 mg/kg/dose IV/IM ×1
  Maintenance: 1—2 mg/kg/24 hr ÷ Q4—6 hr; **max. dose:** 16 mg/24 hr

Continued

DEXAMETHASONE *continued*

Ophthalmic use (infant, child, and adult):

Solution: Instill 1—2 drops into the conjunctival sac(s) of the affected eye(s) Q1 hr during the day and Q2 hr during the night as initial therapy. When a favorable response is achieved, reduce dosage to Q3—4 hr. Further dose reduction to 1 drop TID—QID may be sufficient to control symptoms.

Suspension: Shake well before using. Instill 1—2 drops in the conjunctival sac(s) of the affected eye(s) up to 4—6 times/24 hr. For severe disease, drops may be used Q1 hr, being tapered to discontinuation as inflammation subsides. For mild disease, drops may be used ≤4—6 times/24 hr.

Not recommended for systemic therapy in the prevention or treatment of chronic lung disease in infants with very low birth weight because of increased risk for adverse events. Dexamethasone is a substrate of CYP P450 3A3/4 and P-glycoprotein, and a moderate inducer of CYP P450 3A4.

Compared to prednisone, dexamethasone has no mineralocorticoid effects with greater glucocorticoid effects. Consider use of alternative low glucocorticoid systemic steroid for patients with hyperglycemia. **Contraindicated** in active untreated infections and fungal, viral, and mycobacterial ocular infections.

Oral peak serum levels occur 1—2 hr and within 8 hr following IM administration. **For other uses, doses based on body surface area, and dose equivalence to other steroids, see Chapter 10.**

OPHTHALMIC USE: Use ophthalmic preparation only in consultation with an ophthalmologist. **Use with caution** in corneal/scleral thinning and glaucoma. Consider the possibility of persistent fungal infections of the cornea after prolonged use. Ophthalmic solution/suspension may be used in otitis externa.

DEXMEDETOMIDINE
Precedex and generics
α adrenergic agonist, sedative

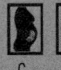   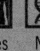

C ? No Yes No

Injection (Precedex and generics): 200 mCg/2 mL (2 mL); preservative free

Multidose injection: 400 mCg/4 mL (4 mL), 1000 mCg/10 mL (10 mL); contains methyl- and propyl-parabens

Premixed injection in NS (Precedex and generics): 80 mCg/20 mL (20 mL), 200 mCg/50 mL (50 mL), 400 mCg/100 mL (100 mL), 1000 mCg/250 mL (250 mL); preservative free

NOTE: Maintenance infusion rate dosing metric is mCg/kg/HR.

ICU sedation:

Child (limited data): 0.5—1 mCg/kg/dose IV × 1 over 10 min followed by 0.2—1 mCg/kg/hr infusion titrated to effect. Children <1 yr of age may require higher dosages.

Adult: 1 mCg/kg/dose IV × 1 over 10 min, followed by 0.2—0.7 mCg/kg/hr infusion and titrated to effect.

Procedural sedation:

Child (limited data):

IV: 2 mCg/kg/dose × 1 IV followed by 1.5 mCg/kg/hr was administered to children with autism/pervasive developmental disorders for sedation for electroencephalography (EEG).

IM: 1—4.5 mCg/kg/dose × 1 IM was administered to children for sedation for EEG. Extremely anxious, inconsolable, aggressive, and noncompliant children received doses >2.5 mCg/kg, and calm and relatively compliant children received doses ≤2.5 mCg/kg. A second lower repeat dose (~2 mCg/kg/dose IM) was administered when adequate sedation was not achieved after 10 min of the first dose.

Intranasal route (limited data): 1—2 mCg/kg/dose × 1 for premedication 30—60 min prior to anesthesia induction

Adult: 0.5—1 mCg/kg/dose IV × 1 over 10 min, followed by 0.6 mCg/kg/hr titrated to effect; dosage has ranged from 0.2—1 mCg/kg/hr

DEXMEDETOMIDINE *continued*

Use with caution with other vasodilating or negative chronotropic agents (additive pharmacodynamic effects), hepatic impairment (decrease drug clearance; consider dose reduction), advanced heart block, hypovolemia, diabetes mellitus, chronic hypertension, and severe ventricular dysfunction. Prolonged use >24 hr may be associated with tolerance and tachyphylaxis and dose-related side effects (ARDS, respiratory failure, and agitation). Withdrawal symptoms within 24 hr after discontinuing dexmedetomidine have been reported in ∼5% of adults receiving the medication up to 7 days regardless of dosage; no withdrawal symptoms were seen in adults after discontinuing therapy lasting <6 hr in duration.

Hypotension and bradycardia are common side effects; may be more pronounced in hypovolemia, diabetes, or chronic hypertension. Transient hypertension has been observed during loading doses. QT prolongation, hypernatremia, sinus arrest, and polyuria have been reported. **Do not** abruptly withdraw therapy, as withdrawal symptoms (nausea, vomiting, and agitation) are possible; taper the dose when discontinuing use. May cause hyperthermia or pyrexia, which may be resistant to administration of cooled IV fluids and antipyretics; may require discontinuing dexmedetomidine.

Use with anesthetics, sedatives, hypnotics, and opioids may lead to enhanced effects; consider dosage reduction of dexmedetomidine. Dexmedetomidine is a CYP 450 2A6 substrate and a weak inhibitor of CYP 450 1A2, 2C9, and 3A4.

Onset of action for procedural sedation: IV or IM: 15 min, intranasal: 15–30 min. Duration of action for procedural sedation: IM: 1 hr, intranasal: 1–1.5 hr

This drug should be administered by individuals skilled in the management of patients in the ICU and OR. Concentrated IV solution (100 mCg/1 mL) must be diluted with NS to a concentration of 4 mCg/mL prior to administration. See Chapter 6 for additional information.

DEXMETHYLPHENIDATE
Focalin, Focalin XR, and generics
CNS stimulant

   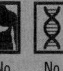

| C | 3 | No | No | No |

Tab, immediate release (Focalin and generics): 2.5, 5, 10 mg
Extended release caps (Focalin XR and generics): 5, 10, 15, 20, 25, 30, 35, 40 mg

Attention deficit/hyperactivity disorder:
METHYLPHENIDATE NAÏVE:

Age/Dosage Form	Initial Dose	Dosage Increase at Weekly Intervals, if Needed	Daily Maximum Dose
≥6 YR AND ADOLESCENT			
Immediate release tabs[a]	2.5 mg PO BID	2.5–5 mg/24 hr	20 mg/24 hr (10 mg BID)
Extended release caps[b]	5 mg PO once daily	5 mg/24 hr	30 mg/24 hr (some may require and be able to tolerate up to 50 mg/24 hr)
ADULT			
Immediate release tabs[a]	2.5 mg PO BID	2.5–5 mg/24 hr	20 mg/24 hr (10 mg BID)
Extended release caps[b]	10 mg PO once daily	10 mg/24 hr	40 mg/24 hr

[a]BID dosing (at least 4 hr apart).
[b]Once-daily dosing.

Continued

DEXMETHYLPHENIDATE *continued*

CONVERTING FROM METHYLPHENIDATE:

≥6 yr and adult: Start at 50% of the total daily dose of racemic methylphenidate with the following max. doses:

Immediate release tabs (BID dosing): 20 mg/24 hr; some may require and be able to tolerate 50 mg/24 hr

Extended release caps (once daily dosing):

≥6 yr—adolescent: 30 mg/24 hr (some may require and be able to tolerate 50 mg/24 hr)

Adult: 40 mg/24 hr

CONVERTING FROM IMMEDIATE RELEASE TABS (BID) TO EXTENDED RELEASE CAPS (ONCE DAILY) DEXMETHYLPHENIDATE:

Use the equivalent mg dosage amount.

Dexmethylphenidate is the d-enantiomer of methylphenidate and accounts for the majority of clinical effects for methylphenidate. **Contraindicated** in glaucoma, anxiety disorders, motor tics, and Tourette syndrome. **Do not** use with monoamine oxidase (MAO) inhibitor; hypertensive crisis may occur if used within 14 days of discontinuation of MAO inhibitor. When used in combination with risperidone, any dosage change to either medication may increase the risk for extrapyramidal symptoms. See Methylphenidate for additional warnings and drug interactions.

Common side effects include abdominal pain, indigestion, appetite suppression, nausea, headache, insomnia, and anxiety. Peripheral vasculopathy, including Raynaud phenomenon, and priapism have been reported. Monitor for long-term growth suppression in children and assess for risk of abuse and dependence prior to prescribing.

Immediate release tablets are dosed BID (minimum 4 hr between doses), and extended release capsules are dosed once daily. Contents of the extended release capsule may be sprinkled on a spoonful of applesauce and consumed immediately for those who are unable to swallow capsules.

DEXTROAMPHETAMINE ± AMPHETAMINE
Dexedrine, ProCentra, Zenzedi, Xelstrym, and many generics
In combination with amphetamine: Adderall, Adderall XR, Mydayis, and generics
CNS stimulant, amphetamine

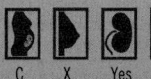 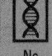

C   X   Yes   Yes   No

Tabs, immediate release:
Generics: 5, 10 mg
Zenzedi: 2.5, 5, 7.5, 10, 15, 20, and 30 mg
Sustained release caps:
Generics: 5, 10, 15 mg
Dexedrine: 10, 15 mg
Oral solution (ProCentra and generics): 1 mg/mL (473 mL); may contain benzoic acid and saccharin
Transdermal patch (Xelstrym): 4.5 mg/9 hr (4.76 cm^2 patch), 9 mg/9 hr (9.52 cm^2 patch), 13.5 mg/9 hr (14.29 cm^2 patch), and 18 mg/9 hr (19.02 cm^2 patch) (30s)
In combination with amphetamine (Adderall): Available as 1:1:1:1 mixture of dextroamphetamine sulfate, dextroamphetamine saccharate, amphetamine aspartate, and amphetamine sulfate salts (e.g., 5 mg tablet contains 1.25 mg dextroamphetamine sulfate, 1.25 mg dextroamphetamine saccharate, 1.25 mg amphetamine aspartate, and 1.25 mg amphetamine sulfate; 5 mg of the mixture is equivalent to 3.1 mg amphetamine base):

DEXTROAMPHETAMINE ± AMPHETAMINE *continued*

Tabs (Adderall and generics): 5, 7.5, 10, 12.5, 15, 20, 30 mg
Caps, extended release:
  Adderal XR and generics: 5, 10, 15, 20, 25, 30 mg
  Mydayis: 12.5, 25, 37.5, 50 mg
Oral suspension: 1 mg/mL

Dosages are in terms of mg of dextroamphetamine when using dextroamphetamine
alone OR in terms of mg of the total dextroamphetamine and amphetamine salts
(e.g., Adderall, Mydayis, or generic equivalent).
Attention deficit/hyperactivity disorder (PO):

	Dextroamphetamine	Dextroamphetamine + Amphetamine
Immediate release dosage forms[a]	**Zenzedi and generics**	**Adderall and generics**
3—5 yr	Start at 2.5 mg QAM; increase by 2.5 mg/24 hr at weekly intervals PRN to a **max. dose** of 40 mg/24 hr ÷ BID-TID (first dose in the morning)	Start at 2.5 mg QAM; increase by 2.5 mg/24 hr at weekly intervals PRN to a **max. dose** of 40 mg/24 hr ÷ QAM-TID (first dose in the morning)
6—17 yr	Start at 5 mg QAM or BID (first dose in the morning); increase by 5 mg/24 hr at weekly intervals PRN to a **max. dose** of 40 mg/24 hr ÷ BID-TID (first dose in the morning)	Start at 5 mg QAM or BID (first dose in the morning); increase by 5 mg/24 hr at weekly intervals PRN to a **max. dose** of 40 mg/24 hr ÷ QAM-TID (first dose in the morning). **Max. dose** of 60 mg/24 hr has been used in patients >50 kg.
Extended/sustained release dosage forms[b]	**Dexedrine and generics**	**Adderall XR and generics**
6—12 yr	Start at 5 mg QAM or BID (first dose in the morning); increase by 5 mg/24 hr at weekly intervals PRN to a **max. dose** of 40 mg/24 hr ÷ QAM or BID (first dose in the morning). **Max. dose** of 60 mg/24 hr has been used in patients >50 kg.	Start at 5 or 10 mg QAM; increase by 5 or 10 mg/24 hr at weekly intervals PRN to a **max. dose** of 30 mg/24 hr. **Max. dose** of 60 mg/24 hr has been used in patients >50 kg.
13—17 yr	Similar dosing as 6—12 yr (see above)	Start at 10 mg QAM; if needed after 1 week, may increase to 20 mg QAM. **Max. dose:** 20 mg/24 hr. **Max. dose** of 60 mg/24 hr has been used in patients >50 kg.

[a]Usually given PO BID-TID; first dose upon awakening and subsequent doses at intervals of 4—6 hr later.
[b]Usually given PO once daily, sometimes BID (6—8 hr between doses).

Continued

DEXTROAMPHETAMINE ± AMPHETAMINE *continued*

Mydayis (extended release capsules):

   13—17 yr: Start at 12.5 mg PO QAM; increase by 12.5 mg/24 hr PRN at weekly intervals to a **max. dose** of 25 mg/24 hr QAM.

   Adult: Start at 12.5 mg PO QAM; increase by 12.5 mg/24 hr PRN at weekly intervals to a **max. dose** of 50 mg/24 hr QAM.

Transdermal patch (Xelstrym; see remarks): Apply to the hip, upper arm, chest, upper back, or flank 2 hr before the effect is desired and remove within 9 hr. Patch may be removed before 9 hr if shorter duration of effect is desired.

   6—17 yr: Start with 4.5 mg/9 hr patch. Dose may be adjusted in weekly increments of 4.5 mg up to a **maximum** of 18 mg/9 hr.

   Adult: Start with 9 mg/9 hr patch. **Maximum dose:** 18 mg/9 hr

Narcolepsy (divide daily dosage once daily—TID for immediate release dosage form and once daily—BID for extended release dosage form; PO):

   6—12 yr: 5 mg/24 hr ÷ once daily-TID; increase by 5 mg/24 hr at weekly intervals to a **max. dose** of 60 mg/24 hr

   >12 yr and adult: 10 mg/24 hr ÷ once daily-TID; increase by 10 mg/24 hr at weekly intervals to a **max. dose** of 60 mg/24 hr

Use with caution in presence of hypertension, cardiovascular disease, and renal or hepatic impairment (drug elimination may be decreased). **Avoid** use in known serious structural cardiac abnormalities, cardiomyopathy, serious heart rhythm abnormalities, coronary artery disease, or other serious cardiac problems that may increase risk of sympathomimetic effects of amphetamines (sudden death, stroke, and MI have been reported). **Do not** give with MAO inhibitors (also within 14 days of discontinuance) or general anesthetics. Use with proton pump inhibitors (PPIs) may reduce the effectiveness of either dextroamphetamine or the combination with amphetamine.

DEXTROAMPHETAMINE AND AMPHETAMINE: Serotonin syndrome may occur when used with serotonergic neurotransmitter medications such as MAO inhibitors, SSRIs, serotonin and norepinephrine reuptake inhibitors (SNRIs), triptans, and TCAs. CYP 450 2D6 inhibitors may increase the effects/toxicity of the combination medication.

Not recommended for children <3 yr. Medication should generally **not** be used in children <5 yr old, as diagnosis of attention deficit and hyperactivity disorder (ADHD) in this age group is extremely difficult (use in consultation with a specialist). Interrupt administration occasionally to determine need for continued therapy. Many side effects, including insomnia (**avoid** dose administration within 6 hr of bedtime), restlessness/irritability, anorexia, psychosis, visual disturbances, headache, vomiting, abdominal cramps, dry mouth, and growth failure. Paranoia, mania, peripheral vasculopathy (including Raynaud phenomenon), priapism, bruxism, intestinal ischemia, and auditory hallucination have been reported. Assess for risk of abuse and dependence prior to prescribing. Tolerance develops. Same guidelines as for methylphenidate apply. See Amphetamine for amphetamine-containing products.

DIAZEPAM
Valium, Diastat, Diastat AcuDial, Valtoco, and generics
Benzodiazepine; anxiolytic, anticonvulsant

    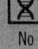

| D | X | Yes | Yes | No |

Tabs: 2, 5, 10 mg

Oral solution: 1 mg/mL, 5 mg/mL; contains 19% alcohol

Injection: 5 mg/mL (2, 10 mL); contains 40% propylene glycol, 10% alcohol, 5% sodium benzoate, and 1.5% benzyl alcohol

Intramuscular auto-injector: 5 mg/mL (2 mL); contains 40% propylene glycol, 10% alcohol, 5% sodium benzoate, and 1.5% benzyl alcohol

DIAZEPAM *continued*

Rectal gel:

> **Pediatric rectal gel (Diastat and generics):** 2.5 mg (5 mg/mL concentration with 4.4 cm rectal tip delivery system; contains 10% alcohol, 1.5% benzyl alcohol, sodium benzoate, and propylene glycol); in twin packs

> **Pediatric/Adult rectal gel (Diastat AcuDial and generics):**

>> **4.4 cm rectal tip delivery system (pediatric/adult):** 10 mg (5 mg/mL, delivers set doses of either 5, 7.5, or 10 mg); contains 10% alcohol, 1.5% benzyl alcohol, sodium benzoate, and propylene glycol; in twin packs

>> **6 cm rectal tip delivery system (adult):** 20 mg (5 mg/mL, delivers set doses of either 12.5, 15, 17.5, 20 mg); contains 10% alcohol, 1.5% benzyl alcohol, sodium benzoate, and propylene glycol; in twin packs

Nasal spray:

> **Valtoco:** 5 mg/0.1 mL, 7.5 mg/0.1 mL, 10 mg/0.1 mL (in 2 individual blister packs with one nasal spray device in each blister pack); contains alcohol and benzyl alcohol

---

Sedative/muscle relaxant:

> **Child:**

>> **IM or IV:** 0.05—0.2 mg/kg/dose Q6—12 hr; **max. dose:** 0.6 mg/kg within an 8-hr period

>> **PO:** 0.12—0.8 mg/kg/24 hr ÷ Q6—12 hr; **max. dose:** 10 mg/dose

> **Adult:**

>> **IM or IV:** 5—10 mg/dose Q3—4 hr PRN

>> **PO:** 2—10 mg/dose Q6—8 hr PRN

Status epilepticus:

> **Neonate (use only after failed therapy of other agents; note the excipients of the IV dosage forms):** 0.1—0.3 mg/kg/dose IV Q15—30 min × 2—3 doses up to **max. total dose** of 2 mg

> **Child >1 mo—<5 yr:** 0.2—0.5 mg/kg/dose IV Q2—5 min up to **max. total dose** of 5 mg. May repeat dosing in 2—4 hr as needed.

> **Child ≥5 yr:** 1 mg/kg/dose IV Q2—5 min up to **max. total dose** of 10 mg. May repeat dosing in 2—4 hr as needed.

> **Adult:** 5—10 mg/dose IV Q10—15 min; **max. total dose:** 30 mg in an 8-hr period. May repeat dosing in 2—4 hr as needed.

Acute seizures:

> **Nasal spray:** Administer one dose using the dosing table below. If needed, a second dose may be administered 4 hr after the first dose. **Max. dose:** 2 doses per single seizure episode. Do not use more than once every 5 days and no more than 5 times per month.

> **Child >6 yr and adult:**

Dose Based on Age and Weight			Administration	
6—11 yr (0.3 mg/kg/dose) Weight (kg)	≥12 yr (0.2 mg/kg/dose) Weight (kg)	Dose (mg)	Number of Nasal Spray Devices	Number of Sprays
10—18	14—27	5	One 5 mg device	One spray in only one nostril
19—37	28—50	10	One 10 mg device	One spray in only one nostril
38—55	51—75	15	Two 7.5 mg devices	One spray in each nostril
56—74	>76	20	Two 10 mg devices	One spray in each nostril

Continued

DIAZEPAM *continued*

Rectal dose (using IV dosage form): 0.5 mg/kg/dose followed by 0.25 mg/kg/dose in 10 min PRN; **max. dose:** 20 mg/dose

Rectal gel: All doses rounded up to the nearest 2.5 mg increment; repeat dose in 4—12 hr PRN. **Do not use** more than once every 5 days and no more than 5 times per month.

2—5 yr: 0.5 mg/kg/dose
6—11 yr: 0.3 mg/kg/dose
≥12 yr and adult: 0.2 mg/kg/dose
Max. dose (all ages): 20 mg/dose

Contraindicated in myasthenia gravis, severe respiratory insufficiency, severe hepatic failure, and sleep apnea syndrome. Hypotension and respiratory depression may occur.
Use with caution in hepatic and renal dysfunction, glaucoma, shock, and depression.
Do not use in combination with protease inhibitors. Concurrent use with CNS depressants, cimetidine, erythromycin, itraconazole, and valproic acid may enhance the effects of diazepam. Use with opioids may result in profound sedation, respiratory depression, coma, and mortality. Diazepam is a substrate for CYP 450 2B6, 2C8, 2C9, and 3A5-7, and minor substrate and inhibitor for CYP 450 2C19 and 3A3/4. The active desmethyldiazepam metabolite is a CYP 450 2C19 substrate.
Nasal discomfort, dysgeusia, and epistaxis may occur with the intranasal route of administration.
Ataxia, headache, dizziness, sedation, and rash have been reported with use of the the rectal gel.
Administer the conventional IV product undiluted no faster than 2 mg/min and **do not** mix with IV fluids. **Do not** test or prime the nasal spray dosage form as each device sprays one time only.
In status epilepticus, diazepam must be followed by long-acting anticonvulsants. Onset of anticonvulsant effect: 1—3 min with IV route; 2—10 min with rectal route; and <5 min with intranasal route. **For management of status epilepticus, see Chapter 1.**

DIAZOXIDE
Proglycem and generics
Antihypoglycemic agent

C	?	Yes	No	No

Oral suspension: 50 mg/mL (30 mL); contains 7.25% alcohol

Hyperinsulinemic hypoglycemia (due to insulin-producing tumors; start at the lowest dose; see remarks):
Newborn and infant: Start at 5 mg/kg/24 hr ÷ Q8—12 hr PO and gradually titrate if needed; usual range of 8—15 mg/kg/24 hr with reported range of 5—20 mg/kg/24 hr ÷ Q8—12 hr
Child and adolescent: Start at 5 mg/kg/24 hr ÷ 8 hr PO and gradually titrate if needed; usual range: 3—8 mg/kg/24 hr ÷ Q8—12 hr PO

Hypoglycemia should be treated initially with IV glucose; diazoxide should be introduced only if refractory to glucose infusion. Should **not** be used in patients hypersensitive to thiazides unless benefit outweighs risk. Thiazides may enhance diazoxide's hyperglycemic effects.
Use with caution in renal impairment (clearance of drug is reduced); consider dosage reduction.
Sodium and fluid retention is common in young infants and adults and may precipitate congestive heart failure (CHF) in patients with compromised cardiac reserve (usually responsive to diuretics). Hirsutism (reversible), GI disturbances, transient loss of taste, tachycardia, ketoacidosis, palpitations, rash, headache, weakness, and hyperuricemia may occur. Pulmonary hypertension in newborns/infants treated for hypoglycemia (especially at doses ≥10 mg/kg/24 hr) has been reported, and resolution/improvement of the condition was achieved after discontinuing diazoxide. Monitor BP closely for hypotension.
Hyperglycemic effect with PO administration occurs within 1 hr, with a duration of 8 hr.

DIGOXIN
Lanoxin, Lanoxin Pediatric, Digitek, and generics
Antiarrhythmic agent, inotrope

C   2   Yes   No   No

Tabs:
    Digitek: 125, 250 mCg
    Lanoxin and generics: 62.5, 125, 250 mCg
Oral solution: 50 mCg/mL (60 mL); may contain 10% alcohol
Injection:
    Lanoxin Pediatric: 100 mCg/mL (1 mL); may contain propylene glycol and alcohol
    Lanoxin and generics: 250 mCg/mL (2 mL); may contain propylene glycol and alcohol

Digitalizing: Total digitalizing dose (TDD) and maintenance doses in mCg/kg/24 hr (see the following table):

DIGOXIN DIGITALIZING AND MAINTENANCE DOSES

	TDD		Daily Maintenance	
Age	**PO**	**IV/IM**	**PO**	**IV/IM**
Premature neonate	20	15	5	3—4
Full-term neonate	30	20	8—10	6—8
1 mo—<2 yr	40—50	30—40	10—12	7.5—9
2—10 yr	30—40	20—30	8—10	6—8
>10 yr and <100 kg	10—15	8—12	2.5—5	2—3

TDD, Total digitalizing dose.

Initial: $\frac{1}{2}$ TDD, then $\frac{1}{4}$ TDD Q8—18 hr × 2 doses; obtain electrocardiogram (ECG) 6 hr after dose to assess for toxicity
Maintenance:
    <10 yr: Give maintenance dose ÷ BID.
    ≥10 yr: Give maintenance dose once daily.

Contraindicated in patients with ventricular dysrhythmias. Use should be **avoided** in patients with preserved left ventricular systolic function. **Use with caution** in renal failure, with calcium channel blockers (may result in heart block), and with adenosine (enhanced depressant effects on sinoatrial [SA] and atrioventricular [AV] nodes). May cause AV block or dysrhythmias. In patients treated with digoxin, cardioversion, or calcium infusion, may lead to ventricular fibrillation (pretreatment with lidocaine may prevent this). Patients with beri beri heart disease may not respond to digoxin if underlying thiamine deficiency is not treated concomitantly. Decreased serum potassium and magnesium, or increased magnesium and calcium may increase risk for digoxin toxicity. For signs and symptoms of toxicity, see Chapter 3.

Excreted via the kidney; **adjust dose in renal failure (see Chapter 31).** Therapeutic concentration: 0.8—2 ng/mL. Higher doses may be required for supraventricular tachycardia. Neonates, pregnant women, and patients with renal, hepatic, or heart failure may have falsely elevated digoxin levels due to the presence of digoxin-like substances.

Digoxin is a CYP450 3A4 and P-glycoprotein substrate. Calcium channel blockers, captopril, carvedilol, amiodarone, quinidine, cyclosporine, itraconazole, tetracycline, and macrolide antibiotics may increase digoxin levels. Use with β-blockers and ivabradine may increase risk for bradycardia. Succinylcholine may cause arrhythmias in digitalized patients.

$T_{1/2}$: Premature infants, 61—170 hr; full-term neonates, 35—45 hr; infants, 18—25 hr; and children, 35 hr.

Recommended serum sampling at steady state: Obtain a single level from 6 hr postdose to just before the next scheduled dose following 5—8 days of continuous dosing. Levels obtained prior to steady state may be useful in preventing toxicity.

DIGOXIN IMMUNE FAB (OVINE)
DigiFab
Antidigoxin antibody

 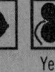 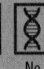

C   ?   Yes   No   No

Injection: 40 mg; derived from the blood of healthy sheep immunized with digoxin derivative

Dosing based on known amounts of digoxin acutely ingested:
  First, determine total body digoxin load (TBL):
    TBL (mg) = mg digoxin ingested × 0.8
  Then, calculate digoxin immune Fab dose:
    Dose in number of digoxin immune Fab vials (DigiFab): # of vials = TBL ÷ 0.5
Dosing based on steady-state serum digoxin levels:
DigiFab dose (mg) from steady-state digoxin levels

Patient Weight (kg)	Serum Digoxin Concentration (ng/mL)						
	1	**2**	**4**	**8**	**12**	**16**	**20**
1	0.4 mg[a]	1 mg[a]	1.5 mg[a]	3 mg[a]	5 mg	6.5 mg	8 mg
3	1 mg[a]	2.5 mg[a]	5 mg	10 mg	14 mg	19 mg	24 mg
5	2 mg[a]	4 mg	8 mg	16 mg	24 mg	32 mg	40 mg
10	4 mg	8 mg	16 mg	32 mg	48 mg	64 mg	80 mg
20	8 mg	16 mg	32 mg	64 mg	96 mg	128 mg	160 mg
40	20 mg	40 mg	80 mg	120 mg	200 mg	280 mg	320 mg
60	20 mg	40 mg	120 mg	200 mg	280 mg	400 mg	480 mg
70	40 mg	80 mg	120 mg	240 mg	360 mg	440 mg	560 mg
80	40 mg	80 mg	120 mg	280 mg	400 mg	520 mg	640 mg
100	40 mg	80 mg	160 mg	320 mg	480 mg	640 mg	800 mg

[a]Use 1 mg/mL DigiFab concentration for dose accuracy.

Dosage administration:
  Reconstitute each vial with 4 mL NS for a 10 mg/mL concentration and infuse IV dose over 30 min. If an infusion rate reaction occurs, stop infusion and restart at a slower rate. In situations of cardiac arrest, DigiFab can be administered as a bolus injection, but expect an increased risk for infusion-related reactions. For smaller doses, vials may be reconstituted with 36 mL NS for a 1 mg/mL concentration.

Contraindicated if hypersensitive to sheep products. **Use with caution** in renal **or** cardiac failure. May cause rapidly developing severe hypokalemia, decreased cardiac output (from withdrawal of digoxin's inotropic effects), rash, edema, and phlebitis. Digoxin therapy may be reinstituted in 3–7 days, when toxicity has been corrected. Digoxin-immune FAB will interfere with digitalis immunoassay measurements to result in misleading concentrations.

DILTIAZEM
Cardizem, Cardizem CD, Cardizem LA, Cartia XT,
Matzim LA, Taztia XT, Tiazac, and many
others including generics
Calcium channel blocker, antihypertensive

    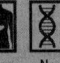

C   2   Yes   Yes   No

DILTIAZEM *continued*

Tabs: 30, 60, 90, 120 mg
Extended release tabs (for Q24 hr dosing):
    Various generics: 180, 240, 300, 360, 420 mg
    Cardizem LA: 120, 180, 240, 300, 360, 420 mg
    Matzim LA: 180, 240, 300, 360, 420 mg
Extended release caps (for Q12 hr dosing): 60, 90, 120 mg
Extended release caps (for Q24 hr dosing):
    Various generics: 120, 180, 240, 300, 360, 420 mg
    Cardizem CD, Taztia XT: 120, 180, 240, 300, 360 mg
    Cartia XT: 120, 180, 240, 300 mg
    Tiazac: 120, 180, 240, 300, 360, 420 mg
Oral liquid: 12 mg/mL
Injection: 5 mg/mL (5, 10, 25 mL)

Hypertension:
    Child: 1.5—2 mg/kg/24 hr PO ÷ TID—QID; **max. dose:** 3.5 mg/kg/24 hr; alternative **max. dose** of 6 mg/kg/24 hr up to 360 mg/24 hr has been recommended
    Adolescent and adult:
        Immediate release: 30—120 mg/dose PO TID—QID; usual range 180—360 mg/24 hr
        Extended release: 120—360 mg/24 hr PO ÷ once daily—BID (BID dosing with Q12 hr extended release generic capsule; once daily dosing with extended release tab, Cardizem CD, Cartia XT, Cardizem LA, Matzim LA, Taztia XT, Tiazac, and Q24 hr generic extended release capsule or tab); **max. dose:** 540 mg/24 hr

Contraindicated in acute myocardial infarction (MI) with pulmonary congestion, second- or third-degree heart block, and sick sinus syndrome. **Use with caution** in CHF or renal and hepatic impairment. Dizziness, headache, edema, nausea, vomiting, heart block, and arrhythmias may occur. Acute hepatic injury and severe skin reactions have been reported. Monitor heart rate with concurrent clonidine use (sinus bradycardia has been reported).

Diltiazem is a substrate and inhibitor of the CYP 450 3A4 enzyme system. May increase levels and effects/toxicity of buspirone, cyclosporine, carbamazepine, fentanyl, digoxin, ivabradine, quinidine, tacrolimus, benzodiazepines, and β-blockers. Cimetidine and statins may increase diltiazem serum levels. Rifampin may decrease diltiazem serum levels.

Maximal antihypertensive effect seen within 2 wk. Extended release dosage forms should be swallowed whole and NOT crushed or chewed. Cardizem immediate release tablets should be swallowed whole, as crushing or chewing them may alter their pharmacokinetics.

DIMENHYDRINATE
Dramamine, Diminate, and generics
Antiemetic, antihistamine

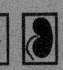

| B | 3 | No | No | No |

Tabs (OTC): 50 mg
Chewable tabs (OTC): 50 mg; contains 0.75 mg phenylalanine
Injection: 50 mg/mL; contains benzyl alcohol and propylene glycol

Child (<12 yr): 5 mg/kg/24 hr ÷ Q6 hr PO/IM/IV; alternative oral dosing by age:
    2—5 yr: 12.5—25 mg/dose Q6—8 hr PRN PO with the max. dosage below

Continued

DIMENHYDRINATE *continued*

6–12 yr: 25–50 mg/dose Q6–8 hr PRN PO with the max. dosage below
≥12 yr and adult: 50–100 mg/dose Q4–6 hr PRN PO/IM/IV
MAX. PO DOSE:
  2–5 yr: 75 mg/24 hr
  6–12 yr: 150 mg/24 hr
  ≥12 yr and adult: 400 mg/24 hr
MAX. IM DOSE:
  Child: 300 mg/24 hr

Causes drowsiness and anticholinergic side effects. May mask vestibular symptoms and cause CNS excitation in young children. **Caution** when taken with ototoxic agents or history of seizures. **Use should be limited to management of prolonged vomiting of known etiology. Not recommended** in children <2 yr. Toxicity resembles anticholinergic poisoning.

DIPHENHYDRAMINE
Benadryl, many other brand names, and generics
Antihistamine

B   3   Yes   No   No

Elixir (OTC): 12.5 mg/5 mL; may contain 5.6% alcohol
Oral liquid/solution (OTC): 12.5 mg/5 mL
Caps/tabs (OTC): 25, 50 mg
Chewable tabs (OTC): 12.5 mg; contains aspartame, phenylalanine
Injection: 50 mg/mL (1, 10 mL)
Topical cream (OTC): 2% (28, 35, 42 g); may contain zinc acetate
Topical gel (OTC): 2% (103, 118 mL); contains parabens
Topical stick (OTC): 2% (14 mL); contains alcohol

Severe allergic reaction (anaphylaxis) and dystonic reactions (including phenothiazine toxicity) (PO/IM/IV):
  Child: 1–2 mg/kg/dose Q6 hr; usual dose: 5 mg/kg/24 hr ÷ Q6 hr. **Max. dose:** 50 mg/dose and 300 mg/24 hr
  Adult: 25–50 mg/dose Q4–8 hr; **max. dose:** 400 mg/24 hr
Sleep aid (PO/IM/IV): Administer dose 30 min before bedtime.
  2–11 yr: 0.5–1 mg/kg/dose; **max. dose:** 50 mg/dose
  ≥12 yr: 25–50 mg
Topical (cream, gel, stick):
  ≥2 yr–adult: Apply to affected area no more than TID–QID.

Contraindicated with concurrent MAO inhibitor use, acute attacks of asthma, GI or urinary obstruction. **Use with caution** in infants and young children, and **do not use** in neonates due to potential CNS effects. Side effects include sedation, nausea, vomiting, xerostoma, blurred vision, and other reactions common to antihistamines. CNS side effects more common than GI disturbances. May cause paradoxical excitement in children. False-positive test for urine phencyclidine (PCP) screen may occur. **Adjust dose in renal failure (see Chapter 31).**
TOPICAL USE: Side effects include rash, urticaria, and photosensitivity.

DIVALPROEX SODIUM
Depakote, Depakote Sprinkles, Depakote ER, and
generics
Anticonvulsant

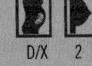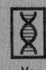

D/X 2 No Yes Yes

Delayed release tabs: 125, 250, 500 mg
Extended release tabs (for Q24 hr dosing):
  Depakote ER and generics: 250, 500 mg
Sprinkle caps (Depakote Sprinkles and generics): 125 mg

Dose: See Valproic Acid.

See Valproic Acid. Preferred over valproic acid for patients on ketogenic diet. **Contraindicated**
  with known urea cycle disorders. Depakote ER is prescribed by a once-daily interval, whereas
  Depakote is typically prescribed BID. Depakote and Depakote ER are not bioequivalent; see package
  insert for dose conversion.
Efficacy was not established in separate randomized double-blinded, placebo-controlled trials for the
  treatment of pediatric bipolar disorder (10—17 yr old) and migraine prophylaxis (12—17 yr old).
Pregnancy category is "X" when used for migraine prophylaxis and is "D" for all other indications.

DOBUTAMINE
Various generics; previously available as
Dobutrex
Sympathomimetic agent

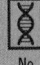

B ? No No No

Injection: 12.5 mg/mL (20 mL); contains sulfites
Prediluted injection in D₅W: 1 mg/mL (250 mL), 2 mg/mL (250 mL), 4 mg/mL (250 mL)

Continuous IV infusion (all ages): 2—20 mCg/kg/min
  Recommended max. dose: 40 mCg/kg/min
To prepare infusion: See page iii.

Contraindicated in idiopathic hypertrophic subaortic stenosis (IHSS). Tachycardia, arrhythmias
  (premature ventricular contractions [PVCs]), and hypertension may occasionally occur
  (especially at higher infusion rates). Correct hypovolemic states before use. Increases AV conduction
  and may precipitate ventricular ectopic activity.
Dobutamine has been shown to increase cardiac output and systemic pressure in pediatric patients of
  every age group. However, in premature neonates, dobutamine is less effective than dopamine in
  raising systemic blood pressure without causing undue tachycardia, and dobutamine has not been
  shown to provide any added benefit when given to such infants already receiving optimal infusions
  of dopamine.
Monitor BP and vital signs. T₁/₂: 2 min. Peak effects in 10—20 min. Use with linezolid
  may potentially increase blood pressure. Use with catechol-O-methyltransferase (COMT)
  inhibitors (e.g., entacapone) may increase heart rate and risk for arrhythmias and changes in blood
  pressure.

DOCUSATE
Colace, DocuSol Kids, DocuSol Mini, Enemeez
Mini, and many other brands
Stool softener, laxative

C 1 No No No

Continued

DOCUSATE *continued*

Available as docusate sodium:
Caps (OTC): 100, 250 mg; sodium content (100 mg cap: ~5 mg)
Tabs (OTC): 100 mg
Syrup (OTC): 20 mg/5 mL (473 mL); may contain alcohol
Oral liquid (OTC): 10 mg/mL (118, 473 mL); contains 1 mg/mL sodium
Rectal enema:
  DocuSol Kids (OTC): 100 mg/5 mL (5 mL); contains polyethylene glycol
  Enemeez Mini, and DocuSol Mini (OTC): 283 mg/5 mL (5 mL); DocuSol Plus product contains
    benzocaine
Available as docusate calcium:
Caps (OTC): 240 mg

PO (take with liquids; see remarks):
  <3 yr: 10—40 mg/24 hr ÷ once daily—QID
  3—6 yr: 20—60 mg/24 hr ÷ once daily—QID
  6—12 yr: 40—150 mg/24 hr ÷ once daily—QID
  >12 yr and adult: 50—400 mg/24 hr ÷ once daily—QID
Rectal (see remarks):
  2—<12 yr: 100 mg/5 mL or 283 mg/5 mL PR once daily
  ≥12 yr and adult: 283 mg/5 mL PR once daily—TID. Alternatively, 50—100 mg of oral liquid (not syrup)
    mixed in enema fluid (saline or oil retention enemas) may be used.

Oral dosage effective only after 1—3 days of therapy, whereas the enema has an onset of
  action in 2—15 min. Reassess therapy if no response seen after 7 days of continuous use.
Incidence of side effects is exceedingly low. Rash, nausea, and throat irritation have been reported.
  Oral liquid is bitter; give with milk, fruit juice, or formula to mask taste.
A few drops of the 10 mg/mL oral liquid may be used in the ear as a cerumenolytic. Effect is usually
  seen within 15 min.

DOLASETRON
Anzemet
Antiemetic agent, 5-HT3 antagonist

| B | ? | Yes | Yes | No |

Tabs: 50 mg
Oral suspension: 10 mg/mL

Chemotherapy-induced nausea and vomiting prevention:
  2 yr—adult: 1.8 mg/kg/dose PO up to a **max. dose** of 100 mg. Administer PO dose 60 min
    prior to chemotherapy. IV route of administration is considered **contraindicated** for this indication
    due to increased risk for QTc prolongation and is no longer available.

May cause hypotension and prolongation of cardiac conduction intervals, particularly QTc
  interval (dose-dependent effect). Common side effects include dizziness, headache, sedation,
  blurred vision, fever, chills, and sleep disorders. Rare cases of sustained supraventricular and
  ventricular arrhythmias, fatal cardiac arrest, and MI have been reported in children and adolescents.
Avoid use in patients with congenital long QTc syndrome, hypomagnesemia, hypokalemia, or with
  concurrent use with other drugs that increase QTc interval (e.g., erythromycin, cisapride). Drug's
  active metabolite (hydrodolasetron) is a substrate for CYP 450 2D6 and 3A3/4 isoenzymes;
  concomitant use of enzyme inhibitors (e.g., cimetidine) may increase risk for side effects, and use of
  enzyme inducers (e.g., rifampin) may decrease dolasetron's efficacy. Serotonin syndrome has been
  associated with concurrent use of SSRIs (e.g., fluoxetine, sertraline), SNRIs (e.g., duloxetine,
  venlafaxine), MAO inhibitors, mirtazapine, fentanyl, lithium, tramadol, and IV methylene blue.

DOLASETRON *continued*

Although no dosage adjustments are necessary, hydrodolasetron's clearance decreases 42% with severe hepatic impairment and 44% with severe renal impairment.

ECG monitoring is recommended in patients with electrolyte abnormalities, CHF, bradyarrhythmias, or renal impairment.

DOPAMINE
Various generics; previously available as Intropin
Sympathomimetic agent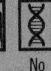

C ? No No No

Injection: 40 mg/mL (5, 10 mL)
Prediluted injection in D₅W: 0.8, 1.6, 3.2 mg/mL (250, 500 mL)

All ages:
 Low dose: 2–5 mcg/kg/min IV; increases renal blood flow; minimal effect on heart rate and cardiac output
 Intermediate dose: 5–15 mcg/kg/min IV; increases heart rate, cardiac contractility, cardiac output, and to a lesser extent, renal blood flow
 High dose: >15 mcg/kg/min IV; α adrenergic effects are prominent; decreases renal perfusion
 Max. dose recommended: 20–50 mcg/kg/min IV
 To prepare infusion: See page iii.

Do not use in pheochromocytoma, tachyarrhythmias, or hypovolemia. Monitor vital signs and blood pressure continuously. Correct hypovolemic states. Tachyarrhythmias, ectopic beats, hypertension, vasoconstriction, and vomiting may occur. **Use with caution** with phenytoin because hypotension and bradycardia may be exacerbated. Use with linezolid may potentially increase blood pressure.

Newborn infants may be more sensitive to the vasoconstrictive effects of dopamine. Children <2 yr of age clear dopamine faster, and high variability in neonates is exhibited.

Should be administered through a central line or large vein. Extravasation may cause tissue necrosis; treat with phentolamine. **Do not** administer into an umbilical arterial catheter.

DORNASE ALFA/DNASE
Pulmozyme
Inhaled mucolytic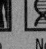

B 1 No No No

Inhalation solution: 1 mg/mL (2.5 mL; in boxes of 30s)

Cystic fibrosis:
 Child 3 mo–<5 yr (limited data from 65 patients receiving 2 wk of therapy): 2.5 mg via nebulizer once daily
 Child ≥5 yr and adult: 2.5 mg via nebulizer once daily. Some patients may benefit from 2.5 mg BID.

Contraindicated in patients with hypersensitivity to epoetin alfa. Voice alteration, pharyngitis, laryngitis may result. These are generally reversible without dose adjustment. Safety and efficacy have not been demonstrated in patients >1 yr of continuous use.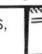

Has been used intranasally via the Pari Sinus device for chronic rhinosinusitis in cystic fibrosis (>5 yr and adult); 2.5 mg intranasally once daily (limited data).

Do not mix with other nebulized drugs. An inhaled β-agonist may be useful before administration to enhance drug distribution. Chest physiotherapy should be incorporated into treatment regimen. The following nebulizer compressor systems have been recommended for use: Pulmo-Aide, Pari-Proneb, Mobilaire, Porta-Neb, or PariBaby. Use of the "Sidestream" nebulizer cup can significantly reduce the medication administration time.

Continued

DOXYCYCLINE
Acticlate, Vibramycin, Doxy, Doryx, Monodox,
Oracea, many others, and generics
Antibiotic, tetracycline derivative

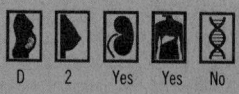

D   2   Yes   Yes   No

Caps: 50, 75, 100, 150 mg
Tabs (Acticlate and generics): 20, 50, 75, 100, 150 mg
Delayed release caps (Oracea): 40 mg
Delayed release tabs (Doryx and generics): 50, 75, 80, 100, 150, 200 mg
Syrup: 50 mg/5 mL (473 mL); contains parabens and propylene glycol
Oral suspension: 25 mg/5 mL (60 mL)
Injection (Doxy and generics): 100 mg

**General dosing, Lyme disease, rickettsial disease, Rocky Mountain spotted fever, and
skin/soft tissue infection** (see remarks):
  ≤45 kg: 2.2 mg/kg/dose BID PO/IV; **max. dose:** 200 mg/24 hr
  >45 kg: 100 mg/dose BID PO/IV
  Max. dose: 200 mg/24 hr
PID (see latest CDC STI treatment guidelines):
  Inpatient: 100 mg IV Q12 hr with cefotetan or cefoxitin, or ceftriaxone + metronidazole. Convert to oral
  therapy 24 hr after patient improves on IV to complete a 14-day total course (IV and PO).
  Outpatient: 100 mg PO Q12 hr × 14 days with ceftriaxone single IM dose with metronidazole, or
  cefoxitin single IM dose + probenecid single PO dose with metronidazole, or other parenteral third-
  generation cephalosporin with metronidazole
Anthrax (inhalation/systemic/cutaneous; see remarks): Initiate therapy with IV route and convert to
  PO route when clinically appropriate. Duration of therapy is 60 days (IV and PO combined):
  ≤8 yr or ≤45 kg: 2.2 mg/kg/dose BID IV/PO; **max. dose:** 200 mg/24 hr
  >8 yr and >45 kg: 100 mg/dose BID IV/PO
**Malaria prophylaxis (start 1–2 days prior to exposure and continue for 4 wk after leaving endemic
area):**
  ≥8 yr: 2.2 mg/kg/24 hr PO once daily; **max. dose:** 100 mg/24 hr and max. duration of 4 mo
  Adult 100 mg PO once daily
Acne:
  ≥8 yr and adolescent: 50-100 mg BID PO or 150 mg once daily PO
Periodontitis:
  Adult: 20 mg BID PO × ≤9 mo

Use with caution in hepatic and renal disease. Generally **not recommended** for use in children
  <8 yr due to risk for tooth enamel hypoplasia and discoloration. However, the AAP Red Book
  recommends doxycycline as the drug of choice for rickettsial disease regardless of age and the use
  in children <8 yr for short treatment courses (≤21 days). May cause GI symptoms, photosensitivity,
  hemolytic anemia, rash, and hypersensitivity reactions. Increased intracranial pressure (pseudotumor
  cerebri), TEN, DRESS, erythema multiforme, and Stevens-Johnson syndrome have been reported.
Doxycycline is approved for the treatment of anthrax (*Bacillus anthracis*) in combination with one or two
  other antimicrobials. If meningitis is suspected, consider using an alternative agent because of poor
  CNS penetration. Consider changing to high-dose amoxicillin (25–35 mg/kg/dose TID PO) for penicillin-
  susceptible strains. See www.cdc.gov/anthrax/treatment/index.html for the latest information.
Rifampin, barbiturates, phenytoin, and carbamazepine may increase clearance of doxycycline.
  Doxycycline may enhance the hypoprothrombinemic effect of warfarin. See Tetracycline for additional
  drug/food interactions and remarks.
Infuse IV over 1–4 hr. **Avoid** prolonged exposure to direct sunlight.
For periodontitis, take tablets ≥1 hr prior to or 2 hr after meals.

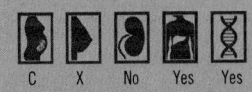

DRONABINOL
Marinol, Syndros, Tetrahydrocannabinol, THC,
and generics
Antiemetic

C　X　No　Yes　Yes

Caps (Marinol and generics): 2.5, 5, 10 mg; may contain sesame oil
Oral solution (Syndros): 5 mg/mL (30 mL); contains alcohol (50% w/w), parabens, and polyethylene
glycol

**Oral capsule and solution dosage forms are NOT bioequivalent and should not be used
interchangeably.**
ORAL CAPSULES:
Antiemetic:
　Child and adult (PO capsules): 5 mg/m^2/dose 1—3 hr prior to chemotherapy, then Q2—4 hr up to a
　max. dose of 4—6 doses/24 hr; doses may be gradually increased by 2.5 mg/m^2/dose increments up
　to a **max. dose** of 15 mg/m^2/dose if needed and tolerated.
Appetite stimulant:
　Adult (PO capsules): 2.5 mg BID 1 hr before lunch and dinner; if not tolerated, reduce dose to 2.5 mg
　once daily 1 hr before dinner or QHS. **Max dose:** 20 mg/24 hr (use **caution** when increasing doses
　because of increased risk of dose-related adverse reactions at higher dosages)
ORAL SOLUTION:
Antiemetic:
　Adult (PO oral solution): 4.2 mg/m^2/dose 1—3 hr prior to chemotherapy, then Q2—4 hr up to a **max.
　dose** of 4—6 doses/24 hr; doses may be gradually increased by 2.1 mg/m^2/dose increments up to a
　max. dose of 12.6 mg/m^2/dose if needed and tolerated.
Appetite stimulant:
　Adult (PO oral solution): 2.1 mg BID 1 hr before lunch and dinner; if not tolerated, reduce dose to 2.1
　mg once daily 1 hr before dinner or QHS. Dose may be gradually increased, if needed and tolerated,
　by increasing the pre-dinner dose to 4.2 mg 1 hr before dinner. Further increase to 4.2 mg BID 1 hr
　before lunch and dinner if needed and tolerated. **Max. dose:** 16.8 mg/24 hr

Contraindicated in patients with history of substance abuse and mental illness and allergy to
sesame oil (capsules only). **Use with caution** in heart disease, seizures, hepatic disease
(reduce dose if severe), and in patients who operate motor vehicles or dangerous machinery. Side
effects: euphoria, dizziness, difficulty concentrating, anxiety, mood change, sedation, hallucinations,
ataxia, paresthesia, hypotension, excessively increased appetite, and habit-forming potential.
Exacerbation of mania, depression, schizophrenia, and seizures have been reported. **Avoid use** with
other medications that can produce similar side effects.
Dronabinol is a substrate for CYP 450 2C9 and 3A4. Individuals with poor CYP 450 2C9 activity may
have reduced clearance of dronabinol, which may increase effects/toxicity.
Onset of action: 0.5—1 hr; duration of psychoactive effects 4—6 hr, appetite stimulation 24 hr

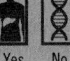

DROPERIDOL
Generics; previously available as Inapsine
Sedative, antiemetic

C　3　Yes　Yes　No

Injection: 2.5 mg/mL (2 mL)

Antiemetic/sedation:
　Child: 0.03—0.07 mg/kg/dose IM or IV over 2—5 min; if needed, may give 0.1—0.15
　mg/kg/dose; **initial max. dose:** 0.1 mg/kg/dose and subsequent **max. dose:** 2.5 mg/dose

Continued

DROPERIDOL *continued*

> **Dosage interval:**
> **Antiemetic:** PRN Q4—6 hr
> **Sedation:** Repeat dose in 15—30 min if necessary.
> **Adult:** 2.5—5 mg IM or IV over 2—5 min; **initial max. dose** is 2.5 mg
> **Dosage interval:**
> **Antiemetic:** PRN Q3—4 hr
> **Sedation:** Repeat dose in 15—30 min if necessary.

Use with caution in renal and hepatic impairment; 75% of metabolites are excreted renally, and drug is extensively metabolized in the liver. Side effects include hypotension, tachycardia, extrapyramidal side effects such as dystonia, feeling of motor restlessness, laryngospasm, and bronchospasm. May lower seizure threshold. **Fatal arrhythmias and QT interval prolongation have been associated with use.**

Onset in 3—10 min. Peak effects within 10—30 min. Duration of 2—4 hr. Often given as adjunct to other agents.

DYMISTA

See Azelastine and Fluticasone.

E

ELEXACAFTOR/TEZACAFTOR/IVACAFTOR
Trikafta
Cystic fibrosis transmembrane conductance regulator corrector and potentiator

    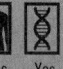

C   ?   Yes   Yes   Yes

Tabs:
> **Morning dose:**
> **Light orange colored:** Elexacaftor 50 mg + tezacaftor 25 mg + ivacaftor 37.5 mg
> **Orange colored:** Elexacaftor 100 mg + tezacaftor 50 mg + ivacaftor 75 mg
> **Evening dose (light blue colored):** Ivacaftor 75 mg or 150 mg
> Available as an 84-tablet carton containing 4 wallets for a 28-day supply; each wallet contains 14 morning-dose tablets and 7 evening-dose tablets for a 7-day supply of the following combinations:
> > Light orange colored morning tablets (elexacaftor 50 mg + tezacaftor 25 mg + ivacaftor 37.5 mg) and light blue colored evening tablets (ivacaftor 75 mg)
> > Orange colored morning tablets (elexacaftor 100 mg + tezacaftor 50 mg + ivacaftor 75 mg) and light blue colored evening tablets (ivacaftor 150 mg)

Morning and evening doses should be taken (PO) ~12 hr apart with fat-containing food; see remarks.

Child 6—11 yr weighing <30 kg:
> **Morning dose:** 2 morning-dose tablets (elexacaftor 50 mg + tezacaftor 25 mg + ivacaftor 37.5 mg each tablet) every morning
> **Evening dose:** 1 evening-dose tablet (75 mg ivacaftor) every evening

Child 6—11 yr weighing ≥30 kg, and child ≥12 yr and adult:
> **Morning dose:** 2 morning-dose tablets (elexacaftor 100 mg + tezacaftor 50 mg + ivacaftor 75 mg each tablet) every morning

ELEXACAFTOR/TEZACAFTOR/IVACAFTOR *continued*

Evening dose: 1 evening-dose tablet (150 mg ivacaftor) every evening
Dose Adjustment for Hepatic Impairment:

	Mild (Child-Pugh Class A)	[a]Moderate (Child-Pugh Class B)	Severe (Child-Pugh Class C)
Morning dose	Use regular dosage	Day 1: Use regular AM dosage (2 tablets) Day 2: Use one AM tablet Then continue alternating Day 1 and Day 2 dosing thereafter and closely monitor liver function tests	Should not be used
Evening dose	Use regular dosage	No evening dosage	Should not be used

[a]Use not recommended unless benefit exceeds risk.

Dose Adjustment for Moderate CYP 450 3A inhibitors (e.g., fluconazole, erythromycin): Administer all doses in the morning.
  Child 6—11 yr weighing <30 kg:
    Day 1: 2 morning-dose tablets of elexacaftor 50 mg + tezacaftor 25 mg + ivacaftor 37.5 mg each tablet (light orange tabs)
    Day 2: 1 evening-dose tablet (ivacaftor 75 mg) in the morning
    Then continue alternating Day 1 and Day 2 regimens QAM thereafter.
  Child 6—11 yr weighing ≥30 kg, and child ≥12 yr and adult:
    Day 1: 2 morning-dose tablets of elexacaftor 100 mg + tezacaftor 50 mg + ivacaftor 75 mg each tablet (orange tabs)
    Day 2: 1 evening-dose tablet (ivacaftor 150 mg) in the morning
    Then continue alternating Day 1 and Day 2 regimens QAM thereafter.
Dose Adjustment for Strong CYP 450 3A inhibitors (e.g., ketoconazole, itraconazole, posaconazole, voriconazole, telithromycin, and clarithromycin): Administer all doses in the morning twice weekly.
  Child 6—11 yr weighing <30 kg:
    Day 1: 2 morning-dose tablets of elexacaftor 50 mg + tezacaftor 25 mg + ivacaftor 37.5 mg each tablet (light orange tabs)
    Days 2 and 3: No dose
    Day 4: Use day 1 regimen (2 morning-dose tablets), then continue the same dosage twice a week (approximately 3—4 days apart).
  Child 6—11 yr weighing ≥30 kg, and child ≥12 yr and adult:
    Day 1: 2 morning-dose tablets of elexacaftor 100 mg + tezacaftor 50 mg + ivacaftor 75 mg each tablet (orange tabs)
    Days 2 and 3: No dose
    Day 4: Use Day 1 regimen (2 morning-dose tablets), then continue the same dosage twice a week (approximately 3—4 days apart).

Works on CFTR trafficking defects with two correctors (elexacaftor and tezacaftor) and a potentiator (ivacaftor). Indicated for individuals with at least one F508del CFTR mutation. Common side effects include headache, URI, abdominal pain, diarrhea, rash, nasal congestion, rhinorrhea, rhinitis, influenza sinusitis, and increases in liver enzymes (ALT/AST, bilirubin) and serum creatine phosphokinase. Monitor baseline ALT/AST and bilirubin at baseline and repeat every 3 mo for the first year followed by annual assessments. Ocular exams should be obtained at baseline and annually as cataracts have been reported in children. May cause a false-positive urine drug screen for cannabinoids.

Continued

ELEXACAFTOR/TEZACAFTOR/IVACAFTOR *continued*

Do **not use** in severe hepatic impairment (Child-Pugh C) and use is not recommended, unless the benefit outweighs the risk, for moderate hepatic impairment (Child-Pugh B). Liver failure resulting in transplantation has been reported in a patient with cirrhosis and portal hypertension. Mental status changes (e.g., fogginess, memory issues) have been reported within the first 3 months of therapy. **Use with caution** with CrCl ≤30 mL/min and ESRD because of lack of data.

All three components of this medication are substrates of CYP 450 3A. **Avoid use** in combination with strong inducers of CYP 450 3A (e.g., rifampin, rifabutin, phenobarbital, carbamazepine, phenytoin, and St. John's wort). Use with moderate and strong CYP 3A inhibitors requires dose reductions; see dosing section. Elexacaftor/tezacaftor/ivacaftor may increase the effects/toxicity of digoxin, cyclosporine, everolimus, glimepiride, glipizide, glyburide, nateglinide, repaglinide, sirolimus, tacrolimus, and warfarin. Always evaluate the potential drug-drug interactions.

Avoid food or drink containing grapefruit or Seville oranges.

Administer all doses with high-fat foods to ensure absorption. If a dose is missed within 6 hr of a scheduled dose, administer the respective morning or evening dose immediately and resume usual dosing. However, if the missed dose is >6 hr, the following are recommended:

Missed morning dose: Take missed dose as soon as possible and do not take evening dose for that day, then resume usual dosing the next day.

Missed evening dose: Do not take the missed dose, then resume usual dosing the next day.

Never take a double dose for a missed dose.

EMLA

See Lidocaine and Prilocaine.

ENALAPRIL MALEATE (PO), ENALAPRILAT (IV)
Enalapril: Vasotec, Epaned, and generics
Enalaprilat: generics; previously available as
Vasotec IV
Angiotensin-converting enzyme inhibitor,
antihypertensive

    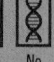

D   2   Yes   No   No

Enalapril:
Tabs (Vasotec and generics): 2.5, 5, 10, 20 mg (scored)
Oral solution (Epaned and generics): 1 mg/mL (150 mL); may contain sodium benzoate
Oral suspension: 0.1, 1 mg/mL

Enalaprilat:
Injection: 1.25 mg/mL (1, 2 mL); contains benzyl alcohol

Hypertension:

Infant and child:

> **PO:** 0.08 mg/kg/24 hr up to 5 mg/24 hr once daily; increase PRN over 2 wk
> **Max. dose (higher doses have not been evaluated):** 0.58 mg/kg/24 hr up to 40 mg/24 hr
> **IV:** 0.005–0.01 mg/kg/dose Q8–24 hr; **max. dose:** 1.25 mg/dose

Adolescent and adult:

> **PO:** 2.5–5 mg/24 hr once daily initially to **max. dose** of 40 mg/24 hr ÷ once daily–BID
> **IV:** 0.625–1.25 mg/dose IV Q6 hr; doses as high as 5 mg Q6 hr are reported to be tolerated for up to 36 hr

---

Contraindicated with hypersensitivity to ACE inhibitors and use in combination with a neprilysin inhibitor (e.g., sacubitril). **Use with caution** in bilateral renal artery stenosis. **Avoid use** in dialysis with high-flux membranes because anaphylactoid reactions have been reported. Side effects: nausea, diarrhea, headache, dizziness, hyperkalemia, hypoglycemia, hypotension, and hypersensitivity. Cough is a reported side effect of ACE inhibitors.

ENALAPRIL MALEATE (PO), ENALAPRILAT (IV) *continued*

Risk for angioedema increases with enalapril and coadministration of rapamycin or sacubitril.
Enalapril (PO) is converted to its active form (Enalaprilat) by the liver. Administer IV over 5 min. **Adjust dose in renal impairment (see Chapter 31).**

Nitritoid reactions have been seen in patients receiving concomitant IV gold therapy. Enalapril/enalaprilat should be discontinued as soon as possible when pregnancy is detected. If oliguria or hypotension occurs in a neonate with in utero exposure with enalapril/enalaprilat, exchange transfusions or dialysis may be needed to reverse hypotension and/or support renal function.

ENOXAPARIN
Lovenox and generics
Anticoagulant, low-molecular-weight heparin

   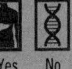

| B | 1 | Yes | Yes | No |

Injection: 100 mg/mL (3 mL); contains pork proteins and 15 mg/mL benzyl alcohol
Injection (prefilled syringes with 27-gauge × $\frac{1}{2}$-inch needle): 30 mg/0.3 mL, 40 mg/0.4 mL, 60 mg/0.6 mL, 80 mg/0.8 mL, 100 mg/1 mL, 120 mg/0.8 mL, 150 mg/1 mL; preservative free and may contain pork proteins
Approximate anti–factor Xa activity: 100 IU per 1 mg

Initial empiric dosage; patient-specific dosage defined by therapeutic drug monitoring when indicated (see remarks)

DVT treatment:

    Premature neonate: 2 mg/kg/dose Q12 hr SC

    Full-term neonate: 1.7 mg/kg/dose Q12 hr SC

    1–<2 mo: 1.5 mg/kg/dose Q12 hr SC

    ≥2 mo–adult: 1 mg/kg/dose Q12 hr SC; alternatively, 1.5 mg/kg/dose Q24 hr SC can be used in adults

    Dosage adjustment for DVT treatment to achieve target anti–factor Xa low-molecular-weight heparin (LMWH) levels of 0.5–1 units/mL (see the following table):

Anti-factor Xa Level LMWH (units/mL)	Hold Next Dose?	Dose Change	Repeat Anti-factor Xa Level LMWH?
<0.4	No	Increase by 25%	4 hr after the second new dose
0.4	No	Increase by 10%	4 hr after the second new dose
0.5	No	No	4 hr after the next dose; if within therapeutic range recheck 1 wk later (4 hr after the dose)
0.6–0.7	No	No	1 wk later (4 hr after the dose)
0.8–1	No	No	4 hr after the next dose; if within therapeutic range recheck 1 wk later (4 hr after the dose)
1.1–1.5	No	Decrease by 20%	4 hr after the second new dose

Continued

ENOXAPARIN *continued*

Anti-factor Xa Level LMWH (units/mL)	Hold Next Dose?	Dose Change	Repeat Anti-factor Xa Level LMWH?
1.6—2	Hold dose for 3 hr and measure level (goal <0.5 units/mL) prior to next new dose.	Decrease by 30%	4 hr after the second new dose
>2	Hold dose until anti-factor Xa LMWH reaches 0.5 units/mL (levels can be measured Q12 hr until it reaches ≤0.5 units/mL).	When anti-factor Xa LMWH reaches ≤0.5 units/mL, dose may be restarted at a dose 40% less than the previous dose.	4 hr after the second new dose

DVT prophylaxis:

Infant <2 mo: 0.75 mg/kg/dose Q12 hr SC

Infant ≥2 mo—child 18 yr: 0.5 mg/kg/dose Q12 hr SC; **max. dose:** 30 mg/dose

Patients with indwelling epidural catheters/neuraxial anesthesia (≥2 mo—child 18 yr): 1 mg/kg/dose Q24 hr SC; **max. dose:** 40 mg/dose. Twice-daily dosing is contraindicated for these patients. See remarks.

Adult: 40 mg Q24 hr SC

Dosage adjustment for DVT prophylaxis to achieve target anti—factor Xa low-molecular-weight heparin (LMWH) levels of 0.1—0.4 units/mL for all children (see the following table):

Anti-Xa Level LMWH (units/mL)	Hold Next Dose?	Dose Change	Repeat Anti-factor Xa Level LMWH?
<0.1	No	Increase by 20%—30%	4 hr after the second new dose
0.1-0.4	No	No	1 wk later (4 hr after the dose)
0.5-0.7	No	Decrease by 20%	4 hr after the second new dose
0.7-1	No	Decrease by 30%—40%	4 hr after the second new dose
>1	Hold dose until anti-factor Xa LMWH is <0.5 units/mL.	When anti-factor Xa LMWH reaches <0.5 units/mL, dose may be restarted at a dose 40% less than the previous dose.	4 hr after the second new dose

---

Inhibits thrombosis by inactivating factor Xa without significantly affecting bleeding time, platelet function, PT, or aPTT at recommended doses. Dosages of enoxaparin, heparin, or other LMWHs **CANNOT** be used interchangeably on a unit-for-unit (or mg-for-mg) basis because of differences in pharmacokinetics and activity. Peak anti—factor Xa LMWH activity is achieved 4 hr after a SC dose. **Anti—factor Xa LMWH is NOT THE SAME as unfractionated heparin anti—factor Xa level** (used for monitoring heparin therapy).

ENOXAPARIN *continued*

Contraindicated in major bleeding, drug-induced thrombocytopenia, and pork hypersensitivity. Relative contraindications include: platelets ≤ 50,000/mm³ and IM injections. **Use with caution** in uncontrolled arterial hypertension, bleeding diathesis, history of recurrent GI ulcers, diabetic retinopathy, and severe renal dysfunction (reduce dose by increasing the dosage interval from Q12 hr to Q24 hr if GFR <30 mL/min). Prophylactic use is not recommended in patients with prosthetic heart valves (especially in pregnant women) due to reports of fatalities in patients and fetuses. **Concurrent use with spinal or epidural anesthesia or spinal puncture has resulted in long-term or permanent paralysis; potential benefits must be weighed against the risks.** May cause fever, confusion, edema, nausea, hemorrhage, thrombocytopenia (including heparin-induced thrombocytopenia ± thrombosis [HIT/HITTS]), hypochromic anemia, and pain/erythema at injection site. Allergic reactions, headache, eosinophilia, alopecia, hepatocellular and cholestatic liver injury, and osteoporosis (long-term use) have been reported. **Protamine sulfate is the antidote**; 1 mg protamine sulfate neutralizes 1 mg enoxaparin.

DVT prophylaxis for patients with epidural catheters/neuraxial anesthesia: If placing needle, hold anticoagulation for 12 hr and restart dosing ≥ 4 hr after needle insertion. If removing catheter, hold anticoagulation for 12 hr and restart dosing ≥ 2 hr after catheter removal.

Recommended anti–factor Xa LMWH levels obtained 4 hr after subcutaneous dose after the third consecutive dose for children (anti–factor Xa LMWH response in children is highly variable compared to adults):

DVT treatment: 0.5–1 units/mL

DVT prophylaxis: 0.1–0.4 units/mL

Administer by deep SC injection by having the patient lie down. Alternate administration between the left and right anterolateral and left and right posterolateral abdominal wall. See package insert for detailed SC administration recommendations. To minimize bruising, do not rub the injection site. IM route of administration is not recommended.

For additional information, see *Chest* 2008;133:887–968 and *Regional Anesthesia and Pain Medicine* 2003;28(3):172–197.

EPINEPHRINE HCL
Adrenalin, EpiPen, Auvi-Q, Symjepi, Epinephrine
SNAP, Primatene Mist, and generics
Sympathomimetic agent

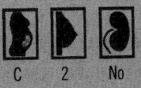 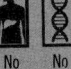

C   2   No   No   No

Injection:
1:1000 (aqueous): 1 mg/mL (1, 30 mL); may contain chlorobutanol and metabisulfite

Injection, in prefilled syringe:
1:10,000 (aqueous): 0.1 mg/mL (10 mL prefilled syringes with either 18-G 3.5-inch or 20-G 1.5-inch needles)

Autoinjector:
EpiPen and generics: Delivers a single 0.3 mg (0.3 mL) dose (2 pack; EpiPen and some generic products include a training device)

EpiPen Jr and generics: Delivers a single 0.15 mg (0.3 mL) dose (2 pack; EpiPen Jr and some generic products include a training device)

Auvi-Q: Delivers a single 0.1 mg (0.1 mL) dose, 0.15 mg (0.15 mL) dose, or 0.3 mg (0.3 mL) dose (2 pack with training device; each unit provides voice instructions when activated)

Symjepi: Delivers a single 0.15 mg (0.3 mL) dose or 0.3 mg (0.3 mL) dose (1 or 2 pack)

Syringe Kit for Anaphylaxis (for specific weight-based dosages for any size patient):
EpinephrineSNAP: 1 mg/mL (1 mL single use vial in a box of 25 vials, 30 mL multi-use vial as a single vial or box of 10 vials)

Continued

EPINEPHRINE HCL *continued*

Many preparations may contain sulfites.
Aerosol inhaler (HFA):
Primatene Mist [OTC]: 0.125 mg per spray (160 sprays per inhaler) (11.7 g); contains 1% alcohol and polysorbate 80

CARDIAC USE:

Neonate:
Asystole and bradycardia: 0.01—0.03 mg/kg of 1:10,000 solution (0.1—0.3 mL/kg) IV/IO Q3—5 min PRN
Infant and child:
Bradycardia/asystole and pulseless arrest: See page ii and PALS algorithms in the back of the book.
Bradycardia, asystole, and pulseless arrest (see remarks):
First dose: 0.01 mg/kg of 1:10,000 solution (0.1 mL/kg) IO/IV; **max. dose:** 1 mg (10 mL).
Subsequent doses Q3—5 min PRN should be the same. High-dose epinephrine after failure of standard dose has not been shown to be effective (see remarks). Must circulate drug with CPR. For ET route, see below.
All ET doses: 0.1 mg/kg (**max. dose:** 2.5 mg) of 1:1000 solution (0.1 mL/kg; **max. dose** 2.5 mL) ET Q3—5 min
Adult:
Asystole: 1 mg IV or 2—2.5 mg ET Q3—5 min
IV drip (all ages): 0.1—1 mCg/kg/min; titrate to effect; to prepare infusion, see p. iii.
HYPERSENSITIVITY/ANAPHYLACTIC REACTIONS:
Recommended IM administration via the anterolateral aspect of the thigh through clothing if necessary; see remarks for IV dosing.
Infant, child, and adolescent: 0.01 mg/kg/dose IM (**max. dose:** 0.3 mg/dose for prepubertal child, 0.5 mg/dose for adolescent) Q5—15 min PRN
Auvi-Q (administer the following dosage IM ×1; an additional dose may be repeated in 5—15 min):
7.5 to <15 kg: 0.1 mg
15 to <30 kg: 0.15 mg
≥30 kg: 0.3 mg
EpiPen/EpiPen Jr, Adrenaclick, Symjepi, or equivalent generic autoinjector (administer the following dosage IM ×1; an additional dose may be repeated in 5—15 min):
7.5 to <30 kg: 0.15 mg
≥30 kg: 0.3 mg
Adult: Start with 0.2—0.5 mg IM Q5—15 min PRN. If using EpiPen, Adrenaclick, Symjepi, or equivalent generic autoinjector, use 0.3 mg IM ×1; an additional dose may be repeated in 5—15 min.
RESPIRATORY BRONCHODILATOR USE:
SC Injection (use 1:1000 or 1 mg/mL aqueous injection):
Infant and child: 0.01 mL/kg/dose SC (**max. single dose** 0.5 mL); repeat Q15 min × 3—4 doses or Q4 hr PRN
Adult: 0.3—0.5 mg (0.3—0.5 mL)/dose SC Q20 min × 3 doses
Nebulization (alternative to racemic epinephrine): 0.5 mL/kg of 1:1000 solution diluted in 3 mL NS; **max. doses:** ≤4 yr: 2.5 mL/dose; >4 yr: 5 mL/dose
Aerosol inhaler (Primatene Mist):
≥12 yr and adult: 1 inhalation PO, may repeat 1 inhalation if needed one minute after the first dose. Wait >4 hours between additional doses PRN; **max. dose:** 8 inhalations/24 hr

High-dose rescue therapy for in-hospital cardiac arrest in children after failure of an initial standard dose has been reported to be of no benefit compared to standard dose (*N Engl J Med* 2004;350:1722—1730).

EPINEPHRINE HCL *continued*

May produce arrhythmias, tachycardia, hypertension, headaches, nervousness, nausea, vomiting, and rare cases of stress cardiomyopathy. Necrosis may occur at site of repeated local injection. Rare cases of serious skin and soft tissue infections, including necrotizing fasciitis and myonecrosis, have been reported with IM or deep SC injections.

Concomitant use of noncardiac selective β-blockers, MAO inhibitors, COMT inhibitors, levothyroxine, diphenhydramine, chlorpheniramine, clonidine, or tricyclic antidepressants may enhance epinephrine's pressor response. Chlorpromazine, diuretics, ergot alkaloids, nitrates, or α-blockers may reverse the pressor response. β-blockers may antagonize epinephrine's cardiostimulating and bronchodilating effects. Cardiac arrhythmias may develop for those who receive epinephrine while concomitantly taking cardiac glycosides, diuretics, or anti-arrhythmics. **Do not** use products containing chlorobutanol for ophthalmic use, as it may be harmful to the corneal endothelium.

ETT doses should be diluted with NS to a volume of 3–5 mL before administration. Follow with several positive pressure ventilations.

Hypersensitivity reactions: For bronchial asthma and certain allergic manifestations (e.g., angioedema, urticaria, serum sickness, anaphylactic shock), use epinephrine SC. Patients with anaphylaxis may benefit from IM administration. The adult IV dose for hypersensitivity reactions or to relieve bronchospasm usually ranges from 0.1 to 0.25 mg injected slowly over 5–10 min Q5–15 min as needed. Neonates may be given a dose of 0.01 mg/kg body weight; for infants, 0.05 mg is an adequate initial dose, and this may be repeated at 20- to 30-min intervals in the management of asthma attacks.

Due to the inconsistent availability of autoinjector products, periodic reeducation of available device may be necessary. See respective autoinjector product for proper dose administration methods, including methods to prevent injury and/or inadvertent dose administration to the individual administering the dose. Accidental injection into the digits, hand, or feet may result in the loss of blood flow to the affected area. **Do not** inject into the buttock area.

EPINEPHRINE, RACEMIC
Asthmanefrin and S-2
Sympathomimetic agent

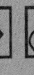   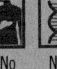

C   2   No   No   No

Solution for inhalation (OTC): 2.25% (1.25% epinephrine base) (0.5 mL) (30s)
Contains edetate disodium and may contain sulfites

<4 yr:
   Croup (using 2.25% solution): 0.05 mL/kg/dose up to a **max. dose** of 0.5 mL/dose diluted to 3 mL with NS. Given via nebulizer over 15 min PRN but **not** more frequently than Q1–2 hr
≥4 yr: 0.5 mL/dose diluted to 3 mL with NS via nebulizer over 15 min Q3–4 hr PRN

Tachyarrhythmias, headache, nausea, palpitations have been reported. Rebound symptoms may occur. Cardiorespiratory monitoring should be considered if administered more frequently than Q1–2 hr.

EPOETIN ALFA
Epogen, Procrit, Retacrit, and Erythropoietin
Recombinant human erythropoietin

    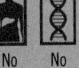

C   2   Yes   No   No

Injection (single-dose, preservative-free vials): 2000, 3000, 4000, 10,000, 40,000 U/mL (1 mL)
Injection (multidose vials): 10,000 U/mL (2 mL), 20,000 U/mL (1 mL); contains 1% benzyl alcohol
All dosage forms contain 2.5 mg albumin per 1 mL.
NOTE: Epoetin alfa-epbx (Retacrit) is a biosimilar product.

Continued

EPOETIN ALFA *continued*

Single-dose preservative-free vials: 2000, 3000, 4000, 10,000, 40,000 U/mL (1 mL) and contains phenylalanine

Multidose vials: 10,000 U/mL (2 mL), 20,000 U/mL (1 mL); contains benzyl alcohol

Anemia in chronic renal failure (see remarks for dosage adjustment and withholding therapy): SC/IV (IV preferred for hemodialysis patients)

Initial dose:

Child and adolescent: Start at 50 U/kg/dose 3 times per week. Reported dosage range for children (3 mo—20 yr) not requiring dialysis, 50—250 U/kg/dose 3 times per week. Reported dosage range for children receiving hemodialysis, 50—450 U/kg/dose 2—3 times per week

Adult: Start at 50—100 U/kg/dose 3 times per week.

Maintenance dose: Dose is individualized to achieve and maintain the lowest Hgb level sufficient to avoid transfusions and **not to exceed** the following levels:

Child ≤16 yr (receiving or not receiving dialysis): 12 g/dL

>16 yr :

Receiving dialysis: 11 g/dL

Not receiving dialysis: 10 g/dL

Anemia in cancer (use until chemotherapy is completed; see remarks for dosage reduction and withholding therapy):

Initial dose:

Child (5—18 yr): Start at 600 U/kg (**max. dose:** 40,000 U) IV once weekly.

Adult: Start at 150 U/kg/dose SC 3 times per week or 40,000 U SC once every week.

Increasing doses (if needed):

Three-times-a-week dosing regimen (adult): If no increase in Hgb >1 g/dL and Hgb remains <10 g/dL after initial 4 wk of therapy, increase dosage to 300 U/kg/dose 3 times per week.

Weekly dosing regimen: If no increase in Hgb >1 g/dL and Hgb remains <10 g/dL after initial 4 wk of therapy:

Child: Increase dose to 900 U/kg/dose IV (**max. dose:** 60,000 U) once weekly.

Adult: 60,000 U SC once weekly

For all ages, discontinue use after 8 wk of therapy if transfusions are still required or no hemoglobin response is observed.

AZT-treated HIV patients (Hgb should not exceed 12 g/dL): SC/IV

Child: Reported dosage range in children (≥3 mo—17 yr), 50—400 U/kg/dose 2—3 times per wk

Adult (with serum erythropoietin ≤500 milliunits/mL and receiving ≤4200 mg AZT per week): Start at 100 U/kg/dose 3 times per wk × 8 wk. If response is NOT satisfactory in reducing transfusion requirements or increasing Hgb levels after 8 wk of therapy, dose may be increased by 50—100 U/kg/dose given 3 times per wk and reevaluated every 4—8 wk thereafter. Patients are unlikely to respond to doses >300 U/kg/dose 3 times per wk.

For all ages, withhold therapy if Hgb >12 g/dL and resume therapy by decreasing dosage by 25% once Hgb falls below 11 g/dL. For adults, discontinue therapy if Hgb does not increase after 8 wk of the 300 U/kg/dose 3 times per wk dosage.

Anemia of prematurity (many regimens exist):

250 U/kg/dose SC 3 times per wk × 10 doses; alternatively, 200—400 U/kg/dose IV/SC 3—5 times per wk for 2—6 wk (total dose per wk is 600—1400 U/kg). Administer with supplemental iron at 3—6 mg elemental iron/kg/24 hr.

Use the lowest dose to avoid transfusions.

Increased risk for death, serious cardiovascular events, and thrombosis/stroke have been reported in patients treated with chronic kidney disease and hemoglobin levels >11 g/dL.

Increased risk for death, shortened survival and/or shortened time to tumor progression/regression, serious cardiovascular events, and thrombosis in various cancer patients, especially with Hgb levels >12 g/dL, have been reported with epoetin alfa and other erythropoiesis-stimulating agents.

Evaluate serum iron, ferritin, TIBC before therapy. Iron supplementation recommended during therapy unless iron stores are already in excess. Monitor Hct, BP, clotting times, platelets, BUN, serum creatinine. Peak effect in 2—3 wk.

DOSAGE ADJUSTMENT FOR ANEMIA IN CHRONIC RENAL FAILURE:

Reduce dose by ≥25%: When Hgb increases >1 g/dL in any 2-wk period. Dose reductions can be made more frequently than once every 4 wk if needed.

Increase dose by 25%: When Hgb does not increase by 1 g/dL after 4 wk of therapy. Dosage increments should not be made more frequently than once every 4 wk.

Withholding therapy: When Hgb exceeds the age and dialysis-specific maximum level; restart therapy at a 25% lower dose after Hgb decreases below the age and dialysis-specific maximum level.

Inadequate response after a 12-week dose escalation: Use minimum effective dosage that will maintain hemoglobin levels to avoid the need for recurrent blood transfusions and evaluate other causes of anemia. Discontinue use if patient remains transfusion dependent.

DOSAGE REDUCTION ADJUSTMENT/WITHHOLDING THERAPY FOR ANEMIA IN CANCER:

If Hgb exceeds a level needed to avoid blood transfusion: Withhold dose and resume therapy at a reduced dosage by 25% when Hgb approaches a level where blood transfusions may be needed.

If Hgb increases >1 g/dL in any 2-wk period or Hgb reaches a level to avoid blood transfusion: Reduce dose by 25%.

May cause hypertension, seizure, hypersensitivity reactions, headache, edema, dizziness. SC route provides sustained serum levels compared to IV route. For IV administration, infuse over 1—3 min.

Do not use multidose vial preparation for neonates, infants, and pregnant/breastfeeding mothers because of concerns for benzyl alcohol.

EPOPROSTENOL
Flolan, Veletri, and generics, PGI$_2$, PGX, prostacyclin
Prostaglandin I$_2$, vasodilator

B ? No No No

Injection: 0.5, 1.5 mg

Flolan: Reconstitute with provided pH 12 sterile diluent for Flolan (50 mL).

Veletri (available only via designated specialty outpatient pharmacies): Reconstitute with sterile water for injection or 0.9% sodium chloride.

Generic: Reconstitute with provided sterile diluent for epoprostenol sodium (50 mL) or with sterile water for injection or 0.9% sodium chloride (product specific).

Pulmonary Hypertension (limited data):

IV Infusion via central-line and 0.22-micron filter: Start at 1—2 **nanograms**/kg/min IV. Increase by 0.5—2 **nanograms**/kg/min Q45 min as needed and tolerated. **Avoid** abrupt withdrawal, interruptions in delivery, or sudden large decreases in dosage.

  Usual effective dose:

  Neonate: 20—40 **nanograms**/kg/min

  Infant, child, and adolescent: 40 to >150 **nanograms**/kg/min (average 80 **nanograms**/kg/min) Down-titration of dosage is required in the presence of high-output state (hyperdynamic right ventricle).

Inhalation route (very limited data):

  Neonate: 50 **nanograms**/kg/min via continuous nebulization at a rate of 8 mL/hr, OR 50 **nanograms**/kg/min diluted in 3 mL Q2 hr via intermittent nebulization has been reported.

  Child: 20—50 **nanograms**/kg/min via continuous nebulization has been reported.

Continued

EPOPROSTENOL *continued*

Contraindicated in heart failure caused by decreased left ventricular ejection fraction. **Use with caution** in bleeding disorders; inhibits platelet aggregation.

Dose-dependent side effects of nausea, diarrhea, jaw pain, bone pain, and headaches are common. Other common side effects include hypotension, flushing, diarrhea, loss of appetite, and chest and musculoskeletal pain. Reported complications include sepsis, local site infection, and catheter dislodgement resulting in severe sepsis or rebound pulmonary hypertension (**avoid** abrupt dose withdrawal and monitor for IV line interruptions). Hypoxia, flushing, and tachycardia may suggest an overdose.

Use with medications exhibiting antiplatelet effects (e.g., SSRI antidepressants, desvenlafaxine, venlafaxine, duloxetine, NSAIDs, and anticoagulants) may increase risk for bleeding. May increase digoxin levels.

Systemic $T_{1/2}$ is 2–5 min. Continuous IV infusion is administered via central venous catheter with a 0.22-micron filter. Medication temperature stability requirements and the use of icepacks are product specific; consult with a pharmacist.

ERGOCALCIFEROL
Calcidol, Drisdol, Ergocal, and generics
Vitamin D₂

   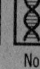

A/C   2   No   No   No

Caps:
Ergocal: 2500 IU
Drisdol and generics: 50,000 IU (1.25 mg)
Tabs [OTC]: 400, 2000, 2400 IU
Drops [OTC]: 8000 IU/mL (200 mCg/mL) (60 mL); contain propylene glycol
Conversion: 1 mg = 40,000 IU vitamin D activity

Dietary supplementation (see Chapter 21 for additional information):
Preterm neonate: 200–400 IU/24 hr PO
Term neonate and infant (<1 yr) (breastfed or receiving <32 oz formula): 400 IU/24 hr PO
Child (≥1 yr) and adolescent: 400–600 IU/24 hr PO
Renal failure (CKD stages 2–5) and 25-OH vitamin D levels <30 ng/mL (monitor serum 25-OH vitamin D and corrected calcium/phosphorus 1 mo after initiation and Q3 mo thereafter):
25-OH vitamin D <5 ng/mL:
 Child: 8000 IU/24 hr × 4 wk followed by 4000 IU/24 hr × 2 mo; or 50,000 IU weekly × 4 wk followed by 50,000 IU twice monthly for 2 mo
25-OH vitamin D 5–15 ng/mL:
 Child: 4000 IU/24 hr PO × 12 wk or 50,000 IU every other wk × 12 wk
25-OH vitamin D 16–30 ng/mL:
 Child: 2000 IU/24 hr PO × 3 mo or 50,000 IU every mo × 3 mo
Vitamin D dependent rickets:
Child: 3000–5000 IU/24 hr PO; **max. dose:** 60,000 IU/24 hr
Nutritional rickets:
Child and adult with normal GI absorption: 2000–5000 IU/24 hr PO × 6–12 wk
Malabsorption:
 Child: 10,000–25,000 IU/24 hr PO
 Adult: 10,000–300,000 IU/24 hr PO
Vitamin D resistant rickets (with phosphate supplementation):
Child: Initial dose 40,000–80,000 IU/24 hr PO; increase daily dose by 10,000–20,000 IU PO Q3–4 mo if needed

ERGOCALCIFEROL *continued*

Adult: 10,000—60,000 IU/24 hr PO
Hypoparathyroidism (with calcium supplementation):
Child: 50,000—200,000 IU/24 hr PO
Adult: 25,000—200,000 IU/24 hr PO

Consider using cholecalciferol instead; cholecalciferol has shown to be more biologically potent with better absorption than ergocalciferol. Vitamin D_2 is activated by 25-hydroxylation in liver and 1-hydroxylation in kidney to the active form, calcitriol.

Monitor serum Ca^{2+}, PO_4, 25-OH vitamin D (goal level for infant and child: ≥20 ng/mL), and alkaline phosphate. Serum Ca^{2+}, PO_4 product should be <70 mg/dL to avoid ectopic calcification. Titrate dosage to patient response. Watch for symptoms of hypercalcemia: weakness, diarrhea, polyuria, metastatic calcification, nephrocalcinosis.

Serum 25-OH vitamin D level of ≥35 ng/mL has been suggested in cystic fibrosis patients to decrease the risk of hyperparathyroidism and bone loss.

Pregnancy category changes to "C" if used in doses above the U.S. RDA.

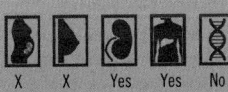

ERGOTAMINE TARTRATE ± CAFFEINE
Ergomar
In combination with caffeine: Cafergot, Migergot, and generics
Ergot alkaloid

X X Yes Yes No

Sublingual tabs (Ergomar): 2 mg
In combination with caffeine:
Tabs (Cafergot and generics): 1 mg and 100 mg caffeine
Suppository (Migergot): 2 mg and 100 mg caffeine (12s)

ERGOTAMINE:
Adolescent and adult:
SL: 2 mg at onset of migraine attack, then 2 mg Q30 min PRN up to **max. dose** of 6 mg/24 hr; **do not exceed** 10 mg/wk

ERGOTAMINE PLUS CAFFEINE:
Doses based on mg of ergotamine
Oral tablet:
Adolescent and adult: 1 or 2 mg PO at onset of migraine attack, then 1 mg Q30 min up to 6 mg per attack, **not to exceed** 10 mg/wk
Suppository:
Adolescent: 1 mg (0.5 suppository) at first sign of attack; follow with second 1 mg dose after 45 min if needed; **max. dose:** 2 mg per attack, 4 mg/24 hr, **not to exceed** 8 mg/wk
Adult: 2 mg at first sign of attack; follow with second 2 mg dose after 1 hr if needed; **max. dose:** 4 mg per attack, **not to exceed** 10 mg/wk

Use with caution in renal or hepatic disease. May cause paresthesias, GI disturbance, angina-like pain, rebound headache with abrupt withdrawal, or muscle cramps.
Contraindicated in pregnancy and has **not been recommended** in breastfeeding. Concurrent administration with protease inhibitors, clarithromycin, erythromycin, other CYP 450 3A4 inhibitors, and nitroglycerin are **contraindicated** owing to risk of ergotism (nausea, vomiting, vasospastic ischemia leading to cerebral and peripheral ischemia).
For sublingual administration, place tablet under the tongue and do not crush.

ERTAPENEM
Invanz and generics
Antibiotic, carbapenem

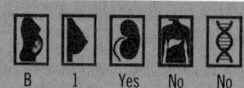

B   1   Yes   No   No

Injection: 1 g
Contains ~6 mEq Na/g drug

≥1 mo–12 yr: 15 mg/kg/dose IV/IM Q12 hr; **max. dose:** 1 g/24 hr
Adolescent and adult: 1 g IV/IM Q24 hr
Recommended duration of therapy (all ages):
    Complicated intra-abdominal infection: 5–14 days or 4–7 days with source control
    Complicated skin/subcutaneous tissue infections: 7–14 days
    Diabetic foot infection without osteomyelitis: 14–28 days
    Community-acquired pneumonia, complicated UTI/pyelonephritis: 10–14 days
    Acute pelvic infection: 3–10 days
Surgical prophylaxis:
    Child and adolescent: 15 mg/kg (**max. dose:** 1 g/dose) IV 1 hr before procedure
    Adult (colorectal surgery): 1 g IV 1 hr before procedure

Ertapenem has poor activity against *P. aeruginosa, Acinetobacter,* MRSA, and Enterococcus.
    Do not use in meningitis due to poor CSF penetration. **Use with caution** with CNS disorders
    including seizures. **Adjust dosage in renal impairment; see Chapter 31.**
Diarrhea, infusion complications, nausea, headache, vaginitis, phlebitis/thrombophlebitis, and
    vomiting are common. Seizures (primarily with renal insufficiency and/or CNS disorders such as
    brain lesions and seizures), decreased consciousness, muscle weakness, gait disturbance,
    abnormal coordination, teeth staining, hypersensitivity vasculitis, and DRESS syndrome have been
    reported. Increased ALT, AST, and neutropenia have been reported in pediatric clinical trials.
    Decreases valproic acid levels. Probenecid may increase ertapenem levels.
IM route requires reconstitution with 1% lidocaine and **should not** be administered by IV. **Do not**
    reconstitute or co-infuse with dextrose-containing solutions.

ERYTHROMYCIN PREPARATIONS
Erythromycin, EES, EryPed, Ery-Tab, and generics
Ophthalmic ointment: Generics; previously
available as Ilotycin
Topical gel: Ery, Erygel, and generics
Antibiotic, macrolide

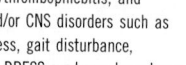

B   2   Yes   Yes   No

Erythromycin base:
    Tabs: 250, 500 mg
    Delayed release tabs (Ery-Tab and generics): 250, 333, 500 mg
    Delayed release caps: 250 mg
    Topical gel (Erygel and generics): 2% (30, 60 g); contains alcohol 92%
    Topical solution: 2% (60 mL); may contain 44%–66% alcohol
    Topical pad/swab (Ery): 2% (60s); may contain propylene glycol and alcohol
    Ophthalmic ointment: 0.5% (1, 3.5 g)
Erythromycin ethyl succinate (EES):
    Oral suspension (EES, EryPed, and generics): 200 mg/5 mL (100, 200 mL), 400 mg/5 mL (100 mL)
    Tabs (EES and generics): 400 mg
Erythromycin stearate (Erythrocin):
    Tabs: 250 mg

ERYTHROMYCIN PREPARATIONS *continued*

Erythromycin lactobionate (Erythrocin and generics):
  Injection: 500 mg

Oral:
  Neonate (use EES preparation; see remarks for safety concerns):
    <1.2 kg: 20 mg/kg/24 hr ÷ Q12 hr PO
    ≥1.2 kg:
      0—7 days: 20 mg/kg/24 hr ÷ Q12 hr PO
      >7 days:
        1.2—2 kg: 30 mg/kg/24 hr ÷ Q8 hr PO
        ≥2 kg: 30—40 mg/kg/24 hr ÷ Q6—8 hr PO
    Chlamydial conjunctivitis and pneumonia: 50 mg/kg/24 hr ÷ Q6 hr PO × 14 days; **max. dose:** 2 g/24 hr
  Child (use base, EES, or stearate preparation): 30—50 mg/kg/24 hr ÷ Q6—8 hr; **max. dose:** 4 g/24 hr
  Pertussis: 40—50 mg/kg/24 hr ÷ Q6 hr PO × 14 days (**max. dose:** 2 g/24 hr); use azithromycin for infants <1 mo old
  Adult: 2 g/24 hr ÷ Q6 hr PO × 14 days
Parenteral:
  Child and adult: 15—20 mg/kg/24 hr ÷ Q6 hr IV; **max. dose:** 4 g/24 hr
Ophthalmic:
  Neonatal gonococcal ophthalmia prophylaxis: Apply 1-cm ribbon to both eyes × 1.
  Conjunctivitis:
    Infant, child, and adolescent: Apply 1-cm ribbon to affected eye(s) several times a day up to 6 times daily.
Preoperative bowel prep: 20 mg/kg/dose (**max. dose:** 1000 mg/dose) PO erythromycin base × 3 doses, with neomycin, 1 day before surgery
Prokinetic agent:
  Infant and child: 10—20 mg/kg/24 hr PO ÷ TID—QID (QAC or QAC and QHS)
Topical (administer doses after washing skin with warm water and soap and patting it dry):
  Acne (≥7 yr—adolescent; typically not used as monotherapy):
    Topical gel: Apply to affected area once daily—BID; discontinue use after 8 wk if no improvement or worsening of condition.
    Topical solution or pad: Apply to affected area BID (morning and evening).

Avoid use in patients with known QT prolongation, proarrhythmic conditions (e.g., hypokalemia, hypomagnesemia, significant bradycardia), and receiving class IA or class III antiarrhythmic agents, HMG CoA reductase inhibitors metabolized by CYP 450 3A4 (e.g., lovastatin or simvastatin; increases risk for myopathy and rhabdomyolysis), cisapride, or pimozide. Hypertrophic pyloric stenosis in neonates receiving prophylactic therapy for pertussis; life-threatening episodes of ventricular tachycardia associated with prolonged QTc interval; and exacerbation of myasthenia gravis have been reported. May produce false-positive urinary catecholamines, 17-hydroxycorticosteroids, and 17-ketosteroids.

GI side effects common (nausea, vomiting, abdominal cramps). Cardiac dysrhythmia, anaphylaxis, interstitial nephritis, and hearing loss have been reported. Use with **caution** in liver disease. Estolate formulation may cause cholestatic jaundice, although hepatotoxicity is uncommon (2% of reported cases). Inhibits CYP 450 1A2, 3A3/4 isoenzymes. May produce elevated digoxin, theophylline, carbamazepine, clozapine, cyclosporine, and methylprednisolone levels. **Adjust dose in renal failure (see Chapter 31).** Use ideal body weight for obese patients when calculating doses.

Continued

ERYTHROMYCIN PREPARATIONS *continued*

Oral therapy should replace IV as soon as possible. Give oral doses after meals. Because of different absorption characteristics, higher oral doses of EES are needed to achieve therapeutic effects. **Avoid** IM route (pain, necrosis). For ophthalmic use, **avoid** contact of ointment tip with eye or skin.

ERYTHROPOIETIN

See Epoetin Alfa.

ESCITALOPRAM
Lexapro and generics
Antidepressant, selective serotonin reuptake inhibitor

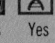

C   3   Yes   Yes   Yes

Tabs: 5, 10, 20 mg
Oral solution: 1 mg/mL (240 mL); contains parabens and propylene glycol

Depression:
   <12 yr: Limited data, only one placebo-controlled RCT did not demonstrate efficacy
   ≥12 yr and adolescent: Start with 10 mg PO once daily. If needed after 3 wk, dose may be increased to 20 mg once daily.
   Adult: Start with 10 mg PO once daily. If needed after 1 wk, dose may be increased to 20 mg once daily.

Autism and pervasive developmental disorders (PDD; limited data)
   6–17 yr: A 10-wk open-label trial in which 28 subjects were given a weekly PRN increasing PO dosage regimen of 2.5, 5, 10, 15, and 20 mg/24 hr. Mean dosage of responders with significant improvement at 11.1 ± 6.5 mg/24 hr. 25% of subjects responded at doses <10 mg/24 hr, and 36% responded at doses ≥10 mg/24 hr. Seven of the 17 (41%) responders and 25% of all treated subjects could not tolerate the 10 mg/24 hr dose.

Social Anxiety Disorder (limited data):
   10–17 yr: A 12-wk open-label trial in which 20 subjects were given an initial PO dosage of 5 mg once daily × 7 days followed by 10 mg once daily. If needed and tolerated, increase by 5 mg/24 hr at weekly intervals up to a **maximum** of 20 mg/24 hr. Two subjects did not complete the trial due to lack of efficacy and tolerability. Sixty-five percent of the remaining subjects met the response criteria with a mean final dose of 13 ± 4.1 mg/24 hr. Common adverse events included somnolence (25%), insomnia (20%), flu symptoms (15%), increased appetite (15%), and decreased appetite (15%).

Increased risk for serotonin syndrome when used with MAO inhibitors (or within 14 days of discontinuance), linezolid, or methylene blue; concurrent use considered **contraindicated.**
   Do not use with pimozide because of risk for increased QTc interval. **Use with caution** with hepatic or severe renal impairment; dosage adjustment may be needed. **Avoid** abrupt discontinuation to prevent withdrawal symptoms.
Diaphoresis, GI discomfort, xerostomia, dizziness, headache, insomnia, somnolence, sexual dysfunction, and fatigue are common side effects. Abnormal bleeding, depression, QTc prolongation, and suicidal ideation (especially during initiation of therapy and with any dosage change) have been reported.
   Mixed/manic episode may occur when treating a depressive episode in patients with bipolar disorders.
Primarily metabolized by the CYP 450 2C19 and 3A4 enzymes and is a weak inhibitor for CYP 450 2D6 enzyme. Consider an alternative medication (not significantly metabolized by CYP 450 2C19) for individuals with ultrarapid CYP 450 2C19 activity. Poor CYP450 2C19 metabolizers can either initiate therapy at 50% the usual dose and titrate to response or consider alternative therapy.

ESCITALOPRAM *continued*

Taking with other medications with QTc prolongation may further increase that risk. Omeprazole may increase the toxicity of escitalopram. Doses may be administered with or without food.

ESMOLOL HCL
Brevibloc and generics
β₁ selective adrenergic blocking agent, anti-hypertensive agent, class II antiarrhythmic

C   ?   No   No   No

Injection: 10 mg/mL (10 mL); preservative free
Injection, premixed infusion in iso-osmotic sodium chloride: 2000 mg/100 mL (100 mL), 2500 mg/250 mL (250 mL); preservative free
Injection, premixed infusion in iso-osmotic water for injection: 2000 mg/100 mL (100 mL), 2500 mg/250 mL (250 mL); contains ethanol, propylene glycol

Postoperative hypertension: Titrate to response (limited information):
  Loading dose: 500 mCg/kg IV over 1 min
  Maintenance dose: 50–250 mCg/kg/min IV as infusion. Titrate doses upward 50–100 mCg/kg/min Q 5–10 min as needed. Heart surgery patients may require higher doses (~700 mCg/kg/min). Dosages as high as 1000 mCg/kg/min have been reported in children 1–12 yr.
SVT: Titrate to response (limited information):
  Loading dose: 100–500 mCg/kg IV over 1 min
  Maintenance dose: 25–100 mCg/kg/min IV as infusion. Titrate doses upward 50–100 mCg/kg/min Q5–10 min as needed. Dosages as high as 1000 mCg/kg/min have been reported.

Contraindicated in sinus bradycardia, >first-degree heart block, and cardiogenic shock or heart failure. Short duration of action; $T_{1/2}$ = 2.9–4.7 min for children and 9 min for adults. May cause bronchospasm, congestive heart failure, hypotension (at doses >200 mCg/kg/min), nausea, and vomiting. May increase digoxin (by 10%–20%) and theophylline levels. Morphine may increase esmolol level by 46%. Theophylline may decrease esmolol's effects.
Administer only in a monitored setting. Concentration for administration is typically ≤10 mg/mL, but 20 mg/mL has been administered in pediatric patients.

ESOMEPRAZOLE
Nexium, Nexium 24HR, and generics
Gastric acid proton pump inhibitor

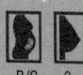 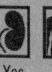

B/C   2   Yes   Yes   No

Caps, delayed release (Nexium and generics): 20, 40 mg; contains magnesium (some generic products may contain strontium instead)
  Nexium 24 HR [OTC]: 20 mg
  Nexium 24 HR Clear Minis [OTC]: 20 mg
Tab, delayed release (Nexium24HR; [OTC]): 20 mg; contains magnesium
Powder for oral suspension:
  Nexium: 2.5, 5, 10, 20, 40 mg packets (30s); contains magnesium
  Generics: 10, 20, 40 mg packets (30s)
Injection (Nexium and generics): 40 mg; contains EDTA

Child (PO):
  GERD (use for 4–8 wk):
    Weight-based dosage: 0.7–3.3 mg/kg/24 hr once daily; **max. dose:** 40 mg/24 hr
    <20 kg: 10 mg once daily

Continued

ESOMEPRAZOLE *continued*

≥**20 kg:** 20 mg once daily

Erosive esophagitis in GERD:

Infant (1 mo to <1 yr; use for up to 6 wk):

3–5 kg: 2.5 mg once daily

>5 to 7.5 kg: 5 mg once daily

>7.5 kg: 10 mg once daily

1–11 yr (use for 8 wk):

<20 kg: 10 mg once daily

≥**20 kg:** 10 or 20 mg once daily

12–17 yr: 20 or 40 mg once daily for 4–8 wk

Child (IV):

GERD with erosive esophagitis:

Infant: 0.5–1 mg/kg/dose once daily

Child 1–17 yr:

<55 kg: 10 mg once daily

≥**55 kg:** 20–40 mg once daily

Adult (PO/IV):

GERD: 20 mg once daily

GERD with erosive esophagitis: 20 or 40 mg once daily × 4–8 wk

Prevention of NSAID-induced gastric ulcers: 20 or 40 mg once daily for up to 6 mo

Pathological hypersecretory conditions (e.g., Zollinger-Ellison syndrome): 40 mg BID; doses up to 240 mg/24 hr have been used

Hepatic impairment: Patients with severe hepatic function impairment (Child-Pugh class C) should not exceed 20 mg/24 hr (40 mg/24 hr for pathological hypersecretory conditions).

Cross-allergic reactions with other proton pump inhibitors (e.g., lansoprazole, pantoprazole, rabeprazole). **Use with caution** in liver impairment (see dosage adjustment recommendation in dosing section). GI disturbances and headache are common. Hypomagnesemia may occur with continuous use and may lead to hypocalcemia and/or hypokalemia. Anaphylaxis, angioedema, bronchospasm, acute interstitial nephritis, erythema multiforme, urticaria, Stevens-Johnson syndrome, TEN, pancreatitis, and fractures of the hip, wrist, and spine (in adults >50 yr old receiving high doses or prolonged therapy >1 yr) have been reported. Fundic gland polyps have been associated with long-term use of >1 yr.

Drug is a substrate and inhibitor of CYP 450 2C19 and substrate of CYP 450 3A4. May decrease the absorption or effects of atazanavir, clopidogrel, ketoconazole, itraconazole, mycophenolate mofetil, and iron salts. May increase the effect/toxicity of diazepam, midazolam, digoxin, carbamazepine, and warfarin. Voriconazole may increase the effects of esomeprazole.

May be used in combination with clarithromycin and amoxicillin for *Helicobacter pylori* infections.

Pregnancy category is a "B" for the magnesium-containing product and a "C" for the strontium-containing product.

Administer all oral doses before meals and 30 min before sucralfate (if receiving). **Do not** crush or chew capsules. IV doses may be given as fast as 3 min or infused over 10–30 min.

ETANERCEPT
Enbrel, Enbrel SureClick, Enbrel Mini
*Antirheumatic, immunomodulatory agent, tumor
necessary factor receptor p75 Fc fusion protein*

 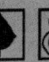

B   ?   No   Yes   No

ETANERCEPT *continued*

Prefilled injection (single use): 25 mg (0.5 mL), 50 mg (1 mL); contains sucrose, L-arginine (preservative free) (carton of 4 prefilled syringes)

Injection (powder; multidose vial): 25 mg with diluent (1 mL bacteriostatic water containing 0.9% benzyl alcohol); contains mannitol, sucrose, tromethamine (carton of 4 vials)

Injection (single dose vial): 25 mg (0.5 mL); contains sucrose, L-arginine (preservative free) (carton of 4 vials)

Autoinjector:

Enbrel SureClick (single use): 50 mg (1 mL); contains sucrose, L-arginine (preservative free) (carton of 4 autoinjectors)

Prefilled injection cartridge to be used with Auto Touch reusable autoinjector device:

Enbrel Mini: 50 mg (1 mL); contains sucrose, L-arginine (preservative free) (carton of 4 cartridges)

Juvenile idiopathic arthritis:

Child 2–17 yr: 0.4 mg/kg/dose SC twice weekly administered 72–96 hr apart; **max. dose:** 25 mg. Alternative once-weekly dose of 0.8 mg/kg/dose SC (**max. dose:** 50 mg/wk and **max. single injection site dose** of 25 mg) may be used.

Rheumatoid arthritis, psoriatic arthritis, ankylosing spondylitis:

Adult: 25 mg SC twice weekly administered 72–96 hr apart. Alternative once weekly dose of 50 mg SC (**max. single injection site dose** of 25 mg) may be used.

Plaque psoriasis:

Child and adolescent (4–17 yr): 0.8 mg/kg/dose (**max. dose:** 50 mg) SC once weekly

Adult: Start with 50 mg SC twice weekly administered 72–96 hr apart × 3 mo, followed by a reduced maintenance dose of 50 mg SC per wk. Starting doses of 25 mg or 50 mg/wk have also been shown to be effective.

Max. single injection site dose: 25 mg

Contraindicated in serious infections, sepsis, or hypersensitivity to any of medication components. **Use with caution** in patients with history of recurrent infections (including hepatitis B) or underlying conditions that may predispose them to infections (including concomitant immunosuppressive therapy), CNS demyelinating disorders, malignancies, immune-related diseases, and latex allergy. Use in patients with granulomatosis with polyangiitis receiving immunosuppressive therapy is not recommended due to the risk for noncutaneous solid malignancies and no improved clinical outcomes.

Common adverse effects in children include headache, abdominal pain, vomiting, and nausea. Injection site reactions (e.g., discomfort, itching, swelling), rhinitis, dizziness, rash, depression, infections (varicella, aseptic meningitis, rare cases of TB, and fatal/serious infections and sepsis), bone marrow suppression (e.g., aplastic anemia), sarcoidosis, vertigo, and CNS demyelinating disorder have also been reported. Malignancies (some fatal and ∼50% were lymphomas) have been reported in children and adolescents.

Do not administer live vaccines concurrently with this drug. In JRA, it is recommended that before initiating therapy, the patient be brought up to date with all immunizations in agreement with current immunization guidelines.

Onset of action is 1–4 wk, with peak effects usually within 3 mo.

Patients must be properly instructed on preparing and administering the medication (see specific product information). For multidose vial, reconstitute vial by gently swirling its contents with the supplied diluent (**do not** shake or vigorously agitate), as some foaming will occur. Reconstituted solutions should be clear and colorless; unused portions must be stored in the refrigerator and used within 14 days. Do not store Auto Touch autoinjector device in the refrigerator.

Drug is administered subcutaneously by rotating injection sites (thigh, abdomen, or upper arm) with a **max. single injection site dose** of 25 mg. Administer new injections ≥1 inch from an old site and NEVER where the skin is tender, bruised, red, or hard.

ETHAMBUTOL HCL
Myambutol and generics
Antituberculosis drug

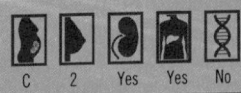

C   2   Yes   Yes   No

Tabs: 100, 400 mg; 400 mg tabs may be scored
Oral suspension: 50, 100 mg/mL

Tuberculosis (use in combination with other medications; see remarks):
  Infant, child, adolescent, and adult (see latest CDC guidelines as additional dosing schedules exist):
    <15 yr and <40 kg: 15–25 mg/kg/dose (**max. dose:** 1 g/24 hr) PO once daily or 50 mg/kg/dose PO twice weekly (**max. dose:** 2.5 g/week)
    <15 yr and ≥40 kg, or ≥15 yr:
      40–55 kg: 800 mg PO once daily or 5 times weekly
      56–75 kg: 1200 mg PO once daily or 5 times weekly
      76–90 kg: 1600 mg PO once daily or 5 times weekly
Nontuberculous mycobacterial infection; and *Mycobacterium avium* complex in AIDS (recurrence prophylaxis or treatment; use in combination with other medications):
  Infant, and child: 15–25 mg/kg/24 hr PO once daily; **max. dose:** 2.5 g/24 hr
  Adolescent: 15 mg/kg/24 hr PO once daily; **max. dose:** 2.5 g/24 hr

May cause reversible optic neuritis, especially with larger doses. Obtain baseline ophthalmologic studies before beginning therapy and then monthly. Follow visual acuity, visual fields, and (red-green) color vision. **Do not use** in optic neuritis and in children whose visual acuity cannot be assessed. **Discontinue** if any visual deterioration occurs. Monitor uric acid, liver function, heme status, and renal function. Hyperuricemia, GI disturbances, and mania are common. Erythema multiforme and hepatotoxicity have been reported.
Dosing should be based on lean body weight. Coadministration with aluminum hydroxide can reduce ethambutol's absorption; space administration by 4 hr. Give with food. **Adjust dose with renal failure (see Chapter 31).**

ETHOSUXIMIDE
Zarontin and generics
Anticonvulsant

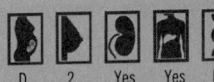

D   2   Yes   Yes   No

Caps: 250 mg
Oral solution: 250 mg/5 mL (473 mL); may contain sodium benzoate

Oral:
  ≤6 yr:
    Initial: 10 mg/kg/24 hr up to 250 mg/24 hr ÷ BID-TID; increase by 5–10 mg/kg/24 hr as needed Q4–7 days
    Usual maintenance dose: 15–40 mg/kg/24 hr ÷ BID-TID
  >6 yr and adult: 10 mg/kg/24 hr up to 500 mg/24 hr ÷ BID-TID; increase by 250 mg/24 hr as needed Q4–7 days
    Usual maintenance dose: 20–40 mg/kg/24 hr ÷ BID-TID
  Max. dose (all ages): The lesser of 60 mg/kg/24 hr or 2 g/24 hr

Drug of choice for absence seizures. **Use with caution** in hepatic and renal disease. Ataxia, anorexia, drowsiness, sleep disturbances, rashes, and blood dyscrasias are rare idiosyncratic reactions. May cause lupus-like syndrome; may increase frequency of grand mal seizures in patients with mixed-type seizures. Serious dermatological reactions (e.g., Stevens-Johnson and DRESS) and

ETHOSUXIMIDE *continued*

immune thrombocytopenia have been reported. May increase risk of suicidal thoughts/behavior. Cases of birth defects have been reported; ethosuximide crosses the placenta.

Carbamazepine, phenytoin, primidone, phenobarbital, valproic acid, nevirapine, and ritonavir may decrease ethosuximide levels.

Therapeutic levels: 40–100 mg/L. $T_{1/2}$ = 24–42 hr. Recommended serum sampling time at steady state: obtain trough level within 30 min prior to the next scheduled dose after 5–10 days of continuous dosing.

To minimize GI distress, may administer with food or milk. Abrupt withdrawal of drug may precipitate absence status.

ETOMIDATE
Amidate and generics
General anesthetic

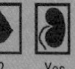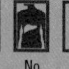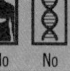

C 2 Yes No No

Injection: 2 mg/mL (10, 20 mL); may be preservative free or contain propylene glycol

Rapid Sequence Intubation (infuse dose over 30–60 sec):
  Normotensive patient: 0.3 mg/kg/dose IV/IO ×1; **max. dose:** 20 mg/dose
  Hypotensive patient (see remarks): 0.15 mg/kg/dose IV/IO ×1; **max. dose:** 20 mg/dose

Not recommended for patients in septic shock due to transient adrenocortical suppression and increased risk for mortality. **Avoid use** with benznidazole and metronidazole due to the risk for disulfiram-like reaction. **Use with caution** in renal impairment (higher risk for toxicity) and in heart failure (may exacerbate condition).

Injection site pain, myoclonus (pretreatment with midazolam may reduce risk), nausea, and vomiting are reported common side effects for indications other than rapid-sequence intubation.

F

FAMCICLOVIR
Generics; previously available as Famvir
Antiviral

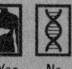

B ? Yes Yes No

Tabs: 125, 250, 500 mg

Adult:

Herpes zoster: 500 mg Q8 hr PO × 7–10 days; initiate therapy promptly as soon as diagnosis is made (initiation within 48 hr after rash onset is ideal; currently no data for starting treatment >72 hr after rash onset)

Genital herpes (first episode):
  Immunocompetent: 250 mg Q8 hr PO × 7–10 days
  Immunocompromised: 500 mg Q12 hr PO × 5–10 days

Recurrent genital herpes (initiate therapy within 1 day of lesion onset):
  Immunocompetent: 1000 mg Q12 hr PO × 1 day or 125 mg Q12 hr PO × 5 days
  Immunocompromised: 500 mg Q12 hr PO × 5–7 days

Suppression of recurrent genital herpes (immunocompetent): 250 mg Q12 hr PO up to 1 yr, then reassess for HSV infection recurrence

Continued

FAMCICLOVIR *continued*

Recurrent herpes labialis:
 Immunocompetent: 1500 mg PO × 1
 Immunocompromised: 500 mg Q12 hr PO × 7 days
Recurrent mucocutaneous herpes in HIV: 500 mg Q12 hr PO × 7 days

Drug is converted to its active form (penciclovir). Hepatic impairment may impair/reduce the
 conversion of famciclovir to penciclovir. Better absorption than PO acyclovir.
May cause headache, diarrhea, nausea, and abdominal pain. Serious skin reactions (e.g., TEN and
 Stevens-Johnson), angioedema, hypersensitivity vasculitis, seizure, palpitations, cholestatic
 jaundice, and abnormal LFTs have been reported. Concomitant use with probenecid and other drugs
 eliminated by active tubular secretion may result in decreased penciclovir clearance. **Reduce dose
 in renal impairment (see Chapter 31).**
Safety and efficacy in suppression of recurrent genital herpes have not been established beyond 1 yr.
 No efficacy data are available for children 1–<12 yr to support its use for genital herpes, recurrent
 herpes labialis, and varicella. Furthermore, efficacy has not been established for recurrent herpes
 labialis for children 12–<18 yr. May be administered with or without food.

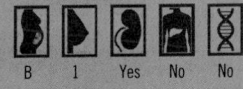

FAMOTIDINE
Pepcid, Pepcid AC [OTC], Pepcid AC Maximum
Strength [OTC], Pepcid Complete [OTC], Zantac
360 [OTC], Zantac 360 Maximum Strength
[OTC], and generics
Histamine-2-receptor antagonist

B   1   Yes   No   No

Injection: 10 mg/mL (2, 4, 20 mL); multidose vials contain 0.9% benzyl alcohol
Premixed injection: 20 mg/50 mL in iso-osmotic sodium chloride
Oral suspension: 40 mg/5 mL (50 mL); may contain parabens and sodium benzoate
Tabs:
 Pepcid AC, Zantac 360, and generics [OTC]: 10 mg
 **Pepcid, Pepcid AC Maximum Strength, Zantac 360 Maximum Strength, and generics [OTC and by
 prescription]:** 20 mg
 Pepcid and generics: 40 mg
Chewable tabs:
 Pepcid Complete (OTC): 10 mg famotidine with 800 mg calcium carbonate and 165 mg magnesium
 hydroxide (25s, 50s, 100s)

Neonate and <3 mo:
 IV: 0.25–0.5 mg/kg/dose Q24 hr
 PO: 0.5–1 mg/kg/dose Q24 hr
≥3 mo–1 yr (GERD):
 IV (limited to PK data): 0.25 mg/kg/dose Q12 hr
 PO: 0.5 mg/kg/dose Q12 hr
Child (1–12 yr):
 IV: Initial: 0.5–1 mg/kg/24 hr ÷ Q12 hr up to a **max.** of 40 mg/24 hr
 PO: Initial: 1–1.2 mg/kg/24 hr ÷ Q12 hr up to a **max.** of 40 mg/24 hr
 Peptic ulcer: 0.5–1 mg/kg/24 hr PO/IV QHS or ÷ Q12 hr up to a **max. dose** of 40 mg/24 hr
 GERD:
  IV: 0.5–1 mg/kg/24 hr ÷ Q12 hr up to a **max. dose** of 40 mg/24 hr
  PO: 1–2 mg/kg/24 hr ÷ Q12 hr up to a **max. dose** of 80 mg/24 hr

FAMOTIDINE *continued*

Adolescent and adult:
  Duodenal ulcer:
    PO: 20 mg BID or 40 mg QHS × 4–8 wk, then maintenance therapy at 20 mg QHS
    IV: 20 mg BID
  GERD: 20 mg BID PO × 6 wk
  Esophagitis: 20–40 mg BID PO × 12 wk

A Q12-hr dosage interval is generally recommended; however, infants and young children may require a Q8-hr interval because of enhanced drug clearance. Headaches, dizziness, constipation, diarrhea, and drowsiness have occurred. **Dosage adjustment is required in severe renal failure (see Chapter 31)**; prolonged QT interval has been reported very rarely in patients with renal impairment whose dosage had not been adjusted appropriately. Rhabdomyolysis has been reported. Shake oral suspension well prior to each use. Oral doses may be administered with or without food.

FELBAMATE
Felbatol and generics
Anticonvulsant

 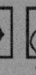

C   3   Yes   Yes   No

Tabs: 400, 600 mg
Oral suspension: 600 mg/5 mL (240, 473 mL)

Lennox-Gastaut for child 2–14 yr (adjunctive therapy):
Start at 15 mg/kg/24 hr PO ÷ TID–QID; increase dosage by 15 mg/kg/24 hr increments at weekly intervals up to a **max. dose** of 45 mg/kg/24 hr or 3600 mg/24 hr (whichever is less). See remarks for adjusting concurrent anticonvulsants.

Child ≥14 yr–adult:
  Adjunctive therapy: Start at 1200 mg/24 hr PO ÷ TID–QID; increase dosage by 1200 mg/24 hr at weekly intervals up to a **max. dose** of 3600 mg/day. See remarks for adjusting concurrent anticonvulsants.
  Monotherapy (as initial therapy): Start at 1200 mg/24 hr PO ÷ TID–QID. Increase dose under close clinical supervision at 600 mg increments Q2 wk to 2400 mg/24 hr. **Max. dose:** 3600 mg/24 hr
  Conversion to monotherapy: Start at 1200 mg/24 hr ÷ PO TID–QID for 2 wk; then increase to 2400 mg/24 hr for 1 wk. At wk 3, increase to 3600 mg/24 hr. Reduce dose of other anticonvulsants by 33% at the initiation of felbamate, then an additional 33% of original dose at wk 2 and continue to reduce other anticonvulsants as clinically indicated at wk 3 and beyond.

Drug should be prescribed under strict supervision by a specialist. **Contraindicated** in blood dyscrasias or hepatic dysfunction (prior or current), and hypersensitivity to meprobamate. Aplastic anemia and hepatic failure leading to death have been associated with drug. May cause headache, fatigue, anxiety, GI disturbances, gingival hyperplasia, increased liver enzymes, and bone marrow suppression. Suicidal behavior or ideation have been reported. **Obtain serum levels of concurrent anticonvulsants.** Monitor liver enzymes, bilirubin, CBC with differential, platelets at baseline, and every 1–2 wk. Doses should be decreased by 50% in renally impaired patients.

When initiating adjunctive therapy (all ages), reduce doses of other antiepileptic drugs (AEDs) by 20% to control plasma levels of concurrent phenytoin, valproic acid, phenobarbital, and carbamazepine. Further reductions of concomitant AED dosage may be necessary to minimize side effects caused by drug interactions.

When converting to monotherapy, reduce other AEDs by one-third at the start of felbamate therapy. Then after 2 wk and at the start of increasing the felbamate dosage, reduce other AEDs by an additional one-third. At wk 3, continue to reduce other AEDs as clinically indicated.

Continued

FELBAMATE continued

Carbamazepine levels may be decreased; however, phenytoin and valproic acid levels may be increased. Phenytoin and carbamazepine may increase felbamate clearance; valproic acid may decrease its clearance.

Doses can be administered with or without food.

FENTANYL
Sublimaze, Fentora, Actiq, generics; previously available as Duragesic
Narcotic; analgesic, sedative

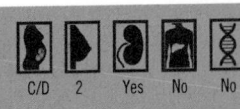

C/D   2   Yes   No   No

Injection: 50 mCg/mL (1, 2, 5, 10, 20, 50 mL)
SR transdermal patch: 12.5, 25, 37.5, 50, 62.5, 75, 87.5, 100 mCg/hr (5s)
Tabs for buccal administration:
Fentora and generics: 100, 200, 400, 600, 800 mCg (28s)
Lozenge on a stick:
Actiq and generics: 200, 400, 600, 800, 1200, 1600 mCg (30s)

Titrate dose to effect.
Neonate and younger infant:
Sedation/analgesia: 1—4 mCg/kg/dose (**max. dose:** 100 mCg/dose) IV Q2—4 hr PRN
Continuous IV infusion: 1—5 mCg/kg/hr; tolerance may develop
Older infant and child:
Sedation/analgesia: 1—2 mCg/kg/dose (**max. dose:** 100 mCg/dose) IV/IM Q30—60 min PRN
Continuous IV infusion: 1 mCg/kg/hr; titrate to effect; usual infusion range 1—3 mCg/kg/hr
To prepare infusion, use the following formula:

$$50 \times \frac{\text{Desired dose(mCg/kg/hr)}}{\text{Desired infusion rate(mL/hr)}} \times \text{Wt(kg)} = \frac{\text{mCg Fentanyl}}{\text{50 mL fluid}}$$

Oral, breakthrough cancer pain for opioid-intolerant patients (see remarks):
Buccal tabs (≥18 yr NOT previously using Actiq): Start with 100 mCg by placing tablet in the buccal cavity (above a rear molar, between the upper cheek and gum) and letting the tablet dissolve for 15—25 min. A second 100 mCg dose, if needed, may be administered 30 min after the start of the first dose. If needed, increase dose initially in multiples of 100 mCg tablets when patients require >1 dose per breakthrough pain episode for several consecutive episodes. Must wait at least 4 hr before treating another episode with buccal tabs. If titration requires >400 mCg/dose, use 200 mCg tabs.
Lozenges (≥16 yr): Start with 200 mCg by placing lozenge in the mouth between the cheek and lower gum. If needed, may repeat dose 15 min after the completion of the first dose (30 min after start of prior dose). If therapy requires >1 lozenge per episode, consider increasing the dose to the next higher strength. **Do not** give more than 2 doses for each episode of breakthrough pain and reevaluate long-acting opioid therapy if patient requires >4 doses/24 hr. **Must wait at least 4 hr before treating another episode with lozenges.**
Transdermal (see remarks): Safety has not been established in children <2 yr and should be administered in children ≥2 yr who are opioid tolerant. Use is **contraindicated** in acute or postoperative pain in opiate-naïve patients.
Opioid-tolerant child receiving at least 60 mg morphine equivalents/24 hr: Use 25 mCg/hr patch Q72 hr. Patch titration should not occur before 3 days of administration of the initial dose or more frequently than every 6 days thereafter.
See Chapter 6 for equianalgesic dosing and PCA dosing.

FENTANYL *continued*

Intranasal route for acute and pre-procedure analgesia (use IV dosage form; see remarks):
≥1 yr—adolescent: 1—2 mCg/kg/dose intranasally via an automizer (**max. dose:** 100 mCg/dose) Q1 hr PRN

Use with caution in bradycardia, respiratory depression, and increased intracranial pressure.
Adjust dose in renal failure (see Chapter 31). Fatalities and life-threatening respiratory
depression have been reported with inappropriate use (overdoses, use in opioid-naïve patients,
changing the patch too frequently, and exposing the patch to a heat source) of the transdermal
route.

Highly lipophilic and may deposit into fat tissue. IV onset of action 1—2 min with peak effects
in 10 min. IV duration of action 30—60 min. Give IV dose over 3—5 min. Rapid infusion may
cause respiratory depression and chest wall rigidity. Respiratory depression may persist
beyond the period of analgesia. Transdermal onset of action 6—8 hr with a 72-hr duration of action.
See Chapter 6 for pharmacodynamic information with transmucosal and transdermal routes.

Buccal tabs and oral lozenges are indicated only for the management of breakthrough cancer pain in
patients who are already receiving and who are tolerant to opioid therapy. Buccal tabs (Fentora),
transdermal patches (Duragesic), and lozenge (Actiq) dosage forms are available through a restricted
distribution program (REMS) and are **NOT bioequivalent** (see package insert for conversion).

Intranasal route of administration for analgesia has an onset of action at 10—30 min. Pediatric
studies have demonstrated that the intranasal fentanyl is equivalent to and better than morphine
(PO/IV/IM) and equivalent to intravenous fentanyl for providing analgesia.

Fentanyl is a substrate for the CYP 450 3A4 enzyme. Be aware of medications that inhibit or induce
this enzyme, for they may increase or decrease the effects of fentanyl, respectively.

Pregnancy category changes to "D" if drug is used for prolonged periods or in high doses at term.

FERRIC GLUCONATE

See Iron—Injectable Preparations.

FERROUS SULFATE

See Iron—Oral Preparations.

FEXOFENADINE ± PSEUDOEPHEDRINE
Allegra [OTC], Children's Allegra Allergy [OTC],
Allegra-D 12 Hour [OTC], Allegra-D 24 Hour
[OTC], and generics
Antihistamine, less-sedating ± decongestant

C | 2 | Yes | No | No

Tabs: 60 mg [OTC], 180 mg [OTC]
Tabs, orally disintegrating (Children's Allegra Allergy; ODT) [OTC]: 30 mg; contains phenylalanine
Oral suspension [OTC]: 6 mg/mL (120, 240 mL); contains parabens
Extended release tab in combination with pseudoephedrine (PE):
Allegra-D 12 Hour and generics [OTC]: 60 mg fexofenadine + 120 mg pseudoephedrine
Allegra-D 24 Hour and generics [OTC]: 180 mg fexofenadine + 240 mg pseudoephedrine

Fexofenadine:
6 mo—<2 yr: 15—30 mg PO BID
2—11 yr: 30 mg PO BID
≥12 yr—adult: 60 mg PO BID; 180 mg PO once daily may be used in seasonal rhinitis

Continued

FEXOFENADINE ± PSEUDOEPHEDRINE *continued*

Extended release tabs of fexofenadine and pseudoephedrine:
  ≥12 yr—adult:
    Allegra-D 12 Hour: 1 tablet PO BID
    Allegra-D 24 Hour: 1 tablet PO once daily

May cause drowsiness, fatigue, headache, dyspepsia, nausea, and dysmenorrhea. Has not
  been implicated in causing cardiac arrhythmias when used with other drugs that are
  metabolized by hepatic microsomal enzymes (e.g., ketoconazole, erythromycin). **Reduce dose
  to 15 mg PO once daily for child 6 mo—<2 yr, 30 mg PO once daily for child 6—11 yr old, and 60
  mg PO once daily for ≥12 yr old for any degree of renal impairment. For use of Allegra-D 12
  Hour and decreased renal function (CrCl <80 mL/min), an initial dose of 1 tablet PO once daily is
  recommended. **Avoid use** of Allegra-D 24 Hour in renal impairment. See Pseudoephedrine for
  additional remarks if using the combination product.
Medication as the single agent may be administered with or without food. **Do not** administer antacids
  with or within 2 hr of fexofenadine dose. The extended release combination product should be
  swallowed whole without food.

FIDAXOMICIN
Dificid
Antibiotic, macrolide

   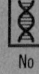

B   ?   No   No   No

Oral suspension: 40 mg/mL (136 mL); contains sodium benzoate
Tabs: 200 mg; contains soybean lecithin

C. difficile **treatment (PO):**
  Child >6 mo: 16 mg/kg/dose (**max. dose:** 200 mg/dose) BID × 10 days; or alternative fixed
    dosage by weight:
    4—<7 kg: 80 mg BID
    7—<9 kg: 120 mg BID
    9—<12.5 kg: 160 mg BID
    ≥12.5 kg: 200 mg BID
  Adult: 200 mg BID × 10 days

Minimally absorbable macrolide antibiotic with bactericidal activity against *C. difficile*; inhibits
  RNA polymerase sigma subunit resulting in inhibition of protein synthesis and cell death.
  Fidaxomicin use in children <18 yr is currently indicated as a second-line agent following
  recurrent courses of oral vancomycin, whereas it is the recommended first-line initial episode
  therapy for adults.
Acute hypersensitivity reactions such as angioedema, dyspnea, pruritus, and rash have been reported,
  and individuals with a history of macrolide allergies may be at risk. Common side effects include
  abdominal pain, nausea, vomiting, anemia, and neutropenia. Bowel obstruction and GI hemorrhage have
  been reported.
Fidaxomicin and its main metabolite (OP-118) are substrates of the P-gp efflux transporter in the GI
  tract. Use with cyclosporine, a P-gP inhibitor, may increase systemic levels of fidaxomicin and OP-
  118 without affecting the safety and efficacy for treating *C. difficile* in adult clinical trials.
Doses may be administered with or without food.

FILGRASTIM
Neupogen, G-CSF
Colony-stimulating factor

  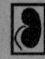 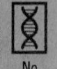

C   2   Yes   No   No

FILGRASTIM *continued*

Injection (Neupogen): 300 mCg/mL (1, 1.6 mL vials)

Injection, prefilled syringes with 27-gauge ½-inch needles (Neupogen: 600 mCg/mL (300 mCg per 0.5 mL and 480 mCg per 0.8 mL) (10s)

All dosage forms contain polysorbate 80 and are preservative free.

NOTE: The following biosimilar products are available (all contain polysorbate 80 and are preservative free).

    Single-dose vials [Nivestym (filgrastim-aafi), Granix (tbo-filgrastim), Releuko (filgrastim-ayow)]: 300 mCg/1 mL and 480 mCg/1.6 mL (10s)

    Prefilled syringes [Nivestym (filgrastim-aafi), Zarxio (filgrastim-sndz), Releuko (filgrastim-ayow)]: 300 mCg/ 0.5 mL and 480 mCg/0.8 mL (1 or 10s); may be attached with a 27-gauge, ½-inch needle

Individual protocols may direct dosing.

Myelosuppressive chemotherapy recipients with non-myeloid malignancies:

    IV/SC: 5 mCg/kg/dose once daily × 14 days or until ANC >10,000/mm³. Dosage may be increased by 5 mCg/kg/24 hr if desired effect is not achieved within 7 days.

    Discontinue therapy when ANC >10,000/mm³.

Contraindicated for patients sensitive to *E. coli*–derived proteins. **Avoid** simultaneous administration with chemotherapy and radiation and do not administer 24 hr before or after administration of chemotherapy. May cause bone pain, fever, and rash. Monitor CBC, uric acid, and LFTs. Aortitis, sickle cell crisis, serious allergic reactions, glomerulonephritis, and thrombocytopenia have been reported. Decreased bone density/osteoporosis has been reported in pediatric patients with severe chronic neutropenia. **Use with caution** in patients with malignancies with myeloid characteristics. Myelodysplastic syndrome and acute myeloid leukemia have been associated with the filgrastim in conjunction with chemotherapy and/or radiotherapy in patients with breast and lung cancer.

Safety and effectiveness have been established for nonmyeloid malignancies receiving myelosuppressive chemotherapy in children ≥1 mo–<17 yr old. The safety profile was similar to adults.

SC routes of administration are preferred because of prolonged serum levels over IV route. If used via IV route and G-CSF final concentration <15 mCg/mL, add 2 mg albumin/1 mL of IV fluid to prevent drug adsorption to the IV administration set.

FLECAINIDE ACETATE
Generics; previously available as Tambocor
Antiarrhythmic, class Ic

   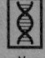

C   2   Yes   Yes   Yes

Tabs: 50, 100, 150 mg
Oral suspension: 20 mg/mL

Child: Initial: 1–3 mg/kg/24 hr ÷ Q8 hr PO; usual range: 3–6 mg/kg/24 hr ÷ Q8 hr PO, monitor serum levels to adjust dose if needed

Adult:

    Sustained V tach: 100 mg PO Q12 hr; may increase by 50 mg Q12 hr (100 mg/24 hr) every 4 days to **max. dose** of 400 mg/24 hr

    Paroxysmal SVT/paroxysmal AF: 50 mg PO Q12 hr; may increase dose by 50 mg Q12 hr every 4 days to **max. dose** of 300–400 mg/24 hr

May aggravate LV failure, sinus bradycardia, preexisting ventricular arrhythmias. May cause AV block, dizziness, blurred vision, dyspnea, nausea, headache, and increased PR or QRS intervals. **Reserve for life-threatening cases. Use with caution** in renal and/or hepatic impairment.

Continued

FLECAINIDE ACETATE *continued*

Flecainide is a substrate for the CYP P-450 2D6 enzyme. Be aware of medications that inhibit (e.g., certain SSRIs) or induce this enzyme, for it may increase or decrease the effects of flecainide, respectively. 50% and 25% dose reductions with ECG and serum level monitoring have been recommended for poor and intermediate CYP2D6 metabolizers, respectively.

Therapeutic trough level: 0.2—1 mg/L. Recommended serum sampling time at steady state: Obtain trough level within 30 min prior to the next scheduled dose after 2—3 days of continuous dosing for children; after 3—5 days for adults. **Adjust dose in renal failure (see Chapter 31).**

FLUCONAZOLE Diflucan and generics *Antifungal agent*	 
	C/D 2 Yes Yes No

Tabs: 50, 100, 150, 200 mg
Injection: 2 mg/mL (50, 100, 200 mL); contains 9 mEq Na/2 mg drug
Oral suspension: 10 mg/mL (35 mL), 40 mg/mL (35 mL)

Neonate (IV/PO):
  Loading dose: 12—25 mg/kg
    Thrush: 6 mg/kg
  Maintenance dose: 6—12 mg/kg with the following dosing intervals (see following table); use higher doses for severe infections of *Candida* strains with MICs >4—8 mcG/mL.
    Thrush: 3—6 mg/kg/dose with the following dosing intervals (see following table) for at least 2 wk

Postconceptional Age (wk)	Postnatal Age (days)	Dosing Interval (hr) and Time (hr) to Start First Maintenance Dose After Load
≤29	0—14	48
	>14	24
≥30	0—7	48
	>7	24

Child ≥1 mo (IV/PO):

Indication	Dosage Q24 hr	Maximum Dose
Oropharyngeal candidiasis	6—12 mg/kg	400 mg/dose
Esophageal candidiasis	6—12 mg/kg	600 mg/dose
Invasive systemic candidiasis (e.g., endocarditis) and cryptococcal meningitis	12 mg/kg	800 mg/dose
Suppressive therapy for HIV infected with cryptococcal meningitis	6 mg/kg	200 mg/dose

Adult:
  Oropharyngeal candidiasis: Loading dose of 200 mg PO/IV followed by 100—200 mg Q24 hr (24 hr after load) for 7—14 days; doses up to 400 mg/24 hr have been used
  Esophageal candidiasis: Loading dose of 400 mg PO/IV followed by 200—400 mg Q24 hr (24 hr after load); doses up to 800 mg/24 hr have been used
  Systemic candidiasis: Loading dose of 800 mg PO/IV, followed by 400—800 mg Q24 hr (24 hr after load)

FLUCONAZOLE *continued*

Bone marrow transplant prophylaxis: 400 mg PO/IV Q24 hr
Suppressive therapy in for HIV infected with cryptococcal meningitis: 200—400 mg PO/IV Q24 hr
Vaginal candidiasis: 150 mg PO × 1
  Severe infection in immunocompromised: 150 mg Q72 hr × 2—3 doses

Use with other medications known to prolong the QT interval and that are metabolized via the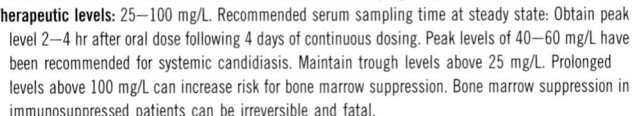
  CYP 450 3A4 enzyme (e.g., erythromycin) are considered **contraindicated.** May cause nausea,
  headache, rash, vomiting, abdominal pain, hepatitis, cholestasis, and diarrhea. Neutropenia,
  agranulocytosis, thrombocytopenia, exfoliative skin disorders (e.g., SJS, TEN, DRESS), and adrenal
  insufficiency (reversible) have been reported. **Use with caution** in hepatic or renal dysfunction and
  in patients with hypokalemia, proarrhythmic conditions, or advanced cardiac failure.
Inhibits CYP 450 2C9/10 and CYP 450 3A3/4 (weak inhibitor). May increase effects, toxicity, or
  levels of cyclosporine, midazolam, phenytoin, rifabutin, tacrolimus, theophylline, warfarin, oral
  hypoglycemics, AZT, and medicines containing ivacaftor. Rifampin increases fluconazole
  metabolism. May increase the risk of myopathy and rhabomyolysis when co-administered with
  HMG-CoA reductase inhibitors (statins); statin dosage reduction may be needed.
Consider using higher doses in morbidly obese patients. **Adjust dose in renal failure (see Chapter 31).**
Pregnancy category is "C" for single 150 mg use for vaginal candidiasis, but a Danish study reports a
  higher risk for miscarriages for during weeks 7—22 of gestation. Pregnancy category "D" is for all
  other indications (high-dose use during first trimester of pregnancy may result in birth defects).

FLUCYTOSINE
Ancobon, 5-FC, 5-Fluorocytosine, and generics
Antifungal agent

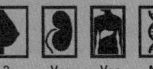 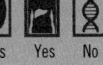

C   3   Yes   Yes   No

Caps: 250, 500 mg
Oral suspension: 10, 50 mg/mL

Neonate (monitor serum concentrations):
  <1 kg:
    ≤14 days old: 75 mg/kg/24 hr ÷ Q8 hr PO
    15—28 days old: 75 mg/kg/24 hr ÷ Q6 hr PO
  1—2 kg:
    ≤7 days old: 75 mg/kg/24 hr ÷ Q8 hr PO
    8—28 days old: 75 mg/kg/24 hr ÷ Q6 hr PO
  >2 kg and ≤60 days old: 75 mg/kg/24 hr ÷ Q6 hr PO
Dosages of 75—100 mg/kg/24 hr have been used in neonates (preterm and term) for candidal
meningitis.
Child and adult (monitor serum concentrations): 50—150 mg/kg/24 hr ÷ Q6 hr PO

Monitor CBC, BUN, serum creatinine, alkaline phosphatase, AST, and ALT. Common side
  effects: nausea, vomiting, diarrhea, rash, CNS disturbance, anemia, leukopenia, and
  thrombocytopenia. **Use with caution** in hepatic and renal impairment and in hematologic
  disorders. Use is **contraindicated** in the first trimester of pregnancy.
Therapeutic levels: 25—100 mg/L. Recommended serum sampling time at steady state: Obtain peak
  level 2—4 hr after oral dose following 4 days of continuous dosing. Peak levels of 40—60 mg/L have
  been recommended for systemic candidiasis. Maintain trough levels above 25 mg/L. Prolonged
  levels above 100 mg/L can increase risk for bone marrow suppression. Bone marrow suppression in
  immunosuppressed patients can be irreversible and fatal.
Flucytosine interferes with creatinine assay tests using the dry-slide enzymatic method (Kodak
  Ektachem analyzer). **Adjust dose in renal failure (see Chapter 31).**

FLUDROCORTISONE ACETATE
Generics (previously available as Florinef);
9-fluorohydrocortisone
Corticosteroid

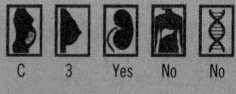

C 3 Yes No No

Tabs: 0.1 mg
Oral suspension: 0.1 mg/mL 🔖

Infant and child: 0.05–0.1 mg/24 hr once daily PO
  Congenital adrenal hyperplasia: 0.05–0.3 mg/24 hr once daily PO
Adult: 0.05–0.2 mg/24 hr once daily PO

Contraindicated in CHF and systemic fungal infections. Has primarily mineralocorticoid activity.
  Use with caution in hypertension, edema, or renal dysfunction. May cause hypertension,
  hypokalemia, acne, rash, bruising, headaches, GI ulcers, and growth suppression.
Monitor BP and serum electrolytes. See Chapter 10 for steroid potency comparison.
Drug interactions: Drug's hypokalemic effects may induce digoxin toxicity; phenytoin and rifampin
  may increase fludrocortisone metabolism.
Doses 0.2–2 mg/24 hr have been used in the management of severe orthostatic hypotension in
  adults. Use a gradual dosage taper when discontinuing therapy.

FLUMAZENIL
Generics; previously available as Romazicon
Benzodiazepine antidote

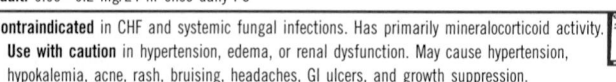

C ? No Yes No

Injection: 0.1 mg/mL (5, 10 mL); contains parabens

Benzodiazepine overdose (IV, see remarks):
  Child and adolescent (limited data): 0.01 mg/kg (**max. dose:** 0.2 mg) IV over 15 seconds
  Q1 minute PRN up to a **max. total cumulative dose** of 1 mg. As an alternative for repeat
  bolus doses, a continuous infusion of 0.005–0.01 mg/kg/hr has been used.
  Adult: Initial dose: 0.2 mg over 30 sec, if needed, give 0.3 mg 30 sec later over 30 sec. Additional
  doses of 0.5 mg given over 30 sec Q1 min PRN up to a cumulative dose of 3 mg (usual cumulative
  dose: 1–3 mg). Patients with only partial response to 3 mg may require additional slow titration to
  a total of 5 mg. Patients who have not responded 5 min after receiving a cumulative dose of 5 mg
  should be reassessed for other causes of sedation from non-benzodiazepines.
Reversal of benzodiazepine sedation (IV):
  Child and adolescent: Initial dose: 0.01 mg/kg (**max dose:** 0.2 mg) given over 15 sec; if needed after
  45 sec, 0.01 mg/kg (**max. dose:** 0.2 mg) Q1 min to a **max. total cumulative dose** of 0.05 mg/kg or 1
  mg, whichever is lower. Usual total dose: 0.08–1 mg (average 0.65 mg)
  Adult: Initial dose: 0.2 mg over 15 sec; if needed after 45 sec, give 0.2 mg Q1 min to a **max. total
  cumulative dose** of 1 mg. Doses may be repeated at 20 min interval (**max. dose** of 1 mg per 20 min
  interval) up to a **max. dose** of 3 mg in 1 hr.

Does not reverse narcotics. Onset of benzodiazepine reversal occurs in 1–3 min. Reversal
  effects of flumazenil ($T_{1/2}$ approximately 1 hr) may wear off sooner than benzodiazepine
  effects. If patient does not respond after cumulative 1–3 mg dose, suspect agent other than
  benzodiazepines.
May precipitate seizures, especially in patients taking benzodiazepines for seizure control or in patients
  with tricyclic antidepressant overdose. Fear and panic attacks in patients with history of panic
  disorders have been reported.

FLUMAZENIL *continued*

Use with caution in liver dysfunction; flumazenil's clearance is significantly reduced. Use normal dose for initial dose and decrease the dosage and frequency for subsequent doses.
See Chapter 3 for complete management of suspected ingestions.

FLUNISOLIDE
Generics; previously available as Nasarel or Nasalide
Corticosteroid

   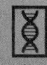

C   1   No   No   No

Nasal solution: 25 mCg/spray (200 sprays/bottle) (25 mL); contains propylene glycol and benzalkonium chloride

---

After symptoms are controlled, reduce to lowest effective maintenance dose (e.g., 1 spray each nostril once daily) to control symptoms.
Nasal solution:
  Child (6—14 yr):
    Initial: 1 spray per nostril TID or 2 sprays per nostril BID; **max. dose:** 4 sprays per nostril/24 hr
  ≥15 yr and adult:
    Initial: 2 sprays per nostril BID; if needed in 4—7 days, increase to 2 sprays per nostril TID; **max. dose:** 8 sprays per nostril/24 hr

---

Nasal burning and stinging is common. Nasal congestion, sneezing, epistaxis, watery eyes, sore throat, nausea/vomiting, and headaches may also occur. May cause a reduction in growth velocity. Nasal septal perforations have been reported. Flunisolide is a minor substrate of CYP 450 3A4.

Shake nasal solution well before use and clear nasal passages before use. Priming of the nasal spray is recommended when using a new bottle or if the bottle has not been used for ≥5 days.

FLUORIDE
NaFrinse, Fluoritab, many others, and generics
Mineral

    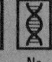

B   2   No   No   No

Concentrations and strengths based on fluoride ion:
  Oral drops/solution:
    Fluoritab NaFrinse, and generics: 0.125 mg/drop (30 mL)
    Generics: 0.5 mg/mL (50 mL)
  Chewable tabs:
    Fluoritab, NaFrinse, and generics: 1 mg
    Generics: 0.25, 0.5 mg

All doses/24 hr (see table below):
Recommendations from American Academy of Pediatrics and American Dental Association for prevention of dental caries.

Age	Concentration of Fluoride in Drinking Water (ppm)		
	<0.3	**0.3—0.6**	**>0.6**
Birth—6 mo	0	0	0
6 mo—3 yr	0.25 mg	0	0
3—6 yr	0.5 mg	0.25 mg	0
6—16 yr	1 mg	0.5 mg	0

Continued

FLUORIDE *continued*

Contraindicated in areas where drinking water fluoridation is >0.7 ppm. **Acute overdose:** GI distress, salivation, CNS irritability, tetany, seizures, hypocalcemia, hypoglycemia, and cardiorespiratory failure. Chronic excess use may result in mottled teeth or bone changes.

Take with food, but **not** milk, to minimize GI upset. The doses have been decreased owing to concerns over dental fluorosis.

FLUOXETINE HYDROCHLORIDE
Prozac and generics
Antidepressant, selective serotonin reuptake inhibitor

C   X   Yes   Yes   No

Oral solution: 20 mg/5 mL (120 mL); may contain alcohol
Caps: 10, 20, 40 mg
Delayed release caps: 90 mg
Tabs: 10, 20, 60 mg

All dosages are with immediate release dosage forms.
Depression:
  Child, 8—<12 yr: Start at 5 or 10 mg once daily PO. Usual dose: 10 mg once daily. May increase dose every 1—2 weeks as needed up to a **maximum dose** of 40 mg/24 hr (some patients may require higher doses)
  Adolescent ≥12 yr: Start at 10 or 20 mg once daily PO. May increase increase by 10—20 mg increments every 1—2 weeks as needed up to a **maximum dose** of 60 mg/24 hr. Usual effective dose: 20—40 mg once daily
  Adult: Start at 20 mg once daily in the morning PO. May increase after several weeks by 20 mg/24 hr increments to **max. dose** of 80 mg/24 hr. Doses >20 mg/24 hr should be divided BID.
Obsessive-compulsive disorder:
  Child, 7—18 yr:
    Lower-weight child: Start at 5 or 10 mg once daily PO. May increase after several weeks. Usual dose range: 20—30 mg/24 hr. There is very minimal experience with doses >20 mg/24 hr and no experience with doses >60 mg/24 hr.
    Higher-weight child and adolescent: Start at 10 mg once daily PO and increase dose to 20 mg/24 hr after 2 wk. May further increase dose after several weeks. Usual dose range: 20—60 mg/24 hr
Bulimia:
  Adolescent (PO; limited data): 20 mg QAM × 3 days, then 40 mg QAM × 3 days, then 60 mg QAM
  Adult: 60 mg QAM PO; it is recommended to titrate up to this dose over several days

Contraindicated in patients taking MAO inhibitors (e.g., linezolid) due to possibility of seizures, hyperpyrexia, and coma. **Use with caution** in patients with angle-closure glaucoma, receiving diuretics, or with liver (reduce dose with cirrhosis) or renal impairment. May increase the effects of tricyclic antidepressants. May cause headache, insomnia, nervousness, drowsiness, GI disturbance, sexual dysfunction, and weight loss. Increased bleeding diathesis with unaltered prothrombin time may occur with warfarin. Hyponatremia has been reported. Monitor for clinical worsening of depression and suicidal ideation/behavior following the initiation of therapy or after dose changes.

May displace other highly protein-bound drugs. Inhibits CYP 450 2C19, 2D6, and 3A3/4 drug metabolism isoenzymes, which may increase the effects or toxicity of drugs metabolized by these enzymes. For example, use with pimozide or thioridazine may increase the risk for prolonged cardiac QTc interval and is considered **contraindicated.** Use with serotonergic drugs (e.g., triptans, methylene blue) and drugs that impair serotonin metabolism (MAOIs) may increase the risk for serotonin syndrome. Carefully review the patients' medication profile for potential interactions.

FLUOXETINE HYDROCHLORIDE *continued*

Delayed release capsule is currently indicated for depression and is dosed at 90 mg Q7 days. It is unknown if weekly dosing provides the same protection from relapse as does daily dosing.

Breastfeeding is not recommended by the manufacturer, as adverse events to nursing infants have been reported. Fluoxetine and metabolite are variable and are higher when compared with other SSRIs. Maternal use of SSRIs during pregnancy and postpartum may result in more difficult breastfeeding. Infants exposed to SSRIs during pregnancy may also have an increased risk for persistent pulmonary hypertension of the newborn.

FLUTICASONE FUROATE + VILANTEROL
Breo Ellipta and generics
Corticosteroid and long-acting β₂ adrenergic agonist

    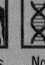 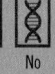

C   2   No   Yes   No

Breath-activated aerosol powder for inhalation; contains lactose and milk proteins:
   100 mCg fluticasone furoate + 25 mCg vilanterol per actuation (28, 60 doses)
   200 mCg fluticasone furoate + 25 mCg vilanterol per actuation (28, 60 doses)
For Fluticasone Furoate (Arnuity Ellipta) as a single agent, see Fluticasone Preparations.

Asthma (see remarks):
   Adult: One inhalation of 100 mCg fluticasone furoate + 25 mCg vilanterol OR 200 mCg fluticasone furoate + 25 mCg vilanterol once daily
   Max. dose: One inhalation/24 hr for either dosage strength (25 mCg vilanterol/24 hr)

Contraindicated with hypersensitivity to milk proteins. See Fluticasone Preparations for remarks. Vilanterol is a long-acting β₂ adrenergic agonist with a faster onset and longer duration of action compared to salmeterol.

Hypersensitivity reactions, hyperglycemia, muscle spasms, and tremor have been reported.

Titrate to the lowest effective strength after asthma is adequately controlled. This dosage form's breath-activated device requires a minimum inspiratory flow rate of 60 mL/min for proper dose activation. Proper patient education including dosage administration technique is essential; see patient package insert for detailed instructions. Rinse mouth after each use.

FLUTICASONE PREPARATIONS
Fluticasone propionate: Flonase, Flovent Diskus,
Flovent HFA, ArmonAir Digihaler, and generics
Fluticasone furoate: Flonase Sensimist and
Arnuity Ellipta
Corticosteroid

    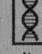

C   2   No   Yes   No

FLUTICASONE PROPIONATE:
Nasal spray (Flonase and generics; OTC): 50 mCg/actuation (9.9 mL = 60 doses, 15.8 mL = 120 doses); contains benzalkonium chloride and polysorbate 80
Topical cream: 0.05% (15, 30, 60 g)
Topical ointment: 0.005% (15, 30, 60 g)
Topical lotion: 0.05% (60 mL); contains parabens and propylene glycol
Aerosol inhaler (MDI) (Flovent HFA and generics): 44 mCg/actuation (10.6 g), 110 mCg/actuation (12 g), 220 mCg/actuation (12 g); each inhaler provides 120 metered inhalations

Continued

FLUTICASONE PREPARATIONS *continued*

Dry-powder inhalation (DPI) (Flovent Diskus): 50 mCg/dose, 100 mCg/dose, 250 mCg/dose; all strengths come in a package of 15 Rotadisks; each Rotadisk provides 4 doses for a total of 60 doses per package. Contains lactose.

Breath-activated aerosol powder inhaler (ArmonAir Digihaler): 55 mCg/inhalation, 113 mCg/inhalation, 232 mCg/inhalation; each inhaler contains 0.9 g of formulation and provides 60 doses. Contains lactose. Digihaler device contains a built-in electronic module that detects, records, and stores usage events, including peak inspiratory flow rate (L/min).

FLUTICASONE FUROATE:

Nasal spray (Flonase Sensimist [OTC]): 27.5 mCg/actuation (5.9 mL = 60 doses); contains benzalkonium chloride and polysorbate 80

Breath-activated aerosol powder inhaler (Arnuity Ellipta): 50 mCg/actuation, (30 doses), 100 mCg/actuation (14, 30 doses), 200 mCg/actuation dose (14, 30 doses); contains lactose

Allergic rhinitis (Intranasal):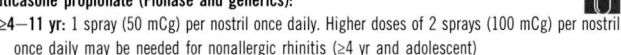

Fluticasone propionate (Flonase and generics):

≥4—11 yr: 1 spray (50 mCg) per nostril once daily. Higher doses of 2 sprays (100 mCg) per nostril once daily may be needed for nonallergic rhinitis (≥4 yr and adolescent)

≥12 yr and adult: Initial 200 mCg/24 hr [2 sprays (100 mCg) per nostril once daily; OR 1 spray (50 mCg) per nostril BID]. Reduce to 1 spray per nostril once daily when symptoms are controlled.

Max. dose (4 yr—adult): 2 sprays (100 mCg) per nostril/24 hr

Fluticasone furoate (Veramyst):

2—11 yr: 1 spray (27.5 mCg) per nostril once daily. If needed, dose may be increased to 2 sprays each nostril once daily. Reduce to 1 spray per nostril once daily when symptoms are controlled.

≥12 yr and adult: 2 sprays (55 mCg) each nostril once daily. Reduce to 1 spray per nostril once daily when symptoms are controlled.

Max. dose (2 yr—adult): 2 sprays (55 mCg) per nostril/24 hr

Asthma maintenance therapy (oral inhalation; see remarks):

Fluticasone propionate (Flovent HFA and Diskus): Divide all 24 hr doses BID. If desired response is not seen after 2 wk of starting therapy, increase dosage. Then reduce to the lowest effective dose when asthma symptoms are controlled. Administration of MDI (HFA) with aerochamber enhances drug delivery.

Recommended dosages for asthma (see following table):

Age	Previous Use of Bronchodilators Only: (Max. Dose)	Previous Use of Inhaled Corticosteroid: (Max. Dose)	Previous Use of Oral Corticosteroid: (Max. Dose)
Child (4—11 yr)	MDI: 88 mCg/24 hr (176 mCg/24 hr) DPI: 100 mCg/24 hr (200 mCg/24 hr)	MDI: 88 mCg/24 hr (176 mCg/24 hr) DPI: 100 mCg/24 hr (200 mCg/24 hr)	Dose not available
≥12 yr and adult	MDI: 176 mCg/24 hr (880 mCg/24 hr) DPI: 200 mCg/24 hr (2000 mCg/24 hr)	MDI: 176—440 mCg/24 hr (880 mCg/24 hr) DPI: 200—500 mCg/24 hr (2000 mCg/24 hr)	MDI: 880 mCg/24 hr (1760 mCg/24 hr) DPI: 1000—2000 mCg/24 hr (2000 mCg/24 hr)

DPI, Dry-powder inhaler (breath activated); *MDI,* metered dose inhaler.

FLUTICASONE PREPARATIONS *continued*

Fluticasone propionate (ArmonAir Digihaler; breath-activated aerosol powder inhaler):
≥12 yr and adult:
No prior inhaled corticosteroids: Start with 55 mCg inhaled BID; **max. dose:** 232 mCg BID
Prior treatment with inhaled corticosteroids: Start with low (55 mCg), medium (113 mCg), or high (232 mCg) inhaled BID based on the strength of previous inhaled corticosteroid and disease severity; **max. dose:** 232 mCg BID

Fluticasone furoate (Arnuity Ellipta; breath-activated inhaler aerosol powder inhaler):
5–11 yr: Inhale 50 mCg once daily.
≥12 yr and adult: Inhale 100–200 mCg once daily; **max. dose:** 200 mCg/24 hr

Eosinophilic esophagitis (limited data and other regimens exist; use oral fluticasone propionate HFA dosage form without spacer for PO administration as doses are swallowed):
Induction (short-term):
Child (1–10 yr): 220 mCg QID × 4 wk, then 220 mCg TID × 3 wk, then 220 mCg BID × 3 wk, and 220 mCg once daily × 2 wk
Child ≥11 yr and adolescent: 440 mCg QID × 4 wk, then 440 mCg TID × 3 wk, then 440 mCg BID × 3 wk, and 440 mCg once daily × 2 wk
Maintenance (long-term):
Child 2–4 yr: 88 mCg BID
Child 5–10 yr: 220 mCg BID
Child ≥11 yr and adolescent: 440 mCg BID

Atopic dermatitis (topical fluticasone propionate; reassess diagnosis if no improvement in 2 wk):
Cream (see Chapter 8 for topical steroid comparisons):
≥3 mo and adult: Apply thin film to affected areas once daily—BID; then reduce to a less potent topical agent when symptoms are controlled. Safety and efficacy have not been evaluated longer than 4 wk.
Lotion (see remarks):
≥3 mo and adult: Apply thin film to affected areas once daily. Safety and efficacy have not been evaluated longer than 4 wk.
Ointment:
Adult: Apply thin film to affected areas BID.

Fluticasone propionate and fluticasone furoate do not have equivalent potencies; follow specific dosing regimens for the respective products.

For mild asthma exacerbation in patients with mild/moderate disease, no history of life-threatening exacerbations, and a good asthma self-management plan, limited data in adolescents (>16 yr) and adults suggest a temporary quadrupling of the maintenance dosage when asthma control starts to deteriorate. Revert back to baseline maintenance dose after symptoms stabilize or up to a maximum of 14 days of the quadrupled dose, whichever comes first. **DO NOT** use this management strategy for children <12 years of age due to the lack of efficacy and increased risk for decreasing linear growth.

Concurrent administration with ritonavir and other CYP 450 3A4 inhibitors may increase fluticasone levels, resulting in Cushing syndrome and adrenal suppression. **Use with caution** and monitor closely in hepatic impairment.

Intranasal: Clear nasal passages prior to use. May cause epistaxis and nasal irritation, which are usually transient. Taste and smell alterations, rare hypersensitivity reactions (angioedema, pruritis, urticaria, wheezing, dyspnea), and nasal septal perforation have been reported in postmarketing studies.

Oral inhalation: DO NOT USE a spacer or volume holding chamber with breath-activated dosage forms. Specific breath-activated dosage forms require the following minimum inspiratory flow rates for proper dose activation:
Arnuity Ellipta: 60 L/min

Continued

FLUTICASONE PREPARATIONS *continued*

ArmonAir Digihaler: 30 L/min

Rinse mouth after each use. May cause dysphonia, oral thrush, and dermatitis. Esophageal candidiasis and hypersensitivity reactions have been reported. Compared to beclomethasone, has been shown to have less of an effect on suppressing linear growth in asthmatic children. Eosinophilic conditions may occur with the withdrawal or decrease of oral corticosteroids after the initiation of inhaled fluticasone.

TOPICAL USE: Irritation, folliculitis, acneiform eruptions, hypopigmentation, perioral dermatitis, allergic contact dermatitis, secondary infection, skin atrophy, striae, hypertrichosis, miliaria, cataracts, and glaucoma have been reported. **Avoid** contact with topical dosage forms to the eyes.

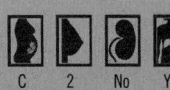

FLUTICASONE PROPIONATE AND SALMETEROL
Advair Diskus, Advair HFA, AirDuo Digihaler,
AirDuo RespiClick, and generics
***Corticosteroid and long-acting β2-adrenergic
agonist***

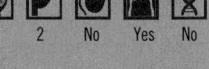

C   2   No   Yes   No

Aerosol inhaler (MDI) (Advair HFA):
 45 mCg fluticasone propionate + 21 mCg salmeterol per inhalation (8 g delivers 60 doses, 12 g delivers 120 doses)
 115 mCg fluticasone propionate + 21 mCg salmeterol per inhalation (8 g delivers 60 doses, 12 g delivers 120 doses)
 230 mCg fluticasone propionate + 21 mCg salmeterol per inhalation (8 g delivers 60 doses, 12 g delivers 120 doses)

Breath-activated DPI (Advair Diskus and generics; contains lactose and milk proteins):
 100 mCg fluticasone propionate + 50 mCg salmeterol per inhalation (14, 60 doses)
 250 mCg fluticasone propionate + 50 mCg salmeterol per inhalation (14, 60 doses)
 500 mCg fluticasone propionate + 50 mCg salmeterol per inhalation (14, 60 doses)

Breath-activated aerosol powder inhaler (AirDuo Digihaler, AirDuo RespiClick and generics; contains lactose):
 55 mCg fluticasone propionate + 14 mCg salmeterol per inhalation (0.45 g delivers 60 doses)
 113 mCg fluticasone propionate + 14 mCg salmeterol per inhalation (0.45 g delivers 60 doses)
 232 mCg fluticasone propionate + 14 mCg salmeterol per inhalation (0.45 g delivers 60 doses)
 Digihaler device contains a built-in electronic module that detects, records, and stores usage events, including peak inspiratory flow rate (L/min).

Asthma:

 Without prior inhaled steroid use:
  Breath-activated (DPI; Advair Diskus; see remarks):
   4—11 yr: Start with one inhalation BID of 100 mCg fluticasone propionate + 50 mCg salmeterol.
   ≥12 yr and adult: Start with one inhalation BID of 100 mCg fluticasone propionate + 50 mCg salmeterol, OR 250 mCg fluticasone propionate + 50 mCg salmeterol; **max. dose:** one inhalation BID of 500 mCg fluticasone propionate + 50 mCg salmeterol
  Aerosol inhaler (MDI; Advair HFA):
   ≥12 yr and adult: Start with 2 inhalations BID of 45 mCg fluticasone + 21 mCg salmeterol, OR 115 mCg fluticasone + 21 mCg salmeterol; **max. dose:** 2 inhalations BID of 230 mCg fluticasone + 21 mCg salmeterol
  Breath-activated aerosol powder inhaler (AirDuo Digihaler, AirDuo RespiClick; see remarks):
   ≥12 yr and adult: Start with 1 inhalation BID of 55 mCg fluticasone + 14 mCg salmeterol; **max. dose:** one inhalation BID of 232 mCg fluticasone propionate + 14 mCg salmeterol

FLUTICASONE PROPIONATE AND SALMETEROL *continued*

With prior inhaled steroid use (conversion from other inhaled steroids; see following table and below):

Inhaled Corticosteroid	Current Daily Dose	Recommended Strength of Fluticasone Propionate + Salmeterol Diskus (DPI) (Advair Diskus) Administered at One Inhalation BID	Recommended Strength of Fluticasone Propionate + Salmeterol Aerosol Inhaler (MDI) (Advair HFA) Administered at Two Inhalations BID
Beclomethasone dipropionate (Qvar Redihaler)	160 mCg	100 mCg + 50 mCg	45 mCg + 21 mCg
	320 mCg	250 mCg + 50 mCg	115 mCg + 21 mCg
	640 mCg	500 mCg + 50 mCg	230 mCg + 21 mCg
Budesonide	≤400 mCg	100 mCg + 50 mCg	45 mCg + 21 mCg
	800—1200 mCg	250 mCg + 50 mCg	115 mCg + 21 mCg
	1600 mCg	500 mCg + 50 mCg	230 mCg + 21 mCg
Fluticasone propionate aerosol (HFA)	≤176 mCg	100 mCg + 50 mCg	45 mCg + 21 mCg
	440 mCg	250 mCg + 50 mCg	115 mCg + 21 mCg
	660—880 mCg	500 mCg + 50 mCg	230 mCg + 21 mCg
Fluticasone propionate dry powder (DPI)	≤200 mCg	100 mCg + 50 mCg	45 mCg + 21 mCg
	500 mCg	250 mCg + 50 mCg	115 mCg + 21 mCg
	1000 mCg	500 mCg + 50 mCg	230 mCg + 21 mCg
Mometasone furoate	220 mCg	100 mCg + 50 mCg	45 mCg + 21 mCg
	440 mCg	250 mCg + 50 mCg	115 mCg + 21 mCg
	880 mCg	500 mCg + 50 mCg	230 mCg + 21 mCg

DPI, Dry powder inhaler (breath activated); *MDI,* metered dose inhaler.

Breath-activated aerosol powder inhaler (AirDuo Digihaler, AirDuo RespiClick): Select low (55 mCg fluticasone + 14 mCg salmeterol), medium (113 mCg fluticasone + 14 mCg salmeterol), or high (232 mCg fluticasone + 14 mCg salmeterol) dose strength based on the previous inhaled corticosteroid product or the strength of the inhaled corticosteroid from a combination product and disease severity. All dosage strengths are administered as one inhalation BID.

Max. doses:

Breath-activated (DPI; Advair Diskus): One inhalation BID of 500 mCg fluticasone propionate + 50 mCg salmeterol

Aerosol inhaler (MDI; Advair HFA): Two inhalations BID of 230 mCg fluticasone propionate + 21 mCg salmeterol

Breath-activated aerosol powder inhaler (AirDuo RespiClick): One inhalation BID of 232 mCg fluticasone propionate + 14 mCg salmeterol

Contraindicated with hypersensitivity to milk proteins. See Fluticasone Preparations and Salmeterol for remarks. Titrate to the lowest effective strength after asthma is adequately controlled.

Continued

FLUTICASONE PROPIONATE AND SALMETEROL *continued*

DO NOT USE a spacer or volume holding chamber with breath-activated dosage forms. Specific breath-activated dosage forms require the following minimum inspiratory flow rates for proper dose activation:

Advair Diskus: 60 L/min

AirDuo Digihaler, AirDuo RespiClick: 30 L/min

Proper patient education including dosage administration technique is essential; see patient package insert to specific dosage form for detailed instructions. Rinse mouth after each use.

FLUVOXAMINE
Generics; previously available as Luvox and Luvox CR
Antidepressant, selective serotonin reuptake inhibitor

| C | 2 | No | Yes | Yes |

Tabs: 25, 50, 100 mg
Extended release capsules: 100, 150 mg

Obsessive compulsive disorder (use immediate release tablets unless noted otherwise, see remarks):

Child 8—12 yr: Start at 12.5—25 mg PO QHS. Dose may be increased by 25 mg/24 hr Q7—14 days (slower titration at Q2—4 wk may be used for minimizing behavioral side effects). Total daily doses >50 mg/24 hr should be divided BID. Female patients may require lower dosages compared to males.

Max. dose: Child: 8—11 yr: 200 mg/24 hr; and child 12 yr: 300 mg/24 hr

Adolescent: Start at 25—50 mg PO QHS. Dose may be increased by 25 mg/24 hr Q7—14 days (slower titration at Q2—4 wk may be used for minimizing behavioral side effects). Total daily doses >50 mg/24 hr should be divided BID with the larger dose at bedtime. **Max. dose:** 300 mg/24 hr

Adult: Start at 50 mg PO QHS. Dose may be increased by 50 mg/24 hr Q4—7 days to a **max. dose** of 300 mg/24 hr. Total daily doses >100 mg/24 hr should be divided BID with larger dose at bedtime.

Extended release capsule (adult): Start at 100 mg PO QHS. Dose may be increased by 50 mg/24 hr Q7 days up to a **max. dose** of 300 mg/24 hr.

Contraindicated with coadministration of cisapride, pimozide, thioridazine, tizanidine, or MAO inhibitors. **Use with caution** in hepatic disease (dosage reduction may be necessary as drug is extensively metabolized by the liver) and in combination with serotonergic drugs (e.g., TCAs, triptans, fentanyl, lithium, tramadol, amphetamines, tryptophan, and St. John's wort). Monitor for clinical worsening of depression and suicidal ideation/behavior following the initiation of therapy or after dose changes.

Major substrate for CYP 450 1A2 and 2D6. Poor metabolizers of CYP 450 2D6 should consider an initial dose reduction of 25%—50% and titrate to response or use an alternative medication not metabolized by this enzyme.

Inhibits CYP 450 1A2, 2C19, 2C9, 2D6, and 3A3/4, which may increase the effects or toxicity of drugs metabolized by these enzymes. Dose-related use of thioridazine with fluvoxamine may cause prolongation of QT interval and serious arrhythmias. May increase warfarin plasma levels by 98% and prolong PT. May increase toxicity and/or levels of theophylline, caffeine, and tricyclic antidepressants. Side effects include: headache, insomnia, somnolence, nausea, diarrhea, dyspepsia, dry mouth, and sexual dysfunction.

Titrate to lowest effective dose. Use a gradual taper when discontinuing therapy to prevent withdrawal symptoms.

Consider the benefits to potential risk for maternal use in breastfeeding. Maternal use during pregnancy and postpartum may result in breastfeeding difficulties.

FOLIC ACID
FA-8 and many generics; previously available as Folvite
Water-soluble vitamin

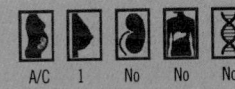

A/C 1 No No No

Tabs [OTC]: 0.4, 0.8, 1 mg
Caps:
  FA-8: 0.8 mg [OTC]
  Generics: 5 mg, 20 mg
Oral solution: 0.05 mg/mL 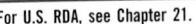, 1 mg/mL
Injection: 5 mg/mL (10 mL); contains 1.5% benzyl alcohol

For U.S. RDA, see Chapter 21.
Folic acid deficiency PO, IM, IV, SC:
  Infant: 0.1 mg/24 hr once daily
  Child <4 yr: 0.1—0.3 mg/24 hr once daily
  Child ≥4 yr and adolescent: 0.1—0.4 mg/24 hr once daily
  Adult: 0.4 mg/24 hr once daily
  Pregnant and lactating women: 0.8 mg/24 hr once daily

Normal levels: See Chapter 28. May mask hematologic effects of vitamin B_{12} deficiency but will not prevent progression of neurologic abnormalities. High-dose folic acid may decrease the absorption of phenytoin.

Women of childbearing age considering pregnancy should take at least 0.4 mg once daily before and during pregnancy to reduce risk of neural tube defects in the fetus. Pregnancy category changes to "C" if used in doses above the RDA.

FOMEPIZOLE
Generics; previously available as Antizol
Antidote for ethylene glycol or methanol toxicity

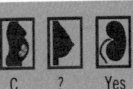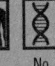

C ? Yes No No

Injection: 1 g/mL (1.5 mL); preservative free

Child and adult not requiring hemodialysis (IV, all doses administered over 30 min):
  Load: 15 mg/kg/dose × 1
  Maintenance: 10 mg/kg/dose Q12 hr × 4 doses, then 15 mg/kg/dose Q12 hr until ethylene glycol or methanol level decreases to <20 mg/dL and the patient is asymptomatic with normal pH
Child and adult requiring hemodialysis (IV following the recommended doses at the intervals indicated here. Fomepizole is removed by dialysis. All doses administered IV over 30 min):
  Dosing at the beginning of hemodialysis:
    If <6 hr since last fomepizole dose: DO NOT administer dose.
    If ≥6 hr since last fomepizole dose: Administer next scheduled dose upon beginning dialysis.
  Dosing during hemodialysis: Administer Q4 hr or, alternatively, 10—20 mg/kg loading dose, followed by a continuous infusion of 1—1.5 mg/kg/hr.
  Dosing at the time hemodialysis is completed (based on the time between last dose and end of hemodialysis):
    <1 hr: DO NOT administer dose at end of hemodialysis.
    1—3 hr: Administer $^{1}/_{2}$ of next scheduled dose at the end of hemodialysis.
    >3 hr: Administer next scheduled dose at the end of hemodialysis.

Continued

FOMEPIZOLE *continued*

Maintenance dose off hemodialysis: Give next scheduled dose 12 hr from last dose administered.

Works by competitively inhibiting alcohol dehydrogenase. Safety and efficacy in pediatrics have not been established. **Contraindicated** in hypersensitivity to any components or other pyrazole compounds. Most frequent side effects include headache, nausea, and dizziness. Fomepizole is extensively eliminated by the kidneys (**use with caution** in renal failure) and removed by hemodialysis.

Drug product may solidify at temperatures <25°C (77°F); vial can be liquefied by running it under warm water (efficacy, safety, and stability are not affected). All doses must be diluted with at least 100 mL of D5W or NS to prevent vein irritation. **DO NOT** use polycarbonate syringe or polycarbonate-containing needles when diluting or administering this medication.

FOSCARNET
Foscavir and generics
Antiviral agent

  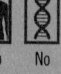

C   3   Yes   No   No

Injection: 24 mg/mL (250 mL); preservative free
Contains 10 mEq Na/g drug

HIV positive or exposed with the following infection (IV):
  CMV disease:
    Infant, child, and adolescent:
      Induction: 180 mg/kg/24 hr ÷ Q8–12 hr in combination with ganciclovir; continue until symptom improvement and convert to maintenance therapy
      Maintenance: 90–120 mg/kg/dose Q24 hr
  CMV retinitis (disseminated disease; IV):
    Infant and child:
      Induction: 180 mg/kg/24 hr ÷ Q8–12 hr × 14–21 days with or without ganciclovir
      Maintenance: 90–120 mg/kg/24 hr once daily
    Adolescent and adult:
      Induction: 180 mg/kg/24 hr ÷ Q8–12 hr × 14–21 days
      Maintenance: 90–120 mg/kg/24 hr once daily
  Acyclovir-resistant herpes simplex (limited data; IV):
    Infant and child: 40 mg/kg/dose Q8 hr or 60 mg/kg/dose Q12 hr for up to 3 wk or until lesions heal
    Adolescent and adult: 40 mg/kg/dose Q8–12 hr × 14–21 days or until lesions heal
  Varicella zoster unresponsive to acyclovir (IV):
    Infant and child: 40–60 mg/kg/dose Q8 hr × 7–10 days
    Adolescent: 90 mg/kg/dose Q12 hr
  Varicella zoster, progressive outer retinal necrosis (IV):
    Infant, child, and adolescent: 90 mg/kg/dose Q12 hr in combination with ganciclovir IV and intravitreal foscarnet with or without ganciclovir
  Intravitreal route for progressive outer retinal necrosis (HIV positive or exposed):
    Child and adolescent: 1.2 mg/0.05 mL or 2.4 mg/0.1 mL per dose 2–3 times weekly in combination with IV foscarnet and ganciclovir and/or intravitreal ganciclovir

Use with caution in patients with renal insufficiency and hypernatremia (large sodium content). **Discontinue** use in adults if serum Cr ≥2.9 mg/dL. **Adjust dose in renal failure** (see Chapter 31).

FOSCARNET *continued*

May cause peripheral neuropathy, seizures, neutropenia, esophageal ulceration, hallucinations, GI disturbance, increased LFTs, hypertension, chest pain, ECG abnormalities (QT interval prolongation has been reported), coughing, dyspnea, bronchospasm, and renal failure (adequate hydration and avoiding nephrotoxic medications may reduce risk). Hypocalcemia (increased risk if given with pentamidine), hypokalemia, and hypomagnesemia may also occur. Hypersensitivity reactions have been reported. Use with ciprofloxacin may increase risk for seizures.

Correction of dehydration and adequate hydration reduces the risk for nephrotoxicity. 10—20 mL/kg IV (**max. dose:** 1000 mL) of NS or D$_5$W should be administered prior to the first dose and concurrently with subsequent doses. For lower foscarnet dosage regimens of 40—60 mg/kg, use 50% of the aforementioned hydration recommendations. Actual hydration may need to be reduced when clinically indicated. Oral hydration methods may also be considered in patients who are able to tolerate.

For peripheral line IV administration, the concentration must be diluted to 12 mg/mL in NS or D$_5$W.

FOSPHENYTOIN
Cerebyx and generics
Anticonvulsant

    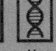

D   2   Yes   Yes   Yes

Injection: 50 mg phenytoin equivalent (75 mg fosphenytoin)/1 mL (2, 10 mL)
1 mg phenytoin equivalent provides 0.0037 mmol phosphate

All doses are expressed as phenytoin sodium equivalents (PE) (see remarks for dose administration information):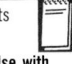
  Neonate, child, and adolescent: See Phenytoin and use the conversion of 1 mg phenytoin = 1 mg PE
  Adult:
    Loading dose:
      Status epilepticus: 20 mg PE/kg IV (**max. dose:** 1500 mg PE/dose)
      Nonemergent loading: 10—20 mg PE/kg IV/IM
      Nonemergent initial maintenance dose (initiated 12 hr after loading dose): 4—7 mg PE/kg/24 hr IV/IM ÷ Q6—12 hr

All doses should be prescribed and dispensed in terms of mg phenytoin sodium equivalents (PE) to avoid medication errors. Safety in pediatrics has not been fully established.

Contraindicated in patients with history of phenytoin or other hydantoin hypersensitivity. **Use with caution** in patients with renal or hepatic impairment and porphyria (consider amount of phosphate delivered by fosphenytoin in patients with phosphate restrictions). Drug is also metabolized to liberate small amounts of formaldehyde, which is considered clinically insignificant with short-term use (e.g., 1 wk). Side effects: hypokalemia (with rapid IV administration), slurred speech, dizziness, ataxia, rash, exfoliative dermatitis (e.g., TEN, SJS; increased risk with patients with HLA-B*1502 allele), nystagmus, diplopia, and tinnitus. Angioedema, macrocytosis, megaloblastic anemia, and pure red cell aplasia have been reported. Increased unbound phenytoin concentrations may occur in patients with renal disease or hypoalbuminemia; measure "free" or "unbound" phenytoin levels in these patients. Patients with reduced CYP 2C9 activity (CYP2C*3) have decreased clearance of phenytoin, resulting in increased phenytoin levels.

Abrupt withdrawal may cause status epilepticus. BP and ECG monitoring should be present during IV loading dose administration. **Max. IV infusion rate:** 2 mg PE/kg/min up to a **max.** of 150 mg PE/min. Administer IM via 1 or 2 injection sites, and IM route is not recommended in status epilepticus.

Therapeutic levels: 10—20 mg/L (free and bound phenytoin) OR 1—2 mg/L (free only). Recommended peak serum sampling times: 4 hr following an IM dose or 2 hr following an IV dose.

Continued

FOSPHENYTOIN *continued*

See Phenytoin remarks for drug interactions and additional side effects. Drug is more safely
administered via peripheral IV than phenytoin.

FUROSEMIDE
Lasix and generics
Loop diuretic

C/D   3   Yes   Yes   No

Tabs: 20, 40, 80 mg
Injection: 10 mg/mL (2, 4, 10 mL)
Oral solution: 10 mg/mL (60, 120 mL), 40 mg/5 mL (500 mL)

IM, IV:
   Neonate (see remarks): 0.5—1 mg/kg/dose Q12—24 hr; **max. dose:** 2 mg/kg/dose
   Infant and child: 0.5—2 mg/kg/dose Q6—12 hr; **max. dose:** 6 mg/kg/dose not to exceed 200 mg/dose
   Adult: 20—40 mg/24 hr ÷ Q6—12 hr; **max. dose:** 200 mg/dose
PO:
   Neonate: Bioavailability by this route is poor; doses of 1—3 mg/kg/dose once daily to BID have been
      used.
   Infant and child: Start at 2 mg/kg/dose; may increase by 1—2 mg/kg/dose no sooner than 6—8 hr
      following the previous dose. **Max. dose:** 6 mg/kg/dose. Dosages have ranged from 1—6 mg/kg/dose
      Q12—24 hr.
   Adult: 20—80 mg/dose Q6—12 hr; **max. dose:** 600 mg/24 hr
Continuous IV infusion:
   Infant and child: 0.1 mg/kg IV bolus followed by 0.05—0.4 mg/kg/hr infusion and titrate to effect
   Adult: 40—100 mg IV bolus followed by 10—40 mg/hr infusion and titrate to effect

Contraindicated in anuria and hepatic coma. **Use with caution** in hepatic disease (hepatic
   encephalopathy has been reported); cirrhotic patients may require higher than usual doses.
   Ototoxicity may occur in presence of renal disease (especially when used with aminoglycosides and
   other nephrotoxic drugs), with rapid IV injection (do not infuse >4 mg/min in adults), or with
   hypoproteinemia. May cause hypokalemia, alkalosis, dehydration, hyperuricemia, and increased
   calcium excretion. Rash with eosinophilia and systemic symptoms and acute generalized
   exanthematous pustulosis have been reported. Prolonged use in premature infants and in children
   <4 yr may result in nephrocalcinosis. May increase risk for PDA in premature infants during the first
   week of life. Premature infants <31 wk post conceptual age receiving doses >1 mg/kg/24 hr may
   develop plasma levels that could be associated with potential ototoxicity.
Furosemide-resistant edema in pediatric patients may benefit with the addition of metolazone. Some
   of these patients may have an exaggerated response leading to hypovolemia, tachycardia, and
   orthostatic hypotension requiring fluid replacement. Severe hypokalemia has been reported with a
   tendency for diuresis persisting for up to 24 hr after discontinuing metolazone, prolonged use of
   laxatives, or concomitant use of corticosteroids, ACTH, and large amounts of licorice.
High doses of furosemide may inhibit binding of thyroid hormones to carrier proteins and result in
   transient increase in free thyroid hormones followed by an overall decrease in total thyroid hormone
   levels.
Max. rate of intermittent IV dose: 0.5 mg/kg/min. For patients receiving ECMO, **do not** administer IV
   doses directly into the ECMO circuit as the medication is absorbed in the circuit, which may result in
   diminished effects and the need for higher doses.
Pregnancy category changes to "D" if used in pregnancy-induced hypertension.

G

GABAPENTIN
Neurontin, Gralise, Horizant, and generics
Anticonvulsant

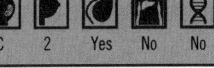
C   2   Yes   No   No

Caps: 100, 300, 400 mg
Tabs: 300, 600, 800 mg
Slow release/extended release tabs (these dosage forms are **not interchangeable** with other
gabapentin products due to different pharmacokinetic profiles affecting the dosing interval; see
specific product information for specific indications for use and dosage):
Gralise: 300, 600 mg
Horizant (Gabapentin Enacarbil): 300, 600 mg
Oral solution: 250 mg/5 mL (470 mL)

Seizures, adjunctive therapy (maximum time between doses should not exceed 12 hr):
  3—<12 yr (PO, see remarks):
    Day 1: 10—15 mg/kg/24 hr ÷ TID, then gradually titrate dose upward to the following
      dosages over a 3-day period:
      3—4 yr: 40 mg/kg/24 hr ÷ TID
      ≥5—<12 yr: 25—35 mg/kg/24 hr ÷ TID
      Dosages up to 50 mg/kg/24 hr have been well tolerated.
  ≥12 yr and adult (PO, see remarks): Start with 300 mg TID; if needed, increase dose up to 1800 mg/
    24 hr ÷ TID. Usual effective doses: 900—1800 mg/24 hr ÷ TID. Doses as high as 3.6 g/24 hr have
    been tolerated.
Neuropathic pain (see remarks):
  Child (PO; limited data):
    Day 1: 5 mg/kg/dose (**max.** 300 mg/dose) at bedtime
    Day 2: 5 mg/kg/dose (**max.** 300 mg/dose) BID
    Day 3: 5 mg/kg/dose (**max.** 300 mg/dose) TID; then titrate dose to effect with TID schedule. A
      dosage range of 8—35 mg/kg/24 hr ÷ TID has been reported in patients taking concurrent
      analgesics.
    Maximum daily dose of 3600 mg/24 hr has been suggested but not formally evaluated.
  Adult (PO):
    Day 1: 300 mg at bedtime
    Day 2: 300 mg BID
    Day 3: 300 mg TID; then titrate dose to effect with TID schedule. Usual dosage range: 1800—2400
      mg/24 hr; **max. dose:** 3600 mg/24 hr
    Postherpetic neuralgia: The above dosage regimen may be titrated up PRN for pain relief to a daily
      dose of 1800 mg/24 hr ÷ TID (efficacy has been shown from 1800 to 3600 mg/24 hr; however, no
      additional benefit has been shown for doses >1800 mg/24 hr). The Gralise dosage form is designed
      for once-daily administration with the evening meals, whereas the Horizant dosage form is
      dosed once daily—BID. These slow release/extended release dosage forms are NOT interchangeable
      due to different pharmacokinetic profiles. See specific product information for details.

Generally used as adjunctive therapy for partial and secondary generalized seizures, and
neuropathic pain.
Somnolence, dizziness, ataxia, fatigue, and nystagmus were common when used for seizures (≥12 yr).
Viral infections, fever, nausea and/or vomiting, somnolence, and hostility have been reported in
patients 3—12 yr receiving other antiepileptics. Dizziness, somnolence, and peripheral edema are

Continued

GABAPENTIN *continued*

common side effects in adults with postherpetic neuralgia. Suicidal behavior or ideation, agitation, and multiorgan hypersensitivity (e.g., anaphylaxis, angioedema, or drug reaction with eosinophilia and systemic symptoms [DRESS]) have been reported. Life-threatening or fatal respiratory depression in patients taking gabapentin with opioids or other CNS depressants, or with an underlying respiratory impairment, has been reported.

Do not withdraw medication abruptly (gradually over a minimum of 1 wk). Drug is not metabolized by the liver and is primarily excreted in the urine unchanged. Higher doses may be required for children <5 yr because of faster clearance in this age group.

May be taken with or without food. In TID dosing schedule, **interval between doses should not exceed 12 hr. Adjust dose in renal impairment (see Chapter 31).**

GANCICLOVIR
Cytovene, Zirgan, and generics
Antiviral agent

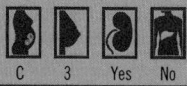

C   3   Yes   No   No

Injection (Cytovene and generics): 500 mg; contains 4 mEq Na per 1 g drug
Injection in solution: 500 mg/10 mL (10 mL)
Premixed injection in 0.8% sodium chloride: 500 mg/250 mL (250 mL); preservative free
Ophthalmic gel (drops):
  Zirgan: 0.15% (5 g); contains benzalkonium chloride

Cytomegalovirus (CMV) infections:
  Neonate (congenital CMV): 12 mg/kg/24 hr ÷ Q12 hr IV with transition to oral
    valganciclovir to complete a total 6 mo course
  Child >3 mo and adult:
    Induction therapy (duration 14–21 days): 10 mg/kg/24 hr ÷ Q12 hr IV
    IV maintenance therapy: 5 mg/kg/dose once daily IV for 7 days/wk or 6 mg/kg/dose once daily IV for
      5 days/wk
Prevention of CMV in transplant recipients:
  Child and adult:
    Induction therapy (duration 5–7 days): 10 mg/kg/24 hr ÷ Q12 hr IV
    IV maintenance therapy: 5 mg/kg/dose once daily IV for 7 days/wk or 6 mg/kg/dose once daily IV for
      5 days/wk for 100–120 days posttransplant
**CMV in HIV-infected individuals: See www.aidsinfo.nih.gov for latest recommendations and
  guidelines for CMV treatment and prophylaxis.**
Herpetic keratitis (ophthalmic gel/drops):
  ≥2 yr and adult: Apply 1 drop onto affected eye(s) 5 times a day (∼Q3 hr while awake) until corneal
    ulcer is healed, then 1 drop TID × 7 days.

Limited experience with use in children <12 yr old. **Contraindicated** in severe neutropenia (ANC <500/microliter) or severe thrombocytopenia (platelets <25,000/microliter). **Use with extreme caution. Reduce dose in renal failure (see Chapter 31).** Has not been evaluated in hepatic impairment. For oral route of administration, see Valganciclovir.

Common side effects: neutropenia, thrombocytopenia, retinal detachment, and confusion. Drug reactions alleviated with dose reduction or temporary interruption. Ganciclovir may increase didanosine and zidovudine levels, whereas didanosine and zidovudine may decrease ganciclovir levels. Immunosuppressive agents may increase hematologic toxicities. Amphotericin B, cyclosporine, and tacrolimus increase risk for nephrotoxicity. Imipenem/cilastatin may increase risk for seizures. May cause female and male infertility.

Minimum dilution is 10 mg/mL and should be infused IV over ≥1 hr. IM and SC administration are **contraindicated** because of high pH of 11.

GATIFLOXACIN
Zymaxid and generics
Antibiotic, quinolone

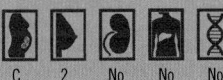

C   2   No   No   No

Ophthalmic solution: 0.5% (2.5 mL); may contain benzalkonium chloride
Previously available as a 0.3% ophthalmic solution (Zymar)

Conjunctivitis:

≥1 yr–adult: Instill 1 drop to affected eye(s) Q2 hr while awake (up to 8 times/24 hr) for the
first day, then 1 drop BID–QID while awake on days 2–7.

Worsening of conjunctivitis, decreased visual acuity, excessive tear production, and keratitis
are common side effects. Conjunctival hemorrhage has been reported.

Avoid touching the applicator tip to eye, fingers, or other surfaces, and **do not** wear contact lenses
during treatment of ocular infections. Apply pressure to the lacrimal sac during and for 1–2 min
after dose administration to reduce risk of systemic absorption.

GCSF

See Filgrastim.

GENTAMICIN
Gentak and generics; previously available as
Garamycin
Antibiotic, aminoglycoside

   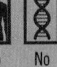

C/D   2   Yes   No   No

Injection: 10 mg/mL (2 mL, preservative free), 40 mg/mL (2, 20 mL); some products may contain
sodium metabisulfite
Premixed injection in NS: 60 mg (50 mL), 80 mg (50, 100 mL), 100 mg (50, 100 mL), 120 mg (100 mL)
Ophthalmic ointment (Gentak and generics): 0.3% (3.5 g); may contain parabens
Ophthalmic drops: 0.3% (5 mL)
Topical ointment: 0.1% (15, 30 g)
Topical cream: 0.1% (15, 30 g)

**Initial empiric dosage; patient-specific dosage defined by therapeutic drug monitoring
(see remarks).**

Parenteral (IM or IV):
Neonate/Infant (see table below):

Postconceptional Age (wk)	Postnatal Age (days)	Dose (mg/kg/dose)	Interval (hr)
≤29[a]	0–7	5	48
	8–28	4	36
	>28	4	24
30–34	0–7	4.5	36
	>7	4	24
≥35	ALL	4	24[b]

[a]Or significant asphyxia, patent ductus arteriosus (PDA), indomethacin use, poor cardiac output, reduced renal function.
Alternatively, dosing by levels may be necessary for situations of unstable renal function.
[b]Use Q36 hr interval for hypoxic-ischemic encephalopathy (HIE) patients receiving whole-body therapeutic cooling.

Continued

GENTAMICIN *continued*

Child (eGFR >75 mL/min/1.73m²): 7.5 mg/kg/24 hr ÷ Q8 hr
Adult (eGFR >75 mL/min/1.73m²): 3—6 mg/kg/24 hr ÷ Q8 hr
Cystic fibrosis (eGFR >75 mL/min/1.73m²): 7.5—10.5 mg/kg/24 hr ÷ Q8 hr
Intrathecal/intraventricular (use preservative-free product only):
  Newborn: 1 mg once daily
  >3 mo: 1—2 mg once daily
  Adult: 4—8 mg once daily
Ophthalmic ointment: Apply 0.5-inch ribbon to the conjunctival sac of the affected eye(s) Q8—12 hr.
Ophthalmic drops: Instill 1—2 drops to affected eye(s) Q4 hr; up to 2 drops Q1 hr for severe infections.
Topical cream or ointment:
  >1 yr and adult: Apply to affected area TID—QID.

Use with caution in patients receiving anesthetics or neuromuscular blocking agents and in patients with neuromuscular disorders. May cause nephrotoxicity and ototoxicity. Ototoxicity may be potentiated with the use of loop diuretics. Eliminated more quickly in patients with cystic fibrosis, neutropenia, and burns. **Adjust dose in renal failure (see Chapter 31).** Monitor peak and trough levels.

Therapeutic peak levels are 6—10 mg/L in general, and 8—10 mg/L in pulmonary infections, cystic fibrosis, neutropenia, osteomyelitis, and severe sepsis.

To maximize bactericidal effects, an individualized peak concentration to target a peak/minimal inhibitory concentration (MIC) ratio of 8—10:1 may be applied.

Therapeutic trough levels: <2 mg/L. Recommended serum sampling time at steady state: trough within 30 min prior to the 3rd consecutive dose and peak 30—60 min after the administration of the 3rd consecutive dose.

For initial dosing in obese patients, use an adjusted body weight (ABW). ABW = Ideal Body Weight + 0.4 (Total Body Weight − Ideal Body Weight)

Pregnancy category is a "C" for ophthalmic use, a "D" with IV use, and not classified for topical use.

GLUCAGON HCL
GlucaGen, Glucagon Emergency Kit, Gvoke,
Baqsimi, and generics
Antihypoglycemic agent

B   1   No   No   No

Injection: 1 mg vial (requires reconstitution)
Injection kit:
  GlucaGen Hypokit and generics: 1 mg vial with 1 mL syringe of sterile water for injection
  Gvoke Kit: 1 mg/0.2 mL vial with syringe; for subcutaneous injection only
Injection in prefilled syringe (Gvoke PFS): 0.5 mg/0.1 mL (1 or 2 pack), 1 mg/0.2 mL (1 or 2 pack); for subcutaneous injection only
Injection in autoinjector (Gvoke HypoPen): 0.5 mg/0.1 mL (1 or 2 pack), 1 mg/0.2 mL (1 or 2 pack); for subcutaneous injection only
Nasal powder (Baqsimi): 3 mg/dose (1 or 2 pack); contains betadex and dodecylphosphocholine
1 unit = 1 mg

Hypoglycemia (see remarks):
  Injectable route (IM, IV, SC; see remarks):
    Neonate, infant, and child <20 kg: 0.5 mg/dose (or 0.02—0.03 mg/kg/dose) Q15—20 min PRN
    Child ≥20 kg and adult: 1 mg/dose Q15—20 min PRN
  Intranasal route (see remarks):
    ≥4 yr and adult: Actuate 3 mg (1 actuation) intranasally into one nostril × 1. If no response after 15 min, an additional 3 mg dose may be given.

GLUCAGON HCL *continued*

β-blocker or calcium channel blocker overdose (for hypotension that is unresponsive to fluid boluses; limited data):
    Infant and child: Load with 0.05 mg/kg IV × 1; if no response, may repeat dose. Some recommend initiating a continuous IV infusion of 0.05–0.1 mg/kg/hr at the time of the responsive dose.
    Adolescent: Loading dose of 5–10 mg IV × 1, followed by a continuous IV infusion of 1–5 mg/hr

Contraindicated in insulinoma, pheochromocytoma, glucagonoma, and history of hypersensitivity to glucagon and components. Drug product is genetically engineered and identical to human glucagon. High doses have a cardiac stimulatory effect and have been used with some success in β-blocker and calcium channel blocker overdose. May increase myocardial oxygen demand, blood pressure, and pulse, which may be life-threatening in patients with cardiac disease. May cause nausea, vomiting, urticaria, and respiratory distress. Necrolytic migratory erythema (NME) has been reported with continuous IV infusion; assess benefit/risk for continued use.

Do not delay glucose infusion; dose for hypoglycemia is 2–4 mL/kg of dextrose 25%.

Glucagon may increase the effects/toxicity of warfarin. Indomethacin use may decrease the effects of glucagon.

Sufficient hepatic glycogen is necessary for effect; patients in states of starvation, with adrenal or chronic hypoglycemia, may not have adequate levels of glycogen. Onset of action: IM: 8–10 min; SC: ~10 min; IV: 1 min. Duration of action: IM: 12–27 min; SC: up to 90 min; IV: 9–17 min.

INTRANASAL USE: See product information for dose administration instructions. Dose does not need to be inhaled and can be administered if the patient has nasal congestion or the common cold. Common side effects include nausea, vomiting, headache, rhinorrhea, nasal discomfort/congestion, cough, epistaxis, and irritation to the eyes, nose, and throat. In type 1 pediatric diabetes trials, the time to increase glucose ≥20 mg/dL from nadir was 11–15 min, and peak plasma levels were achieved in 15–20 min with a median $T_{1/2}$ of 21–31 min.

GLYCERIN
Pedia-Lax, Fleet Liquid Glycerin Supp, and
others, including generics
Osmotic laxative

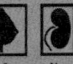 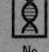
C   ?   No   No   No

Rectal liquid suppository [OTC]:
    Pedia-Lax: 4 mL with average 2.7 mL (2.8 g) dose delivered (6s)
    Fleet Liquid Glycerin: 7.5 mL with average 5.4 mL (5.4 g) dose delivered (4s)
Suppository [OTC]:
    Infant/pediatric:
        Pedia-Lax and generics: 1 g (12s)
        Generics: 1.2 g (12s, 25s)
    Adult:
        Generics: 2 g (12s, 25s, 50s, 100s)

Constipation:
    Neonate: 0.5 mL/kg/dose rectal solution PR as an enema once daily PRN or sliver/chip of infant/pediatric suppository PR once daily PRN
    Child <6 yr: 2–5 mL rectal solution PR as an enema or 1 infant/pediatric suppository PR once daily PRN
    >6 yr–adult: 5–15 mL rectal solution PR as an enema or 1 adult suppository PR once daily PRN

Continued

GLYCERIN *continued*

Onset of action: 15—30 min. May cause rectal irritation, abdominal pain, bloating, and dizziness. Insert suppository high into rectum and retain for 15 min.

GLYCOPYRROLATE
Robinul, Glycate, Glyrx-PF, Cuvposa, and generics
Anticholinergic agent

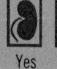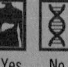

B/C   3   Yes   Yes   No

Tabs (Robinul, Glycate, and generics): 1, 1.5, 2 mg
Oral solution (Cuvposa and generics): 1 mg/5 mL (473 mL); contains propylene glycol and parabens
Injection (Glyrx-PF and generics): 0.2 mg/mL (1, 2, 5, 20 mL); some multidose vials contain 0.9% benzyl alcohol

Respiratory antisecretory:
  IM/IV:
    Child: 0.004—0.01 mg/kg/dose TID—QID
    Adult: 0.1—0.2 mg/dose TID—QID
    Max. dose: 0.2 mg/dose or 0.8 mg/24 hr
  Oral:
    Child: 0.04—0.1 mg/kg/dose TID—QID
    Alternative dosage for 3—16 yr old with chronic severe drooling secondary to neurologic conditions: Start with 0.02 mg/kg/dose PO TID and titrate in increments of 0.02 mg/kg/dose every 5—7 days as needed and tolerated up to a **max. dose** of 0.1 mg/kg/dose TID not to exceed 1.5—3 mg/dose.
    Adult: 1—2 mg/dose BID—TID
Reverse neuromuscular blockade:
  Child and adult: 0.2 mg IV for every 1 mg neostigmine or 5 mg pyridostigmine

Use with caution in hepatic and renal disease, ulcerative colitis, asthma, glaucoma, ileus, or urinary retention. Atropine-like side effects: tachycardia, nausea, constipation, confusion, blurred vision, and dry mouth. These may be potentiated if given with other drugs with anticholinergic properties.
Onset of action: PO: within 1 hr; IM/SC: 15—30 min; IV: 1 min. Duration of antisialagogue effect: PO: 8—12 hr; IM/SC/IV: 7 hr. Oral doses should be administered 1 hr before and 2 hr after meals.
Pregnancy category is "B" for the injection and tablet dosage forms and "C" for the oral solution.

GRANISETRON
Sancuso, Sustol, and generics; previously available as Kytril
Antiemetic agent, 5-HT$_3$ antagonist

B   ?   No   Yes   No

Injection: 1 mg/mL (1, 4 mL); 4 mL multidose vials contain benzyl alcohol
Prefilled syringe for subcutaneous extended release injection (Sustol): 10 mg/0.4 mL (0.4 mL); contains polyethylene glycol
Tabs: 1 mg
Oral suspension: 0.2 mg/mL , 50 mCg/mL
Transdermal patch (Sancuso): 3.1 mg/24 hr

Chemotherapy-induced nausea and vomiting prevention (used in combination with dexamethasone):

GRANISETRON *continued*

IV:
> **Child ≥2 yr and adult:** 10—20 mCg/kg/dose 15—60 min before chemotherapy; the same dose may be repeated 2—3 times at ≥10-min intervals following chemotherapy (within 24 hr after chemotherapy) as a treatment regimen. **Max. dose:** 3 mg/dose or 9 mg/24 hr. Alternatively, a single 40 mCg/kg/dose 15—60 min before chemotherapy has been used.

SC (Sustol, extended release):
> **Adult:** 10 mg at least 30 min prior to first dose of moderately emetogenic chemotherapy. **Do not** administer more frequently than Q7 days.

PO:
> **Infant, child, and adolescent:** 40 mCg/kg/dose BID is recommended for moderately or low emetogenic chemotherapy; initiate first dose 1 hr prior to chemotherapy
> **Adult:** 2 mg/24 hr ÷ once daily—BID; initiate first dose 1 hr prior to chemotherapy

Postoperative nausea and vomiting prevention (dosed prior to anesthesia or immediately before anesthesia reversal) and treatment (IV; see remarks):
> **Adult:** 1 mg × 1

Radiation-induced nausea and vomiting prevention:
> **Adult:** 2 mg once daily PO administered within 1 hr of radiation

Transdermal patch (see remarks):
> **Prophylaxis for chemotherapy-induced nausea and vomiting (adult):** Apply 1 patch 24—48 hr prior to chemotherapy. Patch removal at a minimum of 24 hr after completion of chemotherapy. Patch may be worn up to 7 days, depending on the chemotherapy regimen duration.

Use with caution in liver disease, recent abdominal surgery, and preexisting cardiac conduction disorders and arrhythmias. May cause hypertension, hypotension, progressive ileus, gastric distention, arrhythmias, agitation, and insomnia. QT prolongation has been reported. Inducers or inhibitors of the CYP 450 3A3/4 drug metabolizing enzymes may increase or decrease, respectively, the drug's clearance. Serotonin syndrome has been reported with concomitant use of 5-HT3 antagonists and other serotonergic drugs.

Safety and efficacy in pediatric patients for the prevention of postoperative nausea and vomiting have not been established due to lack of efficacy and QT prolongation in a prospective multicenter, randomized double-blinded trial in 157 patients aged 2—16 yr.

Avoid external heat sources (e.g., heating pads) on and around the transdermal patch dosage form as heat may increase the rate of drug release. Application site reactions of pain, pruritus, rash, irritation, vesicles, and discoloration have been reported with transdermal patch use. Covering the application site of the transdermal system with clothing (while wearing the patch and 10 days following removal) is recommended to prevent potential phototoxic skin reactions.

Onset of action: IV: 4—10 min. Duration of action: IV: ≤24 hr.

GRISEOFULVIN
Microsize: Generics; previously available as Grifulvin V, Griseofulvin Microsize
Ultramicrosize: Generics; previously available as Gris-PEG
Antifungal agent

    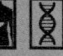

| X | 3 | No | Yes | No |

Microsize:
> **Tabs:** 250, 500 mg
> **Oral suspension:** 125 mg/5 mL (120 mL); contains 0.2% alcohol, parabens, and propylene glycol

Ultramicrosize:

Continued

GRISEOFULVIN *continued*

Tabs: 125, 250 mg
250 mg ultramicrosize is approximately 500 mg microsize.

Microsize:
   Child >2 yr and adolescent: 20—25 mg/kg/24 hr PO ÷ once daily—BID; give with milk,
   eggs, fatty foods
   Adult: 500—1000 mg/24 hr PO ÷ once daily—BID
   Max. dose (all ages): 1 g/24 hr
Ultramicrosize:
   Child >2 yr and adolescent: 10—15 mg/kg/24 hr PO ÷ once daily—BID
   Adult: 375 mg/dose PO once daily or BID
   Max. dose (all ages): 750 mg/24 hr

Contraindicated in porphyria, pregnancy, and hepatic disease. Monitor hematologic, renal, and
hepatic function. May cause leukopenia, rash, headache, paresthesias, and GI symptoms.
Severe skin reactions (e.g., Stevens-Johnson, TEN), erythema multiforme, LFT elevations (AST, ALT,
bilirubin), and jaundice have been reported. Possible cross-reactivity in penicillin-allergic patients.
Usual treatment period is 8 wk for tinea capitis and 4—6 mo for tinea unguium. Photosensitivity
reactions may occur. May reduce effectiveness or decrease level of oral contraceptives, warfarin,
and cyclosporine. Induces CYP 450 1A2 isoenzyme. Phenobarbital may enhance clearance of
griseofulvin. Coadministration with fatty meals will increase the drug's absorption.

GUANFACINE
Intuniv and generics
α_2 *adenergic agonist*

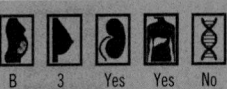

| B | 3 | Yes | Yes | No |

Tabs: 1, 2 mg
Extended release tabs (Intuniv and generics): 1, 2, 3, 4 mg

Attention-deficit hyperactivity disorder (see remarks):
Immediate release tab:
   ≥6 yr and adolescent:
      ≤45 kg: Start at 0.5 mg QHS; if needed and tolerated, increase dose every 3—4 days at 0.5 mg/24
      hr increments by increasing the dosing frequency to BID, TID, QID. **Max. dose:** 27—40.5 kg: 2
      mg/24 hr and 40.5—45 kg: 3 mg/24 hr
      >45 kg: Start at 1 mg QHS; if needed and tolerated, increase dose every 3—4 days at 1 mg/24 hr
      increments by increasing the dosing frequency to BID, TID, QID. **Max. dose:** 4 mg/24 hr
Extended release tab:
   6—17 yr: Start at 1 mg Q24 hr; if needed and tolerated, increase dose no more than 1 mg per week
   up to the **max. dose** of 4 mg/24 hr for 6—12 yr and 7 mg/24 hr for 13—17 yr.
Use with strong CYP 450 3A4 inhibitors or inducers:

CYP 450 3A4 Characteristic	Adding Guanfacine With Respective CYP 450 3A4 Inducer/Inhibitor Already on Board	Adding Respective CYP 450 3A4 Inducer/Inhibitor With Guanfacine Already on Board
Strong inducer (e.g., carbamazepine, phenytoin, rifampin, St. John's wort)	Guanfacine may be titrated up to double the recommended target dose.	Consider increasing guanfacine dose up to double the recommended target dose over 1—2 wk

GUANFACINE *continued*

CYP 450 3A4 Characteristic	Adding Guanfacine With Respective CYP 450 3A4 Inducer/Inhibitor Already on Board	Adding Respective CYP 450 3A4 Inducer/Inhibitor With Guanfacine Already on Board
		as tolerated. If the strong inducer is discontinued, decrease guanfacine dose to target dose over 1—2 wk.
Strong inhibitor (e.g., clarithromycin, azole antifungals)	Decrease guanfacine dose to 50% of recommended target dose.	Decrease guanfacine dose to 50% of recommended target dose. If the strong inhibitor is discontinued, increase guanficine dose to recommended target dose.

Use with caution in patients at risk for hypotension, bradycardia, heart block, and syncope. A dose-dependent hypotension and bradycardia may occur. Somnolence, fatigue, insomnia, dizziness, and abdominal pain are common side effects. Orthostatic hypotension, hallucinations, syncope, and erectile dysfunction have been reported.

Drug is a substrate for CYP 450 3A4. See dosing section for dosage adjustment with inhibitors and inducers.

Do not abruptly discontinue therapy (may cause rebound hypertension); taper of no more than 1 mg Q3—7 days has been recommended. Dose reductions may be required with clinically significant renal or hepatic impairment. When converting from an immediate release tab to the extended release tab, **do not** covert on a mg per mg basis (due to differences in pharmacokinetic profiles) but discontinue the immediate release and titrate with the extended release product using the recommended dosing schedules.

H

HALOPERIDOL
Haldol, Haldol Decanoate, and generics
Antipsychotic agent

    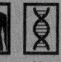

C   3   Yes   Yes   Yes

Injection (IM use only):
Lactate: 5 mg/mL (1, 10 mL)
Decanoate (long acting): 50, 100 mg/mL (1, 5 mL); in sesame oil with 1.2% benzyl alcohol
Tabs: 0.5, 1, 2, 5, 10, 20 mg
Oral solution: 2 mg/mL (15, 120 mL)

Child 3—12 yr (limited data; see remarks):
PO: Initial dose at 0.5 mg/24 hr ÷ BID—TID. If necessary, increase daily dosage by 0.25—0.5 mg/24 hr Q5—7 days PRN. Benefits are not to be expected for doses beyond 6 mg/24 hr. Usual maintenance doses for specific indications include the following:
Agitation: 0.01—0.03 mg/kg/24 hr once daily PO
Psychosis: 0.05—0.15 mg/kg/24 hr ÷ BID—TID PO

Continued

HALOPERIDOL *continued*

Tourette's syndrome: 0.05—0.075 mg/kg/24 hr ÷ BID—TID PO; may increase daily dose by 0.5 mg Q5—7 days

IM, as lactate, for 6—12 yr: 1—3 mg/dose Q4—8 hr; **max. dose:** 0.15 mg/kg/24 hr

>12 yr (limited data):

Acute agitation: 2—5 mg/dose IM as lactate or 1—15 mg/dose PO; repeat in 1 hr PRN

Psychosis: 2—5 mg/dose Q4—8 hr IM PRN or 1—15 mg/24 hr ÷ BID—TID PO

Tourette's syndrome: 0.5—2 mg/dose BID—TID PO; 3—5 mg/dose BID—TID PO may be used for severe symptoms

Contraindicated in severe toxic CNS depression, comas, Parkinson disease, and dementia Lewy bodies. **Use with caution** in patients with cardiac disease (risk of hypotension), cerebrovascular adverse reaction risk, renal or hepatic dysfunction, thyrotoxicosis, and in patients with epilepsy since the drug lowers the seizure threshold. Extrapyramidal symptoms, drowsiness, headache, tachycardia, ECG changes, nausea, and vomiting can occur. Higher-than-recommended doses are associated with a higher risk of QT prolongation and torsades de pointes. Leukopenia/ neutropenia, including agranulocytosis and rhabdomyolysis (IM route), and transient dyskinetic signs (following abrupt withdrawal from maintenance therapies) have been reported.

Drug is metabolized by CYP 450 1A2, 2D6, and 3A3/4 isoenzymes. May also inhibit CYP 450 2D6 and 3A3/4 isoenzymes. Serotonin-specific reuptake inhibitors (e.g., fluoxetine) may increase levels and effects of haloperidol. Carbamazepine and phenobarbital may decrease levels and effects of haloperidol. Monitor for encephalopathic syndrome when used in combination with lithium.

For poor metabolizers of CYP 450 2D6, consider a 50% reduction of initial dose and titrate to response, OR use an alternative medication not metabolized by this enzyme system.

Acutely aggravated patients may require doses as often as Q60 min. **Decanoate salt is given every 3—4 wk in doses that are 10—15 times the individual patient's stabilized oral dose.**

HEPARIN SODIUM Various generics ***Anticoagulant***	 C · · · 1 · · · No · · · Yes · · · No

Injection:

Porcine intestinal mucosa: 1000, 5000, 10,000, 20,000 U/mL (some products may be preservative free; multidosed vials contain benzyl alcohol)

Lock flush solution (porcine based): 10, 100 U/mL (some products may be preservative free or contain benzyl alcohol)

Injection for IV infusion (porcine based):

D_5W: 40 U/mL (500 mL), 50 U/mL (250, 500 mL), 100 U/mL (100, 250 mL); contains bisulfite

NS (0.9% NaCl): 2 U/mL (500, 1000 mL)

0.45% NaCl: 50 U/mL (250, 500 mL), 100 U/mL (250 mL); contains EDTA

120 U = approximately 1 mg

Anticoagulation empiric dosage:

Continuous IV infusion (initial doses for goal unfractionated heparin [UFH] anti-Xa level of 0.3—0.7 units/mL):

Age	Loading Dose (IV)[a]	Initial IV infusion Rate (units/kg/hr)
Neonate and infant <1 yr	75 U/kg IV	28
Child age 1—18 yr	75 U/kg IV (max. dose: 8000 U)	20 (max. initial rate: 1650 U/hr)
>18 yr	70 U/kg IV (max. dose: 8000 U)	18 (max. initial rate: 1650 U/hr)

[a]Do not give loading dose for patients with stroke or significant bleeding risk and obtain aPPT 4 hr after loading dose.

HEPARIN SODIUM *continued*

DVT or PE prophylaxis:
  Adult: 5000 U/dose SC Q8—12 hr until ambulatory
Heparin flush (doses should be less than heparinizing dose):
  Younger child: Lower doses should be used to avoid systemic heparinization.
  Older child and adult:
    Peripheral IV: 1—2 mL of 10 U/mL solution Q4 hr
    Central lines: 2—3 mL of 100 U/mL solution Q24 hr
    TPN (central line) and arterial line: Add heparin to make final concentration of 0.5—1 U/mL.

Contraindicated in active major bleeding, known or suspected HIT, and concurrent epidural
  therapy. **Use with caution** if platelets <50,000/mm^3. **Avoid** IM injections and other
  medications affecting platelet function (e.g., NSAIDs and ASA). Toxicities include bleeding,
  allergy, alopecia, and thrombocytopenia. May increase serum aminotransferases (AST and ALT).
Adjust dose with one of the following laboratory goals:
  Unfractionated heparin (UFH) anti-Xa level: 0.3—0.7 units/mL
  aPTT level (reagent specific to reflect anti-Xa level of 0.3—0.7 units/mL): 50—80 sec
These laboratory measurements are best measured 4—6 hr after initiation or changes in infusion rate.
  Do not collect blood levels from the heparinized line or same extremity as site of heparin infusion. If
  unfractionated heparin anti-Xa or aPTT levels are not available, a ratio of aPPT 1.5—2.5 times
  control value has been used in the past. Unfractionated heparin anti-Xa level is NOT THE SAME as
  low-molecular-weight heparin anti-Xa (used for monitoring low-molecular-weight heparin products
  such as enoxaparin).
Use with IV nitroglycerin may decrease the partial thromboplastin time (PTT) with subsequent rebound
  upon discontinuation of nitroglycerin. Antithrombin III (human) and NSAIDs may increase heparin's
  anticoagulant effects and bleeding risk.
Use preservative-free heparin in neonates. **Note:** Heparin flush doses may alter aPTT in smaller
  patients; consider using more dilute heparin in these cases. Multiple strengths of heparin exist, and
  do not use the more concentrated injectable product as flushes.
Use actual body weight when dosing obese patients. Due to recent regulatory changes to the
  manufacturing process, heparin products may exhibit decreased potency.
Antidote: Protamine sulfate (1 mg per 100 U heparin in previous 4 hr). For low-molecular-weight
  heparin (LMWH), see Enoxaparin.

HYALURONIDASE
Amphadase, Hylenex, and Vitrase
Antidote, extravasation
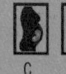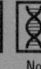
C ? No No No

Injection:
  Amphadase: 150 U/mL (1 mL); bovine source; contains edetate disodium and thimerosal
  Hylenex: 150 U/mL (1 mL); recombinant human source; contains 1 mg albumin, 1.5 mg L-methionine,
    and 0.2 mg polysorbate 80 per 150 U
  Vitrase: 200 U/mL (1.2 mL); ovine source containing lactose, preservative free
  Pharmacy can make a 15 U/mL dilution.

Extravasation:
  Infant and child: Give 1 mL (150 U) by injecting 5 separate injections of 0.2 mL (30 U) at
    borders of extravasation site SC or intradermal using a 25- or 26-gauge needle. Alternatively, a
    diluted 15 U/mL concentration has been used with the same dosing instructions.

Continued

HYALURONIDASE *continued*

Contraindicated in dopamine and alpha-agonist extravasation and hypersensitivity to the respective product sources (bovine or ovine). May cause urticaria. Patients receiving large amounts of salicylates, cortisone, ACTH, estrogens, or antihistamines may decrease the effects of hyaluronidase (larger doses may be necessary). Administer as early as possible (minutes to 1 hr) after IV extravasation.

Hylenex product is chemically incompatible with sodium metabisulfite, furosemide, benzodiazepines, and phenytoin.

HYDRALAZINE HYDROCHLORIDE
Generics; previously available as Apresoline
Antihypertensive, vasodilator

C · 1 · Yes · No · Yes

Tabs: 10, 25, 50, 100 mg
Injection: 20 mg/mL (1 mL)
Oral liquid: 4 mg/mL
Some dosage forms may contain tartrazines or sulfites.

Acute severe hypertension (may result in severe and prolonged hypotension; see Chapter 1, Table 1.7 for alternatives):
  Child: 0.1–0.2 mg/kg/dose IM or IV Q4–6 hr PRN; **max. dose:** 20 mg/dose. Usual IV/IM dosage range is 0.2–0.6 mg/kg/dose Q4–6 hr.
  Adult: 10–20 mg IM or IV Q4–6 hr PRN; may increase to **max. dose** of 40 mg/dose if needed
Chronic hypertension:
  Infant and child: Start at 0.75–1 mg/kg/24 hr PO ÷ Q6–12 hr (**max. initial dose:** 10 mg/dose). If necessary, increase dose over 3–4 wk up to a **max. dose** of 5 mg/kg/24 hr for infants and 7.5 mg/kg/24 hr for children; or 200 mg/24 hr.
  Adult: 10–50 mg/dose PO QID; **max. dose:** 300 mg/24 hr

Use with caution in severe renal and cardiac disease. Slow acetylators, patients receiving high-dose chronic therapy, and those with renal insufficiency are at highest risk of lupus-like syndrome (generally reversible). May cause reflex tachycardia, palpitations, dizziness, headaches, and GI discomfort. MAO inhibitors and β-blockers may increase hypotensive effects. Indomethacin may decrease hypotensive effects.

Drug undergoes first-pass metabolism. Onset of action: PO: 20–30 min; IV: 5–20 min. Duration of action: PO: 2–4 hr; IV: 2–6 hr. **Adjust dose in renal failure (see Chapter 31).**

HYDROCHLOROTHIAZIDE
Generics; previously available as HydroDiuril and Microzide
Diuretic, thiazide

B/D · 2 · Yes · No · No

Tabs: 12.5, 25, 50 mg
Caps: 12.5 mg
Oral suspension: 5 mg/mL, 10 mg/mL

Edema:
  Neonate and infant <6 mo: 1–3 mg/kg/24 hr ÷ once daily–BID PO; **max. dose:** 37.5 mg/24 hr
  ≥6 mo, child, and adolescent: 1–2 mg/kg/24 hr ÷ once daily–BID PO; **max. dose:** <2 yr: 37.5 mg/24 hr, child 2–12 yr: 100 mg/24 hr, and adolescent: 200 mg/24 hr
  Adult: 25–100 mg/24 hr ÷ once daily–BID PO; **max. dose:** 200 mg/24 hr

HYDROCHLOROTHIAZIDE *continued*

Hypertension:
Infant and child: Start at 1—2 mg/kg/24 hr ÷ once daily—BID PO; **max. dose:** <6 mo: 37.5 mg/24 hr,
child ≥6 mo—12 yr: 100 mg/24 hr (37.5 mg/24 hr has been recommended by some experts)
Adult: 12.5—25 mg/dose once daily—BID PO; doses >50 mg/24 hr often result in hypokalemia

See Chlorothiazide. May cause fluid and electrolyte imbalances and hyperuricemia. Drug may
not be effective when creatinine clearance is less than 25—50 mL/min/1.73m^2. Use with
carbamazepine may result in symptomatic hyponatremia.

Hydrochlorothiazide is also available in combination with potassium-sparing diuretics (e.g.,
spironolactone), ACE inhibitors, angiotensin II receptor antagonists, hydralazine, methyldopa,
reserpine, and β-blockers.

Pregnancy category is "D" if used in pregnancy-induced hypertension.

HYDROCORTISONE
Systemic dosage forms: Solu-Cortef, Cortef,
Alkindi Sprinkle, and generics
Topical: Anusol HC, Cortifoam, Cortenema,
MiCort-HC, NuCort, Proctocort, and many others
including generics
Corticosteroid

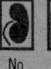 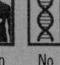

C   2   No   No   No

Hydrocortisone base:
Tabs (Cortef and generics): 5, 10, 20 mg
Oral granules in capsules (Alkindi sprinkle): 0.5, 1, 2, 5 mg
Oral suspension: 2 mg/mL
Rectal cream: 1% (30 g)
Anusol HC and generics: 2.5% (30 g)
Rectal suspension as an enema (Cortenema): 100 mg/60 mL; may contain parabens
Topical ointment: 0.5% [OTC], 1% [OTC], 2.5%
Topical cream: 0.5% [OTC], 1% [OTC], 2.5%
Topical lotion: 1% [OTC], 2%, 2.5%
Na Succinate (Solu-Cortef):
Injection: 100, 250, 500, 1000 mg/vial; contains benzyl alcohol
Acetate:
Topical cream: 1% [OTC]
MiCort-HC: 2.5% (4, 28.4 g); contains parabens
Topical lotion (NuCort): 2% (60 g); contains benzyl alcohol
Suppository:
Anusol HC and generics: 25 mg
Proctocort and generics: 30 mg
Rectal foam aerosol (Cortifoam): 10% (90 mg/dose) (15 g); may contain parabens

Status asthmaticus:
Child:
Load (optional): 4—8 mg/kg/dose IV; **max. dose:** 250 mg
Maintenance: 8 mg/kg/24 hr ÷ Q6 hr IV
Adult: 100—500 mg/dose Q6 hr IV
Physiologic replacement: See Chapter 10 for dosing.
Antiinflammatory/immunosuppressive:
Child:

Continued

HYDROCORTISONE *continued*

> **PO:** 2.5—10 mg/kg/24 hr ÷ Q6—8 hr
> **IM/IV:** 1—5 mg/kg/24 hr ÷ Q12—24 hr
> **Adolescent and adult:**
> > **PO/IM/IV:** 15—240 mg/dose Q12 hr

Acute adrenal insufficiency: See Chapter 10 for dosing.

Topical use:
> **Child and adult:** Apply to affected areas BID—QID, depending on severity and specific indication for use.

Ulcerative colitis, induction for mild/moderate case:
> **Child, adolescent, and adult:** Insert 1 application of 100 mg rectal enema once daily—BID × 2—3 wk.

Hemorrhoids:
> **Adult:**
> > **Rectal cream:** Apply sparingly up to BID with either 1% or 2.5% strength.
> > **Suppository:** 25 or 30 mg PR BID × 2 wk

Use with caution in immunocompromised patients, as they should avoid exposure to chickenpox or measles. Hypertrophic cardiomyopathy has been reported in premature infants.

Alkindi sprinkle product: Administered by sprinkling the capsule's contents directly onto the tongue or mixed with soft food. **DO NOT** swallow capsules. Different hydrocortisone exposure may occur when converting to Alkindi sprinkle from other oral manipulated oral formulations (e.g., split or crushed tabs, compounded formulations).

For potency comparisons of topical preparations, see Chapter 8. For doses based on body surface area, see Chapter 10.

HYDROMORPHONE HCL
Dilaudid and generics
Narcotic, analgesic

   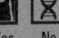

C/D　3　Yes　Yes　No

Tabs: 2, 4, 8 mg
Extended release tabs: 8, 12, 16, 32 mg
Injection: 1, 2, 4 mg/mL (1 mL), 10 mg/mL (1, 5, 50 mL); may be preservative free
Prefilled injectable syringes: 0.2 mg/mL (1 mL), 1 mg/mL (0.5, 1 mL), 2 mg/mL (1 mL)
Suppository: 3 mg (6s)
Oral solution: 1 mg/mL; may contain parabens and metasulfite

Analgesia, initial doses with immediate release dosage forms to opioid-naïve (titrate to effect):
> **Child (<50 kg):**
> > **IV:** 0.015 mg/kg/dose Q3—6 hr PRN
> > **PO:** 0.03—0.08 mg/kg/dose Q3—4 hr PRN; **max. dose:** 5 mg/dose
> **Child and adolescent (≥50 kg; NOTE: doses are NOT weight based):**
> > **IV:** 0.2—0.6 mg/dose Q2—4 hr PRN
> > **IM, SC (not preferred route; absorption is erratic):** 0.8—1 mg/dose Q4—6 hr PRN
> > **PO:** 1—2 mg/dose Q3—4 hr PRN
> > **PR:** 3 mg/dose Q6—8 hr PRN
> **Adult:**
> > **IV:** 0.2—0.5 mg/dose Q2—4 hr PRN
> > **IM, SC (not preferred route; absorption is erratic):** 0.2—0.5 mg/dose Q2—3 hr PRN
> > **PO:** 1—2 mg/dose Q4—6 hr PRN
> > **PR:** 3 mg Q6—8 hr PRN

HYDROMORPHONE HCL *continued*

Refer to Chapter 6 for equianalgesic doses and for patient-controlled analgesia dosing. Less pruritus than morphine. Similar profile of side effects to other narcotics. **Use with caution** in infants and young children, and **do not use** in neonates due to potential CNS effects. Dose reduction recommended in renal insufficiency or severe hepatic impairment. Pregnancy category changes to "D" if used for prolonged periods or in high doses at term.

The FDA has assigned a Risk Evaluation and Mitigation Strategy (REMS) for this medication, which involves an education program for provision of safety information. See www.opioidanalgesicrems.com.

HYDROXYCHLOROQUINE SULFATE
Plaquenil and generics
Antimalarial, antirheumatic agent

   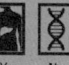

?   2   Yes   Yes   No

Tabs: 200 mg (155 mg base)
Oral suspension: 25 mg/mL (19.375 mg/mL base)

All doses expressed in mg of hydroxychloroquine base.
Malaria prophylaxis (start 2 wk prior to exposure and continue for 4 wk after leaving endemic area):
  Child: 5 mg/kg/dose PO once weekly; **max. dose:** 310 mg
  Adult: 310 mg PO once weekly
Malaria treatment (acute uncomplicated cases):
  For treatment of malaria, consult with ID specialist or see the latest edition of the AAP Red Book.
    Child: 10 mg/kg/dose (**max. dose:** 620 mg) PO × 1 followed by 5 mg/kg/dose (**max. dose:** 310 mg) 6 hr later. Then 5 mg/kg/dose (**max. dose:** 310 mg) Q24 hr × 2 doses starting 24 hr after the first dose.
    Adult: 620 mg PO × 1 followed by 310 mg 6 hr later. Then 310 mg Q24 hr × 2 doses starting 24 hr after the first dose.
Systemic lupus erythematosus (limited data):
  Child: 3.1–5 mg/kg/24 hr (base) PO ÷ once daily–BID; **max. dose:** 310 mg/24 hr

Contraindicated in psoriasis, porphyria, retinal or visual field changes, and 4-aminoquinoline hypersensitivity. **Use with caution** in liver disease, G6PD deficiency, concomitant hepatic toxic drugs, renal impairment, metabolic acidosis, or hematologic disorders. Long-term use in children is **not recommended.** May cause headaches, myopathy, GI disturbances, skin and mucosal pigmentation, agranulocytosis, visual disturbances, and increased digoxin serum levels. Hypoglycemia, cardiomyopathy with phospholipidosis without inflammation, proximal myopathy/ neuropathy, and suicidal behavior have been reported. Baseline ocular exam is recommended within the first year of initiating long-term therapy, as retinal damage has been reported.

Use with aurothioglucose may increase risk for blood dyscrasias. When used in combination with other immunosuppressive agents for SLE and JRA, lower doses of hydroxychloroquine can be used.

Pregnancy category has not been formally assigned by the FDA. The only situation where use is recommended during pregnancy is during the suppression or treatment of malaria, when the benefits outweigh the risks.

HYDROXYZINE
Vistaril and generics
Antihistamine, anxiolytic, antiemetic

   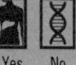

C   3   No   Yes   No

Tabs (HCl salt): 10, 25, 50 mg
Caps (pamoate salt): 25, 50, 100 mg

Continued

HYDROXYZINE *continued*

Oral syrup (HCl salt): 10 mg/5 mL (120, 473 mL); may contain alcohol, parabens, and propylene glycol
Oral solution (HCl salt): 10 mg/5 mL (473 mL); may contain sodium benzoate
Injection for IM use (HCl salt): 25 mg/mL (1 mL), 50 mg/mL (1, 2 mL); may contain benzyl alcohol
NOTE: Pamoate and HCL salts are equivalent in regard to mg of hydroxyzine.

Pruritus and anxiety:
  Oral:
    Child and adolescent: 2 mg/kg/24 hr ÷ Q6—8 hr PRN; **max. single dose:** <6 yr: 12.5 mg, 6—12 yr: 25 mg, and >12 yr: 100 mg
      Alternative dosing by age:
      <6 yr: 50 mg/24 hr ÷ Q6—8 hr PRN
      ≥6 yr: 50—100 mg/24 hr ÷ Q6—8 hr PRN
    Adult: 25—100 mg/dose TID—QID PRN
  IM:
    Child and adolescent: 0.5—1 mg/kg/dose Q4—6 hr PRN; **max. single dose:** 100 mg
    Adult: 25—100 mg/dose Q4—6 hr PRN
Antiemetic (excluding use during pregnancy):
  Child and adolescent: 1.1 mg/kg/dose IM; **max. single dose:** 100 mg
  Adult: 25—100 mg IM

Contraindicated in prolonged QT interval. May potentiate barbiturates, meperidine, and other CNS depressants. **Use with caution** with concomitant use of other medications known to prolong the QT interval. May cause dry mouth, drowsiness, tremor, convulsions, blurred vision, and hypotension. May cause pain at injection site. Fixed drug eruptions have been reported with use of the oral dosage form.
Increase dosage interval to Q24 hr or longer in the presence of liver disease (e.g., primary biliary cirrhosis).
Onset of action within 15—30 min. Duration of action: 4—6 hr. IV administration is **NOT recommended.**

IBUPROFEN
PO: Motrin, Advil, Children's Advil, Children's Motrin, and generics
IV: NeoProfen, Caldolor
Nonsteroidal antiinflammatory agent

C/X   1   Yes   Yes   No

Oral suspension [OTC]: 100 mg/5 mL (120, 240, 473 mL); may contain propylene glycol and sodium benzoate
Oral drops [OTC]: 40 mg/mL (15, 30 mL); may contain sodium benzoate
Chewable tabs [OTC]: 100 mg; contains aspartame
Caplets [OTC]: 100, 200 mg
Tabs: 200 [OTC], 400, 600, 800 mg
Capsules [OTC]: 200 mg
Injection:
  NeoProfen and generic (lysine salt): 10 mg ibuprofen base/1 mL (2 mL); preservative-free
  Caldolor:

IBUPROFEN *continued*

100 mg/mL (8 mL); contains 78 mg/mL arginine
Ready to use: 4 mg/mL (200 mL)

PO:

Infant and child (≥6 mo):

Analgesic/antipyretic: 5—10 mg/kg/dose Q6—8 hr PO; **max. dose:** the lesser of 40 mg/kg/24 hr or 3200 mg/24 hr (analgesic), or 2400 mg/24 hr (antipyretic)

JRA (6 mo—12 yr): 30—50 mg/kg/hr ÷ Q6 hr PO; **max. dose:** 800 mg/dose or 2400 mg/24 hr

Adult:

Inflammatory disease: 400—800 mg/dose Q6—8 hr PO; **max. dose:** 800 mg/dose or 3.2 g/24 hr

Pain/fever/dysmenorrhea: 200—400 mg/dose Q4—6 hr PRN PO; **max. dose:** 3.2 g/24 hr

IV:

6 mo—<12 yr:

Analgesic and antipyretic: 10 mg/kg/dose up to 400 mg/dose Q4—6 hr PRN; **max. dose:** the lesser of 40 mg/kg/24 hr or 2400 mg/24 hr

12—17 yr:

Analgesic and antipyretic: 400 mg/dose Q4—6 hr PRN; **max. dose:** 2400 mg/24 hr

≥18 yr and adult:

Analgesic (see remarks): 400—800 mg/dose Q6 hr PRN; **max. dose:** 3200 mg/24 hr

Antipyretic (see remarks): 400 mg/dose Q4—6 hr or 100—200 mg/dose Q4 hr PRN; **max. dose:** 3200 mg/24 hr

Closure of ductus arteriosus:

<32 wks' gestation and 0.5—1.5 kg (use birth weight to calculate all doses and infuse all doses over 15 min; see remarks): 10 mg/kg/dose IV × 1 followed by two doses of 5 mg/kg/dose each, 24 and 48 hr after the initial dose. Hold second or third dose if urinary output is <0.6 mL/kg/hr; dosing should resume when laboratory studies indicate the return of normal renal function. If the ductus arteriosus fails to close or reopens, a second course of ibuprofen, the use of IV indomethacin, or surgery may be necessary.

Contraindicated with active GI bleeding and ulcer disease. **Use caution** with aspirin hypersensitivity, hepatic/renal insufficiency, heart disease (risk for MI and stroke with prolonged use), or dehydration, and in patients receiving anticoagulants. GI distress (lessened with milk), rashes, ocular problems, hypertension, granulocytopenia, and anemia may occur. Inhibits platelet aggregation. Consumption of more than three alcoholic beverages per day or use with corticosteroids or anticoagulants may increase risk for GI bleeding. False-positive test for urine cannabinoid and phencyclidine (PCP) screen may occur.

May increase serum levels and effects of digoxin, methotrexate, and lithium. May decrease the effects of antihypertensives, aspirin (antiplatelet effects), furosemide, and thiazide diuretics.

Pregnancy category is "C" for prior to 30 wks' gestation and "X" for 30 wk and greater. **Avoid use** at >30 wks' gestation due to increased risk for premature closure of the fetal ductus arteriosus. Limit dose and duration of use at 20—30 wks' gestation for concerns of fetal renal dysfunction and oligohydramnios.

IV USE for analgesia/antipyretic: Hydrate patient well before use. Doses must be diluted to a concentration ≤4 mg/mL with NS, D_5W, or LR and infused over ≥30 min for adults and ≥10 min for children. Most common reported side effects in clinical trials include nausea, flatulence, vomiting, and headache.

IV USE for PDA: Contraindicated in untreated infections, congenital heart diseases requiring a patent ductus arteriosus to facilitate satisfactory pulmonary and systemic blood flow, active intracranial or gastrointestinal bleeds, thrombocytopenia, coagulation defects, suspected/active NEC, and significant renal impairment. **Use with caution** in hyperbilirubinemia. Not indicated for IVH prophylaxis. Renal side effects are generally less frequent and severe when compared with IV indomethacin. NEC, GI perforation, and pulmonary hypertension have been reported. NeoProfen doses must be administered within 30 min of preparation and infused intravenously over 15 min.

ILOPROST
Ventavis, synthetic PGI$_2$
Prostaglandin I$_2$, vasodilator

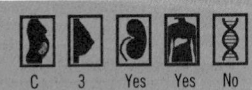

C	3	Yes	Yes	No

Inhalation solution: 10 mCg/mL (1 mL), 20 mCg/mL (1 mL); contains ethanol and tromethamine

Pulmonary arterial hypertension (limited data):
   Intermittent inhalation via nebulization: Start at 2.5 mCg/dose (some recommend
      1.25 mCg/dose for infant and small child). If tolerated, increase dose to 5 mCg/dose at
      intervals of 6 to 9 times daily (Q2–3 hr while awake; Q3–4 hr may be considered for patients
      with moderate/severe hepatic impairment).

Use with caution in bleeding disorders, respiratory diseases, and hypotension.
   Headache, nausea, cough, flu-like symptoms, and flushing are common side effects.
   Bronchospasm, hypotension, and AKI have been reported. May increase the effects/toxicity of
   anticoagulants and antiplatelet, antihypertensive, and vasodilating medications.
Administer by nebulization, which may take 10–15 min. **Avoid** contact with skin or eyes and do not
   ingest by mouth.

IMIPENEM AND CILASTATIN
Primaxin IV and generics
Antibiotic, carbapenem

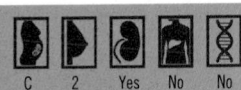

C	2	Yes	No	No

Injection: 250, 500 mg; each 1 mg drug contains 1 mg imipenem and 1 mg cilastatin
Contains 3.2 mEq Na/g drug

Dosages based on imipenem component.
Neonate (see remarks):
   <1 kg:
      ≤14 days old: 40 mg/kg/24 hr ÷ Q12 hr IV
      15–28 days old: 50 mg/kg/24 hr ÷ Q12 hr IV
   1–2 kg:
      ≤7 days old: 40 mg/kg/24 hr ÷ Q12 hr IV
      8–28 days old: 50 mg/kg/24 hr ÷ Q12 hr IV
   >2 kg:
      ≤7 days old: 50 mg/kg/24 hr ÷ Q12 hr IV
      8–28 days old: 75 mg/kg/24 hr ÷ Q8 hr IV
Child (4 wk–3 mo): 100 mg/kg/24 hr ÷ Q6 hr IV
Child (>3 mo): 60–100 mg/kg/24 hr ÷ Q6 hr IV; **max. dose:** 4 g/24 hr
   Cystic fibrosis:
      Pulmonary exacerbation: 100 mg/kg/24 hr ÷ Q6 hr IV; **max. dose:** 4 g/24 hr
      Non-tuberculosis mycobacterium: 30–40 mg/kg/24 hr ÷ Q12 hr IV; **max. dose:** 2 g/24 hr
Adult: 0.5–1 g/dose Q6–8 hr IV; **max. dose:** 4 g/24 hr or 50 mg/kg/24 hr, whichever is less

For IV use, give slowly over 30–60 min at a concentration ≤5 mg/mL to reduce risk for
   nausea (lowering the rate may reduce severity). Adverse effects: thrombophlebitis, pruritus,
   urticaria, GI symptoms, seizures, dizziness, hypotension, elevated LFTs, blood dyscrasias, and
   penicillin allergy. Greater risk for seizures may occur with CNS infections, concomitant use with
   ganciclovir, higher doses, and renal impairment. CSF penetration is variable but best with inflamed
   meninges. Not recommended in CNS infections for neonates due to cilastatin accumulation and
   seizure risk.

IMIPENEM AND CILASTATIN *continued*

Do not administer with probenecid (increases imipenem/cilastatin levels) and ganciclovir (increased risk for seizures). May significantly reduce valproic acid levels.
Adjust dose in renal insufficiency (see Chapter 31).

IMIPRAMINE
Tofranil and generics
Antidepressant, tricyclic

C   2   Yes   Yes   Yes

Tabs (HCl): 10, 25, 50 mg
Caps (pamoate): 75, 100, 125, 150 mg; strengths are expressed as imipramine HCl equivalent

Antidepressant (see remarks):
  Child (≥8 yr):
    Initial: 1.5 mg/kg/24 hr ÷ BID–TID PO; increase 1 mg/kg/24 hr Q3–4 days to a **max. dose** of 5 mg/kg/24 hr
  Adolescent:
    Initial: 25–50 mg/24 hr ÷ once daily–TID PO; **max. dose:** 200 mg/24 hr. Dosages exceeding 100 mg/24 hr are generally not necessary.
  Adult:
    Initial: 75–100 mg/24 hr ÷ TID PO
    Maintenance: 50–300 mg/24 hr QHS PO; **max. dose:** 300 mg/24 hr
Enuresis (≥6 yr):
  Initial: 10–25 mg QHS PO
  Increment if needed: 10–25 mg/dose at 1- to 2-wk intervals until **max. dose** for age or desired effect achieved. Continue × 2–3 mo, then taper slowly.
  Max. dose:
    6–12 yr: The lesser of 2.5 mg/kg/24 hr or 50 mg/24 hr
    ≥12 yr: 75 mg/24 hr
Augment analgesia for chronic pain:
  Initial: 0.2–0.4 mg/kg/dose QHS PO; increase 50% every 2–3 days PRN to a **max. dose** of 1–3 mg/kg/dose QHS PO

Contraindicated in narrow-angle glaucoma and patients who used MAO inhibitors within 14 days. See Chapter 3 for management of toxic ingestion. Monitor for clinical worsening of depression and suicidal ideation/behavior following the initiation of therapy or after dose changes. **Use with caution** in renal or hepatic impairment. Side effects include sedation, urinary retention, constipation, dry mouth, dizziness, drowsiness, and arrhythmia. QHS dosing during first weeks of therapy will reduce sedation. Monitor ECG, BP, CBC at start of therapy and with dose changes. Tricyclics may cause mania. False-positive test for urine PCP screen may occur.

Therapeutic reference range for depression (sum of imipramine and desipramine) = 150–250 ng/mL. Levels >1000 ng/mL are toxic; however, toxicity may occur at >300 ng/mL.

Recommended serum sampling times at steady-state: Obtain trough level within 30 min prior to the next scheduled dose after 5–7 days of continuous therapy.

Imipramine is a major substrate for CYP 450 2C19 and 2D6. See the remarks in amitriptyline for pharmacogenomic dosing considerations. Carbamazepine may reduce imipramine levels, and cimetidine, fluoxetine, fluvoxamine, labetalol, quinidine may increase imipramine levels.

Onset of antidepressant effects: 1–3 wk. **Do not discontinue** abruptly in patients receiving long-term high-dose therapy.

Pregnancy category has not been officially assigned by the FDA as congenital abnormalities have been reported in humans with the causal relationship not being established.

IMMUNE GLOBULIN
Immune globulins

C   ?   Yes   No   No

IM preparations:
   GamaSTAN: 150—180 mg/mL (2, 10 mL); contains 0.16—0.26 M glycine; preservative free
IV preparations in solution (preservative free):
   Asceniv: 10% (100 mg/mL) (50 mL); contains polysorbate 80, 0.2—0.29 M glycine and <200 mCg/mL
      IgA; sucrose free
   Bivigam: 10% (100 mg/mL) (50, 100 mL); contains polysorbate 80, 0.2—0.29 M glycine and <200
      mCg/mL IgA; sucrose free
   Flebogamma DIF:
      5% (50 mg/mL) (10, 50, 100, 200, 400 mL); contains 50 mg/mL sorbitol, ≤3 mg/mL polyethylene
         glycol, and <50 mCg/mL IgA; sucrose free
      10% (100 mg/mL) (50, 100, 200 mL); contains 50 mg/mL sorbitol, ≤6 mg/mL polyethylene glycol
         and <100 mCg/mL IgA; sucrose free
   Gamunex-C: 10% (100 mg/mL) (10, 25, 50, 100, 200, 400 mL); contains 0.16—0.24 M glycine and
      ~46 mCg/mL IgA; sucrose free
   Gammagard liquid: 10% (100 mg/mL) (10, 25, 50, 100, 200, 300 mL); contains 0.25 M glycine and
      ~37 mCg/mL IgA; sucrose free
   Gammaked: 10% (100 mg/mL) (10, 25, 50, 100, 200 mL); contains 0.16—0.24 M glycine and ~46
      mCg/mL IgA; sucrose free
   Gammaplex:
      5% (50 mg/mL) (100, 200, 400 mL); contains polysorbate 80, 50 mg/mL D-sorbitol, 6 mg/mL
         glycine, and <10 mCg/mL IgA; sucrose free
      10% (100 mg/mL) (50, 100, 200 mL); contains polysorbate 80, 2—3 mM/mL glycine, and <20 mCg/
         mL IgA; sucrose free
   Octagam: 5% (50 mg/mL) (20, 50, 100, 200, 500 mL), 10% (100 mg/mL) (20, 50, 100, 200, 300 mL);
      contains ~100 mg/mL maltose and ≤0.2 mg/mL IgA; sucrose free
   Panzyga 10%: (100 mg/mL) (10, 25, 50, 100, 200, 300 mL); contains 15—19.5 mg/mL glycine and
      ~100 mCg/mL IgA; sucrose free
   Privigen 10% (100 mg/mL) (50, 100, 200, 400 mL); contains 210—290 mmol/L L-proline and <25
      mCg/mL IgA; sucrose free
IV preparations in powder for reconstitution (sucrose and preservative free):
   Gammagard S/D: 5, 10 g (when diluted at 5% or 50 mg/mL, contains <1 mCg/mL of IgA, 3 mg/mL
      albumin, 22.5 mg/mL glycine, 20 mg/mL glucose, 2 mg/mL polyethylene glycol, 1 mCg/mL tri-n-
      butyl phosphate, 1 mCg/mL octoxynol 9, and 100 mCg/mL polysorbate 80); may be diluted to 5% or
      10%
Subcutaneous (SC) preparations (sucrose and preservative free):
   Hizentra: 20% (200 mg/mL) (5, 10, 20, 50 mL); contains 210—290 mmol/L L-proline, 8—30 mg/L
      polysorbate 80, and ≤50 mCg/mL IgA
   Cutaquig: 16.9% (169 mg/mL) (6, 10, 12, 20, 24, 48 mL); contains 30 mEq/L sodium, polysorbate 80,
      and~0.206 mg/mL IgA
   Cuvitru: 20% (200 mg/mL) (5, 10, 20, 40, 50 mL); contains 0.25 M glycine, ~80 mCg/mL IgA, and
      polysorbate 80
   Xembify: 20% (200 mg/mL) (5, 10, 20, 50 mL); contains 0.16—0.26 M glycine, 10—40 mCg/mL
      polysorbate 80, and IgA

IMMUNE GLOBULIN *continued*

Intravenous (IV) preparations:

Kawasaki disease (should be initiated within first 10 days of symptoms): 2 g/kg × 1 dose over 8—12 hr infusion. If signs and symptoms persist, infliximab monotherapy as second line therapy is recommended by a meta-analysis. If a second IVIG dose is used instead, consider using a different drug brand or lot number.

Immune thrombocytopenia (ITP) (see RH$_o$[D] immune globulin intravenous for Rh-positive patients):

  Acute therapy: 400—1000 mg/kg/dose once daily for 2—5 days for a total cumulative dose 2000 mg/kg

  Maintenance therapy: 400—1000 mg/kg/dose Q3—6 wk based on clinical response

Replacement therapy for antibody-deficient disorders: Start at 400—500 mg/kg/dose Q4 wk and adjust dose based on clinical response and to maintain a trough IgG level ≥500 mg/dL. For severe hypogammaglobulinemia (<100 mg/dL), patients may benefit with a loading dose of 400 mg/kg/dose once daily × 2, followed by 400—500 mg/kg/dose Q4 wk.

Pediatric HIV with IgG <400 mg/dL: See replacement therapy for antibody-deficient disorder from above.

Bone marrow transplantation (may decrease risk for infection and death but not acute graft-versus-host disease): Start at 400—500 mg/kg/dose to maintain IgG levels ≥400 mg/dL resulting in dosage intervals ranging from once weekly to Q3—4 wk.

Measles, postexposure prophylaxis for individuals with primary humoral immunodeficiency or without evidence of measles immunity (6—16 yr): 400 mg/kg/dose as soon as possible and within 6 days after exposure.

General guidelines for administration (see package insert of specific products):

  IV: Begin infusion at 0.01 mL/kg/min, double rate every 15—30 min, up to **max.** of 0.08 mL/kg/min. If adverse reactions occur, stop infusion until side effects subside and may restart at rate that was previously tolerated.

Subcutaneous (SC) preparations:

  Converting to SC route from previous IV dosage for patients receiving IV immune globulin (IVIG) infusions at regular intervals for at least 3 mo (≥2 yr):

  Initial weekly dose (start 1 wk after last IV dose):

SC Product	Dose Calculation (mg)	Dose Calculation (mL)
Hizentra	Dose (g) = 1.37 × Previous IVIG dose in grams (g) ÷ number of weeks between IVIG doses	mL = multiply dose (g) by 5
Cutaquig	Dose (g) = 1.30 × Previous IVIG dose in grams (g) ÷ number of weeks between IVIG doses	mL = multiply dose (g) by 6
Cuvitru	Dose (g) = 1.30 × Previous IVIG dose in grams (g) ÷ number of weeks between IVIG doses	mL = multiply dose (g) by 5

Adjust dose over time by clinical response and serum IgG trough levels. Obtain a previous trough level from IVIG therapy prior to SC conversion and repeat trough level 2—3 mo after initiating the SC route. A goal trough with the SC route of ∼290 mg/dL higher than a trough with the IV route has been recommended. A Q2 wk dosing interval may be used after establishing the patient individualized weekly dosage by multiplying the weekly dosage by 2.

Measles, postexposure prophylaxis for high-risk patients:

  Hizentra: 0.2 g/kg/dose SC Q7 days × 2, or 0.4 g/kg/dose SC × 1

SC administration: Injection sites include the abdomen, thigh, upper arm, and/or lateral hip. Doses may be administered into multiple sites (spaced ≥2 inches apart) simultaneously. See following table.

Continued

IMMUNE GLOBULIN *continued*

SC Product	Max. Simultaneous Injection Sites	Max. Infusion Rate	Max. Infusion Volume
Hizentra	8	First infusion: 15 mL/hr per infusion site for primary immunodeficiency (PI) or 20 mL/hr per infusion site for chronic inflammatory demyelinating polyneuropathy (CIDP) Subsequent infusions: 25 mL/hr per infusion site for PI or 50 mL/hr per infusion site for CIDP	First infusion: 15 mL per infusion site for PI or 20 mL per infusion site for CIDP Subsequent infusions: 25 mL per infusion site for PI or 50 mL per infusion site for CIDP
Cutaquig	6	Child 2–<18 yr: First 2 infusions: ≤15 mL/hr per infusion site Subsequent infusions: Gradually increase as tolerated by 5–10 mL/hr per infusion site Q2–4 wk up to a **maximum rate** of 25 mL/hr per infusion site. 18 yr and older: First 2 infusions: ≤20 mL/hr per infusion site Subsequent infusions: Gradually increase as tolerated by 10 mL/hr per infusion site Q2–4 wk up to a **maximum rate** of 52 mL/hr per infusion site.	Child 2–6 yr: First 2 infusions: ≤10 mL per infusion site Subsequent infusions: Gradually increase as tolerated by 5–10 mL per infusion site Q2–4 wk up to a **maximum** of 15.5 mL per infusion site. Child >6–<17 yr: First 2 infusion: ≤15 mL per infusion site Subsequent infusions: Gradually increase as tolerated by 5–10 mL per infusion site Q2–4 wk up to a **maximum** of 29 mL per infusion site. 17 yr and older: First 2 infusion: ≤25 mL per infusion site Subsequent infusions: Gradually increase as tolerated by 10 mL per infusion site Q2–4 wk up to a **maximum** of 40 mL per infusion site.
Cuvitru	4	First 2 infusions: 10–20 mL/hr per infusion site Subsequent infusions: Gradually increase as tolerated to 60 mL/hr per infusion site.	First 2 infusions: <40 kg: ≤20 mL per infusion site; ≥40 kg: ≤60 mL per infusion site Subsequent infusions (all weights): ≤60 mL per infusion site

IMMUNE GLOBULIN *continued*

Intramuscular (IM) preparations:
Measles, postexposure prophylaxis for high-risk patients: 0.5 mL/kg/dose (**max. dose:** 15 mL) IM × 1 within 6 days of exposure
IM administration: Administer in the anterolateral aspects of the upper thigh or deltoid muscle of the upper arm. **Avoid** gluteal region due to risk of injury to sciatic nerve. Consider splitting doses for multiple injection sites to address age-specific maximum IM injection volumes.

Use with caution in patients with increased risk of thrombosis (e.g., hypercoagulable states, prolonged immobilization, indwelling catheters, estrogen use, thrombosis history, cardiovascular risks, and hyperviscosity) or hemolysis (e.g., non-O blood type, associated inflammatory conditions, and receiving high cumulative doses of immune globulins over several days).

May cause flushing, chills, fever, headache, and hypotension. Hypersensitivity reaction may occur when IV form is administered rapidly. Maltose-containing products may cause an osmotic diuresis. May cause **anaphylaxis** in IgA-deficient patients due to varied amounts of IgA. Some products are IgA depleted; consult a pharmacist.

To decrease risk of renal dysfunction, including acute renal failure, IV preparations containing sucrose should not be infused at a rate such that the amount of sucrose exceeds 3 mg/kg/min.

SC route provides higher serum trough levels, lower rate of adverse reactions, and shorter administration time when compared with the IV route. Use of adjusted body weight (ABW = Ideal Body Weight + 0.5 [Actual Body Weight − Ideal Body Weight]) for dosing in obese patients has been recommended.

Delay immunizations after immune globulin administration (see latest AAP Red Book for details).

INDOMETHACIN
Indocin, Tivorbex, and generics
Nonsteroidal antiinflammatory agent

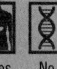

| C/X | 1 | Yes | Yes | No |

Caps: 20, 25, 50 mg
 Tivorbex: 20, 40 mg
Sustained release caps: 75 mg
Oral suspension: 25 mg/5 mL (237 mL); contains 1% alcohol
Suppositories: 50 mg (30s)
Injection: 1 mg; preservative free

Antiinflammatory/rheumatoid arthritis:
 Child (≥2 yr):
  Immediate release: Start at 1—2 mg/kg/24 hr ÷ TID—QID PO; **max. dose:** the lesser of 4 mg/kg/24 hr or 200 mg/24 hr
  Sustained release caps (≥15 yr): Start with 75 mg once daily PO, may increase to 75 mg BID; **max. dose:** 150 mg/24 hr
 Adult (immediate release): 50—150 mg/24 hr ÷ BID—QID PO; **max. dose:** 200 mg/24 hr
  Tivorbex: 20 mg TID PO or 40 mg BID—TID PO
  Sustained release caps: Start with 75 mg once daily PO, may increase to 75 mg BID; max. dose: 150 mg/24 hr

Continued

INDOMETHACIN *continued*

Closure of ductus arteriosus:
Infuse intravenously over 20—30 min:

Postnatal Age at Time of 1st Dose	Dose (mg/kg/dose Q12—24 hr)[a]		
	#1	#2	#3
<48 hr	0.2	0.1	0.1
2—7 days	0.2	0.2	0.2
>7 days	0.2	0.25	0.25

[a]Do not administer if urine output is <0.6 mL/kg/hr or anuric.

For infants <1500 g, 0.1—0.2 mg/kg/dose IV Q24 hr may be given for an additional 3—5 days.
Intraventricular hemorrhage prophylaxis: 0.1 mg/kg/dose IV Q24 hr × 3 doses, initiated at 6—12 hr of age (give in consultation with a neonatologist)

Contraindicated in active bleeding, coagulation defects, necrotizing enterocolitis, and renal insufficiency (urine output <0.6 mL/kg/hr). **Use with caution** in cardiac dysfunction, hypertension, heart disease (risk for MI and stroke with prolonged use), and renal or hepatic impairment. May cause (especially in neonates) decreased urine output, thrombocytopenia, and decreased GI blood flow, and a reduction in the antihypertensive effects of β-blockers, hydralazine, and ACE inhibitors. **Fatal hepatitis reported in JRA treatment.** Pancreatitis has been reported. Thrombotic events have been observed in adults receiving high doses or prolonged duration of therapy. Monitor renal and hepatic function before and during use. False-positive test for urine cannabinoid screen may occur.
Reduction in cerebral blood flow associated with rapid IV infusion; infuse all IV doses over 20—30 min.
Sustained-release capsules are dosed once daily—BID.
Pregnancy category is "C" for prior to 30 wks' gestation and "X" for 30 wk and greater. **Avoid use** at >30 wks' gestation due to increased risk for premature closure of the fetal ductus arteriosus. Limit dose and duration of use at 20—30 wks' gestation for concerns of fetal renal dysfunction and oligohydramnios.

INSULIN PREPARATIONS
Pancreatic hormone

| B | 1 | Yes | Yes | No |

Many preparations, at concentrations of 100, 500 Units/mL. See Chapter 10, Table 10.3.
Diluted concentrations of 1 Unit/mL or 10 Units/mL may be necessary for smaller doses in neonates and infants.

Hyperkalemia: See Resuscitation Medications Table in the front matter of the book.
DKA: See Chapter 10, Figure 10.1.

Accidental mix-ups between insulin products have been reported. Always check the insulin label before each use or injection.
When using insulin drip with new IV tubing, fill the tubing with the insulin infusion solution and wait for 30 min (before connecting tubing to the patient). Then flush the line and connect the IV line to the patient to start the infusion. This will ensure proper drug delivery. **Adjust dose in renal failure (see Chapter 31). Use with caution** and monitor closely in hepatic impairment.

IODIDE

See Potassium Iodide.

IODIXANOL
Visipaque and generics
Radiopaque agent, contrast media

B   3   Yes   Yes   No

Injection: 270 mg/mL, 320 mg/mL (50, 100, 150, 200 mL); may contain EDTA and tromethamine (some products are preservative free)

Consult with your local radiologist for specific dosing and administration recommendations.
IV contrast for CT scans: Use Visipaque 320 mg/mL, check for contraindications, and all patients should be encouraged to drink extra fluids for 8 hr after the exam as allowed.
eGFR ≥60 mL/min/1.73 m²: 2 mL/kg/dose
eGFR 30—60 mL/min/1.73 m²: Administered a reduced dose with IV fluids + acetylcysteine to reduce risk for nephropathy
eGFR <30 mL/min/1.73 m²: Avoid use unless life-threatening situation where benefits outweigh the risk.
PO contrast for CT scans: See Iohexol.

Contraindicated in children with prolonged fasting and the administration of a laxative before use. **Avoid use** via intrathecal route (serious life-threatening reactions may occur) and previous hypersensitivity reactions with contrast agents. **Use with caution** in asthma, hay fever, food allergy, congestive heart failure, severe liver or renal impairment, diabetic nephropathy, multiple myeloma, pheochromocytoma, hyperthyroidism, and sickle cell disease.
Common side effects include general discomfort, sensations of warmth, and pain. Cardiac arrest, dysrhythmia, heart failure, shock, severe dermatologic reactions (e.g., SJS, TEN), sickle cell crisis, thromboembolic disorder, acute kidney injury, and hypersensitivity reactions have been reported.
Children at higher risk for adverse events with contrast medium administration may include those having asthma, sensitivity to medication and/or allergens, congestive heart failure, or serum creatinine >1.5 mg/dL, and those aged <12 mo. Hypothyroidism or transient thyroid suppression following single or multiple exposures has been reported in children 0—3 yr old.
Avoid use with metformin as lactic acidosis and acute renal failure may occur. Postpone IV administration in patients who have recently received an oral cholecystographic contrast agent as renal toxicity may occur.
Visipaque 320 mg/mL has an osmolality of 290 mOsmol/kg than Omnipaque 350 mg/mL (884 mOsmol/kg) for a lower risk of contrast nephropathy. See product information for intravenous and intra-arterial administration guidelines.

IOHEXOL
Iohexol: Omnipaque 140, Omnipaque 180, Omnipaque 240, Omnipaque 300, Omnipaque 350, Omnipaque oral solution 9, Omnipaque oral solution 12, Oraltag
Iodixanol: see Visipaque
Radiopaque agent, contrast media

    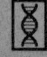

B   3   Yes   Yes   No

Injection:
Omnipaque 140: 302 mg iohexol equivalent to 140 mg iodine/mL (50 mL)

Continued

IOHEXOL *continued*

Omnipaque 180: 388 mg iohexol equivalent to 180 mg iodine/mL (10, 20 mL)

Omnipaque 240: 518 mg iohexol equivalent to 240 mg iodine/mL (10, 20, 50, 100, 150, 200 mL)

Omnipaque 300: 647 mg iohexol equivalent to 300 mg iodine/mL (10, 30, 50, 75, 100, 125, 150, 200, 500 mL)

Omnipaque 350: 755 mg iohexol equivalent to 350 mg iodine/mL (50, 75, 100, 125, 150, 200, 250, 500 mL)

Oral solution:

Omnipaque, Oraltag: 9 mg iodine/mL (19 mg/mL iohexol equivalent; 500 mL)

Omnipaque: 12 mg iodine/mL (26 mg iohexol equivalent; 500 mL)

All preparations contain tromethamine and edetate calcium disodium.

Consult with your local radiologist for specific dosing and administration recommendations.

Oral contrast for CT scans: Use oral Omnipaque 9 mg iodine/mL solution. If oral solution not available, mix 13 mL of the Omnipaque 350 injection with 500 mL of noncarbonated beverage to make an Omnipaque 9 mg iodine/mL solution. Administer dose all at once or over a period of up to 45 min. The more contrast the patient consumes, the better the CT study.

1–7 kg: 40–60 mL

8–11 kg: 110–160 mL

12–15 kg: 165–240 mL

16–42 kg: 250–360 mL

>42 kg: ≥480 mL

IV contrast for CT scans: See Iodixanol.

Use in hysterosalpingography is **contraindicated** in pregnant women due to the potential risk to the fetus from an intrauterine procedure. **Avoid** use with history of severe cutaneous reactions to iohexol. **Use with caution** in dehydration, previous allergic reaction to a contrast medium, iodine sensitivity, asthma, hay fever, food allergy, congestive heart failure, severe liver or renal impairment, diabetic nephropathy, multiple myeloma, pheochromocytoma, hyperthyroidism, and sickle cell disease. Allergic reactions, arrhythmias, hypothyroidism, transient thyroid suppression, and nephrotoxicity have been reported.

Children at higher risk for adverse events with contrast medium administration may include those having asthma, sensitivity to medication and/or allergens, congestive heart failure, serum creatinine >1.5 mg/dL, or those aged <12 mo. Hypothyroidism or transient thyroid suppression following single or multiple exposures has been reported in children 0–3 yr old.

Use **NOT** recommended with drugs that lower seizure threshold (e.g., phenothiazines), amiodarone (increased risk of cardiotoxicity), and metformin (lactic acidosis and acute renal failure).

Many other uses exist; see package insert for additional information. Iohexol is particularly useful when barium sulfate is **contraindicated** in patients with suspected bowel perforation or those in whom aspiration of contrast medium is of concern. Oral dose is poorly absorbed from the normal GI tract (0.1%–0.5%); absorption increases with bowel perforation or bowel obstruction. Concentrations 302–755 mg iohexol/mL have osmolalities from 1.1 to 3 times that of plasma (285 mOsm/kg) and CSF (301 mOsm/kg) and may be hypertonic.

IPRATROPIUM BROMIDE ± ALBUTEROL
Atrovent HFA and generics
In combination with albuterol: Combivent
Respimat and generics; previously available as
DuoNeb
Anticholinergic agent

   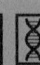

B/C 1 No No No

IPRATROPIUM BROMIDE ± ALBUTEROL *continued*

Aerosol oral inhaler (Atrovent HFA): 17 mCg/dose (200 actuations per canister, 12.9 g); contains alcohol

Nebulized solution: 0.02% (500 mCg/2.5 mL) (25s, 30s, 60s)

Nasal spray: 0.03% (21 mCg per actuation, 30 mL provides 345 sprays); 0.06% (42 mCg per actuation, 15 mL provides 165 sprays)

In combination with albuterol:

Nebulized solution (generic; previously available as DuoNeb): 0.5 mg ipratropium bromide and 2.5 mg albuterol in 3 mL (30s, 60s)

Inhalation spray (Combivent Respimat): 20 mCg ipratropium and 100 mCg albuterol per actuation (120 actuations per canister, 4 g); contains benzalkonium chloride

Ipratropium:

Acute use in the ED or ICU for moderate/severe asthma exacerbations:

Nebulizer treatments:

<12 yr: 250–500 mCg/dose Q20 min × 3, then Q2–4 hr PRN

≥12 yr: 500 mCg/dose Q20 min × 3, then Q2–4 hr PRN

Inhaler:

<12 yr: 4–8 puffs Q20 min PRN up to 3 hr

≥12 yr: 8 puffs Q20 min PRN up to 3 hr

Nonacute use:

Inhaler:

<12 yr: 1–2 puffs Q6 hr; **max. dose:** 12 puffs/24 hr

≥12 yr: 2–3 puffs Q6 hr; **max. dose:** 12 puffs/24 hr

Nebulized treatments:

Infant: 125–250 mCg/dose Q8 hr

Child ≤12 yr: 250–500 mCg/dose Q6–8 hr

>12 yr and adult: 250–500 mCg/dose Q6 hr

Nasal spray:

0.03% strength (21 mCg/spray):

Allergic and nonallergic rhinitis (≥6 yr and adult): 2 sprays (42 mCg) per nostril BID–TID

0.06% strength (42 mCg/spray):

Rhinitis associated with common cold (use up to a total of 4 days; safety and efficacy have not been evaluated >4 days):

2–<5 yr (limited data): 2 sprays (84 mCg) per nostril TID

5–11 yr: 2 sprays (84 mCg) per nostril TID

12 yr–adult: 2 sprays (84 mCg) per nostril TID–QID

Rhinitis associated with seasonal allergies:

2–<5 yr (limited data): 1 spray (42 mCg) per nostril TID × 14 days

≥5 yr–adult: 2 sprays (84 mCg) per nostril QID; use up to a total of 3 weeks (safety and efficacy have not been evaluated for >3 weeks)

Ipratropium in combination with albuterol:

Acute use in the ED or ICU for severe asthma exacerbations:

Nebulizer treatments:

<12 yr: 1.5 or 3 mL (0.25 mg ipratropium and 1.25 mg albuterol or 0.5 mg ipratropium and 2.5 mg albuterol) Q20 min × 3 then PRN for up to 3 hr

≥12 yr: 3 mL (0.5 mg ipratropium and 2.5 mg albuterol) Q20 min × 3 then PRN for up to 3 hr

Continued

IPRATROPIUM BROMIDE ± ALBUTEROL *continued*

Inhalation spray (Combivent Respimat):
<12 yr: 4—8 sprays Q20 min × 3 then PRN for up to 3 hr
≥12 yr: 8 sprays Q20 min × 3 then PRN for up to 3 hr

Contraindicated in atropine hypersensitivity. **Use with caution** in narrow-angle glaucoma or bladder neck obstruction, though ipratropium has fewer anticholinergic systemic effects than atropine. May cause anxiety, dizziness, headache, GI discomfort, and cough with inhaler or nebulized use. Epistaxis, nasal congestion, and dry mouth/throat have been reported with the nasal spray. Reversible anisocoria may occur with unintentional aerosolization of drug to the eyes, particularly with mask nebulizers. Proven efficacy of nebulized solution in pediatrics is currently limited to reactive airway disease management in the emergency room and intensive care unit areas.

Current aerosol inhaler product does not contain soy products. Combination ipratropium and albuterol products are currently approved for use only in adults and have not been formally studied in children. See albuterol for additional remarks if using the combination product.

Bronchodilation onset of action is 1—3 min with peak effects within 1.5—2 hr and duration of action of 4—6 hr.

Shake inhaler well prior to use with spacer. Nebulized solution may be mixed with albuterol (or use the combination product).

Pregnancy category is "C" for Combivent Respimat. Breastfeeding safety **extrapolated** from safety of atropine.

IRON DEXTRAN

See Iron—Injectable Preparations.

IRON—INJECTABLE PREPARATIONS
Ferric gluconate: Ferrlecit and generics
Iron dextran: INFeD
Iron sucrose: Venofer
Parenteral iron

B/C   2   No   No   No

Injection:
Ferric gluconate (Ferrlecit and generics): 62.5 mg/mL (12.5 mg elemental Fe/mL) (5 mL); contains 9 mg/mL benzyl alcohol and 20% sucrose
Iron dextran (INFeD): 50 mg/mL (50 mg elemental Fe/mL) (2 mL); products containing phenol 0.5% are only for IM administration; products containing sodium chloride 0.9% can be administered via the IM or IV route
Iron sucrose (Venofer): 20 mg/mL (20 mg elemental Fe/mL) (2.5, 5, 10 mL); contains 300 mg/mL sucrose; preservative free

FERRIC GLUCONATE (IV):
Iron deficiency anemia in patients undergoing chronic hemodialysis who are receiving supplemental erythropoietin therapy (most require 8 doses at 8 sequential dialysis treatments to achieve a favorable response):
Child ≥6 yr: 1.5 mg/kg elemental Fe (0.12 mL/kg) IV; **max. dose:** 125 mg elemental Fe/dose. Dilute dose in 25 mL NS and infuse over 1 hr.
Adult: 125 mg elemental Fe in 100 mL NS IV; infuse over 1 hr. Most require a minimum cumulative dose of 1 g elemental Fe administered over 8 sessions.

IRON—INJECTABLE PREPARATIONS *continued*

IRON DEXTRAN (IV OR IM):
Iron deficiency anemia (≥4 mo, child, adolescent):
   Test dose (IV over 5 min or IM; may initiate treatment dose 1 hr after test dose):
      <10 kg: 10 mg
      10—20 kg: 15 mg
      ≥20 kg: 25 mg
   Total replacement dose of iron dextran (mL) = 0.0442 × lean body wt (kg) × (desired Hb [g/dL] − measured Hb [g/dL]) + (0.26 × lean body wt [kg]). For patients weighing 5—15 kg, use actual body weight instead lean body weight. Total replacement dose is divided into smaller daily doses if exceeds respective IV or IM daily **max. doses** (see below).
Acute blood loss: Total replacement dose of iron dextran (mL) = 0.02 × blood loss (mL) × hematocrit expressed as decimal fraction. Assumes 1 mL of RBC = 1 mg elemental iron
If no reaction to test dose, give remainder of replacement dose ÷ over 2—3 daily doses.
Max. daily IV dose: 100 mg
Max. daily IM dose:
   <5 kg: 0.5 mL (25 mg)
   5—10 kg: 1 mL (50 mg)
   >10 kg: 2 mL (100 mg)
IM administration: Use "Z-track" technique.
IV administration: Dilute in NS at a **max. concentration** of 50 mg/mL and infuse over 1—6 hr at a **max. rate** of 50 mg/min.
IRON SUCROSE (IV):
Test dose (optional): Infuse 25% of first day dose up to a max. of 25 mg undiluted over 30 min.
Iron deficiency anemia in patients with chronic kidney disease:
   Child:
      ESRD on hemodialysis: (limited data from 14 children): 1 mg/kg/dialysis was adequate for correcting ferritin levels and 0.3 mg/kg/dialysis was successful in maintaining ferritin levels between 193 and 250 mCg/L. Doses were administered during the last hr of each dialysis and are recommended at a frequency of 3 times a week. A 10 mg test dose was administered.
      Nonrenal iron deficiency, refractory to PO therapy (limited data): Calculate total iron replacement dose (mg) = 0.6 × wt (kg) × (100 − [measured Hb ÷ desired Hb × 100]). Replacement dose is administered by giving an initial dose of 5—7 mg/kg (**max. dose:** 100 mg/24 hr) followed by a maintenance dose of 5—7 mg/kg/dose (**max. dose:** 300 mg/24 hr) Q3—7 days until total iron replacement dose is achieved.
   Adult:
      Hemodialysis-dependent: 100 mg elemental Fe 1—3 times a wk during dialysis up to a total cumulative dose of 1000 mg. May continue to administer at lowest dose to maintain target Hb, Hct, and iron levels.
      Nonhemodialysis-dependent: 200 mg elemental Fe on 5 different days over a 2 wk period (total cumulative dose: 1000 mg)
   IV administration: May administer undiluted over 2—5 min. For an infusion, dilute each 100 mg with a **max.** of 100 mL NS and infuse over at least 15 min.

Oral therapy with iron salts is preferred; injectable routes are painful. Gluconate and sucrose salts may be better tolerated than iron dextran. Adverse effects include hypotension, GI disturbances, fever, rash, myalgia, arthralgias, cramps, and headaches. Hypersensitivity reactions have been reported for iron dextran and sucrose products; use of test dose prior to first therapeutic dose is recommended.

Continued

IRON—INJECTABLE PREPARATIONS *continued*

IM administration is only possible with iron dextran salt product. Follow infusion recommendations for specific product. Monitor vital signs during IV infusion. TIBC levels may not be meaningful within 3 wk after dosing.

Efficacy and safety of iron sucrose for maintenance therapy have been evaluated in children 2 yr and older with CKD and receiving erythropoietin therapy. Common side effects include headache, respiratory tract viral infection, peritonitis, vomiting, pyrexia, dizziness, and cough.

Pregnancy category is "B" for ferric gluconate and iron sucrose and "C" for iron dextran.

IRON—ORAL PREPARATIONS
Ferrous sulfate: Fer-In-Sol, Slow FE, Slow Iron, and many generics
Ferrous gluconate: Ferate and generics
Ferrous fumarate: Ferretts, Ferrimin 150, and generics
Polysaccharide-iron complex: EZFE 200, Poly-Iron 150, iFerex 150, NovaFerrum, NovaFerrum Pediatric Drops, and many other brands; previously available as Niferex
Oral iron supplements

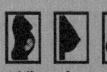 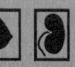 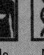

A/?   2   No   No   No

Ferrous sulfate (20% elemental Fe):
   Drops and oral solution (Fer-In-Sol and generics; OTC): 75 mg (15 mg Fe)/1 mL (50 mL); may contain 0.2% alcohol and sodium bisulfite
   Oral elixir and liquid (OTC): 220 mg (44 mg Fe)/5 mL (473 mL); may contain 5% alcohol
   Oral syrup (OTC): 300 mg (60 mg Fe)/5 mL
   Tabs (OTC): 325 mg (65 mg Fe)
   Extended release tabs (Slow FE, Slow Iron, and generics; OTC): 142 mg (45 mg Fe), 160 mg (50 mg Fe), 324 mg (65 mg Fe), and 325 mg (65 mg Fe)
Ferrous gluconate (12% elemental Fe):
   Tabs (Ferate and generics; OTC): 240 mg (27 mg Fe), 324 mg (37.5 mg Fe)
Ferrous fumarate (33% elemental Fe):
   Tabs (all OTC):
      Generics: 90 mg (29.5 mg Fe), 324 mg (106 mg Fe)
      Ferretts: 325 mg (106 mg Fe)
      Ferrimin 150: 456 mg (150 mg Fe)
Polysaccharide-iron complex and ferrous bis-glycinate chelate (expressed in mg elemental Fe):
   Caps (OTC): 50 mg (NovaFerrum 50), 150 mg (Poly-Iron 150, iFerex 150, and others), 200 mg (EZFE 200); 150 mg strength may contain 50 mg vitamin C
   Oral liquid (NovaFerrum 125; OTC): 125 mg/5 mL (180 mL); contains sodium benzoate and 100 units cholecalciferol/5 mL
   Oral drops (NovaFerrum Pediatric Drops; OTC): 15 mg/mL (120 mL); contains sodium benzoate

---

Iron deficiency anemia, treatment:
   Premature infant: 2—4 mg elemental Fe/kg/24 hr ÷ once daily—BID PO; **max. dose:**
      15 mg elemental Fe/24 hr
   Child: 3—6 mg elemental Fe/kg/24 hr ÷ BID—TID PO
   Adult: 60—100 mg elemental Fe BID PO up to 60 mg elemental Fe QID
Prophylaxis:
   Child: Give dose below PO ÷ once daily—TID

IRON—ORAL PREPARATIONS *continued*

Premature infant: 2 mg elemental Fe/kg/24 hr; **max. dose:** 15 mg elemental Fe/24 hr
Full-term infant: 1—2 mg elemental Fe/kg/24 hr; **max. dose:** 15 mg elemental Fe/24 hr
Child 2—12 yr: 2 mg elemental Fe/kg/24 hr; **max. dose:** 30 mg elemental Fe/24 hr
Adolescent and adult: 60 mg elemental Fe/24 hr PO once daily

Contraindicated in hemolytic anemia and hemochromatosis. **Avoid** use in GI tract
inflammation. May produce constipation, dark stools (false-positive guaiac is controversial),
nausea, and epigastric pain. Iron and tetracycline inhibit each other's absorption. Antacids may
decrease iron absorption.

Iron preparations are variably absorbed. Less GI irritation when given with or after meals. Vitamin C,
200 mg per 30 mg iron, may enhance absorption. Liquid iron preparations may stain teeth. Give
with dropper or drink through straw.

Pregnancy category is "A" for ferrous sulfate and is unknown for the other salt forms.

IRON SUCROSE

See Iron—Injectable Preparations.

ISONIAZID
Generics, INH; previously available as Nydrazid
and Laniazid
Antituberculous agent

C   1   Yes   Yes   No

Tabs: 100, 300 mg
Syrup: 50 mg/5 mL (473 mL); contains parabens
Injection: 100 mg/mL (10 mL); contains 0.25% chlorobutanol

See most recent edition of the AAP Red Book for details and length of therapy.
TB Treatment (other dosing regimens exist; see remarks):
Infant and child:
10—15 mg/kg (**max. dose:** 300 mg) PO once daily or 20—30 mg/kg (**max. dose:** 900 mg) per dose
three times weekly with rifampin for uncomplicated pulmonary tuberculosis in compliant patients.
Additional drugs are necessary in complicated disease.
Adult:
5 mg/kg (**max. dose:** 300 mg) PO once daily or 15 mg/kg (**max. dose:** 900 mg) per dose three times
weekly with rifampin. Additional drugs are necessary in complicated disease.
For INH-resistant TB: Discuss with Health Department or consult ID specialist.

Should not be used alone for treatment. Contraindicated in acute liver disease and previous
isoniazid-associated hepatitis. Peripheral neuropathy, optic neuritis, seizures, encephalopathy,
psychosis, and hepatic side effects may occur with higher doses, especially in combination with
rifampin. Severe liver injury has been reported in children and adults treated for latent TB. Follow
LFTs monthly. Pancreatitis, toxic epidermal necrolysis, and DRESS have been reported. May cause
false-positive urine glucose test.

Supplemental pyridoxine (1—2 mg/kg/24 hr) is recommended for prevention of neurologic side effects.
Inhibits CYP 450 1A2, 2C9, 2C19, and 3A3/4 microsomal enzymes; decrease dose of carbamazepine,
diazepam, phenytoin, and prednisone. Prednisone may decrease isoniazid's effects. Also a substrate
and inducer of CYP 450 2E1 and may potentiate acetaminophen hepatotoxicity. **Avoid** daily alcohol
use to reduce risk for isoniazid-induced hepatitis.

Continued

ISONIAZID *continued*

May be given IM (same as oral doses) when oral therapy is not possible. Administer oral doses 1 hr prior to and 2 hr after meals. Aluminum salts may decrease absorption. **Adjust dose in renal failure (see Chapter 31).**

ISOPROTERENOL
Generics; previously available as Isuprel
Adrenergic agonist

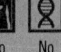

C   ?   Yes   No   No

Injection: 0.2 mg/mL (1, 5 mL); preparations may be preservative free or contain disodium EDTA

NOTE: The dosage units for adults are in mCg/min, compared to mCg/kg/min for children.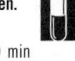
IV infusion:
  Neonate—child: 0.05—2 mCg/kg/min; start at minimum dose and increase every 5—10 min by 0.1 mCg/kg/min until desired effect or onset of toxicity; **max. dose:** 2 mCg/kg/min
  Adult: 2—20 mCg/min; titrate to desired effect

Use with caution in diabetes, hyperthyroidism, renal disease, CHF, ischemia, or aortic stenosis. May cause flushing, ventricular arrhythmias, profound hypotension, anxiety, and myocardial ischemia. Monitor heart rate, respiratory rate, and blood pressure. **Not** for treatment of asystole or for use in cardiac arrests, unless bradycardia is due to heart block.
Continuous infusion for bronchodilatation must be gradually tapered over a 24—48 hr period to prevent rebound bronchospasm. Tolerance may occur with prolonged use. Clinical deterioration, myocardial necrosis, congestive heart failure, and **death** have been reported with continuous infusion use in refractory asthmatic children.

ISOTRETINOIN
Absorica, Absorica LD, Accutane, Amnesteem,
Claravis, Myorisan, Zenatane, and generics
Retinoic acid, vitamin A derivative

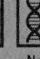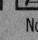

X   3   No   Yes   No

Caps, standard formulation (all products contain soybean oil):
  Absorica: 10, 20, 25, 30, 35, 40 mg
  Amnesteem: 10, 20, 40 mg; contains EDTA
  Accutane, Claravis, Myorisan, Zenatane: 10, 20, 30, 40 mg; may contain EDTA
  Generics: 10, 20, 25, 30, 35, 40 mg
Caps, micronized formulation (not substitutable with standard formulation due to different bioavailability):
  Absorica LD: 8, 16, 20, 24, 28, 32 mg; contains soybean oil and polysorbate 80

Cystic acne/severe recalcitrant nodular acne (see remarks):
  Child (>12 yr) and adult:
    Standard formulation: 0.5—2 mg/kg/24 hr ÷ BID PO × 15—20 wk or until the total cyst count decreases by 70%, whichever comes first. Dosages as low as 0.05 mg/kg/24 hr have been reported to be beneficial.
    Micronized formulation (Absorica LD): 0.4—0.8 mg/kg/24 hr ÷ BID PO × 15—20 wk or until the total cyst count decreases by 70%, whichever comes first. Dosages as high as 1.6 mg/kg/24 hr ÷ BID have been used for severe cases in adults.

ISOTRETINOIN *continued*

Micronized (Absorica LD) and standard formulations are not bioequivalent and are **NOT** substitutable.

Contraindicated during pregnancy; known teratogen. Use with caution in females during childbearing years. May cause conjunctivitis, xerosis, pruritus, photosensitivity reactions (**avoid** exposure to sunlight and use sunscreen), epistaxis, anemia, hyperlipidemia, pseudotumor cerebri (especially in combination with tetracyclines; **avoid** this combination), cheilitis, bone pain, muscle aches, skeletal changes, lethargy, nausea, vomiting, elevated ESR, mental depression, aggressive/ violent behavior, and psychosis. Serious skin reactions (e.g., Stevens-Johnson syndrome, TEN) have been reported.

Elevation of liver enzymes may occur during treatment; a dosage reduction or continued treatment may result in normalization. Discontinue use if liver enzymes do not normalize or if hepatitis is suspected.

To avoid additive toxic effects, **do not** take vitamin A concomitantly. Increases clearance of carbamazepine. Hormonal birth control (oral, injectable, and implantable) failures have been reported with concurrent use. Monitor CBC, ESR, triglycerides, and LFTs.

Prescribers, site pharmacists, patients, and wholesalers must register with the iPLEDGE system (a risk minimization program) at www.ipledgeprogram.com or 1-866-495-0654 before doses are dispensed. Prescriptions may not be written for more than a 1-mo supply.

ITRACONAZOLE Sporanox, Tolsura, and generics *Antifungal agent*					
	C	3	Yes	Yes	No

Caps:
   Sporanox and generics: 100 mg
   Tolsura: 65 mg
Oral solution (Sporanox and generics): 10 mg/mL (150 mL); contains hydroxypropyl-β-cyclodextrin, propylene glycol, and saccharin

Neonate (limited data in full-term neonates treated for tinea capitis): 5 mg/kg/24 hr PO once daily × 6 wk

Child (limited data): 3—5 mg/kg/24 hr PO ÷ once daily—BID; dosages as high as 5—10 mg/kg/24 hr have been used for *Aspergillus* prophylaxis in chronic granulomatous disease. Population pharmacokinetic data in pediatric cystic fibrosis and bone marrow transplant patients suggest an oral liquid dosage of 10 mg/kg/24 hr PO ÷ BID or oral capsule dosage of 20 mg/kg/24 hr PO ÷ BID to be more reliable for achieving trough plasma levels between 500 and 2000 ng/mL.

   Prophylaxis for recurrence of opportunistic disease in HIV:
      Coccidioides spp.: 2—5 mg/kg/dose PO Q12 hr; **max. dose:** 400 mg/24 hr
      Cryptococcal meningitis: 5 mg/kg/dose PO Q24 hr; **max. dose:** 200 mg/24 hr
      Histoplasmosis: 5—10 mg/kg/dose PO once daily; **max. dose:** 200 mg/dose
   Treatment of opportunistic disease in HIV:
      Candidiasis: 5 mg/kg/24 hr PO ÷ Q12—24 hr; **max. dose:** 400 mg/24 hr
      ***Coccidioides* spp. pneumonia:** 2—5 mg/kg/dose (**max. dose:** 200 mg/dose) PO TID × 3 days, followed by 2—5 mg/kg/dose PO BID; **max. dose:** 400 mg/24 hr
      Cryptococcal meningitis: 2.5—5 mg/kg/dose (**max. dose:** 200 mg/dose) PO TID × 3 days, followed by 5—10 mg/kg/24 hr (**max. dose:** 400 mg/24 hr) ÷ once to twice daily for a minimum of 8 wk

Continued

ITRACONAZOLE *continued*

    Histoplasmosis: 2—5 mg/kg/dose (**max. dose:** 200 mg/dose) PO TID × 3 days, followed by 2—5
       mg/kg/dose (**max. dose:** 200 mg/dose) PO BID × 12 mo
Adult:
    Blastomycosis and nonmeningeal histoplasmosis: 200 mg PO TID × 3 days, followed by 200 mg PO
       once daily or BID depending on severity
    Aspergillosis and severe infections (use oral solution): 600 mg/24 hr PO ÷ TID × 3—4 days,
       followed by 200—400 mg/24 hr ÷ BID; **max. dose:** 600 mg/24 hr ÷ TID

Oral solution and capsule dosage form should NOT be used interchangeably; oral solution
is more bioavailable. Only the oral solution has been demonstrated effective for oral and/or
esophageal candidiasis. **Contraindicated** in CHF and certain interacting drugs (see below). **Use
with caution** in hepatic and/or renal impairment, cardiac dysrhythmias, and azole hypersensitivity.
May cause GI symptoms, headaches, rash, liver enzyme elevation, hepatitis, and hypokalemia.
Double/blurred vision, dizziness, and tremor have been reported.

Like ketoconazole, it inhibits the activity of the CYP450 3A4 drug metabolizing isoenzyme. Thus, the
coadministration of cisapride, dofetilide, felodipine, methadone, nisoldipine, pimozide, quinidine,
triazolam, lovastatin, simvastatin, ergot derivatives, and oral midazolam is contraindicated. May
increase systemic hormone concentrations of oral contraceptives. See remarks in Ketoconazole for
additional drug interaction information.

Steady-state serum concentrations of >0.25 mg/L itraconazole and >1 mg/L hydroxyitraconazole
(metabolite) have been recommended. Recommended serum sampling time at steady state: any
time after 2 wk after continuous dosing. Itraconazole has a 34—42-hour $T_{1/2}$.

Administer oral solution on an empty stomach but administer capsules with food. Oral
capsule bioavailability has been shown to be reduced in immunocompromised patients. Achlorhydria
reduces absorption of the drug. **Do not** oral liquid dosage form in patients with GFR
<30 mL/min because hydroxypropyl-β-cyclodextrin excipient has reduced clearance with renal
failure.

IVACAFTOR
Kalydeco
*Cystic fibrosis transmembrane conductance
regulator potentiator*

  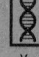

B   ?   Yes   Yes   Yes

Oral granules: 25 mg (56 packets), 50 mg (56 packets), 75 mg (56 packets)
Tabs: 150 mg (56 tabs)

Cystic fibrosis (see remarks):
    4—<6 mo and ≥5 kg (use oral granules): 25 mg PO Q12 hr
    ≥6 mo and child <6 yr (use oral granules):
       5—<7 kg: 25 mg PO Q12 hr
       7—<14 kg: 50 mg PO Q12 hr
       ≥14 kg: 75 mg PO Q12 hr
    ≥6 yr, adolescent, and adult: 150 mg PO Q12 hr
    Dosage modification with hepatic impairment:
       Child-Pugh class B: Use above dosage with a once-daily dosage interval.
       Child-Pugh class C: Studies have not been completed but exposure is expected to be higher than
         class B; use above dosage with caution once daily or with a less frequent dosage interval.
    Hepatotoxicity (ALT or AST > 5× ULN) during therapy: Hold doses and reinitiate therapy after
       resolution of enzyme elevation if the benefits outweigh the risks.

IVACAFTOR *continued*

Dosage modification when used with CYP 450 3A inhibitors:

Age	Weight (kg)	Dosed With Strong CYP 450 3A Inhibitor (e.g., Ketoconazole, Itraconazole, Voriconazole, Posaconazole, Clarithromycin)	Dosed With Moderate CYP 450 3A Inhibitor (e.g., Erythromycin, Fluconazole)
4—<6 mo	≥5 kg	Use not recommended	Use not recommended
≥6 mo and <6 yr	5—<7 kg	25 mg PO twice weekly	25 mg PO once daily
	7—<14 kg	50 mg PO twice weekly	50 mg PO once daily
	≥14 kg	75 mg PO twice weekly	75 mg PO once daily
≥6 yr, adolescent, and adult	All	150 mg PO twice weekly	150 mg PO once daily

Works as a CFTR potentiator on class 3 CFTR mutations. Originally indicated for G551D CFTR mutation but has since been approved for many other mutations; see product information for list of approved mutations. Use is not recommended in children 4—<6 mo with hepatic impairment (due to variability of CYP enzyme maturation) and/or taking moderate or strong CYP 450 3A inhibitors.

Common side effects include rash, abdominal pain, diarrhea, nausea, dizziness, headache, nasal congestion, pharyngitis, and URIs. Increased liver enzymes and cataracts may occur; monitor baseline AST/ALT and ocular exam. Repeat AST/ALT every 3 months for the first year followed by annual assessments. Repeat ocular exams annually. May cause a false-positive urine drug screen test for cannabinoids. **Use with caution** in patients with CrCl ≤30 mL/min; has not been studied.

Ivacaftor is CYP 450 3A substrate; see dose modification table in the dosing section. Use with strong CYP 450 3A inducers (e.g., rifampin, rifabutin, carbamazepine, St. John's wort) is not recommended. Ivacaftor may inhibit CYP 450 2C9 and increase the effects/toxicity of warfarin. Always evaluate potential drug-drug interactions; see https://www.kalydecohcp.com/drug-interactions. **Avoid** food or drink containing grapefruit or Seville oranges.

Administer all doses with high-fat foods to ensure absorption. Oral granules can be mixed with 5 mL of soft foods or liquids such as puréed fruits or vegetables, yogurt, applesauce, water, breast milk, infant formula, milk, or juice. Once mixed, it should be consumed within an hour. If a dose (all dosage forms) is missed within 6 hr of a scheduled dose, administer a dose immediately. However, if the missed dose is >6 hr, skip that dose and resume therapy at the next scheduled dose. Never take a double dose for a missed dose.

IVERMECTIN
Stromectol and generics; previously available as
Sklice and Soolantra
Anthelmintic

 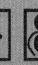   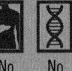

C   2   No   No   No

Tab (Stromectol and generics): 3 mg
Topical lotion (OTC and prescription; previously available as Sklice): 0.5% (117 g); contains parabens

Continued

IVERMECTIN *continued*

Topical cream (previously available as Soolantra): 1% (45 g); contains cetyl alcohol, EDTA, parabens, and propylene glycol

Systemic use:

Cutaneous lava migrans or strongyloidiasis: 0.2 mg/kg/dose PO once daily × 1–2 days for cutaneous lava migrans and × 2 days for strongyloidiasis; dosing by body weight (see first table)

Scabies: 0.2 mg/kg/dose PO × 1, followed by repeat second dose in 7 or 10–14 days, dosing by body weight as follows:

Weight (kg)	Oral Dose
15–24	3 mg
25–35	6 mg
36–50	9 mg
51–65	12 mg
66–79	15 mg
≥80	0.2 mg/kg

Onchocerciasis: 0.15 mg/kg/dose PO × 1; may repeat dose every 6–12 mo until asymptomatic; dosing by body weight as follows:

Weight (kg)	Single Oral Dose
15–25	3 mg
26–44	6 mg
45–64	9 mg
65–84	12 mg
≥85	0.15 mg/kg

Topical use:

Lotion:

Head lice infestation (≥6 mo to adult): Apply lotion to dry hair in sufficient amounts (up to one full tube) to thoroughly coat the hair and scalp for 10 min. Then rinse off with water.

Cream:

Rosacea (Adult): Apply cream to each affected area once daily.

Systemic Use: Rare fatal encephalopathy may occur in onchocerciasis with a concurrent heavy *Loa loa* infection. Reactions experienced with strongyloidiasis include diarrhea, nausea, vomiting, pruritus, rash, dizziness, and drowsiness. Adverse reactions experienced in onchocerciasis include cutaneous or systemic allergic/inflammatory reactions of varying severity (Mazzotti reaction) and ophthalmologic reactions. Neurotoxicity ranging from somnolence/drowsiness, stupor, and coma has been reported in patients without onchocerciasis or in patients with onchocerciasis in the absence of *Loa loa*. Specific reactions may include arthralgia/synovitis, lymph node enlargement and tenderness, pruritus, edema, fever, orthostatic hypotension, and tachycardia. Therapy for postural hypotension may include oral hydration, recumbency, IV normal saline, and/or IV steroids. Antihistamines or aspirin, or both, have been used for most mild-to-moderate cases.

Ivermectin may increase the effects/toxicity of warfarin. Administer oral doses on an empty stomach with water.

Topical Use: Safety and efficacy have not been established for children <6 mo. Common side effects include conjunctivitis, ocular hyperemia, eye irritation, dandruff, dry skin, and skin burning. Contact dermatitis has been reported. Not for oral, ophthalmic, or intravaginal use. Use of lotion for children should be supervised by an adult to prevent oral ingestion.

K

KALYDECO

See Ivacaftor.

KETAMINE
Ketalar and generics
General anesthetic

   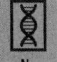

?   3   No   Yes   No

Injection: 10 mg/mL (20 mL), 50 mg/mL (10 mL), 100 mg/mL (5, 10 mL); contains benzethonium chloride

Child (see remarks):
  Sedation:
    PO: 5 mg/kg × 1
    IV: 0.5—1 mg/kg; **max. dose:** 150 mg/dose
    IM: 2—5 mg/kg × 1
    Intranasal (≥3 mo; limited data): 3—6 mg/kg × 1, administering half of total dose per nostril using a mucosal automizer device

Adult:
  Analgesia with sedation:
    IV (see remarks): 0.2—1 mg/kg
    IM: 0.5—4 mg/kg

Contraindicated in significant hypertension and known hypersensitivity to the drug. **Use with caution** in elevated ICP, aneurysms, thyrotoxicosis, CHF, angina, and psychotic disorders. May cause hypertension, hypotension, emergence reactions, tachycardia, laryngospasm, respiratory depression, and stimulation of salivary secretions. Cystitis has been reported with chronic use/abuse. Intravenous use may induce general anesthesia. Hepatobiliary dysfunction with or without biliary obstruction has also been reported with recurrent use. Diplopia and nystagmus have been noted following IV administration. False-positive test for urine phencyclidine (PCP) screen may occur.

Co-administration of an anticholinergic agent may be added in situations of clinically significant hypersalivation in patients with impaired ability to mobilize secretions. Benzodiazepine may be used in the presence of a ketamine-associated recovery reaction (prophylaxis use in adults may be beneficial). Ondansetron prophylaxis can slightly reduce vomiting. See *Ann Emerg Med.* 2001;57:449—461 for additional use information in the emergency department.

Drug is a substrate for CYP 450 2B6, 2C9, and 3A4 isoenzymes. Consider potential drug interactions with respective enzyme inhibitors and inducers, especially with prolonged use. Use with aminophylline or theophylline may increase risk for seizures. Use with sympathomimetics and vasopressin may enhance the sympathomimetic effects of ketamine. Use with CNS depressants may result in profound sedation, respiratory depression, and coma.

Rate of IV infusion should **not** exceed 0.5 mg/kg/min and **should not** be administered in less than 60 sec. For additional information including onset and duration of action, see Chapter 6.

KETOCONAZOLE
Nizoral, Xolegel, Extina, Ketodan, and generics
Antifungal agent, imidazole

    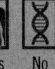

C   2   No   Yes   No

Continued

KETOCONAZOLE continued

Tabs: 200 mg
Oral suspension: 100 mg/5 mL
Cream: 2% (15, 30, 60 g); contains sulfites
Gel: 2% [Xolegel] (45 g); contains 34% alcohol and polyethylene glycol
Topical foam: 2% [Extina, Ketodan, and generics] (50, 100 g); contains alcohol and propylene glycol
Shampoo:
   1% [Nizoral (OTC)] (125, 200 mL)
   2% [generics] (120 mL)

Oral:
   Child ≥2 yr and adolescent: 3.3—6.6 mg/kg/24 hr once daily
   Adult: 200—400 mg/24 hr once daily
   Max. dose (all ages): 400 mg/24 hr
Topical (≥12 yr; see remarks):
   Cream: 1 application to affected area once daily × 2—6 wk. For seborrheic dermatitis, use BID × 4 wk.
   Gel (Xolegel): 1 application to affected area once daily × 2 wk for seborrheic dermatitis
   Foam: 1 application to affected area BID × 4 wk for seborrheic dermatitis
Shampoo:
   1% (Dandruff): Apply to wet hair, generously lather, rinse thoroughly; use every 3—4 days for up to 8 wk PRN.
   2% (Tinea versicolor): Apply to wet hair and leave on for 5 minutes before rinsing × 1.

The systemic dosage form should NOT be first-line treatment for any fungal infection due to concerns of hepatotoxicity and adrenal gland effects (per the FDA).
Monitor LFTs in long-term use and adrenal function for patients at risk. Drugs that decrease gastric acidity will decrease absorption. May cause nausea, vomiting, rash, headache, pruritus, and fever. Hepatotoxicity (including fatal cases) has been reported; use with hepatic impairment is **contraindicated.** High doses may decrease adrenocortical function and serum testosterone levels. Hypersensitivity reactions (including anaphylaxis) have been reported with all dosage forms.
Safety and efficacy with topical use in seborrheic dermatitis for patients >12 yr of age have been established. **Avoid** topical use on breast or nipples in nursing mothers.
Inhibits CYP 450 3A4. **Contraindicated** when used with cisapride, disopyramide, methadone, mefloquine, quinidine, terfenadine, pimozide, or any drug that can prolong the QT interval (because of risk for cardiac arrhythmias), and HMG-CoA reductase inhibitors (e.g., simvastatin and lovastatin). Excessive sedation and prolonged hypnotic effects with triazolam use (also **contraindicated**). May increase levels/effects of phenytoin, digoxin, cyclosporine, corticosteroids, nevirapine, protease inhibitors, and warfarin. Achlorhydria, phenobarbital, rifampin, isoniazid, H₂ blockers, antacids, and omeprazole can decrease levels of oral ketoconazole.
Administering oral doses with food or acidic beverages and 2 hr prior to antacids will increase absorption. For topical products, **avoid contact** with eyes and other mucous membranes.
To use shampoo, wet hair and scalp with water, apply sufficient amount to scalp, and gently massage for about 1 min. Rinse hair thoroughly, reapply shampoo and leave on the scalp for an additional 3 min, and rinse.

KETOROLAC
Many generics (previously available as Toradol),
Acular, Acular LS, Acuvail
Nonsteroidal antiinflammatory agent

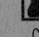

C/X   3   Yes   Yes   No

KETOROLAC *continued*

Injection: 15 mg/mL (1 mL), 30 mg/mL (1, 2 mL); contains 10% alcohol and tromethamine
Tabs: 10 mg; contains tromethamine
Ophthalmic solution (all containing tromethamine):
  Acular and generics: 0.5% (3, 5, 10 mL); contains benzalkonium chloride and EDTA
  Acular LS and generics: 0.4% (5 mL); contains benzalkonium chloride and EDTA
  Acuvail: 0.45% (0.4 mL); 30s); preservative free

Systemic use is not to exceed 3–5 days, regardless of systemic route of administration (IM, IV, PO).
IM/IV:
  Child: 0.5 mg/kg/dose IM/IV Q6–8 hr. **Max. dose:** 30 mg Q6 hr or 120 mg/24 hr
  Adult: 30 mg IM/IV Q6 hr. **Max. dose:** 120 mg/24 hr
PO:
  Child 2–≤16 yr (limited data): 1 mg/kg/dose Q4-6 hr; **max. dose:** 10 mg/dose and 40 mg/24 hr
  Child >16 yr and adult: 10 mg PRN Q4-6 hr; **max. dose:** 40 mg/24 hr
Ophthalmic (see remarks):
  Postoperative cataract surgery:
    ≥2 yr–adult (use 0.5%): 1 drop in each affected eye QID starting 24 hr after surgery × 2 wk
  Postoperative corneal refractive surgery:
    ≥3 yr–adult (use 0.4%): 1 drop in each affected eye QID PRN for up to 4 days after surgery
  Seasonal allergic conjunctivitis:
    ≥2 yr–adult (use 0.5%): 1 drop in each eye QID

May cause GI bleeding, nausea, dyspepsia, drowsiness, decreased platelet function, and interstitial nephritis. **Not recommended** in patients at increased risk of bleeding. **Do not use** in hepatic or renal failure. **Use with caution** in heart disease (risk for MI and stroke with prolonged use). False-positive test for urine cannabinoid screen may occur with systemic use.

Duration of therapy for ophthalmic use: 14 days after cataract surgery, and up to 4 days after corneal refractive surgery. Also indicated for ocular itching associated with seasonal allergic conjunctivitis. Bronchospasm or asthma exacerbations, allergic reactions, corneal erosion/perforation/thinning/melt, and epithelial breakdown have been reported with ophthalmic use. **Avoid** having the tip of the ophthalmic bottle touch the eye or surrounding structures to decrease risk for ocular infections.

Pregnancy category is "C" for prior to 30 wks' gestation and "X" for 30 wk and greater. **Avoid use** at >30 wks' gestation due to increased risk for premature closure of the fetal ductus arteriosus. Limit dose and duration of use at 20–30 wks' gestation for concerns of fetal renal dysfunction and oligohydramnios.

L

LACOSAMIDE
Vimpat and generics
Anticonvulsant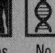

          C   2   Yes   Yes   No

Oral solution: 10 mg/mL (200 mL); contains aspartame, parabens, and propylene glycol
Tabs: 50, 100, 150, 200 mg
Injection: 10 mg/mL (20 mL); preservative free

Continued

LACOSAMIDE *continued*

Partial-onset seizures as monotherapy or adjunctive therapy:
Child (1 mo—<17 yr):

Weight (kg)	Initial Dosage	Titration Regimen	Maintenance Dosage
<6	PO: 1 mg/kg/dose BID IV: 0.66 mg/kg/dose TID	PO: Increase by 1 mg/kg/dose BID every 7 days IV: Increase by 0.66 mg/kg/dose TID every 7 days	PO: 3.75—7.5 mg/kg/dose BID IV: 2.5—5 mg/kg/dose TID
6—<30	PO/IV: 1 mg/kg/dose BID	PO/IV: Increase by 1 mg/kg/dose BID every 7 days	PO/IV: 3—6 mg/kg/dose BID
30—<50	PO/IV: 1 mg/kg/dose BID	PO/IV Increase by 1 mg/kg/dose BID every 7 days	PO/IV: 2—4 mg/kg/dose BID
≥50	PO/IV: 50 mg BID	PO/IV: Increase by 50 mg BID every 7 days	PO/IV: Monotherapy: 150—200 mg BID Adjunctive therapy: 100—200 mg BID

Primary generalized tonic-clonic seizures as adjunctive therapy:
Child (4 yr—<17 yr):

Weight (kg)	Initial Dosage	Titration Regimen	Maintenance Dosage
11—<30	PO/IV: 1 mg/kg/dose BID	PO/IV: Increase by 1 mg/kg/dose BID every 7 days	PO/IV: 3—6 mg/kg/dose BID
30—<50	PO/IV: 1 mg/kg/dose BID	PO/IV Increase by 1 mg/kg/dose BID every 7 days	PO/IV: 2—4 mg/kg/dose BID
≥50	PO/IV: 50 mg BID	PO/IV: Increase by 50 mg BID every 7 days	PO/IV: Monotherapy: 150—200 mg BID Adjunctive therapy: 100—200 mg BID

**Partial-onset seizures as monotherapy or adjunctive therapy, and primary generalized tonic-clonic
seizures as adjunctive therapy:**
17 yr and adult:

Initial Dosage (PO/IV)	Titration Regimen (PO/IV)	Maintenance Dosage (PO/IV)
Monotherapy: 100 mg BID[a] Adjunctive therapy: 50 mg BID[a]	Increase by 50 mg BID every 7 days	Monotherapy: 150—200 mg BID Adjunctive therapy: 100—200 mg BID Doses up to 300 mg BID may provide benefit for some patients for both indications

[a]Alternative initial dosage (under medical supervision due to increased risk for CNS side effects): 200 mg × 1 and start 12 hr later, 100 mg BID × 7 days then titrate to the respective monotherapy or adjunctive therapy goal.

LACOSAMIDE *continued*

Converting from other single antiepileptic drug (AED) to lacosamide monotherapy: administer lacosamide in combination with the established single AED for at least 3 days before tapering. Gradually withdrawing the concomitant AED over 6 wk is recommended.

IV use: Use same dose when converting from PO to IV and vice versa; except for pediatric patients <6 kg (see above table). IV use should be considered for short-term use as clinical treatment evaluations have been limited to 5 days of consecutive use.

Use with caution with known cardiac conduction problems (e.g., second-degree AV block), severe cardiac disease (e.g., MI or heart failure), concomitant use with drugs known to prolong PR interval, and renal (see Chapter 31) and hepatic impairment. Lacosamide undergoes 95% renal excretion; a reduction of 25% of the **maximum** dosage is recommended for adult and pediatric patients with severe renal impairment (CrCl <30 mL/min and ESRD), or with mild/moderate hepatic impairment. Use is **not recommended** in severe hepatic impairment. Dose reduction may be also necessary with concurrent strong inhibitor of CYP 450 3A4 or 2C9 medication. Patients with mild/moderate hepatic impairment should be observed closely during dose titration. Oral bioavailability is approximately 100%.

Most common side effects in adults include diplopia, headache, dizziness, and nausea. Somnolence and irritability were frequently reported in pediatric studies. Patients should be advised of potential dizziness, ataxia, and syncope with use. Multiorgan hypersensitivity reactions (including DRESS, affecting the skin, kidney, and liver), worsening of seizures, agranulocytosis, and euphoria (high doses) have been reported. As with other AEDs, monitor for suicidal behavior and ideation.

Oral doses may be administered with or without food. Swallow tablets whole; **do not** cut tablets. IV doses should be administered over 30–60 min. **Do not** abruptly withdraw therapy; gradually taper to prevent potential seizures.

Lacosamide is present in human milk as increased sleepiness in breastfed infants has been reported.

LABETALOL
Generics; previously available as Normodyne and Trandate
Adrenergic antagonist (α and β), antihypertensive

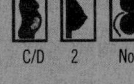   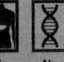

| C/D | 2 | No | Yes | No |

Tabs: 100, 200, 300 mg
Injection: 5 mg/mL (4, 20, 40 mL); contains parabens
Injection, premixed:
　In 0.72% NaCl: 1 mg/mL (100, 200, 300 mL)
　In D₅W: 1 mg/mL (200 mL)
Oral suspension: 10 mg/mL, 40 mg/mL

Child (see remarks):
　PO: Initial: 1–3 mg/kg/24 hr ÷ BID. May increase up to a **maximum** of 12 mg/kg/24 hr up to 1200 mg/24 hr
　IV: Hypertensive emergency (start at lowest dose and titrate to effect; see Chapter 4 for additional information):
　　Intermittent dose: 0.2–1 mg/kg/dose Q10 min PRN; **max. dose:** 40 mg/dose
　　Infusion (hypertensive emergencies): 0.4–1 mg/kg/hr to a **max. dose** of 3 mg/kg/hr; may initiate with a 0.2–1 mg/kg bolus; **max. bolus:** 40 mg
Adult (see remarks):
　PO: 100 mg BID, increase by 100 mg/dose Q2–3 days PRN to a **max. dose** of 2.4 g/24 hr. Usual range: 200–800 mg/24hr ÷ BID

Continued

LABETALOL *continued*

IV: Hypertensive emergency (start at lowest dose and titrate to effect with a **max. total dose** of 300 mg for both methods of administration):

Intermittent dose: 10—20 mg/dose Q10 min PRN; **max. dose:** 80 mg/dose

Infusion: 0.5—2 mg/min, increase to titrate to response; may initiate with a 10—20 mg bolus over 2 min

Contraindicated in asthma, pulmonary edema, cardiogenic shock, and heart block. May cause orthostatic hypotension, edema, CHF, bradycardia, AV conduction disturbances, bronchospasm, urinary retention, and skin tingling. **Use with caution** in hepatic disease (dose reduction may be necessary), diabetes, liver function test elevation, hepatic necrosis, and hepatitis. Cholestatic jaundice has been reported. Use with digitalis glycosides may increase risk for bradycardia. False-positive test for urine amphetamine screen may occur.

Patient should remain supine for up to 3 hr after IV administration. Pregnancy category changes to "D" if used in second or third trimesters.

Onset of action: PO: 1—4 hr; IV: 5—15 min

LACTULOSE
Constulose, Enulose, Generlac, Kristalose, and generics
Ammonium detoxicant, hyperosmotic laxative

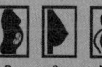 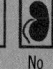 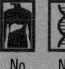 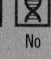

B   ?   No   No   No

Oral syrup: 10 g/15 mL (15, 30, 237, 473, 946 mL); contains galactose, lactose, and other sugars
Crystals for reconstitution (Kristalose and generics): 10 g (15s, 30s), 20 g (30s)

Constipation:
Child: 1.5—3 mL/kg/24 hr PO ÷ once daily—BID; **max. dose:** 90 mL/24 hr
Adult: 15—30 mL/24 hr PO once daily × 1—2 days; may increase to 60 mL/24 hr if needed
Portal systemic encephalopathy (adjust dose to produce 2—3 soft stools/day):
Infant: 2.5—10 mL/24 hr PO ÷ TID—QID
Child and adolescent: 40—90 mL/24 hr PO ÷ TID—QID
Adult: 30—45 mL/dose PO TID—QID; acute episodes 30—45 mL Q1—2 hr until 2—3 soft stools/day
Rectal (adult): 300 mL diluted in 700 mL water or NS in 30—60 min retention enema; may give Q4—8 hr

Contraindicated in galactosemia. **Use with caution** in diabetes mellitus. GI discomfort and diarrhea may occur. For portal systemic encephalopathy, monitor serum ammonia, serum potassium, and fluid status.

Do not use with antacids. Dissolve crystal dosage form with 4 ounces of water or juice. All doses may be administered with juice, milk, or water.

LAMIVUDINE
Epivir, Epivir-HBV, 3TC, and generics
Antiviral agent, nucleoside analogue reverse transcriptase inhibitor

C   2   Yes   Yes   No

Tabs:
Epivir-HBV and generics: 100 mg
Epivir and generics: 150, 300 mg
Oral solution:
Epivir-HBV: 5 mg/mL (240 mL) contains parabens

LAMIVUDINE *continued*

Epivir and generics: 10 mg/mL (240 mL); contains parabens

HIV: See https://clinicalinfo.hiv.gov/en/guidelines
HIV vertical transmission and presumptive treatment during high-risk situations (mothers who received no antepartum antiretroviral therapy, mothers who received only intrapartum antiretroviral therapy, mothers who receive antepartum antiretroviral therapy, but with suboptimal viral suppression (≥50 copies/mL) within 4 weeks prior to delivery, or mothers with acute or primary HIV infection during pregnancy or breastfeeding (immediately discontinue breastfeeding). Transition to a treatment regimen if positive HIV diagnosis is confirmed and discontinue use after a negative diagnosis; see **Chapter 17** for additional information:

Neonate ≥32 wks' gestation (use in combination with zidovudine and either raltegravir or nevirapine): 2 mg/kg/dose PO BID within 6—12 hr after birth. Increase dose to 4 mg/kg/dose PO BID at 4 wk of age.

Chronic hepatitis B, non—HIV exposed or infected (see remarks):
2—17 yr: 3 mg/kg/dose PO once daily up to a **max. dose** of 100 mg/dose
18 and adult: 100 mg/dose PO once daily

See https://clinicalinfo.hiv.gov/en/guidelines for remarks for use in HIV. Oral tablet dosage form is preferred over oral solution for children ≥14 kg treated for HIV because subjects in the ARROW clinical trial receiving oral solution had lower rates of HIV viral suppression and lower plasma lamivudine exposure, and developed viral resistance more frequently.

May cause headache, fatigue, GI disturbances, rash, and myalgia/arthralgia. Lactic acidosis, severe hepatomegaly with steatosis, posttreatment exacerbations of hepatitis B and ALT elevations, pancreatitis, and emergence of resistant viral strains have been reported. Treatment should be suspended in any patient developing clinical or laboratory signs of lactic acidosis or hepatotoxicity.

Avoid use with sorbitol-containing medicines, as sorbitol reduces lamivudine exposure. Concomitant use with co-trimoxazole (TMP/SMX) may result in increased lamivudine levels.

Use Epivir-HBV product for chronic hepatitis B indication only. Safety and effectiveness beyond 1 yr have not been determined. If serum HBV DNA remains detectable after 24 wk of lamivudine monotherapy, consider switching to an alternative therapy. Patients with both HIV and hepatitis B should use the higher HIV doses along with an appropriate combination regimen.

May be administered with food. **Adjust dose in renal impairment (see Chapter 31).**

LAMOTRIGINE
Lamictal, Subvenite, Lamictal ODT, Lamictal XR, and generics
Anticonvulsant

   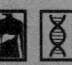
C   2   Yes   Yes   No

Tabs (Lamictal, Subvenite, and generics): 25, 100, 150, 200 mg
Extended release tabs (Lamictal XR and generics): 25, 50, 100, 200, 250, 300 mg
Chewable tabs (Lamictal and generics): 5, 25 mg
Orally disintegrated tabs (Lamictal ODT and generics): 25, 50, 100, 200 mg
Oral suspension: 1 mg/mL

Infant and child <2 yr adjunctive seizure therapy (limited data; use immediate release dosage forms):
WITH enzyme-inducing AEDs (e.g., carbamazepine, phenytoin, phenobarbital, primidone) and WITHOUT valproic acid:

Continued

LAMOTRIGINE *continued*

Wk 1 and 2: 0.6 mg/kg/24 hr PO ÷ once daily—BID

Wk 3 and 4: 1.2 mg/kg/24 hr PO ÷ once daily—BID

Usual maintenance dose (>wk 4): Titrate dose to effect PRN by increasing dosage every week by no more than 1.2 mg/kg/24 hr up to a **maximum** of 15.6 mg/kg/24 hr ÷ TID **not to exceed** 400 mg/24 hr.

WITH AEDs containing valproic acid or non-enzyme-inducing AEDs:

Wk 1 and 2: 0.15 mg/kg/24 hr PO ÷ once daily—BID

Wk 3 and 4: 0.3 mg/kg/24 hr PO ÷ once daily—BID

Usual maintenance dose (>wk 4): Titrate dose to effect PRN by increasing dosage every week by no more than 0.3 mg/kg/24 hr up to a **maximum** of 5.1 mg/kg/24 hr ÷ TID **not to exceed** 200 mg/24 hr.

Child 2—12 yr adjunctive seizure therapy (maintenance doses for patients <30 kg may need to be increased as much as 50%; use immediate release dosage forms; see remarks):

WITH AEDs other than carbamazepine, phenytoin, phenobarbital, primidone, or valproic acid:

Wk 1 and 2: 0.3 mg/kg/24 hr PO ÷ once daily—BID; rounded down to the nearest whole tablet

Wk 3 and 4: 0.6 mg/kg/24 hr PO ÷ BID; rounded down to the nearest whole tablet

Usual maintenance dose (>wk 4): 4.5—7.5 mg/kg/24 hr PO ÷ BID; titrate to effect. To achieve the usual maintenance dose, increase doses Q1—2 wk by 0.6 mg/kg/24 hr (rounded down to the nearest whole tablet) as needed.

Max. dose: 300 mg/24 hr ÷ BID

WITH enzyme-inducing AEDs WITHOUT valproic acid:

Wk 1 and 2: 0.6 mg/kg/24 hr PO ÷ BID; rounded down to the nearest whole tablet

Wk 3 and 4: 1.2 mg/kg/24 hr PO ÷ BID; rounded down to the nearest whole tablet

Usual maintenance dose (>wk 4): 5—15 mg/kg/24 hr PO ÷ BID; titrate to effect. To achieve the usual maintenance dose, increase doses Q1—2 wk by 1.2 mg/kg/24 hr (rounded down to the nearest whole tablet) as needed.

Max. dose: 400 mg/24 hr ÷ BID

WITH AEDs WITH valproic acid:

Wk 1 and 2: 0.15 mg/kg/24 hr PO ÷ once daily—BID; rounded down to the nearest whole tablet (see following table)

Wk 3 and 4: 0.3 mg/kg/24 hr PO ÷ once daily—BID; rounded down to the nearest whole tablet (see following table)

Weight (kg)	Weeks 1 and 2	Weeks 3 and 4
6.7—14	2 mg every other day	2 mg once daily
14.1—27	2 mg once daily	4 mg/24 hr ÷ once daily—BID
27.1—34	4 mg/24 hr ÷ once daily—BID	8 mg/24 hr ÷ once daily—BID
34.1—40	5 mg once daily	10 mg/24 hr ÷ once daily—BID

Usual maintenance dose: 1—5 mg/kg/24 hr PO ÷ once daily—BID; titrate to effect. To achieve the usual maintenance dose, increase doses Q1—2 wk by 0.3 mg/kg/24 hr (rounded down to the nearest whole tablet) as needed. If adding lamotrigine with valproic acid alone, usual maintenance dose is 1—3 mg/kg/24 hr.

LAMOTRIGINE *continued*

Max. dose: 200 mg/24 hr

>12 yr and adult adjunctive therapy:

WITH AEDs other than carbamazepine, phenytoin, phenobarbital, primidone, or valproic acid (use immediate release dosage forms):

Wk 1 and 2: 25 mg once daily PO

Wk 3 and 4: 50 mg once daily PO

Usual maintenance dose (>wk 4): 225—375 mg/24 hr ÷ BID PO; titrate to effect. To achieve the usual maintenance dose, increase doses Q1—2 wk by 50 mg/24 hr as needed.

WITH enzyme-inducing AEDs WITHOUT valproic acid (use immediate release dosage forms):

Wk 1 and 2: 50 mg once daily PO

Wk 3 and 4: 50 mg BID PO

Usual maintenance dose (>wk 4): 300—500 mg/24 hr ÷ BID PO; titrate to effect. To achieve the usual maintenance dose, increase doses Q1—2 wk by 100 mg/24 hr as needed. Doses as high as 700 mg/24 hr ÷ BID have been used.

WITH AEDs WITH valproic acid: (use immediate release dosage forms)

Wk 1 and 2: 25 mg every other day PO

Wk 3 and 4: 25 mg once daily PO

Usual maintenance dose (>wk 4): 100—400 mg/24 hr ÷ once daily—BID PO, titrate to effect. To achieve the usual maintenance dose, increase doses Q1—2 wk by 25—50 mg/24 hr as needed. If adding lamotrigene to valproic acid alone, usual maintenance dose is 100—200 mg/24 hr.

Extended release dosage form (Lamictal XR):

≥13 yr and adult adjunctive therapy (dose increases at wk 8 or later should not exceed 100 mg/24 hr at weekly intervals; see remarks):

	Weeks 1 and 2	Weeks 3 and 4	Week 5	Week 6	Week 7	Maintenance Dose
Patient NOT receiving enzyme-inducing drugs (e.g., carbamazepine) OR valproic acid	25 mg once daily	50 mg once daily	100 mg once daily	150 mg once daily	200 mg once daily	300—400 mg once daily
Patients receiving enzyme-inducing drugs (e.g., carbamazepine) WITHOUT valproic acid	50 mg once daily	100 mg once daily	200 mg once daily	300 mg once daily	400 mg once daily	400—600 mg once daily
Patients receiving valproic acid	25 mg every other day	25 mg once daily	50 mg once daily	100 mg once daily	150 mg once daily	200—250 mg once daily

Continued

LAMOTRIGINE *continued*

Converting Adjunctive Therapy to Lamotrigine Monotherapy:

	Immediate Release Lamotrigine Dosage Form Regimen (≥16 Yr and Adult)	Extended Release Tabs (≥13 Yr and Adult)
Patient NOT receiving enzyme-inducing drugs (e.g., carbamazepine) OR valproic acid	No specific dosing guidelines provided	After achieving a maintenance dose of 250—300 mg/24 hr with the above recommendations, withdraw the concomitant AED by 20% decrements each week over a 4-wk period.
Patients receiving enzyme-inducing drugs (e.g., carbamazepine) WITHOUT valproic acid	After achieving a maintenance dose of 500 mg/24 hr with the above recommendations, withdraw the concomitant enzyme-inducing AED by 20% decrements each week over a 4-wk period.	After achieving a maintenance dose of 500 mg/24 hr with the above recommendations, withdraw the concomitant enzyme-inducing AED by 20% decrements each week over a 4-wk period. After 2 wk of the complete withdrawal of enzyme-inducing AED, lamotrigine may be decreased no faster than 100 mg/24 hr each week to the maintenance dose of 250—300 mg/24 hr.
Patients receiving valproic acid	*Step 1*: Achieve maintenance dose of 200 mg/24 hr with the above recommendations. *Step 2*: Decrease valproic acid by decrements no greater than 500 mg/24 hr per week to reach 500 mg/24 hr and maintain for 1 wk. *Step 3*: Increase lamotrigine to 300 mg/24 hr and decrease valproic acid to 250 mg/24 hr; maintain both for 1 wk. *Step 4*: Increase lamotrigine by 100 mg/24 hr Q7 days until reaching maintenance dose of 500 mg/24 hr and discontinue valproic acid.	*Step 1*: Achieve maintenance dose of 150 mg/24 hr with the above recommendations. *Step 2*: Decrease valproic acid by decrements no greater than 500 mg/24 hr per week to reach 500 mg/24 hr and maintain for 1 wk. *Step 3*: Increase lamotrigine to 200 mg/24 hr and decrease valproic acid to 250 mg/24 hr; maintain both for 1 wk. *Step 4*: Increase lamotrigine to 250—300 mg/24 hr and discontinue valproic acid.

LAMOTRIGINE *continued*

Bipolar disease (use immediate release dosage forms; see remarks):
  ≥18 yr and adult (PO; see table below):

	Weeks 1 and 2	Weeks 3 and 4	Week 5	Weeks 6 and Thereafter
Patient NOT receiving enzyme-inducing drugs (e.g., carbamazepine) OR valproic acid	25 mg/24 hr	50 mg/24 hr ÷ once daily—BID	100 mg/24 hr ÷ once daily—BID	200 mg/24 hr ÷ once daily—BID (target dose); some patients may require 400 mg/24 hr
Patents receiving enzyme-inducing drugs (e.g., carbamazepine) WITHOUT valproic acid	50 mg/24 hr ÷ once daily—BID	100 mg/24 hr ÷ once daily—BID	200 mg/24 hr ÷ once daily—BID	Week 6: 300 mg/24 hr ÷ once daily—BID Week 7 and thereafter: may increase to 400 mg/24 hr ÷ once daily—BID[a]
Patients receiving valproic acid	25 mg every other day	25 mg once daily	50 mg/24 hr ÷ once daily—BID	100 mg/24 hr ÷ once daily—BID (target dose)[b]

[a]If carbamazepine or other enzyme-inducing drug is discontinued, maintain current lamotrigine dose for 1 wk, then decrease daily lamotrigine dose in 100 mg increments at weekly intervals until 200 mg/24 hr.
[b]If valproic acid is discontinued, increase by 50 mg at weekly intervals, up to 200 mg/24 hr.

Enzyme-inducing AEDs include carbamazepine, phenytoin, and phenobarbital. Stevens-Johnson syndrome, toxic epidermal necrolysis, and other potentially life-threatening rashes have been reported in children (0.3%—0.8%) and adults (0.08%—0.3%) for adjunctive therapy in seizures. Reported rates for adults treated for bipolar/mood disorders as monotherapy and adjunctive therapy are 0.08% and 0.13%, respectively. May cause fatigue, drowsiness, ataxia, rash (especially with valproic acid), headache, nausea, vomiting, and abdominal pain. Diplopia, nystagmus, aseptic meningitis, hemophagocytic lymphohistiocytosis, aggression, and alopecia have also been reported. False-positive test for urine phencyclidine (PCP) screen may occur.

Use during the first 3 mo of pregnancy may result in a higher chance for cleft lip or cleft palate in the newborn. Suicidal behavior or ideation has been reported. In vitro studies show lamotrigine having Class IB antiarrhythmic activity; access the benefit/risk for use in patients with clinically significant structural or functional heart disease, including cardiac channelopathies.

If converting from immediate release to extended release dosage form, match the initial dose of extended release to the total daily dose of the immediate release dosage and administer once daily. Adjust dose as needed with the recommended dosage guidelines.

Reduce maintenance dose in renal failure. Reduce all doses (initial, escalation, and maintenance) in liver dysfunction defined by the Child-Pugh grading system as follows:
  Grade B: Moderate dysfunction; decrease dose by ~50%
  Grade C: Severe dysfunction; decrease dose by ~75%

Withdrawal symptoms may occur if discontinued suddenly. A stepwise dose reduction over ≥2 wk (~50% per week) is recommended unless safety concerns require a more rapid withdrawal.

Continued

LAMOTRIGINE *continued*

Lamotrigine is metabolized by uridine 5'-diphospho-glucuronyl transferases (UGT). Strong and moderate inducers of CYP 450 3A4 are known to induce UGT to increase lamotrigine clearance. Acetaminophen, carbamazepine, oral contraceptives (ethinylestradiol), phenobarbital, primidone, phenytoin, and rifampin may decrease levels of lamotrigine. Valproic acid may increase levels. Use with sodium channel blockers may increase the risk of arrhythmias. False-positive urine drug screen for phencyclidine (PCP) has been reported.

Safety and efficacy for maintenance therapy for bipolar disorder in 10—17 yr olds were not established in an RCT with 301 subjects.

LANSOPRAZOLE
Prevacid, Prevacid SoluTab, First-Lansoprazole, and generics
Gastric acid pump inhibitor

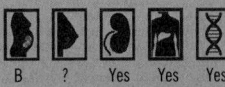

B   ?   Yes   Yes   Yes

Caps, delayed release: 15 mg (OTC and Rx), 30 mg
Tabs, disintegrating delayed release (Prevacid SoluTab and generics): 15 mg (OTC and Rx), 30 mg; contains aspartame
Oral suspension (First-Lansoprazole): 3 mg/mL (90, 150, 300 mL); contains benzyl alcohol

---

Neonate: 0.5—1.5 mg/kg/24 hr PO ÷ once daily—BID
Short-term treatment of GERD and erosive esophagitis, for up to 12 wk (see remarks):
Infant ≥3 mo: 15 mg/24 hr PO ÷ once daily—BID
Child 1—11 yr (initial dose using fixed dosing):
  ≤30 kg: 15 mg PO once daily
  >30 kg: 30 mg PO once daily
  Subsequent dosage increase (if needed): May be increased up to 30 mg PO BID after ≥2 wk of therapy without response at initial dose level
Alternative weight-based dosing:
  Infant: 1—2 mg/kg/24 hr PO once daily
  Child and adolescent: 0.7—3 mg/kg/24 hr PO ÷ once daily—BID; **max. dose:** 30 mg/24 hr
12 yr—adult:
  GERD: 15 mg PO once daily for up to 8 wk
  Erosive esophagitis: 30 mg PO once daily × 8—16 wk; maintenance dose: 15 mg PO once daily
  Duodenal ulcer: 15 mg PO once daily × 4 wk; maintenance dose: 15 mg PO once daily
  Gastric ulcer and NSAID-induced ulcer:
    Prophylaxis: 15 mg PO once daily for up to 12 wk
    Treatment: 30 mg PO once daily for up to 8 wk
  Hypersecretory conditions: 60 mg PO once daily; dosage may be increased up to 90 mg PO BID, where doses >120 mg/24 hr are divided BID

Common side effects include GI discomfort, headache, fatigue, rash, and taste perversion. Hypersensitivity reactions may result in anaphylaxis, angioedema, severe cutaneous reactions, bronchospasm, interstitial nephritis, and urticaria. Prolonged use may result in vitamin B_{12} deficiency (≥2 yr) or hypomagnesemia (>1 yr; sometimes leading to hypocalcemia, tetany, arrhythmias, and seizures). Microscopic colitis, resulting in watery diarrhea, has been reported, and switching to an alternative proton pump inhibitor may be beneficial in resolving diarrhea. Increased risk for fundic gland polyps has been associated with long-term use >1 yr.

Drug is a substrate for CYP 450 2C19 and 3A3/4. Ultrarapid metabolizers of CYP 450 2C19 may experience reduced efficacy and may require a 4-fold higher dosage. Lansoprazole may decrease levels of itraconazole, ketoconazole, iron salts, mycophenolate, nelfinavir, and ampicillin esters; and

LANSOPRAZOLE *continued*

increase the levels/effects of methotrexate, tacrolimus, and warfarin. Theophylline clearance may be enhanced. **Reduce dose in severe hepatic impairment.** May be used in combination with clarithromycin and amoxicillin for *H. pylori* infections.

A multicenter, double-blind, parallel-group study in infants (1 mo–1 yr) with GERD was no more effective than placebo.

Administer all oral doses before meals and 30 min prior to sucralfate. **Do not** crush or chew the granules (all dosage forms). Capsule may be opened and intact granules may be administered in an acidic beverage or food (e.g., apple or cranberry juice, applesauce). **Do not** break or cut the orally disintegrating tablets. Use of oral disintegrating tablets dissolved in water has been reported to clog and block oral syringes and feeding tubes (gastric and jejunostomy). For IV use, use a 1.2-micron in-line filter.

LEVALBUTEROL
Xopenex, Xopenex HFA, and generics
β₂ adrenergic agonist

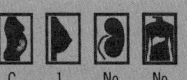

C   1   No   No   No

Prediluted nebulized solution: 0.31 mg in 3 mL, 0.63 mg in 3 mL, 1.25 mg in 3 mL (30s)
Concentrated nebulized solution: 1.25 mg/0.5 mL (0.5 mL) (30s)
Aerosol inhaler (MDI; Xopenex HFA and generics): 45 mCg/actuation (15 g delivers 200 doses)

Nonacute exacerbation symptom relief:
  Nebulizer:
    ≤4 yr (limited data): Start at 0.31 mg inhaled Q4–6 hr PRN; dose may be increased up to 1.25 mg Q4–6 hr PRN.
    5–11 yr: Start at 0.31 mg inhaled Q8 hr PRN; dose may be increased to 0.63 mg Q8 hr PRN.
    ≥12 yr and adult: Start at 0.63 mg inhaled Q6–8 hr PRN; dose may be increased to 1.25 mg inhaled Q6–8 hr PRN.
  Aerosol inhaler (MDI):
    ≥4 yr and adult: 2 puffs Q4–6 hr PRN
For use in acute exacerbations, more aggressive dosing may be used.

R-isomer of racemic albuterol. Side effects include tachycardia, palpitations, tremor, insomnia, nervousness, nausea, and headache.

Clinical data in children demonstrate levalbuterol is as effective as albuterol with fewer cardiac side effects at equipotent doses (0.31–0.63 mg levalbuterol ∼ 2.5 mg albuterol). However, when higher doses of levalbuterol (1.25 mg) were compared to 2.5 mg albuterol, changes in heart rate were similar.

More frequent dosing may be necessary in asthma exacerbation.

LEVETIRACETAM
Keppra, Keppra XR, Elepsia XR, Roweepra,
Spritam, and generics
Anticonvulsant

    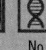

C   2   Yes   No   No

Tabs: 250, 500, 750, 1000 mg
Extended release tabs (Q24 hr dosing; see remarks):
  Keprra XR and generics: 500, 750 mg
  Elepsia XR: 1000, 1500 mg
Tabs, disintegrating (Spritam; see remarks): 250, 500, 750, 1000 mg

Continued

LEVETIRACETAM *continued*

Oral solution: 100 mg/mL (480 mL); dye free and contains parabens

Injection: 100 mg/mL (5 mL); contains 45 mg sodium chloride and 8.2 mg sodium acetate trihydrate per 100 mg drug

Premixed injection: 500 mg/100 mL in 0.82% sodium chloride, 1000 mg/100 mL in 0.75% sodium chloride, 1500 mg/100 mL in 0.54% sodium chloride

Partial seizures (mono or adjunctive therapy; using immediate release dosage forms and IV):

> **Infant (1—5 mo):** Start at 7 mg/kg/dose PO/IV BID; increase by 7 mg/kg/dose BID every 2 wk as tolerated to the recommended dose of 21 mg/kg/dose BID. An average daily dose of 35 mg/kg/24 hr was reported in clinical trials.

> **Infant ≥6 mo—child 3 yr (>20 kg):** Start at 10 mg/kg/dose PO/IV BID; increase by 10 mg/kg/dose BID every 2 wk as tolerated to the recommended dose of 25 mg/kg/dose BID. An average daily dose of 47 mg/kg/24 hr was reported in clinical trials.

> **Child 4—15 yr:** Start at 10 mg/kg/dose PO/IV BID; increase by 10 mg/kg/dose BID every 2 wk as tolerated up to the recommended dose of 30 mg/kg/dose BID or up to a **max. dose** of 3000 mg/24 hr. An average daily dose of 44 mg/kg/24 hr was reported in clinical trials.

>> **Alternative dosing with oral tablets:**

>>> **20—40 kg:** Start at 250 mg PO BID; increase by 250 mg BID every 2 wk as tolerated up to a **maximum** of 750 mg BID.

>>> **>40 kg:** Start at 500 mg PO BID; increase by 500 mg BID every 2 wk as tolerated up to a **maximum** of 1500 mg BID.

> **16 yr—adult:** Start at 500 mg PO/IV BID; may increase by 500 mg/dose BID every 2 wk as tolerated up to a **max. dose** of 1500 mg BID.

> **Extended release tabs (>12 yr and adult):** Start at 1000 mg PO once daily; increase by 1000 mg/24 hr every 2 wk as tolerated up to a **maximum** of 3000 mg/24 hr once daily.

Myoclonic seizure (adjunctive therapy; using immediate release dosage forms and IV):

> **≥12 yr and adult:** Start at 500 mg PO/IV BID; then increase dosage by 500 mg/dose BID every 2 wk as tolerated to reach the target dosage of 1500 mg BID.

Tonic-clonic seizure (primary generalized, adjunctive therapy; use immediate release dosage forms and IV):

> **Child 6—15 yr:** Start at 10 mg/kg/dose PO/IV BID; increase by 10 mg/kg/dose BID every 2 wk as tolerated to reach the target dosage of 30 mg/kg/dose BID.

>> **Alternative fixed dosing with oral disintegrating tabs (Spritam):**

>>> **20—40 kg:** Start at 250 mg PO BID; increase by 250 mg BID every 2 wk as tolerated up to a **maximum** of 750 mg BID.

>>> **>40 kg:** Start at 500 mg PO BID; increase by 500 mg BID every 2 wk as tolerated up to a **maximum** of 1500 mg BID.

> **16 yr—adult:** Start at 500 mg PO/IV BID; then increase dosage by 500 mg/dose BID every 2 wk as tolerated to reach the target dosage of 1500 mg BID.

Refractory status epilepticus (limited data):

> **Infant, child, and adolescent:** 60 mg/kg (**max. dose:** 4500 mg/dose) IV/IO over 10 min × 1, then start maintenance therapy based on clinical response and seizure type

Do not abruptly withdraw therapy, to reduce risk for seizures. **Use with caution** in renal impairment (**reduce dose; see Chapter 31**), hemodialysis, and neuropsychiatric conditions.

May cause loss of appetite, vomiting, dizziness, headaches, somnolence, agitation, depression, and mood swings. Drowsiness, fatigue, nervousness, and aggressive behavior have been reported in children. Nonpsychotic behavioral symptoms reported in children are approximately 3 times greater than in adults (37.6% vs. 13.3%). Suicidal behavior or ideation, serious dermatologic reactions

LEVETIRACETAM *continued*

(e.g., Stevens-Johnson and TEN), hematologic abnormalities (e.g., anemia, leukopenia), reversible alopecia, hyponatremia, hypertension, and worsening of seizures have been reported. Levetiracetam may decrease carbamazepine's effects. Ginkgo may decrease levetiracetam's effects.

Drug has excellent PO absorption. For IV use, use similar immediate release PO dosages only when the oral route of administration is not feasible. Extended release tablet is designed for once-daily administration at similar daily dosage of the immediate release forms (e.g., 1000 mg once daily of the extended release tablet is equivalent to 500 mg BID of the immediate release tablet). Disintegrating tabs (Spritam) may be administered by allowing the tablet to disintegrate in the mouth when taken with a sip of liquid or made into a suspension (see package insert); **do not** swallow this dosage form whole.

LEVOCARNITINE

See Carnitine.

LEVOFLOXACIN
Generics; previously available as Levaquin and Quixin
Antibiotic, quinolone

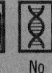

C   2   Yes   No   No

Tabs: 250, 500, 750 mg
Oral solution: 25 mg/mL (100, 200, 480 mL)
Injection: 25 mg/mL (20, 30 mL)
Premixed injection in D₅W: 250 mg/50 mL, 500 mg/100 mL, 750 mg/150 mL
Ophthalmic drops (generics previously available as Quixin): 0.5% (5 mL)

Child:
  General dosing:
    6 mo—<5 yr: 10 mg/kg/dose IV/PO Q12 hr; **max. dose:** 500 mg/24 hr
    ≥5 yr: 10 mg/kg/dose IV/PO Q24 hr; **max. dose:** 750 mg/24 hr
  Recurrent or persistent acute otitis media (6 mo—<5 yr): 10 mg/kg/dose PO Q12 hr × 10 days; **max. dose:** 500 mg/24 hr
  Community-acquired pneumonia (IDSA/Pediatric Infectious Disease Society):
    6 mo—<5 yr: 8—10 mg/kg/dose PO/IV Q12 hr; **max. dose:** 750 mg/24 hr
    5—16 yr: 8—10 mg/kg/dose PO/IV Q24 hr; **max. dose:** 750 mg/24 hr
  Inhalational anthrax (postexposure) and plague:
    ≥6 mo and <50 kg: 8 mg/kg/dose PO/IV Q12 hr; **max. dose:** 500 mg/24 hr
    >50 kg: 500 mg PO/IV once daily
    Duration of therapy:
      Inhalational anthrax (postexposure): 60 days
      Plague: 10—14 days
Adult:
  Community-acquired pneumonia: 750 mg PO/IV Q24 hr × 5 days
  Complicated UTI/acute pyelonephritis: 750 mg PO/IV Q24 hr × 5—7 days
  Acute bacterial sinusitis: 500 mg PO/IV Q24 hr × 10—14 days; OR 750 mg PO/IV Q24 hr × 5 days
  Inhalational anthrax (postexposure): 750 mg PO/IV Q24 hr × 60 days
  Plague: 500 mg PO/IV Q24 hr × 10—14 days

Continued

LEVOFLOXACIN *continued*

Conjunctivitis:
    ≥1 yr and adult: Instill 1−2 drops of the 0.5% solution to affected eye(s) Q2 hr up to 8 times/24 hr
        while awake for the first 2 days, then Q4 hr up to 4 times/24 hr while awake for the next 5 days.

Contraindicated in hypersensitivity to other quinolones. **Avoid** in patients with history of QTc
    prolongation or taking QTc prolonging drugs, and excessive sunlight exposure. **Use with
    caution** in diabetes, seizures, myasthenia gravis, children <18 yr, and renal impairment **(adjust
    dose, see Chapter 31).** May cause GI disturbances, headache, and blurred vision with the
    ophthalmic solution. Musculoskeletal disorders (e.g., arthralgia, arthritis, tendinopathy, and gait
    abnormality) may occur. Peripheral neuropathy and uveitis have been reported. Safety in pediatric
    patients treated more than 14 days has not been evaluated. Like other quinolones, tendon rupture
    can occur during or after therapy (risk increases with concurrent corticosteroids). Psychiatric
    adverse events, increased intracranial pressure, seizures, and blood glucose disturbances have
    been reported. Use with NSAIDs may increase risk of CNS stimulation and seizures.
Infuse IV over 1−1.5 hr; **avoid** IV push or rapid infusion because of risk of hypotension. **Do not**
    administer antacids or other divalent salts with or within 2 hr of oral levofloxacin dose; otherwise
    may be administered with or without food.

LEVOTHYROXINE (T₄)
Synthroid, Euthyrox, Levoxyl, Tirosint, Thyquidity,
Tirosint-Sol, Unithroid, and generics
Thyroid product

    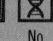

A   1   No   No   No

Tabs: 25, 50, 75, 88, 100, 112, 125, 137, 150, 175, 200, 300 mCg
Caps (Tirosint): 13, 25, 50, 75, 88, 100, 112, 125, 137, 150, 175, 200 mCg
Injection: 100, 200, 500 mCg; preservative free
Oral solution:
    Thyquidity: 100 mcg/5 mL (100 mL); contains parabens
    Tirosint-Sol: 13, 25, 37.5, 44, 50, 62.5, 75, 88, 100, 112, 125, 137, 150, 175, 200 mCg/1 mL
        (30 ampules per box)
Oral suspension: 25 mCg/mL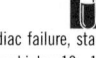

Hypothyroidism:
    Child PO dosing (see remarks):
        1−3 mo: 10−15 mCg/kg/dose once daily. If patient is at risk for developing cardiac failure, start
            with lower dose of 25 mCg/24 hr; and if patient has very low T₄ (<5 mCg/dL), use higher 12−17
            mCg/kg/24 hr dose.
        >3−6 mo: 8−10 mCg/kg/dose once daily
        >6−12 mo: 6−8 mCg/kg/dose once daily
        1−5 yr: 5−6 mCg/kg/dose once daily
        6−12 yr: 4−5 mCg/kg/dose once daily
        >12 yr:
            Incomplete growth and prepuberty: 2−3 mCg/kg/dose once daily
            Complete growth and puberty: 1.7 mCg/kg/dose once daily
    Child IM/IV dose: 50%−75% of oral dose once daily
    Adult:
        PO: Start with 12.5−25 mCg/dose once daily. Increase by 12.5−25 mCg/24 hr at intervals of Q2−4
            wk until euthyroid. Usual adult dose: 100−200 mCg/24 hr
        IM/IV dose: 50% of oral dose once daily

LEVOTHYROXINE (T4) *continued*

Myxedema coma or stupor:
  Adult: 300—500 mCg IV × 1, then 50—100 mCg IV once daily; convert to oral therapy once patient is stabilized

Contraindications include acute MI, thyrotoxicosis, and uncorrected adrenal insufficiency. May cause hyperthyroidism, rash, growth disturbances, hypertension, worsening of diabetic control, decreased bone mineral density (primarily in postmenopausal females), arrhythmias, diarrhea, and weight loss. Pseudotumor cerebri and slipped capital femoral epiphysis have been reported in children. Overtreatment may cause craniosynostosis in infants and premature closure of the epiphyses in infants who have not undergone complete closure of the fontanelles.

Total replacement dose may be used in children unless there is evidence of cardiac disease; in that case, begin with one-fourth of maintenance and increase weekly. Titrate dosage with clinical status and serum T_4 and TSH.

Increases the effects of warfarin. Phenytoin, rifampin, carbamazepine, iron and calcium supplements, antacids, grapefruit juice, and orlistat may decrease levothyroxine levels. Tricyclic antidepressants and SSRIs may enhance toxic effects. Use with ketamine may cause hypertension and tachycardia. High doses of propranolol or dexamethasone, and amiodarone may decrease the conversion of T_4 to T_3.

100 mCg levothyroxine = 65 mg thyroid USP. Administer oral doses on an empty stomach and tablets with a full glass of water. Iron and calcium supplements and antacids may decrease absorption; **do not** administer within 4 hr of these agents. Excreted in low levels in breast milk; preponderance of evidence suggests no clinically significant effect in infants.

LIDOCAINE
Xylocaine, L-M-X, Lidoderm, Gen7T Plus, many different brands of topical products, and generics
Antiarrhythmic class Ib, local anesthetic

   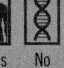

B   1   Yes   Yes   No

Injection: 0.5%, 1%, 1.5%, 2%, 4% (1% sol = 10 mg/mL)
IV infusion (in D₅W): 0.4% (4 mg/mL) (250, 500 mL); 0.8% (8 mg/mL) (250 mL)
Injection with epinephrine (some preparations may contain metasulfite and parabens or are preservative free):
  Injection with 1:100,000 epinephrine: 1%, 2% lidocaine
  Injection with 1:200,000 epinephrine: 0.5%, 1%, 1.5%, 2% lidocaine
Ointment: 4% (50 g), 5% (30, 50 g)
Cream, topical: 3% (30, 85 g), 4% (L-M-X-4 and generics) [OTC] (5, 15, 30, 45 g), 5% (L-M-X-5 and generics) [OTC] (15, 30 g); may contain benzyl alcohol
Cream, rectal: 5% (L-M-X-5 and others; 15, 30 g); contains benzyl alcohol
Gel (external): 2% (5, 10, 20, 30 mL), 3% (10, 30 mL), 4% (10, 30 , 113 g), 5% (10, 30, 113 g); may contain benzyl alcohol, EDTA
Lotion: 3% (118, 177 mL), 4% (88 mL)
Solution (external): 4% (50 mL); may contain parabens
Aerosol spray (external): 4% (104 mL)
Transdermal patch:
  Gen7T Plus and generics: 3.5% (5s, 10s, 15s); may contain menthol
  Lidocaine Pain Relief and generics [OTC]: 4% (5s, 10s); may contain menthol, capsaicin, and methyl salicylate
  Lidoderm and generics: 5% (1s, 15s, 30s)

Continued

LIDOCAINE continued

Oral solution (mouth/throat): 2% (15, 100 mL), 4% (4 mL)

Topical cream or gel 2.5% with 2.5% prilocaine: See Lidocaine and Prilocaine.

Anesthetic:

Injection (local): Use <2% concentration. Dosage varies with procedure, degree and duration of analgesia, tissue vascularity, and patient condition.

Without epinephrine: max. dose of 4.5 mg/kg/dose (up to 300 mg); do not repeat within 2 hr.

With epinephrine: max. dose of 7 mg/kg/dose (up to 500 mg); do not repeat within 2 hr.

Topical:

Cream (child ≥2 yr and adult): Apply to affected intact skin areas BID—QID; **max. dose:** 4.5 mg/kg/dose up to 300 mg/dose

Gel, lotion, or ointment (child ≥2 yr and adult): Apply to affected intact skin areas once daily—QID (BID—TID for lotion); **max. dose:** 4.5 mg/kg/dose up to 300 mg/dose

Patch:

4% (≥12 yr and adult): Apply patch to painful area and leave in place for up to 12 hr; **max. dose:** one patch/24 hr

5% (adult): Apply to most painful area with up to 3 patches at a time. Patch(es) may be left in place for up to 12 hr in any 24 hr period.

Antiarrhythmic (infant, child, adolescent):

Bolus: 1 mg/kg/dose (**max. dose:** 100 mg) slowly IV; may repeat in 10—15 min × 2; **max. total dose:** 3—5 mg/kg within the first hr. ETT dose = 2—3 × IV dose.

Continuous infusion: 20—50 mCg/kg/min IV/IO (**do not exceed** 20 mCg/kg/min for patients with shock, CHF, hepatic disease, or cardiac arrest); see inside cover for infusion preparation. Administer a 1 mg/kg bolus when infusion is initiated if bolus has not been given within previous 15 min.

Oral use (2% viscous liquid):

Child (≥3 yr): Up to the lesser of 4.5 mg/kg/dose or 300 mg/dose, swish and spit Q3 hr PRN up to a **max. dose** of 4 doses per 12 hr period

Adult: 15 mL, swish and spit Q3 hr PRN up to a **max. dose** 4.5 mg/kg/dose or 300 mg/dose up to 8 doses/24 hr

For cardiac arrest, amiodarone is the preferred agent over lidocaine; lidocaine may be used only when amiodarone is not available.

Contraindicated in Stokes-Adams or Wolff-Parkinson-White syndromes and SA, AV, or intraventricular heart block without a pacemaker. Solutions containing dextrose may be contraindicated in patients with known allergy to corn or corn products. Side effects include hypotension, asystole, seizures, and respiratory arrest. Anaphylactic reactions have been reported. Local anesthetic use has been associated with methemoglobinemia.

CYP 450 2D6 and 3A3/4 substrate. **Use with caution** in severe liver or renal disease. Decrease dose in hepatic failure or decreased cardiac output. **Do not use** topically for teething. Prolonged infusion may result in toxic accumulation of lidocaine, especially in infants. **Do not use** epinephrine-containing solutions for treatment of arrhythmias.

Therapeutic levels 1.5—5 mg/L. Toxicity occurs at >7 mg/L. Toxicity in neonates may occur at >5 mg/L due to reduced protein binding of drug. Elimination $T_{1/2}$: premature infant: 3.2 hr, adult: 1.5—2 hr.

When using the topical patch, **avoid** exposing the application site to external heat sources as this may increase the risk for toxicity.

LIDOCAINE AND PRILOCAINE

Many brand names, Oraqix, Eutectic mixture of lidocaine and prilocaine; previously available as EMLA

Topical analgesic

B   ?   Yes   Yes   No

Cream: Lidocaine 2.5% + prilocaine 2.5% (5, 30 g)
Peridontal gel (Oraqix): Lidocaine 2.5% + prilocaine 2.5% (1.7 g in dental cartridges; 20s)

See Chapter 6 for general use information.
Neonate:
   <37 wk gestation (limited data):
      Painful procedures (e.g., IM injections): 0.5 g/site for 60 min
   ≥37 wk gestation and <5 kg:
      Painful procedures (e.g., IM injections): 1 g/site for 60 min. **Max. dose:** 1 g for all sites combined with a **max.** application area of 10 cm^2 and **max.** application time of 1 hr
      Circumcision: 1–2 g and cover with occlusive dressing for 60–90 min
Infant and child: The following are the recommended **maximum doses** based on the child's age and weight.

Age and Weight	Maximum Total EMLA Dose (g)	Maximum Application Area (cm^2)	Maximum Application Time
Birth–<3 mo or <5 kg	1	10	1 hr
3–12 mo and >5–10 kg[a]	12	20	4 hr
1–6 yr and >10 kg	10	100	4 hr
7–12 yr and >20 kg	20	200	4 hr

[a]If patient is >3 mo and is not >5 kg, use the **maximum** total dose which corresponds to the patient's weight.
EMLA, Eutectic mixture of local anesthetics.

Adolescent and adult:
   Minor procedures: 2.5 g/site over 20–25 cm^2 of skin for at least 60 min
   Painful procedures: 2 g/10 cm^2 of skin for at least 2 hr

Should not be used in neonates <37 wk of gestation or in infants <12 mo old receiving treatment with methoglobin-inducing agents (e.g., sulfa drugs, acetaminophen, nitrofurantoin, nitroglycerin, nitroprusside, phenobarbital, phenytoin). **Use with caution** in patients with G6PD deficiency, patients treated with class I or III antiarrhythmic drugs (additive or toxic cardiac effects), and in patients with renal and hepatic impairment. Prilocaine has been associated with methemoglobinemia. Long duration of application, large treatment area, small patients, or impaired elimination may result in high blood levels.
Apply topically to intact skin and cover with occlusive dressing; **avoid** mucous membranes or the eyes. Wipe cream off before procedure.

LINDANE
Gamma benzene hexachloride and various generics
Scabicidal agent, pediculocide

C   3   No   No   No

Shampoo: 1% (60 mL)

Pediculosis capitis (second-line therapy; see remarks):
   Child and adult: Apply ≤30 mL (amount depends on length and density of hair; **max. dose:** 60 mL) shampoo to dry hair without adding water. Work shampoo thoroughly into hair and allow to remain in place for 4 min. Then add small amounts of water to the hair until a good lather forms. Immediately rinse all the lather away and **avoid** contact of lather to other body surfaces. Towel dry and comb hair with fine-tooth comb to remove nits. **Do not re-treat.**

Continued

LINDANE *continued*

Lindane is now considered a second-line therapy owing to side effect risk and reports of resistance. **Contraindicated** in premature infants and seizure disorders. **Use with caution** with drugs that lower seizure threshold. Systemically absorbed. Risk of toxic effects is greater in young children; use other agents (permethrin) in infants, young children (<2 yr), and during pregnancy.

May cause a rash; rarely may cause seizures or aplastic anemia. For scabies, change clothing and bed sheets after starting treatment and treat family members. For pediculosis pubis, treat sexual contacts.

Avoid contact with face, urethral meatus, damaged skin, or mucous membranes. **Do not use** any covering that does not breathe (e.g., plastic lining or clothing) over the applied lindane.

LINEZOLID
Zyvox and generics
Antibiotic, oxazolidinone

   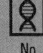

C   2   Yes   Yes   No

Tabs: 600 mg; contains ~0.45 mEq Na per 200 mg drug
Oral suspension: 100 mg/5 mL (150 mL); contains phenylalanine and sodium benzoate and 0.8 mEq Na per 200 mg drug
Injection, premixed: 200 mg in 100 mL, 600 mg in 300 mL; contains 1.7 mEq Na per 200 mg drug

Neonate:
  <1 kg:
    <14 days old: 10 mg/kg/dose IV Q12 hr
    ≥14 days old: 10 mg/kg/dose IV Q8 hr
  ≥1–2 kg:
    <7 days old: 10 mg/kg/dose IV/PO Q12 hr
    ≥7–28 days old: 10 mg/kg/dose IV/PO Q8 hr
  >2 kg: 10 mg/kg/dose IV/PO Q8 hr
  Alternate dosing by gestational age:
    <34 wk's gestation:
      <7 days old: 10 mg/kg/dose IV/PO Q12 hr
      ≥7–28 days old: 10 mg/kg/dose IV/PO Q8 hr
    ≥34 wk's gestation and 0–28 days old: 10 mg/kg/dose IV/PO Q8 hr
Infant and child <12 yr old:
  Pneumonia, bacteremia, bone/joint infections, septic thrombosis (MRSA), complicated skin/skin structure infections, vancomycin-resistant *E. faecium* (VRE) infections (including endocarditis): 10 mg/kg/dose IV/PO Q8 hr
  Uncomplicated skin/skin structure infections:
    <5 yr: 10 mg/kg/dose IV/PO Q8 hr
    5–11 yr: 10 mg/kg/dose IV/PO Q12 hr
  Max. dose for all indications <12 yr: 600 mg/dose
≥12 yr and adult: 600 mg Q12 hr IV/PO; 400 mg Q12 hr IV/PO may be used for adults with uncomplicated infection.

Most common side effects include diarrhea, headache, and nausea. Anemia, leukopenia, pancytopenia, and thrombocytopenia may occur in patients who are at risk for myelosuppression and who receive regimens >2 wk. Complete blood count monitoring is recommended in these individuals. Pseudomembranous colitis, neuropathy (peripheral and optic), hyponatremia, hypoglycemia, and severe cutaneous adverse reactions (e.g., TEN and SJS) have also been reported. CSF penetration is variable in patients with VP shunts.

LINEZOLID *continued*

Do not use with SSRIs (e.g., fluoxetine, paroxetine), tricyclic antidepressants, venlafaxine, and trazodone; may cause serotonin syndrome. **Avoid** use with monoamine oxidase inhibitors (e.g., phenelzine); and in patients with uncontrolled hypertension, pheochromocytoma, or thyrotoxicosis, and taking sympathomimetics or vasopressive agents (may elevate blood pressure). **Use caution** when consuming large amounts of foods and beverages containing tyramine; may increase blood pressure. Use in severe hepatic impairment (e.g., cirrhosis) or kidney impairment may increase risk for thrombocytopenia.

Protect all dosage forms from light and moisture. Oral suspension product must be gently mixed by inverting the bottle 3—5 times prior to each use **(do not shake).** All oral doses may be administered with or without food.

LIRAGLUTIDE
Saxenda, Victoza
Antidiabetic agent, glucagon-like peptide-1
(GLP-1) receptor agonist

 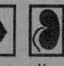 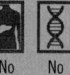

X   ?   Yes   No   No

Subcutaneous pen-injector:
  Saxenda and Victoza: 18 mg/3 mL (3 mL); contains phenol, propylene glycol

Type 2 diabetes mellitus (adjunctive therapy with diet and exercise):
  Victoza (child >10 yr and adolescent): Start with 0.6 mg SC once daily × 1 wk, if needed, increase by 0.6 mg increments on a weekly basis PRN up to a **maximum dose** of 1.8 mg/24 hr. In clinical trials, metformin was also prescribed with some receiving insulin (those receiving insulin had their insulin dose reduced by ~20%).

Chronic weight management (adjunctive therapy with diet and exercise):
  Saxenda (child >12 yr and adolescent): Start with 0.6 mg SC once daily × 1 wk, then increase dose by 0.6 mg/24 hr at weekly increments up to the target dose of 3 mg once daily. If unable to tolerate 3 mg once daily, may reduce dose to 2.4 mg once daily (discontinue use if 2.4 mg dose is not tolerated). Pediatric patients who are unable to tolerate the dose escalation may use the lower dose, and the targeted escalation could take up to 8 wk. Discontinue therapy if the patient has a <1% reduction in BMI after 12 weeks of therapy.

A bioengineered analog of human GLP-1 in *Saccharomyces cerevisiae* and acts as a GLP-1 receptor agonist. **Contraindicated** in patients with a family history of medullary thyroid carcinoma and in patients with multiple endocrine neoplasia syndrome type 2.

Common side effects include hypoglycemia, constipation, diarrhea, nausea, vomiting, indigestion, and headache. Pancreatitis, cholelithiasis/cholecystitis, hypersensitivity reactions (e.g., anaphylaxis and angioedema), and acute renal failure have been reported. Use with **caution** with other medications that could cause hypoglycemia (e.g., sulfonylurea, insulin, fluoroquinolones, beta-blockers, and SSRIs).

Doses are injected subcutaneously in the abdomen, thigh, or upper arm any time of the day without regard to meals. Each new prefilled pen requires priming before the first injection. Use a new needle for each dose administration. **Do not share** pens between patients despite changing needles. **Do not mix** with insulin and **do not administer** adjacent to insulin. If a dose is missed more than 3 days, reinitiate the dosage titration at 0.6 mg/24 hr. **Never administer** extra or doubled doses.

LISDEXAMFETAMINE
Vyvanse
CNS stimulant

   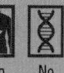

C   X   Yes   No   No

Capsules: 10, 20, 30, 40, 50, 60, 70 mg
Chewable tabs: 10, 20, 30, 40, 50, 60 mg; contains mannitol and sucralose

Continued

LISDEXAMFETAMINE *continued*

Attention-deficit hyperactivity disorder: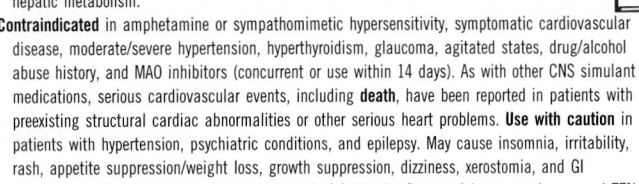

  Child ≥6 yr and adult: Start with 20—30 mg PO QAM (adult, start at 30 mg). May increase
    dose by 10—20 mg/24 hr at weekly intervals if needed, up to a **max. dose** of 70 mg/24 hr. Lower
    maximum dosages for renal insufficiency include the following:
    GFR ≥30 mL/min/1.73 m²: 70 mg/24 hr
    GFR 15—<30 mL/min/1.73 m²: 50 mg/24 hr
    GFR <15 mL/min/1.73 m² or ESRD on hemodialysis: 30 mg/24 hr
Binge eating disorder (moderate to severe):
  Adult: Start with 30 mg PO once daily. Increase in increments of 20 mg at weekly intervals to achieve
    the recommended dosage of 50—70 mg PO once daily; **max. dose:** 70 mg/24 hr; discontinue use if
    no improvement.

Lisdexamfetamine is a prodrug of dextroamphetamine that requires activation by intestinal/
  hepatic metabolism.
Contraindicated in amphetamine or sympathomimetic hypersensitivity, symptomatic cardiovascular
  disease, moderate/severe hypertension, hyperthyroidism, glaucoma, agitated states, drug/alcohol
  abuse history, and MAO inhibitors (concurrent or use within 14 days). As with other CNS simulant
  medications, serious cardiovascular events, including **death**, have been reported in patients with
  preexisting structural cardiac abnormalities or other serious heart problems. **Use with caution** in
  patients with hypertension, psychiatric conditions, and epilepsy. May cause insomnia, irritability,
  rash, appetite suppression/weight loss, growth suppression, dizziness, xerostomia, and GI
  disturbances. Dermatillomania, bruxism, intestinal ischemia, Stevens-Johnson syndrome, and TEN
  have been reported.
Urinary acidifying agents may reduce levels of amphetamines, and urinary alkalinizing agents may
  increase levels. May increase the effects of TCAs; increase or decrease the effects of guanfacine and
  phenytoin, and phenobarbital; and decrease the effects of adrenergic blockers, antihistamines, and
  antihypertensives. Norepinephrine may increase the effects of amphetamines.
Chewable tablets must be completely chewed before swallowing. Chewable tablet and capsule dosage
  forms can be converted on an equal mg-per-mg basis.
See Dextroamphetamine ± Amphetamine for additional remarks.

LISINOPRIL
Qbrelis, Zestril, and generics; previously available as Prinivil
Angiotensin-converting enzyme inhibitor,
antihypertensive

    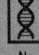

| X | 3 | Yes | Yes | No |

Tabs: 2.5, 5, 10, 20, 30, 40 mg
Oral solution (Qbrelis): 1 mg/mL (150 mL); contains sodium benzoate
Oral suspension: 1 mg/mL
Oral syrup: 2 mg/mL

Hypertension (see remarks):
  Child (<6 yr; limited data): Use 6—16 yr dosing below.
    6—16 yr: Start with 0.07—0.1 mg/kg/dose PO once daily; **max. initial dose:** 5 mg/dose. If needed,
      titrate dose upward at 1—2 wk intervals to doses up to 0.61 mg/kg/24 hr or 40 mg/24 hr (higher
      doses have not been evaluated).
    Adult: Start with 10 mg PO once daily (use 5 mg if using a diuretic). If needed, increase dose by 5—10
      mg/24 hr at 1—2 wk intervals. Usual dosage range: 20—40 mg/24 hr; **max. dose:** 80 mg/24 hr.

LISINOPRIL *continued*

Use lower initial dose (50% of recommended dose) if using with a diuretic or with the presence of hyponatremia, hypovolemia, severe CHF, or decreased renal function.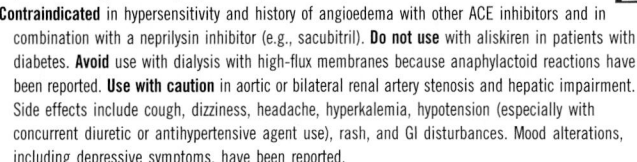

Contraindicated in hypersensitivity and history of angioedema with other ACE inhibitors and in combination with a neprilysin inhibitor (e.g., sacubitril). **Do not use** with aliskiren in patients with diabetes. **Avoid** use with dialysis with high-flux membranes because anaphylactoid reactions have been reported. **Use with caution** in aortic or bilateral renal artery stenosis and hepatic impairment. Side effects include cough, dizziness, headache, hyperkalemia, hypotension (especially with concurrent diuretic or antihypertensive agent use), rash, and GI disturbances. Mood alterations, including depressive symptoms, have been reported.

Dual blockade of the renin-angiotensin system with lisinopril and angiotensin receptor antagonists (e.g., losartin) or aliskiren is associated with increased risk for hypotension, syncope, hyperkalemia, and renal impairment. Diabetic patients on lisinopril treated with oral antidiabetic agents should be monitored for hypoglycemia, especially during the first month of use. NSAIDs (e.g., indomethacin) may decrease linsinopril's effects. Use with mTOR inhibitors (e.g., sirolimus, everolimus) may increase risk for angioedema. **Adjust dose in renal impairment (see Chapter 31).**

Onset of action: 1 hr with maximal effect in 6—8 hr. Long-term blood pressure monitoring is recommended at Q2—4 wk until good control is achieved, followed by Q3—4 mo.

Additional indications with limited data in children include proteinuria associated with mild IgA nephropathy, and renal protection for diabetes or renal parenchymal disease.

Lisinopril should be discontinued as soon as possible when pregnancy is detected as it can cause fetal harm especially when used during the second and third trimesters.

LITHIUM Lithobid and many generics; previously available as Eskalith *Antimanic agent*	 D	 X	 Yes	 No  No

Carbonate salt:
300 mg carbonate = 8.12 mEq lithium
Caps: 150, 300, 600 mg
Tabs: 300 mg
Extended release tabs: 300 mg (Lithobid and generics), 450 mg
Citrate salt:
Syrup: 8 mEq/5 mL (500 mL); 5 mL is equivalent to 300 mg lithium carbonate

Child (see remarks):
Initial (immediate release dosage forms): 15—60 mg/kg/24 hr ÷ TID—QID PO. Adjust as needed (weekly) to achieve therapeutic levels.

Adolescent: 600—1800 mg/24 hr ÷ TID—QID PO (divided BID—TID using extended-release tablets)
Adult:
Initial: 300 mg TID PO. Adjust as needed to achieve therapeutic levels. Usual dose is about 300 mg TID—QID with immediate release dosage form. For extended release tablets, 900—1800 mg/24 hr PO ÷ BID—TID

Contraindicated in severe cardiovascular disease (including Brugada syndrome) or renal disease. Decreased sodium intake, increased sodium wasting, or significant renal or cardiovascular disease may increase lithium levels, resulting in toxicity. May cause goiter, nephrogenic diabetes insipidus, hypothyroidism, arrhythmias, or sedation at therapeutic doses. Nephrotic syndrome and dermatologic reactions (e.g., alopecia, acne, psoriasis, and DRESS) have been reported.

Continued

LITHIUM *continued*

Coadministration with diuretics, metronidazole, ACE inhibitors, angiotensin receptor antagonists (e.g., losartan), or NSAIDs may increase risk for lithium toxicity. Use with iodine may increase risk for hypothyroidism. If used in combination with haloperidol, closely monitor neurologic toxicities because an encephalopathic syndrome followed by irreversible brain damage has been reported.

Safety and efficacy for monotherapy for acute mania or mixed episodes of bipolar I disorder and maintenance monotherapy of bipolar I disorder in children 7—17 yr have been established from a clinical trial. Common adverse effects observed in this study included nausea/vomiting, polyuria, thyroid abnormalities, tremor, polydipsia, dizziness, rash/dermatitis, ataxia/gait disturbance, anorexia, and blurry vision.

Therapeutic levels: 0.6—1.5 mEq/L. In either acute or chronic toxicity, confusion and somnolence may be seen at levels of 2—2.5 mEq/L. **Seizures or death** may occur at levels >2.5 mEq/L. Recommended serum sampling: trough level within 30 min prior to the next scheduled dose. Steady-state is achieved within 4—6 days of continuous dosing. **Adjust dose in renal failure (see Chapter 31).**

LODOXAMIDE
Alomide
Antiallergic agent, mast cell stabilizer

B   ?   No   No   No

Ophthalmic solution: 0.1% (10 mL); contains benzalkonium chloride

≥2 yr and adult: Instill 1—2 drops to affected eye(s) QID for up to 3 mo.

Transient burning, stinging, or discomfort of the eye and headache are common side effects. Itching/pruritus, blurred vision, dry eye, tearing, hyperemia, crystalline deposits, and foreign body sensation may also occur.

Do not wear soft contact lenses during treatment because medication contains benzalkonium chloride.

LOPERAMIDE
Imodium, Imodium A—D, and generics
Antidiarrheal

    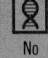

C   1   No   No   No

Caps (OTC): 2 mg
Tabs (OTC): 2 mg
Oral solution (OTC): 1 mg/7.5 mL (120, 240 mL); may contain propylene glycol and sodium benzoate; each 30 mL contains 16 mg of sodium

Acute diarrhea (see remarks):
   Child (initial doses within the first 24 hr):
      2—5 yr (13—<21 kg): 1 mg PO TID
      6—8 yr (21—27 kg): 2 mg PO BID
      9—11 yr (>27—43 kg): 2 mg PO TID
      Max. single dose: 2 mg
      Follow initial day's dose with 0.1 mg/kg/dose after each loose stool (not to exceed the aforementioned initial doses).
   ≥12 yr and adult: 4 mg/dose × 1, followed by 2 mg/dose after each stool up to **max. dose** of 8 mg/24 hr for 12—<18 yr and 16 mg/24 hr for adult

LOPERAMIDE *continued*

Chronic diarrhea (see remarks):
    Infant—child (limited data): 0.08–0.24 mg/kg/24 hr PO ÷ BID—TID; **max. dose:** 2 mg/dose

Contraindicated in acute dysentery; acute ulcerative colitis; bacterial enterocolitis caused by *Salmonella, Shigella, Campylobacter,* and *Clostridium difficile;* and abdominal pain in the absence of diarrhea. **Avoid** use in children <2 yr due to reports of paralytic ileus associated with abdominal distention. Rare hypersensitivity reactions including anaphylactic shock have been reported. May cause nausea, rash, vomiting, constipation, cramps, dry mouth, and CNS depression. Use of higher than recommended dosages via abuse or misuse can cause serious cardiac events (e.g., Torsades de Pointes, arrhythmias, cardiac arrest, and QT prolongation).

Discontinue use if no clinical improvement is observed within 48 hr. Naloxone may be administered for CNS depression.

LORATADINE ± PSEUDOEPHEDRINE
Alavert, Claritin, Claritin Children's Allergy, Claritin
RediTabs, many others and generics
In combination with pseudoephedrine:
Claritin-D 12 Hour, Claritin-D 24 Hour, Alavert D-12 Hour Allergy and Congestion,
Loratadine-D 12 Hour, Loratadine-D 24 Hour, Allergy Relief-D, and generics
Antihistamine, less sedating ± decongestant

B/C   2   Yes   Yes   No

Tabs [OTC]: 10 mg
Caps, liquid filled [OTC]: 10 mg; contains polysorbate 80
Chewable tabs (Claritin Children's Allergy and others) [OTC]: 5 mg; contains aspartame
Disintegrating tabs (Claritin RediTabs and others) [OTC]: 5, 10 mg; contains aspartame
Oral solution or syrup [OTC]: 1 mg/mL (120 mL); contains propylene glycol and sodium benzoate; some preparations may contain metasulfite
Time-release tabs in combination with pseudoephedrine (PE):
    Claritin-D 12 Hour, Alavert D-12 Hour Allergy and Congestion, Loratadine-D 12 Hour, and generics [OTC]: 5 mg loratadine + 120 mg PE
    Claritin-D 24 Hour, Loratadine-D 24 Hour, Allergy Relief-D and generics [OTC]: 10 mg loratadine + 240 mg PE

Loratadine:
    2—5 yr: 5 mg PO once daily
    ≥6 yr and adult: 10 mg PO once daily. Disintegrating tablet may be dosed at 5 mg PO BID or 10 mg PO once daily.
Time-release tabs of loratidine and pseudoephedrine:
    ≥12 yr and adult (see remarks):
        Claritin-D 12 Hour and generics: 1 tablet PO BID
        Claritin-D 24 Hour and generics: 1 tablet PO once daily

May cause drowsiness, fatigue, dry mouth, headache, bronchospasms, palpitations, dermatitis, and dizziness. Has not been implicated in causing cardiac arrhythmias when used with other drugs that are metabolized by hepatic microsomal enzymes (e.g., ketoconazole, erythromycin). May be administered safely in patients who have allergic rhinitis and asthma.

In hepatic and renal function impairment (GFR <30 mL/min), prolong loratadine (single agent) dosage interval to every other day. **Adjust dose in renal failure (see Chapter 31).**

For time-release tablets of the combination product (loratadine and pseudoephedrine), prolong dosage interval in renal impairment (GFR <30 mL/min) as follows: Claritin-D 12 Hour: 1 tablet PO once daily; Claritin-D 24 Hour: 1 tablet PO every other day. **Do not** use the combination product in hepatic

Continued

LORATADINE ± PSEUDOEPHEDRINE *continued*

impairment because drugs cannot be individually titrated. Pregnancy category changes to "C" for the combination product (loratadine and pseudoephedrine).

Administer doses on an empty stomach. For use of RediTabs, place tablet on tongue and allow it to disintegrate in the mouth with or without water. For Claritin-D products, also see remarks in Pseudoephedrine.

LORAZEPAM
Ativan, Loreev XR, and generics
Benzodiazepine anticonvulsant

D   2   Yes   Yes   No

Tabs: 0.5, 1, 2 mg
Extended release capsules (Loreev XR): 1, 1.5, 2, 3 mg
Injection: 2, 4 mg/mL (1, 10 mL); each contains 2% benzyl alcohol and propylene glycol
Oral solution: 2 mg/mL (30 mL); some dosage forms may be alcohol and dye free, and contain propylene glycol

DOSAGES ARE FOR IMMEDIATE RELEASE DOSAGE FORMS (TABS, INJECTION, AND ORAL SOLUTION):

Status epilepticus (IV route is preferred but may use IM route if IV is not available):
   Neonate, infant, child, and adolescent: 0.05—0.1 mg/kg/dose IV over 2—5 min. May repeat dose in 10—15 min. **Max. dose:** 4 mg/dose. If IV access not available, 0.1 mg/kg/dose (**max.** 4 mg/dose) may be administered intranasally.
   Adult: 4 mg/dose IV given slowly over 2—5 min. May repeat in 10—15 min. Usual total **max. dose** in 12-hr period is 8 mg.

Antiemetic adjunct therapy:
   Child: 0.025—0.05 mg/kg/dose IV Q6 hr PRN; **max. single dose:** 2 mg

Anxiolytic/sedation:
   Infant and child: 0.05 mg/kg/dose Q4—8 hr PO/IV; **max. dose:** 2 mg/dose
   May also give IM for preprocedure sedation
   Adult: 0.5—2 mg/dose PO/IV Q4-6 hr PRN up to 10 mg/24 hr

Contraindicated in narrow-angle glaucoma and severe hypotension. **Use with caution** in renal insufficiency (glucoronide metabolite clearance is reduced), hepatic insufficiency (may worsen hepatic encephalopathy; decrease dose with severe hepatic impairment), compromised pulmonary function, and use of CNS depressant medications. May cause respiratory depression, especially in combination with opioids and other sedatives. May also cause sedation, dizziness, mild ataxia, mood changes, rash, and GI symptoms. Paradoxical excitation has been reported in children (10%—30% of patients <8 yr old).

When compared to diazepam for status epilepticus (3 mo—17 yr), lorazepam was found to be more sedating with a longer time to return to baseline mental status.

Significant respiratory depression and/or hypotension has been reported when used in combination with loxapine. Probenecid and valproic acid may increase the effects/toxicity of lorazepam, and oral contraceptive steroids may decrease lorazepam's effects.

Injectable product may be given rectally. Benzyl alcohol and propylene glycol may be toxic to newborns at higher doses.

Onset of action for sedation: PO, 20—30 min; IM, 30—60 min; IV, 1—5 min. Duration of action: 6—8 hr.

Extended release capsules (Loreev XR) may be swallowed whole or its content may be opened and sprinkled over a tablespoon of applesauce followed by drinking water; **DO NOT** crush or chew. See product information for dose conversion from immediate release dosage forms.

Flumazenil is the antidote.

LOSARTAN
Cozaar and generics
Angiotensin II receptor antagonist

    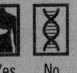

X 3 Yes Yes No

Tabs: 25, 50, 100 mg
Oral suspension: 2.5 mg/mL
Contains 2.12 mg potassium per 25 mg drug

Hypertension (see remarks):
  6–16 yr: Start with 0.7 mg/kg/dose (**max. dose:** 50 mg/dose) PO once daily. Adjust dose
   to desired blood pressure response and daily dose may be divided BID. **Max. dose** (higher doses
   have not been evaluated): 1.4 mg/kg/24 hr or 100 mg/24 hr
  ≥17 yr and adult: Start with 50 mg PO once daily (use lower initial dose of 25 mg PO once daily if
   patient receiving diuretics, experiencing intravascular volume depletion, or has hepatic
   impairment). Usual maintenance dose is 25–100 mg/24 hr PO ÷ once daily–BID.

Use with caution in angioedema (current or past), excessive hypotension (volume depletion),
  hepatic (use lower starting dose) or renal (contains potassium) impairment, hyperkalemia
  (including use with medications that can cause hyperkalemia), renal artery stenosis, and severe
  CHF. Not recommended in patients <6 yr or in children with GFR <30 mL/min/1.73 m², owing to
  lack of data.
Discontinue use as soon as possible when pregnancy is detected because injury and death to
  developing fetus may occur; especially during the second and third trimesters.
Diarrhea, asthenia, dizziness, fatigue, and hypotension are common. Thrombocytopenia,
  rhabdomyolysis, hallucinations, and angioedema have been rarely reported.
Losartan is a substrate for CYP 450 2C9 (major) and 3A4. Fluconazole and cimetidine may increase
  losartan's effects/toxicity. Rifampin, phenobarbital, and indomethacin may decrease its effects.
  Losartan may increase the risk of lithium toxicity. **Do not use** with aliskiren in patients with diabetes
  or with renal impairment (GFR <60 mL/min). Dual blockade of the renin-angiotensin system with
  losartan and ACE inhibitors (e.g., captopril) or aliskiren is associated with increased risk for
  hypotension, syncope, hyperkalemia, and renal impairment.

LOW-MOLECULAR-WEIGHT HEPARIN

See Enoxaparin.

LUCINACTANT

See Surfactant, pulmonary.

LUMACAFTOR AND IVACAFTOR
Orkambi
*Cystic fibrosis transmembrane conductance
regulator corrector and potentiator*

    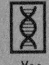

B 2 Yes Yes Yes

Oral granules (Lumacaftor:Ivacaftor): 75 mg:94 mg (14 packets), 100 mg:125 mg (56 packets), 150
  mg:188 mg (56 packets)

Continued

LUMACAFTOR AND IVACAFTOR *continued*

Tabs (Lumacaftor:Ivacaftor): 100 mg:125 mg (112 tabs), 200 mg:125 mg (112 tabs)

Child 1—<2 yr:
    7—<9 kg: One lumacaftor 75 mg/ivacaftor 94 mg granule packet PO Q12 hr
    9—<14 kg: One lumacaftor 100 mg/ivacaftor 125 mg granule packet PO Q12 hr
    ≥14 kg: One lumacaftor 150 mg/ivacaftor 188 mg granule packet PO Q12 hr
Child ≥2—5 yr:
    <14 kg: One lumacaftor 100 mg/ivacaftor 125 mg granule packet PO Q12 hr
    ≥14 kg: One lumacaftor 150 mg/ivacaftor 188 mg granule packet PO Q12 hr
Child ≥6—11 yr: Two lumacaftor 100 mg/ivacaftor 125 mg tablets PO Q12 hr
Child ≥12, adolescent, and adult: Two lumacaftor 200 mg/ivacaftor 125 mg tablets PO Q12 hr
Dosage modification for hepatic impairment:

Level of Hepatic Impairment (Child-Pugh Class)	Age Group	Morning Dose	Evening Dose
A. Mild	1—5 yr	No dose adjustment; use usual dose	No dose adjustment; use usual dose
	≥6 yr	No dose adjustment; use usual dose	No dose adjustment; use usual dose
B. Moderate	1—5 yr	1 packet of granules	1 packet of granules every other day
	≥6 yr	2 tablets	1 tablet
C. Severe	1—5 yr	1 packet of granules[a]	No dose
	≥6 yr	1 tablet[a]	1 tablet[a]

[a]or less frequently as studies have not been conducted in severe hepatic impairment.

Dosage modification when used with CYP 450 3A inhibitors:
    Already taking Orkambi and initiating a strong CYP 450 3A inhibitor (e.g., itraconazole): No dosage adjustment
    Already taking a strong CYP 450 3A inhibitor and initiating Orkambi: Reduce Orkambi dosage to 1 tablet or 1 packet of granules every other day × the first week followed by the recommended daily dose. If Orkambi is interrupted for >1 wk and reinitiated while taking strong CYP 450 3A inhibitors, Orkambi should be reintroduced with the reduced dosage of 1 tablet or 1 packet of granules every other day × 1 wk followed by the recommended daily dose.

Works on CFTR trafficking defect by acting as a CFTR corrector (lumacaftor) and in combination with a CFTR potentiator (ivacaftor). Indicated for individuals with homozygous F508del CFTR mutation.

Respiratory events, such as chest discomfort, dyspnea, and abnormal respiration, may occur during the initiation of therapy and may vary from transient to severe (requiring discontinuation). Common side effects include rash, diarrhea, nausea, flatulence, fatigue, nasal discharge, and URIs. Increased liver enzymes and cataracts may occur; monitor AST/ALT and ocular exam at baseline. Repeat AST/ALT every 3 mo for the first year followed by annual assessments. Repeat ocular exams annually. Hypertension has been reported. May cause a false-positive urine drug screen for cannabinoids.

Use with **caution** with CrCl ≤30 mL/min and ESRD. Reduce dose with moderate/severe hepatic impairment (see dosage section) or when initiating therapy while taking a strong CYP 450 3A4 inhibitor.

LUMACAFTOR AND IVACAFTOR *continued*

Lumecaftor is a strong inducer of CYP 450 3A and ivacaftor is a CYP 450 3A substrate; see dose modification table in the dosage section. Use with strong CYP 450 3A inducers (e.g., rifampin, rifabutin, carbamazepine, St. John's wort) is not recommended. Lumecaftor/ivacaftor may reduce the efficacy of hormonal contraceptives and increase the incidence of menstruation-associated side effects (e.g., amenorrhea, dysmenorrhea, and irregular menses). Always evaluate potential drug-drug interactions; see https://www.orkambihcp.com/drug-interactionsddi—tool. **Avoid** food or drink containing grapefruit or Seville oranges.

Administer all doses with high-fat foods to ensure absorption. Oral granules can be mixed with 5 mL of soft foods or liquids, such as puréed fruits or vegetables, yogurt, applesauce, water, breast milk, infant formula, milk, or juice. Once mixed, it should be consumed within an hour. If a dose (all dosage forms) is missed within 6 hr of a scheduled dose, administer a dose immediately. However, if the missed dose is >6 hr, skip that dose and resume therapy at the next scheduled dose. Never take a double dose for a missed dose.

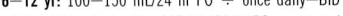

M

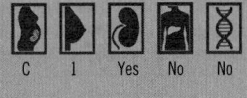

MAGNESIUM CITRATE
Various generics
16.17% Elemental Magnesium
Laxative/cathartic

C · 1 · Yes · No · No

Oral solution (OTC): 1.75 g/30 mL (300 mL); 5 mL = 3.9—4.7 mEq Mg
Tabs: 100 mg

Constipation:
  2—<6 yr: 2—4 mL/kg/24 hr PO ÷ once daily—BID; *OR* 60—90 mL/24 hr PO ÷ once daily—BID
  6—12 yr: 100—150 mL/24 hr PO ÷ once daily—BID
  >12 yr and adult: 150—300 mL/24 hr PO ÷ once daily—BID
Bowel prep:
  Child >6 yr and adolescent: 4—6 mL/kg/24 hr (**max.** 300 mL/24 hr) PO × 1 as a single or divided dose the day prior to surgery

Use with caution in renal insufficiency (monitor magnesium level) and patients receiving digoxin. May cause hypermagnesemia, diarrhea, muscle weakness, hypotension, and respiratory depression. Up to approximately 30% of dose is absorbed. May decrease absorption of H₂ antagonists, phenytoin, iron salts, tetracyclines, steroids, benzodiazepines, and quinolone antibiotics.

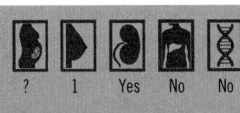

MAGNESIUM HYDROXIDE
Milk of Magnesia, Pedia-Lax, and various generics
41.69% Elemental Magnesium
Antacid, laxative

? · 1 · Yes · No · No

Oral liquid (OTC): 400 mg/5 mL (Milk of Magnesia and others) (355, 473 mL)
Concentrated oral liquid (OTC): 2400 mg/10 mL (Milk of Magnesia concentrate) (10 mL)

Continued

MAGNESIUM HYDROXIDE *continued*

Chewable tabs [Pedia-Lax, see remarks [OTC]): 400 mg
400 mg magnesium hydroxide is equivalent to 166.76 mg elemental magnesium.
Combination product with aluminum hydroxide: See Aluminum Hydroxide.

Laxative (all liquid mL doses based on 400 mg/5 mL magnesium hydroxide, unless noted otherwise):

Dose/24 hr ÷ once daily—QID PO

<2 yr: 0.5 mL/kg
2—5 yr: 5—15 mL *OR* 400—1200 mg (1—3 chewable tabs)
6—11 yr: 15—30 mL *OR* 1200—2400 mg (3—6 chewable tabs)
≥12 yr and adult: 30—60 mL *OR* 2400—4800 mg (6—12 chewable tabs)

Antacid:
Child:
Liquid: 2.5—5 mL/dose once daily—QID PO
Tabs: 400 mg once daily—QID PO
Adult:
Liquid: 5—15 mL/dose once daily—QID PO
Concentrated liquid (800 mg/5 mL): 2.5—7.5 mL/dose once daily—QID PO
Tabs: 400—1200 mg/dose once daily—QID PO

See Magnesium Citrate. **Use with caution** in renal insufficiency (monitor magnesium level) and patients receiving digoxin. Drink a full 8 oz of liquid with each dose of the chewable tablets.
Pedia-Lax chewable tablet is magnesium hydroxide. However, other dosage forms bearing the Pedia-Lax name (e.g., oral liquid, suppository, and enema) contain different active ingredients.

MAGNESIUM OXIDE
Mag-200, Mag-Ox 400, and other generics
60.32% Elemental Magnesium
Oral magnesium salt

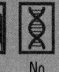

A/? 1 Yes No No

Tabs (OTC): 100, 200, 250, 400, 420, 500 mg
Caps (OTC): 300, 500 mg
400 mg magnesium oxide is equivalent to 241.3 mg elemental Mg or 20 mEq Mg.

Doses expressed in magnesium oxide salt.
Magnesium supplementation:
Child: 5—10 mg/kg/24 hr ÷ TID—QID PO
Adult: 400—800 mg/24 hr ÷ BID—QID PO
Hypomagnesemia:
Child: 65—130 mg/kg/24 hr ÷ QID PO
Adult: 2000 mg/24 hr ÷ QID PO

See Magnesium Citrate. **Use with caution** in renal insufficiency (monitor magnesium level) and patients receiving digoxin. **For dietary recommended intake (U.S. recommended daily allowance (RDA)) for magnesium, see Chapter 21.**
Pregnancy category is an "A" for doses up to 400 mg/24 hr.

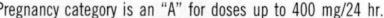

MAGNESIUM SULFATE
Epsom salts, many others, and generics
9.9% Elemental Magnesium
Magnesium salt

D 2 Yes No No
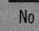

MAGNESIUM SULFATE *continued*

Injection: 500 mg/mL (4 mEq/mL) (2, 10, 20, 50 mL); must be diluted before use
Injection, prediluted in sterile water for injection; ready to use: 40 mg/mL (0.325 mEq/mL) (50, 100, 500, 1000 mL); 80 mg/mL (0.65 mEq/mL) (50 mL)
Injection, prediluted in D₅W; ready to use: 10 mg/mL (0.081 mEq/mL) (100 mL)
Granules (Epsom salts and generics): Approx. 40 mEq Mg per 5 g (454, 1810 g)
500 mg magnesium sulfate is equivalent to 49.3 mg elemental Mg or 4.1 mEq Mg.

All doses expressed in magnesium sulfate salt.
Cathartic:
  Child: 0.25 g/kg/dose PO Q4–6 hr
  Adult: 10–30 g/dose PO Q4–6 hr
Hypomagnesemia or hypocalcemia:
  IV/IM: 25–50 mg/kg/dose Q4–6 hr × 3–4 doses; repeat PRN. **Max. single dose:** 2 g
  PO: 100–200 mg/kg/dose QID PO
Daily maintenance for parenteral nutrition:
  30–60 mg/kg/24 hr or 0.25–0.5 mEq/kg/24 hr IV; **max. dose:** 1 g/24 hr
Adjunctive therapy for moderate to severe reactive airway disease exacerbation (bronchodilation); some recommend an IV saline bolus prior to magnesium administration to prevent hypotension:
  Child: 25–75 mg/kg/dose (**max. dose:** 2 g) × 1 IV over 20 min
  Adult: 2 g/dose × 1 IV over 20 min

When magnesium sulfate is given IV, **beware** of hypotension, bradycardia, respiratory depression, complete heart block, and/or hypermagnesemia. Calcium gluconate (IV) should be available as **antidote. Use with caution** in patients with renal insufficiency (monitor magnesium levels) and with patients on digoxin. **Serum level dependent toxicity** includes the following: >3 mg/dL: CNS depression; >5 mg/dL: decreased deep tendon reflexes, flushing, somnolence; and >12 mg/dL: respiratory paralysis, heart block.
Max. IV intermittent infusion rate:
  Emergent situations: 1 mEq/kg/hr or 125 mg MgSO₄ salt/kg/hr
  Asymptomatic hypomagnesemia: 0.1 mEq/kg/hr or 12.5 mg MgSO₄ salt/kg/hr
Pregnancy category is "D" because hypocalcemia, osteopenia, and fractures in the developing baby or fetus have been reported in pregnant women receiving magnesium >5–7 days for preterm labor.

MANNITOL
Osmitrol and generics; inhalation: Bronchitol
Osmotic diuretic

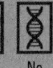
C   ?   Yes   No   No

Injection: 100, 150, 200, 250 mg/mL (10%, 15%, 20%, 25%, respectively)
Inhalation powder in capsules:
  Bronchitol: 40 mg (10s, 140s, 560s with 1, 1, and 4 inhalers, respectively)

Oliguria (child and adult):
  Test dose to assess renal function: 0.2 g/kg/dose (**max. dose:** 12.5 g) IV over 3–5 min.
    If there is no diuresis within 2 hr, discontinue mannitol.
  Initial: 0.5–1 g/kg/dose IV over 2–6 hr
  Maintenance: 0.25–2 g/kg/dose Q4–6 hr IV over 2–6 hr
Intracranial pressure reduction (see remarks): 0.25–1 g/kg/dose IV/IO over 20–30 min; may repeat dose if needed
Inhalational use:
  Cystic fibrosis maintenance (Bronchitol; after passing tolerance test):

Continued

MANNITOL *continued*

> Child ≥6 yr and adult (limited data <18 yr): Inhale the contents of 10 capsules (400 mg) BID (every morning and 2—3 hr before bedtime). Use an inhaled short-acting bronchodilator 5—15 min prior to each dose.

Contraindicated in severe renal disease, active intracranial bleed, dehydration (especially severe hypovolemia), prior hypersensitivity to mannitol, and pulmonary edema. May cause circulatory overload and electrolyte disturbances. For hyperosmolar therapy, keep serum osmolality at 310—320 mOsm/kg. **Do not use** with aminoglycosides as this may enhance nephrotoxicity risk. Larger doses may require fluid bolus to prevent hypotension. May cause hypovolemia, headache, acute kidney injury, and polydipsia. Reduction in ICP occurs in 15 min and lasts 3—6 hr.

Caution: Drug may crystallize at low temperatures with concentrations ≥15%; redissolve crystals by warming solution up to 70°C with agitation. Use an in-line filter (≤5 micron).

INHALED USE (Bronchitol): Do not puncture the capsule more than once and **do not** swallow capsule. Use an inhaled bronchodilator prior to each dose. Patients are instructed to exhale fully first, then place inhaler device in the mouth by closing the lips around the mouthpiece, and take a steady, deep breath, inhaling the contents of the capsule, followed by holding the breath for 5 sec before exhaling. Repeat the process again if powder is still left. Each inhaler device should be replaced after 7 days of use. Use of this product is **contraindicated** if the patient fails the Bronchitol Tolerance Test (BTT); see product information for testing procedure and passing criteria. Common side effects from the BTT include: nausea, retching, chest discomfort, dizziness, headache, cough, dyspnea, respiratory tract pain, nasal discharge, throat irritation, and wheezing. Common side effects during maintenance therapy include arthralgia, cough, throat pain, pulmonary bacterial infection (positive sputum), and fever.

MEBENDAZOLE
Emverm; previously available as Vermox
Anthelmintic

C	1	No	Yes	No

Chewable tabs: 100 mg (may be swallowed whole or chewed)

Child (≥2 yr) and adult:
Pinworms (*Enterobius*): 100 mg PO × 1, repeat in 2 wk if not cured.
Hookworms, roundworms (*Ascaris*), and whipworm (*Trichuris*): 100 mg PO BID × 3 days. Repeat in 3—4 wk if not cured. Alternatively, may administer 500 mg PO × 1 and repeat in 3—4 wk if not cured.
Capillariasis: 200 mg PO BID × 20—30 days
Visceral larva migrans (toxocariasis): 100—200 mg PO BID × 5 days
Trichinellosis (*Trichinella spiralis*): 200—400 mg PO TID × 3 days, then 400—500 mg PO TID × 10 days; use with steroids for severe symptoms
Eosinophilic enterocolitis: 100 mg PO BID × 3 days
See latest edition of the AAP Red Book for additional information.

Experience in children <2 yr and pregnancy is limited. May cause rash, headache, diarrhea, and abdominal cramping in cases of massive infection. Liver function test elevations and hepatitis have been reported with prolonged courses; monitor hepatic function with prolonged therapy.

Family may need to be treated as a group. Therapeutic effect may be decreased if administered to patients receiving aminoquinolones, carbamazepine, or phenytoin. Cimetidine may increase the effects/toxicity of mebendazole. **Avoid** taking with metronidazole as this my cause serious skin reactions. Administer with food. Tablet may be crushed and mixed with food, swallowed whole, chewed, or turned into a soft mass by adding 2—3 mL of water to a spoon, then placing the tablet into the water (which can then be swallowed).

MEDROXYPROGESTERONE
Depo-Provera, Provera, Depo-Sub Q Provera 104,
and generics
Contraceptive, progestin

    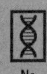

| X | 2 | No | Yes | No |

Tabs (Provera and generics): 2.5, 5, 10 mg
Injection, suspension as acetate:
    Depo-Provera and generics, for IM use only: 150 mg/mL (1 mL and 1 mL prefilled syringe), 400 mg/
    mL (2.5 mL); may contain parabens and polyethylene glycol
Injection, prefilled syringe as acetate:
    Depo-Sub Q Provera 104, for SC use only: 104 mg (0.65 mL of 160 mg/mL); contains parabens and
    polyethylene glycol

Adolescent and adult:
    Contraception: Initiate therapy during the first 5 days after onset of a normal menstrual
    period; within 5 days postpartum if not breastfeeding; or if breastfeeding, at 6 wk postpartum.
    When converting contraceptive method to Depo-Sub Q Provera, administer dose within 7 days after
    the last day of using the previous method (pill, ring, patch).
      IM (Depo-Provera and generics): 150 mg Q3 mo (every 13 wk)
      SC (Depo-Sub Q Provera 104): 104 mg Q3 mo (every 12—14 wk)
    Amenorrhea: 5—10 mg PO once daily × 5—10 days
    Abnormal uterine bleeding: 5—10 mg PO once daily × 5—10 days initiated on the 16th or 21st day of
    the menstrual cycle
    Endometriosis-associated pain (Depo-Sub Q Provera 104): 104 mg SC Q3 mo. Do not use longer than
    2 yr due to impact on bone mineral density.

Consider patient's risk for osteoporosis because of the potential for decrease in bone mineral
density with long-term use. Contraception use >2 yr for is NOT recommended.
    Contraindicated in pregnancy, breast or genital cancer, liver disease, missed abortion,
thrombophlebitis, thromboembolic disorders, cerebral vascular disease, and undiagnosed vaginal
bleeding. **Use with caution** in patients with family history of breast cancer, depression, diabetes,
and fluid retention. May cause dizziness, headache, insomnia, fatigue, nausea, weight increase,
appetite changes, amenorrhea, and breakthrough bleeding. Cholestatic jaundice, adrenal
suppression, anaphylaxis, and increased intracranial pressure have been reported. Injection site
reactions may include pain/tenderness, persistent atrophy/indentation/dimpling, lipodystrophy,
sterile abscess, skin color change, and node/lump.
Drug is a substrate to CYP 450 3A4 isoenzyme. Aminoglutethimide may decrease medroxyprogesterone
levels. May alter thyroid and liver function tests, prothrombin time, factors VII, VIII, IX, and X, and
metyrapone test.
The WHO recommends the use of injectable depot medroxyprogesterone should not be used before 6
weeks postpartum.
Do not inject IM or SC product intravenously. Shake IM injection vial well before use, and administer in
the upper arm or buttock. Administer SC injection product into the anterior thigh or abdomen.
Administer oral doses with food.

MEFLOQUINE HCL
Generics; previously available as Lariam
Antimalarial

    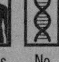

| B | 2 | No | Yes | No |

Tabs: 250 mg (228 mg base)

Continued

MEFLOQUINE HCL *continued*

Doses expressed in mg mefloquine HCl salt.

Malaria prophylaxis (start 2 wk prior to exposure and continue for 4 wk after leaving endemic area; see remarks):

Child (PO, administered Q7 days):

<10 kg: 5 mg/kg

10—19 kg: 62.5 mg (1/4 tablet)

20—30 kg: 125 mg (1/2 tablet)

31—45 kg: 187.5 mg (3/4 tablet)

>45 kg: 250 mg (1 tablet)

Adult: 250 mg PO Q7 days

Malaria treatment (uncomplicated/mild infection, chloroquine-resistant *Plasmodium vivax*; used in combination with other agents):

Child ≥6 mo and >5 kg: 15 mg/kg (**max. dose:** 750 mg) × 1 PO followed by 10 mg/kg (**max. dose:** 500 mg) × 1 PO 6—12 hr later

Adult: 750 mg × 1 PO followed by 500 mg × 1 PO 6—12 hr later

See latest edition of the Red Book for additional information.

Contraindicated in active or recent history of depression, anxiety disorders, psychosis or schizophrenia, seizures, or hypersensitivity to quinine or quinidine. **Use with caution** in cardiac dysrhythmias and neurologic disease. May cause dizziness, ringing of the ears, headache, syncope, psychiatric symptoms (e.g., anxiety, paranoia, depression, hallucinations, and psychotic behavior), seizures, ocular abnormalities, GI symptoms, leukopenia, and thrombocytopenia. If neurologic or psychiatric side effects occur, discontinue therapy and use an alternative medication. Most adverse events occur within 3 doses with prophylaxis use. Monitor liver enzymes and ocular exams for therapies >1 yr.

Mefloquine is a substrate and inhibitor of P-glycoprotein and may reduce valproic acid levels. ECG abnormalities may occur when used in combination with quinine, quinidine, chloroquine, halofantrine, and β-blockers. If any of the aforementioned antimalarial drugs is used in the initial treatment of severe malaria, initiate mefloquine at least 12 hr after the last dose of any of these drugs. **Do not** initiate halofantrine or ketoconazole within 15 days of the last dose of mefloquine. Use with chloroquine may increase risk for seizures. Rifampin may decrease mefloquine levels.

Do not take on an empty stomach. Administer with at least 240 mL (8 oz) water. Treatment failures in children may be related to vomiting of administered dose. If vomiting occurs less than 30 min after the dose, administer a second full dose. If vomiting occurs 30—60 min after the dose, administer an additional half-dose. If vomiting continues, monitor patient closely and consider alternative therapy.

MEROPENEM
Generics; previously available as Merrem
Carbapenem antibiotic

B	2	Yes	Yes	No

Injection: 0.5, 1 g; contains 3.92 mEq Na/g drug

Injection, in a duplex chamber to be diluted in supplied sodium chloride for injection:

500 mg in 50 mL; contains 10.7 mEq Na per 500 mg drug when diluted

1000 mg in 50 mL; contains 12.6 mEq Na per 1000 mg drug when diluted

Neonate and infant <3 mo (IV):

Non-CNS general dosing (meropenem MIC <4):

≤2 kg:

≤14 days old: 20 mg/kg/dose Q12 hr

MEROPENEM *continued*

- **15–28 days old:** 20 mg/kg/dose Q8 hr
- **29–60 days old:** 30 mg/kg/dose Q8 hr
- **>2 kg:**
  - **≤14 days old:** 20 mg/kg/dose Q8 hr
  - **15–60 days old:** 30 mg/kg/dose Q8 hr

Non-CNS infection with moderately resistant meropenem isolate (MIC 4–8 mCg/mL; from a single-dose PK simulation study):
- **>30 wks' gestation and >7 days old:** 40 mg/kg/dose IV Q8 hr

Intra-abdominal infection (meropenem MIC <4 mCg/mL):
- **<32 wks' gestation:**
  - **<14 days old:** 20 mg/kg/dose Q12 hr
  - **≥14 days old:** 20 mg/kg/dose Q8 hr
- **≥32 wks' gestation:**
  - **<14 days old:** 20 mg/kg/dose Q8 hr
  - **≥14 days old:** 30 mg/kg/dose Q8 hr

Meningitis (limited data):
- **≤2 kg:**
  - **≤14 days old:** 40 mg/kg/dose Q12 hr
  - **15–60 days old:** 40 mg/kg/dose Q8 hr
- **>2 kg:**
  - **≤60 days old:** 40 mg/kg/dose Q8 hr
- **1–3 mo, IV; recommendation from 2004 IDSA meningitis practice guidelines:** 40 mg/kg/dose Q8 hr

Infant (≥3 mo), child, and adolescent (IV):
- **Meningitis, severe infections, and cystic fibrosis pulmonary exacerbations:** 40 mg/kg/dose (**max. dose:** 2 g/dose) Q8 hr
- **Complicated skin and skin structure infection:** 10 mg/kg/dose (**max. dose:** 500 mg/dose) Q8 hr. For severe or necrotizing infections or *Pseudomonas aeruginosa* infection (suspected or confirmed), use 20 mg/kg/dose (**max. dose:** 1 g/dose) Q8 hr.
- **Intra-abdominal and mild/moderate infections, and fever/neutropenia empiric therapy:** 20 mg/kg/dose (**max. dose:** 1 g/dose) Q8 hr

Adult (IV):
- **Skin and subcutaneous tissue infections:** 500 mg Q8 hr; use 1 g Q8 hr for suspected or confirmed *Pseudomonas aeruginosa*
- **Intra-abdominal and mild/moderate infections; and fever/neutropenia empiric therapy:** 1 g Q8 hr
- **Meningitis and severe infections:** 2 g Q8 hr

Contraindicated in patients sensitive to carbapenems, or with a history of anaphylaxis to β-lactam antibiotics. **Use with caution** in meningitis and CNS disorders (may cause seizures) and renal impairment (**adjust dose; see Chapter 31**). Drug penetrates well into the CSF.

May cause diarrhea, rash, nausea, vomiting, oral moniliasis, glossitis, pain and irritation at the IV injection site, and headache. Hepatic enzyme and bilirubin elevation, dermatologic reactions (including Stevens-Johnson, DRESS, and TEN), leukopenia, thrombocytopenia (in renal dysfunction), and neutropenia have been reported. Probenecid may increase serum meropenem levels. May reduce valproic acid levels.

Lengthening the IV drug administration time to 4 hr will improve the meropenem concentration time above the MIC and may be useful in situations of resistant organisms.

MESALAMINE
Apriso, Asacol HD, Canasa, Delzicol, Lialda,
Pentasa, Rowasa, SfRowasa, and generics;
5-aminosalicylic acid, 5-ASA
Salicylate, GI antiinflammatory agent

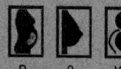

B 2 Yes Yes No

Caps, controlled release:
　Pentasa and generics: 250, 500 mg
　Delzicol and generics: 400 mg
　Apriso and generics (for Q24 hr dosing): 375 mg; contains aspartame
Tabs, delayed release:
　Asacol HD and generics: 800 mg
　Lialda and generics: 1200 mg
Suppository (Canasa and generics): 1000 mg (1, 6s, 30s)
Rectal suspension enema (Rowasa, SfRowasa, and generics): 4 g/60 mL; contains sulfites
　(SfRowasa is sulfite free) and sodium benzoate

Child and adolescent (ulcerative colitis):
　Caps (controlled release) and tabs (delayed release): 60–80 mg/kg/24 hr ÷ once
　　daily–BID (defined by dosage form used); **max. dose:** 4.8 g/24 hr
　Delzicol (mild/moderate ulcerative colitis treatment for 6 wk; ≥5–18 yr; see remarks):
　　17–32 kg: 800 mg QAM and 400 mg Q afternoon PO
　　33–53 kg: 1200 mg QAM and 800 mg Q afternoon PO
　　54–90 kg: 1200 mg QAM and Q afternoon PO
　Lialda (mild/moderate ulcerative colitis; child and adolescent ≥24 kg):
　　24–35 kg: 2400 mg once daily PO × 8 weeks, then decrease to 1200 mg once daily PO
　　>35–50 kg: 3600 mg once daily PO × 8 weeks, then decrease to 2400 mg once daily PO
　　>50 kg: 4800 mg once daily PO × 8 weeks, then decrease to 2400 mg once daily PO
Older child and adolescent (mild/moderate ulcerative colitis; see remarks):
　Enema (Rowasa): 25 mg/kg/dose (**max. dose:** 1 g/dose) PR once daily; doses greater than 1 g are not
　　more effective
Adult (mild/moderate ulcerative colitis; see remarks):
　Caps, controlled release:
　　Initial therapy: 1 g QID PO × 3–8 wk
　　Delzicol: 800 mg TID PO × 6 wk
　　Maintenance therapy for remission:
　　　Apriso: 1.5 g QAM PO
　　　Delzicol: 1.6 g/24 hr PO divided BID–QID
　　　Pentasa: 1 g QID PO
　Tabs, delayed release:
　　Initial therapy:
　　　Asacol HD: 1.6 g TID PO × 6 wk
　　　Lialda: 2.4–4.8 g once daily PO up to 8 wk
　　Maintenance therapy for remission:
　　　Generic: At least 2 g PO once daily
　　　Lialda: 2.4 g PO once daily
Suppository (ulcerative proctitis): 1000 mg QHS PR × 3–6 wk; retain each dose in the rectum for
　1–3 hr or longer, if possible
Rectal suspension (ulcerative colitis or proctitis): 60 mL (4 g) QHS × 3–6 wk, retaining each dose
　for about 8 hr; lie on left side during administration to improve delivery to the sigmoid colon

MESALAMINE *continued*

Generally **not recommended** in children <16 yr with chickenpox or flu-like symptoms (risk of Reye syndrome). **Contraindicated** in active peptic ulcer disease, severe renal failure, and salicylate hypersensitivity. Rectal suspension should not be used in patients with history of sulfite allergy. **Use with caution** in sulfasalazine hypersensitivity, impaired hepatic or renal function, pyloric stenosis, nephrotoxic medications, and concurrent thrombolytics. May cause headache, GI discomfort, pancreatitis, pericarditis, and rash. Angioedema, Stevens-Johnson syndrome, DRESS, fatal infections (e.g., sepsis and pneumonia; discontinue use), interstitial nephritis, renal failure, nephrolithiasis, and photosensitivity have been reported. May cause a false-positive urinary normetanephrine test.

Safety and efficacy of Delzicol in children 5—17 yr for mild/moderate acute ulcerative colitis have been established over a 6-wk period; safety and efficacy for maintenance of remission of ulcerative colitis in children have not been established. Safety and efficacy of Canasa suppositories have not been demonstrated for mild/moderate active ulcerative proctitis in a 6-wk open-label study in 49 patients 5—17 yr old.

Do not administer with lactulose or other medications that can lower intestinal pH. Use with myelosuppressive drugs (e.g., azathioprine, 6-mercaptopurine) may increase risk for blood disorders, bone marrow failure, and associated complications.

Two Delzicol 400-mg capsules have not been shown to be interchangeable or substitutable with one mesalamine 800-mg delayed release tablet. Oral capsules are designed to release medication throughout the GI tract, and oral tablets release medication at the terminal ileus and beyond. 400 mg PO mesalamine is equivalent to 1 g sulfasalazine PO. Tablets should be swallowed whole.

METFORMIN
Glumetza, Fortamet, Riomet, and generics;
previously available as Glucophage and
Glucophage XR
Antidiabetic, biguanide

B 2 Yes Yes No

Tabs: 500, 850, 1000 mg
Tabs, extended release:
   Generics: 500, 750, 1000 mg
   Fortamet and Glumetza: 500, 1000 mg
Oral suspension (Riomet and generics): 100 mg/mL (120, 480 mL); may contain saccharin and propylene glycol

Type 2 diabetes: Administer all doses with meals (e.g., BID: morning and evening meals).
   Child (10—16 yr; PO) (see remarks):
      Immediate release dosage forms: Start with 500 mg BID; may increase dose every 1—2 wk as tolerated by 500 mg/24 hr in 2 divided doses up to a **max. dose** of 2000 mg/24 hr.
      Extended release tabs: Start with 500—1000 mg once daily × 7—14 days; may increase dose every 1—2 wk as tolerated by 500—1000 mg/24 hr as once daily or divided doses up to a **max. dose** of 2000 mg/24 hr.
   Child ≥17 yr and adult (see remarks):
      500 mg immediate release tabs: Start with 500 mg PO BID; may increase dose weekly by 500 mg/24 hr in 2 divided doses up to a **max. dose** of 2500 mg/24 hr. Administer 2500 mg/24 hr doses by dividing daily dose TID with meals.
      850 mg immediate release tabs: Start with 850 mg PO once daily with morning meal; may increase by 850 mg every 2 wk up to a **max. dose** of 2550 mg/24 hr (first dosage increment: 850 mg PO BID; second dosage increment: 850 mg PO TID).

Continued

METFORMIN *continued*

Extended release tabs: Start with 500 mg PO once daily with evening meal; may increase by 500 mg every week up to a **max. dose** of 2000 mg/24 hr (if glycemic control is not achieved at **max. dose**, divide dose to 1000 mg PO BID). If using Fortamet, **max. dose** is 2500 mg/24 hr. If a dose >2000 mg is needed, consider switching to non—extended release tablets in divided doses and increase dose to a **max. dose** of 2550 mg/24 hr.

Assess patient's eGFR prior to initiating therapy. **Contraindicated** in severe renal impairment (<30 mL/min/1.73 m^2), hepatic impairment (increased risk for lactic acidosis), CHF, and metabolic acidosis and during radiology studies using iodinated contrast media. **Use with caution** when transferring patients from chlorpropamide therapy (potential hypoglycemia risk), excessive alcohol intake, hypoxemia, dehydration, surgical procedures, mild/moderate renal impairment, hepatic disease, anemia, and thyroid disease.

Fatal lactic acidosis (diarrhea; severe muscle pain, cramping; shallow and fast breathing; unusual weakness and sleepiness) and decrease in vitamin B$_{12}$ levels have been reported. May cause GI discomfort (~50% incidence), anorexia, and vomiting. Transient abdominal discomfort or diarrhea has been reported in 40% of pediatric patients. Organic cationic transporter-2 (OCT2) and multidrug and toxin extrusion (MATE) inhibitors (e.g., cimetidine), furosemide, and nifedipine may increase the effects/toxicity of metformin. In addition to monitoring serum glucose and glycosylated hemoglobin, monitor renal function and hematologic parameters (baseline and annual).

Adult patients initiated on 500 mg PO BID may also have their dose increased to 850 mg PO BID after 2 wk.

COMBINATION THERAPY WITH SULFONYLUREAS: If patient has not responded to 4 wk of **maximum** doses of metformin monotherapy, consider gradual addition of an oral sulfonylurea with continued **maximum** metformin dosing (even if failure with sulfonylurea has occurred). Attempt to identify the minimum effective dosage for each drug (metformin and sulfonylurea) because the combination can increase risk for sulfonylurea-induced hypoglycemia. If patient does not respond to 1—3 mo of combination therapy with maximum metformin doses, consider discontinuing combination therapy and initiating insulin therapy.

Administer all doses with food.

METHADONE HCL
Methadose and generics; previously available as Dolophine
Narcotic, analgesic

| C | 2 | Yes | Yes | No |

Tabs: 5, 10 mg
Tabs, dispersible (Methadose and generics): 40 mg
Oral solution: 5 mg/5 mL (500 mL), 10 mg/5 mL (500 mL); contains 8% alcohol
Concentrated oral solution (Methadose and generics): 10 mg/mL (30 mL); may contain propylene glycol and parabens and may be sugar free
Injection: 10 mg/mL (20 mL), contains 0.5% chlorobutanol

Analgesia (initial doses; see remarks):
Child: 0.7 mg/kg/24 hr ÷ Q4—6 hr PO, SC, IM, or IV PRN pain; **max. dose:** 10 mg/dose
Adult: 2.5—10 mg/dose Q8—12 hr PO, SC, IM, or IV PRN pain
Detoxification or maintenance: See package insert.

Unintentional overdoses have resulted in fatalities and severe adverse events such as respiratory depression and cardiac arrhythmias. **Use with caution** in hepatic (**avoid** in severe cases) and biliary tract impairment. May cause respiratory depression, sedation, increased intracranial pressure, hypotension, and bradycardia. Cardiac QT interval prolongation and serious

Chapter 30 Drug Dosages **1025**

METHADONE HCL *continued*

arrhythmias have occurred mostly with higher doses; **avoid use** with other medications that may prolong QT interval. Nystagmus, strabismus, hypoglycemia, hypokalemia, hypomagnesemia, and weight gain have been reported.

Average $T_{1/2}$: Children 19 hr, and adults 35 hr. Duration of action PO is 6—8 hr initially and 22—48 hr after repeated doses. Respiratory effects last longer than analgesia. Accumulation may occur with continuous use, making it necessary to adjust dose.

Nevirapine may decrease serum levels of methadone. Fatalities have been reported with abuse in combination with benzodiazepines. Serotonin syndrome has been reported with use with selective serotonin reuptake inhibitors (SSRIs), serotonin norepinephrine reuptake inhibitor (SNRIs), TCAs, 5-HT3 antagonists, MAO inhibitors, and drugs that affect the serotonergic neurotransmitter system (e.g., trazodone, tramadol). Methadone is a substrate for CYP 450 3A3/4, 2D6, and 1A2 and inhibitor of 2D6.

See Chapter 6 for equianalgesic dosing and onset of action. **Adjust dose in renal failure (see Chapter 31).**

A Risk Evaluation and Mitigation Strategy (REMS) is required for healthcare providers to ensure the benefits outweigh the risks of addiction, abuse, and misuse. See www.fda.gov/OpioidAnalgesicREMSBlueprint or call 1-800-503-0784.

METHIMAZOLE Generics; previously available as Tapazole *Antithyroid agent*	
	D 2 No Yes No

Tabs: 5, 10 mg

Hyperthyroidism:
  Child:
    Initial: 0.4—0.7 mg/kg/24 hr or 15—20 mg/m²/24 hr PO ÷ Q8 hr
    Maintenance: 1/3—2/3 of initial dose PO ÷ Q8 hr
    Max. dose: 30 mg/24 hr
  Adult:
    Initial: 15—60 mg/24 hr PO ÷ Q8 hr
    Maintenance: 5—15 mg/24 hr PO ÷ Q8 hr

Readily crosses placental membranes and distributes into breast milk (maternal doses ≤20 mg/24 hr are considered safe, but there are insufficient data to support safe use with maternal doses >20 mg/24 hr). Blood dyscrasias, dermatitis, hepatitis, arthralgia, CNS reactions, pruritus, nephritis, hypoprothrombinemia, agranulocytosis, headache, fever, and hypothyroidism may occur. Acute hepatic failure and hepatitis have been reported.

May increase the effects of oral anticoagulants. When correcting hyperthyroidism, consider whether existing β-blocker, digoxin, and theophylline doses need to be reduced to avoid potential toxicities.

Switch to maintenance dose when patient is euthyroid. Administer all doses with food.

METHYLENE BLUE ProvayBlue and generics *Antidote, drug-induced methemoglobinemia,* *and cyanide toxicity*	
	X ? Yes No No

Injection: 10 mg/mL (1%) (10 mL)
Intravenous solution (ProvayBlue): 50 mg/10 mL (2, 10 mL; see remarks)

Continued

METHYLENE BLUE *continued*

Methemoglobinemia:
Child and adult: 1–2 mg/kg/dose or 25–50 mg/m^2/dose IV/IO over 5 min. May repeat in 30–60 min if needed.

At high doses, may cause methemoglobinemia. **Avoid** subcutaneous or intrathecal routes of administration. **Use with caution** in G6PD deficiency or renal insufficiency (methylene blue concentrations have increased in subjects with renal impairment). May cause nausea, vomiting, dizziness, headache, diaphoresis, stained skin, and abdominal pain. Causes blue-green discoloration of urine and feces.

Serotonin syndrome has been reported with the coadministration of SSRI, SNRI, or clomipramine. Use with bupropion, paroxetine, sertraline, duloxetine, vilazodone, venlafaxine, fluoxetine, or desipramine is considered **contraindicated**.

ProvayBlue (50 mg/10 mL) dosage form is hypotonic and may be diluted in 50 mL D$_5$W to prevent local infusion pain. **Avoid** diluting in sodium chloride as this may reduce the solubility of methylene blue.

METHYLPHENIDATE HCL
Ritalin, Adhansia XR, Aptensio XR, Jornay PM, Methylin, Metadate ER, Methylin ER, Concerta, Relexxii, QuilliChew ER, Quillivant XR, Ritalin LA, Cotempla XR-ODT, Daytrana, and generics
CNS stimulant

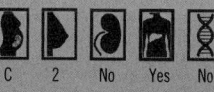

C   2   No   Yes   No

Tabs (Ritalin and generics): 5, 10, 20 mg
Chewable tabs (generics): 2.5, 5, 10 mg; contains phenylalanine
Extended release chewable tabs (dosed once daily in the morning):
　QuilliChew ER: 20, 30, 40 mg; contains phenylalanine
Oral solution (Methylin and generics): 1 mg/mL, 2 mg/mL; may contain propylene glycol
Oral suspension, extended release (dosed once daily in the morning):
　Quillivant XR: 25 mg/5 mL (60, 120, 150, 180 mL); contains sodium benzoate
Extended release tabs:
　8-hr duration (Metadate ER): 20 mg; dosed BID–TID
　24-hr duration:
　　Concerta and generics: 18, 27, 36, 54 mg
　　Relexxii and generics: 72 mg
Extended release oral disintegrating tabs:
　Cotempla XR-ODT (dosed once daily in the morning): 8.6, 17.3, 25.9 mg; contains polyethylene glycol
Extended release caps:
　24-hr duration:
　　Ritalin LA, and generics: 10, 20, 30, 40, 50, 60 mg
　　Adhansia XR: 25, 35, 45, 55, 70, 85 mg
　　Aptensio XR: 10, 15, 20, 30, 40, 50, 60 mg
　　Jornay PM: 20, 40, 60, 80, 100 mg (dosed only in the evening)
Transdermal patch (Daytrana and generics): 10 mg/9 hr (each 12.5 cm^2 patch contains 27.5 mg), 15 mg/9 hr (each 18.75 cm^2 patch contains 41.3 mg), 20 mg/9 hr (each 25 cm^2 patch contains 55 mg), 30 mg/9 hr (each 37.5 cm^2 patch contains 82.5 mg) (30s)

Attention-deficit/hyperactivity disorder (ADHD):
Immediate release oral dosage forms (Methylin, Ritalin; ≥6 yr):

METHYLPHENIDATE HCL *continued*

Initial: 0.3 mg/kg/dose (or 2.5—5 mg/dose) given before breakfast and lunch. May increase by 0.1 mg/kg/dose PO (or 5—10 mg/24 hr) weekly until maintenance dose achieved. May give extra afternoon dose if needed.

Maintenance dose range: 0.3—1 mg/kg/24 hr

Max. dose: 2 mg/kg/24 hr or 60 mg/24 hr for those weighing ≤50 kg and 100 mg/24 hr >50 kg

Extended release once-daily oral dosage form (Concerta; ≥6 yr):

Methylphenidate-naïve patients: Start with 18 mg PO QAM for children and adolescents and 18—36 mg PO QAM for adults; dosage may be increased at weekly intervals at 18 mg increments up to the following **max. dose:**

6—12 yr: 54 mg/24 hr

13—17 yr: 72 mg/24 hr **not to exceed** 2 mg/kg/24 hr

Patients weighing >50 kg: Higher **max. dose** of 108 mg/24 hr may be used.

Patients currently receiving methylphenidate: See following table.

RECOMMENDED DOSE CONVERSION FROM METHYLPHENIDATE REGIMENS TO CONCERTA

Previous Methylphenidate Daily Dose	Recommended Concerta Dose
5 mg PO BID—TID or 20 mg SR PO once daily	18 mg PO QAM
10 mg PO BID—TID or 40 mg SR PO once daily	36 mg PO QAM
15 mg PO BID—TID or 60 mg SR PO once daily	54 mg PO QAM
20 mg PO BID—TID	72 mg PO QAM

After a week of receiving the above-recommended Concerta dose, dose may be increased in 18 mg increments at weekly intervals PRN up to a **maximum** of 54 mg/24 hr for 6—12 yr and 72 mg/24 hr (**not to exceed** 2 mg/kg/24 hr) for 13—17 yr.

Other extended release oral dosage forms (see specific product information if converting from another product or dosage form):

Product (Dosage Form)	Initial Dose (≥6 yr)[a]	Dosage Adjustment	Max. Dose
Adhansia XR (extended release caps)	25 mg PO once daily in the AM	Increase at 10—15 mg increments at intervals ≥5 days PRN	85 mg/24 hr but doses ≥70 mg/24 hr were associated with higher rate of side effects in children
Aptensio XR (extended release caps)	10 mg PO once daily in the AM	Increase at 10 mg increments Q7 days PRN	60 mg/24 hr
Cotempla XR-ODT (extended release oral disintegrating tabs)[b]	17.3 mg PO once daily in the AM	Increase at 8.6 or 17.3 mg increments Q7 days PRN	51.8 mg/24 hr
Jornay PM (extended release caps)	20 mg PO QHS (between 6:30 and 9:30 PM; 8:00 PM was the most optimal time for 6—12 yr in clinical trials)	Increase at 20 mg increments Q7 days PRN; administered QHS	100 mg/24 hr

Continued

METHYLPHENIDATE HCL *continued*

Product

(Dosage Form)	Initial Dose (≥6 yr)[a]	Dosage Adjustment	Max. Dose
Metadate CD (extended release caps)	20 mg PO once daily	Increase at 10—20 mg increments Q7 days PRN	≤50 kg: 60 mg/24 hr >50 kg: 100 mg/ 24 hr
Quillivant XR (extended release oral suspension)[a]	20 mg PO once daily	Increase at 10—20 mg increments Q7 days PRN	60 mg/24 hr
QuilliChew (extended release chewable tabs)	20 mg PO once daily	Increase by 10, 15, or 20 mg Q7 days PRN	Doses >60 mg/24 hr have not been studied
Relexxii (extended release tabs)	18 mg PO once daily in the AM	Increase by 18 mg Q7 days PRN	6—12 yr[c]: 54 mg/24 hr 13—<18 yr[c]: lesser of 72 mg/24 hr or 2 mg/kg/24 hr ≥18 yr: 72 mg/24 hr
Ritalin LA (extended release caps)	20 mg PO once daily	Increase at 10 mg increments Q7 days PRN	≤50 kg: 60 mg/24 hr >50 kg: 100 mg/ 24 hr

[a]Quillivant XR dosing recommendations for children 6—12 yr.
[b]Cotempla XR ODT dosing recommendations for children 6—17 yr.
[c]Higher doses have not been studied for this age group.

Metadate ER (8-hr duration of action): Convert immediate release tabs when the 8-hr dosage corresponds to the available extended release tablet size. Usual **max. dose:** 60 mg/24 hr for children, but some patients >50 kg may tolerate doses up to 100 mg/24 hr with increased monitoring.

Transdermal patch (Daytrana; see remarks): Apply to the hip 2 hr before the effect is needed and remove 9 hr later. Patch may be removed before 9 hr if shorter duration of effect is desired or if late-day adverse effects appear.

    6—17 yr: Start with 10 mg/9 hr patch once daily. Increase dose PRN Q7 days by increasing to the next dosage strength. Higher starting doses have been reported in patients converting from oral dosage forms >20 mg/24 hr.

Contraindicated in glaucoma, anxiety disorders, motor tics, and Tourette syndrome. Medication should generally not be used in children <5 yr old; diagnosis of ADHD in this age group is extremely difficult and should be done only in consultation with a specialist. Sudden death (children, adolescents, and adults), stroke (adults), and MI (adults) have been reported in patients with preexisting structural cardiac abnormalities or other serious heart problems. **Use with caution** in patients with hypertension, psychiatric conditions, and epilepsy. Insomnia, weight loss, anorexia, rash, nausea, emesis, abdominal pain, hypertension or hypotension, tachycardia, arrhythmias, palpitations, restlessness, headaches, fever, tremor, visual disturbances, and thrombocytopenia may occur. Abnormal liver function (ranging from transaminase elevation to severe hepatic injury), cerebral arteritis and/or occlusion, peripheral vasculopathy (including Raynaud phenomenon), leukopenia and/or anemia, hypersensitivity reactions, transient depressed mood, paranoia, mania, auditory hallucination, priapism, and scalp hair loss have been reported. Skin irritation, chemical leukoderma, and contact dermatitis have been reported with transdermal route. High doses may slow growth by appetite suppression. GI obstruction has been reported with Concerta.

METHYLPHENIDATE HCL *continued*

May increase serum concentrations/effects of tricyclic antidepressants, dopamine agonists (e.g., haloperidol), phenytoin, phenobarbital, and warfarin. May decrease the effects of antihypertensive drugs. Effect of methylphenidate may be potentiated by MAO inhibitors; hypertensive crisis may also occur if used within 14 days of discontinuance of the MAO inhibitor. When used with risperidone, any dosage adjustment (increase/decrease) to either medication can result in extrapyramidal symptoms.

Extended/sustained release dosage forms have either an 8- or 24-hr dosage interval (as stipulated previously). Concerta dosage form delivers 22.2% of its dose as an immediate release product with the remaining amounts as an extended release product (e.g., 18 mg strength: 4 mg as immediate release, and 14 mg as extended release). Jornay PM is dosed only in the evening and should **NOT** be taken in the morning. **Do not** consume alcohol with Ritalin LA dosage form, because it may result in a more rapid release of the drug. **Do not** expose transdermal application site to external heat sources (e.g., electric blankets, heating pads); this may increase drug release.

METHYLPREDNISOLONE
Medrol, Medrol Dosepack, Solu-Medrol,
Depo-Medrol, and generics
Corticosteroid

C   2   No   No   No

Tabs: 2, 4, 8, 16, 32 mg
Tabs, dose pack (Medrol Dosepack and generics): 4 mg (21s)
Injection, Na succinate (Solu-Medrol and generics): 40, 125, 500, 1000 mg (IV or IM use); multidose vials contain benzyl alcohol
Injection, acetate suspension (Depo-Medrol and generics; for IM, intrasynovial, and soft tissue injection): 20 mg (5 mL), 40 mg (1, 5, 10 mL), 80 mg/mL (1, 5 mL); multidose vials contain benzyl alcohol

---

Antiinflammatory/immunosuppressive: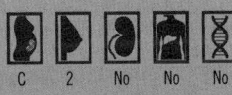
   PO/IM/IV (use succinate salt for IM/IV): 0.5—1.7 mg/kg/24 hr ÷ Q6—12 hr
Asthma exacerbations (2007 National Heart, Lung, and Blood Institute Guideline Recommendations; dose until peak expiratory flow reaches 70% of predicted or personal best):
   Child ≤12 yr (IV/IM/PO; use succinate salt for IV/IM): 1—2 mg/kg/24 hr ÷ Q12 hr (**max. dose:** 60 mg/24 hr). An alternative regimen for ≤5 yr old of 1 mg/kg/dose Q6 hr × 24 hr followed by oral corticosteroids to complete a 3—5 day course has been suggested.
   Child >12 yr and adult (IV/IM/PO; use succinate salt for IV/IM): 40—80 mg/24 hr ÷ Q12—24 hr
Outpatient asthma exacerbation burst therapy (longer durations may be necessary):
   PO:
      Child ≤12 yr: 1—2 mg/kg/24 hr ÷ Q12—24 hr (**max. dose:** 60 mg/24 hr) × 3—10 days
      Child >12 yr and adult: 40—60 mg/24 hr ÷ Q12—24 hr × 3—10 days
   IM (use methylprednisolone acetate product) for patients vomiting or with adherence issues:
      Child ≤4 yr: 7.5 mg/kg (**max. dose:** 240 mg) IM × 1
      Child >4 yr, adolescent, and adult: 240 mg IM × 1
Acute spinal cord injury:
   30 mg/kg IV over 15 min followed in 45 min by a continuous infusion of 5.4 mg/kg/hr × 23 hr

---

See Chapter 10 for relative steroid potencies. Acetate form may also be used for intra-articular and intralesional injection and has longer times to max. effect and duration of action; it should **NOT** be given IV. **Use with caution** with systemic sclerosis. Like all steroids, may cause hypertension, leukocytosis, pseudotumor cerebri, acne, Cushing syndrome, adrenal axis suppression,

Continued

METHYLPREDNISOLONE *continued*

GI bleeding, hyperglycemia, and osteoporosis. Hypertrophic cardiomyopathy has been reported in premature infants.

Barbiturates, phenytoin, and rifampin may enhance methylprednisolone clearance. Erythromycin, itraconazole, and ketoconazole may increase methylprednisolone levels. Methylprednisolone may increase cyclosporine and tacrolimus levels.

METOCLOPRAMIDE
Reglan and generics
Antiemetic, prokinetic agent

    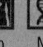

B   2   Yes   No   No

Tabs: 5, 10 mg
Tabs, orally disintegrating (ODT): 5, 10 mg
Injection: 5 mg/mL (2 mL)
Oral solution: 5 mg/5 mL (473 mL)

Gastroesophageal reflux (GER) or GI dysmotility:
    Infant and child: 0.1—0.2 mg/kg/dose up to QID IV/IM/PO; **max. dose:** 0.8 mg/kg/24 hr or 10 mg/dose
    Adult: 10 mg/dose QAC and QHS IV/IM/PO
Antiemetic for chemotherapy-induced nausea and vomiting (child and adolescent): Premedicate with diphenhydramine to reduce extrapyramidal symptoms (EPS).
    1—2 mg/kg/dose Q2—6 hr IV/IM/PO up to 5 doses/24 hr
Postoperative nausea and vomiting:
    Child (limited data): 0.1—0.2 mg/kg/dose Q6—8 hr PRN IV; **max. dose:** 10 mg/dose
    >14 yr and adult: 10 mg Q6—8 hr PRN IV

Contraindicated in GI obstruction, seizure disorder, tardive dyskinesia, pheochromocytoma, or in patients receiving drugs likely to cause EPS. May cause EPS, especially at higher doses. Sedation, headache, anxiety, depression, leukopenia, and diarrhea may occur. Neuroleptic malignant syndrome and tardive dyskinesia (increased risk with prolonged duration of therapy; **avoid use >12 wk**) have been reported.

Metoclopramide is a substrate for CYP 450 2D6; inhibitors to this enzyme may increase risk for metoclopramide toxicity. G6PD deficiency may increase risk for methemoglobinemia; **DO NOT** use methylene blue as it may cause a fatal hemolytic anemia.

For GER, give 30 min before meals and at bedtime. **Reduce dose in renal impairment (see Chapter 31).**

METOLAZONE
Generics; previously available as Zaroxolyn
Diuretic, thiazide-like

   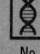 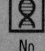

B   2   Yes   Yes   No

Tabs: 2.5, 5, 10 mg
Oral suspension: 0.25 mg/mL , 1 mg/mL

Dosage based on Zaroxolyn (for oral suspension, see remarks):
    Child:
        Edema: 0.2—0.4 mg/kg/24 hr ÷ once daily—BID PO
    Adult:
        Hypertension: 2.5—5 mg once daily PO
        Edema: 2.5—20 mg once daily PO

METOLAZONE *continued*

Contraindicated in patients with anuria, hepatic coma, or hypersensitivity to sulfonamides or thiazides. **Use with caution** in severe renal disease, impaired hepatic function, gout, lupus erythematosus, diabetes mellitus, and elevated cholesterol and triglycerides. Electrolyte imbalance, GI disturbance, hyperglycemia, marrow suppression, chills, hyperuricemia, chest pain, hepatitis, and rash may occur.

Oral suspensions have increased bioavailability; therefore lower doses may be necessary when using these dosage forms. More effective than thiazide diuretics in impaired renal function; may be effective in GFRs as low as 20 mL/min. Furosemide-resistant edema in pediatric patients may benefit with the addition of metolazone.

METOPROLOL
Lopressor, Toprol-XL, Kapspargo Sprinkle, and generics
Adrenergic blocking agent (β_1 selective), class II antiarrhythmic

  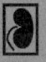 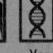

C   1   No   Yes   Yes

Tabs: 25, 37.5, 50, 75, 100 mg
Extended release tabs (Toprol-XL and generics): 25, 50, 100, 200 mg
Extended release caps as sprinkles (Kapspargo Sprinkle): 25, 50, 100, 200 mg; contains corn starch
Oral liquid: 10 mg/mL
Injection: 1 mg/mL (5 mL)

Hypertension:
  Child ≥1 yr and adolescent:
    Non—extended release oral dosage forms: Start at 1—2 mg/kg/24 hr PO ÷ BID (**max. initial dose:** 25 mg/dose); if needed, adjust dose up to a **max. dose** of 6 mg/kg/24 hr **up to** 200 mg/24 hr.
    Extended release tabs or caps (≥6 yr and adolescent): Start at 1 mg/kg/dose (**max. dose:** 50 mg) PO once daily; if needed, adjust dose **up to** a **max. dose** of 2 mg/kg/24 hr or 200 mg/24 hr once daily (higher doses have not been evaluated).
  Adult:
    Non—extended release tabs: Start at 50—100 mg/24 hr PO ÷ once daily—BID; if needed, increase dosage at weekly intervals to desired blood pressure. Usual effective dosage range is 100—200 mg/24 hr. Doses >450 mg/24 hr have not been studied. Patients with bronchospastic diseases should receive the lowest possible daily dose divided TID.
    Extended release tabs or caps: Start at 25—100 mg/24 hr PO once daily; if needed, increase dosage at weekly intervals to desired blood pressure. Usual dosage range is 50—200 mg/24 hr. Doses >400 mg/24 hr have not been studied.

Contraindicated in sinus bradycardia, heart block >1st degree, sick sinus syndrome (except with functioning pacemaker), cardiogenic shock, and uncompensated CHF. **Use with caution** in hepatic dysfunction, peripheral vascular disease, history of severe anaphylactic hypersensitivity drug reactions, pheochromocytoma, and concurrent use with verapamil, diltiazem, or anesthetic agents that may decrease myocardial function. Should not be used with bronchospastic diseases. Reserpine and other drugs that deplete catecholamines (e.g., MAO inhibitors) may increase the effects of metoprolol. Metoprolol is a CYP 450 2D6 substrate. Poor metabolizers and extensive metabolizers who concomitantly use CYP 2D6 inhibitors will have significant increases in metoprolol blood levels to decrease its cardioselectivity.

Continued

METOPROLOL *continued*

Avoid abrupt cessation of therapy in ischemic heart disease; angina, ventricular arrhythmias, and MI have occurred. Common side effects include bradyarrhythmia, heart block, heart failure, pruritus, rash, GI disturbances, dizziness, fatigue, and depression. Bronchospasm, dyspnea, and elevations in transaminase, alkaline phosphatase, and LDH have all been reported.

METRONIDAZOLE
Flagyl, First-Metronidazole, MetroGel, MetroLotion, MetroCream, Rosadan, Noritate, Vandazole, Nuvessa, and generics
Antibiotic, antiprotozoal

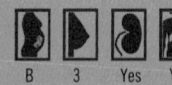
B   3   Yes   Yes   No

Tabs: 250, 500 mg
Caps: 375 mg
Oral suspension: 50 mg/mL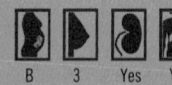
  First-Metronidazole: 50 mg/mL (150 mL); contains sodium benzoate and saccharin
Ready-to-use injection: 5 mg/mL (100 mL); contains 28 mEq Na/g drug
Gel, topical:
  Rosadan and generics: 0.75% (45 g)
  MetroGel and generics: 1% (55, 60 g)
Lotion (MetroLotion and generics): 0.75% (59 mL); contains benzyl alcohol
Cream, topical:
  MetroCream, Rosadan, and generics: 0.75% (45 g); contain benzyl alcohol
  Noritate: 1% (60 g); contains parabens
Gel, vaginal:
  Vandazole and generics: 0.75% (each applicator delivers ~5 g of gel containing ~37.5 mg metronidazole); contains parabens (70 g with 5 applicators)
  Nuvessa: 1.3%: (each applicator delivers ~5 g containing ~65 mg metronidazole); contains parabens and benzyl alcohol (1 prefilled applicator)

Amebiasis:
  Child: 35–50 mg/kg/24 hr PO ÷ Q8 hr × 10 days; **max. dose:** 750 mg/dose
  Adult: 500–750 mg/dose PO Q8 hr × 10 days
Anaerobic infection (see remarks):
  Neonate: PO/IV:
    Loading dose (all ages): 15 mg/kg × 1
    Maintenance dose based on postmenstrual age (PMA):
      PMA 24–25 wk: 7.5 mg/kg/dose Q24 hr
      PMA 26–27 wk: 10 mg/kg/dose Q24 hr
      PMA 28–33 wk: 7.5 mg/kg/dose Q12 hr
      PMA 34–40 wk: 7.5 mg/kg/dose Q8 hr
      PMA >40 wk: 7.5 mg/kg/dose Q6 hr
  Infant/child/adolescent:
    PO: 30–50 mg/kg/24 hr ÷ Q8 hr; **max. dose:** 2250 mg/24 hr
    IV: 22.5–40 mg/kg/24 hr ÷ Q6–8 hr; **max. dose:** 4 g/24 hr
  Adult:
    PO/IV: 30 mg/kg/24 hr ÷ Q6–8 hr; **max. dose:** 4 g/24 hr. A 15 mg/kg/dose IV loading dose over 1 hr is administered 6 hr prior to the aforementioned maintenance dose for IV route.
Bacterial vaginosis:
  Child >45 kg, adolescent, and adult:

METRONIDAZOLE continued

PO:
  Immediate release tabs: 500 mg BID × 7 days
Vaginal:
  Vaginal gel 0.75% (Adolescent and adult): ~37.5 mg (1 applicator full) QHS × 5 days
  Vaginal gel 1.3% (≥12 yr and adult): ~65 mg (1 applicator full) at bedtime × 1

Giardiasis:
  Child: 15–30 mg/kg/24 hr PO ÷ TID × 5–7 days; **max. dose:** 750 mg/24 hr
  Adult: 250 mg PO TID × 5 days

Trichomoniasis: Treat sexual contacts.
  Child <45 kg: 45 mg/kg/24 hr PO ÷ TID × 7 days; **max. dose:** 2000 mg/24 hr
  Child ≥45 kg, adolescent/adult: 2 g PO × 1, or 500 mg PO BID × 7 days

Clostridium difficile **infection (IV may be less efficacious):**
  Child: 30 mg/kg/24 hr ÷ Q6 hr PO/IV × 10–14 days; **max. dose:** 2000 mg/24 hr
  Severe fulminant infection (with oral or rectal vancomycin): 30 mg/kg/24 hr ÷ Q8 hr IV × 10 days; **max. dose:** 500 mg/dose
  Adult: 500 mg TID PO/IV × 10–14 days
  Severe fulminant infection (with oral or rectal vancomycin): 500 mg IV Q8 hr

Helicobacter pylori **infection (use in combination with amoxicillin and acid-suppressing agent with/ without clarithromycin):**
  Child: 20 mg/kg/24 hr (**max. dose:** 1000 mg/24 hr) ÷ BID PO × 10–14 days
  Adult: 250–500 mg TID–QID (QAC and QHS) PO × 10–14 days

Topical use for rosacea: Apply and rub a thin film to affected areas at the following frequencies specific to product concentration.
  0.75% cream: BID
  1% cream: Once daily

Contraindicated in Cockayne syndrome as fatal liver failure has been reported. **Avoid use** in first-trimester pregnancy. **Use with caution** in patients with CNS disease, blood dyscrasias, severe liver (reduce dose by 50% with Child-Pugh C) or **renal disease (GFR <10 mL/min; see Chapter 31).** If using single 2 g dose in a breastfeeding mother, discontinue breastfeeding for 12–24 hr to allow excretion of the drug.

Nausea, diarrhea, urticaria, dry mouth, leukopenia, vertigo, metallic taste, and peripheral neuropathy may occur. Candidiasis may worsen. May discolor urine. Patients **should not** ingest alcohol for 24–48 hr after dose (disulfiram-type reaction). Peripheral neuropathy has been reported with topical use. May interfere with AST, ALT, triglycerides, glucose, and LDH testing.

Single-dose oral regimen no longer recommended in bacterial vaginosis due to poor efficacy. May increase levels or toxicity of phenytoin, lithium, and warfarin. Phenobarbital and rifampin may increase metronidazole metabolism. QT prolongation has been reported when used with other medications with the potential for prolonging the QT interval.

IV infusion must be given slowly over 1 hr. For intravenous use in all ages, some references recommend a 15 mg/kg loading dose.

MICAFUNGIN SODIUM
Mycamine and generics
Antifungal, echinocandin

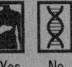

| C | ? | Yes | Yes | No |

Injection: 50, 100 mg; contains lactose

Invasive candidiasis (see remarks):

Continued

MICAFUNGIN SODIUM *continued*

Neonate and infant (based on a multidose pharmacokinetic and safety trial in 13 neonates/infants >48 hr and <120 days old with suspected or invasive candidiasis; minimum of 4–5 days of therapy):
- **<1 kg:** 10 mg/kg/dose IV Q24 hr; additional data from another multidose trial in 12 preterm neonates (median birth weight: 775 g, 27 wks' gestation) suggest 15 mg/kg/dose IV Q24 hr will provide similar AUC drug exposure of approximately 5 mg/kg/dose in adults
- **≥1 kg:** 7–10 mg/kg/dose IV Q24 hr; 10–12 mg/kg/dose IV Q24 hr may be needed for HIV-exposed/infected neonates

Infant (≥1 mo), child, and adolescent: 3 mg/kg/dose IV Q24 hr; **max. dose:** 100 mg/dose
Adult: 100–150 mg IV Q24 hr

Esophageal candidiasis, invasive aspergillosis, candidal endocarditis (see remarks):
Infant (≥1 mo), child, and adolescent: 4 mg/kg/dose IV Q24 hr; **max. dose:** 150 mg/24 hr
Adult: 150 mg IV Q24 hr

Candida **prophylaxis in hematopoietic stem cell transplant:**
Infant (1 mo), child, and adult: 1 mg/kg/dose IV Q24 hr; **max. dose:** 50 mg/dose

Prior hypersensitivity to other echinocandins (anidulafungin, casopofungin) increases risk; anaphylaxis with shock has been reported. **Use with caution** in hepatic and renal impairment.

No dosing adjustments are required based on race or gender, or in patients with severe renal dysfunction or mild to moderate hepatic function impairment. Effect of severe hepatic function impairment on micafungin pharmacokinetics has not been evaluated. Higher dosage requirements in premature and young infants may be attributed to the faster drug clearance due to lower protein binding. Higher treatment doses in infants and children have been reported at 8.6–12 mg/kg/dose IV once daily.

May cause GI disturbances, phlebitis, rash, hyperbilirubinemia, liver function test elevation, headache, fever, and rigor. Anemia, leukopenia, neutropenia, thrombocytopenia, TEN, Stevens-Johnson syndrome, and hemolysis have been reported. Micafungin is CYP 450 3A isoenzyme substrate and weak inhibitor. May increase the effects/toxicity of nifedipine and sirolimus.

Safety and efficacy in children ≤4 mo have been established in patients without meningoencephalitis and/or other dissemination. This is supported by adequate and well-controlled studies in children ≥4 mo with additional pharmacokinetic/safety data in children <4 mo.

MICONAZOLE
Topical products: Micatin, Desenex, Lotrimin AF, and other brands including generics
Vaginal products: Miconazole 7, Miconazole 3, Monistat, Vagistat-3, other brands & generics
Oral buccal tab: Oravig
Antifungal agent

   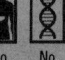

C   2   No   No   No

Cream (OTC): 2% (15, 30, 57, 118 g); may contain benzoic acid
Ointment (OTC): 2% (56, 141 g)
Topical solution (OTC): 2% with alcohol (30 mL); may contain benzyl alcohol
Powder (OTC): 2% (43, 71, 85, 90 g)
Spray, powder (OTC): 2% (85, 113, 133 g); contains alcohol
Vaginal cream (OTC): 2% (45 g); contains benzoic acid
Vaginal suppository (OTC): 100 mg (7s), 200 mg (3s)

MICONAZOLE *continued*

Vaginal combination packs:
Monistat 1 Combination Pack (OTC): 1200 mg vaginal suppository (1) and 2% cream (9 g)
Miconazole 3 Combo Pack, Monistat 3 Combo Pack, Vagistat-3 (OTC): 200 mg (4%) vaginal suppository (3s); and 2% external cream (9 g)
Monistat 7 Combo Pack (OTC): 100 mg vaginal suppository (7s) and 2% cream (9 g)
Oral buccal tab:
Oravig: 50 mg; contains corn starch and milk proteins

Topical (≥2 yr and adolescent): Apply BID × 2—4 wk.
Vaginal (≥12 yr and adult):
7-day regimen: 1 applicator full of 2% cream or 100 mg suppository QHS × 7 days
3-day regimen: 1 applicator full of 4% cream or 200 mg suppository QHS × 3 days
1-day regimen (Monistat 1): 1200 mg suppository × 1 at bedtime or during the day
Mild oropharyngeal candidiasis (adult): Apply 1 tab (50 mg) to the upper gum once daily × 7—14 days.

Use with caution in hypersensitivity to other imidazole antifungal agents (e.g., clotrimazole, ketoconazole). Side effects include pruritus, rash, burning, phlebitis, headaches, and pelvic cramps.

Drug is a substrate and inhibitor of the CYP 450 3A3/4 isoenzymes. Vaginal use with concomitant warfarin use has also been reported to increase warfarin's effect. Vegetable oil base in vaginal suppositories may interact with latex products (e.g., condoms and diaphragms); consider switching to the vaginal cream.

Avoid contact with eyes.

Do not crush, chew, or swallow the buccal tabs. Apply buccal tabs in the morning after brushing teeth by placing the tablet against the upper gum above one of the incisor tooth and hold with slight pressure over the upper lip for 30 sec (alternate sides of the mouth with each application). Placement of the rounded side of the tablet against the gum may be more comfortable, and avoid chewing gum while tablet is in place. If tablet falls off within 6 hr of application, reposition the same tablet immediately. See product information for additional information. Oral discomfort, including mouth and tongue ulceration, dry mouth, toothache, and loss/altered taste, has been reported with use of buccal tabs.

MIDAZOLAM
Generics; previously available as
Versed; intranasal: Nayzilam
Benzodiazepine

   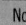

| D | 2 | Yes | Yes | No |

Injection: 1 mg/mL (2, 5, 10 mL), 5 mg/mL (1, 2, 5, 10 mL); some preparations may contain 1% benzyl alcohol
Oral syrup: 2 mg/mL (118 mL); contains sodium benzoate
Nasal solution (Nayzilam): 5 mg per 0.1 mL (2s); contains propylene glycol

Titrate to effect under controlled conditions (see remarks).
See Chapter 6 for additional routes of administration.
Sedation for procedures:
Infant, child, and adolescent:
IM: 0.1—0.15 mg/kg/dose 30—60 min prior to procedure. Higher dose of 0.5 mg/kg/dose has been used for anxious patients. **Max. dose:** 10 mg

Continued

MIDAZOLAM *continued*

IV:

6 mo—5 yr: 0.05—0.1 mg/kg/dose over 2—3 min. May repeat dose PRN in 2—3 min intervals up to a **max. total dose** of 6 mg. A total dose up to 0.6 mg/kg may be necessary for desired effect.

6—12 yr: 0.025—0.05 mg/kg/dose over 2—3 min. May repeat dose PRN in 2—3 min intervals up to a **max. total dose** of 10 mg. A total dose up to 0.4 mg/kg may be necessary for desired effect.

>12—18 yr: 0.5—2.5 mg over 2—3 min. May repeat in 2—3 min intervals up to **max. total dose** of 10 mg

PO:

≥6 mo, child, and adolescent <16 yr: 0.25—0.5 mg/kg/dose × 1; **max. dose:** 20 mg. Younger patients (6 mo—5 yr) may require higher doses of 1 mg/kg/dose, whereas older patients (6—15 yr) may require only 0.25 mg/kg/dose. Use 0.25 mg/kg/dose for patients with cardiac or respiratory compromise, concurrent CNS depressive drug, or high-risk surgery.

Intranasal (limited data; using IV dosage form with nasal atomizer):

Infant, child, and adolescent: 0.2—0.3 mg/kg/dose (**max.** 10 mg/dose) intranasally × 1. Higher doses of 0.4—0.5 mg/kg/dose (**max.** 10 mg/dose) have also been reported.

Adult (Sedation for procedures):

IM: 0.07—0.08 mg/kg/dose 30—60 min prior to procedure; usual dose is 5 mg

IV: 0.5—2 mg/dose over 2 min. May repeat PRN in 2—3 min intervals until desired effect. Usual total dose: 2.5—5 mg. **Max. total dose:** 5 mg

Sedation with mechanical ventilation:

Intermittent:

Infant and child: 0.05—0.15 mg/kg/dose IV Q1—2 hr PRN

Continuous IV infusion (initial doses, titrate to effect):

Neonate:

<32-wks' gestation: 0.5 mCg/kg/min

≥32-wks' gestation: 1 mCg/kg/min

Infant and child: 1—2 mCg/kg/min

Refractory status epilepticus:

≥2 mo and child: Load with 0.2 mg/kg IV × 1 followed by a continuous infusion of 1 mCg/kg/min; titrate dose upward Q5 min to effect (mean dose of 2.3 mCg/kg/min with a range of 1—18 mCg/kg/min has been reported).

Acute treatment of intermittent, stereotypic episodes of frequent seizure activity (i.e., seizure clusters, acute repetitive seizures) that are distinct from a patient's usual seizure pattern in patients with epilepsy:

Infant, child, and adolescent (intranasal using IV dosage form with nasal automizer): Inhale 0.2—0.3 mg/kg/dose (**max. dose:** 10 mg/dose) intranasally by administering half of total dose into each nostril. If no response after 10 min, dose may be repeated once.

≥12 yr and adult (Nayzilam intranasal; see remarks): Administer one spray (5 mg) intranasally into one nostril. If no response in 10 min, administer an additional 5 mg spray into the alternative nostril. **Do not** administer the second dose if patient has trouble breathing or if there is excessive sedation that is uncharacteristic of the patient during a seizure episode. **Max. dose:** 10 mg/dose per episode; **not to exceed** one episode every 3 days and 5 episodes per month.

Contraindicated in patients with narrow-angle glaucoma and shock. **Use with caution** in CHF, renal impairment (**adjust dose; see Chapter 31**), pulmonary disease, hepatic dysfunction, and neonates. Causes respiratory depression, hypotension, and bradycardia. Cardiovascular monitoring is recommended. Use lower doses or reduce dose when given in combination with narcotics or in patients with respiratory compromise.

MIDAZOLAM *continued*

Higher recommended dosage for younger patients (6 mo—5 yr) is attributed to the water-soluble properties of midazolam and the higher percent body water for younger patients.

Drug is a substrate for CYP 450 3A4. Serum concentrations may be increased by cimetidine, clarithromycin, diltiazem, erythromycin, itraconazole, ketoconazole, ranitidine, and protease inhibitors **(use contraindicated)**. Sedative effects may be antagonized by theophylline. **Effects can be reversed by flumazenil.** For pharmacodynamic information, see Chapter 6.

Do not prime Nayzilam intranasal dosage form, because this will promote drug loss.

MILRINONE
Generics; previously available as Primacor
Inotrope, phosphodiesterase inhibitor

   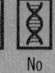

C   ?   Yes   No   No

Injection: 1 mg/mL (10, 20, 50 mL); single-dose use products are preservative free
Premixed injection in D₅W: 200 mCg/mL (100, 200 mL); preservative free

Infant, child, and adolescent (limited data): Optional 50 mCg/kg IV loading dose over 15 min, followed by a continuous infusion of 0.25—0.75 mCg/kg/min and titrate to effect. Loading dose is **NOT recommended** by some due to the risk of hypotension.

Adult: Continuous infusion of 0.125—0.75 mCg/kg/min; titrate to the lowest dose for clinical effect. Prior use of loading dose is **NOT recommended** due to the risk of hypotension.

Contraindicated in severe aortic stenosis, severe pulmonic stenosis, and acute MI. May cause headache, dysrhythmias, hypotension, hypokalemia, nausea, vomiting, anorexia, abdominal pain, hepatotoxicity, and thrombocytopenia. Pediatric patients may require higher mCg/kg/min doses because of a faster elimination $T_{1/2}$ and larger volume of distribution, when compared with adults. Hemodynamic effects can last up to 3—5 hr after discontinuation of infusion in children. **Reduce dose in renal impairment.**

MINERAL OIL
GoodSense Mineral Oil, Kondremul, Fleet Mineral Oil, and generics
Laxative, lubricant

C   2   No   No   No

Liquid, oral (GoodSense Mineral Oil and generics; OTC): 473, 946 mL
Emulsion, oral (Kondremul; OTC): 480 mL; each 5 mL Kondremul contains 2.5 mL mineral oil
Rectal liquid (Fleet Mineral Oil and generics; OTC): 133 mL bottle delivers approximately 120 mL

Constipation:
  Child 6—11 yr (see remarks):
    Oral liquid: 5—15 mL/24 hr ÷ once daily (QHS)—TID PO
    Oral emulsion (Kondremul): 10—30 mL/24 hr ÷ once daily (QHS)—TID PO
    Rectal (2—11 yr): ~60 mL (half-bottle) as single dose
  Child ≥12 yr and adult (see remarks):
    Oral liquid: 15—45 mL/24 hr ÷ once daily (QHS)—TID PO
    Oral emulsion (Kondremul): 30—90 mL/24 hr ÷ once daily (QHS)—TID PO
    Rectal (≥12 yr and adult): ~120 mL (full bottle) as single dose

May cause diarrhea, cramps, and lipid pneumonitis via aspiration. Use as a laxative **should not exceed** >1 wk. Onset of action is approximately 6—8 hr. Higher doses may be necessary to achieve desired effect. **DO NOT** give QHS dose and use with **caution** in children <5 yr to

Continued

MINERAL OIL *continued*

minimize risk of aspiration. May impair the absorption of fat-soluble vitamins, calcium, phosphorus, oral contraceptives, and warfarin. Emulsified preparations are more palatable and are dosed differently than the oral liquid preparation.

For disimpaction, doses up to 1 ounce (30 mL) per year of age (**max. dose** of 240 mL) BID can be given.

MINOCYCLINE
Minocin, CoreMino, Solodyn, Minolira, Ximino,
Amzeeq, and generics
Antibiotic, tetracycline derivative

  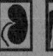 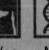

D	2	Yes	Yes	No

Tabs: 50, 75, 100 mg
Caps: 50, 75, 100 mg
Extended release tabs (Q24 hr dosing):
 Solodyn and generics: 55, 65, 80, 105, 115 mg
 CoreMino: 45, 90, 135 mg
 Minolira: 105, 135 mg
 Other generics: 45, 90, 135 mg
Extended release caps (Q24 hr dosing):
 Ximino and generics: 45, 90, 135 mg
Injection (Minocin): 100 mg; may contain 2.2 mEq magnesium/100 mg drug
Topical foam (dispensed in a pressurized container with butane, isobutrane, and propane propellants):
 Amzeeq: 4% (30 g); contains alcohols

General infections:
 Child (8–12 yr): 4 mg/kg/dose (**max. dose:** 200 mg/dose) × 1 IV/PO, then 2 mg/kg/dose Q12 hr IV/PO; **max. dose:** 200 mg/24 hr
 Adolescent and adult: 200 mg/dose × 1 IV/PO, then 100 mg Q12 hr IV/PO
Chlamydia trachomatis/Ureaplasma urealyticum:
 Adolescent and adult: 100 mg IV/PO Q12 hr × 7 days
Acne (≥12 yr–adult):
 Immediate release dosage forms: 50–100 mg PO once daily–BID
 Extended release tabs:
  Solodyn and generics:
   45–49 kg: 45 mg PO once daily
   50–59 kg: 55 mg PO once daily
   60–71 kg: 65 mg PO once daily
   72–84 kg: 80 mg PO once daily
   85–96 kg: 90 mg PO once daily
   97–110 kg: 105 PO once daily
   111–125 kg: 115 mg PO once daily
   126–136 kg: 135 mg PO once daily
  Minolira:
   45–59 kg: 52.5 mg (half of 105 mg tab)
   60–89 kg: 67.5 mg (half of 135 mg tab) PO once daily
   90–125 kg: 105 mg PO once daily
   126–136 kg: 135 mg PO once daily

MINOCYCLINE *continued*

> **Extended release caps:**
> > **Ximino:**
> > > **45—59 kg:** 45 mg PO once daily
> > > **60—90 kg:** 90 mg PO once daily
> > > **91—136 kg:** 135 mg PO once daily
> > **Topical foam (Amzeeq; moderate-to-severe acne vulgaris):**
> > > **≥9 yr and adult (see remarks):** Apply a small amount to affected areas QHS until all areas are treated.

Not recommended for children <8 yr and during the last half of pregnancy due to risk of permanent tooth discoloration. **Use with caution** in renal failure; lower dosage may be necessary. High incidence of vestibular dysfunction (30%—90%). Nausea, vomiting, allergy, increased intracranial pressure (e.g., pseudotumor cerebri), photophobia, and injury to developing teeth may occur. Hepatitis, including autoimmune hepatitis, liver failure, hypersensitivity reactions (e.g., anaphylaxis, Stevens-Johnson syndrome, erythema multiforme), and serum sickness—like and lupus-like syndrome have been reported.

May increase effects/toxicity of warfarin and decrease the efficacy of live attenuated oral typhoid vaccine. May be administered with food but **NOT** with milk or dairy products. See Tetracycline for additional drug/food interactions and comments.

TOPICAL USE: Dosage form is flammable; **avoid** smoking during and immediately after application. Not for oral, ophthalmic, or intravaginal use. Headache is the most common side effect. Hyperpigmentation, erythema, dryness, itching, and headache have also been reported.

MINOXIDIL
Tabs: Generics; previously available as Loniten
Topical: Rogaine Men's/Women's, Minoxidil for Men/Women, Hair Regrowth Treatment Men, Men's Rogaine Extra Strength
Antihypertensive agent, hair growth stimulant

 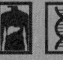

C   2   Yes   Yes   No

Tabs: 2.5, 10 mg
Topical solution:
> **Minoxidil for Men, Minoxidil for Women, Rogaine, and generics (OTC):** 2% (60 mL); contains alcohol and propylene glycol
> **Hair Regrowth Treatment for Men, Men's Rogaine Extra Strength, Minoxidil Extra Strength for Men, and generics (OTC):** 5% (60, 120 mL); contains 30% alcohol
Topical foam:
> **Rogaine Men's, Rogaine Women's, Rogaine Men's Extra Strength (OTC):** 5% (60 g); contains cetyl alcohol

---

Hypertension:
> **Child <12 yr:** Start with 0.1—0.2 mg/kg/24 hr PO once daily; **max. dose:** 5 mg/24 hr. Dose may be increased in increments of 0.1—0.2 mg/kg/24 hr at 3-day intervals. Usual effective range: 0.25—1 mg/kg/24 hr PO ÷ once daily—TID; **max. dose:** 50 mg/24 hr
> **≥12 yr and adult:** Start with 5 mg PO once daily. Dose may be gradually increased at 3-day intervals. Usual effective range: 10—40 mg/24 hr ÷ once daily—TID; **max. dose:** 100 mg/24 hr
Topical (alopecia; see remarks):
> **Adult:**
> > **Solution (2% or 5%):** Apply 1 mL to affected areas of the scalp BID (QAM and QHS).

Continued

MINOXIDIL *continued*

Foam:
Female: Apply $^1/_2$ capful to affected areas of the scalp once daily.
Male: Apply $^1/_2$ capful to affected areas of the scalp BID.

Contraindicated in acute MI, dissecting aortic aneurysm, and pheochromocytoma. Concurrent use with a β-blocker and diuretic is recommended to prevent reflex tachycardia and reduce water retention, respectively. Use with **caution** in hepatic impairment as decrease in drug clearance has been reported in mild cirrhosis for adults. May cause drowsiness, dizziness, CHF, pulmonary edema, pericardial effusion, pericarditis, thrombocytopenia, leukopenia, Stevens-Johnson syndrome, TEN, and hypertrichosis (reversible) with systemic use. Neonatal hypertrichosis has been reported following use during pregnancy.

Concurrent use of guanethidine may cause profound orthostatic hypotension; use with other antihypertensive agents may cause additive hypotension. Patients with renal failure or receiving dialysis may require a dosage reduction. Antihypertensive onset of action within 30 min and peak effects within 2–8 hr.

TOPICAL USE: Local irritation, contact dermatitis may occur. **Do not use** in conjunction with other topical agents, including topical corticosteroids, retinoids or petrolatum, or agents that are known to enhance cutaneous drug absorption. Onset of hair growth is 4 mo. Wash hands thoroughly after each application. The 5% solution is flammable.

MOMETASONE FUROATE ± FOMOTEROL FUMARATE
Asmanex, Nasonex, and other generic nasal and topical products; previously available as Elocon (topical forms)
In combination with fomoterol: Dulera
Corticosteroid

    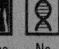

C   2   No   Yes   No

Nasal spray (Nasonex and generics): 0.05%, 50 mCg per actuation (10 mL provides 60 doses [OTC]; 17 g, provides 120 doses)
Aerosol for inhalation (Asmanex HFA): 50 mCg per actuation (13 g, provides 120 actuations), 100 mCg per actuation (13 g, provides 120 actuations), 200 mCg per actuation (13 g, provides 120 actuations)
Powder for inhalation, breath activated (Asmanex Twisthaler; see remarks): 110 mCg per actuation (30 doses), 220 mCg per actuation (14, 30, 60, 120 doses); contains lactose and milk proteins
Topical cream and ointment: 0.1% (15, 45 g)
Topical lotion: 0.1% (30, 60 mL); contains isopropyl alcohol
In combination with fomoterol:
Aerosol inhaler (Dulera):
50 mCg mometasone furoate + 5 mCg fomoterol fumarate dihydrate per inhalation (13 g delivers 120 inhalations)
100 mCg mometasone furoate + 5 mCg fomoterol fumarate dihydrate per inhalation (8.8 g delivers 60 inhalations, 13 g delivers 120 inhalations)
200 mCg mometasone furoate + 5 mCg fomoterol fumarate dihydrate per inhalation (8.8 g delivers 60 inhalations, 13 g delivers 120 inhalations)

MOMETASONE FUROATE:
Intranasal (allergic rhinitis): Patients with known seasonal allergic rhinitis should initiate therapy 2–4 wk prior to anticipated pollen season.
Child 2–11 yr: 50 mCg (1 spray) each nostril once daily (100 mCg/24 hr)
Child ≥12 yr and adult: 100 mCg (2 sprays) each nostril once daily (200 mCg/24 hr)

MOMETASONE FUROATE ± FOMOTEROL FUMARATE *continued*

Oral inhalation:

Asmanex HFA (aerosol for inhalation):

Child 5—<12 yr: 2 inhalations (100 mCg) BID of 50 mCg inhaler (200 mCg/24 hr)

Child ≥12 yr and adult: Max. effects may not be achieved until 2 wk. Titrate doses to lowest effective dose once asthma stabilized.

Previously treated with bronchodilators alone or medium-dose inhaled corticosteroids: 2 inhalations (200 mCg) BID of 100 mCg inhaler (400 mCg/24 hr)

Previously receiving high-dose inhaled or chronic oral corticosteroids: 2 inhalations (400 mCg) BID of 200 mCg inhaler (800 mCg/24 hr)

Max. dose (all ages): 800 mCg/24 hr

Asmanex Twisthaler (breath-activated powder for inhalation; see remarks):

Child 4—11 yr: Start with 110 mCg (1 inhalation) QHS of the 110 mCg inhaler regardless of prior therapy; **max. dose:** 110 mCg/24 hr.

Child ≥12 yr and adult: Max. effects may not be achieved until 1—2 wk or longer. Titrate doses to the lowest effective dose once asthma stabilized.

Previously treated with bronchodilators alone or with inhaled corticosteroids: Start with 220 mCg (1 inhalation) QHS. Dose may be increased up to a **max. dose** of 440 mCg/24 hr ÷ QHS or BID.

Previously treated with oral corticosteroids: Start with 440 mCg BID; **max. dose:** 880 mCg/24 hr.

Topical (see Chapter 8 for topical steroid comparisons):

Cream and ointment:

≥2 yr and adult: Apply a thin film to affected area once daily. Safety and efficacy for >3 wk have not been established for pediatric patients.

Lotion:

≥12 yr and adult: Apply a few drops to affected area and massage lightly into skin once daily until it disappears.

MOMETASONE FUROATE + FOMOTEROL FUMARATE (DULERA):

Child 5—<12 yr: Two inhalations BID of 50 mCg mometasone + 5 mCg fomoterol; **max. dose:** 2 inhalations BID

Child ≥12 yr and adult: Two inhalations BID of either 100 mCg mometasone + 5 mCg formoterol or 200 mCg mometasone + 5 mCg formoterol based on prior asthma therapy (see the following table). If using the lower strength (100 mCg mometasone + 5 mCg formoterol), allow for 2 wk of therapy before increasing to the higher strength if no adequate response. **Max. dose:** Two inhalations BID of 200 mCg mometasone + 5 mCg formoterol.

Previous Therapy	Recommended Starting Dose	Recommended Maximum Daily Dose
Medium-dose inhaled corticosteroids	100 mCg mometasone + 5 mCg formoterol: 2 inhalations BID	400 mCg mometasone + 20 mCg formoterol
High-dose inhaled corticosteroids	200 mCg mometasone + 5 mCg formoterol: 2 inhalations BID	800 mCg mometasone + 20 mCg formoterol

Mometasone is a CYP 450 3A4 substrate; concurrent administration with ketoconazole and other CYP 450 3A4 inhibitors (e.g., protease inhibitors) may increase mometasone levels, resulting in Cushing syndrome and adrenal suppression. Blurred vision, cataracts, and glaucoma have been reported. Use with **caution** with hepatic impairment; increased drug exposure is possible.

Continued

MOMETASONE FUROATE ± FOMOTEROL FUMARATE *continued*

INTRANASAL: Clear nasal passages and shake nasal spray well before each use. Onset of action for nasal symptoms of allergic rhinitis has been shown to occur within 11 hr after the first dose. Nasal burning and irritation, and epistaxis may occur. Nasal septal perforation, localized *Candida* infections, adrenal suppression (using higher than recommended dosages), and taste and smell disturbances have been reported. Monitor linear growth in children; especially with long-term use. A clinical trial in children 6—17 yr old was not able to demonstrate effectiveness for treating nasal polyps. A combination intranasal product of mometasone and olopatadine (Ryaltris) is available for seasonal allergic rhinitis and currently indicated for children ≥12 yr and adults.

ORAL INHALATION (all forms): Rinse mouth after each use. Fever, allergic rhinitis, URI, UTI, GI discomfort, and sore throat have been reported in children. Musculoskeletal pain, oral candidiasis, arthralgia, and fatigue may occur. May potentially worsen tuberculosis, fungal, bacterial, viral or parasitic infection, or ocular herpes simplex. **Do not use** Asmanex Twisthaler if allergic to milk proteins. The Twisthaler dosage form requires a minimum 30—60 L/min inspiratory flow rate to ensure proper dose delivery. Breastfeeding information is currently unknown, but most experts consider use of inhaled corticosteroids acceptable.

MOMETASONE + FOMOTEROL (Dulera): Common side effects include nasopharyngitis, sinusitis, and headache. Angioedema, anaphylaxis, and arrhythmias have been reported. See Formoterol for additional remarks.

TOPICAL USE: HPA axis suppression and skin atrophy have been reported with cream and ointment use in infants 6—23 mo. **Avoid** application/contact to face, eyes, underarms, groin, and mucous membranes. Occlusive dressings and use in diaper dermatitis are not recommended.

MONTELUKAST
Singulair and generics
Antiasthmatic, antiallergy, leukotriene receptor antagonist

B   1   No   Yes   No

Chewable tabs: 4, 5 mg; contain phenylalanine
Tabs: 10 mg
Oral granules: 4 mg per packet (30s)

Asthma and allergic rhinitis:
  Child:
    6—5 yr: 4 mg (oral granules or chewable tablet) PO QHS; minimum age for use in asthma (per product label) is 12 mo
    6—14 yr: 5 mg (chewable tablet) PO QHS
  Adolescent ≥15 yr and adult: 10 mg PO QHS
Prevention of exercise-induced bronchospasm (administer dose at least 2 hr prior to exercise; additional doses should not be administered within 24 hr):
  Child (6—14 yr): 5 mg (chewable tablet) PO
  ≥15 yr and adult: 10 mg PO

Chewable tablet dosage form is **contraindicated** in phenylketonuric patients. Side effects include: headache, abdominal pain, dyspepsia, fatigue, dizziness, cough, and elevated liver enzymes. Diarrhea, enuresis, epistaxis, pulmonary eosinophilia, thrombocytopenia, hypersensitivity reactions (including Stevens-Johnson and TEN), pharyngitis, nausea, otitis, sinusitis, and viral infections have been reported in children. Neuropsychiatric events, including aggression, anxiety, dream abnormalities, obsessive-compulsive symptoms, hallucinations, depression, suicidal behavior, and insomnia, have been reported.

MONTELUKAST *continued*

Drug is a substrate for CYP 450 3A4 and 2C9. Phenobarbital and rifampin may induce hepatic metabolism to increase the clearance of montelukast.

Doses may be administered with or without food.

MORPHINE SULFATE
Duramorph, MS Contin, Avinza, Kadian, and many generics
Narcotic, analgesic

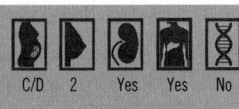

C/D   2   Yes   Yes   No

Oral solution: 10 mg/5 mL, 20 mg/5 mL
Concentrated oral solution: 100 mg/5 mL
Tabs: 15, 30 mg
Extended release tabs:
   MS Contin and generics: 15, 30, 60, 100, 200 mg
Extended release caps:
   Kadian: 10, 20, 30, 40, 50, 60, 80, 100, 200 mg
   Generics: 10, 20, 30, 45, 50, 60, 75, 80, 90, 100, 120 mg
Combination immediate release and extended release caps:
   Avinza (10% of dose as immediate release): 30, 60, 90, 120 mg
Rectal suppository: 5, 10, 20, 30 mg (12s)
Injection: 0.5, 1, 2, 4, 5, 8, 10, 15, 25, 50 mg/mL

Titrate to effect.
Neonate:
   Analgesia/tetralogy (cyanotic) spells: 0.05—0.1 mg/kg/dose IM, slow IV, SC Q4 hr
   Opiate withdrawal: 0.04—0.2 mg/kg/dose PO Q3—4 hr PRN
Infant 1—6 mo:
   Analgesia:
      PO: 0.08—0.1 mg/kg/dose Q3—4 hr PRN
      IV: 0.025—0.03 mg/kg/dose Q2—4 hr PRN
Infant >6 mo and child:
   Analgesia:
      PO: 0.2—0.5 mg/kg/dose (**initial max. dose:** 15—20 mg/dose) Q4—6 hr PRN (immediate release) or 0.3—0.6 mg/kg/dose Q12 hr PRN (controlled release)
      IM/IV/SC: 0.1—0.2 mg/kg/dose Q2—4 hr PRN; **max. initial dose:** infant: 2 mg/dose, 1—6 yr: 4 mg/dose, 7—12 yr: 8 mg/dose, and adolescent: 10 mg/dose
Adult (analgesia):
   PO: 10—30 mg Q4 hr PRN (immediate release) or 15—30 mg Q8—12 hr PRN (controlled release; see specific dosage form product information for additional instructions)
   IM/IV/SC: 2—15 mg/dose Q2—6 hr PRN
Continuous IV infusion and SC infusion: Dosing ranges, titrate to effect.
   Neonate (IV route only): 0.01—0.02 mg/kg/hr
   Infant and child:
      Postoperative pain: 0.01—0.04 mg/kg/hr
      Sickle cell and cancer: 0.04—0.07 mg/kg/hr
   Adult: 0.8—10 mg/hr

Continued

MORPHINE SULFATE *continued*

To prepare infusion for neonates, infants, and children, use the following formula:

$$50 \times \frac{\text{Desired dose (mg/kg/hr)}}{\text{Desired infusion rate (mL/hr)}} \times \text{Wt(kg)} = \frac{\text{mg morphine}}{\text{50 mL fluid}}$$

Dependence, CNS and respiratory depression, nausea, vomiting, urinary retention, constipation, hypotension, bradycardia, increased ICP, miosis, biliary spasm, and allergy may occur.
Be aware of concomitant medications with similar side effect profiles. **Naloxone may be used to reverse effects, especially respiratory depression.** Causes histamine release, resulting in itching and possible bronchospasm. Low-dose naloxone infusion may be used for itching. Inflammatory masses (e.g., granulomas) have been reported with continuous infusions via indwelling intrathecal catheters.

Dosage reduction may be necessary with liver cirrhosis. See Chapter 6 for equianalgesic dosing. Pregnancy category changes to "D" if used for prolonged periods or in higher doses at term. Rectal dosing is same as oral dosing but is not recommended due to poor absorption. Controlled/sustained release oral tablets must be administered whole. Controlled release oral capsules may be opened and the entire contents sprinkled on applesauce immediately prior to ingestion. **Be aware** of the various oral solution concentrations; the concentrated oral solution (100 mg/5 mL) has been associated with accidental overdoses. **Adjust dose in renal failure (see Chapter 31).**

The FDA has assigned a REMS for Opioid Analgesia; see www.fda.gov/OpioidAnalgesicREMSPCG. The REMS strongly encourages the provider to (1) complete a REMS-compliant education program; (2) counsel patients/caregivers on prescription safe use, risks, storage, and disposal; (3) emphasize the importance of reading the Medication Guide provided by pharmacists at all times; and (4) consider other methods for improving patient, household, and community safety.

MUPIROCIN
Centany, Centany AT, and generics; previously
available as Bactroban
Topical antibiotic

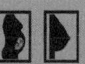

B   2   No   No   No

Ointment (Centany, Centany AT, and generics): 2% (15, 22, 30 g); contains propylene glycol
Cream (Generics): 2% (15, 30 g); may contain benzyl alcohol

Topical (see remarks):
  ≥3 mo–adult: Apply small amount TID to affected area × 5–10 days. Topical ointment may be used in infants ≥2 mo for impetigo.
Intranasal for elimination of nasal colonization of *Staphylococcus aureus*, including MRSA (in the absence of the nasal ointment dosage form, use ointment dosage form):
  Infant and child: Apply small amount intranasally to both nostrils BID × 5–10 days.
  Child ≥12 yr and adult: Apply approximately 500 mg intranasally to both nostrils using a cotton swab BID × 5–10 days.

Avoid contact with the eyes. Topical cream is not intended for use in lesions >10 cm in length or 100 cm² in surface area. **Do not use** topical ointment preparation on open wounds because of concerns about systemic absorption of polyethylene glycol. May cause minor local irritation and dry skin. Intranasal route may cause nasal stinging, taste disorder, headache, rhinitis, and pharyngitis. Severe allergic reactions (e.g., anaphylaxis, urticaria, angioedema, and rash) have been reported.

If clinical response is not apparent in 3–5 days with topical use, reevaluate infection.

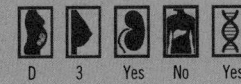

MYCOPHENOLATE
Mycophenolate mofetil: CellCept and generics
Mycophenolic acid: Myfortic and generics
Immunosuppressant agent

D　3　Yes　No　Yes

Mycophenolate mofetil (CellCept and generics):
　Caps: 250 mg
　Tabs: 500 mg
　Oral suspension: 200 mg/mL (160 mL); contains phenylalanine (0.56 mg/mL) and methylparabens
　Injection: 500 mg; may contain polysorbate 80
Mycophenolic acid:
　Delayed release tabs (Myfortic and generics): 180, 360 mg

Infant ≥3 mo, child, and adolescent (see remarks):
　Heart and liver transplant (mycophenolate mofetil):
　　Suspension: Start with 600 mg/m^2/dose PO BID, if tolerated, may increase to 900 mg/m^2/dose BID.
　　　Max. dose: 3000 mg/24 hr
　　Tabs or caps:
　　　BSA 1.25–<1.5 m^2: Start with 750 mg PO BID; if tolerated, may increase dose with BID dosage
　　　　interval up to a **maximum** of 3000 mg/24 hr.
　　　BSA ≥1.5 m^2: Start with 1000 mg PO BID; if tolerated, may increase dose with BID dosage interval
　　　　up to a **maximum** of 3000 mg/24 hr.
　Renal transplant:
　　Caps, tabs, or suspension (mycophenolate mofetil): 600 mg/m^2/dose PO/IV BID up to a **max. dose**
　　　of 2000 mg/24 hr; alternatively, patients with BSAs ≥1.25 m^2 may be dosed as follows:
　　　1.25–1.5 m^2: 750 mg PO BID
　　　>1.5 m^2: 1000 mg PO BID
　　Delayed release tabs (Myfortic; ≥5 yr): 400 mg/m^2/dose PO BID; **max. dose:** 720 mg BID; this
　　　dosage form not recommended in patients with BSAs <1.19 m^2. Alternatively, patients with BSAs
　　　≥1.19 m^2 may be dosed as follows:
　　　1.19–1.58 m^2: 540 mg PO BID
　　　>1.58 m^2: 720 mg PO BID
　Nephrotic syndrome:
　　Frequently relapsing: 12.5–18 mg/kg/dose or 600 mg/m^2/dose PO BID up to a **max. dose** of 2000
　　　mg/24 hr for 1–2 yr and taper prednisone regimen
　　Steroid dependent: 12–18 mg/kg/dose or 600 mg/m^2/dose PO BID up to a **max. dose** of 2000 mg/
　　　24 hr for at least 12 mo
Adult (in combination with corticosteroids and cyclosporine; check specific transplantation
**　protocol for specific dosage):**
　IV: 1000–3000 mg/24 hr ÷ BID
　Oral:
　　Caps, tabs, or suspension: 500–1500 mg PO BID
　　Delayed release tabs (Myfortic): 360–1080 mg PO BID

Check specific transplantation protocol for specific dosage. Mycophenolate mofetil is a
prodrug for mycophenolic acid. Owing to differences in absorption, the delayed release
tablets should **not** be interchanged with other oral dosage forms on an equivalent milligram-to-
milligram basis. Increases risk of first trimester pregnancy loss and increased risk of congenital
malformations (especially external ear and facial abnormalities including cleft lip and palate, and
anomalies of the distal limbs, heart, and esophagus).

Continued

MYCOPHENOLATE *continued*

Common side effects may include headache, hypertension, diarrhea, vomiting, bone marrow suppression, anemia, fever, opportunistic infections, and sepsis. May cause drowsiness and increase the risk for bacterial, fungal, protozoal, and viral infections, and lymphomas or other malignancies. GI bleeds and increased risk for rejection in heart transplant patients switched from calcineurin inhibitors (e.g., cyclosporine and tacrolimus) and CellCept to sirolimus and CellCept have been reported. Cases of progressive multifocal leukoencephalopathy (PML), pure red cell aplasia (PRCA), posttransplant lymphoproliferative disorder (PTLD), acute inflammatory syndrome, and hypogammaglobulinemia have also been reported. The type and frequency of adverse reactions in pediatric heart or kidney transplant patients have been reported to be similar to those observed in pediatric renal transplant patients and in adults.

Use of mycophenolic acid (Myfortic) should be **avoided** in patients with hypoxanthine-guanine phosphoribosyltransferase (HGPRT) deficiency (e.g., Lesch-Nyhan and Kelley-Seegmiller syndrome) because it may exacerbate disease symptoms characterized by increased uric acid, leading to acute arthritis, tophi, nephrolithiasis/urolithiasis, and renal failure.

Use with caution in patients with active GI disease or renal impairment (GFR <25 mL/min/1.73 m^2) outside of the immediate posttransplant period. In adults with renal impairment, **avoid** doses >2 g/24 hr and observe carefully. Dose should be interrupted or reduced in the presence of neutropenia (ANC <1.3 × 10^3/microliter). No dose adjustment is needed for patients experiencing delayed graft function postoperatively.

Drug interactions: (1) Displacement of phenytoin or theophylline from protein-binding sites will decrease total serum levels and increase free serum levels of these drugs. Salicylates displace mycophenolate to increase free levels of mycophenolate. (2) Competition for renal tubular secretion results in increased serum levels of acyclovir, ganciclovir, probenecid, and mycophenolate (when any of these are used together). (3) **Avoid** live and live attenuated vaccines (including influenza); decreases vaccine effectiveness. (4) Proton pump inhibitors, antacids, cholestyramine, cyclosporine, and telmisartan may reduce mycophenolate levels.

Administer oral doses on an empty stomach. Infuse intravenous doses over 2 hr. Oral suspension may be administered via NG tube with a minimum size of 8 Fr.

N

NAFCILLIN
Generics; previously available as Nallpen
Antibiotic, penicillin (penicillinase resistant)

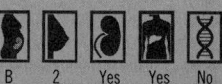

B 2 Yes Yes No

Injection: 1, 2, 10 g; contains 2.9 mEq Na/g drug
Injection, premixed in iso-osmotic dextrose: 1 g in 50 mL, 2 g in 100 mL

Neonate (IM/IV):
  <1 kg:
    ≤14 days old: 50 mg/kg/24 hr ÷ Q12 hr
    15—28 days old: 75 mg/kg/24 hr ÷ Q8 hr
  1—2 kg:
    ≤7 days old: 50 mg/kg/24 hr ÷ Q12 hr
    8—28 days old: 75 mg/kg/24 hr ÷ Q8 hr
  >2 kg:
    ≤7 days old: 75 mg/kg/24 hr ÷ Q8 hr
    8—28 days old: 100 mg/kg/24 hr ÷ Q6 hr

NAFCILLIN *continued*

Meningitis: Use twice the above mg/kg/24 hr dose with the same dosage interval.
Infant and child (IM/IV):
Mild to moderate infections: 100—150 mg/kg/24 hr ÷ Q6 hr
Severe infections: 150—200 mg/kg/24 hr ÷ Q4—6 hr; give 200 mg/kg/24 hr ÷ Q4—6 hr for
staphylococcal endocarditis or meningitis
Max. dose: 12 g/24 hr
Adult:
IV: 1000—2000 mg Q4—6 hr
IM: 500—1000 mg Q4—6 hr
Max. dose: 12 g/24 hr

Allergic cross-sensitivity with penicillin. Solutions containing dextrose may be **contraindicated**
in patients with known allergy to corn or corn products. High incidence of phlebitis with IV
dosing. May cause rash, bone marrow suppression, and false-positive urinary and serum proteins.
Hypokalemia has been reported. Acute interstitial nephritis is rare.
Cerebrospinal fluid (CSF) penetration is poor unless meninges are inflamed. **Use with caution** in
patients with combined renal and hepatic impairment (reduce dose by 33%—50%). Nafcillin may
increase elimination of cyclosporine and warfarin.

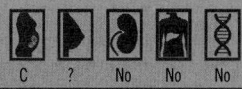

NALOXONE
Narcan, Kloxxado, Zimhi, and generics
Narcotic antagonist

C ? No No No

Injection: 0.4 mg/mL (1, 10 mL); some preparations may contain parabens
Injection, in prefilled syringe:
Generic: 2 mg/2 mL (2 mL)
Zimhi: 5 mg/0.5 mL (0.5 mL)
Injection in single-dose Carpuject: 0.4 mg/mL (1 mL)
Auto-injector: 10 mg/0.4 mL single-dose prefilled auto-injector (box of 10)
Nasal liquid:
Narcan and generics: 4 mg/0.1 mL (1 or 2 each); may contain benzalkonium chloride and EDTA
Kloxxado: 8 mg/0.1 mL (2 each); contains 20% alcohol, EDTA, and propylene glycol

Opiate intoxication (full reversal, IM/IV/IO/SC, use 2—10 times IV dose for ETT route;
see remarks):

Neonate, infant, child ≤20 kg or ≤5 yr (IV/IO route is preferred for faster onset of action):
0.1 mg/kg/dose. May repeat PRN Q2—3 min
Child >20 kg or >5 yr (IV/IO route preferred): 2 mg/dose. May repeat PRN Q2—3 min.
Zimhi (≥12 yr): 5 mg/dose × 1 IM/SC into the anterolateral aspect of the thigh, through clothing if
necessary. May repeat PRN Q2—3 min
Continuous infusion (child and adult): 0.005 mg/kg loading dose followed by infusion of 0.0025 mg/
kg/hr has been recommended. A range of 0.0025—0.16 mg/kg/hr has been reported. Taper gradually
to avoid relapse.
Adult: 0.4—2 mg/dose. May repeat PRN Q2—3 min. Use 0.1 to 0.2 mg increments in opiate-dependent
patients.
Zimhi: 5 mg/dose × 1 IM/SC into the anterolateral aspect of the thigh, through clothing if
necessary. May repeat PRN Q2—3 min
Auto-injector product (10 mg/0.4 mL) for suspected high-potency opiate intoxication:
Child ≥12 yr and adult: Administer one dose (10 mg) into the anterolateral aspect of the thigh,
through clothing if necessary, by pressing the device firmly until you hear a click and hiss sound and

Continued

NALOXONE *continued*

then hold in place for 5 seconds. If the patient symptoms relapse after the first dose, additional
doses may be necessary.

Intranasal route for opiate intoxication (full reversal):

All ages: 4 or 8 mg of nasal liquid dosage form into one nostril Q2–3 min PRN in alternating nostrils.

Opioid-dependent patient at risk for opioid withdrawal: Use lower 2 mg of nasal liquid dosage
form into one nostril Q2–3 min PRN in alternating nostrils. Alternatively, the 2 mg/2 mL
intravenous (IV) syringe dosage form with nasal adapter may be used by administering 1 mg (1
mL) per nostril.

Opiate-induced pruritus (limited data): 0.25–2 mCg/kg/hr IV; a dose-finding study in 59 children
suggests a minimal dose of 1 mCg/kg/hr when used as prophylactic therapy. Doses ≥3 mCg/kg/hr
increase the risk for reduced pain control.

Short duration of action may necessitate multiple doses. For severe intoxication, doses of
0.2 mg/kg may be required. If no response is achieved after a cumulative dose of 10 mg,
reevaluate diagnosis. **In the nonarrest situation, use the lowest dose effective (may start at 0.001
mg/kg/dose). See Chapter 6 for additional information.**

Will produce narcotic withdrawal syndrome in patients with chronic dependence. Use with **caution** in
patients with chronic cardiac disease. Abrupt reversal of narcotic depression may result in nausea,
vomiting, diaphoresis, tachycardia, hypertension, and tremulousness. Aggressive behavior has been
reported in abrupt reversal of an opioid overdose. False-positive test for urine opiates screen may
occur.

IV administration is preferred for faster onset of action. Onset of action may be delayed with other
routes of administration; the intranasal route is slightly delayed compared to IM or or IV routes.

NAPROXEN/NAPROXEN SODIUM
Naprosyn, EC-Naprosyn, Anaprox DS, Naprelan,
Aleve [OTC], and many others, including
generics
Nonsteroidal antiinflammatory agent

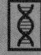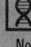

C/X   3   Yes   Yes   No

Naproxen:

Tabs: 250, 375, 500 mg

Delayed release tabs:

EC-Naprosyn: 375, 500 mg

Anaprox DS: 550 mg

Oral suspension (Naprosyn and generics): 125 mg/5 mL; contains 0.34 mEq Na/1 mL and parabens

Naproxen sodium:

Tabs:

Aleve and generics (OTC): 220 mg (200 mg base); contains 0.87 mEq Na

Generics: 275 mg (250 mg base), 550 mg (500 mg base); contains 1 mEq, 2 mEq Na, respectively

Controlled release tabs:

Naprelan and generics: 412.5 mg (375 mg base), 550 mg (500 mg base), 825 mg (750 mg base)

Anaprox DS: 550 mg (500 mg base)

All doses based on naproxen base.

Child >2 yr:

Analgesia: 5–10 mg/kg/dose Q12 hr PO

JRA: 10–20 mg/kg/24 hr ÷ Q12 hr PO

Usual max. dose: 1000 mg/24 hr

NAPROXEN/NAPROXEN SODIUM *continued*

Adolescent and adult:
  Analgesia:
    Over-the-counter dosage forms: 200 mg Q8—12 hr PRN PO (400 mg initial dose may be needed).
      Max. dose: 600 mg/24 hr
    Prescription-strength dosage forms: 250 mg Q8—12 hr PRN (500 mg initial dose may be needed)
    or 500 mg Q12 hr PRN PO. **Max. dose:** 1250 mg/24 hr for first day, then 1000 mg/24 hr
  Rheumatoid arthritis, ankylosing spondylitis:
    Immediate release forms: 250—500 mg BID PO
    Delayed release tabs:
      EC-Naprosyn: 375—500 mg BID PO
      Anaprox DS: 275—550 mg BID PO
    Controlled release tabs (Naprelan): 750—1000 mg once daily PO. For patients converting from
    immediate and delayed release forms, calculate daily dose and administer Naprelan as a single
    daily dose.
    Max. dose (all dosage forms): 1000—1500 mg/24 hr
  Dysmenorrhea:
    500 mg × 1, then 250 mg Q6—8 hr PRN PO or 500 mg Q12 hr PRN PO; **max. dose:** 1250 mg/24 hr
    for first day, then 1000 mg/24 hr

Contraindicated in treating perioperative pain for coronary artery bypass graft surgery. May
cause GI bleeding, thrombocytopenia, heartburn, headache, drowsiness, vertigo, and tinnitus.
Use with caution in patients with GI disease, cardiac disease (risk for thrombotic events,
myocardial infarction [MI], stroke), or renal or hepatic impairment, and those receiving
anticoagulants. drug reaction with eosinophilia and systemic symptoms (DRESS) has been reported.
False-positive test for urine cannabinoid screen may occur.
Use is **NOT** recommended for moderate/severe renal impairment (CrCl <30 mL/min). See Ibuprofen for
other side effects.
Pregnancy category is "C" for prior to 30 weeks' gestation and "X" for 30 wk and greater. **Avoid use** at
>30 weeks' gestation due to increased risk for premature closure of the fetal ductus arteriosus.
Limit dose and duration of use at 20—30 weeks' gestation for concerns of fetal renal dysfunction
and oligohydramnios.
Administer doses with food or milk to reduce GI discomfort.

NEO-POLYMYCIN OPHTHALMIC OINTMENT

See Neomycin/polymyxin B Ophthalmic Products.

NEOSPORIN OPHTHALMIC SOLUTION

See Neomycin/polymyxin B Ophthalmic Products.

NEO-POLYCIN HC

See Neomycin/polymyxin B Ophthalmic Products.

NEOMYCIN SULFATE
Generics
Antibiotic, aminoglycoside; ammonium detoxicant

    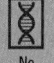

D   2   Yes   No   No

Continued

NEOMYCIN SULFATE *continued*

Tabs: 500 mg
Oral solution: 25 mg/mL ; contains parabens
125 mg neomycin sulfate is equivalent to 87.5 mg neomycin base.

Enteric bacterial eradication (limited data):
    Preterm (>1.2 kg) and newborn: 50—100 mg/kg/24 hr ÷ Q6 hr PO for up to 2 wk
Hepatic encephalopathy (limited data):
    Infant and child: 50—100 mg/kg/24 hr ÷ Q6—8 hr PO × 5—6 days. **Max. dose:** 12 g/24 hr
    Adult: 4—12 g/24 hr ÷ Q4—6 hr PO × 5—6 days
Bowel prep (in combination with erythromycin base; many other regimens exist):
    Child: 90 mg/kg/24 hr PO ÷ Q4 hr × 2—3 days
    Adult: 1 g Q1 hr PO × 4 doses, then 1 g Q4 hr PO × 5 doses

---

Contraindicated in ulcerative bowel disease, intestinal obstruction, or aminoglycoside hypersensitivity. Monitor for nephrotoxicity and ototoxicity. Oral absorption is limited, but levels may accumulate. Consider dosage reduction in the presence of renal failure. May cause itching, redness, edema, colitis, candidiasis, or poor wound healing if applied topically. Prevalence of neomycin hypersensitivity has increased. May decrease absorption of penicillin V, vitamin B_{12}, digoxin, and methotrexate. May potentiate oral anticoagulants and the adverse effects of other neurotoxic, ototoxic, or nephrotoxic drugs.

NEOMYCIN/POLYMYXIN B OPHTHALMIC PRODUCTS
Neomycin/Polymyxin B + Bacitracin:
Neo-Polycin and generics
Neomycin/Polymyxin B + Dexamethasone:
Maxitrol
Neomycin/Polymyxin B + Gramicidin:
Generics
Neomycin/Polymyxin B + Hydrocortisone:
Generics
**Neomycin/Polymyxin B + Bacitracin +
Hydrocortisone:**
Neo-Polycin HC and generics
Ophthalmic antibiotic ± corticosteroid

   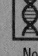 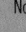 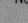

C   2   No   No   No

Neomycin/Polymyxin B + Bacitracin:
    Ophthalmic ointment (Neo-Polycin Ophthalmic Ointment and generics): 3.5 g neomycin, 10,000 U polymyxin B, and 400 U bacitracin per g ointment (3.5 g)
Neomycin/Polymyxin B + Dexamethasone:
    Ophthalmic ointment (Maxitrol): 3.5 mg neomycin, 10,000 U polymyxin B, and 1 mg dexamethasone per 1 g (3.5 g)
    Ophthalmic suspension (Maxitrol): 3.5 mg neomycin, 10,000 U polymyxin B, and 1 mg dexamethasone per 1 mL (5 mL); contains benzalkonium chloride
Neomycin/Polymyxin B + Gramicidin:
    Ophthalmic solution: 1.75 neomycin, 10,000 U polymyxin B, and 0.025 mg gramicidin per 1 mL (10 mL); contains propylene glycol, alcohol, and thimerosal
Neomycin/Polymyxin B + Hydrocortisone:
    Ophthalmic suspension: 3.5 mg neomycin, 10,000 U polymyxin B, and 10 mg hydrocortisone per 1 mL (7.5 mL)

NEOMYCIN/POLYMYXIN B OPHTHALMIC PRODUCTS *continued*

Neomycin/Polymyxin B + Bacitracin + Hydrocortisone:
  Ophthalmic ointment (Neo-Polycin HC and generics): 3.5 mg neomycin, 10,000 U polymyxin B, 400 U bacitracin, and 10 mg hydrocortisone per 1 g (3.5 g)

Neomycin/Polymyxin B + Bacitracin (Neo-Polycin and generics):
  Child and adult: Apply 0.5-inch ribbon to affected eye(s) Q3—4 hr for acute infections or BID—TID for mild/moderate infections × 7—10 days.

Neomycin/Polymyxin B + Dexamethasone (Maxitrol):
  Child (≥2 yr)—adult:
   Ophthalmic suspension: Instill 1—2 drops into the conjunctival sac of the affected eye(s) 4—6 times per day for mild/moderate infections. For severe infections, administer Q1 hr and taper to discontinuation as inflammation subsides. No more than 20 mL should be prescribed initially.
   Ophthalmic ointment: Apply ~0.5-inch ribbon into the conjunctival sac of the affected eye(s) TID—QID. Reevaluate diagnosis if signs and symptoms do not improve in 48 hr. Do not dispense >8 g.

Neomycin/Polymyxin B + Gramicidin:
  Child and adult: Instill 1—2 drops to affected eye(s) Q4 hr or 2 drops every hour for severe infections × 7—10 days.

Neomycin/Polymyxin B + Hydrocortisone:
  Child and adult: Instill 1—2 drops to affected eye(s) Q3—4 hr. More frequent dosing has been used for severe infection in adults.

Neomycin/Polymyxin B + Bacitracin + Hydrocortisone (Neo-Polycin HC and generics):
  Child and adult (limited data): Apply ointment sparingly to inside of lower lid of affected eye(s) Q3—4 hr. Reevaluate diagnosis if signs and symptoms do not improve in 48 hr. Monitor intraocular pressure if use is equal to or greater than 10 days.

Contraindicated if patient is hypersensitive to specific medications (e.g., neomycin, polymyxin B, gramicidin, bacitracin, or hydrocortisone) of respective product. **Use with caution** in glaucoma. Blurred vision, burning, and stinging may occur. Increased intraocular pressure and mycosis may occur with prolonged use. **Avoid** prolonged use with products containing corticosteroids.
Ophthalmic solution/suspension: Shake well before use and **avoid** contamination of tip of eye dropper. Apply finger pressure to lacrimal sac during and 1—2 min after dose application.
Ophthalmic ointment: Do not touch tube tip to eyelids or other surfaces to prevent contamination.

NEOMYCIN/POLYMYXIN B/BACITRACIN
Neosporin Original, Triple Antibiotic, and various
generics
Topical antibiotic

   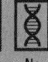
C   ?   No   No   No

Ointment, topical (OTC): 3.5 mg neomycin sulfate, 400 U bacitracin, 5000 U polymyxin B/g (1, 15, 30, 454 g)
For ophthalmic products, see Neomycin/Polymyxin B Ophthalmic Products.

Child and adult: Apply to minor wounds and burns once daily—TID.

Do not use for extended periods. May cause superinfection, delayed healing. See Neomycin for additional remarks. Prevalence of neomycin hypersensitivity has increased.

NEOSTIGMINE
Bloxiverz and generics
Anticholinesterase (cholinergic) agent

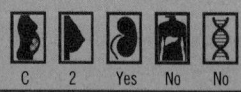

| C | 2 | Yes | No | No |

Injection (Bloxiverz and generics): 0.5, 1 mg/mL (10 mL) (as methylsulfate); contains phenol
Prefilled syringe injection: 1 mg/mL (3 mL); may contain phenol

Myasthenia gravis diagnosis: Use with atropine (see remarks).
  Child: 0.025–0.04 mg/kg IM × 1
  Adult: 1.5 mg IM × 1
Treatment:
  Child: 0.01–0.04 mg/kg/dose IM/IV/SC Q2–4 hr PRN
  Adult: 0.5–2.5 mg/dose IM/IV/SC Q1–3 hr PRN up to **max. dose** of 10 mg/24 hr
Reversal of nondepolarizing neuromuscular blocking agents: Administer with atropine or
  glycopyrrolate.
  All ages: 0.03–0.07 mg/kg/dose IV; **max. dose:** 5 mg/dose

Contraindicated in GI and urinary obstruction. **Caution** in patients with asthma. May cause
  cholinergic crisis, bronchospasm, salivation, nausea, vomiting, diarrhea, miosis, diaphoresis,
  lacrimation, bradycardia, hypotension, fatigue, confusion, respiratory depression, and seizures.
  Titrate for each patient, but **avoid** excessive cholinergic effects.
For reversal of neuromuscular blockade, infants and small children may be at greater risk of complications
  from incomplete reversal of neuromuscular blockade due to decreased respiratory reserve.
For diagnosis of myasthenia gravis (MG), administer atropine 0.011 mg/kg/dose IV immediately before
  or IM (0.011 mg/kg/dose) 30 min before neostigmine. For treatment of MG, patients may need higher
  doses of neostigmine at times of greatest fatigue.
Antidote: Atropine 0.01–0.04 mg/kg/dose. Atropine and epinephrine should be available in the event
  of a hypersensitivity reaction.
Adjust dose in renal failure (see Chapter 31).

NEVIRAPINE
Generics; previously available as Viramune,
Viramune XR; NVP
*Antiviral, nonnucleoside reverse transcriptase
inhibitor*

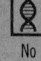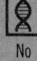

| B | 2 | Yes | Yes | No |

Tabs: 200 mg
Extended release tabs: 100, 400 mg
Oral suspension: 10 mg/mL (240 mL); contains parabens, propylene glycol, and polysorbate 80

HIV treatment: See https://clinicalinfo.hiv.gov/en/guidelines
**Prevention of HIV vertical transmission during high-risk situations (mothers who received
  no antepartum antiretroviral therapy, mothers who received only intrapartum antiretroviral
  therapy, mothers who receive antepartum antiretroviral therapy but with suboptimal viral
  suppression [>50 copies/mL] within 4 weeks prior to delivery, or mothers with acute or primary
  HIV infection during pregnancy or breastfeeding [immediately discontinue breastfeeding]); see
  Chapter 17 for additional information:**
  Newborn: Use in combination with zidovudine within 6-12 hr after birth (discontinue this regimen
    and convert to presumptive treatment regimen if HIV diagnosis is obtained): 3 doses (based on
    birth weight) in the first week of life; dose 1: within 48 hr of birth; dose 2: 48 hr after dose 1; dose 3:
    96 hr after dose 2

NEVIRAPINE *continued*

     Birth weight 1.5—2 kg: 8 mg/dose PO
     Birth weight >2 kg: 12 mg/dose PO

HIV vertical transmission and presumptive treatment during high-risk situations (see above). Use in combination with zidovudine and lamivudine initiated within 6-12 hr after birth; transition to a treatment regimen if positive HIV diagnosis is confirmed and discontinue use after a negative diagnosis (see Chapter 17 for additional information):

     ≥32—<34 weeks' gestation at birth (dosage based on pharmacokinetic modeling and simulation and has not been evaluated in clinical trials):

          Birth to 2 wk old: 2 mg/kg/dose PO BID; first dose within 6—12 hr after delivery
          2—4 wk old: 4 mg/kg/dose PO BID
          4—6 wk old: 6 mg/kg/dose PO BID
          >6 wk old (use this higher dose only if infant has a confirmed HIV diagnosis): 200 mg/m^2/dose PO BID

     ≥34—<37 weeks' gestation at birth (dosage based on pharmacokinetic and safety data):

          Birth to 1 week old: 4 mg/kg/dose PO BID; first dose within 6—12 hr after delivery
          1—4 weeks old: 6 mg/kg/dose PO BID
          >4 weeks old (use this higher dose only if infant has a confirmed HIV diagnosis): 200 mg/m^2/dose PO BID

     ≥37 weeks' gestation at birth (dosage based on pharmacokinetic and safety data):

          Birth to 4 wk old: 6 mg/kg/dose PO BID; first dose within 6—12 hr after delivery
          >4 wk old (use this higher dose only if infant has a confirmed HIV diagnosis): 200 mg/m^2/dose PO BID

See https://clinicalinfo.hiv.gov/en/guidelines for additional remarks.

Use with caution in patients with hepatic or renal dysfunction. **Contraindicated** in moderate/severe hepatic impairment (Child-Pugh Class B or C) and postexposure (occupational or nonoccupational) prophylactic regimens. Most frequent side effects with continuous therapy include skin rash (may be life threatening, including Stevens-Johnson syndrome and DRESS; permanently discontinue and never restart), fever, abnormal liver function tests, headache, and nausea.

Discontinue therapy if any of the following occurs: severe rash; rash with fever, blistering, oral lesions, conjunctivitis, or muscle aches. Permanently discontinue and do not restart therapy if symptomatic hepatitis, severe transaminase elevations, or hypersensitivity reactions occur.

Life-threatening hepatotoxicity has been reported primarily during the first 12 wk of continuous therapy. Patients with increased serum transaminase or a history of hepatitis B or C infection prior to nevirapine are at greater risk for hepatotoxicity. Women, including pregnant women, with CD$_4$ cell counts >250/mm^3 or men with CD$_4$ cell counts >400/mm^3 are at risk for hepatotoxicity. Monitor liver function tests (obtain transaminases immediately after development of hepatitis signs/symptoms, hypersensitivity reactions, or rash) and complete blood counts. Hypophosphatemia has been reported.

Nevirapine induces the CYP 450 3A4 drug metabolizing isoenzyme to cause an autoinduction of its own metabolism within the first 2—4 wk of therapy and has the potential to interact with many drugs. **Carefully review the patient's drug profile for other drug interactions each time nevirapine is initiated or when a new drug is added to a regimen containing nevirapine.**

Doses can be administered with food and concurrently with didanosine.

NIACIN/VITAMIN B$_3$
Niacor, Niaspan, Slo-Niacin, Nicotinic acid, Vitamin B$_3$, and many generics
Vitamin, water soluble

A/C   2   Yes   Yes   No

Continued

NIACIN/VITAMIN B₃ *continued*

Tabs:
    Generics (OTC): 50, 100, 250, 500 mg
    Niacor: 500 mg
Timed or extended release tabs:
    Generics: 250 (OTC), 500, 750, 1000 mg
    Slo-Niacin (OTC): 500, 750 mg
    Niaspan: 500, 750, 1000 mg; dosed QHS
Caps (OTC): 100, 500, 1000 mg
Timed or extended release caps (OTC): 250, 500 mg
Powder (OTC): 100, 500, 1000 g

US recommended dietary allowance (RDA): See Chapter 21.
Pellagra (PO): Usual treatment duration is 3—4 wk
    Child: 50—100 mg/dose TID
    Adult: 50—100 mg/dose TID—QID
    Max. dose: 500 mg/24 hr

Contraindicated in hepatic dysfunction, active peptic ulcer, and severe hypotension. **Use with caution** in unstable angina, acute MI (especially if patient is receiving vasoactive drugs), renal dysfunction, and in patients with history of jaundice, hepatobiliary disease, or peptic ulcer. Adverse reactions of flushing, pruritus, or GI distress may occur with oral administration. May cause hyperglycemia, hyperuricemia, blurred vision, abnormal liver function tests, dizziness, and headaches. Burning sensation of the skin, skin discoloration, acanthosis nigricans, hepatitis, and elevated creatine kinase have been reported. May cause false-positive urine catecholamines (fluorometric methods) and urine glucose (Benedict reagent).

Use with statins may increase the risk of myopathy/rhabdomyolysis. Bile acid sequestrants (e.g., cholestyramine) may bind to niacin and should be taken at least 4—6 hr before niacin administration.

Pregnancy category changes to "C" if used in doses above the RDA or for typical doses used for lipid disorders. Breastfeeding should be discontinued when used for the treatment of dyslipidemias for mothers as hepatotoxicity is a potential to the infant. **See Chapter 21 for multivitamin preparations.**

NICARDIPINE
Cardene IV and generics
Calcium channel blocker, antihypertensive

    C   1   Yes   Yes   No

Caps (immediate release): 20, 30 mg
Injection:
    Cardene IV: 0.1 mg/mL (200 mL; premixed in isotonic dextrose or saline), 0.2 mg/mL (200 mL; premixed in isotonic saline)
    Generic: 2.5 mg/mL (10 mL); may contain sorbitol or benzoic acid

Child (see remarks):
    Hypertension:
        Continuous IV infusion for severe hypertension: Start at 0.5—1 mCg/kg/min, dose may be increased as needed every 15—30 min up to a **max.** of 4—5 mCg/kg/min.

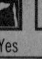 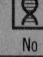

Adult (see remarks):
    Hypertension:
        Oral: 20 mg PO TID; dose may be increased after 3 days to 40 mg PO TID if needed

NICARDIPINE *continued*

Continuous IV infusion: Start at 5 mg/hr, increase dose as needed by 2.5 mg/hr Q5—15 min up to a **max. dose** of 15 mg/hr. Following attainment of desired BP, decrease infusion to 3 mg/hr and adjust rate as needed to maintain desired response.

Reported use in children has been limited to a small number of preterm infants, infants, and children.

Contraindicated in advanced aortic stenosis. **Avoid** systemic hypotension in patients following an acute cerebral infarct or hemorrhage. Use with **caution** in hepatic or renal dysfunction by carefully titrating dose. The drug undergoes significant first-pass metabolism through the liver and is excreted in the urine (60%). Use **caution** when converting to another dosage form; they are NOT equivalent on a milligram-per-milligram basis.

May cause headache, dizziness, asthenia, peripheral edema, and GI symptoms. Nicardipine is a substrate for CYP 450 3A and inhibitor of CYP 450 2 C9/19. Cimetidine increases the effects/toxicity of nicardipine. Nicardipine may increase effect/toxicity of cyclosporine and tacrolimus. **See Nifedipine for additional drug and food interactions.**

Onset of action for orally administered drug is 20 min with peak effects in 0.5 to 2 hr. Onset of action of intravenously administered drug is 1 min. Duration of action following a single IV or PO dose is 3 hr. To reduce the risk for venous thrombosis, phlebitis, and vascular impairment with IV administration, do not use small veins (e.g., dorsum of hand or wrist). **Avoid** intra-arterial administration or extravasation. For additional information, **see Chapter 4.**

NIFEDIPINE
Procardia XL and many generics; previously available as Procardia and Adalat CC
Calcium channel blocker, antihypertensive

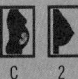   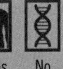

| C | 2 | No | Yes | No |

Caps: 10 mg (0.34 mL), 20 mg (0.45 mL)
Sustained release tabs: (Procardia XL, and generics): 30, 60, 90 mg
Oral suspension: 4 mg/mL

Child (see remarks for precautions):
   Chronic hypertension:
      Sustained release tabs: Start with 0.2—0.5 mg/kg/24 hr (initial **max. dose:** 30—60 mg/24 hr) ÷ Q12—24 hr. May increase to **max. dose:** 3 mg/kg/24 hr up to 120 mg/24 hr
Adult:
   Chronic hypertension or angina:
      Sustained release tabs: Start with 30 or 60 mg PO once daily. May increase to **max. dose** of 120 mg/24 hr. Dosing above 90 mg/24 hr for angina is limited and should be used with caution.

Use of immediate release dosage form in children is controversial and has been abandoned by many. **Use with caution** in children with acute CNS injury due to increased risk for stroke, seizure, hepatic impairment, and altered level of consciousness. To prevent rapid decrease in blood pressure in children, an initial dose of ≤0.25 mg/kg is recommended.

Use with caution in patients with congestive heart failure (CHF), aortic stenosis, GI obstruction/narrowing (bezoar formation), and cirrhosis (reduced drug clearance). May cause severe hypotension, peripheral edema, flushing, tachycardia, headaches, dizziness, nausea, palpitations, and syncope. Acute generalized exanthematous pustulosis has been reported.

Although overall use in adults has been abandoned, the immediate release dosage form is **contraindicated** in adults with severe obstructive coronary artery disease or recent MI and in hypertensive emergencies.

Continued

NIFEDIPINE *continued*

Nifedipine is a substrate for CYP 450 3A3/4, and 3A5-7. **Do not administer** with grapefruit juice; may increase bioavailability and effects. Itraconazole and ketoconazole may increase nifedipine levels and/or effects. CYP 3A inducers (e.g., rifampin, rifabutin, phenobarbital, phenytoin, carbamazepine) may reduce nifedipine's effects. Nifedipine may increase phenytoin, cyclosporine, and digoxin levels. For hypertensive emergencies, **see Chapter 4.**

For sublingual (SL) administration, capsule must be punctured and liquid expressed into the patient's mouth. A small amount is absorbed via the SL route. Most effects are due to swallowing and oral absorption. **Do not** crush or chew sustained release tablet dosage form.

NITROFURANTOIN
Macrodantin, Macrobid, and generics; previously
available as Furadantin
Antibiotic

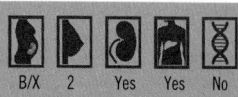

B/X   2   Yes   Yes   No

Caps (macrocrystals; Macrodantin and generics): 25, 50, 100 mg
Caps (dual release; Macrobid and generics): 100 mg (25 mg macrocrystal/75 mg monohydrate)
Oral suspension: 25 mg/5 mL (230 mL); may contain parabens, sorbitol, and saccharin

Child (>1 mo; oral suspension or macrocrystals):
  UTI treatment: 5–7 mg/kg/24 hr ÷ Q6 hr PO; **max. dose:** 400 mg/24 hr
  UTI prophylaxis: 1–2 mg/kg/dose QHS PO; **max. dose:** 100 mg/24 hr
≥12 yr and adult:
  UTI treatment:
    Macrocrystals: 50–100 mg/dose Q6 hr PO
    Dual release (Macrobid): 100 mg/dose Q12 hr PO
  UTI prophylaxis (macrocrystals): 50–100 mg/dose PO QHS

Contraindicated in severe renal disease, infants younger than 1 mo of age, glomerular filtration rate (GFR) below 60 mL/min (reduced drug distribution in the urine), active/previous cholestatic jaundice/hepatic dysfunction, and pregnant women at term. **Use with caution** in G6PD deficiency, anemia, lung disease, and peripheral neuropathy. May cause nausea, hypersensitivity reactions (including vasculitis), vomiting, cholestatic jaundice, headache, hepatotoxicity, polyneuropathy, and hemolytic anemia.

Anticholinergic drugs and high-dose probenecid may increase nitrofurantoin toxicity. Magnesium salts may decrease nitrofurantoin absorption. Causes false-positive urine glucose with Clinitest. Administer doses with food or milk.

Pregnancy category changes to "X" at term (38–42 weeks' gestation). Breastfeeding in mothers receiving nitrofurantoin is not recommended for infants younger than 1 mo and those with G6PD deficiency; use in infants 1 mo and without G6PD deficiency is compatible.

NITROGLYCERIN
Nitro-Bid, Nitrostat, Nitro-Time, Nitro-Dur,
Nitrolingual, Nitromist, Rectiv, and generics
Vasodilator, antihypertensive

C   ?   Yes   Yes   No

Injection: 5 mg/mL (10 mL); contains alcohol or propylene glycol
Prediluted injection in D₅W: 100 mCg/mL (250 mL), 200 mCg/mL (250 mL), 400 mCg/mL (250 mL); contains alcohol and propylene glycol
Sublingual tabs (Nitrostat and generics): 0.3, 0.4, 0.6 mg

NITROGLYCERIN *continued*

Sustained release caps (Nitro-Time): 2.5, 6.5, 9 mg
Ointment, topical (Nitro-Bid): 2% (1, 30, 60 g)
Ointment, rectal (Rectiv): 0.4% (30 g); contains propylene glycol
Patch (Nitro-Dur and generics): 2.5 mg/24 hr (0.1 mg/hr), 5 mg/24 hr (0.2 mg/hr), 7.5 mg/24 hr (0.3 mg/hr), 10 mg/24 hr (0.4 mg/hr), 15 mg/24 hr (0.6 mg/hr), 20 mg/24 hr (0.8 mg/hr) (30s, 100s)
Spray, translingual (Nitrolingual and generics): 0.4 mg per metered spray (4.9, 12 g; delivers 60 and 200 doses, respectively); contains 20% alcohol (flammable)
Aerosol spray, translingual (Nitromist): 0.4 g per spray (4.1, 8.5 g; delivers 90 and 230 doses, respectively); contains peppermint oil and menthol

---

NOTE: The IV dosage units for children are in mCg/kg/min, compared with mCg/min for adults (see remarks).

Infant/child:

    Continuous IV infusion: Begin with 0.25—0.5 mCg/kg/min; may increase by 0.5—1 mCg/kg/min Q3—5 min PRN. Usual dose: 1—5 mCg/kg/min. **Max. dose:** 20 mCg/kg/min

    Treatment of sympathomimetic/vasopressor extravasation (alternative to phentolamine; very limited data): Apply 4 mm/kg of the 2% ointment as a thin ribbon to the affected areas. If no improvement seen after 8 hr, apply another dose. Monitor patient's blood pressure for hypotension.

Adult:

    Continuous IV infusion: 5 mCg/min IV, then increase Q3—5 min PRN by 5 mCg/min up to 20 mCg/min. If no response, increase by 10—20 mCg/min Q3—5 min PRN up to a **max.** of 200 mCg/min for hypertension and 400 mCg/min for acute angina.

    Acute angina:

        Sublingual tabs: 0.3—0.4 mg Q5 min. **Max.** of three doses in 15 min

    Angina prophylaxis:

        Sustained release oral caps: 2.5—6.5 mg TID—QID; up to 26 mg QID

        Sublingual tabs: 0.3—0.4 mg 5—10 min before activity that might induce an attack

        Translingual spray (0.4 mg/spray): 1—2 sprays 5—10 min before activity that might induce an attack

        Ointment: Apply ½ inch upon rising in the morning and another ½ inch 6 hr later if needed, double the dose to 1 inch with the same dosing schedule the next day and subsequently to 2 inches if needed. Max. recommended dose: 2 doses/24 hr. Provide 10—12 hr/day of nitrate-free period to minimize tolerance.

        Patch: 0.2—0.4 mg/hr initially, then titrate to 0.4—0.8 mg/hr; apply new patch daily (tolerance is minimized by removing patch for 10—12 hr/24 hr)

Contraindicated in glaucoma, with increased ICP, cerebral hemorrhage, traumatic brain injury, shock, severe anemia, concurrent phosphodiesterase-5 inhibitor (e.g., sildenafil), and concurrent guanylate cyclase stimulator (e.g., riociguat). In small doses (1—2 mCg/kg/min), acts mainly on systemic veins and decreases preload. At 3—5 mCg/kg/min, acts on systemic arterioles to decrease resistance. May cause headache, flushing, hypersensitivity reactions, hypotension, GI upset, blurred vision, and methemoglobinemia. **Use with caution** in severe renal impairment and hepatic failure. IV nitroglycerin may antagonize anticoagulant effect of heparin. Tachyphylaxis develops within 24—48 hr of continuous IV administration; 10—12 hr/day of nitrate-free period has been recommended to prevent tachyphylaxis in adults.

Decrease dose gradually in patients receiving drug for prolonged periods to avoid withdrawal reaction. Must use polypropylene infusion sets to avoid adsorption of drug to plastic tubing. Use in heparinized patients may result in a decrease of PTT with subsequent rebound effect on discontinuation of nitroglycerin.

Continued

NITROGLYCERIN *continued*

Onset (duration) of action: IV: 1—2 min (3—5 min); sublingual: 1—3 min (30—60 min); PO sustained release: 40 min (4—8 hr); topical ointment: 20—60 min (2—12 hr); and transdermal patch: 40—60 min (18—24 hr).

NITROPRUSSIDE
Nipride RTU and generics
Vasodilator, antihypertensive

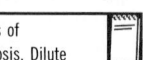

C   X   Yes   Yes   No

Injection: 25 mg/mL (2 mL)
Prediluted injection in 0.9% sodium chloride:
   Nipride RTU: 0.2 mg/mL (100 mL), 0.5 mg/mL (100 mL)

Child, adolescent, and adult: IV, continuous infusion
   Dose: Start at 0.3—0.5 mCg/kg/min, titrate to effect. Usual dose is 3—4 mCg/kg/min.
      Max. dose: 10 mCg/kg/min

Contraindicated in patients with decreased cerebral perfusion and in situations of compensatory hypertension (increased ICP). Monitor for hypotension and acidosis. Dilute with D₅W and protect from light.

Pediatric efficacy is supported by a dose-ranging trial, an open-label trial, and adult trials. No novel safety issues were found in the aforementioned pediatric trials.

Nitroprusside is nonenzymatically converted to cyanide, which is converted to thiocyanate. Cyanide may produce metabolic acidosis and methemoglobinemia; thiocyanate may produce psychosis and seizures. Monitor thiocyanate levels if used for more than 48 hr or in a dose equal to or greater than 4 mCg/kg/min. **Thiocyanate levels should be less than 50 mg/L. Monitor cyanide levels (toxic levels >2 mCg/mL)** in patients with hepatic dysfunction and thiocyanate levels in patients with renal dysfunction.

Onset of action is 2 min with a 1- to 10-min duration of effect.

NOREPINEPHRINE BITARTRATE
Levophed and generics
Adrenergic agonist

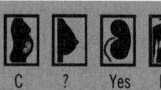

C   ?   Yes   No   No

Injection: 1 mg/mL as norepinephrine base (4 mL); may contain sulfites
Prediluted injection in D₅W or normal saline: 16 mCg/mL (250 mL), 32 mCg/mL (250 mL), 64 mCg/mL (250 mL); contains sulfites

NOTE: The dosage units for children are in mCg/kg/min compared with mCg/min for adults.
Child: Continuous IV infusion doses as norepinephrine base. Start at 0.05—0.1 mCg/kg/min. Titrate to effect. **Max. dose:** 2 mCg/kg/min
Adult: Continuous IV infusion **doses as norepinephrine base.** Start at 8—12 mCg/min and titrate to effect. Usual maintenance dosage range: 2—4 mCg/min

May cause cardiac arrhythmias, hypertension, hypersensitivity, headaches, vomiting, uterine contractions, and organ ischemia. May cause decreased renal blood flow and urine output.
   Avoid extravasation into tissues; may cause severe tissue necrosis. If this occurs, treat locally with phentolamine.

NORTRIPTYLINE HYDROCHLORIDE
Pamelor and generics
Antidepressant, tricyclic

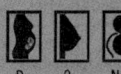   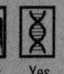

D   2   No   Yes   Yes

Caps: 10, 25, 50, 75 mg; may contain benzyl alcohol, parabens, or EDTA
Oral solution: 10 mg/5 mL (473 mL); contains up to 4% alcohol, benzoic acid, and sorbitol

Depression (see remarks):
  Child 6–12 yr: 1–3 mg/kg/24 hr ÷ TID–QID PO or 10–20 mg/24 hr ÷ TID–QID PO
  Adolescent: 1–3 mg/kg/24 hr ÷ TID–QID PO or 30–50 mg/24 hr ÷ TID–QID PO
  Adult: 75–100 mg/24 hr ÷ TID–QID PO
  Max. dose (all ages): 150 mg/24 hr
Nocturnal enuresis (see remarks):
  6–7 yr (20–25 kg): 10 mg PO QHS
  8–11 yr (26–35 kg): 10–20 mg PO QHS
  >11 yr (36–54 kg): 25–35 mg PO QHS

See imipramine for contraindications and common side effects. Also **contraindicated** with
  linezolid or IV methylene blue due to increased risk for serotonin syndrome. **Avoid** use in
  patients with Brugada syndrome. Fewer CNS and anticholinergic side effects than with
  amitriptyline. May cause mild pupillary dilation, which can lead to narrow angle glaucoma.
Lower doses and slower dose titration are recommended in hepatic impairment. Therapeutic
  antidepressant effects occur in 7–21 days. Monitor for clinical worsening of depression and
  suicidal ideation/behavior following the initiation of therapy or after dose changes. **Do not**
  discontinue abruptly. Nortriptyline is a substrate for the CYP 450 1A2 and 2D6 drug-metabolizing
  enzymes. Use and dosing considerations have been recommended based on the following CYP 450
  2D6 phenotypes:
  Ultrarapid metabolizer: Use of alternative drug not metabolized by CYP 2D6. If use is warranted, titrate
    to the highest target dose and monitor serum levels.
  Intermediate metabolizer: Reduce recommended initial dose by 25% and monitor serum levels.
  Poor metabolizer: **Avoid use** to prevent potential side effect and use alternative drug not metabolized
    by CYP 2D6. If use is warranted, reduce recommended initial dose by 50% and monitor serum
    levels.
Rifampin may increase the metabolism of nortriptyline.
Therapeutic nortriptyline levels for depression: 50–150 ng/mL. Recommended serum sampling time:
  Obtain a single level 8 or more hours after an oral dose (following 4 days of continuous dosing for
  children and after 9–10 days for adults).
Administer with food to decrease GI upset.

NYSTATIN
Nyamyc, Nystop, and generics; previously
available as Mycostatin and Nilstat
Antifungal agent

    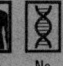

C   2   No   No   No

Tabs: 500,000 U
Oral suspension: 100,000 U/mL (5, 60, 480 mL)
Topical cream and ointment: 100,000 U/g (15, 30 g)
Topical powder (Nyamyc, Nystop, and generics): 100,000 U/g (15, 30, 60 g)

Oropharyngeal candidiasis:
  Preterm infant: 0.5 mL (50,000 U) to each side of mouth QID

Continued

NYSTATIN *continued*

Term infant: 1—4 mL (100,000—400,000 U) to each side of mouth QID
Child, adolescent, and adult: 4—6 mL (400,000—600,000 U) swish and swallow QID
Nonesophageal mucous membrane GI candidiasis:
  Adult (oral tabs): 500,000—1,000,000 U PO Q8 hr until 48 hr after clinical cure
Topical (all topical dosage forms):
  All ages: Apply to affected areas BID-QID.

May produce diarrhea and GI side effects. Local irritation, contact dermatitis, and
  Stevens-Johnson syndrome have been reported. Treat until 48—72 hr after resolution of
  symptoms. Drug is poorly absorbed through the GI tract. Oral suspension should be swished about
  the mouth and retained in the mouth as long as possible before swallowing.

O

OCTREOTIDE ACETATE
Sandostatin, Sandostatin LAR Depot, and
generics
Somatostatin analog, antisecretory agent

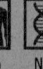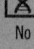

B   2   Yes   No   No

Injection (amps and single dose vials): 0.05, 0.1, 0.5 mg/mL (1 mL); preservative free
Injection (multidose vials): 0.2, 1 mg/mL (5 mL); contains phenol
Injection, microspheres for suspension (Sandostatin LAR Depot; see remarks): 10, 20, 30 mg (in
  kits with 2 mL diluent and 1.5-inch 20-gauge needles)

Infant and child:
  Intractable diarrhea (very limited data):
    IV/SC: 1—10 mCg/kg/24 hr ÷ Q12—24 hr. Dose may be increased within the recommended range
      by 0.3 mCg/kg/dose every 3 days as needed. **Max. dose:** 1500 mCg/24 hr
    IV continuous infusion: Bolus of 1 mCg/kg/dose followed by 1 mCg/kg/hr; this has been used in
      diarrhea associated with graft-versus-host disease.
  Esophageal varices (limited data): Bolus of 1—2 mCg/kg/dose followed by 1—2 mCg/kg/hr. Use was
    reported as safe and effective over a 2—5 day duration with major adverse effects in one subject
    each receiving higher dose or longer duration of therapy. Therapy is typically discontinued 24 hr
    after bleeding has ceased or when no clinical response is seen after 12 hr of use.

Cholelithiasis, hyperglycemia, hypoglycemia, hypothyroidism, nausea, diarrhea, abdominal
  discomfort, headache, dizziness, and pain at injection site may occur. Growth hormone
  suppression may occur with long-term use. Bradycardia, thrombocytopenia, and increased risk for
  pregnancy in patients with acromegaly and pancreatitis have been reported. Cyclosporine levels may
  be reduced in patients receiving this drug. May increase the effects/toxicity of bromocriptine.
Patients with severe renal failure requiring dialysis may require dosage adjustments due to an
  increase in half-life. Effects of hepatic dysfunction on octreotide have not been evaluated.
  Octreotide may interfere with the efficacy of lutetium Lu 177 dotatate; discontinue octreotide at
  least 24 hr prior to each lutetium Lu 177 dotatate dose. May decrease the effects of cyclosporine
  and increase the effect/toxicity of bromocriptine. **Use with caution** with medications that are
  primarily metabolized via CYP 450 3A4 with low therapeutic index (e.g., quinidine) as somatostatin
  analogs may decrease CYP 450 activity via growth hormone suppression.
Sandostatin LAR Depot is administered once every 4 wk **only** by the IM route and is currently indicated
  for use in adults who have been stabilized on IV/SC therapy. See package insert for details.

OFLOXACIN (OTIC AND OPHTHALMIC)
Ocuflox, and generics; previously available as
Floxin and Floxin Otic
Antibiotic, quinolone

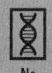

C 2 No No No

Otic solution: 0.3% (5, 10 mL); contains benzalkonium chloride
Ophthalmic solution (Ocuflox and generics): 0.3% (5, 10 mL); contains benzalkonium chloride

Otic use:
  Otitis externa (acute):
    6 mo—12 yr: 5 drops to affected ear(s) once daily × 7 days
    ≥13 yr—adult: 10 drops to affected ear(s) once daily × 7 days
  Chronic suppurative otitis media:
    ≥12 yr—adult: 10 drops to affected ear(s) BID × 14 days
  Acute otitis media with tympanostomy tubes:
    1—12 yr: 5 drops to affected ear(s) BID × 10 days
Ophthalmic use (>1 yr—adult):
  Conjunctivitis: 1—2 drops to affected eye(s) 2—4 hr while awake × 2 days, then QID × 5 additional
  days
  Corneal ulcer: 1—2 drops to affected eye(s) Q30 min while awake and Q4—6 hr while asleep at night
  × 2 days, followed by Q1 hr while awake × 5 days, and then QID until treatment has been
  completed

Pruritus, local irritation, taste perversion, dizziness, and earache have been reported with
  otic use. Ocular burning/discomfort is frequent with ophthalmic use. Consult with
  ophthalmology in corneal ulcers.
When otic solution is being used, the solution should be warmed by holding the bottle in the hand for
  1—2 min. The use of cold solutions may result in dizziness. For otitis externa, the patient should lie
  with the affected ear upward before instillation and remain in the same position after dose
  administration for 5 min to enhance drug delivery. For acute otitis media with tympanostomy
  tubes, the patient should lie in the same position prior to instillation and the tragus should be
  pumped
  4 times after the dose to assist in drug delivery to the middle ear.
Systemic use of ofloxacin is typically replaced by levofloxacin, its S-isomer, which has a more favorable
  side effect profile than ofloxacin. See **Levofloxacin**.

OLANZAPINE
Zyprexa, Zyprexa Zydis, Zyprexa Relprevv, and
generics
Antipsychotic, atypical second generation

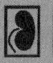

C 2 No Yes No

Tabs: 2.5, 5, 7.5, 10, 15, 20 mg
Orally disintegrating tabs (Zyprexa Zydis and generics): 5, 10, 15, 20 mg; contain phenylalanine and
  parabens
IM injection:
  Short-acting: 10 mg; contains tartaric acid
  Long-acting pamoate salt (Zyprexa Relprevv):
    Every 2 wk dosing: 210, 300 mg; contains mannitol, polysorbate 80
    Every 4 wk dosing: 405 mg; contains mannitol, polysorbate 80

Continued

OLANZAPINE *continued*

PO DOSING

Severe or refractory agitation for psychiatric emergencies in developmental delay, autism, or oppositional defiant/conduct disorder (very limited data; oral disintegrating tab is preferred):

Child <12 yr: 2.5 mg PO

Child ≥12 yr and adolescent: 5—10 mg PO

Bipolar I disorder (manic or mixed episodes; not first-line therapy):

Child 4—6 yr of age (limited data, based on an open-label trial in 15 subjects): Start at 1.25 mg PO once daily × 7 days, then increase dose Q7 days PRN as tolerated to a target dose of 10 mg once daily.

Child 6—12 yr of age (limited data): Start at 2.5 mg PO once daily × 7 days, then increase dose in 2.5 or 5 mg increments Q7 days to a target dose of 10 mg once daily. Suggested **max. dose:** 20 mg/24 hr

Adolescent (see remarks): Start at 2.5 or 5 mg PO once daily × 7 days, then increase dose in 2.5 or 5 mg increments Q7 days to a target dose of 10 mg once daily. Suggested **max. dose:** 20 mg/24 hr (doses >20 mg/24 hr have not been evaluated)

Adult: Start at 10 or 15 mg PO once daily (use 10 mg if used with lithium or valproate). If needed, increase or decrease dose by 5 mg daily at intervals not <24 hr. Maintenance dosage range: 5—20 mg/24 hr. Suggested **max. dose:** 20 mg/24 hr (doses >20 mg/24 hr have not been evaluated)

Schizophrenia:

Child ≥8 yr of age and adolescent (see remarks): Start with 2.5 or 5 mg PO once daily, then increase dose in 2.5 or 5 mg increments Q7 days to the target dose of 10 mg once daily (doses >20 mg/24 hr have not been evaluated).

Adult: Start with 5 or 10 mg PO once daily (use 5 mg for individuals who are debilitated, predisposed to hypotension, pharmacodynamically sensitive to olanzapine, or nonsmoking females ≥65 yr old) with a target dose of 10 mg once daily within 5—7 days. If needed, increase or decrease dose by 5 mg daily at weekly intervals. Usual dosage range: 10—15 mg once daily. Additional clinical assessment is recommended for doses >10 mg/24 hr (doses >20 mg/24 hr have not been evaluated).

Chemotherapy-induced nausea and vomiting (refractory breakthrough; limited data):

Child ≥3 yr and adolescent: 0.1—0.14 mg/kg/dose (rounded to the nearest 1.25 mg dosage increment) PO once daily—BID. Many report use in combination with other antiemetics such as aprepitant, dexamethasone, ondansetron, or granisetron.

IM DOSING

Short-acting IM injection:

Severe or refractory agitation for psychiatric emergencies in developmental delay, autism, or oppositional defiant/conduct disorder (PO administration is preferred; limited data):

Child <12 yr: 1.25—5 mg IM

Child ≥12 yr and adolescent: 5—10 mg IM; dose may be repeated after 2 hr if needed

Acute agitation associated with bipolar I or schizophrenia:

Child and adolescent (limited retrospective data in 15 children and 35 adolescents): ≤12 yr: 5 mg and adolescent (13—17 yr): 10 mg. Dosing frequencies and max. doses were not reported.

Adult: 10 mg (5 mg for geriatric patients and 2.5 mg for individuals who are debilitated, predisposed to hypotension, or pharmacodynamically sensitive to olanzapine). If needed, additional doses × 2 may be given; second dose 2 hr after the first dose and third dose 4 hr after the second dose. Recommended max. dose is 30 mg/24 hr (10 mg × 3 given 2—4 hr apart); safety of doses >30 mg/24 hr has not been evaluated.

OLANZAPINE *continued*

Long-acting pamoate salt (Zyprexa Relprevv):
 Schizophrenia (adult): See remarks and package insert for specific dosage based on established oral dosage.

Use with caution in cardiovascular or cerebrovascular disease, hypotensive conditions, diabetes/hyperglycemia, elevated serum lipids and cholesterol, paralytic ileus, hepatic impairment, seizure disorders, narrow angle glaucoma, and prostatic hypertrophy. Medication exhibits anticholinergic effects.

Common side effects include orthostatic hypotension, peripheral edema, hypercholesterolemia, hyperprolactinemia, appetite simulation, weight gain (greater in adolescents than adults; monitoring is recommended), hypertriglyceridemia, constipation, xerostomia, akathisia, asthenia, dizziness, somnolence, tremor, and personality disorder. Neuroleptic malignant syndrome, dystonia, cognitive and motor impairment, tardive dyskinesia (irreversible with cumulative high doses), neutropenia, leukopenia, agranulocytosis, suicidal intent, acute pancreatitis, pulmonary embolism, increases in liver function tests (ALT, AST, GGT), DRESS, salivary hypersecretion, and hyperthermia have been reported.

Olanzapine is a major substrate for CYP 450 1A2 and minor substrate for 2D6. It also is a weak inhibitor to CYP 450 1A2, 2C9/19. Do not use in combination with alcohol, benzodiazepines, or opiates due to increased risk for sedation and cardiopulmonary depression. Caution is also indicated with anticholinergic agents (e.g., azelastine, glycopyrrolate), as olanzapine may enhance the anticholinergic effects. Use with QTc-prolonging medications may further increase the risk for QTc prolongation. Metoclopramide may enhance neurologic side effects of olanzapine. Do not use oral disintegrating tablets in phenylketonuria.

$T_{1/2}$: 37 hr for children and 21–54 hr for adults via PO route. Short-acting IM $T_{1/2}$ in adults is similar to PO route, but long-acting IM $T_{1/2}$ is ∼30 days in adults.

Maintenance treatment for bipolar I disorder and schizophrenia has not been systematically evaluated in adolescents. Therefore it is recommended to utilize the lowest dose to maintain efficacy and to reassess the need for maintenance treatment periodically for this age group.

All oral dosages may be taken either with or without food. For orally disintegrating tabs, tablet must be placed in patient's mouth immediately after removing it from the foil pack (by peeling off the foil, not by pushing the tablet through the foil) and allowed to dissolve in saliva; then swallowed with or without liquids.

Zyprexa Relprevv (long-acting IM injection): Postinjection delirium and sedation syndrome have been reported with this dosage form. Patients must be observed by a healthcare provider at a healthcare facility for at least 3 hr after administration. The FDA REMS program requires prescribers, healthcare facilities, and pharmacies to register with the Zyprexa Relprevv Patient Care Program at 1-877-772-9390 for use of this product.

OLOPATADINE
Patanol, Pataday, Patanase, and generics
Antihistamine

    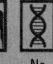

C   2/?   No   No   No

Ophthalmic solution (products may contain benzalkonium chloride):
 Patanol, Pataday, and generics (OTC): 0.1% (5 mL)
 Pataday and generics (OTC): 0.2% (2.5 mL)
 Pataday: 0.7% (2.5 mL)
Nasal spray (Patanase and generics): 0.6% (30.5 g provides 240 metered spray doses); contains benzalkonium chloride and EDTA

Continued

OLOPATADINE *continued*

Ophthalmic use for allergic conjunctivitis (≥2 yr old and adult):
  0.1% solution: 1 drop in affected eye(s) BID (spaced 6—8 hr apart)
  0.2% or 0.7% solution: 1 drop in affected eye(s) once daily
Intranasal use of allergic rhinitis:
  Patients 6—11 yr old: Inhale 1 spray into each nostril BID.
  Patients ≥12 yr old and adult: Inhale 2 sprays into each nostril BID.

Ocular use: DO NOT use while wearing contact lenses; wait at least 10 min after instilling
drops before inserting lenses. Ocular side effects include burning or stinging, dry eye,
foreign body sensation, hyperemia, keratitis, lid edema, and pruritus. May also cause headaches,
asthenia, pharyngitis, rhinitis, and taste perversion. Use with caution in lactation with the ocular
route of administration.
Nasal use: Common side effects include bitter taste and headaches. Somnolence, impaired mental
alertness, nasal ulceration, epistaxis, nasal septal perforation, throat pain, and postnasal drip have
been reported. Diarrhea was reported more frequently (9%) in an allergic rhinitis clinical trial for
2—5 yr old children compared to 6—11 yr old (<1%). Breastfeeding information is unknown with
the intranasal route of administration.
To reduce the risk of drug being systemically absorbed with ophthalmic use, place pressure on the tear
duct by the corner of the eye for ≥1 min, then remove the excess solution with an absorbent tissue.
A combination intranasal product of olopatadine and mometasone (Ryaltris) is available for
seasonal allergic rhinitis and currently indicated for children >12 yr and adults.

OMEPRAZOLE
Prilosec, Prilosec OTC, First-Omeprazole, and generics
In combination with sodium bicarbonate:
Zegerid, Zegerid OTC, and generics
Gastric acid pump inhibitor

C   2   Yes   Yes   Yes

Caps, sustained release: 10, 20, 40 mg; may contain magnesium
Tabs, delayed release (Prilosec OTC and generics; OTC): 20 mg; may contain magnesium
Oral suspension:
  First-Omeprazole: 2 mg/mL (90, 150, 300 mL); contains benzyl alcohol
  Compounded formulation: 2 mg/mL; contains ~0.5 mEq sodium bicarbonate per 1 mg drug
Granules for oral suspension (Prilosec): 2.5 and 10 mg packets (30s); contains magnesium
In combination with sodium bicarbonate:
  Powder for oral suspension (Zegerid and generics): 20, 40 mg packets (30s); each packet
    (regardless of strength) contains 1680 mg (20 mEq) sodium bicarbonate
  Caps, immediate release (Zegerid, Zegerid OTC, and generics): 20 mg (OTC), 40 mg; each capsule
    (regardless of strength) contains 1100 mg (13.1 mEq) sodium bicarbonate
  Chewable tabs (Zegerid): 20 and 40 mg; each tab (regardless of strength) contains 600 mg (7.1 mEq)
    sodium bicarbonate and 700 mg magnesium hydroxide

Infant and child:
  Esophagitis, GERD, or ulcers: Start at 1 mg/kg/24 hr PO ÷ once daily—BID (**max. dose:**
    20 mg/24 hr). Reported effective range for GERD: 0.7—4 mg/kg/24 hr. Children 1—6 yr may require
    higher doses due to enhanced drug clearance. Alternative dosing by weight category:
    3—<5 kg: 2.5 mg PO once daily
    5—<10 kg: 5 mg PO once daily
    10—<20 kg: 10 mg PO once daily
    20 kg and above: 20 mg PO once daily

OMEPRAZOLE *continued*

Adult:

> **Duodenal ulcer or GERD:** 20—40 mg/dose PO once daily × 4—8 wk; may give up to 12 wk for erosive esophagitis
>
> **Gastric ulcer:** 20—40 mg/24 hr PO ÷ once daily—BID × 4—8 wk
>
> **Pathologic hypersecretory conditions:** Start with 60 mg/24 hr PO once daily. If needed, dose may be increased up to 120 mg/24 hr PO ÷ TID. Daily doses >80 mg should be administered in divided doses.

Common side effects: Headache, diarrhea, nausea, and vomiting. Allergic reactions (discontinue use immediately) including anaphylaxis, acute interstitial nephritis, severe skin reactions, hypomagnesemia, and vitamin B$_{12}$ deficiency (with prolonged use) have been reported. Fundic gland polyps have been associated with long-term use of PPIs. Has been associated with increased risk for *Clostridium difficile*—associated diarrhea.

Drug induces CYP 450 1A2 (decreases theophylline levels) and is also a substrate and inhibitor of CYP 2C19. Recommended dosage modification for ultrarapid metabolizers of CYP 2C19 is to increase the usual dose by threefold. Increases T$_{1/2}$ of citalopram, diazepam, phenytoin, and warfarin. May decrease the effects of itraconazole, ketoconazole, clopidogrel, iron salts, and ampicillin esters. St. John's wort and rifampin may decrease omeprazole effects. May be used in combination with clarithromycin and amoxicillin for *Helicobacter pylori* infections. Omeprazole may interfere with serum chromogranin A (CgA) diagnostic test for neuroendocrine tumors; discontinue use at least 14 days prior to testing.

Bioavailability may be increased with hepatic dysfunction or in patients of Asian descent. Safety and efficacy for GERD in children <1 mo have not been established.

Administer all doses before meals. Administer 30 min prior to sucralfate. Capsules contain enteric-coated granules to ensure bioavailability. Do not chew or crush capsule. For doses unable to be divided by 10 mg, capsule may be opened and intact pellets may be administered in an acidic beverage (e.g., apple juice, cranberry juice) or applesauce. The extemporaneously compounded oral suspension product may be less bioavailable due to the loss of the enteric coating.

OMNIPAQUE

See Iohexol.

ONDANSETRON
Zofran, Zofran ODT, and generics
Antiemetic agent, 5-HT3 antagonist

    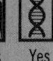

| B | 2 | No | Yes | Yes |

Injection: 2 mg/mL (2, 20 mL); single dose vials are preservative free and multidose vials contain parabens

Tabs: 4, 8. 24 mg

Tabs, orally disintegrating (ODT): 4, 8 mg; contain aspartame

Oral solution: 4 mg/5 mL (50 mL); contains sodium benzoate

Preventing nausea and vomiting associated with chemotherapy:

> **Oral (give initial dose 30 min before chemotherapy):**
>
> > **Child (≥2 yr of age and adolescent), dose based on body surface area:**
> >
> > > **<0.3 m²:** 1 mg TID PRN nausea
> > >
> > > **0.3—0.6 m²:** 2 mg TID PRN nausea
> > >
> > > **0.6—1 m²:** 3 mg TID PRN nausea

Continued

ONDANSETRON *continued*

>**1 m²:** 4—8 mg TID PRN nausea
Dose based on age:
  <4 yr of age: Use dose based on body surface area from preceding dosages
  4—11 yr of age: 4 mg TID PRN nausea
  >11 yr of age and adult: 8 mg TID or 24 mg once daily PRN nausea
IV (child and adult):
  Moderately emetogenic drugs: 0.15 mg/kg/dose (**max. dose:** 8 mg/dose for child and 16 mg/dose adult) at 30 min before and 4 and 8 hr after emetogenic drugs. Then same dose Q4 hr PRN
  Highly emetogenic drugs: 0.15 mg/kg/dose (**max. dose:** 16 mg/dose) 30 min before 4 and 8 hr after emetogenic drugs. Then 0.15 mg/kg/dose (**max. dose:** 16 mg/dose) Q4 hr PRN
Preventing nausea and vomiting associated with surgery (additional doses for controlling nausea and vomiting may not provide any benefits):
  IV/IM (administered prior to anesthesia over 2—5 min):
    Child (1 mo—12 yr of age):
      <40 kg: 0.1 mg/kg/dose × 1
      ≥40 kg: 4 mg × 1
    Adult: 4 mg × 1
  Oral:
    Adult: 16 mg × 1, 1 hr prior to induction of anesthesia
Preventing nausea and vomiting associated with radiation therapy:
  Child: Use above dosage for preventing nausea and vomiting associated with chemotherapy and give initial dose 1—2 hr prior to radiation.
  Adult:
    Total body irradiation: 8 mg PO 1—2 hr prior to radiation once daily—BID
    Single high-dose fraction radiation to abdomen: 8 mg PO 1—2 hr prior to radiation with subsequent doses Q8 hr after first dose × 1—2 days after completion of radiation
    Daily fractionated radiation to abdomen: 8 mg PO 1—2 hr prior to radiation with subsequent doses Q8 hr after first dose for each day radiation is given
Vomiting in acute gastroenteritis (oral route is preferred; use IV route when oral administration is not possible):
  Oral (child 6 mo—10 yr old and weighing ≥8 kg; use oral disintegrating tablet):
    8—15 kg: 2 mg × 1
    >15 and ≤30 kg: 4 mg × 1
    >30 kg: 8 mg × 1
  IV (≥1 mo): 0.15—0.3 mg/kg/dose × 1; **max. dose:** 8 mg/dose

---

Avoid use in congenital long-QTc syndrome. Bronchospasm, tachycardia, hypokalemia, seizures, headaches, lightheadedness, constipation, diarrhea, and transient increases in AST, ALT, and bilirubin may occur. Transient blindness (resolution within a few min up to 48 hr), arthralgia, Stevens-Johnson syndrome, TEN, hepatic dysfunction, masking of progressive ileus and gastric distention, myocardial ischemia (primarily with IV route) and rare/transient ECG changes (including QTc-interval prolongation) have been reported. Data limited for use in children below 3 yr of age.

ECG monitoring is recommended in patients with electrolyte abnormalities, CHF, or bradyarrhythmias. Drug clearance is higher for surgical and cancer patients <18 yr as compared with adults. Clearance is slower for children 1—4 mo old compared with children >4—24 mo old.

Ondansetron is a substrate for CYP 450 1A2, 2D6, 2E1, and 3A3/4 drug metabolizing enzymes. It is likely that the inhibition/loss of one of the previously listed enzymes will be compensated by others and may result in insignificant changes to the elimination of ondansetron, which may be affected by CYP 450 enzyme inducers. Ultrarapid metabolizers of CYP 450 2D6 are associated with decreased response, and use of an alternative drug not predominantly metabolized by CYP 2D6

ONDANSETRON *continued*

(e.g., granisetron) is recommended. Follow theophylline, phenytoin, or warfarin levels closely, if used in combination. Use with apomorphine may result in profound hypotension and loss of consciousness and is **contraindicated.**

To administer the oral film dosage form (Zuplenz), film must be placed on top of patient's tongue, allowed to dissolve completely in 4—20 sec, and swallowed with or without liquid.

ORKAMBI

See Lumacaftor and Ivacaftor.

OSELTAMIVIR PHOSPHATE
Tamiflu and generics
Antiviral, neurominidase inhibitor

   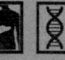 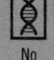

| C | 2 | Yes | Yes | No |

Caps: 30, 45, 75 mg
Oral suspension: 6 mg/mL (60 mL); may contain saccharin and sodium benzoate
May also be extemporaneously compounded from capsules (6 mg/mL)

Treatment of influenza (initiate therapy within 2 days of onset of symptoms):
  Preterm neonate (limited data): Usual duration of therapy for 5 days
    Postmenstrual age (PMA) neonate <38 wk: 1 mg/kg/dose PO BID
    PMA 38—40 wk: 1.5 mg/kg/dose PO BID
  Full-term neonate (PMA >40 wk)—child 1 yr: 3 mg/kg/dose PO BID × 5 days
  Child <1 yr alternative dosing based on age: See following table.

Age (mo)	Dosage for 5 days	Volume of Oral Suspension (6 mg/mL)
<3	12 mg PO BID	2 mL
3—5	20 mg PO BID	3.33 mL
6—11	25 mg PO BID	4.2 mL

Child ≥1—12 yr: See following table.

Weight (kg)	Dosage for 5 days	Volume of Oral Suspension (6 mg/mL)
≤15	30 mg PO BID	5 mL
>15—23	45 mg PO BID	7.5 mL
>23—40	60 mg PO BID	10 mL
>40	75 mg PO BID	12.5 mL

≥13 yr old and adult: 75 mg PO BID × 5 days
Prophylaxis of influenza (initiate therapy within 2 days of exposure; see remarks):
  Child 3 mo—<1 yr: 3 mg/kg/dose PO once daily; alternative dosage based on age:
    3—5 mo: 20 mg PO once daily
    6—11 mo: 25 mg PO once daily

Continued

OSELTAMIVIR PHOSPHATE *continued*

Child 1—12 yr:
  ≤15 kg: 30 mg PO once daily
  16—23 kg: 45 mg PO once daily
  24—40 kg: 60 mg PO once daily
  >40 kg: 75 mg PO once daily
  ≥13 yr old and adult: 75 mg PO once daily for a minimum of 7 days and up to 6 wk; initiate therapy within 2 days of exposure.

Currently indicated for the treatment of influenza A and B strains. Use in children <1 yr of age has not been recommended due to concerns of excessive CNS penetration and fatalities in 7-day-old rats.

Nausea and vomiting generally occur within the first 2 days and are the most common adverse effects. Insomnia, vertigo, seizures, hypothermia, neuropsychiatric events (may result in fatal outcomes), arrhythmias, rash, and toxic epidermal necrolysis have also been reported. If the glomerular filtration rate (GFR) is 10—30 mL/min, reduce treatment dose to 75 mg PO once daily × 5 days for adults. (See Chapter 31.)

PROPHYLACTIC USE: Oseltamivir is not a substitute for annual flu vaccination. Safety and efficacy have been demonstrated for ≤6 wk of therapy; duration of protection lasts for as long as dosing is continued. Adjust prophylaxis dose if GFR is 10—30 mL/min by extending the dosage interval to once every other day.

Probenecid increases oseltamivir levels. Oseltamivir decreases the efficacy of the nasal influenza vaccine (live attenuated influenza vaccine, FluMist); **avoid** administration of vaccine within 2 wk before or 48 hr after oseltamivir administration unless medically indicated.

Dosage adjustments in hepatic impairment, severe renal disease, and dialysis have not been established for either treatment or prophylactic use. The safety and efficacy of repeated treatment or prophylaxis courses have not been evaluated. Doses may be administered with or without food.

OXACILLIN
Various generics
Antibiotic, penicillin (penicillinase resistant)

    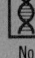

B   2   Yes   Yes   No

Injection: 1, 2, 10 g
Injection, premixed in iso-osmotic dextrose: 1 g/50 mL, 2 g/50 mL
Injectable products contain 2.8—3.1 mEq Na per 1 g drug

Neonate (IM/IV):

  Usual dose: 25 mg/kg/dose; following the dosage interval below
  Meningitis or severe infection: 50 mg/kg/dose; following the dosage interval below
  Postmenstrual age:
    ≤29 wk:
      ≤28 days old: Q12 hr
      >28 days old: Q8 hr
    30—36 wk:
      ≤14 days old: Q12 hr
      >14 days old: Q8 hr
    37—44 wk:
      ≤7 days old: Q12 hr
      >7 days old: Q8 hr
    ≥45 wk (all postnatal ages): Q6 hr

OXACILLIN *continued*

Infant and child (IM/IV): 100—200 mg/kg/24 hr ÷ Q4—6 hr (**max. dose:** 12 g/24 hr); use 200 mg/kg/24 hr for endocarditis and severe infections and Q4 hr dosing for severe/CNS infections
Adult (IM/IV): 250—2000 mg/dose Q4—6 hr; use higher dosage range for endocarditis or severe infections and Q4 hr dosing for severe/CNS infections
Max. dose (all ages): 12 g/24 hr

Rash and GI disturbances are common. Leukopenia, reversible hepatotoxicity, and acute interstitial nephritis have been reported. Hematuria and azotemia have occurred in neonates and infants with high doses. May cause false-positive urinary and serum proteins.
Probenecid increases serum oxacillin levels. Tetracyclines may antagonize the bactericidal effects of oxacillin.
CSF penetration is poor unless meninges are inflamed. Use the lower end of the usual dosage range for patients with creatinine clearances <10 mL/min. **Adjust dose in renal failure (see Chapter 31).**

OXCARBAZEPINE
Trileptal, Oxtellar XR, and generics
Anticonvulsant

   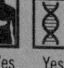

| C | 2 | Yes | Yes | Yes |

Tabs: 150, 300, 600 mg
Extended release tabs (Oxtellar XR): 150, 300, 600 mg
Oral suspension: 300 mg/5 mL (250 mL); contains saccharin, ethanol, and propylene glycol

Child (2—<4 yr old):
Adjunctive therapy for partial-onset seizures (limited data): Start with 8—10 mg/kg/24 hr PO ÷ BID up to a **max. dose** of 600 mg/24 hr. For children <20 kg, may consider using a starting dose of 16—20 mg/kg/24 hr PO ÷ BID; gradually increase the dose over a 2—4 wk period and **do not exceed** 60 mg/kg/24 hr ÷ BID.
Child (4—16 yr old, see remarks):
Adjunctive therapy for partial-onset seizures: Start with 8—10 mg/kg/24 hr PO ÷ BID up to a **max. dose** of 600 mg/24 hr. Then gradually increase the dose over a 2-wk period to the following maintenance doses:
20—29 kg: 900 mg/24 hr PO ÷ BID
29.1—39 kg: 1200 mg/24 hr PO ÷ BID
>39 kg: 1800 mg/24 hr PO ÷ BID
Conversion to monotherapy for partial-onset seizures: Start with 8—10 mg/kg/24 hr PO ÷ BID and simultaneously initiate dosage reduction of concomitant AEDs and withdrawal completely over 3—6 wk. Dose may be increased at weekly intervals, as clinically indicated, by a **maximum** of 10 mg/kg/24 hr to achieve the recommended monotherapy maintenance dose as described in the following table.
Initiation of monotherapy for partial-onset seizures (with no concomitant AEDs): Start with 8—10 mg/kg/24 hr PO ÷ BID. Then increase by 5 mg/kg/24 hr Q3 days up to the recommended monotherapy maintenance dose as described in the following table:

RECOMMENDED MONOTHERAPY MAINTENANCE DOSES FOR CHILDREN BY WEIGHT

Weight (kg)	Daily Oral Maintenance Dose (mg/24 hr) Divided BID
20—<25	600—900
25—<35	900—1200

Continued

OXCARBAZEPINE *continued*

Weight (kg)	Daily Oral Maintenance Dose (mg/24 hr) Divided BID
35—<45	900—1500
45—<50	1200—1500
50—<60	1200—1800
60—<70	1200—2100
≥70	1500—2100

Adult:

Adjunctive therapy for partial-onset seizures: Start with 600 mg/24 hr PO ÷ BID. Dose may be increased at weekly intervals, as clinically indicated, by a **maximum** of 600 mg/24 hr. Usual maintenance dose is 1200 mg/24 hr PO ÷ BID. Doses ≥2400 mg/24 hr are generally not well tolerated due to CNS side effects.

Conversion to monotherapy for partial-onset seizures: Start with 600 mg/24 hr PO ÷ BID and simultaneously initiate dosage reduction of concomitant AEDs. Dose may be increased at weekly intervals as clinically indicated, by a **max** of 600 mg/24 hr to achieve a dose of 2400 mg/24 hr PO ÷ BID. Concomitant AEDs should be terminated gradually over approximately 3—6 wk.

Initiation of monotherapy for partial-onset seizures: Start with 600 mg/24 hr PO ÷ BID. Then increase by 300 mg/24 hr every 3 days up to 1200 mg/24 hr PO ÷ BID.

EXTENDED RELEASE TABS (Oxtellar XR; see remarks):

Child 6—17 yr of age:

Adjunctive therapy for partial-onset seizures: Start with 8—10 mg/kg/24 hr PO once daily up to a **max. dose** of 600 mg/24 hr. Then gradually increase at weekly intervals in increments of 8—10 mg/kg/24 hr (**max. dosage** increment: 600 mg) to the following maintenance doses:

20—29 kg: 900 mg PO once daily

29.1—39 kg: 1200 mg PO once daily

>39 kg: 1800 mg PO once daily

Adult:

Adjunctive therapy for partial-onset seizures: Start with 600 mg PO once daily (consider using 900 mg if patient is receiving concomitant enzyme-inducing AEDs). Then gradually increase at weekly intervals in 600 mg/24 hr increments to the maintenance dose of 1200—2400 mg once daily.

Clinically significant hyponatremia may occur; generally seen within the first 3 mo of therapy. May also cause headache, dizziness, drowsiness, ataxia, fatigue, nystagmus, urticaria, diplopia, abnormal gait, and GI discomfort. About 25%—30% of patients with carbamazepine hypersensitivity will experience a cross-reaction with oxcarbazepine. Serious dermatologic reactions (Stevens-Johnson syndrome [SJS] and TEN), multiorgan hypersensitivity reactions (e.g., DRESS), bone marrow depression, osteoporosis, pancreatitis, folic acid deficiency, hypothyroidism, rare cases of anaphylaxis and angioedema, and suicidal behavior or ideation have been reported. Increased risk for severe dermatologic reactions (e.g., SJS and TEN) has been associated with the HLA-B*1502 (prevalent among persons of Asian descent) alleles.

Inhibits CYP 450 2C19 and induces CYP 450 3A4/5 drug metabolizing enzymes. Carbamazepine, cyclosporine, phenobarbital, phenytoin, rifampin, valproic acid, and verapamil may decrease oxcarbazepine levels. Oxcarbazepine may increase phenobarbital and phenytoin levels. Oxcarbazepine can decrease the effects of oral contraceptives, cyclosporine, felodipine, and lamotrigine.

If GFR <30 mL/min, adjust dosage by administering 50% of the normal starting dose (**max. dose:** 300 mg/24 hr) followed by a slower than normal increase in dose if necessary (**see Chapter 31**). No dosage adjustment is required in mild/moderate hepatic impairment. Use is **not recommended** in severe hepatic impairment due to lack of information.

Extended release and immediate release products are not bioequivalent, as higher doses of the extended release product may be necessary. Doses may be administered with or without food.

OXYBUTYNIN CHLORIDE
Ditropan XL, Oxytrol, Oxytrol for Women, and
generics; previously available as Ditropan
Anticholinergic agent, antispasmodic

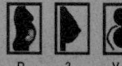 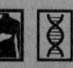

B   ?   Yes   Yes   No

Tabs: 5 mg
Tabs, extended release (Ditropan XL and generics): 5, 10, 15 mg
Syrup: 1 mg/mL (473 mL); contains parabens
Transdermal system (Oxytrol, Oxytrol for Women [OTC]): Delivers 3.9 mg/24 hr (1, 4, 8s); contains 36 mg per system

Child ≤5 yr:
   Immediate release: 0.2 mg/kg/dose BID–TID PO; **max. dose:** 15 mg/24 hr
Child >5 yr:
   Immediate release: 5 mg/dose BID–TID PO; **max. dose:** 20 mg/24 hr
   Extended release (≥6 yr): Start with 5 mg/dose once daily PO; if needed, increase as tolerated by 5 mg weekly increments up to a **maximum** of 20 mg/24 hr.
Adult:
   Immediate release: 5 mg/dose BID–TID PO; **max. dose:** 5 mg QID
   Extended release (Ditropan XL): 5–10 mg/dose once daily PO, adjust in 5-mg weekly increments if needed, up to a **max. dose** of 30 mg/dose once daily PO
   Transdermal system:
      Female: 1 patch (3.9 mg/24 hr) every 4 days
      Male: 1 patch (3.9 mg/24 hr) every 3–4 days (twice weekly)

Use with caution in hepatic or renal disease, hyperthyroidism, GE reflux, IBD, concurrent use of bisphosphonates, or cardiovascular disease. Anticholinergic side effects may occur, including drowsiness, confusion, and hallucinations. **Contraindicated** in glaucoma, GI obstruction, megacolon, myasthenia gravis, severe colitis, hypovolemia, and GU obstruction. Memory impairment, angioedema, and QT-interval prolongation have been reported. Oxybutynin is a CYP 450 3A4 substrate; inhibitors and inducers of CYP 450 3A4 may increase and decrease the effects of oxybutynin, respectively. May antagonize the effects of metoclopramide.

Dosage adjustments for the extended release dosage form are at weekly intervals. The extended release tablets **should not** be crushed, chewed, or divided. Apply transdermal system on dry intact skin on the abdomen, hip, or buttock; rotate the site and avoiding same-site application within 7 days.

OXYCODONE
OxyContin, Roxicodone, RoxyBond, Oxaydo,
Xtampza ER, and many others, including
generics
Narcotic, analgesic

   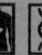

B/D   2   Yes   Yes   No

Expressed as hydrochloride salt unless indicated otherwise.
Oral solution: 1 mg/mL (5, 15, 473 mL); contains alcohol
Concentrated oral solution: 20 mg/mL (30 mL); may contain saccharin
Tabs:
   Generics: 5, 10, 15, 20, 30 mg
   Roxicodone and RoxyBond: 5, 15, 30 mg
   Oxaydo: 5, 7.5 mg
Controlled release tabs (OxyContin and generics): 10, 15, 20, 30, 40, 60, 80 mg (80 mg strength for opioid-tolerant patients only)

Continued

OXYCODONE *continued*

Caps: 5 mg

Extended release caps (Xtampza ER): 9, 13.5, 18, 27, 36 mg oxycodone base; equivalent to 10, 15, 20, 30, and 40 mg oxycodone hydrochloride salt, respectively

Opioid-naïve doses based upon oxycodone hydrochloride salt (limited data):

Infant ≤6 mo: 0.025—0.05 mg/kg/dose Q4—6 hr PRN PO

Infant >6 mo, child, and adolescent <50 kg: 0.05—0.15 mg/kg/dose Q4—6 hr PRN up to 5 mg/dose PO

Adolescent (≥50 kg) and adult: 5—10 mg Q4—6 hr PRN PO; see remarks for use of controlled release tablets

There is a potential for abuse; CNS and respiratory depression, increased ICP, histamine release, constipation, and GI distress may occur. **Use with caution** in severe renal impairment (increases $T_{1/2}$) and mild/moderate hepatic dysfunction (use of one-third to one-half of usual dose has been recommended). **Naloxone is the antidote.** See Chapter 6 for equianalgesic dosing. Check dosages of acetaminophen or aspirin when using combination products (e.g., Percocet, Percodan). Oxycodone is metabolized by the CYP 450 3A4 (major) and 2D6 (minor) isoenzyme.

When controlled release tablets (e.g., Oxycontin) are being used, patient's total 24-hr requirement should be determined and divided by 2 to administer on a Q12 hr dosing interval. Oxycontin 80-mg tablet is **USED ONLY** for opioid-tolerant patients; this strength can cause fatal respiratory depression in opioid-naïve patients. Controlled release dosage form should not be used as a PRN analgesic and must be swallowed whole.

Pregnancy category changes to "D" if used for prolonged periods or in high doses at term.

The FDA has assigned a Risk Evaluation and Mitigation Strategy (REMS) for opioid analgesia; see www.fda.gov/OpioidAnalgesicREMSPCG. The REMS strongly encourages to (1) complete a REMS-compliant education program; (2) counsel patients/caregivers on prescription safe use, risks, storage, and disposal; (3) emphasize the importance of reading the medication guide provided by pharmacists at all times; and (4) consider other methods for improving patient, household, and community safety.

OXYCODONE AND ACETAMINOPHEN
Endocet, Percocet, Roxicet, Prolate, and many
others, including generics
Combination analgesic with a narcotic

C   2   Yes   Yes   No

Tabs (Percocet, Endocet, and others, including generics):

Most common strength: Oxycodone HCl 5 mg + acetaminophen 325 mg

Other strengths:

Oxycodone HCl 2.5 mg + acetaminophen 325 mg

Oxycodone HCl 7.5 mg + acetaminophen 325 mg

Oxycodone HCl 10 mg + acetaminophen 325 mg

Oral solution:

Roxicet: Oxycodone HCl 5 mg + acetaminophen 325 mg/5 mL (500 mL); contains 0.4% alcohol, EDTA, and saccharin

Prolate and generics: Oxycodone HCl 10 mg + acetaminophen 300 mg/5 mL (120, 500 mL); contain EDTA, propylene glycol, and saccharin

Dose based on amount of oxycodone and acetaminophen. **Do not exceed** 4 g/24 hr of acetaminophen.

OXYCODONE AND ACETAMINOPHEN *continued*

See oxycodone and acetaminophen. Check dosages of acetaminophen and oxycodone when using these combination products.

The FDA has assigned a Risk Evaluation and Mitigation Strategy (REMS) for Opioid Analgesia; see www.fda.gov/OpioidAnalgesicREMSPCG. The REMS strongly encourages to (1) complete a REMS-compliant education program; (2) counsel patients/caregivers on prescription safe use, risks, storage and disposal; (3) emphasize the importance of reading the Medication Guide provided by pharmacists at all times; and (4) consider other methods for improving patient, household, and community safety.

OXYCODONE AND ASPIRIN
Various generics; previously available as
Percodan and Endodan
Combination analgesic (narcotic and salicylate)

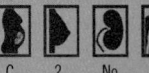 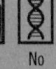

C   2   No   No   No

Tabs: Oxycodone 4.8355 mg and aspirin 325 mg

Dose based on amount of oxycodone and aspirin. **Do not exceed** 4 g/24 hr of aspirin.

See oxycodone and aspirin. **Must not be used** in children <16 yr of age because of risk for Reye syndrome. Check dosages of aspirin and oxycodone when using these combination products.

The FDA has assigned a Risk Evaluation and Mitigation Strategy (REMS) for Opioid Analgesia; see www.fda.gov/OpioidAnalgesicREMSPCG. The REMS strongly encourages to (1) complete a REMS-compliant education program; (2) counsel patients/caregivers on prescription safe use, risks, storage and disposal; (3) emphasize the importance of reading the Medication Guide provided by pharmacists at all times; and (4) consider other methods for improving patient, household, and community safety.

OXYMETAZOLINE
Afrin 12 Hour, Vicks Sinex 12 Hour , Nostrilla,
and many others, including generics
Nasal decongestant, vasoconstrictor

   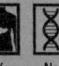 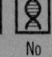

D   2   Yes   Yes   No

Nasal spray (OTC): 0.05% (15 mL); may contain benzalkonium chloride, EDTA, and propylene glycol

Nasal decongestant (not to exceed 3 days in duration):
  ≥**6 yr of age to adult:** 2–3 sprays or 2–3 drops in each nostril BID (separated by 10–12 hr). **Do not exceed** 2 doses/24 hr.

Contraindicated in patients on MAO inhibitor therapy. Rebound nasal congestion may occur with excessive use (>3 days) via the nasal route. Systemic absorption may occur. Headache, insomnia, hypertension, transient burning, stinging, dryness, nasal mucosal ulceration, and sneezing have occurred.

Accidental ingestion in children <5 yr of age has been reported and required hospitalization for adverse events (nausea, vomiting, lethargy, tachycardia, respiratory depression, bradycardia, hypotension, hypertension, sedation, mydriasis, stupor, hypothermia, drooling, and coma).

P

PALIVIZUMAB
Synagis
Monoclonal antibody

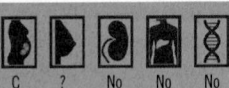

C   ?   No   No   No

Injection, solution: 100 mg/mL (0.5, 1 mL; single use); contains glycine and histidine

RSV prophylaxis during RSV season for the following age and clinical criteria (see latest edition of Red Book for most recent indications).

Following recommendations are from *Pediatrics* 2014;134(2):415—420.

Candidates for recommended use:

<12 mo of age (one of the following):

Born at <29 wks' gestation; OR

With chronic lung disease (CLD) of prematurity (<32 wks' gestation requiring >21% oxygen for at least 28 days after birth); OR

With hemodynamically significant congenital heart disease

<24 mo of age:

Born at ≤32 wks' gestation with CLD requiring medical therapy (e.g., ≥28 days of supplemental oxygen, bronchodilator, diuretics, or chronic steroids) within 6 mo prior to start of RSV season

Candidates for consideration:

<12 mo of age (one of the following):

With congenital airway abnormalities or neuromuscular disorders that decrease ability to manage airway secretions; OR

With cystic fibrosis with clinical evidence of CLD and/or nutritional compromise

≤24 mo of age (one of the following):

With cystic fibrosis with severe lung disease (previous pulmonary exacerbation in first year of life or abnormal chest x-ray) or weight for length less than the 10th percentile; OR

Profoundly immunocompromised; OR

Undergoing cardiac transplantation during RSV season

DOSE:

≤24 mo old: 15 mg/kg/dose IM Q monthly just prior to and during the RSV season. **Maximum** of five doses per RSV season is recommended by the AAP. Therapy should be discontinued if child experiences breakthrough RSV hospitalization.

RSV season typically November through April in the northern hemisphere but may begin earlier or persist later in certain communities. This infection pattern was significantly altered in 2020—2022 due to the implementation of COVID-19 prevention strategies of masking and social distancing. Check with state and county health departments and the CDC for the current RSV activity in your region.

IM is currently the only route of administration, so **use with caution** in patients with thrombocytopenia or any coagulation disorder. The following adverse effects have been reported at slightly higher incidences when compared with placebo: rhinitis, rash, pain, increased liver enzymes, pharyngitis, cough, wheeze, diarrhea, vomiting, conjunctivitis, and anemia. Rare acute hypersensitivity reactions have been reported (first or subsequent doses).

Does not interfere with the response to routine childhood vaccines. May interfere with immunologic-based RSV diagnostic tests (some antigen detection—based assays and viral culture assays) but not with reverse transcriptase-polymerase chain reaction (PCR)—based assays.

Palivizumab is currently indicated for RSV prophylaxis in high-risk infants only. Efficacy and safety have not been demonstrated for treatment of RSV.

PALIVIZUMAB *continued*

Cardiopulmonary bypass and ECMO will significantly reduce serum concentrations; administer a dose immediately after the bypass procedure or ECMO even if it is <1 mo from the previous dose.

Each dose should be administered IM in the anterolateral aspect of the thigh. It is recommended to divide doses with total injection volumes >1 mL. **Avoid** injection in the gluteal muscle because of risk for damage to the sciatic nerve.

PANCRELIPASE/PANCREATIC ENZYMES
Creon, Pancreaze, Pertzye, Ultresa, Viokace, and Zenpep
Pancreatic enzyme

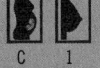   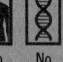

C   1   No   No   No

Delayed release enterically coated beads, microspheres, or minitabs in capsules (porcine derived):

Product	Lipase (USP) Units	Amylase (USP) Units	Protease (USP) Units
Creon[a]			
3	3,000	15,000	9,500
6	6,000	30,000	19,000
12	12,000	60,000	38,000
24	24,000	120,000	76,000
36	36,000	180,000	114,000
Pancreaze[b]			
MT 2	2,600	15,200	8,800
MT 4	4,200	24,600	14,200
MT 10	10,500	61,500	35,500
MT 16	16,800	98,400	56,800
MT 20	21,000	83,900	54,700
MT 37	37,000	149,900	97,300
Pertzye[a,c]			
4	4,000	15,125	14,375
8	8,000	30,250	28,750
16	16,000	60,500	57,500
24	24,000	90,750	86,250
Zenpep[d]			
3	3,000	14,000	10,000
5	5,000	24,000	17,000
10	10,000	42,000	32,000
15	15,000	63,000	47,000
20	20,000	84,000	63,000
25	25,000	105,000	79,000
40	40,000	168,000	126,000

[a]Enteric coated microspheres.
[b]Enteric coated minitabs.
[c]Contains bicarbonate.
[d]Enteric coated beads.

Continued

PANCRELIPASE/PANCREATIC ENZYMES *continued*

Tabs (porcine derived):

Product	Lipase (USP) Units	Amylase (USP) Units	Protease (USP) Units
Viokace			
10	10,440	39,150	39,150
20	20,880	78,300	78,300

Initial doses (actual requirements are patient specific):
Enteric coated microspheres and microtabs:
    Infant: 2000—4000 U lipase per 120 mL (formula or breast milk)
    Child <4 yr: 1000 U lipase/kg/meal
    Child ≥4 yr and adult: 500 U lipase/kg/meal
    Max. dose (child—adult): 2500 U lipase/kg/meal, or 10,000 U lipase/kg/24 hr, or 4000 U lipase/g
    fat/24 hr
Total daily dose should include approximately three meals and two to three snacks per day. Snack
    doses are approximately half of meal doses, depending on the amount of fat and food consumed.

May cause occult GI bleeding, allergic reactions to porcine proteins, hyperuricemia, and
hyperuricosuria with high doses. Dose should be titrated to eliminate diarrhea and to
minimize steatorrhea. **Do not** chew microspheres or microtabs. Concurrent administration with H_2
antagonists or gastric acid pump inhibitors may enhance enzyme efficacy. Doses higher than 6000
U lipase/kg/meal have been associated with colonic strictures in children <12 yr. Non—enteric
coated dosage forms (e.g., powder and tablet) are not preferred, owing to potential GI mucosal
ulceration. Patients who are unable to swallow capsules intact may mix the contents with small
amount of acidic soft foods (pH ≤4.5; such as applesauce), swallow immediately after mixing, and
follow with infant formula, breast milk, or fluids to ensure complete ingestion of the medication.
Avoid use of generic pancreatic enzyme products because they have been associated with treatment
failures. Products not approved by the FDA are no longer allowed to be distributed in the United
States.
Patients requiring enzyme supplementation who receive enteral feeding via a feeding tube may
alternatively use a digestive enzyme cartridge (RELiZORB).

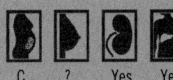

PANCURONIUM BROMIDE
Generics; previously available as Pavulon
Nondepolarizing neuromuscular blocking agent

C   ?   Yes   Yes   No

Injection: 1 mg/mL (10 mL); contains benzyl alcohol

Intermittent dosing (see remarks):
Neonate:
    Initial: 0.02 mg/kg/dose IV
    Maintenance: 0.05—0.1 mg/kg/dose IV Q0.5—4 hr PRN
1 mo—adult:
    Initial: 0.04—0.1 mg/kg/dose IV
    Maintenance: 0.015—0.1 mg/kg/dose IV Q30—60 min
Continuous **IV infusion (see remarks):**
Neonate: 0.02—0.04 mg/kg/hr
Child: 0.03—1 mg/kg/hr

PANCURONIUM BROMIDE *continued*

Adolescent and adult: 0.02—0.04 mg/kg/hr

Onset of action is 1—2 min. May cause tachycardia, salivation, and wheezing. Severe anaphylactic reactions have been reported; cross-reactivity between neuromuscular blocking agents has been reported. Hypoventilation and hypotension have been reported in mechanically ventilated infants.

Drug effects may be accentuated by hypothermia, acidosis, neonatal age, decreased renal function, halothane, succinylcholine, hypokalemia, hyponatremia, hypocalcemia, clindamycin, tetracycline, and aminoglycoside antibiotics. Drug effects may be antagonized by alkalosis, hypercalcemia, peripheral neuropathies, diabetes mellitus, demyelinating lesions, carbamazepine, phenytoin, theophylline, anticholinesterases (e.g., neostigmine, pyridostigmine), and azathioprine. For obese patients, use of lean body weight for dose calculation has been recommended to prevent intense block of long duration and possible overdose.

Antidote is neostigmine (with atropine or glycopyrrolate). **Avoid** use in severe renal impairment (<10 mL/min). Patients with cirrhosis may require a high initial dose to achieve adequate relaxation, but muscle paralysis will be prolonged.

PANTOPRAZOLE
Protonix and generics
Gastric acid pump inhibitor

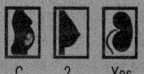 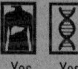

C   2   Yes   Yes   Yes

Tab, delayed release: 20, 40 mg
Injection: 40 mg; contains edetate sodium
Oral suspension: 2 mg/mL ; contains 0.25 mEq sodium bicarbonate per 1 mg drug
Enterically coated granules for delayed release oral suspension: 40 mg packets (30s); may contain polysorbate 80

Child (see remarks):
  GERD (limited data):
    Infant, child, and adolescent: 1—2 mg/kg/24 hr PO once daily; **max. dose:** 40 mg/24 hr × 4—8 weeks
  GERD with erosive esophagitis:
    1—5 yr (limited data): 0.3, 0.6, or 1.2 mg/kg/24 hr PO once daily all improved GERD symptoms in an 8-wk multicenter, randomized placebo control trial for 60 subjects with GERD and histologic/ erosive esophagitis
    ≥5 yr (up to 8 wk of therapy):
      15—<40 kg: 20 mg PO once daily
      ≥40 kg: 40 mg PO once daily
  IV (when PO route not feasible; data limited to pharmacokinetic trials):
    Infant, child, and adolescent: Some doses ranging from 0.32—1.88 mg/kg/dose have been reported from three separate trials (total $N = 31$; 0.01—16.4 yr). Patients with systemic inflammatory response syndrome (SIRS) cleared the drug more slowly, resulting in higher $T_{1/2}$ and AUC, than patients without. Despite limited data, 1—2 mg/kg/24 hr ÷ Q12—24 hr have been used. Additional studies are needed.
Adult:
  GERD with erosive esophagitis:
    PO: 40 mg once daily × 8—16 wk
    IV: 40 mg once daily × 7—10 days
  Peptic ulcer: 40—80 mg PO once daily × 4—8 wk

Continued

PANTOPRAZOLE *continued*

Hypersecretory conditions:

PO: 40 mg BID; dose may be increased as needed up to a **max. dose** of 240 mg/24 hr

IV: 80 mg Q12 hr; dose may be increased as needed to Q8 hr (**max. dose:** 240 mg/24 hr). Therapy >7 days at 240 mg/24 hr has not been evaluated.

Convert from IV to PO therapy as soon as patient is able to tolerate PO. Common side effects include diarrhea and headache. May cause transient elevation in LFTs. Like other PPIs, may increase risk for *Clostridium difficile*—associated diarrhea. Hypomagnesemia has been reported with long-term use. Hypersensitivity reactions (e.g., anaphylaxis, shock, angioedema, bronchospasm, acute interstitial nephritis, TEN, DRESS, and urticaria), agranulocytosis, pancytopenia, hypomagnesemia, and taste disorders have been reported. Fundic gland polyps have been associated with long-term use of PPIs.

May interfere with serum chromogranin A (CgA) diagnostic test for neuroendocrine tumors; discontinue use at least 14 days prior to testing. False-positive test for urine cannabinoid screen may occur.

Drug is a substrate for CYP 450 2C19 (major), 2D6 (minor), and 3A3/4 (minor) isoenzymes. Recommended dosage modification for ultrarapid metabolizers of CYP 2C19 is to increase the usual dose by fivefold. May decrease the absorption of itraconazole, ketoconazole, iron salts, and ampicillin esters. May increase the effect/toxicity of methotrexate. May cause false-positive elevated serum chromogranin A levels.

Children 1—2 yr of age have demonstrated more rapid clearance of pantoprazole in pharmacokinetic studies; this age group may require higher doses. All oral doses may be taken with or without food. **Do not** crush or chew tablets. The extemporaneously compounded oral suspension may be less bioavailable owing to the loss of the enteric coating. Granules for delayed release oral suspension product may be mixed with 5 mL apple juice (administer immediately followed by rinsing container with more apple juice), or sprinkled on 1 teaspoonful of applesauce (administer within 10 min); see package insert for NG administration.

For IV infusion, doses may be administered over 15 min at a concentration of 0.4—0.8 mg/mL or over 2 min at a concentration of 4 mg/mL. Midazolam and zinc are **not compatible** with the IV dosage form. Parenteral routes other than IV are **not recommended.**

PAROMOMYCIN SULFATE
Humatin and generics
Amebicide, antibiotic (aminoglycoside)

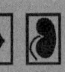

C   1   No   No   No

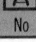

Caps: 250 mg

Intestinal amebiasis (*Entamoeba histolytica*), *Dientamoeba fragilis*, and *Giardia lamblia* infection:
Child and adult: 25—35 mg/kg/24 hr PO ÷ Q8 hr × 5—10 days

Cryptosporidial diarrhea with HIV:
Adult (limited data): 500 mg PO QID for 14—21 days

Contraindicated in intestinal obstruction. **Use with caution** in ulcerative bowel lesions to avoid renal toxicity via systemic absorption. Drug is generally poorly absorbed and therefore not indicated for sole treatment of extraintestinal amebiasis. Side effects include GI disturbance, hematuria, rash, ototoxicity, and hypocholesterolemia. Bacterial overgrowth of nonsusceptible organisms, including fungi, may occur. May decrease the effects of digoxin.

PAROXETINE
Paxil, Pexeva, Paxil CR, and generics
Antidepressant, selective serotonin reuptake inhibitor

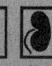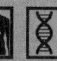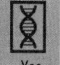

D   2   Yes   Yes   Yes

Tabs (Paxil, Pexeva, and generics): 10, 20, 30, 40 mg
Caps: 7.5 mg
Controlled release tabs (Paxil CR and generics): 12.5, 25, 37.5 mg
Oral suspension (Paxil and generics): 10 mg/5 mL (250 mL); contains saccharin and parabens

Child:
Depression: Well-controlled clinical trials have failed to demonstrate efficacy in children.
The FDA recommends paroxetine not be used for this indication.
Obsessive-compulsive disorder (limited data, based on a 10-wk randomized controlled trial in 207 children 7–17 yr; mean age 11.1 + 3.03 yr): Start with 10 mg PO once daily. If needed, adjust upward by increasing dose no more than 10 mg/24 hr no more frequently than Q7 days up to a **max. dose** of 60 mg/24 hr. Mean doses of 20.3 mg/24 hr (children) and 26.8 mg/24 hr (adolescents) were used.
Social anxiety disorder (limited data; 8–17 yr): Start with 10 mg PO once daily. If needed, increase dose by 10 mg/24 hr no more frequently than Q7 days up to a **max. dose** of 50 mg/24 hr.
Adult:
Depression:
Immediate release dosage forms: Start with 20 mg PO QAM × 4 wk. If no clinical improvement, increase dose by 10 mg/24 hr Q7 days PRN up to a **max. dose** of 50 mg/24 hr.
Controlled release tabs (Paxil CR and generics): Start with 25 mg PO QAM × 4 wk. If no improvement, increase dose by 12.5 mg/24 hr Q7 days PRN up to a **max. dose** of 62.5 mg/24 hr.
Obsessive-compulsive disorder (immediate release): Start with 20 mg PO once daily; increase dose by 10 mg/24 hr Q7 days PRN up to a **max. dose** of 60 mg/24 hr. Usual dose is 40 mg PO once daily. Rapid metabolizers may require doses as high as 100 mg/24 hr.
Panic disorder:
Immediate release dosage forms: Start with 10 mg PO QAM; increase dose by 10 mg/24 hr Q7 days PRN up to a **max. dose** of 60 mg/24 hr.
Paxil CR: Start with 12.5 mg PO QAM; increase dose by 12.5 mg/24 hr Q7 days PRN up to a **max. dose** of 75 mg/24 hr.

Contraindicated in patients taking MAO inhibitors (within 14 days of discontinuing MAO inhibitors), linezolid, methylene blue, pimozide, or thioridazine. **Use with caution** in patients with history of seizures, renal or hepatic impairment, cardiac disease, suicidal concerns, mania/hypomania, concurrent use with other serotonergic drugs (e.g., triptans, fentanyl, lithium, tramadol, amphetamines, or St. John's wort), and diuretic use. Patients with severe renal or hepatic impairment should initiate therapy at 10 mg/24 hr and increase dose as needed up to a **max.** of 40 mg/24 hr.
Common side effects include anxiety, nausea, anorexia, sexual dysfunction, and decreased appetite. Monitor for clinical worsening of depression and suicidal ideation/behavior following the initiation of therapy or after dose changes. Stevens-Johnson syndrome has been reported.
Paroxetine is an inhibitor and substrate for CYP 450 2D6. Ultrametabolizers of CYP 2D6 should avoid use of paroxetine and use an alternative medication not metabolized by this enzyme system. A 50% initial dose reduction for poor CYP 2D6 metabolizers has been recommended. May increase the effects/toxicity of tricyclic antidepressants, theophylline, and warfarin. May decrease the effects of tamoxifen. Cimetidine, ritonavir, MAO inhibitors (fatal serotonin syndrome), dextromethorphan, phenothiazines, and type 1C antiarrhythmics may increase the effect/toxicity of paroxetine. Weakness, hyperreflexia, and poor coordination have been reported when taken with sumatriptan.

Continued

PAROXETINE *continued*

Do not discontinue therapy abruptly; may cause sweating, dizziness, confusion, and tremor. May be taken with or without food.

PENICILLIN G PREPARATIONS—AQUEOUS POTASSIUM AND SODIUM
Pfizerpen and generics
Antibiotic, aqueous penicillin

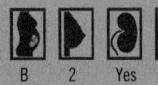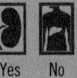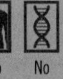

B   2   Yes   No   No

Injection (K$^+$): 5, 20 million units (contains 1.7 mEq K and 0.3 mEq Na/1 million units penicillin G)
Premixed frozen injection (K$^+$): 1 million units in 50 mL dextrose 4%; 2 million units in 50 mL dextrose 2.3%; 3 million units in 50 mL dextrose 0.7% (contains 1.7 mEq K and 0.3 mEq Na/1 million units penicillin G)
Injection (Na$^+$): 5 million units (contains 2 mEq Na/1 million units penicillin G)
Conversion: 250 mg = 400,000 units

Neonate (IM/IV; use higher end of dosage range for meningitis and severe infections):
≤34 wks' gestation:
   ≤7 days old: 100,000—200,000 units/kg/24 hr ÷ Q12 hr
   8—28 days old: 150,000—300,000 units/kg/24 hr ÷ Q8 hr
>34 wks' gestation:
   ≤7 days old:
      General dosing: 100,000 units/kg/24 hr ÷ Q12 hr
      Meningitis and severe infection: 300,000 units/kg/24 hr ÷ Q8 hr
   8—28 days old:
      General dosing: 150,000 units/kg/24 hr ÷ Q8 hr
      Meningitis and severe infection: 400,000 units/kg/24 hr ÷ Q6 hr
Group B streptococcal meningitis:
   ≤7 days old: 450,000 units/kg/24 hr ÷ Q8 hr
   8—28 days old: 500,000 units/kg/24 hr ÷ Q4—6 hr
Congenital syphilis (total of 10 days of therapy; if >1 day of therapy is missed, restart the entire course):
   ≤7 days old: 100,000 units/kg/24 hr ÷ Q12 hr IV; increase to the following dosage at day 8 of life
   8—28 days old: 150,000 units/kg/24 hr ÷ Q8 hr IV
   >28—60 days old: 200,00 units/kg/24 hr ÷ Q6 hr IV; if full-term neonate, may receive higher dose of 300,000 units/kg/24 hr ÷ Q4 hr IV
Infant, child, and adolescent:
   IM/IV (use higher end of dosage range and Q4 hr interval for meningitis and severe infections): 100,000—400,000 units/kg/24 hr ÷ Q4—6 hr; **max. dose:** 24 million units/24 hr
   Neurosyphilis:
      Infant and child: 200,000—300,000 units/kg/24 hr ÷ Q4—6 hr IV × 10—14 days; **max. dose:** 24 million units/24 hr
      Adolescent: 3—4 million units Q4 hr IV × 10—14 days; **max. dose:** 24 million units/24 hr
Adult:
   Moderate/severe infection (IM/IV): 12—24 million units/24 hr ÷ Q4—6 hr; lower doses may be indicated for other indications
   Neurosyphilis: 18—24 million units/24 hr ÷ Q4 hr IV × 10—14 days

---

Use penicillin V potassium for oral use. Side effects: anaphylaxis, urticaria, hemolytic anemia, interstitial nephritis, Jarisch-Herxheimer reaction (syphilis). Preparations containing potassium and/or sodium salts may alter serum electrolytes. $T_{1/2}$ = 30 min; may be prolonged by

PENICILLIN G PREPARATIONS—AQUEOUS POTASSIUM
AND SODIUM *continued*

concurrent use of probenecid. For meningitis, use higher daily dose at shorter dosing intervals. For
the treatment of anthrax (*Bacillus anthracis*), see www.bt.cdc.gov for additional information.
Adjust dose in renal impairment (see Chapter 31).

Tetracyclines, chloramphenicol, and erythromycin may antagonize penicillin's activity. Probenecid
increases penicillin levels. May cause false-positive or false-negative urinary glucose (Clinitest
method), false-positive direct Coombs test, and false-positive urinary and/or serum proteins.

PENICILLIN G PREPARATIONS—BENZATHINE
Bicillin L-A
Antibiotic, penicillin (very-long-acting IM)

    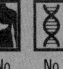

B 2 Yes No No

Injection: 600,000 units/mL (1, 2, 4 mL); contains parabens and povidone
Injection should be IM only.

Group A streptococci:
    Infant and child: 25,000–50,000 units/kg/dose IM × 1. **Max. dose:** 1.2 million units/dose **OR:**
    >1 mo and <27 kg: 600,000 units/dose IM × 1
    ≥27 kg and adult: 1.2 million units/dose IM × 1
Rheumatic fever prophylaxis (Q3 wk administration is recommended for high-risk situations):
    Infant and child (>1 mo and <27 kg): 600,000 units/dose IM Q3–4 wk
    Child ≥27 kg and adult: 1.2 million units/dose IM Q3–4 wk
Congenital syphilis (for cases of low probability of disease; aqueous penicillin is the drug of choice):
    Neonate: 50,000 units/kg/dose IM × 1
**Syphilis (if >1 day of therapy is missed, restart the entire course; divided total dose into two
injection sites):**
    Infant and child:
        Primary, secondary, and early latent syphilis (<1-yr duration): 50,000 units/kg/dose × 1
        Late latent syphilis or latent syphilis of unknown duration: 50,000 units/kg/dose Q7 days × 3
        doses
        Max. dose: 2.4 million units/dose
    Adult:
        Primary, secondary, and early latent syphilis: 2.4 million units/dose IM × 1
        Late latent syphilis or latent syphilis of unknown duration: 2.4 million units/dose IM Q7 days × 3 doses

Provides sustained levels for 2–4 wk. **Use with caution** in renal failure, asthma, G6PD
deficiency (risk for methemoglobinemia), and cephalosporin hypersensitivity. Side effects
and drug interactions same as for Penicillin G Preparations—Aqueous Potassium and Sodium. Injection
site reactions are common. Severe cutaneous reactions (e.g., SJS, TEN, and DRESS) have been reported.
Deep IM administration only. Do not administer intravenously (cardiac arrest and death may occur),
and **do not inject** into or near an artery or nerve (may result in permanent neurologic damage and
necrosis/sloughing at the injection site).

**PENICILLIN G PREPARATIONS—PENICILLIN G BENZATHINE
AND PENICILLIN G PROCAINE**
Bicillin C-R, Bicillin C-R 900/300
Antibiotic, penicillin (very-long-acting IM)

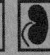 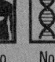

B 2 Yes No No

Bicillin CR: 300,000 units penicillin G procaine + 300,000 units penicillin G benzathine/mL to provide
600,000 units penicillin per 1 mL (2 mL Tubex syringe)

Continued

PENICILLIN G PREPARATIONS—PENICILLIN G BENZATHINE
AND PENICILLIN G PROCAINE *continued*

Bicillin CR (900/300): 150,000 units penicillin G procaine + 450,000 units penicillin G benzathine/mL
(2 mL Tubex syringe)
All preparations contain parabens and povidone.
Injection should be for IM use only.

Dosage based on total amount of penicillin.
Group A streptococci (see remarks):
  Infant and child (Bicillin CR):
    <14 kg: 600,000 units/dose IM × 1
    14—27 kg: 900,000—1,200,000 units/dose IM × 1
  Child >27 kg and adult:
    Bicillin C-R: 2,400,000 units/dose IM × 1
    Bicillin C-R 900/300: 1,200,000 units/dose IM × 1
Pneumococcal infection (non-CNS): Dosed Q2—3 days until afebrile for 48 hr (see remarks)
  Child (Bicillin C-R): 600,000 units/dose IM
  Adult (Bicillin C-R or Bicillin C-R 900/300): 1,200,000 units/dose IM

This preparation provides early peak levels in addition to prolonged levels of penicillin in the
blood. **Do not use this product to treat syphilis; treatment failure can occur. Use with
caution** in renal failure, asthma, significant allergies, G6PD deficiency (risk for
methemoglobinemia), and cephalosporin hypersensitivity. Severe cutaneous reactions (e.g., SJS,
TEN, and DRESS) have been reported. The addition of procaine penicillin has not been shown to be
more efficacious than benzathine alone. However, it may reduce injection discomfort.

Deep IM administration only. Do not administer intravenously (cardiac arrest and death may occur),
and **do not** inject into or near an artery or nerve (may result in permanent neurologic damage and
necrosis/sloughing at the injection site).

Side effects and drug interactions same as for Penicillin G Preparations—Aqueous Potassium and
Sodium. Immune hypersensitivity reaction has been reported.

PENICILLIN G PREPARATIONS—PROCAINE
Generics; previously available as Wycillin
Antibiotic, penicillin (long-acting IM)

B	2	Yes	No	No

Injection: 600,000 units/mL (1, 2 mL); may contain parabens, phenol, povidone, and formaldehyde)
Contains 120 mg procaine per 300,000 units penicillin
Injection should be for IM use only.

General dosing:
  Newborn: 50,000 units/kg/24 hr IM once daily
  Infant, child, adolescent: 50,000 units/kg/24 hr ÷ Q12—24 hr IM. **Max. dose:** 1.2 million units/24 hr
  Adult: 0.6—1 million units/24 hr ÷ Q12—24 hr IM
**Congenital syphilis, syphilis (if >1 day of therapy is missed, restart the entire course; see
remarks):**
  Neonate, infant, child: 50,000 units/kg/dose once daily IM × 10 days; **max. dose:** 2.4 million units/24
    hr
Neurosyphilis (see remarks):
  Adolescent and adult: 2.4 million units IM once daily and probenecid 500 mg Q6 hr PO × 10—14 days
    (both medications)

PENICILLIN G PREPARATIONS—PROCAINE *continued*

Inhaled anthrax: Postexposure prophylaxis (not the preferred drug of choice but total duration of therapy with all forms of therapy is 60 days; switch to an alternative form of therapy after 2 wk of procaine penicillin because of the risk for adverse effects; see remarks):

Child and adolescent: 25,000 units/kg/dose (**max. dose:** 1.2 million units/dose) IM Q12 hr
Adult: 1.2 million units IM Q12 hr

Provides sustained levels for 2—4 days. **Use with caution** in renal failure, asthma, significant allergies, cephalosporin hypersensitivity, G6PD deficiency (risk for methemoglobinemia), and neonates (higher incidence of sterile abscess at injection site and risk of procaine toxicity). Side effects and drug interactions similar to Penicillin G Preparations—Aqueous Potassium and Sodium. In addition, may cause CNS stimulation and seizures. Immune hypersensitivity reaction has been reported.

Deep IM administration only. Do not administer intravenously (cardiac arrest and death may occur), and **do not inject** into or near an artery or nerve (may result in permanent neurologic damage). Large doses may be administered in two injection sites. No longer recommended for empiric treatment of gonorrhea due to resistant strains.

PENICILLIN V POTASSIUM
Generics; previously available as Veetids
Antibiotic, penicillin

B   2   Yes   No   No

Tabs: 250, 500 mg
Oral solution: 125 mg/5 mL, 250 mg/5 mL (100, 200 mL); may contain saccharin
Contains 0.7 mEq potassium/250 mg drug
Conversion: 250 mg = 400,000 units

Infant and child: 25—75 mg/kg/24 hr ÷ Q6—8 hr PO; **max. dose:** 2 g/24 hr
Adolescent and adult: 125—500 mg/dose PO Q6—8 hr
Acute group A streptococcal pharyngitis (use BID dosing regimen ONLY if good compliance is expected):
Child <27 kg: 250 mg PO BID—TID × 10 days
Child ≥27 kg, adolescent, and adult: 500 mg PO BID—TID × 10 days
Rheumatic fever prophylaxis, and pneumococcal prophylaxis for sickle cell disease and functional or anatomic asplenia (regardless of immunization status):
2 mo—<3 yr: 125 mg PO BID
3—5 yr: 250 mg PO BID; for sickle cell and asplenia, use may be discontinued after 5 yr of age if child received recommended pneumococcal immunizations and did not experience invasive pneumococcal infection
Recurrent rheumatic fever prophylaxis:
Child and adult: 250 mg PO BID

See Penicillin G Preparations—Aqueous Potassium and Sodium for side effects and drug interactions. GI absorption is better than penicillin G. **Note:** Must be taken 1 hr before or 2 hr after meals. Penicillin will prevent rheumatic fever if started within 9 days of the acute illness.
Adjust dose in renal failure (see Chapter 31).

PENTAMIDINE ISETHIONATE
Pentam 300, NebuPent, and generics
Antibiotic, antiprotozoal

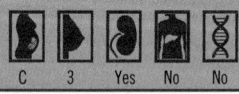

C   3   Yes   No   No

Injection (Pentam 300 and generics): 300 mg
Inhalation (NebuPent and generics): 300 mg

Treatment (child and adult):
  Pneumocystis jiroveci (carinii): 4 mg/kg/24 hr IM/IV once daily × 14—21 days (IV is the preferred route)
  Trypanosomiasis (*Trypanosoma gambiense*, *Trypanosoma rhodesiense* without CNS involvement): 4 mg/kg/24 hr IM/IV once daily × 7—10 days
  Visceral leishmaniasis (*Leishmania donovani, L. infantum, L. chagasi*): 2—4 mg/kg/dose IM/IV once daily, or once every other day × 15—30 doses
  Cutaneous leishmaniasis (*Leishmania [Viannia] panamensis*): 2—4 mg/kg/dose IM/IV once or twice a week until lesions healed
Prophylaxis (child and adult):
  P. jiroveci (carinii):
    IM/IV (IV is the preferred route): 4 mg/kg/dose Q4 wk (Q2—4 wk for hematopoietic stem cell transplant); **max. single dose:** 300 mg
    Inhalation (use with Respigard II nebulizer):
      <5 yr: 9 mg/kg (**max. dose:** 300 mg/dose) Q month
      ≥5 yr: 300 mg Q month

Use with caution in ventricular tachycardia, Stevens-Johnson syndrome, and daily doses >21 days. May cause hypoglycemia, hyperglycemia, hypotension (both IV and IM administration), nausea, vomiting, fever, mild hepatotoxicity, pancreatitis, megaloblastic anemia, nephrotoxicity, hypocalcemia, and granulocytopenia. Additive nephrotoxicity with aminoglycosides, amphotericin B, cisplatin, and vancomycin may occur. Aerosol administration may also cause bronchospasm, cough, oxygen desaturation, dyspnea, and loss of appetite. Infuse IV over 1—2 hr to reduce the risk of hypotension. Sterile abscess may occur at IM injection site.
Adjust dose in renal impairment (see Chapter 31) with systemic use.

PENTOBARBITAL
Nembutal and generics
Barbiturate

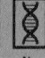

D   3   No   Yes   No

Injection: 50 mg/mL (20, 50 mL); contains propylene glycol and 10% alcohol

Hypnotic
  Child:
    IM: 2—6 mg/kg/dose. **Max. dose:** 100 mg
  Adult:
    IM: 150—200 mg
Reduction in elevated ICP (adjunct therapy; patient must be intubated): Barbiturate coma may be used if needed.
  Child and adolescent:
    IV/IO: 1—3 mg/kg/dose
    IM/PR: 2—6 mg/kg/dose
    Max. dose: 100 mg/dose

PENTOBARBITAL *continued*

Barbiturate coma
Child and adult:
IV: Loading dose: 10—15 mg/kg given slowly over 1—2 hr
Maintenance: Begin at 1 mg/kg/hr. Usual range: 0.5—5 mg/kg/hr as needed

Contraindicated in liver failure and history of porphyria. Use in preprocedure sedation has been replaced by other agents. **Use with caution** in hypovolemic shock, CHF, hypotension, and hepatic impairment. No advantage over phenobarbital for control of seizures. May cause drug-related isoelectric EEG. **Do not administer** for >2 wk in treatment of insomnia. May cause hypotension, arrhythmias, hypothermia, respiratory depression, and dependence.
Onset of action: IM: 10—15 min; IV: 1 min. Duration of action: IV: 15 min.
Administer IV at a rate of <50 mg/min.
Therapeutic serum levels: sedation: 1—5 mg/L; hypnosis: 5—15 mg/L; coma: 20—40 mg/L (steady state is achieved after 4—5 days of continuous IV dosing).

PERMETHRIN
Nix and generics; previously available as Elimite
Scabicidal agent

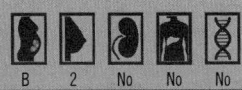

B   2   No   No   No

Cream (generics): 5% (60 g); contains 0.1% formaldehyde
Liquid cream rinse/lotion (Nix Lice-Killing Crème Rinse—OTC and generics) [OTC]: 1% (59 mL with comb); may contain 20% isopropyl alcohol (1 or 2 bottles)
Additional OTC permethrin products for use on bedding, furniture, and garments include the following:
Liquid spray (Nix Lice Control Spray): 0.25% (150 mL)
Spray (Rid Home Lice, Bedbug, and Dust Mite Spray): 0.5% (141.8 g)

Pediculus humanus capitis, Phthirus pubis (>2 mo, child, and adolescent):
Head lice: Saturate hair and scalp and apply behind the ears and at the base of the neck with 1% cream rinse/lotion after shampooing, rinsing, and towel drying hair. Leave on for 10 min, then rinse. May repeat in 7 days. May be used for lice in other areas of the body (e.g., pubic lice) in same fashion. If the 1% cream rinse is resistant, the 5% cream may be used after shampooing, rinsing, and towel drying hair. Leave on for 8—14 hr overnight under a shower cap; then rinse off. May repeat in 7 days.
Scabies: Apply 5% cream from neck to toe (head to toe for infants and toddlers); wash off with water in 8—14 hr. May repeat in 14 days if mites appear. Use in full-term infants <1 mo is safe and effective when applied for a 6-hr period.

Ovicidal activity generally makes single-dose regimen adequate. However, resistance to permethrin has been reported. May cause pruritus, hypersensitivity, burning, stinging, erythema, and rash. For either lice or scabies, instruct patient to launder bedding and clothing. For lice, treat symptomatic contacts only. For scabies, treat all contacts even if asymptomatic.
Avoid contact with eyes during application. **Do not use** near eyes, inside of nose, mouth, or vagina, or for lice in eyebrows/eyelashes. Topical cream dosage form contains formaldehyde. Dispense 60 g per one adult or two small children.

PHENAZOPYRIDINE HCL
Pyridium, Azo-Urinary Pain Relief [OTC], Azo-
Urinary Pain Relief Maximum Strength [OTC],
many other brands and generics
Urinary analgesic

 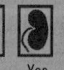 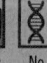

| B | 3 | Yes | Yes | No |

Tabs: 95 mg [OTC] (12s, 30s), 99.5 mg [OTC] (24s, 72s), 100 mg, 200 mg
Oral suspension: 10 mg/mL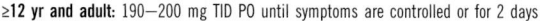

UTI (use with an appropriate antibacterial agent):
  Child 6—<12 yr: 12 mg/kg/24 hr ÷ TID PO until symptoms of lower urinary tract irritation
    are controlled or for 2 days. **Max. dose:** 200 mg/dose
  ≥12 yr and adult: 190—200 mg TID PO until symptoms are controlled or for 2 days

May cause pruritus, rash, GI distress, vertigo, and headache. Anaphylactoid-like reaction,
  methemoglobinemia, hemolytic anemia, and renal and hepatic toxicity have been reported,
  usually at overdosage levels. Colors urine orange; stains clothing. May also stain contact lenses and
  interfere with urinalysis tests based on spectrometry or color reactions. Give doses with or after
  meals.
**Avoid use in moderate/severe renal impairment; adjust dose in mild renal impairment
(see Chapter 31).**

PHENOBARBITAL
Generics; previously available as Luminal
Barbiturate

   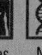 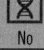

| D | 2 | Yes | Yes | No |

Tabs: 15, 16.2, 30, 32.4, 60, 64.8, 97.2, 100 mg
Oral elixir or solution: 20 mg/5 mL (473 mL); may contain 15% alcohol
Injection: 65, 130 mg/mL (1 mL); may contain 10% alcohol and propylene glycol

Status epilepticus:
  Loading dose, IV:
    Neonate, infant, and child: 15—20 mg/kg/dose (**max. loading dose:** 1000 mg) in a single or divided
      dose. May give additional 5 mg/kg doses Q20 min to a **max. total** of 30 mg/kg
  Seizures maintenance therapy (PO/IV): Monitor levels.
    Neonate: 3—5 mg/kg/24 hr ÷ once daily—BID
    Infant: 5—6 mg/kg/24 hr ÷ once daily—BID
    Child 1—5 yr: 6—8 mg/kg/24 hr ÷ once daily—BID
    Child 6—12 yr: 4—6 mg/kg/24 hr ÷ once daily—BID
    >12 yr: 1—3 mg/kg/24 hr ÷ once daily—-BID
Hyperbilirubinemia (limited data; <12 yr): 3—8 mg/kg/24 hr PO ÷ BID—TID. Doses up to 12 mg/kg/
  24 hr have been used. Not recommended for biliary cirrhosis.
Preoperative sedation (child): 1—3 mg/kg/dose IM/IV/PO × 1. Give 60—90 min before procedure.

Contraindicated in porphyria, severe respiratory disease with dyspnea, or obstruction. **Use with
caution** in hepatic or renal disease (reduce dose). IV administration may cause respiratory
arrest or hypotension. Side effects include drowsiness, cognitive impairment, ataxia, hypotension,
hepatitis, rash, respiratory depression, apnea, megaloblastic anemia, and anticonvulsant
hypersensitivity syndrome. Paradoxic reaction in children (not dose related) may cause hyperactivity,
irritability, or insomnia. Induces several liver enzymes (CYP 450 1A2, 2A6, 2B6, 2C8/9, 3A4),
P-glycoprotein, and glucoronidation (UGT1A1), and thus decreases blood levels of many drugs
(e.g., anticonvulsants). **IV push not to exceed 1 mg/kg/min.**

PHENOBARBITAL *continued*

$T_{1/2}$ is variable with age: neonates, 45—100 hr; infants, 20—133 hr; children, 37—73 hr. Owing to long half-life, consider other agents for sedation for procedures.

Therapeutic levels: 15—40 mg/L. Recommended serum sampling time at steady state: trough level obtained within 30 min prior to the next scheduled dose after 10—14 days of continuous dosing.

Adjust dose in renal failure (see Chapter 31).

PHENTOLAMINE MESYLATE
OraVerse and generics; previously available as Regitine
Adrenergic blocking agent (α); antidote, extravasation

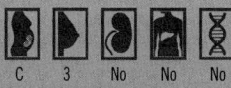

C   3   No   No   No

Injection: 5 mg vial; may contain mannitol
Injection in solution for submucosal use:
  OraVerse: 0.4 mg/1.7 mL (1.7 mL in dental cartridges) (10s); contains edetate disodium

Treatment of α-adrenergic drug extravasation (most effective within 12 hr of extravasation):
  All doses are five doses administered SC around the site of extravasation within 12 hr of extravasation. Monitor for hypotension (BP) Q15 min $\times$ 4 then Q1 hr $\times$ 2. See the following table for weight-based dosing and recommended drug concentration.

Patient Weight	Drug Concentration (Diluted With Preservative-Free NS)	Dose for Each Syringe $\times$ 5 Syringes	Total Dose From All 5 Syringes
<2.5 kg	0.2 mg/mL	0.1 mL	0.1 mg
2.5—<5 kg	0.2 mg/mL	0.25 mL	0.25 mg
5—<10 kg	1 mg/mL	0.1 mL	0.5 mg
10—<20 kg	1 mg/mL	0.2 mL	1 mg
20—<30 kg	1 mg/mL	0.4 mL	2 mg
30—<40 kg	1 mg/mL	0.6 mL	3 mg
40—<50 kg	1 mg/mL	0.8 mL	4 mg
≥50 kg	1 mg/mL	1 mL	5 mg

Max. total dose:
  Neonate: 2.5 mg
  Infant, child, adolescent, and adult: 0.1—0.2 mg/kg/dose or 5 mg
Diagnosis of pheochromocytoma, IM/IV:
  Child: 0.05—0.1 mg/kg/dose up to a **max. dose** of 5 mg
  Adult: 5 mg/dose
Hypertension, prior to surgery for pheochromocytoma, IM/IV:
  Child: 0.05—0.1 mg/kg/dose up to a **max. dose** of 5 mg 1—2 hr *before* surgery, repeat Q2—4 hr PRN
  Adult: 5 mg/dose 1—2 hr *before* surgery, repeat Q2—4 hr PRN

Contraindicated in MI, coronary insufficiency, and angina. **Use with caution** in hypotension, arrhythmias, and cerebral vascular spasm/occlusion.

For diagnosis of pheochromocytoma, patient should be resting in a supine position. A blood pressure reduction of more than 35 mm Hg systolic and 24 mm Hg diastolic is considered a positive test for pheochromocytoma. For treatment of extravasation, use 27- to 30-gauge needle with multiple small injections, and monitor site closely because repeat doses may be necessary.

PHENYLEPHRINE HCL
Vazculep, Neo-Synephrine, Biorphen, many
others, and generics
Adrenergic agonist

C   3   No   No   No

Injection:
  Vazculep and generics: 10 mg/mL (1%) (1, 5, 10 mL); may contain metasulfites
  Biorphen and generics: 10 mg/mL (1%) (1 mL ampules); preservative and sulfite free
Ready-to-use injection:
  Biorphen: 0.1 mg/mL (5 mL ampules); preservative and sulfite free
Nasal spray/drops (OTC; may contain benzalkonium chloride):
  0.125% (Little Remedies Decongestant Nose Drops): 0.125% (15 mL)
  0.25% (Neo-Synephrine Mild Strength, Rhinall): 0.25% (15, 30, 40 mL)
  0.5% (Neo-Synephrine Regular Strength): 0.5% (15 mL)
  1% (4-Way Fast Acting, Nasal Four, Neo-Synephrine Extra Strength, and generics): 1% (15, 30 mL)
  NOTE: For Neo-Synephrine 12-hr Nasal, see Oxymetazoline.
Ophthalmic drops (Altafrin and generics): 2.5% (2, 10, 15 mL), 10% (5 mL); contains benzalkonium
  chloride
Tabs (Sudafed PE Sinus Congestion and others) [OTC]: 10 mg
Oral solution (Sudafed PE Children's) [OTC]: 2.5 mg/5 mL (118 mL)

Hypotension:
  To prepare infusion: See p. iii.

  Child:
    IV bolus: 5—20 mCg/kg/dose (**initial max. dose:** 500 mCg/dose, **subsequent max. dose:** 1000 mCg/
      dose) Q10—15 min PRN
    IV drip: Start at 0.1—0.5 mCg/kg/min; titrate to effect.
    IM/SC: 0.1 mg/kg/dose Q1—2 hr PRN; **max. dose:** 5 mg
  Adult:
    IV drip: 0.5—6 mCg/kg/min; titrate to effect
Pupillary dilation (see remarks):
  <1 yr: 2.5% ophthalmic solution; 1 drop in each eye 15—30 min before exam
  Child (≥1 yr) and adult: 2.5% or 10% ophthalmic solution; 1 drop in each eye 10—60 min before exam
Nasal decongestant (in each nostril; give up to 3 days):
  Child 2—<6 yr: 1—3 drops to each nostril of 0.125% solution Q4 hr PRN
  Child 6—12 yr: 1—3 sprays/drops to each nostril of 0.25% solution Q4 hr PRN
  >12 yr—adult: 1—3 sprays/drops to each nostril of 0.25%, 0.5%, or 1% solution Q4 hr PRN
Oral decongestant (see remarks):
  4—<6 yr: 2.5 mg (5 mL) PO Q4 hr PRN, up to 15 mg (30 mL)/24 hr
  ≥6—<12 yr: 5 mg (10 mL) PO Q4 hr PRN up to 30 mg (60 mL)/24 hr
  ≥12 yr and adult: 10 mg PO Q4 hr PRN up to 60 mg/24 hr

Use with caution in presence of arrhythmias, hyperthyroidism, or hyperglycemia. May cause
  tremor, insomnia, or palpitations. Metabolized by MAO. **Contraindicated** in pheochromocytoma
  and severe hypertension. Injectable product may contain sulfites.
Nasal decongestants may cause rebound congestion with excessive use (>3 days). The 1% nasal
  spray can be used in adults with extreme congestion.
Oral phenylephrine is found in a variety of combination cough and cold products and has replaced
  pseudoephedrine and phenylpropanolamine. Over-the-counter (OTC or nonprescription) use of
  this product is **not recommended** for children younger than age 6; reports of serious adverse effects
  (cardiac and respiratory distress, convulsions, and hallucinations) and fatalities (from unintentional
  overdosages, including combined use of other OTC products containing the same active
  ingredients) have been made.

PHENYLEPHRINE HCL *continued*

Ophthalmic use: Apply pressure to the lacrimal sac during and 2 min after administering drops to minimize systemic absorption.

PHENYTOIN
Dilantin, Dilantin Infatab, Phenytoin Infatab,
Phenytek, and generics
Anticonvulsant, class Ib antiarrhythmic

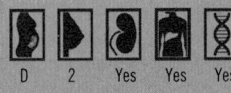

D   2   Yes   Yes   Yes

Chewable tabs (Dilantin Infatab and generics): 50 mg; may contain saccharin
Extended release caps:
  Dilantin: 30, 100 mg
  Phenytek: 200, 300 mg
  Generics: 100, 200, 300 mg
Oral suspension (Dilantin and generics): 125 mg/5 mL (240 mL); contains ≤0.6% alcohol and sodium benzoate
Injection: 50 mg/mL (2, 5 mL); contains alcohol and sodium benzoate

Status epilepticus: See Chapter 1 and remarks.
  Loading dose (all ages): 20 mg/kg IV; **max. dose:** 1500 mg/24 hr
  Maintenance for seizure disorders (initiate 12 hr after administration of loading dose; use once-daily or BID dosing with extended release caps):
    Neonate: Start with 5 mg/kg/24 hr PO/IV ÷ Q12 hr; usual range 4—8 mg/kg/24 hr PO/IV ÷ Q8—12 hr
    Infant/child: Start with 5 mg/kg/24 hr ÷ BID—TID PO/IV; usual dose range (doses divided BID—TID):
      6 mo—3 yr: 8—10 mg/kg/24 hr
      4—6 yr: 7.5—9 mg/kg/24 hr
      7—9 yr: 7—8 mg/kg/24 hr
      10—16 yr: 6—7 mg/kg/24 hr
    Adult: Start with 100 mg/dose Q8 hr IV/PO and carefully titrate (if needed) by 100 mg increments Q2—4 wk to 300—600 mg/24 hr (or 6—7 mg/kg/24 hr) ÷ Q8—24 hr IV/PO.

Contraindicated in patients with heart block or sinus bradycardia; those who are receiving delavirdine (decrease virologic response); and history of hydantoin hypersensitivity. **Use with caution** in patients with pacemakers or cardiac dysrhythmias because of its class IB antiarrhythmic properties. IM administration is **not recommended** because of erratic absorption and pain at injection site; consider fosphenytoin. Side effects include gingival hyperplasia, hirsutism, dermatitis, blood dyscrasia, ataxia, lupus-like and Stevens-Johnson syndromes, lymphadenopathy, liver damage, and nystagmus. Suicidal behavior or ideation, bradycardia, cardiac arrest, red cell aplasia, and multiorgan hypersensitivity (DRESS) have been reported. An increased risk for serious skin reactions (e.g., TEN and Stevens-Johnson) may occur in patients with the HLA-B*1502 allele; do not use this medication in individuals who carry this genotype.
Many drug interactions: Levels may be increased by cimetidine, chloramphenicol, INH, sulfonamides, trimethoprim, etc. Levels may be decreased by some antineoplastic agents. Phenytoin induces hepatic microsomal enzymes (CYP 450 1A2, 2C8/9/19, and 3A3/4), leading to decreased effectiveness of oral contraceptives, direct thrombin inhibitors (e.g., dabigatran, rivaroxaban), fosamprenavir (used without ritonavir), quinidine, lacosamide, valproic acid, theophylline, and other substrates to the previously listed CYP 450 hepatic enzymes. May increase levels of amprenavir when administered with fosamprenavir and ritonavir. May cause resistance to neuromuscular blocking action of nondepolarizing neuromuscular blocking agents (e.g., pancuronium, vecuronium,

Continued

PHENYTOIN *continued*

rocuronium, and cisatracurium) and decrease concentrations of T_4 and T_3 (typically without clinical hypothyroidism). May increase risk for hyperammonemia when used with valproic acid.

The following initial maintenance dose modifications for HLA-B*1502 allele noncarriers and CYP 450 2C9 phenotypes have been recommended:

CYP 2C9 intermediate metabolizer: 25% reduction with therapeutic drug monitoring

CYP 2C9 poor metabolizer: 50% reduction with therapeutic drug monitoring

Some recommend avoiding use for those who are positive for HLA-B*1502 or CYP2C9*3 carriers.

Ideal body weight should be used for calculating dosages. Suggested dosing intervals for specific oral dosage forms: extended release caps (once daily—BID); chewable tablets, and oral suspension (TID). Oral absorption reduced in neonates. $T_{1/2}$ is variable (7—42 hr) and dose dependent. Drug is highly protein bound; free fraction of drug will be increased in patients with hypoalbuminemia.

For seizure disorders, therapeutic levels: 10—20 mg/L (free and bound phenytoin) *OR* 1—2 mg/L (free only). Monitor free phenytoin levels in hypoalbuminemia or renal insufficiency. Recommended serum sampling times: trough level (PO/IV) within 30 min prior to the next scheduled dose; peak or postload level (IV) 1 hr after the end of IV infusion. Steady state is usually achieved after 5—10 days of continuous dosing. For routine monitoring, measure trough.

IV push/infusion rate: **Not to exceed** 0.5 mg/kg/min in neonates, or 1 mg/kg/min in infants, children, and adults with **maximum** of 50 mg/min; may cause cardiovascular collapse. Consider fosphenytoin in situations of tenuous IV access and risk for extravasation.

PHOSPHORUS SUPPLEMENTS
K-PHOS Neutral, Phospho-Trin 250 Neutral,
Phospha 250 Neutral, PHOS-NaK, Sodium
Phosphate, Potassium Phosphate, and many
generics
Electrolyte supplement

   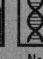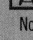

C   2   Yes   No   No

Oral:

Na and K phosphate:

PHOS-NaK and generics; powder: 250 mg (8 mM) P, 6.96 mEq (160 mg) Na, 7.16 mEq (280 mg) K per packet of powder (100s); reconstitute with 75 mL water or juice per packet

K-PHOS Neutral, Phospho-Trin 250 Neutral, Phospha 250 Neutral, and generics; tabs: 250 mg P (8 mM), 13 mEq Na, 1.1 mEq K; administer each dose with a full glass of water

K-PHOS No. 2; tabs: 250 mg P (8 mM), 5.8 mEq Na, 2.3 mEq K; administer each dose with a full glass of water

K phosphate:

K-Phos Original; tabs: 500 mg potassium acid phosphate (114 mg phosphorus and 3.7 mEq K); dissolve each tab in 3—4 oz water

Injection:

Na phosphate: 3 mM (93 mg) P, 4 mEq Na/mL (5, 15, 50 mL)

K phosphate: 3mM (93 mg) P, 4.4 mEq K/mL (5, 15 mL)

Conversion: 31 mg P = 1 mM P

Acute hypophosphatemia: 0.16—0.32 mM/kg/dose (or 5—10 mg/kg/dose) IV over 6 hr

Maintenance/replacement:

Child:

IV: 0.5—1.5 mM/kg (or 15—45 mg/kg) over 24 hr

PO: 30—90 mg/kg/24 hr (or 1—3 mM/kg/24 hr) ÷ TID—QID

PHOSPHORUS SUPPLEMENTS *continued*

Adult:
    IV: 50—65 mM (or 1.5—2 g) over 24 hr
    PO: 3—4.5 g/24 hr (or 100—150 mM/24 hr) ÷ TID—QID
Recommended IV infusion rate: ≤0.1 mM/kg/hr (or 3.1 mg/kg/hr) of phosphate. When potassium salt is used, the rate will be limited by the **max.** potassium infusion rate. **Do not** co-infuse with calcium-containing products.

May cause tetany, hyperphosphatemia, hyperkalemia, or hypocalcemia. **Use with caution** in patients with renal impairment. Be aware of sodium and/or potassium load when supplementing phosphate. IV administration may cause hypotension and renal failure, or arrhythmias, heart block, and cardiac arrest with potassium salt. PO dosing may cause nausea, vomiting, abdominal pain, or diarrhea. See Chapter 21 for daily requirements and Chapter 11 for additional information on hypophosphatemia and hyperphosphatemia.

PHYSOSTIGMINE SALICYLATE
Generics; previously available as Antilirium
Cholinergic agent

  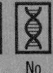

C   ?   No   No   No

Injection: 1 mg/mL (2 mL); contains 2% benzyl alcohol and 0.1% sodium metabisulfite

Reversal of toxic anticholinergic effects from antihistamine or anticholinergic agents:
    Child: 0.02 mg/kg/dose (**max. dose:** 0.5 mg/dose) IM or IV (administered no >0.5 mg/min), dose may be repeated every 5—10 min if no response or return of anticholinergic symptoms up to a **max. total** of 2 mg
    Adult: 0.5—2 mg IM or IV (administered no >1 mg/min); if needed, repeat dose every 10—30 min until response is seen or when adverse effects occur

Physostigmine antidote: Atropine always should be available. **Contraindicated** in asthma, gangrene, diabetes, cardiovascular disease, GI or GU tract obstruction, any vagotonic state, and patients receiving choline esters or depolarizing neuromuscular blocking agents (e.g., decamethonium, succinylcholine). May cause seizures, arrhythmias, bradycardia, GI symptoms, and other cholinergic effects. Rapid IV administration can cause bradycardia and hypersalivation leading to respiratory distress and seizures.

PHYTONADIONE/VITAMIN K₁
Mephyton and generics
Vitamin, fat soluble

    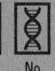

C   2   No   No   No

Tabs (Mephyton and generics): 5 mg
Oral suspension: 1 mg/mL
Injection, emulsion (contains no more than 500 mCg/L aluminum):
    2 mg/mL (0.5 mL); some preparations may be preservative free but may contain propylene glycol
    10 mg/mL (1 mL); contains 0.9% benzyl alcohol

Vitamin K deficiency bleeding (neonatal hemorrhagic disease): Preservative-free dosage form is preferred.
    Prophylaxis (IM, administered 1 hr within 1 hr after birth):
        <1 kg: 0.5 mg/kg/dose × 1
        1—1.5 kg: 0.5 mg × 1
        >1.5 kg: 1 mg × 1
    Treatment: 1—2 mg/24 hr IM/SC/IV

Continued

PHYTONADIONE/VITAMIN K1 *continued*

Warfarin overdose (see remarks):
  No significant bleeding:
    INR 4—4.5: Consider PO vitamin K at dosage indicated for INR >4.5—<10 below and monitor INR Q24 hr. Lower or hold warfarin dose.
    INR >4.5—<10: Repeat INR and hold warfarin dose. Monitor INR Q24 hr until INR <4. Give PO vitamin K for patients with high bleeding risk:
      <40 kg: 0.03 mg/kg PO × 1
      ≥40 kg: 1—2.5 mg PO × 1
    INR ≥10: Repeat INR and hold warfarin dose . Monitor INR Q12 hr and give PO vitamin K (dose may be repeated Q12—24 hr PRN):
      <40 kg: 0.06 mg/kg PO × 1
      ≥40 kg: 5—10 mg PO × 1
  Minor bleeding (any elevated INR): Hold warfarin and monitor INR Q12—24 hr, administer single vitamin K dose and repeat vitamin K dose in 24 hr if full correction not achieved and bleeding persists.
    PO:
      <40 kg: 0.03 mg/kg × 1
      ≥40 kg: 1—2.5 mg × 1
    IV: 0.5—2.5 mg ×1
  Significant or life-threatening bleeding (any elevated INR): Hold warfarin and give vitamin K 5—10 mg IV ×1 in combination with FFP (10—15 mL/kg) or prothrombin complex concentrate (KCentra). Monitor INR Q4—6 hr, repeat vitamin K dose if full correction not achieved at 12—24 hr and bleeding persists.
Vitamin K deficiency:
  Liver disease (infant, child, and adolescent): 2.5—5 mg/24 hr PO
  Cholestasis (infant, child, and adolescent): 2.5—15 mg/24 hr PO

IV or IM doses may cause flushing, dizziness, cardiac/respiratory arrest, hypotension, and anaphylaxis. IV or IM administration is indicated only when other routes of administration are not feasible (or in emergency situations).

Monitor PT/PTT. Large doses (10—20 mg) in newborns may cause hyperbilirubinemia and severe hemolytic anemia. Blood coagulation factors increase within 6—12 hr after oral doses and within 1—2 hr following parenteral administration. Use of higher doses for warfarin overdose may cause warfarin resistance for ≥1 wk. Concurrent administration of oral mineral oil may decrease GI absorption of oral vitamin K.

IV injection rate **not to exceed** 3 mg/m²/min or 1 mg/min. Protect product from light. **See Chapter 21 for multivitamin preparations.**

PILOCARPINE HCL
Vuity, Salagen, and generics; previously
available as Isopto Carpine
Cholinergic agent

    C   3   No   Yes   No

Ophthalmic solution:
  Generics: 1% (15 mL), 2% (15 mL), 4% (15 mL); may contain benzalkonium chloride
  Vuity: 1.25% (2.5 mL); contains benzalkonium chloride
Tab (Salagen and generics): 5, 7.5 mg

For elevated intraocular pressure:
  Infant and child <2 yr: Instill 1 drop of the 1% solution into each affected eye(s) TID.

PILOCARPINE HCL *continued*

Child ≥2 yr, adolescent, and adult: Instill 1–2 drop(s) in each affected eye up to 4 times a day; concentration and dosage frequency are dependent on the degree of elevated pressure and miotic response.

Xerostomia:
Adult: 5 mg/dose PO TID, dose may be titrated to 10 mg/dose PO TID in patients who do not respond to lower dose and who are able to tolerate the drug. 5 mg/dose PO QID has been used in Sjögren syndrome.

OPHTHALMIC USE: Contraindicated in acute iritis or anterior chamber inflammation and uncontrolled asthma. May cause transient blurred or dim/dark vision, stinging, burning, lacrimation, headache, and retinal detachment. **Use with caution** in patients with corneal abrasion or significant cardiovascular disease. Use with topical NSAIDs (e.g., ketorolac) may decrease topical pilocarpine effects.

ORAL USE: Sweating, nausea, rhinitis, chills, flushing, urinary frequency, dizziness, asthenia, and headaches have also been reported. Reduce oral dosing in the presence of mild hepatic insufficiency (Child-Pugh score of 5–6); **avoid use** in severe hepatic insufficiency.

PIMECROLIMUS
Elidel and generics
Topical immunosuppressant, calcineurin inhibitor

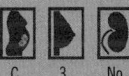 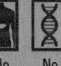

C   3   No   No   No

Cream: 1% (30, 60, 100 g); contains benzyl alcohol and propylene glycol

Atopic dermatitis (second-line therapy):
Child ≥2 yr, adolescent, and adult (see remarks): Apply a thin layer to affected area BID and rub in gently and completely. Reevaluate patient in 6 wk if lesions are not healed.

Do not use in children <2 yr (higher rate of upper respiratory infections), in immunocompromised patients, or with occlusive dressings (promotes systemic absorption). **Avoid use** on malignant or premalignant skin conditions as rare cases of lymphoma and skin malignancy have been reported with topical calcineurin inhibitors. Approved as a second-line therapy for atopic dermatitis for patients who fail to respond, or do not tolerate, other approved therapies. Use medication for short periods of time by using the minimum amounts to control symptoms; long-term safety is unknown. **Avoid** contact with eyes, nose, mouth, and cut, infected, or scraped skin. Minimize and **avoid** exposure to natural and artificial sunlight, respectively.

Most common side effects include burning at the application site, headache, viral infections, and pyrexia. Skin discoloration, skin flushing associated with alcohol use, anaphylactic reactions, ocular irritation after application to the eyelids or near the eyes, angioneurotic edema, and facial edema have been reported. Drug is a CYP 450 3A3/4 substrate.

PIPERACILLIN WITH TAZOBACTAM
Zosyn and generics
Antibiotic, penicillin (extended spectrum with
β-lactamase inhibitor)

   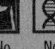

B   2   Yes   No   No

8:1 ratio of piperacillin to tazobactam:
Injection, powder: 2 g piperacillin and 0.25 g tazobactam; 3 g piperacillin and 0.375 g tazobactam; 4 g piperacillin and 0.5 g tazobactam; 12 g piperacillin and 1.5 g tazobactam; 36 g piperacillin and 4.5 g tazobactam

Continued

PIPERACILLIN WITH TAZOBACTAM *continued*

Injection, premixed in iso-osmotic dextrose: 2 g piperacillin and 0.25 g tazobactam in 50 mL; 3 g
piperacillin and 0.375 g tazobactam in 50 mL; 4 g piperacillin and 0.5 g tazobactam in 100 mL
Contains 2.84 mEq Na/g piperacillin

All doses based on piperacillin component.

Neonate and infant (IV; limited data):

  ≤2 kg:

    ≤7 days old: 100 mg/kg/dose Q8 hr

    8—28 days old:

      ≤30 wk postmenstrual age: 100 mg/kg/dose Q8 hr

      >30 wk postmenstrual age: 80 mg/kg/dose Q6 hr

    29—60 days old: 80 mg/kg/dose Q6 hr

  >2 kg:

    ≤60 days old: 80 mg/kg/dose Q6 hr

NOTE: For patients with a postmenstrual age of >35 wk, a pharmacokinetic study suggests using 80
mg/kg/dose IV Q4 hr to achieve targeted drug concentration time above the MIC.

Child and adolescent:

  **Severe infections and nosocomial pneumonia (lengthening the dose administration time to 4 hr
[see remarks] may enhance the pharmacodynamic properties):**

    2—9 mo: 80 mg/kg/dose IV Q6 hr

    >9 mo, child, and adolescent: 100 mg/kg/dose (**max. 4000 mg/dose**) IV Q6 hr

    Max. dose (all ages): 16 g/24 hr

  **Appendicitis or peritonitis (dosing interval may be shortened to Q6 hr to enhance
pharmacodynamic properties):**

    2—9 mo: 80 mg/kg/dose IV Q8 hr

    >9 mo—adolescent:

      ≤40 kg: 100 mg/kg/dose (**max. 3000 mg/dose**) IV Q8 hr

      >40 kg: 3 g/dose IV Q6 hr

    Max. dose (all ages): 16 g/24 hr

Adult:

  Intra-abdominal or soft tissue infections: 3 g IV Q6 hr

  Nosocomial pneumonia: 4 g IV Q6 hr

Cystic fibrosis (antipseudomonal; see remarks):

  All ages: 350—600 mg/kg/24 hr IV ÷ Q4—6 hr; **max. dose:** 24 g/24 hr

---

Tazobactam is a β-lactamase inhibitor, thus extending the spectrum of piperacillin. Like other
penicillins, CSF penetration occurs only with inflamed meninges. GI disturbances, pruritus,
rash, and headaches are common. Abnormal platelet aggregation and prolonged bleeding,
hemophagocytic lymphohistiocytosis, and serious skin reactions (e.g., Stevens-Johnson, DRESS,
acute generalized exanthematous pustulosis, and TEN) have been reported. Cystic fibrosis patients
have an increased risk for fever and rash. Increases in renal failure risk (in critically ill adults) and
incidence of acute kidney injury (in combination with IV vancomycin) have been reported.

Coagulation parameters should be tested more frequently and monitored regularly with high doses of
heparin, warfarin, or other drugs affecting blood coagulation or thrombocyte function. May falsely
decrease aminoglycoside serum levels if the drugs are infused close to one another; allow a
minimum of 2 hr between infusions to prevent this interaction. May prolong the neuromuscular
blockade effects of vecuronium.

Prolonging the dose administration time to 4 hr will maximize the pharmacokinetic/pharmacodynamic
properties by prolonging the time of drug concentration above the MIC; especially for pathogens with
piperacillin MICs of 8—16 mcg/mL. **Adjust dose in renal impairment (see Chapter 31).**

POLYCITRA

See Citrate Mixtures.

POLYETHYLENE GLYCOL—ELECTROLYTE SOLUTION
Bowel cleansing products: GoLYTELY, NuLYTELY, and generics
Laxative products: MiraLax, GaviLAX, GlycoLax, HealthyLax, and many others, including generics
Bowel evacuant, osmotic laxative

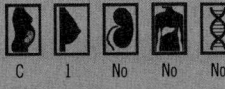

C   1   No   No   No

Powder for oral solution:
Bowel cleansing products:
   GoLYTELY and others: Polyethylene glycol 3350 236 g; contains Na sulfate 22.74 g, Na bicarbonate 6.74 g, NaCl 5.86 g, KCl 2.97 g (mixed with water to 4 L). Contents vary somewhat. See package insert for specific contents of other products.
Laxative products:
   MiraLax [OTC], GaviLAX [OTC], Glycolax [OTC], HealthyLax [OTC], and generics [OTC and Rx]: Polyethylene glycol 3350 (17, 119, 238, 255, 510, 527, 765, 850 g)

Bowel cleansing (using products containing supplemental electrolytes for bowel cleansing such as GoLYTELY, NuLYTELY, and generics; and patients should be NPO 3—4 hr prior to dosing):
Child:
   Oral/nasogastric: 25—40 mL/kg/hr until rectal effluent is clear (usually in 4—10 hr)
Adult:
   Oral: 240 mL PO Q10 min up to 4 L or until rectal effluent is clear
   Nasogastric: 20—30 mL/min (1.2—1.8 L/hr) up to 4 L or until rectal effluent is clear
Bowel cleansing (using MiraLax or equivalent product):
   ≥2 yr and adolescent: 1.5 g/kg/24 hr (**max. dose:** 100 g/24 hr) × 4 days
Constipation (using MiraLax or equivalent product):
   Child (limited data in 20 children with chronic constipation, 18 mo—11 yr; see remarks): A mean effective dose of 0.84 g/kg/24 hr PO ÷ BID for 8 wk (range: 0.25—1.42 g/kg/24 hr) was used to yield 2 soft stools per day. Do not exceed 17 g/24 hr. If stool >20 kg, use adult dose.
   Adult: 17 g (one heaping tablespoonful) mixed in 240 mL of water, juice, soda, coffee, or tea PO once daily
Fecal impaction:
   GoLYTELY and others:
      ≥2 yr (PO/NG tube): 20 mL/kg/hr up to a **maximum** of 1 L/hr × 4 hr per 24 hr for 2 days
   Miralax and others:
      >3 yr: 1—1.5 g/kg/24 hr (**max. dose:** 100 g/24 hr) PO × 3—6 days. Following disimpaction, give a maintenance dose of 0.4—1 g/kg/24 hr for ≥2 mo followed by a gradual decrease in dose.

Contraindicated in polyethylene glycol hypersensitivity. Monitor electrolytes, BUN, serum glucose, and urine osmolality with prolonged administration. Seizures resulting from electrolyte abnormalities have been reported.

BOWEL CLEANSING (GoLYTELY and others): Contraindicated in toxic megacolon, gastric retention, toxic colitis, ileus, and bowel perforation. **Use with caution** in patients prone to aspiration or with impaired gag reflex. **Do not mix** with starch-based thickeners as it may reduce their viscosity and increase the risk of choking and aspiration for patients who have trouble swallowing. Effect should occur within 1—2 hr. Solution generally more palatable if chilled.

Continued

POLYETHYLENE GLYCOL—ELECTROLYTE SOLUTION *continued*

CONSTIPATION (MiraLax and others): **Contraindicated** in bowel obstruction.

Child: Dilute powder using the ratio of 17 g powder to 240 mL of water, juice, or milk. An onset of action within 1 wk in 12 of 20 patients, with the remaining 8 patients reporting improvement during the second week of therapy. Side effects reported in this trial included diarrhea, flatulence, and mild abdominal pain. (See *J Pediatr* 2001;139[3]:428—432 for additional information.)

Adult: 2—4 days may be required to produce a bowel movement. Most common side effects include nausea, abdominal bloating, cramping, and flatulence. Use beyond 2 wk has not been studied.

POLYMYXIN B SULFATE AND BACITRACIN

See Bacitracin ± Polymyxin B.

POLYMYXIN B SULFATE AND TRIMETHOPRIM SULFATE
Polytrim Ophthalmic Solution and generics
Topical antibiotic (ophthalmic preparations listed)

C   2   No   No   No

Ophthalmic solution: Polymyxin B sulfate 10,000 U/mL, and trimethoprim sulfate 1 mg/mL (10 mL); some preparations may contain 0.04 mg/mL benzalkonium chloride

≥2 mo, child, adolescent, and adult: Instill 1 drop in the affected eye(s) Q3 hr (**max. of 6 doses/24 hr**) × 7—10 days

Active against susceptible strains of *Staphylococcus aureus*, *Staphylococcus epidermidis*, *Streptococcus pneumoniae*, *Streptococcus viridans*, *Haemophilus influenzae*, and *Pseudomonas aeruginosa*. **Not indicated** for the prophylaxis or treatment of ophthalmia neonatorum. Local irritation consisting of redness, burning, stinging, and/or itching is common. Hypersensitivity reactions consisting of lid edema, itching, increased redness, tearing, and/or circumocular rash have been reported.

Apply finger pressure to lacrimal sac during and for 1—2 min after dose application.

POLYMYXIN B SULFATE, NEOMYCIN SULFATE, HYDROCORTISONE OTIC
Generics; previously available as Cortisporin Otic
Topical otic antibiotic

C   2   No   No   No

Otic solution or suspension: Polymyxin B sulfate 10,000 U/mL, neomycin sulfate 5 mg/mL (3.5 mg/mL neomycin base), hydrocortisone 10 mg/mL (10 mL); some preparations may contain thimerosol and metabisulfite

For ophthalmic suspension, see Neomycin/Polymyxin B Ophthalmic Products.

Otitis externa:

≥2 yr, child, and adolescent: 3 drops TID—QID × 7—10 days. If preferred, a cotton wick may be saturated and inserted into ear canal. Moisten wick with antibiotic every 4 hr. Change wick Q24 hr.

Adult: 4 drops TID—QID × 7—10 days (otic suspension preferred)

Contraindicated in patients with active varicella and herpes simplex and in cases with perforated eardrum (possible ototoxicity). **Use with caution** in chronic otitis media and when the integrity of the tympanic membrane is in question. Metabisulfite-containing products may

POLYMYXIN B SULFATE, NEOMYCIN SULFATE,
HYDROCORTISONE OTIC *continued*

cause allergic reactions to susceptible individuals. Hypersensitivity (itching, skin rash, redness,
swelling, or other sign of irritation in or around the ear) may occur. Neomycin may cause
sensitization. Prolonged treatment may result in overgrowth of nonsusceptible organisms and fungi.
May cause cutaneous sensitization.

Shake suspension well before use. Warm the medication to body temperature prior to use.

POLYSPORIN

See Bacitracin ± Polymyxin B.

POLYTRIM OPHTHALMIC SOLUTION

See Polymyxin B Sulfate and Trimethoprim Sulfate.

PORACTANT ALFA

See Surfactant, pulmonary.

POSACONAZOLE
Noxafil, Noxafil PowderMix, and generics
Antifungal agent

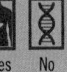

C   3   Yes   Yes   No

Delayed release tabs: 100 mg
Injection: 300 mg/16.7 mL (16.7 mL); contains EDTA and sulfobutyl ether-β-cyclodextrin (SBECD)
Oral suspension: 40 mg/mL (105 mL); contains polysorbate 80 and sodium benzoate
Delayed release oral suspension (Noxafil PowderMix): 300 mg powder packet to be mixed
with 9 mL of mixing liquid to yield a 30 mg/mL oral suspension (8 powder packets); contains
sorbitol

**Prophylaxis for invasive *Aspergillus* and *Candida* in severely immunocompromised
(e.g., hematopoietic stem cell recipients with GVHD or those with hematologic
malignancies with prolonged neutropenia); duration based on recovery from neutropenia or
immunosuppression (see remarks):**
Delayed release oral suspension (Noxafil PowderMIX):
≥2 yr and 10–40 kg:
10–<12 kg: 90 mg (3 mL) PO BID × 1 day, followed by 90 mg PO once daily
12–<17 kg: 120 mg (4 mL) PO BID × 1 day, followed by 120 mg PO once daily
17–<21 kg: 150 mg (5 mL) PO BID × 1 day, followed by 150 mg PO once daily
21–<26 kg: 180 mg (6 mL) PO BID × 1 day, followed by 180 mg PO once daily
26–<36 kg: 210 mg (7 mL) PO BID × 1 day, followed by 210 mg PO once daily
36–40 kg: 240 mg (8 mL) PO BID × 1 day, followed by 240 mg PO once daily
Delayed release tablet:
≥2–<18 yr (>40 kg) and adult: 300 mg PO BID × 1 day, followed by 300 mg PO once daily
Oral suspension:
≥13 yr and adult: 200 mg PO TID

Continued

POSACONAZOLE *continued*

IV:

≥2–<18 yr: 6 mg/kg/dose (**max. dose:** 300 mg/dose) IV BID × 1 day, followed by 6 mg/kg/dose (**max. dose:** 300 mg/dose) IV once daily

Adult: 300 mg IV BID × 1 day, followed by 300 mg IV once daily

Treatment of invasive aspergillosis:

IV or delayed release tablet (switching between these 2 dosage forms is acceptable):

≥13 yr and adult: 300 mg IV/PO BID × 1 day, followed by 300 mg IV/PO once daily for 6–12 weeks

Oropharyngeal candidiasis:

Oral suspension:

≥13 yr and adult: 100 mg PO Q12 hr × 2 doses followed by 100 mg PO Q24 hr × 13 days

Refractory oropharyngeal candidiasis (refractory to itraconazole/fluconazole):

Oral suspension:

≥13 yr and adult: 400 mg PO Q12 hr. Duration of therapy based on severity and response

---

Contraindicated with use of ergot alkaloids (e.g., ergotamine); major substrates for CYP 450 3A4 (e.g., atorvastatin, lovastatin, simvastatin, sirolimus); or CYP 450 3A4 medications that prolong the QTc interval (e.g., pimozide and quinidine). Also **contraindicated** in patients with CLL or SLL who are treated with venetoclax during the initiation and ramp-up phase due to the potential for increased tumor lysis syndrome. **Use with caution** with electrolyte imbalances (correct prior to use), cardiac arrhythmias, and hepatic or renal impairment. Use of IV dosage form is not recommended for eGFR <50 mL/min due to the risk for accumulation of SBECD excipient.

The delayed release oral suspension (Noxafil PowderMix) is not recommended for patients weighing >40 kg (recommended dosage cannot be achieved with this dosage form) and is **contraindicated** for use in patients with hereditary fructose intolerance (dosage form contains sorbitol).

Hypokalemia, diarrhea, nausea, vomiting, headache, and fever are common side effects. Serious reactions include hypersensitivity reactions, arrhythmias, QTc prolongation, and hepatotoxicity (consider discontinuing therapy). Pseudoaldosteronism and pancreatitis have been reported.

Posaconazole is a substrate of UDP-glucoronosyltransferase 1–4 (UGT1A4) and P-gp efflux and strong inhibitor of CYP 450 3A4 (see earlier for contraindicated substrates for concurrent use). Use with vincristine has been associated with neurotoxicity, seizures, peripheral neuropathy, SIADH, and paralytic ileus.

Oral suspension dosage form is **NOT** substitutable with delayed release tablets or delayed release oral suspension. Use respective dosage form for specific indication. Administer delayed release tablets with food to enhance absorption. **Do not** crush or chew delayed release tablets. IV dosage information is currently limited in adults.

POTASSIUM IODIDE
Iosat, SSKI, ThyroShield, ThyroSafe, and others
Antithyroid agent

   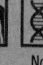

| D | X | Yes | No | No |

Tabs:

Iosat [OTC]: 65 mg (50 mg iodine), 130 mg

ThyroSafe [OTC]: 65 mg

Oral solution:

ThyroShield [OTC] and generics: 65 mg/mL (30 mL); contains parabens and saccharin

Saturated solution (SSKI): 1000 mg/mL (30, 240 mL); 10 drops = 500 mg potassium iodide

Potassium content is 6 mEq (234 mg) K⁺/g potassium iodide.

Neonatal Graves disease: 50–100 mg (about 1–2 drops of SSKI) PO once daily

Thyrotoxicosis:

Child: 50–250 mg (about 1–5 drops of SSKI) PO TID

POTASSIUM IODIDE *continued*

Adult: 50—500 mg (1—10 drops of SSKI) PO TID

Cutaneous or lymphocutaneous sporotrichosis (treat for 4—6 wk after lesions have completely healed; increase dose until either max. dose is achieved or signs of intolerance appear):

Child and adolescent (limited data): 50 mg PO TID. Dose may be gradually increased as tolerated to the **max. dose** of the lesser of 50 mg/kg/dose or 2000—2500 mg PO TID.

Adult: Start with 250 mg PO TID. Doses may be gradually increased as tolerated to the **max. dose** of 2000—2500 mg PO TID.

Contraindicated in pregnancy, hyperkalemia, iodine-induced goiter, and hypothyroidism.

Use with caution in cardiac disease and renal failure. GI disturbance, metallic taste, rash, salivary gland inflammation, headache, lacrimation, and rhinitis are symptoms of iodism. Give with milk or water after meals. Monitor thyroid function tests. Onset of antithyroid effects: 1—2 days.

Lithium carbonate and iodide-containing medications may have synergistic hypothyroid activity. Potassium-containing medications, potassium-sparing diuretics, and ACE inhibitors may increase serum potassium levels.

For use as a thyroid blocking agent in nuclear or radiation emergencies, see https://www.fda.gov/drugs/bioterrorism-and-drug-preparedness/radiation-emergencies

---

POTASSIUM SUPPLEMENTS
Many brand names and generics
Electrolyte

    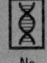

C   1   Yes   No   No

Potassium chloride (40 mEq K = 3 g KCl):
  Sustained release caps: 8, 10 mEq
  Sustained release tabs: 8, 10, 15, 20 mEq
  Powder: 20 mEq/packet (30s, 100s)
  Oral solution/liquid: 10% (6.7 mEq/5 mL), 20% (13.3 mEq/5 mL) (473 mL)
  Concentrated injection: 2 mEq/mL (5, 10, 15, 20 mL)
Potassium gluconate (40 mEq K = 9.4 g K gluconate):
  Tabs: 465 mg (2 mEq), 581 mg (2.5 mEq)
  Caps [OTC as K-99]: 595 mg (2.56 mEq)
Potassium acetate (40 mEq K = 3.9 g K acetate):
  Concentrated injection: 2 mEq/mL (20, 50 mL)
Potassium bicarbonate/citric acid (10 mEq K = 1 g K bicarbonate):
  Effervescent tab for oral solution (Effer-K): 10, 20, 25 mEq; each 10 mEq K contains 0.84 g citric acid
Potassium phosphate:
  See Phosphorus Supplements.

Normal daily requirements: See Chapter 21.

Replacement: Determine based on maintenance requirements, deficit, and ongoing losses. See Chapter 11.

Hypokalemia:
  Oral (mild/moderate hypokalemia):
    Child: 1—4 mEq/kg/24 hr ÷ BID—QID. Monitor serum potassium.
    Adult: 40—100 mEq/24 hr ÷ BID—QID. Limit single doses by 20—25 mEq to minimize GI side effects.
  IV (severe hypokalemia): MONITOR SERUM K CLOSELY.
    Child: 0.5—1 mEq/kg/dose given as an infusion of 0.5 mEq/kg/hr × 1—2 hr

Continued

POTASSIUM SUPPLEMENTS *continued*

Max. IV infusion rate: 1 mEq/kg/hr. This may be used in critical situations (i.e., hypokalemia with arrhythmia).

Adult:

Serum K ≥2.5 mEq/L: Replete at rates up to 10 mEq/hr. **Total dosage not to exceed** 200 mEq/24 hr.

Serum K <2.5 mEq/L: Replete at rates up to 40 mEq/hr. **Total dosage not to exceed** 400 mEq/24 hr.

Max. peripheral IV solution concentration: 40 mEq/L

Max. concentration for central line administration: 150–200 mEq/L

PO administration may cause GI disturbance and ulceration. Oral liquid supplements should be diluted in water or fruit juice prior to administration. Sustained release tablets must be swallowed whole and **NOT** dissolved in the mouth or chewed.

Do not administer IV potassium undiluted. IV administration may cause irritation, pain, and phlebitis at the infusion site. **Rapid or central IV infusion may cause cardiac arrhythmias.** Patients receiving infusion >0.5 mEq/kg/hr (>20 mEq/hr for adults) should be placed on an ECG monitor.

PRALIDOXIME CHLORIDE + ATROPINE
Protopam, 2-PAM, and generics
In combination with atropine: Duodote, ATNAA
Antidote, organophosphate poisoning

 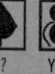 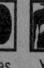
C   ?   Yes   Yes   No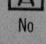

Injection (Protopam): 1000 mg

In combination with atropine (Duodote, ATNNA):

Injection for intramuscular injection in autoinjector device: 600 mg/2 mL of pralidoxime and 2.1 mg/0.7 mL of atropine; contains benzyl alcohol. Duodote or ATNNA must be administered by emergency medical services personnel who have had adequate training in the recognition and treatment of nerve agent or insecticide intoxication.

Organophosphate poisoning (use with atropine):

Child:

IV intermittent: 20–50 mg/kg/dose (**max. dose:** 2000 mg) × 1 IV. May repeat in 1–2 hr if muscle weakness is not relieved, then at Q10–12 hr PRN if cholinergic signs reappear.

IV continuous infusion: Loading dose of 20–50 mg/kg/dose (**max. dose:** 2000 mg) IV over 15–30 min followed by 10–20 mg/kg/hr (**max. dose:** 500 mg/hr)

IM (use when IV route not feasible):

<40 kg: 15 mg/kg/dose × 1 IM. May repeat Q15 min PRN up to a **max. total dose** of 45 mg/kg for mild symptoms; may repeat twice in rapid succession for severe symptoms (**max. total dose** of 45 mg/kg). For persistent symptoms, may repeat another maximum 45 mg/kg series (in 3 divided doses) approximately 1 hr after the last injection.

≥40 kg: 600 mg × 1 IM. May repeat Q15 min PRN up to a **max. total dose** of 1800 mg for mild symptoms; may repeat twice in rapid succession for severe symptoms (**max. total dose** of 1800 mg). For persistent symptoms, may repeat another **max.** 1800 mg series (in 3 divided doses) approximately 1 hr after the last injection.

Adult:

IV intermittent: 1–2 g/dose × 1 IV. May repeat in 1–2 hr if muscle weakness is not relieved, then at Q10–12 hr PRN if cholinergic signs reappear.

IM: Use aforementioned ≥40 kg child IM dosage.

In combination with atropine (Duodote, ATNNA; see remarks for description of symptoms):

Child and adult >41 kg:

PRALIDOXIME CHLORIDE + ATROPINE *continued*

Mild symptoms of nerve agent or insecticide exposure: Inject one prefilled syringe IM × 1 and wait 10—15 min for effect. If severe symptoms emerge at any time after the first dose, inject 2 additional prefilled syringes IM in rapid succession.

Severe symptoms of nerve agent or insecticide exposure: Inject three prefilled syringes IM in rapid succession.

Contraindicated in poisonings due to phosphorus, inorganic phosphates, or organic phosphates without anticholinesterase activity. **Do not use** as an antidote for carbamate classes of pesticides. Removal of secretions and maintaining a patent airway are critical. May cause muscle rigidity, laryngospasm, and tachycardia after rapid IV infusion. Drug is generally ineffective if administered 36—48 hr after exposure. Additional doses may be necessary.

For IV administration, dilute to 50 mg/mL or less and infuse over 15—30 min (**not to exceed** 200 mg/min). Reduce dosage in renal impairment since 80%—90% of the drug is excreted unchanged in the urine 12 hr after administration. Severe hepatic impairment may require less frequent doses after the initial dose for both IV and IM routes.

Pralidoxime and atropine combination (Duodote): Signs of atropine effects/toxicity may occur earlier than when atropine is used alone. Safety and efficacy data are only available for children and adults >41 kg (90 lb). Duodote product information description of mild and severe symptoms:

Mild symptoms: Increased airway secretions, blurred vision, bradycardia, breathing difficulties, chest tightness, drooling, miosis, nausea, vomiting, runny nose, salivation, stomach cramps (acute onset), tachycardia, teary eyes, tremors/muscular twitching, wheezing/coughing

Severe symptoms: Breathing difficulties (severe), confused/strange behavior, convulsions, copious secretions from lung or airways, involuntary urination/defecation, muscular twitching/generalized weakness (severe), unconsciousness

IM injection is via the midlateral thigh.

PREDNISOLONE
Oral products:
Orapred ODT, Pediapred, and generics; previously available as Prelone
Ophthalmic products:
Pred Forte, Pred Mild, Econopred, and generics
Corticosteroid

C/D 2 No No No

Tabs: 5 mg
Oral solution (generics): 15 mg/5 mL (240 mL); may contain alcohol and saccharin
Tablets, orally disintegrating (as Na phosphate) (Orapred ODT and generics): 10, 15, 30 mg
Oral solution/syrup (as Na phosphate):
Pediapred and generics: 5 mg/5 mL (120 mL); alcohol and dye free
Generics: 10 mg/5 mL (237 mL), 15 mg/5 mL (237 mL), 20 mg/5 mL (237 mL), 25 mg/5 mL (237 mL); may contain parabens, alcohol; some preparations may be dye free
Ophthalmic suspension (as acetate; both strengths contain benzalkonium chloride and may contain bisulfites):
Pred Mild: 0.12% (5, 10 mL)
Econopred: 0.125% (5, 10 mL)
PredForte, Econopred Plus, and generics: 1% (5, 10, 15 mL)
Ophthalmic solution (as Na phosphate): 1% (10 mL); may contain benzalkonium chloride

See Prednisone for systemic oral dosing (equivalent dosing).
Ophthalmic (consult ophthalmologist before use; see remarks):

Continued

PREDNISOLONE *continued*

Ophthalmic suspension:

Child (limited data) and adult: 1—2 drops to the conjunctival sac of the affected eye(s) BID—QID (dosage frequency may be increased during initial 24—48 hr if needed). Reevaluate patient if signs and symptoms do not improve after 2 days.

Ophthalmic solution:

Child and adult: Start with 1—2 drops Q1 hr during the day and Q2 hr during the night until favorable response, then reduce dose to 1 drop Q4 hr. Dose may be further reduced to 1 drop TID—QID.

See Prednisone for remarks. See Chapter 10 for relative steroid potencies. Pregnancy category changes to "D" if used in the first trimester.

OPHTHALMIC USE: Contraindicated in viral (e.g., herpes simplex, vaccinia, and varicella), fungal, and mycobacterial infections of the cornea and conjunctiva. Increase in intraocular pressure, cataract formation, eye pain, and delayed wound healing may occur.

PREDNISONE
Deltasone, Rayos, and generics
Corticosteroid

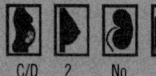 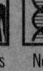

C/D   2   No   Yes   No

Tabs (Deltasone and generics): 1, 2.5, 5, 10, 20, 50 mg
Delayed release tabs (Rayos): 1, 2, 5 mg
Oral solution: 1 mg/mL (120, 500 mL); may contain 5% alcohol and saccharin
Concentrated solution (Prednisone Intensol): 5 mg/mL (30 mL); contains 30% alcohol

Acute asthma:

Child: 2 mg/kg/24 hr PO ÷ once daily—BID × 5—7 days; **max. dose:** 80 mg/24 hr.
Patients may benefit from tapering if therapy exceeds 5—7 days.

Acute exacerbation in emergency care or hospital (2007 National Heart, Lung, and Blood Institute [NHLBI] Guideline Recommendations; dose until peak expiratory flow reaches 70% of predicted or personal best):

Child ≤12 yr: 1—2 mg/kg/24 hr PO ÷ Q12 hr (**max. dose:** 60 mg/24 hr)

Child >12 yr and adult: 40—80 mg/24 hr PO ÷ Q12—24 hr

Outpatient asthma exacerbation burst therapy (2007 NHLBI guidelines; therapy should be continued until symptoms resolve or until peak expiratory flow reaches 80% of personal best; usual therapy duration 3—10 days [average ~5 days]; longer durations may be necessary):

Child ≤12 yr: 1—2 mg/kg/24 hr PO ÷ Q12—24 hr (**max. dose:** 60 mg/24 hr)

Child >12 yr and adult: 40—60 mg/24 hr PO ÷ Q12—24 hr

Acute exacerbation in primary care or acute care facility (2020 Global Initiative for Asthma [GINA] Guidelines):

Infant and child: 1—2 mg/kg/24 hr PO once daily × 3—5 days with the following **maximum dose** by age:

Infant and child ≤2 yr: 20 mg/24 hr

Child 3—5 yr: 30 mg/24 hr

Child 6—11 yr: 40 mg/24 hr

Child >12 yr and adolescent: 1 mg/kg/24 hr (**max. dose:** 50 mg/24 hr) PO once daily × 5—7 days

Antiinflammatory/immunosuppressive:

Child: 0.5—2 mg/kg/24 hr PO ÷ once daily—BID

Nephrotic syndrome:

PREDNISONE *continued*

Child (use ideal body weight for obese patients): Starting dose of 2 mg/kg/24 hr PO (max. dose: 60 mg/24 hr) ÷ once daily—TID is recommended. Further treatment plans are individualized. Consult a nephrologist.

See Chapter 10 for physiologic replacement, relative steroid potencies, and doses based on body surface area.

Despite requiring hepatic metabolism to its active form (prednisolone), patients with liver disease have reported higher prednisolone levels than that of normal patients. Methylprednisolone or prednisolone may be preferable in hepatic disease.

Side effects may include: mood changes, seizures, hyperglycemia, diarrhea, nausea, abdominal distension, GI bleeding, HPA axis suppression, osteopenia, cushingoid effects, and cataracts with prolonged use. Prednisone is a CYP 450 3A3/4 substrate and inducer. Barbiturates, carbamazepine, phenytoin, rifampin, and isoniazid may reduce the effects of prednisone, whereas estrogens may enhance the effects. Pregnancy category changes to "D" if used in the first trimester.

PRIMAQUINE PHOSPHATE
Various generics
Antimalarial

 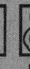

X   3   No   No   No

Tabs: 26.3 mg (15 mg base)
Oral suspension: 10.52 mg (6 mg base)/5 mL

Doses expressed in mg of primaquine base:
Malaria:
Prevention of relapses for *Plasmodium vivax* or *Plasmodium ovale* only (initiate therapy during the last 2 wk of, or following a course of, suppression with chloroquine or comparable drug):
Child: 0.5 mg/kg/dose (**max. dose:** 30 mg/dose) PO once daily × 14 days
Adult: 30 mg PO once daily × 14 days
Prevention of chloroquine-resistant strains (initiate 1 day prior to departure and continued until 7 days after leaving endemic area):
Child: 0.5 mg/kg/dose PO once daily; **max. dose:** 30 mg/24 hr
Adult: 30 mg PO once daily
***P. jirovecii (carinii)* pneumonia (in combination with clindamycin):**
Child: 0.3 mg/kg/dose (**max. dose:** 30 mg/dose) PO once daily × 21 days
Adult: 30 mg PO once daily × 21 days

Contraindicated in granulocytopenia (e.g., rheumatoid arthritis, lupus erythematosus) and bone marrow suppression. **Avoid use** with quinacrine and with other drugs that have a potential for causing hemolysis or bone marrow suppression. **Use with caution** in patients with G6PD and NADH methemoglobin-reductase deficiency due to increased risk for hemolytic anemia and leukopenia, respectively. Monitor ECG for QTc prolongation in patients with cardiac disease, history of arrhythmias, uncorrected hypokalemia and/or hypomagnesemia, bradycardia, and receiving concomitant QTc prolonging medications. Use in pregnancy is **not recommended** by the AAP Red Book. Cross sensitivity with iodoquinol.

May cause headache, visual disturbances, nausea, vomiting, and abdominal cramps. Hemolytic anemia, leukopenia, cardiac arrhythmia, QTc interval prolongation, and methemoglobinemia have been reported. Administer all doses with food to mask bitter taste.

PRIMIDONE
Mysoline and generics
Anticonvulsant, barbiturate

    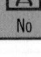

D 2 Yes Yes No

Tabs: 50, 250 mg

Neonate: 12—20 mg/kg/24 hr PO ÷ BID—QID; initiate therapy at the lower dosage range and titrate upward.

Child, adolescent, and adult:

Day of Therapy	<8 Yr	≥8 Yr and Adult
Days 1—3	50 mg PO QHS	100—125 mg PO QHS
Days 4—6	50 mg PO BID	100—125 mg PO BID
Days 7—9	100 mg PO BID	100—125 mg PO TID
Day 10 and thereafter	125—250 mg PO TID or 10—25 mg/kg/ 24 hr ÷ TID—QID	250 mg PO TID-QID; **max. dose:** 2 g/24 hr

Use with caution in renal or hepatic disease and pulmonary insufficiency. Primidone is metabolized to phenobarbital and has the same drug interactions and toxicities (see Phenobarbital). In addition, primidone may cause vertigo, nausea, leukopenia, malignant lymphoma-like syndrome, diplopia, nystagmus, and systemic lupus-like syndrome. Monitor for suicidal behavior or ideation. Acetazolamide may decrease primidone absorption. **Adjust dose in renal failure (see Chapter 31).**

Monitor both primidone and phenobarbital levels. Therapeutic levels: 5—12 mg/L of primidone and 15—40 mg/L of phenobarbital. Recommended serum sampling time at steady state: trough level obtained within 30 min prior to the next scheduled dose after 1—4 days of continuous dosing.

PROBENECID
Various generics
Penicillin therapy adjuvant, uric acid—lowering agent

    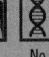

B ? Yes No No

Tabs: 500 mg

To prolong penicillin levels.
   Child (2—14 yr): 25 mg/kg PO × 1, then 40 mg/kg/24 hr ÷ QID; **max. single dose:** 500 mg/dose. Use adult dose if >50 kg.
   Adult: 500 mg PO QID

Hyperuricemia with gout:
   Adult: 250 mg PO BID × 1 wk, then 500 mg PO BID; may increase by 500 mg increments Q4 wk PRN up to a **max. dose** of 2—3 g/24 hr ÷ BID

Gonorrhea, antibiotic adjunct (administer just prior to antibiotic):
   ≤45 kg: 23 mg/kg/dose PO × 1
   >45 kg: 1 g PO × 1

Prevention of nephrotoxicity from cidofovir: See Cidofovir.

Use with caution in patients with peptic ulcer disease. **Contraindicated** in children <2 yr and patients with renal insufficiency. **Do not use** if GFR <30 mL/min.

PROBENECID *continued*

Increases uric acid excretion. Inhibits renal tubular secretion of acyclovir, ganciclovir, ciprofloxacin, levofloxacin, nalidixic acid, moxifloxacin, organic acids, penicillins, cephalosporins, AZT, dapsone, methotrexate, nonsteroidal antiinflammatory agents, and benzodiazepines. Salicylates may decrease probenecid's activity. Alkalinize urine in patients with gout. May cause headache, GI symptoms, rash, anemia, and hypersensitivity. False-positive glucosuria with Clinitest may occur.

PROCHLORPERAZINE
Compro and generics; previously available as
Compazine
Antiemetic, phenothiazine derivative

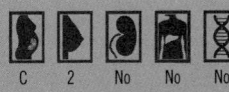

C   2   No   No   No

Tabs (as maleate): 5, 10 mg
Suppository (Compro and generics): 25 mg (12s)
Injection (as edisylate): 5 mg/mL (2 mL); may contain benzyl alcohol

Antiemetic doses:
  Child (≥2 yr and ≥9 kg):
    PO or PR: 0.4 mg/kg/24 hr ÷ TID—QID PRN (**max. dose:** 10 mg/dose) or alternative dosing by
      weight:
      9—13 kg: 2.5 mg once daily—BID PRN; **max. dose:** 7.5 mg/24 hr
      >13—18 kg: 2.5 mg BID—TID PRN; **max. dose:** 10 mg/24 hr
      >18—39 kg: 2.5 mg TID or 5 mg BID PRN; **max. dose:** 15 mg/24 hr
      >39 kg: Use adult dose.
    IM: 0.1—0.15 mg/kg/dose BID—TID PRN; **max. dose:** 10 mg/single dose or 40 mg/24 hr
  Adult:
    PO: 5—10 mg/dose TID—QID PRN; **max. dose:** 40 mg/24 hr
    PR: 25 mg/dose BID PRN
    IM: 5—10 mg/dose Q3—4 hr PRN
    IV: 2.5—10 mg/dose; may repeat Q3—4 hr PRN
    Max. IM/IV dose: 40 mg/24 hr
Psychoses:
  Child 2—12 yr and >9 kg:
    PO: Start with 2.5 mg BID—TID with a **max. first-day dose** of 10 mg/24 hr. Dose may be increased
      as needed to 20 mg/24 hr for children 2—5 yr and 25 mg/24 hr for 6—12 yr.
    IM: 0.13 mg/kg/dose × 1 and convert to PO immediately
  Adult:
    PO: 5—10 mg TID—QID; may be increased as needed to a **max. dose** of 150 mg/24 hr
    IM: 10—20 mg Q2—4 hr PRN; convert to PO immediately
Intractable migraines:
  Child (5—18 yr, limited data): 0.15 mg/kg/dose (**max. dose:** 10 mg/dose) IV over 10 min was effective
    in migraine headaches presenting in the emergency departments (see *Ann Emerg Med.*
    2004;43:256—262).

Toxicity as for other phenothiazines (see Chlorpromazine). Extrapyramidal reactions (reversed by
diphenhydramine) or orthostatic hypotension may occur. May mask signs and symptoms of
overdosage of other drugs and may obscure the diagnosis and treatment of conditions such as
intestinal obstruction, brain tumor, and Reye syndrome. May cause false-positive test for
phenylketonuria, urinary amylase, uroporphyrins, and urobilinogen. **Do not use** IV route in children.
Use only in management of prolonged vomiting of known etiology.

PROMETHAZINE
Phenergan, Promethegan, and generics
*Antihistamine, antiemetic, phenothiazine
derivative*

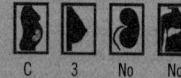

C   3   No   No   No

Tabs: 12.5, 25, 50 mg
Oral solution/syrup: 6.25 mg/5 mL (473 mL); contains alcohol and may contain parabens, sodium
benzoate, or phenol (many formulations exist)
Suppository (Phenadoz, Promethegan, and generics): 12.5, 25, 50 mg (12s)
Injection: 25, 50 mg/mL (1 mL); may contain edetate disodium, sulfites, and phenol

Antihistaminic:
  Child ≥2 yr: 0.1 mg/kg/dose (**max. dose:** 12.5 mg/dose) Q6 hr PO during the day hours and
    0.5 mg/kg/dose (**max. dose:** 25 mg/dose) QHS PO PRN
  Adult: 6.25–12.5 mg PO/PR TID and 25 mg QHS
Nausea and vomiting PO/IM/IV/PR (see remarks):
  Child ≥2 yr: 0.25–1 mg/kg/dose Q4–6 hr PRN; **max. dose:** 25 mg/dose
  Adult: 12.5–25 mg Q4–6 hr PRN
Motion sickness: (1st dose 0.5–1 hr before departure):
  Child ≥2 yr: 0.5 mg/kg/dose Q12 hr PO/PR PRN; **max. dose:** 25 mg/dose
  Adult: 25 mg PO Q8–12 hr PRN

Avoid use in children <2 yr because of risk for fatal respiratory depression. Toxicity similar
  to other phenothiazines (see Chlorpromazine). **Do not** administer SC or intra-arterially
  because of severe local reactions. IV route of administration is **not recommended** (IM preferred) due
  to severe tissue injury (tissue necrosis and gangrene). If using IV route, dilute 25 mg/mL strength
  product with 10–20 mL NS and administer over 10–15 min, consider lower initial doses,
  administer through a large-bore vein and check patency of line before administering, administer
  through an IV line at the port farthest from the patient's vein, and monitor for burning or pain
  during or after injection. Administer oral doses with meals to decrease GI irritation.
May cause profound sedation, blurred vision, respiratory depression (use lowest effective dose in
  children and **avoid** concomitant use of respiratory depressants), and dystonic reactions (reversed by
  diphenhydramine). Cholestatic jaundice and neuroleptic malignant syndrome has been reported.
  May interfere with pregnancy tests (immunologic reactions between hCG and anti-hCG). **For nausea
  and vomiting, use only in management of prolonged vomiting of known etiology.**

PROPRANOLOL
Inderal, Inderal LA, Hemangeol, and generics
*Adrenergic blocking agent (β), class II
antiarrhythmic*

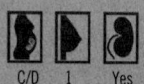 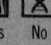

C/D   1   Yes   Yes   No

Tabs: 10, 20, 40, 60, 80 mg
Extended release caps (Inderal LA and others, including generics): 60, 80, 120, 160 mg
Oral solution: 20 mg/5 mL, 40 mg/5 mL; contains parabens and saccharin
  Hemangeol: 4.28 mg/mL (120 mL); alcohol, sugar and paraben free; contains saccharin
Injection: 1 mg/mL (1 mL)

Arrhythmias:
  Child:
    IV: 0.01–0.1 mg/kg/dose IV push over 10 min, repeat Q6–8 hr PRN; **max. dose:** 1 mg/dose for
      infant; 3 mg/dose for child

PROPRANOLOL *continued*

  PO: Start at 0.5—1 mg/kg/24 hr ÷ Q6—8 hr; increase dosage Q3—5 days PRN. Usual dosage range: 2—4 mg/kg/24 hr ÷ Q6—8 hr; **max. dose:** 60 mg/24 hr or 16 mg/kg/24 hr

 Adult:

  IV: 1 mg/dose Q5 min up to total 5 mg

  PO: 10—30 mg/dose TID—QID; increase PRN. Usual range 30—160 mg/24 hr ÷ TID—QID

Hypertension (as alternative therapy):

 Child:

  PO: Initial: 0.5—1 mg/kg/24 hr ÷ Q6—12 hr. May increase dose Q5—7 days PRN; **max. dose:** 8 mg/kg/24 hr

 Adult:

  PO: 40 mg/dose PO BID or 60—80 mg/dose (sustained release capsule) PO once daily. May increase 10—20 mg/dose Q3—7 days; **max. dose:** 640 mg/24 hr

Migraine prophylaxis:

 Child:

  <35 kg: Start with 10 mg PO once daily and increase dose PRN weekly intervals at 10 mg increments. Usual dosage range: 10—20 mg PO TID

  ≥35 kg: 20—40 mg PO TID

 Adult: 80 mg/24 hr ÷ Q6—8 hr PO; increase dose by 20—40 mg/dose Q3—4 wk PRN. Usual effective dose range: 160—240 mg/24 hr

Tetralogy spells:

 IV: 0.15—0.25 mg/kg/dose slow IV push. May repeat in 15 min × 1. See also Chapter 7.

 PO: Start at 2—4 mg/kg/24 hr ÷ Q6 hr PRN. Usual dose range: 4—8 mg/kg/24 hr ÷ Q6 hr PRN. Doses as high as 15 mg/kg/24 hr have been used with careful monitoring.

Thyrotoxicosis:

 Neonate: 0.5—2 mg/kg/24 hr PO ÷ Q6—12 hr

 Infant and child: 0.5—2 mg/kg/24 hr PO ÷ Q8 hr; **max. dose:** 40 mg/dose

 Adolescent and adult:

  IV: 1—3 mg/dose over 10 min. May repeat in 4—6 hr

  PO: 10—40 mg/dose PO Q6 hr

Infantile hemangioma (see remarks):

 Infant (5 wk—5 mo and ≥2 kg; labeled dosing information for Hemangeol product): 0.6 mg/kg/dose BID PO (at least 9 hr apart) × 7 days, then increase to 1.1 mg/kg/dose BID PO × 14 days, followed by 1.7 mg/kg/dose BID PO × 6 mo

 Alternative dosing: Start at 1 mg/kg/24 hr ÷ Q8 hr PO. If tolerated after 1 day, increase dose to 2 mg/kg/24 hr ÷ Q8 hr PO

Contraindicated in asthma, Raynaud syndrome, heart failure, and heart block. **Not indicated** for the treatment of hypertensive emergencies. **Use with caution** in presence of obstructive lung disease, diabetes mellitus, or renal or hepatic disease. May cause hypoglycemia, hypotension, nausea, vomiting, depression, weakness, impotence, bronchospasm, and heart block. Cutaneous reactions, including Stevens-Johnson, TEN, exfoliative dermatitis, erythema multiforme, and urticaria have been reported. Acute hypertension has occurred after insulin-induced hypoglycemia in patients on propranolol.

Therapeutic levels for beta-blockade: 50—100 ng/mL; ventricular arrhythmia: 40—85 ng/mL. Drug is metabolized by CYP 450 1A2, 2C18, 2C19, and 2D6 isoenzymes. Concurrent administration with barbiturates, indomethacin, or rifampin may cause decreased activity of propranolol. Concurrent administration with cimetidine, hydralazine, flecainide, quinidine, chlorpromazine, or verapamil may lead to increased activity of propranolol. **Avoid** IV use of propranolol with calcium channel blockers; may increase effect of calcium channel blocker. Use with amiodarone may increase negative chronotropic effects.

Continued

PROPRANOLOL *continued*

For infantile hemangioma, monitor BP and HR 2 hr after initiating therapy and after dose increases. To reduce risk of hypoglycemia, administer doses during or right after a feeding; hold doses if child is not eating or is vomiting. Infants <6 mo must be fed every 4 hr. Common adverse effects (>10%) reported in clinical trials with Hemangeol include sleep disorders, aggravated respiratory tract infections (e.g., bronchitis and bronchiolitis) associated with cough/fever, diarrhea, and vomiting. Readjust dose periodically with changes (increases) in child's body weight.

Successful use in infantile hepatic hemangiomas has also been reported.

Pregnancy category changes to "D" if used in second or third trimesters.

PROPYLTHIOURACIL
PTU and generics
Antithyroid agent

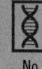

| D | 2 | Yes | Yes | No |

Tabs: 50 mg
Oral suspension: 5 mg/mL
100 mg PTU = 10 mg methimazole

Dosages should be adjusted as required to achieve and maintain T₄, TSH levels in normal ranges.

Neonate: 5–10 mg/kg/24 hr ÷ Q8 hr PO
Child:
  Initial: 5–7 mg/kg/24 hr ÷ Q8 hr PO, OR by age:
    6–10 yr: 50–150 mg/24 hr ÷ Q8 hr PO
    >10 yr: 150–300 mg/24 hr ÷ Q8 hr PO
  Maintenance: Generally begins after 2 mo. Usually 1/3–2/3 the initial dose in divided doses (Q8–12 hr) when the patient is euthyroid
Adult:
  Initial: 300–400 mg/24 hr ÷ Q6–8 hr PO; some may require larger doses of 600–900 mg/24 hr
  Maintenance: 100–150 mg/24 hr ÷ Q8 hr PO

Generally reserved for patients who are unable to tolerate methimazole and for whom radioactive iodine or surgery is not appropriate. May be the antithyroid treatment of choice during or just prior to the first trimester of pregnancy because of risk of fetal abnormalities associated with methimazole.

May cause blood dyscrasias, fever, liver disease, dermatitis, urticaria, malaise, CNS stimulation or depression, and arthralgias. Glomerulonephritis, severe liver injury/failure, agranulocytosis, severe vasculitis, interstitial pneumonitis, exfoliative dermatitis, and erythema nodosum have also been reported. May decrease the effectiveness of warfarin. Monitor thyroid function. A dose reduction of β-blocker may be necessary when the hyperthyroid patient becomes euthyroid.

For neonates, crush tablets, weigh appropriate dose, and mix in formula/breast milk. **Adjust dose in renal failure (see Chapter 31).**

PROSTAGLANDIN E₁

See Alprostadil.

PROTAMINE SULFATE
Various generics
Antidote, heparin

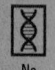

| C | ? | No | No | No |

PROTAMINE SULFATE *continued*

Injection: 10 mg/mL (5, 25 mL); preservative free

Heparin antidote, IV:
1 mg protamine will neutralize 115 U porcine intestinal heparin, or 100 U (1 mg)
low-molecular-weight heparin
Consider time since last heparin dose:
If <0.5 hr: Give 100% of specified dose.
If within 0.5—1 hr: Give 50%—75% of aforementioned dose.
If within 1—2 hr: Give 37.5%—50% of aforementioned dose.
If ≥2 hr: Give 25%—37.5% of aforementioned dose.
Max. dose: 50 mg/dose IV
Max. infusion rate: 5 mg/min
Max. IV concentration: 10 mg/mL
If heparin was administered by deep SC injection, give 1—1.5 mg protamine per 100 U heparin as follows:
Load with 25—50 mg via slow IV infusion followed by the rest of the calculated dose via continuous infusion over 8—16 hr or the expected duration of SC heparin absorption.
Enoxaparin overdosage, IV (see remarks): Approximately 1 mg protamine will neutralize 1 mg enoxaparin.
Consider time since last enoxaparin dose:
If <8 hr: Give 100% of aforementioned dose.
If within 8—12 hr: Give 50% of aforementioned dose.
If >12 hr: Protamine not required but if serious bleeding is present, give 50% of aforementioned dose.
If aPTT remains prolonged 2—4 hr after the first protamine dose or if bleeding continues, a second infusion of 0.5 mg protamine per 1 mg enoxaparin may be given.
Max. dose: 50 mg/dose. See aforementioned heparin antidote IV dosage for **max.** administration concentration and rate.

Risk factors for protamine hypersensitivity include known hypersensitivity to fish and exposure to protamine-containing insulin or prior protamine therapy.
May cause hypotension, bradycardia, dyspnea, and anaphylaxis. Monitor aPTT or ACT. Heparin rebound with bleeding has been reported to occur 8—18 hr later.
Use in enoxaparin overdose may not be complete despite using multiple doses of protamine.

PSEUDOEPHEDRINE
Sudafed, Sudafed 12 Hour, Sudafed 24 Hour, and generics
Sympathomimetic, nasal decongestant

    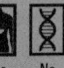

C	2	Yes	No	No

Tabs (OTC): 30, 60 mg
Extended release tab (OTC):
Sudafed 12 Hour and generics: 120 mg
Sudafed 24 Hour: 240 mg
Oral liquid (OTC): 15 mg/5 mL (120 mL); may contain sodium benzoate
Purchases of OTC products are limited to behind the pharmacy counter sales with monthly sale limits due to the methamphetamine epidemic.

Child <12 yr: 4 mg/kg/24 hr ÷ Q6 hr PO or by age:
<4 yr: 4 mg/kg/24 hr ÷ Q6 hr PO; **max. dose:** 60 mg/24 hr
4—5 yr: 15 mg/dose Q4—6 hr PO; **max. dose:** 60 mg/24 hr
6—12 yr: 30 mg/dose Q4—6 hr PO; **max. dose:** 120 mg/24 hr

Continued

PSEUDOEPHEDRINE *continued*

Child ≥12 yr and adult:
   Immediate release: 60 mg/dose Q4–6 hr PO; **max. dose:** 240 mg/24 hr
   Sustained release:
      Sudafed 12 Hour and generics: 120 mg PO Q12 hr
      Sudafed 24 Hour: 240 mg PO Q24 hr

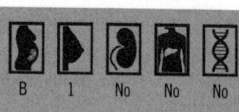

Contraindicated with MAO inhibitor drugs and in severe hypertension and severe coronary artery disease. **Use with caution** in mild/moderate hypertension, hyperglycemia, hyperthyroidism, and cardiac disease. May cause dizziness, nervousness, restlessness, insomnia, and arrhythmias. Pseudoephedrine is a common component of OTC cough and cold preparations and is combined with several antihistamines; these products are not recommended for children <6 yr. Since drug and active metabolite are primarily excreted renally, **doses should be adjusted in renal impairment.** May cause false-positive test for amphetamines (EMIT assay).

PSYLLIUM
Metamucil, Konsyl, Mucilin, and many others,
including some generics
Bulk-forming laxative

B   1   No   No   No

Check specific product label for amount of psyllium per unit of measurement.
Granules [OTC]:
   Konsyl: 4.3 g psyllium per rounded teaspoon or 6 g of granules (300 g); contains maltodextrin and 35 mg potassium for each 6 g dose; sugar and gluten free
Powder [OTC]:
   Metamucil: 3.4 g psyllium per rounded teaspoon; contains 5 mg sodium, 30 mg potassium, and 25 mg phenylalanine for each teaspoon. Other products may contain sucrose or maltodextrin instead of phenylalanine.
3.4 g psyllium hydrophilic mucilloid is equivalent to 2 g soluble fiber

Constipation (granules or powder must be mixed with a full glass [240 mL] of water or juice):
   <6 yr: 1.25–2.5 g/dose PO once daily–TID; **max. dose:** 7.5 g/24 hr
   6–11 yr: 2.5–3.75 g/dose PO once daily–TID; **max. dose:** 15 g/24 hr
   ≥12 yr and adult: 2.5–7.5 g/dose PO once daily–TID; **max. dose:** 30 g/24 hr

Contraindicated in cases of fecal impaction or GI obstruction. **Use with caution** in patients with esophageal strictures and rectal bleeding. Phenylketonurics should be aware that certain preparations may contain aspartame. Should be taken or mixed with a full glass (240 mL) of liquid. Onset of action: 12–72 hr.

PYRANTEL PAMOATE
Reese's Pinworm Medicine, Pin-Away, and many
other generics
Anthelmintic

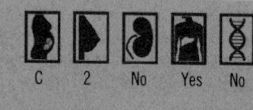

C   2   No   Yes   No

Oral suspension (OTC): 50 mg/mL pyrantel base (144 mg/mL pyrantel pamoate) (30, 60, 473 mL); may contain sodium benzoate, parabens, and saccharin
Tabs (OTC): 62.5 mg pyrantel base (180 mg pyrantel pamoate); scored tablet

All doses expressed in terms of pyrantel base.

PYRANTEL PAMOATE *continued*

Child (≥2 yr), adolescent, and adult:
> *Ascaris* (roundworm) and *Trichostrongylus*: 11 mg/kg/dose PO × 1
> *Enterobius* (pinworm): 11 mg/kg/dose PO × 1. Repeat same dose 2 wk later.
> **Hookworm or eosinophilic enterocolitis:** 11 mg/kg/dose PO once daily × 3 days
> *Moniliformis*: 11 mg/kg/dose PO Q2 wk × 3 doses
> **Max. dose (all indications):** 1 g/dose

Use with caution in liver dysfunction. **Do not use** in combination with piperazine because of antagonism. May cause nausea, vomiting, anorexia, transient AST elevations, headaches, rash, and muscle weakness. Limited experience in children <2 yr. May increase theophylline levels. Drug may be mixed with milk or fruit juice and may be taken with food.

PYRAZINAMIDE
Pyrazinoic acid amide and generics
Antituberculous agent

C   2   Yes   Yes   No

Tabs: 500 mg
Oral suspension: 100 mg/mL
In combination with isoniazid and rifampin (Rifater):
> **Tabs:** 300 mg with 50 mg isoniazid and 120 mg rifampin; contains povidone and propylene glycol

Tuberculosis: Use as part of a multidrug regimen for tuberculosis. See latest edition of the AAP Red Book for recommended treatment for tuberculosis.
Child:
> **<40 kg:**
>> **Daily dose regimen:** 30—40 mg/kg/24 hr PO once daily; **max. dose:** 2 g/24 hr
>> **Twice-weekly dose regimen:** 50 mg/kg/dose PO 2× per week; **max. dose:** 2 g/dose
> **≥40 kg:** Use adult dosage below.

Adult:
> **Daily dose regimen:**
>> **40—55 kg:** 1000 mg PO once daily
>> **56—75 kg:** 1500 mg PO once daily
>> **76—90 kg:** 2000 mg PO once daily
> **Twice-weekly dose regimen:**
>> **40—55 kg:** 2000 mg PO 2× per week
>> **56—75 kg:** 3000 mg PO 2× per week
>> **76—90 kg:** 4000 mg PO 2× per week

See latest edition of the AAP Red Book for recommended treatment for tuberculosis.
Contraindicated in severe hepatic damage and acute gout. The CDC and ATS **do not recommend** the combination of pyrazinamide and rifampin for latent TB infections.
Use with caution in patients with renal failure (dosage reduction has been recommended), gout, or diabetes mellitus. Monitor liver function tests (baseline and periodic) and serum uric acid.
Hepatoxicity is most common dose-related side effect; doses ≤30 mg/kg/24 hr minimize effect. Hyperuricemia, maculopapular rash, arthralgia, fever, acne, porphyria, dysuria, and photosensitivity may occur. Severe hepatic toxicity may occur with rifampin use. May decrease isoniazid levels.

PYRETHRINS WITH PIPERONYL BUTOXIDE
A-200, Pronto Plus, RID, and many others
Pediculicide

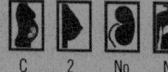

C　2　No　No　No

All products are available OTC without a prescription.
Shampoo (RID, Pronto Plus, A-200): 0.33% pyrethrins and 4% piperonyl butoxide (60, 120, 240 mL);
may contain alcohol

Pediculosis (≥2 yr and adult): Apply to dry hair or affected body area for 10 min, then wash
thoroughly and comb with fine-tooth comb or nit-removing comb; repeat in 7–10 days.

Contraindicated in ragweed hypersensitivity; drug is derived from the chrysanthemum
flowers. For topical use only. **Avoid** use in and around the eyes, mouth, nose, or vagina.
Avoid repeat applications in <24 hr. Low ovicidal activity requires repeat treatment. Dead nits
require mechanical removal. Wash bedding and clothing to eradicate infestation.
Local irritation, including erythema, pruritus, urticaria, edema, and eczema, may occur.

PYRIDOSTIGMINE BROMIDE
Mestinon, Regonol, and generics
Cholinergic agent

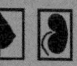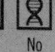

C　1　Yes　No　No

Oral syrup (Mestinon): 60 mg/5 mL (473 mL); contains 5% alcohol and sodium benzoate
Tabs (Mestinon and generics): 30, 60 mg
Sustained release tab (Mestinon and generics): 180 mg; scored tablet
Injection (Regonol): 5 mg/mL (2 mL); may contain 1% benzyl alcohol

Myasthenia gravis:
Neonate:
PO: 1 mg/kg/dose Q4 hr; **max. dose:** 7 mg/kg/24 hr
IM/IV: 0.05–0.15 mg/kg/dose Q4–6 hr; **max.** single IM/IV dose: 10 mg
Child:
PO: 7 mg/kg/24 hr in 5–6 divided doses
IM/IV: 0.05–0.15 mg/kg/dose Q4–6 hr; **max.** single IM/IV dose: 10 mg
Adult:
PO (immediate release): 60 mg TID; increase Q48 hr PRN. Usual effective dose: 60–1500 mg/24 hr
PO (sustained release): 180–540 mg once daily–BID
IM/IV (use when PO therapy is not practical): Give 1/30 of the usual PO

Contraindicated in mechanical intestinal or urinary obstruction. **Use with caution** in patients
with epilepsy, asthma, bradycardia, hyperthyroidism, arrhythmias, or peptic ulcer. May cause
nausea, vomiting, diarrhea, rash, headache, and muscle cramps. Pyridostigmine is mainly excreted
unchanged by the kidney. Therefore, lower doses titrated to effect in renal disease may be necessary.
Changes in oral dosages may take several days to show results. **Atropine is the antidote.**

PYRIDOXINE
Vitamin B$_6$ and various names including generics
Vitamin, water soluble

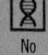

A/C　1　No　No　No

Tabs (HCl) [OTC]: 25, 50, 100, 250, 500 mg
Oral solution (HCl): 1 mg/mL

PYRIDOXINE *continued*

Injection (HCl): 100 mg/mL (1 mL); some products may contain aluminum and 0.5% chlorobutanol

Deficiency, IM/IV/PO (PO preferred):
  Child: 5—25 mg/24 hr × 3 wk, followed by 2.5—5 mg/24 hr as maintenance therapy
    (via multivitamin preparation)
  Adolescent and adult: 10—20 mg/24 hr × 3 wk, followed by 2—5 mg/24 hr as maintenance therapy
    (via multivitamin preparation)
Drug-induced neuritis (PO):
  Prophylaxis:
    Child: 1 mg/kg/24 hr or 10—50 mg/24 hr
    Adolescent and adult: 25—50 mg/24 hr
  Treatment (optimal dose not established):
    Child: 50—200 mg/24 hr
    Adolescent and adult: 50—300 mg/24 hr
Pyridoxine-dependent seizures:
  Neonate and infant:
    Initial: 50—100 mg/dose IM or rapid IV × 1
    Maintenance: 50—100 mg/24 hr PO
Recommended daily allowance: See Chapter 21.

Use caution with concurrent levodopa therapy. Chronic administration has been associated
  with sensory neuropathy. Nausea, headache, increased AST, decreased serum folic acid
  level, and allergic reaction may occur. May lower phenobarbital and phenytoin levels.
  See Chapter 20 for management of neonatal seizures.
Pregnancy category changes to "C" if dosage exceeds U.S. RDA.

PYRIMETHAMINE
Daraprim and generics
Antiparasitic agent

  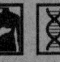

C   2   Yes   Yes   No

Tabs: 25 mg; scored tablet (see remarks for outpatient prescription process)
Oral suspension: 2 mg/mL

Congenital toxoplasmosis (administer with sulfadiazine and leucovorin; see remarks):
  Load: 2 mg/kg/24 hr PO ÷ Q12 hr × 2 days
  Maintenance: 1 mg/kg/24 hr PO once daily × 2—6 mo, then 1 mg/kg/24 hr 3× per wk to complete
    total 12 mo of therapy
Toxoplasmosis (administer with sulfadiazine or trisulfapyrimidines, and leucovorin):
  Child:
    Load: 2 mg/kg/24 hr PO ÷ BID (**max. dose:** 100 mg/24 hr) with the following duration:
      Non—HIV exposed/positive: 2 days
      HIV exposed/positive: 3 days
    Maintenance:
      Non—HIV exposed/positive: 1 mg/kg/24 hr PO once daily (**max. dose:** 25 mg/24 hr) × 6 mo,
        followed by 1 mg/kg/dose (**max. dose:** 25 mg/24 hr) 3 times per week to complete a total 12
        mo therapy
      HIV exposed/positive: 1 mg/kg/24 hr PO once daily (**max. dose:** 25 mg/24 hr) ≥6 wk
  Adult:
    Non—HIV exposed/positive: 50—75 mg/24 hr PO × 1—3 wk. Depending on tolerance and response,
      additional therapy at a 50% reduced dosage is continued × 4—5 wk.
    HIV exposed/positive: 200 mg PO × 1 followed by 50—75 mg/24 hr once daily × ≥6 wk

Continued

PYRIMETHAMINE *continued*

Pyrimethamine is a folate antagonist. Supplementation with folinic acid leucovorin at 5—15 mg/24 hr is recommended. **Contraindicated** in megaloblastic anemia secondary to folate deficiency. **Use with caution** in G6PD deficiency, malabsorption syndromes, alcoholism, pregnancy, and renal or hepatic impairment. Pyrimethamine can cause glossitis, bone marrow suppression, seizures, rash, and photosensitivity. For congenital toxoplasmosis, see *Clin Infect Dis* 1994;18:38—72. Zidovudine and methotrexate may increase risk for bone marrow suppression. Aurothioglucose, trimethoprim, and sulfamethoxazole may increase risk for blood dyscrasias. Administer doses with meals. Most cases of acquired toxoplasmosis do not require specific antimicrobial therapy.

Outpatient prescriptions may need to be processed through a specialty pharmacy program via the manufacturer; see http://www.daraprimdirect.com/healthcare-providers.

Q

QUETIAPINE
Seroquel, Seroquel XR, and generics
Antipsychotic, second generation

  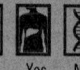

C   2   No   Yes   No

Tabs: 25, 50, 100, 200, 300, 400 mg
Extended release tabs (Seroqul XR and generics): 50, 150, 200, 300, 400 mg
Oral suspension: 10, 40 mg/mL

Bipolar mania (continue therapy at lowest dose to maintain efficacy and periodically assess maintenance treatment needs; PO):
Immediate release dosage forms:

Age	Dose Titration	Usual Effective Dose	Maximum Dose
Child ≥10 yr and adolescent (monotherapy)	Day 1: 25 mg BID Day 2: 50 mg BID Day 3: 100 mg BID Day 4: 150 mg BID Day 5: 200 mg BID ≥Day 6: If needed, additional increases should be ≤100 mg/24 hr up to 600 mg/24 hr. Total daily doses may be divided TID based on response and tolerability.	400—600 mg/24 hr	600 mg/24 hr
Adult (monotherapy or in combination with lithium or divalproex)	Day 1: 50 mg BID Day 2: 100 mg BID Day 3: 150 mg BID Day 4: 200 mg BID ≥Day 5: If needed, additional increases ≤200 mg/24 hr up to 800 mg/24 hr by day 6.	400—800 mg/24 hr	800 mg/24 hr

QUETIAPINE *continued*

Extended release tabs (see remarks):

Age	Dose Titration	Usual Effective Dose	Maximum Dose
Child ≥10 yr and adolescent (monotherapy)	Day 1: 50 mg QHS Day 2: 100 mg QHS Day 3—5: Increase by 100 mg/24 hr increments each day until 400 mg once daily is achieved on day 5.	400—600 mg once daily	600 mg/24 hr
Adult (monotherapy or in combination with lithium or divalproex)	Day 1: 300 mg QHS Day 2: 600 mg QHS Day 3: Adjust dose to 400—800 mg once daily based on efficacy and tolerance.	400—800 mg once daily	800 mg/24 hr (some may require 1200 mg/24 hr)

Schizophrenia (continue therapy at lowest dose to maintain efficacy and periodically assess maintenance treatment needs; PO):
Immediate release dosage forms:

Age	Dose Titration	Usual Effective Dose	Maximum Dose
Adolescent (13—17 yr)	Day 1: 25 mg BID Day 2: 50 mg BID Day 3: 100 mg BID Day 4: 150 mg BID Day 5: 200 mg BID ≥Day 6: If needed, additional increases should be ≤100 mg/24 hr up to 800 mg/24 hr. Total daily doses may be divided TID based on response and tolerability.	400—800 mg/24 hr	800 mg/24 hr
Adult	Day 1: 25 mg BID Day 2 and 3: Increase in increments of 25—50 mg divided 2—3 doses daily to 300—400 mg/24 hr divided BID—TID by day 4. If needed, increase dose by 50—100 mg/24 hr at intervals of at least 2 days.	150—750 mg/24 hr	750 mg/24 hr

Extended release tabs (see remarks):

Age	Dose Titration	Usual Effective Dose	Maximum Dose
Adolescent (13—17 yr)	Day 1: 50 mg once daily Day 2: 100 mg once daily Day 3: 200 mg once daily	400—800 mg once daily	800 mg/24 hr

Continued

QUETIAPINE *continued*

Age	Dose Titration	Usual Effective Dose	Maximum Dose
	Day 4: 300 mg once daily Day 5: 400 mg once daily		
Adult	Day 1: 300 mg QHS If needed, increase dose in increments of up to 300 mg/24 hr.	400—800 mg once daily	800 mg/24 hr

Avoid use in patients with history of cardiac arrhythmias or prolonged QTc syndrome, concurrent medications that can prolong the QTc interval, and alcohol use. **Use with caution** in hypovolemia and diabetes mellitus.

Suicidal ideation/behavior or worsening depression may occur, especially in children and young adults during the first few months of therapy or during dosage changes.

Common side effects in children include hypertension, hyperglycemia, hyperprolactinemia, and significant weight gain. Other common side effects include orthostatic hypotension, tachycardia, hypercholesterolemia, hypertriglyceridemia, abdominal pain, GI disturbances, increased appetite, xerostomia, increased serum transaminases, EPS, headache, dizziness, agitation, and fatigue. Anaphylactic reactions, DRESS, SJS, TEN, SIADH, cardiomyopathy, priapism, DKA, pancreatitis, eosinophilia, agranulocytosis, leukopenia, neutropenia, cataracts, hypothyroidism, neuroleptic malignant syndrome, and seizures have been reported. Anticholinergic side effects (e.g., constipation, urinary retention) may occur due to norquetiapine, its active metabolite, and may be enhanced with concurrent use of anticholinergic medications.

Do not abruptly discontinue medication as acute withdrawal symptoms occur. Dosage adjustment in hepatic impairment may be necessary as it is primarily hepatically metabolized. Quetiapine is a major substrate for CYP 450 3A4 and minor substrate for 2D6. Opioids and other CNS depressants may enhance CNS depressant effects. Carbamazepine may decrease the effects of quetiapine. Quetiapine may decrease dopamine agonist effects (e.g., anti-Parkinson agents) but may enhance the anticholinergic and QTc prolongation effects to those medications processing these risks. Always check for drug interactions as effects can be mild to severe.

Non—extended release dosage forms may be administered with or without food. Extended release tabs must be swallowed whole and administered preferably in the evening without food (a light meal of ≤300 calories is allowed). May convert patients from immediate release to extended release tablets at the equivalent total daily dose and administer once daily; individual dosage adjustments may be necessary.

QUINIDINE
Various generics
Class Ia antiarrhythmic, antimalarial agent

    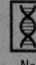

C   2   Yes   Yes   No

As gluconate (62% quinidine):
  Slow-release tabs: 324 mg
As sulfate (83% quinidine):
  Tabs: 200, 300 mg
  Oral suspension: 10 mg/mL
Equivalents: 200 mg sulfate = 267 mg gluconate
NOTE: The intravenous dosage form is no longer available in the United States. Contact the CDC Marlaria Hotline at (770) 488-7788 or (855) 856-4713 for an alternative therapy.

QUINIDINE *continued*

All doses are expressed as salt forms.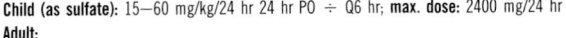
Antiarrhythmic (not first line):
   Child (as sulfate): 15—60 mg/kg/24 hr 24 hr PO ÷ Q6 hr; **max. dose:** 2400 mg/24 hr
   Adult:
     As sulfate: Start at 200 mg/dose Q6 hr and titrate cautiously to desired effect up to 600 mg PO Q6—12 hr.
     As gluconate: 324—648 mg PO Q8—12 hr
Malaria:
   Child and adult (give intravenously as gluconate; see remarks):
     Loading dose: 10 mg/kg/dose IV (**max. dose:** 600 mg) over 1—2 hr followed by maintenance dose. Omit or decrease load if patient has received quinine or mefloquine.
     Maintenance dose: 0.02 mg/kg/min IV as continuous infusion until oral therapy can be initiated. If more than 48 hr of intravenous therapy is required, reduce dose by 30%—50%.

Test dose is given to assess for idiosyncratic reaction to quinidine. Toxicity indicated by increase of QRS interval by ≥0.02 sec (skip dose or stop drug). May cause gastrointestinal (GI) symptoms, hypotension, tinnitus, TTP, rash, heart block, and blood dyscrasias. When used alone, may cause 1:1 conduction in atrial flutter leading to ventricular fibrillation. Patients may develop idiosyncratic ventricular tachycardia with low levels, especially when therapy is being initiated.

Quinidine is a substrate of CYP 450 3A3/4 and 3A5—7 enzymes, and an inhibitor of CYP 450 2D6 and 3A3/4 enzymes. Can cause increase in digoxin levels. Quinidine potentiates the effect of neuromuscular blocking agents, β-blockers, anticholinergics, and warfarin. Amiodarone, antacids, delavirdine, diltiazem, grapefruit juice, saquinavir, ritonavir, verapamil, or cimetidine may enhance the drug's effect. Barbiturates, phenytoin, cholinergic drugs, nifedipine, sucralfate, or rifampin may reduce quinidine's effect. **Use with caution** in renal insufficiency (15%—25% of drug is eliminated unchanged in the urine), myocardial depression, sick sinus syndrome, G6PD deficiency, and hepatic dysfunction.

Therapeutic levels (antiarrhythmic): 3—7 mg/L. Recommended serum sampling times at steady state: trough level obtained within 30 min prior to the next scheduled dose after 1—2 days of continuous dosing (steady state).

MALARIA USE: Continuous monitoring of electrocardiogram, blood pressure, and serum glucose is recommended, especially in pregnant women and young children.

QUINUPRISTIN AND DALFOPRISTIN
Synercid
Antibiotic, streptogramin

   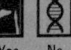

| B | 2 | No | Yes | No |

Injection: 500 mg (150 mg quinupristin and 350 mg dalfopristin)

Doses expressed in mg of combined quinupristin and dalfopristin.
Vancomycin-resistant *Enterococcus faecium* (VREF) and severe infections:
   Child <16 yr (limited data), ≥16 yr, and adult: 7.5 mg/kg/dose IV Q8 hr
     VERF endocarditis duration of therapy: Minimum of 8 weeks
Complicated skin infections:
   Child <16 yr (limited data), ≥16 yr, and adult: 7.5 mg/kg/dose IV Q12 hr for at least 7 days

Not active against *Enterococcus faecalis*. **Use with caution** in hepatic impairment; dosage reduction may be necessary. Most common side effects include pain, burning, inflammation and edema at the intravenous infusion site, thrombophlebitis and thrombosis, GI disturbances,

Continued

QUINUPRISTIN AND DALFOPRISTIN *continued*

rash, arthralgia, myalgia, increased liver enzymes, hyperbilirubinemia, and headache. Dose frequency reductions (Q8 hr—Q12 hr) or discontinuation can improve severe cases of arthralgia and myalgia. Use total body weight for obese patients when calculating dosages.

Drug is an inhibitor to the CYP 450 3A4 isoenzyme. **Avoid use** with CYP 450 3A4 substrates, which can prolong QTc interval. May increase the effects/toxicity of cyclosporine, tacrolimus, sirolimus, delavirdine, nevirapine, indinavir, ritonavir, diazepam, midazolam, carbamazepine, methylprednisolone, vinca alkaloids, docetaxel, paclitaxel, quinidine, and some calcium channel blockers.

Pediatric (<16 yr old) pharmacokinetic studies are incomplete. Reduce dose for patients with hepatic cirrhosis (Child-Pugh A or B).

Drug is compatible with D_5W and incompatible with saline and heparin. Infuse each dose over 1 hr using the following **max. IV concentrations:** peripheral line: 2 mg/mL, central line: 5 mg/mL. If injection site reaction occurs, dilute infusion to <1 mg/mL.

R

RALTEGRAVIR
Isentress and Isentress HD
Antiretroviral agent, integrase inhibitor

 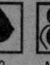 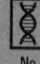

C   2   No   Yes   No

Tabs:
  Isentress: 400 mg
  Isentress HD: 600 mg
Chewable tabs: 25, 100 mg; contains aspartame (100 mg tab is scored)
Oral powder for suspension: 100 mg (60 packets); contains polyethylene glycol

HIV treatment: See https://clinicalinfo.hiv.gov/en/guidelines

HIV vertical transmission and presumptive treatment during high-risk situations (mothers who received no antepartum antiretroviral therapy, mothers who received only intrapartum antiretroviral therapy, mothers who receive antepartum antiretroviral therapy but with suboptimal viral suppression [>50 copies/mL] within 4 weeks prior to delivery, or mothers with acute or primary HIV infection during pregnancy or breastfeeding [immediately discontinue breastfeeding]). Transition to a treatment regimen if positive HIV diagnosis is confirmed and discontinue use after a negative diagnosis; see Chapter 17 for additional information:

≥37 weeks' gestation at birth and ≥2 kg (use 10 mg/mL oral suspension dosage form in combination with zidovudine and lamivudine administered from birth up to 6 weeks; delay first dose of raltegravir 24—48 hr after birth if mother received raltegravir 2 to 24 hours prior to delivery, but initiate zidovudine and lamivudine immediately):

  <7 days old: 1.5 mg/kg/dose PO once daily or by the following weight categories:
    2—<3 kg: 4 mg PO once daily
    3—<4 kg: 5 mg PO once daily
    4—<5 kg: 7 mg PO once daily
  1—4 weeks old: 3 mg/kg/dose PO BID or by the following weight categories:
    2—<3 kg: 8 mg PO BID
    3—<4 kg: 10 mg PO BID
    4—<5 kg: 15 mg PO BID

RALTEGRAVIR *continued*

4—6 weeks old: 6 mg/kg/dose PO BID or by the following weight categories:

3—<4 kg: 25 mg PO BID
4—<6 kg: 30 mg PO BID
6—<8 kg: 40 mg PO BID

Common side effects include nausea, headache, increased ALT and other liver enzymes, insomnia, and fatigue. Severe and life-threatening skin reactions (e.g., SJS, TEN), hypersensitivity reactions characterized by rash, organ dysfunction (including hepatic failure), immune reconstitution syndrome, hyperglycemia, rhabdomyolysis, and autoimmune disorders (e.g., Graves disease and Guillain-Barré syndrome) have been reported.

Raltegravir is ~83% protein bound and primarily metabolized via the UGT1A1 glucuronidation pathway. UGT1A1 activity is low at birth and increases rapidly during the next 4—6 weeks of life. No dosing information is currently available for preterm infants or infants weighing <2 kg at birth and for severe hepatic impairment. Use with antacids containing aluminum or magnesium salts may reduce raltegravir levels and is not recommended. Medications containing polyvalent cations (e.g., supplements containing iron, calcium or magnesium, sucralfate, and laxatives) should be spaced apart by administering raltegravir at least 2 hours before or 6 hours after the administration of polyvalent cation medicine. Use with fosamprenavir may result in reduced levels of amprenavir and raltegravir. Other medications that could decrease raltegravir levels and effects include rifampin, orlistat, and etravirine. Omeprazole may increase raltegravir levels.

Each dosage form has a different pharmacokinetic profile; dosage forms are not interchangeable. Oral tablets must be swallowed whole, and the chewable tablet may be crushed and mixed with ~5 mL of water, juice, or breast milk. The oral suspension must be administered within 30 min after reconstitution. Doses may be administered with or without food; however, the effect of food on the oral suspension has not been evaluated.

RASBURICASE
Elitek
Antihyperuricemic agent

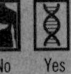

C   ?   No   No   Yes

Injection: 1.5, 7.5 mg; contains mannitol and L-alanine

Hyperuricemia (all ages; see remarks): 0.1—0.2 mg/kg/dose (rounded down to the nearest whole 1.5 mg multiple) IV over 30 min × 1. Patients generally respond to one dose, but if needed dose may be repeated Q24 hr for up to four additional doses.

Contraindicated in G6PD deficiency (risk for acute hemolytic anemia) or history of hypersensitivity, hemolytic reactions, or methemoglobinemia with rasburicase. **Use with caution** in asthma, allergies, hypersensitivity with other medications, and children <2 yr of age (decreased efficacy and increased risk for rash, vomiting, diarrhea, and fever).

Common side effects include nausea, vomiting, abdominal pain, discomfort, diarrhea, constipation, mucositis, fever, and rash. Serious and fatal hypersensitivity reactions have been reported in <1% of patients, including anaphylaxis, and can occur at any time; discontinue use immediately and permanently.

During therapy, uric acid blood samples must be sent to the laboratory immediately. Blood should be collected in prechilled tubes containing heparin and placed in an ice-water bath to avoid potential falsely low uric acid levels (degradation of plasma uric acid occurs in the presence of rasburicase at room temperature). Centrifugation in a precooled centrifuge (4°C) is indicated. Plasma samples must be assayed within 4 hr of sample collection.

RH₀ (D) IMMUNE GLOBULIN INTRAVENOUS (HUMAN)
WinRho-SDF, Rhophylac, HyperRHO S/D
Mini-Dose, HyperRHO S/D Full Dose, RhoGAM Ultra-
Filtered Plus, MICRhoGAM Ultra-Filtered Plus
Immune globulin

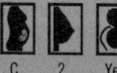 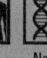 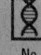

C   2   Yes   No   No

Injection (WinRho-SDF): 1500 IU (1.3 mL), 2500 IU (2.2 mL), 5000 IU (4.4 mL), 15,000 IU (13 mL);
may contain polysorbate 80
Prefilled injection for IV or IM administration:
   Rhophylac: 1500 IU (2 mL); preservative free
Prefilled injection for IM administration:
   HyperRHO S/D Mini-Dose: 250 IU
   HyperRHO S/D Full Dose: 1500 IU
   MICRhoGAM Ultra-Filtered Plus: 250 IU; contains polysorbate 80
   RhoGAM Ultra-Filtered Plus: 1500 IU; contains polysorbate 80
Conversion: 1 mCg = 5 IU
IM route and IM dosage forms: Indicated for prevention of Rh hemolytic disease of newborn by
administering to Rh₀(D) negative mother or prevention of isoimmunization in Rh₀(D)-negative
individuals who have been transfused with Rh₀(D)-positive blood/cell components.

All doses based on international units (IU)
**Immune thrombocytopenic purpura (nonsplenectomized Rh₀[D]-positive patients; see
remarks):**
   WinRho-SDF (child, adolescent, and adult; see remarks):
      Initial dose (may be given in two divided doses on separate days or as a single dose):
         Hemoglobin ≥10 mg/dL: 250 IU/kg/dose IV × 1
         Hemoglobin 8–<10 mg/dL: 125–200 IU/kg/dose IV × 1
         Hemoglobin <8 mg/dL: Use alternative therapy.
      **Subsequent doses (actual dose and frequency of administration is determined by the patient's
      clinical response and subsequent hemoglobin level):**
         Hemoglobin <8 g/dL: Use alternative therapy.
         Hemoglobin 8–10 g/dL: 125–200 IU/kg/dose IV × 1
         Hemoglobin >10 g/dL: 250–300 IU/kg/dose IV × 1
   Rhophylac (child, adolescent, and adult; see remarks): 250 IU/kg/dose IV × 1

Contraindicated in IgA deficiency. **Use with caution** with history of atherosclerosis,
known/suspected hyperviscosity, coagulation disorders, and other thrombotic risks. Adverse
events associated with ITP indication include headache, chills, fever, and reduction in hemoglobin
(due to the destruction of Rh₀[D] antigen-positive red cells). Intravascular hemolysis resulting in
anemia and renal insufficiency has been reported. May interfere with immune response to live virus
vaccines (e.g., MMR, varicella).
Clinical response for ITP therapy requires monitoring of platelet counts, RBC, Hgb, and reticulocyte
count. Rh₀(D)-positive patients should be monitored for signs and symptoms of intravascular
hemolysis, anemia, and renal insufficiency.
Recommended IV administration rate:
   WinRho-SDF: Over 3–5 min
   Rhophylac: Each 1500 IU (2 mL) per 15–60 sec

RIBAVIRIN
Oral: Generics; previously available as Rebetol
Inhalation: Virazole and generics
Antiviral agent

     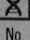

X   3   Yes   Yes   No

RIBAVIRIN *continued*

Oral caps: 200 mg
Tabs: 200, 400, 600 mg
Aerosol (Virazole and generics): 6 g

Hepatitis C (PO, see remarks): Hepatitis C combination therapy is dependent on HCV genotype and treatment status. Specific treatment recommendations are dynamic with newer therapies; see the most recent American Association for the Study of Liver Diseases/Infectious Disease Society of America (AASLD/IDSA) treatment recommendations at www.hcvguidelines.org
  Child: In combination with sofosbuvir for patients with genotypes 2 or 3 with/without cirrhosis:
    Child <12 yr and ≥35 kg, child ≥12 yr and adolescent (see remarks):
      <47 kg: 15 mg/kg/24 hr PO ÷ BID
      47—49 kg: 600 mg/24 hr PO ÷ BID
      50—65 kg: 800 mg/24 hr PO ÷ BID
      66—80 kg: 1000 mg/24 hr PO ÷ BID
      >80 kg: 1200 mg/24 hr PO ÷ BID
  Duration of therapy:
    Genotype 2: 12 weeks
    Genotype 3: 24 weeks
  Adult (see remarks):
    Oral capsules or solution as part of a recommended combination therapy:
      <75 kg: 500 mg PO BID
      ≥75 kg: 600 mg PO BID
Inhalation (see remarks):
  Continuous: Administer 6 g by aerosol over 12—18 hr once daily for 3—7 days. The 6 g ribavirin vial is diluted in 300 mL preservative-free sterile water to a final concentration of 20 mg/mL. Must be administered with Viratek Small Particle Aerosol Generator (SPAG-2).
  Intermittent (for nonventilated patients): Administer 2 g by aerosol over 2 hr TID for 3—7 days. The 6 g ribavirin vial is diluted in 100 mL preservative-free sterile water to a final concentration of 60 mg/mL. The intermittent use is not recommended in patients with endotracheal tubes.

ORAL RIBAVIRIN: Contraindicated in pregnancy, significant or unstable cardiac disease, autoimmune hepatitis, hepatic decompensation (Child-Pugh score >6; class B or C), hemoglobinopathies, and creatinine clearance <50 mL/min. **Use with caution** in preexisting cardiac disease, pulmonary disease, and sarcoidosis. Anemia (most common), insomnia, depression, irritability, and suicidal behavior (higher in adolescent and pediatric patients) have been reported with the oral route.
Combination therapy with peginterferon for Hep C is no longer recommended due to poor efficacy. Tinnitus, hearing loss, vertigo, severe hypertriglyceridemia, and homicidal ideation have been reported in combination with interferon. Suicidal ideation or attempts have been reported more frequently among adolescents compared to adults (2.4% vs. 1%) during treatment and off-therapy follow up. Pancytopenia has been reported in combination with interferon and azathioprine. Increased risk for hepatic decompensation with cirrhotic chronic hepatitis C patients treated with α interferons or with HIV coinfection receiving HAART and interferon alfa-2a. Growth inhibition (delays in weight and height increases) was observed in children (5—17 years old) receiving combination therapy for up to 48 weeks.
May decrease the effects of zidovudine and stavudine and increase the risk for lactic acidosis with nucleoside analogues. **Reduce or discontinue dosage for toxicity as follows:**
Patient with no cardiac disease:
  Hgb <10 g/dL and ≥8.5 g/dL:
    Child: 12 mg/kg/dose PO once daily; may further reduce to 8 mg/kg/dose PO once daily

Continued

RIBAVIRIN *continued*

>   *Adult:* 600 mg PO once daily (capsules or solution) or 200 mg PO QAM and 400 mg PO QPM (tablets)
>
>   *Hgb <8.5 g/dL:* Discontinue therapy permanently.
>   Patient with cardiac disease:
>
> >   *≥2 mg/dL decrease in Hgb during any 4-week period during therapy:*
> >   *Child:* 12 mg/kg/dose PO once daily; may further reduce to 8 mg/kg/dose PO once daily (monitor weekly)
> >   *Adult:* 600 mg PO once daily (capsules or solution) or 200 mg PO QAM and 400 mg PO QPM (tablets)
> >   *Hgb <12 g/dL after 4 weeks of reduced dose:* Discontinue therapy permanently.

INHALED RIBAVIRIN: Use of ribavirin for RSV is controversial and not routinely indicated. Aerosol therapy may be considered for selected infants and young children at high risk for serious RSV disease (see most recent edition of the AAP *Red Book*). Most effective if begun early in course of RSV infection; generally in the first 3 days. May cause worsening respiratory distress, rash, conjunctivitis, mild bronchospasm, hypotension, anemia, and cardiac arrest. **Avoid** unnecessary occupational exposure to ribavirin due to its teratogenic effects. Drug can precipitate in the respiratory equipment.

RIBOFLAVIN
Vitamin B₂ and various brands and generics
Water-soluble vitamin

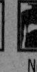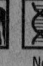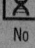

| A/C | 1 | No | No | No |

Tabs [OTC]: 25, 50, 100 mg
Caps [OTC]: 400 mg

Riboflavin deficiency:
  Child: 2.5—10 mg/24 hr ÷ once daily–BID PO
  Adult: 5—30 mg/24 hr ÷ once daily–BID PO
U.S. RDA requirements: See Chapter 21.
Migraine prophylaxis (limited data):
  Child ≥8 yr and adolescent: 200—400 mg PO once daily

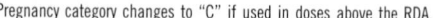

Hypersensitivity may occur. Administer with food. Causes yellow to orange discoloration of urine. For multivitamin information, see Chapter 21.
Pregnancy category changes to "C" if used in doses above the RDA.

RIFABUTIN
Mycobutin and generics
Antituberculous agent

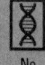

| B | 2 | Yes | Yes | No |

Caps: 150 mg
Oral suspension: 20 mg/mL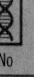

MAC primary prophylaxis for first episode of opportunistic disease in HIV (see remarks for interactions and www.aidsinfo.nih.gov/guidelines):
  Child >5 yr, adolescent, and adult: 300 mg PO once daily; doses may be administered as 150 mg PO BID if gastrointestinal (GI) upset occurs
MAC secondary prophylaxis for recurrence of opportunistic disease in HIV (in combination with ethambutol and a macrolide antibiotic [clarithromycin or azithromycin]):

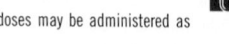

RIFABUTIN *continued*

Infant and child: 5 mg/kg/24 hr PO once daily; **max. dose:** 300 mg/24 hr
Adolescent and adult: 300 mg PO once daily; doses may be administered 150 mg PO BID if GI upset occurs

MAC treatment:
  Child: 10—20 mg/kg/24 hr PO once daily; **max. dose:** 300 mg/24 hr as part of a multidrug regimen for severe disease
  Adult: 300 mg PO once daily; may be used in combination with azithromycin and ethambutol
    Use in combination with HIV antiretroviral agents: See product information for dosage recommendations.

Should not be used for MAC prophylaxis with active TB. May cause GI distress, discoloration of skin and body fluids (brown-orange color), and marrow suppression. Rash, eosinophilia, and bronchospasm have been reported. **Use with caution** in renal and liver impairment. **Adjust dose in renal impairment (see Chapter 31).** May permanently stain contact lenses. Uveitis can occur when using high doses (>300 mg/24 hr in adults) in combination with macrolide antibiotics.
Rifabutin is an inducer of CYP 450 3A enzyme and is structurally similar to rifampin (similar drug interactions, see Rifampin). Clarithromycin, fluconazole, itraconazole, nevirapine, and protease inhibitors increase rifabutin levels. Efavirenz may decrease rifabutin levels. May decrease effectiveness of dapsone, delavirdine, nevirapine, amprenavir, indinavir, nelfinavir, saquinavir, itraconazole, warfarin, oral contraceptives, digoxin, cyclosporine, ketoconazole, and narcotics.
Doses may be administered with food if patient experiences GI intolerance.

RIFAMPIN
Rifadin and generics
Antibiotic, antituberculous agent, rifamycin

  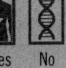

C   2   Yes   Yes   No

Caps: 150, 300 mg
Oral suspension: 10, 25 mg/mL
Injection (Rifadin and generics): 600 mg; contains formaldehyde sulfoxylate

Staphylococcus aureus infections (as part of synergistic therapy with other antistaphylococcal agents):
Neonate, infant, child, and adolescent: 10—20 mg/kg/24 hr ÷ Q12 hr IV/PO; **max. dose:** 600 mg/24 hr
  Prosthetic valve endocarditis:
    Early infection (≤1 yr surgery): 20 mg/kg/24 hr ÷ Q8 hr IV/PO; **max. dose:** 900 mg/24 hr
    Late infection (>1 yr surgery): 15—20 mg/kg/24 hr ÷ Q12 hr IV/PO; **max. dose:** 600 mg/24 hr
    MRSA infection: 15 mg/kg/24 hr ÷ Q8 hr IV/PO; **max. dose:** 900 mg/24 hr
Adult: 600 mg once daily, or 300—450 mg Q12 hr IV/PO
  Prosthetic valve endocarditis: 300 mg Q8 hr IV/PO for a minimum of 6 weeks in combination with antistaphylococcal penicillin with or without gentamicin for first 2 weeks
Tuberculosis (see latest edition of the AAP *Red Book* for duration of therapy and combination therapy): Twice-weekly therapy may be used after 1—2 months of daily therapy.
Infant, child, and adolescent (as part of a combination therapy):
  Daily therapy: 10—20 mg/kg/24 hr ÷ Q12—24 hr IV/PO; higher dose of 20—30 mg/kg/24 hr ÷ Q12—24 hr has been recommended for infants and toddlers and for central nervous system (CNS) and disseminated disease. Max. dose: 600 mg/24 hr
  Twice-weekly therapy: 15—20 mg/kg/24 hr PO twice weekly; higher dose of 20—30 mg/kg/24 hr twice weekly has been recommended for infants and toddlers and for CNS and disseminated disease. **Max. daily dose:** 600 mg/24 hr

Continued

RIFAMPIN *continued*

Adult:
Daily therapy: 10 mg/kg/24 hr IV/PO once daily
Twice-weekly therapy: 10 mg/kg/24 hr IV/PO once daily twice weekly
Max. daily dose: 600 mg/24 hr
TB meningitis (all ages):
PO: 20 mg/kg/dose Q24 hr; **max. dose:** 1200 mg/dose
IV: 15 mg/kg/dose Q24 hr; **max. dose:** 900 mg/dose
Prophylaxis for *Neisseria meningitidis* (see latest edition of the AAP *Red Book* for additional information):
0—<1 mo: 10 mg/kg/24 hr ÷ Q12 hr PO × 2 days
≥1 mo: 20 mg/kg/24 hr ÷ Q12 hr PO × 2 days
Adult: 600 mg PO Q12 hr × 2 days
Max. dose (all ages): 1200 mg/24 hr

Never use as monotherapy except when used for prophylaxis. Patients with latent tuberculosis infection should NOT be treated with rifampin and pyrazinamide because of the risk of severe liver injury. Use is **NOT recommended** in porphyria. **Use with caution** in diabetes.

May cause GI irritation, allergy, headache, fatigue, ataxia, muscle weakness, confusion, fever, hepatitis, transient LFT abnormalities, blood dyscrasias, interstitial nephritis, and elevated BUN and uric acid. Causes red discoloration of body secretions such as urine, saliva, and tears (which can permanently stain contact lenses). Pulmonary toxicity, hepatotoxicity, bleeding, and vitamin K—dependent coagulation disorders have been reported.

Induces several hepatic enzymes and transporters (CYP 450 2C9, 2C19, and 3A4; UGT1A1, P-glycoprotein, and OATP1B1/1B3), which may decrease plasma concentration of digoxin, corticosteroids, buspirone, benzodiazepines, fentanyl, calcium channel blockers, β-blockers, cyclosporine, tacrolimus, itraconazole, ketoconazole, oral anticoagulants, barbiturates, and theophylline. May reduce the effectiveness of oral contraceptives and anti-retroviral agents (protease inhibitors and nonnucleoside reverse transcriptase inhibitors). **Use is contraindicated** with praziquantel due to decreased praziquantel levels; rifampin should be discontinued 4 weeks prior to initiating praziquantel, and rifampin can be restarted 1 day after completion of praziquantel. Hepatotoxicity is a greater concern when used in combination with pyrazinamide and ritonavir-boosted saquinavir **(use is contraindicated).**

Adjust dose in renal failure (see Chapter 31). Reduce dose in hepatic impairment. Give oral doses 1 hr before or 2 hr after meals. Patients should abstain from alcohol, hepatotoxic medications, or herbal products while taking rifampin.

For *Haemophilus influenzae* type b prophylaxis, see latest edition of the *Red Book*.

RIFAXIMIN
Xifaxan
Antibiotic, rifamycin derivative

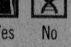
C   ?   No   Yes   No

Tabs: 200, 550 mg; may contain edetate disodium
Oral suspension: 20 mg/mL

Small intestinal bacterial overgrowth (SIBO; limited data):
Child 3—<8 yr: 200 mg PO TID × 7—14 days
Child ≥8 yr and adolescent: 200—550 mg PO TID × 7—14 days
Adult: 550 mg PO TID × 14 days
Irritable bowel syndrome with diarrhea:
Child ≥8 yr and adolescent (limited data): 10—30 mg/kg/24 hr PO ÷ TID; **max. dose:** 1200 mg/24 hr

RIFAXIMIN *continued*

Adult: 550 mg PO TID × 14 days; may repeat up to two times with the same dosage regimen
Travelers' diarrhea (caused by noninvasive strains of *Escherichia coli*):
   Child ≥3—11 yr (limited data): 100 mg PO QID for up to 5 days
   Child ≥12 yr and adult: 200 mg PO TID × 3 days
Recurrent or subsequent *Clostridium difficile* diarrhea (initiated after a 10-day course of oral vancomycin):
   Child <12 yr (limited data): 15—30 mg/kg/24 hr PO ÷ TID × 20 days; **max. dose:** 1200 mg/24 hr
   Child ≥12 yr and adult: 400 mg PO TID × 20 days

Contraindicated with rifamycin hypersensitivity. **Avoid use** in diarrhea complicated by fever
   or blood in the stool. **Use with caution** in severe hepatic impairment (Child-Pugh class C).
   Severe cutaneous reactions (e.g., SJS, TEN) have been reported with use in patients with cirrhosis.
Common side effects include peripheral edema, abdominal pain, nausea, ascites, dizziness, headache,
   and fatigue. Anaphylaxis, angioedema, rhabdomyolysis, and exfoliative dermatitis have been
   reported.
Substrate and inhibitor of OATP1A2/SLCOA2 transporter and substrate of P-glycoprotein ABCB1 and
   OATP1B1/1B3. May decrease the effects of warfarin and immunological effects of cholera and BCG
   vaccines. P-glycoprotein inhibitors (e.g., cyclosporine) may increase the effects/toxicity of rifaximin.
Doses may be administered with or without food.

RIMANTADINE
Generics; previously available as Flumadine
Antiviral agent

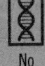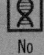

C   3   Yes   Yes   No

Tabs: 100 mg
Oral suspension: 10 mg/1 mL

Influenza A prophylaxis (for at least 10 days after known exposure; usually for 6—8 weeks during influenza A season or local outbreak):
   Child:
      1—9 yr: 5 mg/kg/24 hr PO once daily—BID; **max. dose:** 150 mg/24 hr
      ≥10 yr:
         <40 kg: 5 mg/kg/24 hr PO ÷ BID; **max. dose:** 150 mg/24 hr
         ≥40 kg: 100 mg per dose PO BID
   Adult: 100 mg PO BID
Influenza A treatment (within 48 hr of illness onset; NOT to be used in areas with high resistance rates):
   Use the aforementioned prophylaxis dosage × 7 days.

Resistance to influenza A and recommendations against the use for treatment and
   prophylaxis have been reported by the Centers for Disease Control (CDC). Check with local
   microbiology laboratories and the CDC for seasonal susceptibility/resistance.
Preferred over amantadine for influenza due to lower incidence of adverse events. Individuals
   immunized with live attenuated influenza vaccine (e.g., FluMist) should not receive rimantadine
   prophylaxis for 14 days after the vaccine. Chemoprophylaxis does not interfere with immune
   response to inactivated influenza vaccine.
May cause GI disturbance, xerostomia, dizziness, headache, and urinary retention. CNS disturbances
   are less than with amantadine. **Contraindicated** in amantadine hypersensitivity. **Use with caution**
   in renal or hepatic insufficiency; dosage reduction may be necessary. A dosage reduction of 50%
   has been recommended in severe hepatic or renal impairment. Subjects with severe renal
   impairment have been reported to have an 81% increase in systemic exposure.

RISPERIDONE
Risperdal, Risperdal Consta, Perseris, and generics
Atypical antipsychotic, serotonin (5-HT₂) and dopamine (D₂) antagonist

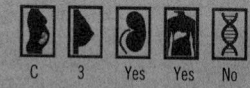

C	3	Yes	Yes	No

Tabs: 0.25, 0.5, 1, 2, 3, 4 mg
Oral solution: 1 mg/mL (30 mL); may contain benzoic acid
Orally disintegrating tabs: 0.25, 0.5, 1, 2, 3, 4 mg; contain phenylalanine
IM injection (Risperdal Consta): 12.5, 25, 37.5, 50 mg (prefilled syringe with 2 mL diluent; includes one 21-gauge 1-in needle for deltoid administration and one 20-gauge 2-in needle for gluteal administration); for IM administration only
Subcutaneous extended release injection (Perseris): 90, 120 mg (prefilled syringe that includes a 18-gauge, 5/8 inch needle)

Irritability associated with autistic disorder:

5–17 yr (PO daily doses may be administered once daily–BID; patients experiencing somnolence may benefit from QHS or BID dosing or dose reduction):

Initial dose:

<20 kg: 0.25 mg/24 hr PO for a minimum of 4 days; use with caution if <15 kg as dosing recommendation is not established

≥20 kg: 0.5 mg/24 hr PO for a minimum of 4 days

Dose increment (if needed) after 4 days of initial dose:

<20 kg: 0.5 mg/24 hr PO for a minimum of 14 days; if additional increments needed, increase dose by 0.25 mg/24 hr at intervals of at least 14 days

≥20 kg: 1 mg/24 hr PO for a minimum of 14 days; if additional increments needed, increase dose by 0.5 mg/24 hr at intervals of at least 14 days

Max. daily dose for plateau of therapeutic effect (from one pivotal clinical trial):

<20 kg: 1 mg/24 hr

≥20–45 kg: 2.5 mg/24 hr

>45 kg: 3 mg/24 hr

Bipolar mania: Oral doses may be administered once or twice daily; patients experiencing somnolence may benefit from QHS or BID dosing or dose reduction. Long-term use beyond 3 weeks and doses (all ages) >6 mg/24 hr have not been evaluated.

Child (10–17 yr): Start with 0.5 mg/24 hr PO once daily (QAM or QHS). If needed, increase dose at intervals ≥24 hr in increments of 0.5 or 1 mg/24 hr, as tolerated, up to a recommended dose of 2.5 mg/24 hr. Although efficacy has been demonstrated between 0.5 and 6 mg/24 hr, no additional benefit was seen above 2.5 mg/24 hr. Higher doses were associated with more adverse effects.

Adult: Start with 2–3 mg PO once. Dosage increases or decreases of 1 mg/24 hr can be made at 24-hr intervals. Dosage range: 4–6 mg/24 hr. *Usual max. dose:* 8 mg/24 hr

Schizophrenia: Oral doses may be administered once daily–BID and patients experiencing somnolence may benefit from BID dosing (see remarks).

Adolescent (13–17 yr): No data are available to support long-term use of >8 wk.

PO: Start with 0.5 mg once daily (QAM or QHS). If needed, increase dose at intervals ≥24 hr in increments of 0.5 to 1 mg/24 hr, as tolerated, to a recommended dose of 3 mg/24 hr. Although efficacy has been demonstrated between 1–6 mg/24 hr, no additional benefit and greater side effects were seen above 3 mg/24 hr. Doses >6 mg/24 hr have not been studied.

Adult:

PO: Start with 1 mg BID on day 1; if tolerated, increase to 2 mg BID on day 2 and to 3 mg BID thereafter. Dosage increases or decreases of 1–2 mg can be made on a weekly basis if needed. Usual effective dose: 2–8 mg/24 hr. Doses above 16 mg/24 hr have not been evaluated.

RISPERIDONE *continued*

IM: Start with 25 mg Q2 wk; if no response, dose may be increased to 37.5 mg or 50 mg at 4-week intervals. **Max. IM dose:** 50 mg Q2 wk. PO risperidone should also be administered with the initial IM dose and continued × 3 weeks and discontinued to provide adequate plasma concentrations during the initial IM dosing period.

Subcutaneous extended release injection (Perseris; establish tolerability with oral therapy first before using this dosage form): 90 or 120 mg SC once every month. 90 mg dose corresponds to a 3 mg/24 hr PO risperidone and 120 mg dose to 4 mg/24 hr PO risperidone. No loading dose nor supplemental oral doses are recommended.

Use with caution in cardiovascular disorders, diabetes, renal or hepatic impairment (dose reduction necessary), hypothermia or hyperthermia, seizures, breast cancer or other prolactin-dependent tumors, and dysphagia. Common side effects include abdominal pain and other GI disturbances, arthralgia, anxiety, dizziness, headache, insomnia, somnolence (use QHS dosing), EPS, cough, fever, pharyngitis, rash, rhinitis, sexual dysfunction, tachycardia, and weight gain. Weight gain, somnolence, and fatigue were common side effects reported in the autism studies. Priapism, QTc prolongation, neuroleptic malignant syndrome, hypothermia, sleep apnea syndrome, sleepwalking, ileus, urinary retention, diabetes mellitus, and hypoglycemia have been reported. Very rare cases of anaphylaxis have been reported with use of the IM dosage form in patients who have previously tolerated the oral dosage form.

In the presence of severe renal or hepatic impairment or risk for hypotension, the following adult dosing has been recommended: Start with 0.5 mg PO BID. Increase dose, if needed and tolerated, in increments no more than 0.5 mg BID. Increases to doses >1.5 mg BID should occur at intervals of at least 1 week; slower titration may be required in some patients.

Limited studies in pediatric related Tourette syndrome, schizophrenia, and aggressive behavior in psychiatric disorders are reported. Autistic disorder safety and efficacy in children <5 years of age have not been established. If therapy has been discontinued for a period of time, therapy should be reinitiated with the same initial titration regimen.

Drug is a CYP 450 2D6 and 3A4 isoenzyme substrate. Concurrent use of isoenzyme inhibitors (e.g., fluoxetine, paroxetine, sertraline, cimetidine) and inducers (e.g., carbamazepine, rifampin, phenobarbital, phenytoin) may increase and decrease the effects of risperidone, respectively. Alcohol, CNS depressants, and St. John's wort may potentiate the drug's side effect. Risperidone may enhance the hypotensive effects of levodopa and dopamine agonists. When used with methylphenidate, an increase risk for extrapyramidal symptoms may occur whenever a dosage change is made to either medication.

Oral dosage forms may be administered with or without food. Oral solution can be mixed in water, coffee, orange juice, or low-fat milk but is incompatible with cola or tea. **Do not split or chew the orally disintegrating tablet.** Use IM suspension preparation within 6 hr after reconstitution.

RIVAROXABAN
Xarelto, Xarelto Starter Pack
Anticoagulant, direct thrombin inhibitor

C   ?   Yes   Yes   No

Tabs: 2.5, 10, 15, 20 mg
Xarelto Starter Pack: 15 mg (42 tabs) and 20 mg (9 tabs); provides 30 days of therapy
Oral suspension: 1 mg/mL (155 mL); contains sodium benzoate

Prevention and treatment venous thromboembolic event (VTE):
Child from birth (≥37 weeks' gestation and ≥2.6 kg) to <18 yr: Prevention and treatment dosages are similar. Initiate therapy after a minimum of 5 days of initial IV anticoagulation therapy.

Continued

RIVAROXABAN *continued*

Neonates and infants <6 months old should have had at least 10 days of oral feedings. Use only the oral suspension dosage form for patients <30 kg and either oral suspension or tablets for patients >30 kg (2.5 mg tablet not recommended in children due to incomplete pharmacokinetic/pharmacodynamic and clinical data). Monitor patient weight regularly (especially those <12 kg) and review dosage level regularly to maintain a therapeutic dose. Administer all doses with feeds or food for VTE treatment but optional for VTE prevention.

2.6—2.9 kg: 0.8 mg PO Q8 hr
3—3.9 kg: 0.9 mg PO Q8 hr
4—4.9 kg: 1.4 mg PO Q8 hr
5—6.9 kg: 1.6 mg PO Q8 hr
7—7.9 kg: 1.8 mg PO Q8 hr
8—8.9 kg: 2.4 mg PO Q8 hr
9—9.9 kg: 2.8 mg PO Q8 hr
10—11.9 kg: 3 mg PO Q8 hr
12—29.9 kg: 5 mg PO Q12 hr
30—49.9 kg: 15 mg PO Q24 hr
≥50 kg: 20 mg PO Q24 hr
Duration of therapy:
  All patients (except for <2 yr old with catheter-related thrombosis): 3—12 months
  <2 yr old with catheter-related thrombosis: 1—3 months
Adult: Administer all doses with food for VTE treatment but optional for VTE prevention.
VTE Treatment: 15 mg PO BID × 21 days followed by 20 mg PO once daily
VTE Prevention: 10 mg PO once daily
Thromboprophylaxis following Fontan procedure:
Child ≥2—<18 yr: Use only the oral suspension dosage form for patients <50 kg and either oral suspension or tablets for patients >50 kg (2.5 mg tablet not recommended in children due to incomplete pharmacokinetic/pharmacodynamic and clinical data). Doses may be administered with or without feeds or food.
  7—7.9 kg: 1.1 mg PO Q12 hr
  8—9.9 kg: 1.6 mg PO Q12 hr
  10—11.9 kg: 1.7 mg PO Q12 hr
  12—19.9 kg: 2 mg PO Q12 hr
  20—29.9 kg: 2.5 mg PO Q12 hr
  30—49.9 kg: 7.5 mg PO Q24 hr
  ≥50 kg: 10 mg PO Q24 hr

Contraindicated in active pathological bleeding and severe hypersensitivity to rivaroxaban and its excipients. **AVOID** use in moderate/severe hepatic impairment (Child-Pugh classes B and C); in those who develop acute renal failure with use; children with moderate/severe renal impairment (eGFR <50 mL/min); adults with severe renal impairment (eGFR <15 m/min); use with medications that are p-glycoprotein (P-gp) and strong CYP3A4 inducers (e.g., carbamazepine, phenytoin, rifampin, and St. John's wort), or use with medications that are P-gp and strong CYP3A4 inhibitors (e.g., ketoconazole, itraconazole, clarithromycin, lopinavir/ritonavir, ritonavir, indinavir/ritonavir). Use is not recommended in triple-positive antiphospholipid syndrome; patients with prosthetic heart valves or transcatheter aortic valve replacement; and with HIV protease inhibitors.

Common side effects include gastroenteritis (13% in children), vomiting (11%—14% in children), cough (16% in children), heavy menstrual bleeding (27% in adolescents), and hemorrhage (5%—36% in children and adults). Spinal hematoma or epidural hemorrhage may occur in patients receiving neuraxial anesthesia or undergoing spinal puncture; if needed, discontinue use of rivaroxaban 72 hours prior to neuraxial intervention and consider checking anti-factor Xa level.

RIVAROXABAN *continued*

Rivaroxaban is a major CYP450 3A4 and minor P-gp/ABC1 and BCRP/ABCG2 substrate. See above for medications to avoid and always assess for other drug interactions.

Administer all dosages with food or feeds as indicated. If anticoagulation needs to be discontinued prior to surgery or other procedures with bleeding risk, discontinue rivaroxaban at least 24 hr before the procedure. If converting from or to another anticoagulant medication, see product information for recommendations. Adjust dosage in renal impairment (see Chapter 31).

RIZATRIPTAN BENZOATE
Maxalt, Maxalt-MLT, and generics
Antimigraine agent, selective serotonin agonist

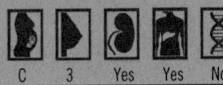

| C | 3 | Yes | Yes | No |

Tabs:
    Generics: 5, 10 mg (12s, 18s)
    Maxalt: 10 mg (18s)
Orally disintegrating tabs (ODT):
    Generics: 5, 10 mg (9s, 12s, 18s); contain aspartame
    Maxalt-MLT: 10 mg (18s); contains aspartame

Treatment of acute migraines with or without aura (tabs and ODT):
    Child 6–17 yr (efficacy and safety with >1 dose within 24 hr has not been established):
        <40 kg: 5 mg PO × 1
        ≥40 kg: 10 mg PO × 1
    ≥18 yr and adult (safety in an average of >4 headaches in a 30-day period has not been established; see remarks): 5–10 mg PO × 1. If needed in 2 hr, a second dose may be administered. **Max. daily dose:** 30 mg/24 hr
    Dosage adjustment if receiving propranolol:
        Child 6–17 yr:
            <40 kg: DO NOT USE
            ≥40 kg: 5 mg PO × 1; **max. dose:** 5 mg/24 hr period
        ≥18 yr and adult: 5 mg PO up to a **maximum** of three doses at 2-hr intervals; **max. dose:** 15 mg/24 hr period

---

Contraindicated in hemiplegic or basilar migraine, coronary artery vasospasm, uncontrolled hypertension, ischemic bowel or coronary artery disease, peripheral vascular disease, history of stroke or transient ischemic attack (TIA), and current or recent use (within 2 weeks) of an MAO inhibitor.

Do not administer within 24 hr with any ergotamine-containing or ergot-type agent, any other 5-HT1 agonist (e.g., triptans), methylene blue, or linezolid.

Use with **caution** in renal and hepatic impairment, as a 44% increase in AUC for patients receiving hemodialysis and a 30% increase in plasma concentration for patients with moderate hepatic dysfunction were reported.

Common adverse effects include nausea, asthenia, dizziness, somnolence, and fatigue. Serious adverse effects include chest pain, coronary artery spasm, hypertension, myocardial infarction (MI), peripheral ischemia, ventricular arrhythmia, ischemic colitis, anaphylaxis, angioedema, cerebrovascular accident, and serotonin syndrome. Transient and permanent vision loss have been reported.

When the ODT is being used, place the whole tablet on the tongue, allow the tablet to dissolve, and swallow with saliva. Administration with liquids is optional. Do not break the ODT tablet.

ROCURONIUM
Generics; previously available as Zemuron
Nondepolarizing neuromuscular blocking agent

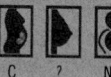

C   ?   No   Yes   No

Injection: 10 mg/mL (5, 10 mL); may be preservative free

Surgical tracheal intubation; use of a peripheral nerve stimulator to monitor drug effect is recommended.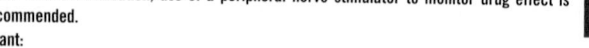
Infant:
   IV: 0.5 mg/kg/dose; may repeat Q20–30 min PRN
Child (3 mo–14 yr):
   IV: 0.6 mg/kg/dose × 1; if needed, give maintenance doses of 0.075–0.125 mg/kg/dose Q20–30 min PRN when neuromuscular blockade returns to 25% of control. Alternatively, a maintenance continuous intravenous infusion may be used starting at 7–12 mCg/kg/min when neuromuscular blockade returns to 10% of control.
Adolescent and adult:
   IV: Start with 0.6–1.2 mg/kg/dose × 1; if needed, maintenance doses at 0.1–0.2 mg/kg/dose Q20–30 min PRN. Alternatively, a maintenance continuous intravenous infusion may be used starting at 10–12 mCg/kg/min (range: 4–16 mCg/kg/min).

Use with caution in hepatic impairment and history of anaphylaxis with other neuromuscular blocking agents. Hypertension, hypotension, arrhythmia, tachycardia, nausea, vomiting, bronchospasm, wheezing, hiccups, rash, and edema at the injection site may occur. Myopathy after long-term use in an intensive care unit (ICU) and QT interval prolongation in pediatric patients receiving general anesthetic agents have been reported. Severe anaphylactic reactions and malignant hypothermia have been reported. Increased neuromuscular blockade may occur with concomitant use of aminoglycosides, clindamycin, tetracycline, magnesium sulfate, quinine, quinidine, succinylcholine, and inhalation anesthetics (for continuous infusion, reduce infusion by 30%–50% at 45–60 min after intubating dose).
Caffeine, calcium, carbamazepine, phenytoin, phenylephrine, azathioprine, and theophylline may reduce neuromuscular blocking effects.
Use must be accompanied by adequate anesthesia or sedation. Peak effects occur in 0.5–1 min for children and in 1–3.7 min for adults. Duration of action: 30–40 min in children and 20–94 min in adults (longer in geriatrics). Recovery time in children 3 months to 1 year of age is similar to that in adults. To prevent residual paralysis, extubate patient **only** after the patient has sufficiently recovered from neuromuscular blockade. In obese patients, use actual body weight for dosage calculation.

RUFINAMIDE
Banzel and generics
Anticonvulsant, triazole derivative

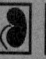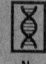

C   3   Yes   Yes   No

Tabs: 200, 400 mg
Oral suspension: 40 mg/mL (460 mL); contains parabens and propylene glycol

Lennox-Gastaut syndrome (adjunctive therapy; it is not known if doses lower than the targeted dosages are effective; see remarks):
Child 1–<17 yr (see remarks): Start at 10 mg/kg/24 hr PO ÷ BID, then increase dose by ~10 mg/kg/24 hr every other day up to the **maximum** targeted dose of 45 mg/kg/24 hr ÷ BID **not to exceed** 3200 mg/24 hr.

RUFINAMIDE *continued*

Child ≥17 yr and adult: Start at 400–800 mg/24 hr PO ÷ BID, then increase dose by 400–800 mg/
24 hr every other day up to the **maximum** targeted dose of 3200 mg/24 hr ÷ BID.
Use with concurrent valproate therapy: Use lower initial dosages; <10 mg/kg/24 hr for child 1–<17
yr and <400 mg/24 hr for ≥17 yr and adult.

Contraindicated in familial short QT syndrome. Use is **not recommended** in severe hepatic
impairment (Child-Pugh 10–15). Use with **caution** when taking other medications that can
shorten the QT interval, performing tasks requiring mental alertness, and in mild/moderate hepatic
impairment (Child-Pugh 5–9).

Common side effects include fatigue, blurred vision, diplopia, ataxia, dizziness, headache,
somnolence, nausea, vomiting, and shortening of cardiac QT interval. Serious side effects of
leukopenia, severe dermatologic reactions (e.g., Stevens-Johnson syndrome), multiorgan
hypersensitivity reactions (e.g., DRESS), and suicidal ideation have been reported.

Rufinamide is a weak inhibitor of CYP 450 2E1 and weak inducer of 3A4. May decrease levels/effects
of nifedipine, nimodipine, piperaquine, calcifediol, clozapine, carbamazepine, lamotrigine,
triazolam, orlistat, and hormonal contraceptives. May increase the levels/effects of phenytoin and
phenobarbital. Primidone, phenobarbital, phenytoin, and carbamazepine may decrease the levels/
effects of rufinamide, whereas valproic acid may increase the levels/effects of rufinamide.

The effectiveness data for 1- to 4-year-old children are based on bridging pharmacokinetic (PK) and
safety data as their PK and safety data are similar to children ≥4 years old and adults.

Consider dose adjustment for drug loss in patients receiving hemodialysis (rufinamide is dialyzable).
For therapy discontinuation, reduce dose by ~25% every 2 days. Tablets may be crushed and all
doses may be administered with or without food.

S

SALMETEROL
Serevent Diskus
β₂ adrenergic agonist (long acting)

 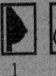

C   1   No   Yes   No

Dry powder inhalation (DPI; Diskus): 50 mCg/inhalation (60 inhalations); contains lactose and milk
protein
In combination with fluticasone: See Fluticasone Propionate and Salmeterol.

Persistent asthma (see remarks):
≥4 yr and adult: 1 inhalation (50 mCg) Q12 hr
Prevention of exercise-induced bronchospasm:
≥4 yr and adult: 1 inhalation 30 to 60 min before exercise. Additional doses should not be used for
another 12 hr. Patients who are already using 12-hr dosing for persistent asthma should NOT
use additional salmeterol doses for this indication and use alternative therapy (e.g., albuterol)
prior to exercise.

For long-term asthma control, should be used in combination with inhaled corticosteroids.
Should not be used to relieve symptoms of acute asthma. It is long acting and has its
onset of action in 10 to 20 min with a peak effect at 3 hr. May be used at QHS (1 inhalation
of the dry powder inhaler [DPI]) for nocturnal symptoms. Salmeterol is a chronic medication and is
not used in similar fashion to short-acting β agonists (e.g., albuterol). Patients already receiving
salmeterol every 12 hr should not use additional doses for prevention of exercise-induced
bronchospasm; consider alternative therapy. Asthma exacerbations or hospitalizations were reported
to be lower when this medication was used with an inhaled corticosteroid.

Continued

SALMETEROL *continued*

WARNING: Long-acting β_2-agonists as monotherapy increase the risks of asthma-related death and asthma-related hospitalizations. Monotherapy without concomitant use of an inhaled corticosteroid is **contraindicated** in asthma. Use salmeterol only as additional therapy for patients not adequately controlled on other asthma-controller medications (e.g., low- to medium-dose inhaled corticosteroids) or whose disease severity clearly requires initiation of treatment with two maintenance therapies. **Contraindicated** in milk allergies; contains milk proteins.

Should not be used in conjunction with an inhaled, long-acting β_2-agonist and is not a substitute for inhaled or systemic corticosteroid. Use with strong CYP450 3A4 inhibitors (e.g., ketoconazole, HIV protease inhibitors, clarithromycin, itraconazole, nefazodone, and telithromycin) is **not recommended** due to risk for cardiovascular adverse events (e.g., QTc prolongation, tachycardia). Salmeterol is a CYP 450 3A4 substrate.

Proper patient education is essential. This dosage form's breath activated device requires a minimum inspiratory flow rate of 60 mL/min for proper dose delivery. Use with caution in hepatic impairment. Side effects are similar to those of albuterol. Hypertension and arrhythmias have been reported. See Chapter 24 for recommendations for asthma controller therapy.

SCOPOLAMINE HYDROBROMIDE
Transderm Scop and generics
Anticholinergic agent

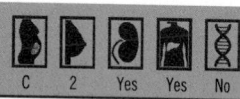

C   2   Yes   Yes   No

Transdermal patch:

Transderm Scop: 1 mg/3 days patch (10s and 24s); delivers ~1 mg over 3 days
Generics: 1 mg/3 days patch (4s, 10s, and 24s); delivers ~1 mg over 3 days

Prevention of postoperative nausea and vomiting (apply patch behind the ear, the evening before surgery and remove patch the morning of the first postoperative day; limited data):

Child <2 yr: $\frac{1}{4}$ patch
Child 2–6 yr: $\frac{1}{2}$ patch
Child 6–12 yr: $\frac{1}{2}$ –1 patch
Child 12 yr and adolescent: 1 patch

Adult indications:

Motion sickness: Apply 1 patch behind the ear at least 4 hr prior to exposure to motion; remove after 72 hr. If additional therapy is needed, apply 1 new patch behind the other ear.

Prevention of postoperative nausea and vomiting (excluding cesarean section): Apply 1 patch behind the ear the evening before surgery. Remove patch 24 hr after surgery.

Antiemetic prior to cesarean section: Apply 1 patch behind the ear 1 hr prior to surgery to minimize infant exposure. Remove patch 24 hr after surgery.

Toxicities similar to those of atropine. **Contraindicated** in closed-angle glaucoma and hypersensitivity to belladonna alkaloids. **Use with caution** in hepatic or renal dysfunction, GI and urinary disorders (discontinue use if there is difficulty in urination), cardiac disease, seizures, or psychosis. May cause dry mouth, drowsiness, and blurred vision. Generalized rash and erythema may indicate hypersensitivity to the medication or other ingredients in the formulation. Hallucinations, amblyopia, and mydriasis have been reported in children.

Drug withdrawal symptoms (nausea, vomiting, headache, and vertigo) have been reported following removal of transdermal patch in patients using the patch for more than 3 days. For perioperative use, the patch should be kept in place for 24 hr following surgery.

SCOPOLAMINE HYDROBROMIDE *continued*

Concurrent use with medications with known CNS adverse reactions or that have anticholinergic properties may potentiate scopolamine's CNS effects. Use of this medication may delay the rate of orally administered drugs and will interfere with the gastric secretion test (discontinue use 10 days prior to testing).

REMOVE transdermal patch before undergoing an MRI; patch contains aluminum.

SELENIUM SULFIDE
Selsun Blue and generics
Topical antiseborrheic agent

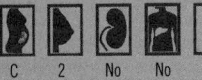

C   2   No   No   No

Shampoo:
  1% (Selsun Blue and others; OTC): 207, 325, 400, 420 mL; some products are available in combination with a conditioner. Be aware of different active ingredients in the Selsun Blue product line.
  2.25%: 180 mL; may contain parabens and propylene glycol
  2.3%: 180 mL; may contain parabens and propylene glycol
Topical lotion: 2.5% (120 mL)

≥2 yr and adult:
  Seborrhea/dandruff:
    Lotion: Massage 5 to 10 mL into wet scalp and leave on scalp for 2 to 3 min. Rinse thoroughly and repeat. Use twice weekly for 2 weeks for control and may be followed by a less frequent maintenance application of once every 1 to 4 wk.
    Shampoo: Massage shampoo into wet scalp then rinse thoroughly. Shampoo at least twice weekly.
    Pityriasis (tinea) versicolor: Apply 2.5% lotion to affected areas of skin. Allow to remain on skin for 10 min. Rinse thoroughly. Repeat once daily for 7 days. Follow with weekly or monthly applications for 3 mo to prevent recurrences.

Rinse hands and body well after treatment. May cause local irritation, hair loss, and hair discoloration. **Avoid** eyes, genital areas, and skin folds. Shampoo may be used for tinea capitis to reduce risk of transmission to others (does not eradicate tinea infection).

For tinea versicolor, 15% to 25% sodium hyposulfite or thiosulfate (Tinver lotion) applied to affected areas twice daily for 2 to 4 wk is an alternative. Topical antifungals (e.g., clotrimazole, miconazole) may be used for small focal infections. **Do not use** for tinea versicolor during pregnancy.

SENNA/SENNOSIDES
Senokot, Senna-Lax, Ex-Lax, Genexa Kids Senna
Laxative, and many others
Laxative, stimulant

C   1   No   No   No

  Based on mg of senna (all products are OTC):
    Oral syrup: 176 mg/5 mL, 218 mg/5 mL (60 mL, 240 mL); may contain parabens and propylene glycol
    Tabs: 187, 217, 374 mg
    187 mg senna extract is approximately 8.6 mg sennosides.
  Based on mg of sennosides (all products are OTC):
    Oral syrup: 8.8 mg/5 mL (237 mL); may contain parabens and propylene glycol
    Tabs: 8.6, 12, 15, 17.2, 25 mg

Continued

SENNA/SENNOSIDES *continued*

Chewable tabs: 8.6 mg
Genexa Kids Senna Laxative: 3 mg
8.6 mg sennosides is approximately 187 mg senna extract.

Constipation (a second-line agent for short-term use; other agents are preferred for maintenance therapy):
Dosing based on mg senna:
Child:
Oral: 10—20 mg/kg/dose PO QHS (**max. dose:** as shown below) or dosage by age:
1 mo—1 yr: 55—109 mg PO QHS to **max. dose:** 218 mg/24 hr
1—5 yr: 109—218 mg PO QHS to **max. dose:** 436 mg/24 hr
5—15 yr: 218—436 mg PO QHS to **max. dose:** 872 mg/24 hr
Adult:
Oral powder: ½ to 1 tsp PO once or twice daily
Syrup: 436—654 mg PO at bedtime; **max. dose:** 654 mg (15 mL) BID
Tabs: 374 mg PO at bedtime; **max. dose:** 748 mg BID
Dosing based on mg sennosides:
Child ≤12 yr:
Syrup:
1 mo—2 yr: 2.2—4.4 mg (1.25—2.5 mL) PO QHS to **max. dose:** 8.8 mg/24 hr
2—5 yr: 4.4—6.6 mg (2.5—3.75 mL) PO QHS to **max. dose:** 6.6 mg BID
6—12 yr: 8.8—13.2 mg (5—7.5 mL) PO QHS to **max. dose:** 13.2 mg BID
Tabs or chewable tabs (8.6 mg):
2—5 yr: 4.3 mg PO QHS to **max. dose:** 8.6 mg BID
6—12 yr: 8.6 mg PO QHS to **max. dose:** 17.2 mg BID
Chewable tabs (Genexa Kids Senna Laxative; 3 mg):
2—5 yr: 3 mg PO once daily or BID
6—12 yr: 6 mg PO once daily or BID
>12 yr and adult:
Granules: 15 mg PO QHS to **max. dose:** 30 mg BID
Syrup: 17.6—26.4 mg (10—15 mL) PO QHS to **max. dose:** 26.4 mg BID
Tabs: 17.2 mg PO QHS to **max. dose:** 34.4 mg BID

Effects occur within 6 to 24 hr after oral administration. Prolonged use (>1 wk) should be **avoided** as it may lead to dependency. May cause nausea, vomiting, diarrhea, and abdominal cramps. Active metabolite stimulates the Auerbach plexus. Syrup may be administered with juice or milk or mixed with ice cream.

SERTRALINE HCL
Zoloft and generics
Antidepressant (selective serotonin reuptake inhibitor)

C   2   Yes   Yes   Yes

Tabs: 25, 50, 100 mg; tablets may be scored
Caps: 150, 200 mg
Oral concentrate solution: 20 mg/mL (60 mL); may contain 12% alcohol and propylene glycol

Depression (see remarks):
Child 6—12 yr: Start at 12.5—25 mg PO once daily. May increase dosage by 12.5—25 mg at weekly intervals up to a **max. dose** of 200 mg/24 hr

SERTRALINE HCL *continued*

> **Child ≥13 yr and adult:** Start at 25—50 mg PO once daily. May increase dosage by 25—50 mg at weekly intervals up to a **max. dose** of 200 mg/24 hr

Obesessive compulsive disorder (see remarks):

> **Child 6—12 yr:** Start at 25 mg PO once daily. May increase dosage by 25—50 mg at weekly intervals up to a **max. dose** of 200 mg/24 hr
>
> **Child ≥13 yr and adult:** Start at 50 mg PO once daily. May increase dosage by 50 mg at weekly intervals up to **max. dose** of 200 mg/24 hr

Drug is **contraindicated** in combination (or within 14 days of discontinuing use) with a monoamine oxidase (MAO) inhibitor (e.g., linezolid or intravenous methylene blue) or pimozide (increases adverse/toxic effects of pimozide). **Use with caution** in patients with abnormal bleeding, syndrome of inappropriate diuretic hormone (SIADH) secretion, and hepatic or renal impairment. Adverse effects include nausea, diarrhea, tremor, sexual dysfunction, and increased sweating. Hyponatremia, diabetes mellitus, rhabdomyolysis, trismus, and platelet dysfunction have been reported. A positive correlation with length of QTc interval and serum sertraline and N-desmethylsertraline levels has been reported.

Monitor for clinical worsening of depression and suicidal ideation/behavior following the initiation of therapy or after dose changes. Use during the late third trimester of pregnancy may increase risk for withdrawal symptoms and persistent pulmonary hypertension in the newborn.

Use with drugs that interfere with hemostasis (e.g., NSAIDs, aspirin, warfarin) may increase risk for GI bleeds. Use with warfarin may increase PT. Inhibits the CYP 450 2D6 drug metabolizing enzyme. Serotonin syndrome may occur when taken with selective serotonin reuptake inhibitors (e.g., amitriptyline, amphetamines, buspirone, dihydroergotamine, sumatriptan, sympathomimetics).

Sertraline is a substrate for CYP 450 2B6, 2C9, 2C19, 2D6, and 3A4. Poor metabolizers of CYP 450 2C19 should initiate therapy at 50% of the recommended dosage and titrate to desired effect *or* consider using an alternative medication not predominantly metabolized by this enzyme. Ultrarapid 2C19 metabolizers should initiate therapy at the recommended starting dose and titrate to the recommended maintenance dosage *or* consider using a drug not predominantly metabolized by this enzyme.

Do not abruptly discontinue use; gradually taper dose (4—6 wk has been recommended) to reduce risk for withdrawal symptoms.

Mix oral concentrate solution with 4 oz of water, ginger ale, lemon/lime soda, lemonade, or orange juice. After mixing, a slight haze may appear; this is normal. This dosage form should be **used cautiously** in patients with latex allergy because the dropper contains dry natural rubber.

SILDENAFIL
Revatio, Viagra, and generics
Phosphodiesterase type-5 (PDE5) inhibitor

    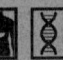

B	2	Yes	Yes	No

Tabs:
> **Revatio and generics:** 20 mg
> **Viagra and generics:** 25, 50, 100 mg

Oral suspension: 2.5 mg/mL
> **Revatio and generics:** 10 mg/mL (112 mL); may contain sodium benzoate

Injection:
> **Revatio and generics:** 0.8 mg/mL (12.5 mL)

Pulmonary hypertension:
> **Neonate (limited data from case reports and small clinical trials):**

Continued

SILDENAFIL *continued*

PO: Several dosages have been reported and have ranged from 0.5 to 3 mg/kg/dose Q6—12 hr PO. A single dose of ~0.3 mg/kg PO has been used in select patients to facilitate weaning from inhaled nitric oxide.

IV (case report from 4 neonates >34 weeks' gestation and <72 hr old): Start with 0.4 mg/kg/dose IV over 3 hr followed by a continuous infusion of 1.6 mg/kg/24 hr (0.067 mg/kg/hr) for up to 7 days.

Infant and child (limited data):

PO: Start at 0.25 mg/kg/dose Q6 hr or 0.5 mg/kg/dose Q8 hr; if needed, titrate dose up to 1—2 mg/kg/dose Q6—8 hr. A single dose of ~0.4 mg/kg PO has been used in select patients to facilitate weaning from inhaled nitric oxide.

Child 1—17 yr (higher doses and long-term use are associated with increased risk for mortality; see remarks):

PO:

≥8—20 kg: 10 mg TID
>20—45 kg: 20 mg TID
>45 kg: 40 mg TID

Pulmonary arterial hypertension:

Adult:

PO: 20 mg TID (take at least 4—6 hr apart)
IV: 10 mg TID

Contraindicated with concurrent use of nitrates (e.g., nitroglycerin) and other nitric oxide donors; potentiates hypotensive effects. **Use with caution** in sepsis (high levels of cGMP may potentiate hypotension), hypotension, sickle cell anemia (use not established), and with concurrent CYP 450 3A4 inhibiting medications (see discussion that follows) and anti-hypertensive medications. Hepatic insufficiency or severe renal impairment (glomerular filtration rate [GFR] <30 mL/min) significantly reduces sildenafil clearance.

Findings from the dose-ranging study in 1- to 17-yr-olds with pulmonary arterial hypertension found an association of increased mortality risk with long-term use (>2 yr). Headache, pyrexia, upper respiratory tract infections (URTIs), vomiting, and diarrhea were the most frequently reported side effects in this study. Optimal dosing based on age and body weight still needs to be determined. Hazard ratios for mortality were 3.95 (95% CI: 1.46—10.65) for high versus low doses and 1.92 (95% CI: 0.65—5.65) for medium versus low doses in follow-up study for those receiving therapy for ≥3 yr. A subsequent extension open-label study on the same population for an additional 16 weeks reported a greater hazard ratio for mortality with high- versus low-dose therapy ($P = 0.007$).

In adults, a transient impairment of color discrimination may occur; this effect could increase risk of severe retinopathy of prematurity in neonates. Common side effects reported in adults have included flushing, rash, diarrhea, indigestion, headache, abnormal vision, and nasal congestion. Hearing loss has been reported.

Sildenafil is substrate for CYP 450 3A4 (major) and 2C8/9 (minor). Azole antifungals, cimetidine, ciprofloxacin, clarithromycin, erythromycin, nicardipine, propofol, protease inhibitors, quinidine, verapamil, and grapefruit juice may increase the effects/toxicity of sildenafil. Bosentan, efavirenz, carbamazepine, phenobarbital, phenytoin, rifampin, St. John's wort, and high-fat meals may decrease sildenafil effects.

SILVER SULFADIAZINE
Silvadene, Thermazene, SSD Cream, and generics
Topical antibiotic

   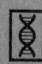

B   3   Yes   Yes   No

SILVER SULFADIAZINE *continued*

Cream: 1% (20, 25, 50, 85, 400, 1000 g); contains methylparabens and propylene glycol

Child (≥2 mo) and adult: Cover affected areas completely once or twice daily. Apply cream to a thickness of 1/16 inch using sterile technique.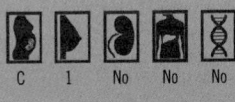

Contraindicated in premature infants and infants up to 2 mo of age due to concerns of kernicterus; also contraindicated in pregnancy (approaching term). **Use with caution** in G6PD and renal and hepatic impairment. Discard product if cream has darkened. Significant systemic absorption may occur in severe burns. Adverse effects include pruritus, rash, bone marrow suppression, hemolytic anemia, hepatitis, interstitial nephritis, and life-threatening cutaneous reactions (e.g., Stevens-Johnson syndrome/toxic epidermal necrolysis [TEN] and exfoliative dermatitis). **Avoid** contact with the eye. Dressing may be used but is not necessary. See Chapter 4 for more information.

SIMETHICONE
Mylicon, Children's Mylicon, Phazyme, Mylanta
Gas, Gas-X, and generics
Antiflatulent

C   1   No   No   No

All dosage forms available OTC
Oral drops and suspension: 40 mg/0.6 mL (15, 30 mL); may contain sodium benzoate and polyethylene glycol
Caps (Phazyme, Gas-X, and generics): 125, 180, 250 mg
Chewable tabs: 80, 125 mg
   Children's Mylicon: 40 mg; contains 400 mg calcium carbonate
Strip, orally disintegrating (Gas-X): 40 mg (16s), 62.5 mg (18s); may contain alcohol

Infant and child <2 yr: 20 mg PO QPC and QHS PRN; **max. dose:** 240 mg/24 hr
2–12 yr: 40 mg PO QPC and QHS PRN; **max. dose:** 480 mg/24 hr
>12 yr and adult: 40–125 mg PO QPC and QHS PRN; **max. dose:** 500 mg/24 hr

Efficacy has not been demonstrated for treating infant colic. **Avoid** carbonated beverages and gas-forming foods. Oral liquid may be mixed with water, infant formula, or other suitable liquids for ease of oral administration.

SIROLIMUS
Rapamune and generics
Immunosuppressant agent

C   3   Yes   Yes   No

Tabs: 0.5, 1, 2 mg
Oral solution: 1 mg/mL (60 mL); contains 1.5%–2.5% ethanol, polysorbate 80, and propylene glycol

Prophylaxis of organ rejection in renal transplantation: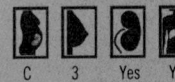
  Child ≥13 yr (tablet and oral solution dosage forms are NOT bioequivalent; see remarks):
    <40 kg: 3 mg/m²/dose PO given once immediately after transplantation, followed by 1 mg/m²/24 hr PO ÷ Q 12–24 hr on the next day. Adjust dose to achieve desired trough blood level.
    ≥40 kg: Use adult (low/moderate immunologic risk) ≥40 kg dosage below and adjust dose to achieve desired trough blood level.
  Adult (tablet and oral solution dosage forms are NOT bioequivalent; see remarks):
    Patients at low/moderate immunologic risk:

Continued

SIROLIMUS *continued*

In combination with cyclosporine (adjust dose to achieve desired trough blood level):
<40 kg: 3 mg/m^2/dose PO given once immediately after transplantation followed by 1 mg/m^2/dose PO once on the next day
≥40 kg: 6 mg PO once immediately after transplantation, followed by 2 mg PO once on the next day
Patients at high immunologic risk:
In combination with cyclosporine (withdrawal of cyclosporine is not recommended): 15 mg PO once immediately after transplantation, followed by 5 mg PO once on the next day. Adjust dose to achieve desired trough blood level.

Increased susceptibility to infection and development of lymphoma may result from immunosuppression. **Fatal** bronchial anastomotic dehiscence has been reported in lung transplantation. Excess mortality, graft loss, and hepatic artery thrombosis have been reported in liver transplantation when used with tacrolimus. Patients with the greatest amount of urinary protein excretion prior to sirolimus conversion were those whose protein excretion increased the most after conversion. Increased risk of BK virus—associated nephropathies has been reported. The following adverse effects have been reported when converting from a calcineurin inhibitor-based regimen to maintenance sirolimus:
Stable liver transplant: increased mortality
Kidney transplant: pneumonia, proteinuria, acute rejection, graft loss, and death
Monitor whole-blood trough levels (just prior to a dose at steady state); especially with pediatric patients; hepatic impairment; concurrent use of CYP 450 3A4 and/or P-gp inducers and inhibitors; and/or if cyclosporine dosage is markedly changed or discontinued. Steady-state is generally achieved after 5 to 7 days of continuous dosing. **Interpretation will vary based on specific treatment protocol and assay methodology (HPLC vs. immunoassay vs. LC/MS/MS). Younger children may exhibit faster sirolimus clearance compared with adolescents.**
Sirolimus is a substrate for CYP 450 3A4 and P-gp. Bromocriptine, cannabidiol, cyclosporine, diltiazem, metoclopramide, protease inhibitors, erythromycin, grapefruit juice, and other inhibitors of CYP 3A4 (e.g., calcium channel blockers) may increase the toxicity of sirolimus. Phenobarbital, carbamazepine, phenytoin, and St John's wort may decrease the effects of sirolimus. Strong inhibitors (e.g., azole antifungals and clarithromycin) and strong inducers (e.g., rifamycins) are **not recommended.**
Hypertension, peripheral edema, increased serum creatinine, dyspnea, epistaxis, headache, anemia, thrombocytopenia, hyperlipidemia, hypercholesterolemia, and arthralgia may occur. Progressive multifocal leukoencephalopathy (PML), diabetes mellitus, posterior reversible encephalopathy syndrome, ovarian cysts, and menstrual disorders have been reported. Urinary tract infections have been reported in pediatric renal transplant patients with high immunologic risk.
Two milligrams of the oral solution have been demonstrated to be clinically equivalent to the 2-mg tablets. However, it is not known whether they are still therapeutically equivalent at higher doses. Reduce maintenance dosage by one-third in the presence of hepatic function impairment. Administer doses consistently with or without food. When administered with cyclosporine, give dose 4 hr after cyclosporine. **Do not** crush or split tablets. Measure the oral liquid dosage form with an amber oral syringe and dilute in a cup with 60 mL of water or orange juice only. Take dose immediately after mixing, add/mix additional 120 mL diluent into the cup, and drink immediately after mixing.

SODIUM BICARBONATE
Generics
Alkalinizing agent, electrolyte

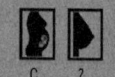

C   ?   Yes   No   No

Injection: 4.2% (0.5 mEq/mL) (5, 10 mL), 7.5% (0.89 mEq/mL) (50 mL), 8.4% (1 mEq/mL) (10, 50 mL)
Tabs: 325 mg (3.8 mEq), 650 mg (7.6 mEq)

SODIUM BICARBONATE *continued*

Powder: 1, 120, 500 g; contains 30 mEq Na$^+$ per 1/2 teaspoon
Each 1 mEq bicarbonate provides 1 mEq Na$^+$.

Cardiac arrest: See inside front cover.
Correction of metabolic acidosis: Calculate patient's dose with the following formulas.
  Neonate, infant, and child:
    HCO_3^- (mEq) = 0.3 × weight (kg) × base deficit (mEq/L), **OR**
    HCO_3^- (mEq) = 0.5 × weight (kg) × [24 − serum HCO_3^- (mEq/L)]
  Adult:
    HCO_3^- (mEq) = 0.2 × weight (kg) × base deficit (mEq/L), **OR**
    HCO_3^- (mEq) = 0.5 × weight (kg) × [24 − serum HCO_3^- (mEq/L)]
  Urinary alkalinization (titrate dose accordingly to urine pH):
    Child: 84—840 mg (1—10 mEq)/kg/24 hr PO ÷ QID
    Adult: 4 g (48 mEq) × 1 followed by 1—2 g (12—24 mEq) PO Q4 hr. Doses up to 16 g (192 mEq)/24
    hr have been used.

Contraindicated in respiratory alkalosis, hypochloremia, and inadequate ventilation during
cardiac arrest. **Use with caution** in congestive heart failure (CHF), renal impairment,
cirrhosis, hypocalcemia, hypertension, and concurrent corticosteroids. Maintain high urine output.
Monitor acid-base balance and serum electrolytes. May cause hypernatremia (contains sodium),
hypokalemia, hypomagnesemia, hypocalcemia, hyperreflexia, edema, and tissue necrosis (extravasation).
Oral route of administration may cause GI discomfort and gastric rupture from gas production.
For direct intravenous administration (cardiac arrest) in neonates and infants, use the 0.5 mEq/mL
(4.2%) concentration or dilute the 1 mEq/mL (8.4%) concentration 1:1 with sterile water for
injection and infuse at a rate **no greater than** 10 mEq/min. The 1 mEq/mL (8.4%) concentration
may be used in children and adults for direct intravenous administration.
For intravenous infusions (for all ages), dilute to a **max. concentration** of 0.5 mEq/mL in dextrose or
sterile water for injection and infuse over 2 hr using a **max. rate** of 1 mEq/kg per hr.
Sodium bicarbonate should not be mixed with or be in contact with calcium, norepinephrine, or
dobutamine.

SODIUM CHLORIDE—INHALED PREPARATIONS
Hypersal, Nebusal, PulmoSal, Simply Saline,
Ocean, Ayr Saline, Ayr Nasal Mist Allergy/Sinus,
many other brands, and generics
Electrolyte, inhalation

Nebulized solution (generics): 0.9% (3, 5, 15 mL), 3% (4, 15 mL), 7% (4 mL), 10% (4, 15 mL)
  Hypersal (preservative-free): 3.5% (4 mL), 7% (4 mL)
  Nebusal: 3% (4 mL), 6% (4 mL)
  PulmoSal: 7% (4 mL)
Nasal solution spray/drops/mist (OTC): 0.65% (15, 30, 45 mL),2.65% (50 mL); may contain
benzalkonium chloride

Intranasal as moisturizer (use 0.65% concentration):
  Child and adult:
    Spray/Mist: 2—6 sprays into each nostril Q2 hr PRN
    Drops: 2—6 drops into each nostril Q2 hr PRN
**Cystic fibrosis (Pretreatment with albuterol is recommended to prevent bronchospasms; see
remarks):**

Continued

SODIUM CHLORIDE—INHALED PREPARATIONS *continued*

≥2 yr and adult: Nebulize 4 mL of 7% solution once or twice daily. If patient is unable to tolerate the 7% strength, lower strengths of 3%, 3.5%, or 5% may be used.

Acute viral bronchiolitis (for hospitalized patients only; pretreatment with albuterol is recommended to prevent bronchospasms; see remarks):

Infant (>34 weeks' gestation up to 18 mo old): Nebulize 4 mL of 3% solution Q2 hr for three doses followed by Q4 hr for five doses followed by Q6 hr dosing until discharge.

INTRANASAL USE: May be used as a nasal wash for sinuses, to restore moisture, to thin nasal secretions, or to relieve dry, crusted, and inflamed nasal membranes from colds, low humidity, allergies, nasal decongestant overuse, minor nosebleeds, and other irritations. Nasal administration instructions:

Nasal drops: Tilt head back and hold bottle upside down.

Nasal spray: Hold head in upright position and give short, firm squeezes into each nostril. Sniff deeply.

NEBULIZATION: Hypertonic solutions lowers sputum viscosity and enhances mucociliary clearance.

Cystic fibrosis: Improves FEV_1 and reduces pulmonary exacerbation frequency. May cause bronchospasm, cough, pharyngitis, hemoptysis, and acute decline in pulmonary function (administer first dose in a medical facility). It is recommended to withhold therapy in the presence of massive hemoptysis.

Acute viral bronchiolitis: Use not recommended in the emergency department but may be administered in hospitalized patients. Reported reduction in length of hospitalization when compared to normal saline is controversial. May cause acute bronchospasm and local irritation.

SODIUM PHENYLACETATE AND SODIUM BENZOATE
Ammonul and generics
Ammonium detoxicant, urea cycle disorder treatment agent

 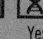

C   ?   Yes   Yes   Yes

Injection: 100 mg sodium phenylacetate and 100 mg sodium benzoate per 1 mL (50 mL)

IV via central line (administered with IV arginine, continue infusion until ammonia levels are in the normal range): See Chapter 13 for dosing information.

Indicated for hyperammonemia due to enzyme deficiencies of the urea cycle (e.g., carbamoyl phosphate synthetase [CPS] and ornithine transcarbamylase deficiency). **Use with caution** in renal and hepatic impairment. Significant amounts of sodium may be administered with prolonged durations of therapy. Ammonia clearance is most efficient with hemodialysis.

Side effects include hypotension, hypokalemia, hyperglycemia, injection site reaction, nausea/vomiting, altered mental status, fever, metabolic acidosis, cerebral edema, seizures, anemia, and disseminated intravascular coagulation. CNS side effects are more frequent with ornithine transcarbamylase (OTC) and CPS. Blood and lymphatic system disorders and hypotension are common in patients 30 days old or younger, whereas nausea, vomiting, and diarrhea are common in patients more than 30 days old. Monitor blood chemistry profiles, blood pH and pCO_2 for hyperventilation and metabolic acidosis.

Although no formal drug interaction studies have been completed, penicillin antibiotics and probenecid may increase serum concentrations of sodium phenylacetate and sodium benzoate by competing for renal tubular secretion. Use of valproic acid or corticosteroids may increase plasma ammonia levels.

Must be diluted and administered IV via central line; peripheral line administration may result in burning and extravasation.

SODIUM PHOSPHATE
Fleet Enema, Fleet Pedia-Lax, Fleet Enema Extra,
GoodSense Enema, LaCrosse Complete,
OsmoPrep, and generics
Laxative, enema/oral

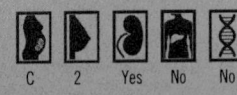

C   2   Yes   No   No

Enema [OTC]:
7 g dibasic sodium phosphate and 19 g monobasic sodium phosphate/118 mL; contains 4.4 g sodium
per 118 mL
   Pediatric size (Fleet Pedia-Lax): 66 mL
   Adult size (Fleet Enema, GoodSense Enema, LaCrosse Complete, and generics): 133 mL
7 g dibasic sodium phosphate and 19 g monobasic sodium phosphate/197 mL; contains 4.4 g sodium
per 197 mL
   Fleet Enema Extra: 230 mL
Oral tablets (OsmoPrep): 1.5 g (1.102 g monobasic sodium and 0.398 g per tablet); gluten free
Injection: See Phosphorus Supplements.

Not to be used for phosphorus supplementation (see Phosphorus Supplements)
Enema (see remarks):
   2–4 yr: 33 mL enema (half of Fleet Pedia-Lax) × 1
   5–11 yr: 66 mL enema (Fleet Pedia-Lax) × 1
   ≥12 yr and adult: 133 mL enema (Fleet Enema or generics) **OR** 230 mL enema (Fleet enema Extra) × 1
Bowel prep prior to colonoscopy:
   Adult (PO):
      Evening prior to colonoscopy: 4 tabs (OsmoPrep) with 8 ounces of clear liquids Q15 min up to a
      total of 5 doses (20 tabs with 40 oz of clear liquids)
      Day of colonoscopy, 3 to 5 hr prior to procedure: 4 tabs (OsmoPrep) with 8 oz of clear liquids Q15
      min up to a total of three doses (12 tabs with 24 oz of clear liquids)

Contraindicated in patients with severe renal failure, megacolon, bowel obstruction, and CHF.
May cause hyperphosphatemia, hypernatremia, hypocalcemia, hypotension, dehydration, and
acidosis. **Avoid** retention of enema solution and **do not exceed** recommended doses, as this may
lead to severe electrolyte disturbances due to enhanced systemic absorption. **Use with caution** in
cardiac arrhythmias. Colonic mucosal aphthous ulceration should be considered when interpreting
colonoscopy findings with use in patients with known or suspected irritable bowel disease (IBD).
Correct electrolyte abnormalities prior to use to minimize electrolyte side effects.
Onset of action: PR, 2–5 min

SODIUM POLYSTYRENE SULFONATE
SPS, and generics; previously available as
Kayexalate and Kionex
Potassium-removing resin

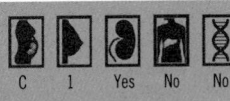

C   1   Yes   No   No

Powder: 15, 454 g
Oral suspension: 15 g/60 mL (60, 120, 473, 500 mL); contains 21.5 mL sorbitol per 60 mL and
0.1%–0.3% alcohol
Contains 4.1 mEq Na$^+$/g drug

Hyperkalemia: Note: Oral suspension may be given PO or PR (PO route is more effective).
Practical exchange ratio is 1 mEq K per 1 g resin. May calculate dose according to desired
exchange (see remarks).

Continued

SODIUM POLYSTYRENE SULFONATE *continued*

Infant and child:
> **PO:** 1 g/kg per dose (**max. dose:** 15 g per dose) Q6 hr
> **PR:** 1 g/kg per dose Q2—6 hr; **max. dose:** 30—50 g per dose. Dosing by practical exchange (1 mEq K per 1 g resin) has been recommended for infants and smaller children.

Adult:
> **PO:** 15 g once daily—QID
> **PR:** 30—50 g Q6 hr

Contraindicated in obstructive bowel disease, neonates with reduced gut motility, and oral administration in neonates. **Use cautiously** in presence of renal failure, CHF, hypertension, or severe edema. May cause hypokalemia, hypernatremia, hypomagnesemia, and hypocalcemia. Cases of colonic necrosis, GI bleeding, ischemic colitis, and perforation have been reported with the concomitant use of sorbitol in patients with GI risk factors (prematurity, history of intestinal disease or surgery hypovolemia, and renal insufficiency/failure). Use in neonates generally **not recommended** due to complication concerns for hypernatremia and NEC.

1 mEq Na delivered for each mEq K removed. **Do not administer** with antacids or laxatives containing Mg^{2+} or Al^{3+}. Systemic alkalosis may result. May reduce absorption of other orally administered medication; administer other oral medications at least 3 hr before or 3 hr after sodium polystyrene sulfonate (patients with gastroparesis may require a 6-hr separation). Enema should be retained in the colon for at least 30—60 min.

SPIRONOLACTONE
Aldactone, CaroSpir, and generics
Diuretic, potassium sparing

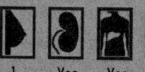

| C/D | 1 | Yes | Yes | No |

Tabs: 25, 50, 100 mg
Oral suspension: 1, 5, 25 mg/mL
CaroSpir: 25 mg/5 mL (118, 473 mL); contains saccharin

Diuretic:
> **Neonate:** 1—3 mg/kg/24 hr ÷ once or twice daily PO
> **Child:** 1—3 mg/kg/24 hr ÷ BID—QID PO; **max. dose by indication:**
>> **Hypertension:** The lesser of 3.3 mg/kg/24 hr or 100 mg/24 hr
>> **Edema:** The lesser of 4—6 mg/kg/24 hr or 400 mg/24 hr
> **Adult:** 25—200 mg/24 hr ÷ once daily—BID PO (see remarks); **max. dose:** 200 mg/24 hr

Diagnosis of primary aldosteronism:
> **Child:** 125—375 mg/m^2/24 hr ÷ once or twice daily PO
> **Adult:** 400 mg once daily PO × 4 days (short test) or 3—4 wk (long test), then 100—400 mg once or twice daily maintenance

Hirsutism in women:
> **Adult:** 50—200 mg/24 hr ÷ once or twice daily PO

Contraindicated in Addison disease, hyperkalemia, use with eplerenone, or severe renal failure (see Chapter 31). **Use with caution** in dehydration, hyponatremia, and renal or hepatic dysfunction. Precipitation of impaired neurologic function, worsening hepatic encephalopathy, and coma may occur with hepatic disease with cirrhosis and ascites. May cause hyperkalemia (especially with severe heart failure), GI distress, rash, lethargy, dizziness, and gynecomastia. May potentiate ganglionic blocking agents and other antihypertensives. Monitor potassium levels and be aware of other K^+ sources, K^+-sparing diuretics, and angiotensin-converting enzyme inhibitors (ACEIs) (all of which can increase K^+).

SPIRONOLACTONE *continued*

Do not use with other medications known to cause hyperkalemia (e.g., ACEIs, angiotensin II antagonists, aldosterone blockers, and other potassium-sparing diuretics). Hyperkalemic metabolic acidosis has been reported with concurrent cholestyramine use. May cause false elevation in serum digoxin levels measured by radioimmunoassay.

Although TID—QID regimens have been recommended, data suggest once- or twice-daily dosing to be adequate. Pregnancy category changes to "D" if used in pregnancy-induced hypertension.

STREPTOMYCIN SULFATE
Generics
Antibiotic, aminoglycoside, antituberculous agent

 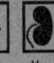 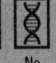

D   2   Yes   No   No

Powder for injection: 1 g

MDR tuberculosis: Use as part of multidrug regimen (see latest edition of AAP *Red Book*). IM route is preferred. Monitor levels.

Infant, child, and adolescent (<15 yr or ≤40 kg):
  Daily therapy: 20—40 mg/kg/24 hr IM/IV once daily
    Max. daily dose: 1 g/24 hr
  Twice weekly therapy (under direct observation): 25—30 mg/kg/dose IM/IV twice weekly
    Max. daily dose: 1 g/24 hr
Child, adolescent, and adult (≥15 yr or >40 kg):
  Daily therapy: 15 mg/kg/24 hr IM/IV once daily; **max. daily dose:** 1 g/24 hr
  Twice-weekly therapy (under direct observation): 15 mg/kg/dose IM/IV twice weekly; **max. daily dose:** 1 g/24 hr

Brucellosis, tularemia, plague, and rat bite fever: See latest edition of the *Red Book*.

Contraindicated with aminoglycoside and sulfite hypersensitivity. **Use with caution** in preexisting vertigo, tinnitus, hearing loss, and neuromuscular disorders. Drug is administered via deep IM injection **only.** Follow auditory status. May cause CNS depression, other neurologic problems, myocarditis, serum sickness, nephrotoxicity, and ototoxicity. Concomitant neurotoxic, ototoxic, or nephrotoxic drugs and dehydration may increase risk for toxicity.

Therapeutic levels: peak 15—40 mg/L; trough: <5 mg/L. Recommended serum sampling time at steady state: trough within 30 min prior to the third consecutive dose and peak at 30—60 min (60 min for IM) after the administration of the third consecutive dose. Therapeutic levels are not achieved in cerebrospinal fluid (CSF).

Adjust dose in renal failure (see Chapter 31).

SUCCIMER
Chemet, DMSA [dimercaptosuccinic acid]
Chelating agent

    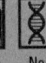

C   3   Yes   Yes   No

Cap: 100 mg

Lead chelation, child:
  10 mg/kg/dose (or 350 mg/m²/dose) PO Q8 hr × 5 days, then 10 mg/kg/dose
  (or 350 mg/m²/dose) PO Q12 hr × 14 days. **Max. dose:** 500 mg per dose
  Manufacturer recommendation (see following table):

Continued

SUCCIMER *continued*

Weight (kg)	Dose (mg) Q8 hr × 5 Days Followed by Same Dose Q12 hr × 14 Days
8—15	100
16—23	200
24—34	300
35—44	400
≥45	500

Use caution in patients with compromised renal or hepatic function. Repeated courses may be necessary. Follow serum lead levels. Allow a minimum of 2 wk between courses unless blood levels require more aggressive management. Side effects: GI symptoms, increased negative liver function tests (LFTs) (10%), rash, headaches, and dizziness. Allergic reactions, such as urticaria and angioedema, and neutropenia have been reported. May cause false-positive urinary ketone readings with nitroprusside reagent tests such as Ketostix and can falsely lower measured serum uric acid and creatine phosphokinase (CPK). **Coadministration with other chelating agents is not recommended.**

Serum transaminases should be monitored at baseline and weekly during therapy. Treatment of iron deficiency is recommended as well as environmental remediation. Contents of capsule may be sprinkled on food for those who are unable to swallow a capsule.

SUCCINYLCHOLINE
Anectine, Quelicin, and generics
Neuromuscular blocking agent

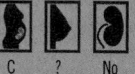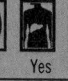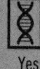

C   ?   No   Yes   Yes

Injection:
    Anectine, Quelicin, and generics: 20 mg/mL (10 mL); may contain parabens
Prefilled syringe injection:
    Generics: 100 mg/5 mL (5 mL); preservative free

Paralysis for intubation (see remarks):
  Infant, child, and adolescent:
    Initial:
      IV:
        Infant: 2—3 mg/kg/dose × 1
        Child: 1—2 mg/kg/dose × 1
        Adolescent: 1—1.5 mg/kg/dose × 1
      IM:
        Infant <6 mo: 4—5 mg/kg/dose × 1
        Infant ≥6 mo and child: 4 mg/kg/dose × 1; **max. dose:** 150 mg per dose
        Adolescent: 3—4 mg/kg/dose × 1; **max. dose:** 150 mg per dose
  Adult:
    Initial:
      IV: 0.3—1.1 mg/kg/dose × 1
    IM: 3—4 mg/kg/dose × 1; **max. dose:** 150 mg/dose
    Maintenance for long surgical procedures: 0.04—0.07 mg/kg/dose IV Q5—10 min PRN. Continuous infusion not recommended.

Contraindicated after the acute phase of an injury following major burns, multiple trauma, extensive denervation of skeletal muscle, or upper motor neuron injury because severe

SUCCINYLCHOLINE *continued*

hyperkalemia and subsequent **cardiac arrest** may occur. Individuals carrying the *RYR1* or *CACNA1S* gene have an increased risk for developing malignant hyperthermia with succinylcholine or halogenated volatile anesthetics; use in these individuals is **contraindicated**. Succinylcholine should be **avoided** in patients who are susceptible to malignant hyperthermia.

Pretreatment with atropine is recommended to reduce incidence of bradycardia. For rapid sequence intubation, see Chapter 1.

Cardiac arrest has been reported in children and adolescents primarily with skeletal muscle myopathies (e.g., Duchenne muscular dystrophy). Identify developmental delays suggestive of a myopathy prior to use. Predose creatine kinase may be useful for identifying patients at risk. Monitoring of the electrocardiogram (ECG) for peaked T waves may be useful in detecting early signs of this adverse effect.

May cause malignant hyperthermia (use dantrolene to treat), bradycardia, hypotension, arrhythmia, and hyperkalemia. Severe anaphylactic reactions have been reported; **use caution** if previous anaphylactic reaction to other neuromuscular blocking agents. **Use with caution** in patients with severe burns, paraplegia, or crush injuries and in patients with preexisting hyperkalemia. Beware of prolonged depression in patients with liver disease, malnutrition, pseudocholinesterase deficiency, hypothermia and those receiving aminoglycosides, phenothiazines, quinidine, β blockers, amphotericin B, cyclophosphamide, diuretics, lithium, acetylcholine, and anticholinesterases. Diazepam may decrease neuromuscular blocking effects. Prior use of succinylcholine may enhance the neuromuscular blocking effect of vecuronium and its duration of action.

Duration of action 4—6 min IV, 10—30 min IM. Must be prepared to intubate within 1 min.

SUCRALFATE
Carafate and generics
Oral antiulcer agent

    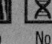

B   1   Yes   No   No

Tabs: 1 g
Oral suspension: 100 mg/mL (420 mL); contains sorbitol and parabens

Child:
  Duodenal or gastric ulcer: 40—80 mg/kg/24 hr ÷ Q6 hr PO; **max. dose:** 1000 mg/dose
  Stomatitis: 5—10 mL (500—1000 mg of suspension), swish and spit or swish and swallow QID
Adult:
  Duodenal ulcer:
    Treatment: 1 g PO QID (1 hr before meals and QHS) or 2 g PO BID × 4—8 wk
    Maintenance/prophylaxis: 1 g PO BID
  Stress ulcer:
    Prophylaxis: 1 g PO QID
  Stomatitis: 10 mL (1000 mg of suspension), swish and spit or swish and swallow QID
  Proctitis (use oral suspension as rectal enema): 20 mL (2 g) PR once or twice daily for at least 4 wk or resolution of symptoms

---

May cause vertigo, constipation, and dry mouth. Hypersensitivity, including anaphylactic reactions, and hyperglycemia in patients with diabetes have been reported. Aluminum may accumulate in patients with renal failure. This may be augmented by the use of aluminum-containing antacids. **Use with caution** in patients with dysphagia or other conditions that may alter gag or cough reflexes or diminish oropharyngeal coordination/motility who are receiving the oral tablet dosage form; cases of tablet aspiration with respiratory complications have been reported.

Continued

SUCRALFATE *continued*

Decreases absorption of phenytoin, digoxin, theophylline, cimetidine, fat-soluble vitamins, ketoconazole, omeprazole, quinolones, and oral anticoagulants. Administer these drugs at least 2 hr before or after sucralfate doses.

Drug requires an acidic environment to form a protective polymer coating for damaged GI tract mucosa. Administer oral doses on an empty stomach (1 hr before meals and QHS).

SUGAMMADEX
Bridion
Neuromuscular blockade reversal agent

   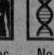

?   1   Yes   Yes   No

Injection: 100 mg/1 mL (2, 5 mL); may be diluted with NS to a concentration of 10 mg/mL to increase the accuracy of smaller doses

Routine reversal of rocuronium-induced moderate blockade (see remarks):
  Infant, child (<2 yr; limited data): 2 or 4 mg/kg/dose IV once over 10 sec; some suggest administering over slow intravenous push to reduce risk for bradycardia or asystole

Reversal rocuronium or vecuronium-induced neuromuscular blockade (see remarks):
  Child ≥2 yr, adolescent, and adult (use actual body weight):
    Deep block (spontaneous recovery of twitch response reaching 1 to 2 post-tetanic counts with no twitch responses to train-of-four stimulation): 4 mg/kg/dose IV × 1 over 10 seconds
    Moderate block (spontaneous recovery of reappearance of the second twitch in response of train-of-four stimulation): 2 mg/kg/dose IV × 1 over 10 seconds

Reversal of neuromuscular blockade 3 min after rocuronium 1.2 mg/kg:
  Adult (use actual body weight): 16 mg/kg/dose IV × 1. The recovery to T_1 of 10% baseline (relative to the time of administration of rocuronium or succinylcholine) was faster with rocuronium/sugammadex than with succinylcholine alone. This dose has not been evaluated for vecuronium-induced neuromuscular blockade.

Sugammadex is a modified gamma cyclodextrin that binds to rocuronium and vecuronium for reduced neuromuscular blockade.

Use is **not recommended** for GFR <30 mL/min or on dialysis. **Use with caution** in hepatic impairment, especially in the presence of coagulopathy or severe edema.

Common side effects include nausea, vomiting, and headache. Serious effects include bradycardia, prolonged QTc interval, hypersensitivity reactions/anaphylaxis, increased creatine kinase, and respiratory arrest. Bronchospasm, laryngospasm, dyspnea, wheezing, and pulmonary edema have been reported. May increase the effects/toxicity of anticoagulants and decrease the effects of hormonal contraceptives. Fusidic acid and toremifene may decrease sugammadex activity.

Limited data in children (especially <2 yr) and dosing in a multicenter, randomized, parallel-group, dose-finding study in 63 children (28 days to 17 yr of age) and 28 adult surgical patients. Doses were well tolerated across all ages with dose-response relationship for those 2 yr of age or older. All had a median recovery time of 1.1 to 1.2 min after a 2 mg/kg dose (*Anesthesiology.* 2009;110:284–294).

SULFACETAMIDE SODIUM OPHTHALMIC
Generics; previously available as Bleph-10
Ophthalmic antibiotic, sulfonamide derivative

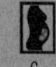   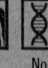

C   ?   No   No   No

Ophthalmic solution: 10% (5, 15 mL); may contain thimerosal or benzalkonium chloride
Ophthalmic ointment: 10% (3.5 g)

SULFACETAMIDE SODIUM OPHTHALMIC *continued*

Conjunctivitis (usual duration of therapy for ophthalmic use is 7—10 days):
≥2 mo and adult:
  Ointment: Apply 0.5-in ribbon into conjunctival sac Q3—4 hr and QHS initially, and reduce the
    dosing frequency with adequate response.
  Drops: 1—2 drops to affected eye(s) Q2—3 hr initially and reduce the dosing frequency with
    adequate response

Hypersensitivity reactions between different sulfonamides can occur regardless of route of
  administration. May cause local irritation, stinging, burning, conjunctival hyperemia,
  excessive tear production, and eye pain. Rare toxic epidermal necrolysis and Stevens-Johnson
  syndrome have been reported. Sulfacetamide preparations are incompatible with silver preparations.
To reduce risk of systemic absorption with ophthalmic solution, apply finger pressure to lacrimal sac
  during and 1—2 min after instillation.

SULFADIAZINE
Various generics
Antibiotic, sulfonamide derivative

C/D   3   Yes   Yes   Yes

Tabs: 500 mg
Oral suspension: 100, 200 mg/mL

General dosing:
  Infant ≥2 mo, child, and adolescent: 75 mg/kg/dose or 2000 mg/m²/dose PO × 1,
    followed by 150 mg/kg/24 hr or 4000 mg/m²/24 hr ÷ Q4—6 hr (**max. dose:** 6000 mg/24 hr)
  Adult: 2—4 g/dose × 1, followed by 2—4 g/24 hr PO ÷ Q4—8 hr
**Congenital toxoplasmosis (administer with pyrimethamine and folinic acid; see Pyrimethamine for
  dosage information):**
  Infant: 100 mg/kg/24 hr PO ÷ BID × 12 mo
**Acquired toxoplasmosis (administer with pyrimethamine and folinic acid; see Pyrimethamine for
  dosage information):**
  Infant ≥2 mo and child: 100—200 mg/kg/24 hr ÷ Q6 hr PO for at least 4—6 wk; **max. dose:** 6000
    mg/24 hr
  Adult: 4—6 g/24 hr PO ÷ Q6 hr for at least 4—6 wk
Rheumatic fever secondary prophylaxis (≥2 mo):
  ≤27 kg: 500 mg PO once daily
  >27 kg: 1000 mg PO once daily

Most cases of acquired toxoplasmosis do not require specific antimicrobial therapy.
  Contraindicated in porphyria and hypersensitivity to sulfonamides. **Use with caution** in
  premature infants and infants below 2 mo of age, because of risk of hyperbilirubinemia,
  and in hepatic or renal dysfunction (30%—44% eliminated in urine). Maintain hydration. May cause
  fever, rash, hepatitis, systemic lupus erythematosus (SLE)—like syndrome, vasculitis,
  bone marrow suppression, and hemolysis in patients with G6PD deficiency, and Stevens-Johnson
  syndrome.
May cause increased effects of warfarin, methotrexate, thiazide diuretics, uricosuric agents,
  and sulfonylureas due to drug displacement from protein binding sites. Large quantities of
  vitamin C or acidifying agents (e.g., cranberry juice) may cause crystalluria. Pregnancy category
  changes from C to D if administered near term. Administer on an empty stomach with plenty
  of water.

SULFAMETHOXAZOLE AND TRIMETHOPRIM
Trimethoprim-sulfamethoxazole, Co-Trimoxazole, TMP-SMX, Bactrim, Bactrin DS, Sulfatrim Pediatric Suspension, and generics; previously available as Septra
Antibiotic, sulfonamide derivative

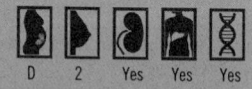

D   2   Yes   Yes   Yes

Tabs (may contain sodium benzoate):
    Reg. strength (Bactrim and generics): 80 mg TMP/400 mg SMX
    Double strength (Bactrim DS and generics): 160 mg TMP/800 mg SMX
Oral suspension (Sulfatrim Pediatric Suspension and generics): 40 mg TMP/200 mg SMX per 5 mL (100, 480 mL)
Injection: 16 mg TMP/mL and 80 mg SMX/mL (5, 10, 30 mL); some preparations may contain propylene glycol and benzyl alcohol

Doses based on TMP component.
Minor/moderate infections (PO or IV):

    Child: 8–12 mg/kg/24 hr ÷ BID; **max. dose:** 160 mg/dose
    Adult (>40 kg): 160 mg/dose BID
Severe infections (PO or IV):
    Child and adult: 20 mg/kg/24 hr ÷ Q6–8 hr
UTI prophylaxis:
    Child: 2–4 mg/kg/24 hr PO once daily
***Pneumocystis jiroveci (carinii)* pneumonia (PCP):**
    Treatment (≥2 mo and adult, PO or IV): 15–20 mg/kg/24 hr ÷ Q6–8 hr × 21 days
    Prophylaxis (PO or IV):
        ≥1 mo and child: 150 mg/m^2/24 hr ÷ BID for 3 consecutive days per wk; **max. dose:** 320 mg/24 hr; see Chapter 17 for use criteria for perinatal HIV PCP prophylaxis.
        Adolescent and adult: 80 or 160 mg once daily or 160 mg 3 days per wk

Not recommended for use in infants below 2 mo of age (excluding PCP prophylaxis). **Contraindicated** in patients with sulfonamide or trimethoprim hypersensitivity, megaloblastic anemia due to folate deficiency, and those who are taking dofetilide. May cause kernicterus in newborns; may cause blood dyscrasias, crystalluria, glossitis, renal or hepatic injury, GI irritation, rash, Stevens-Johnson syndrome, or hemolysis in patients with G6PD deficiency. Severe hyponatremia may occur during treatment of *Pneumocystis jiroveci* pneumonia. Hyperkalemia may appear in HIV/AIDS patients. **Use with caution** in renal and hepatic impairment and in G6PD deficiency. QT prolongation resulting in ventricular tachycardia has been reported. Slow acetylators may be prone to idiosyncratic reactions to sulfonamides. Intravenous dosage form contains propylene glycol and benzyl alcohol, which may result in adverse toxic effects when used at higher dosages, especially in neonates. Use of an adjusted body weight ([ABW] ABW = ideal body weight + 0.4 × [total body weight − ideal body weight]) has been recommended for determining doses for obese patients.

Discontinue use if significant electrolyte abnormality, renal insufficiency, or reduction in CBC occurs.

Epidemiologic studies suggest that use during pregnancy may be associated with increased risk of congenital malformations (particularly neural tube defects), cardiovascular malformations, urinary tract defects, oral clefts, and clubfoot.

Sulfamethoxazole is a CYP 450 2C9 substrate and inhibitor. Trimethoprim is a CYP 450 2C9, 3A4 substrate and an inhibitor or CYP 450 2C8 and OCT2 transporter. **Avoid use** with drugs that are substrates of CYP2C8 and 2C9 or OCT2. **Reduce dose in renal impairment (see Chapter 31).**

SULFASALAZINE
Azulfidine, Azulfidine EN-tabs, Salicylazosulfa-
pyridine, and generics
Anti-inflammatory agent

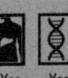

B/D 2 Yes Yes Yes

Tabs (Azulfidine and generics): 500 mg
Delayed release tabs (Azulfidine EN-tabs and generics): 500 mg
Oral suspension: 100 mg/mL

Inflammatory bowel disease:
  Child ≥6 yr:
    Initial dosing:
      Mild: 40–50 mg/kg/24 hr ÷ Q6 hr PO
      Moderate/severe: 50–75 mg/kg/24 hr ÷ Q4–6 hr PO
      Max. initial dose: 4 g/24 hr
    Maintenance: 30–70 mg/kg/24 hr ÷ Q4–8 hr PO; **max. dose:** 4 g/24 hr
  Adult:
    Initial: 3–4 g/24 hr ÷ Q4–8 hr PO
    Maintenance: 2 g/24 hr ÷ Q6 hr PO
    Max. dose: 6 g/24 hr
Juvenile idiopathic arthritis:
  Child 6–16 yr: Start with 10 mg/kg/24 hr ÷ BID PO and increase by 10 mg/kg/24 hr Q7 days until
    planned maintenance dose is achieved. Usual maintenance dose is 30–50 mg/kg/24 hr ÷ BID PO
    up to a **max.** of 2 g/24 hr.

Contraindicated in sulfa or salicylate hypersensitivity, porphyria, and GI or genitourinary (GU)
obstruction. Discontinue use if a serious infection or renal function deterioration develops
while on therapy. **Use with caution** in renal impairment, blood dyscrasias, or asthma. Maintain
hydration. May cause orange-yellow discoloration of urine and skin. May permanently stain contact
lenses. May cause photosensitivity, hypersensitivity (which may result in hepatitis and nephritis),
blood dyscrasias, CNS changes, nausea, vomiting, anorexia, diarrhea, and renal damage.
Hepatotoxicity/hepatic failure, anaphylaxis, angioedema, severe drug rash with eosinophilia and
systemic symptoms (DRESS), and interstitial lung disease have been reported. May cause hemolysis
in patients with G6PD deficiency. Pseudomononucleosis, myocarditis, folate deficiency (decreases
folic acid absorption), nephrolithiasis, and oropharyngeal pain have been reported.
Reduces serum digoxin and cyclosporine levels. Slow acetylators may require lower dosage due to
accumulation of active sulfapyridine metabolite. May cause false-positive test for urinary
normetanephrine if using liquid chromatography methods.
Pregnancy category changes to "D" if drug is administered near term. Bloody stools or diarrhea have
been reported in breastfed infants of mothers receiving sulfasalazine.

SUMATRIPTAN SUCCINATE
Imitrex, Imitrex STAT dose, Sumavel Dose Pro,
Zembrace SymTouch, Tosymra, Onzetra Xsail,
and generics
In combination with naproxen:
Treximet and generics
Antimigraine agent, selective serotonin agonist

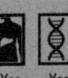

C 2 Yes Yes No

Injection, for subcutaneous use:
  Zembrace SymTouch: 3 mg/0.5 mL (0.5 mL)

Continued

SUMATRIPTAN SUCCINATE *continued*

Imitrex, Imitrex STAT dose, Sumavel DosePro, and generics: 4 mg/0.5 mL (0.5 mL), 6 mg/0.5 mL (0.5 mL)

Tabs: 25, 50, 100 mg

Oral suspension: 5 mg/mL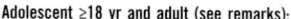

Nasal spray (as a unit-dose spray device):

Imitrex and generics: 5 mg dose in 100 microliters (six units per pack); 20 mg dose in 100 microliters (six units per pack)

Tosymra: 10 mg dose in 100 microliters (six units per pack)

Nasal powder (Onzetra Xsail): 11 mg capsule with nasal inhalation nosepiece (two each per pouch; box of eight pouches)

In combination with naproxen:

Tab (Treximet and generics): 85 mg sumatriptan and 500 mg naproxen sodium (nine tabs)

Child <18 yr:

PO/SC/Nasal: Incomplete clinical trials to establish efficacy with concerns of serious side effects; see remarks

Adolescent ≥18 yr and adult (see remarks):

PO: 25, 50, or 100 mg as soon as possible after onset of headache. If no relief in 2 hr, give 25–100 mg Q2 hr up to a daily **max.** of 200 mg. Safety of treating more than four headaches in a 30-day period has not been established.

Max. single dose: 100 mg/dose

Max. daily dose: 200 mg/24 hr (with exclusive PO dosing or with an initial SC dose and subsequent PO dosing)

SC: 3, 4, or 6 mg × 1 as soon as possible after onset of headache. If no response, may give an additional dose 1 hr later; **max. daily dose:** 12 mg/24 hr. Use lower subsequent dose if side effects occur.

Nasal (safety of treating more than four headaches in a 30-day period has not been established):

Nasal spray (Imitrex, Tosymra, and generics): 5, 10, or 20 mg per dose into one nostril or divided into each nostril after onset of headache. Dose may be repeated in 2 hr up to a **max.** of 40 mg/24 hr.

Nasal powder (Onzetra Xsail): Inhale 22 mg (11 mg per nostril) after onset of headache. Dose may be repeated in 2 hr up to a **max.** of 44 mg/24 hr. If using a combination of different dosage forms, the **max. dose** is one dose of Onzetra Xsail (22 mg) and one dose of another sumatriptan product.

In combination with naproxen sodium:

Treximet and generics:

Child 12–17 yr: 1 tablet (85 mg sumatriptan + 500 mg naproxen sodium) after the onset of headache × 1; **max. dose:** 1 tab/24 hr. Safety of treating more than two headaches in a 30-day period has not been established.

Adult: 1 tablet (85 mg sumatriptan + 500 mg naproxen sodium) after the onset of headache × 1; if response is unsatisfactory in 2 hr, a second dose may be administered. **Max. dose:** 2 tabs/24 hr. Safety of treating more than five headaches in a 30-day period has not been established.

Contraindicated with concomitant administration of ergotamine derivatives, MAO inhibitors (and use within the past 2 wk), other vasoconstrictive drugs, or history of TIA or stroke.

Not for migraine prophylaxis. **Use with caution** in renal or hepatic impairment. **A max. single** PO dose of 50 mg has been recommended in adults with hepatic dysfunction. Acts as selective agonist for serotonin receptor. Induration and swelling at the injection site; flushing; dizziness; as well as chest, jaw, and neck tightness may occur with SC administration. Weakness, hyperreflexia, incoordination, and serotonin syndrome (may be life-threatening) have been reported with use in combination with selective serotonin reuptake inhibitors (e.g., fluoxetine, fluvoxamine, paroxetine, sertraline).

May cause coronary vasospasm if administered intravenously. **Use injectable form SC only!** Onset of action is 10–120 min SC, 60–90 min PO, and 15–120 min intranasal.

SUMATRIPTAN SUCCINATE *continued*

PO, nasal, and SC efficacy studies were not conclusive in clinical trials for children. Some do not recommend use in patients less than 18 yr of age owing to poor efficacy and reports of serious adverse events (e.g., stroke, visual loss, and death) in both children and adults with all dosage forms.

To minimize infant exposure to sumatriptan, **avoid** breastfeeding for 12 hr after treatment. See Naproxen remarks if using the combination sumatriptan and naproxen dosage form.

SURFACTANT, PULMONARY/BERACTANT
Survanta
Bovine lung surfactant

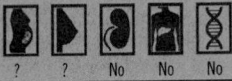

? ? No No No

Suspension for inhalation: 25 mg/mL phospholipids (4, 8 mL); contains 0.5–1.75 mg triglycerides, 1.4–3.5 mg free fatty acids, and <1 mg protein per 1 mL drug

Prophylactic therapy: 4 mL/kg/dose intratracheally as soon as possible; up to four doses may be given at intervals no shorter than Q6 hr PRN during the first 48 hr of life

Rescue therapy (treatment): 4 mL/kg/dose intratracheally immediately following the diagnosis of respiratory distress syndrome (RDS). May repeat dose as needed Q6 hr PRN to a **max.** of four total doses during the first 48 hr of life

Method of administration for previously listed therapies (see remarks): Suction infant prior to administration. Each dose is divided into four aliquots of 1 mL/kg each; administer 1 mL/kg in each of four different positions (slight downward inclination with head turned to the right, head turned to the left; slight upward inclination with the head turned to the right, head turned to the left).

Transient bradycardia, O_2 desaturation, pallor, vasoconstriction, hypotension, endotracheal tube blockage, hypercarbia, hypercapnea, apnea, and hypertension may occur during the administration process. Other side effects may include pulmonary interstitial emphysema, pulmonary air leak, and posttreatment nosocomial sepsis. Monitor heart rate and transcutaneous O_2 saturation during dose administration and arterial blood gases for postdose hyperoxia and hypocarbia after administration.

All doses are administered intratracheally via a 5-french feeding catheter. If the suspension settles during storage, gently swirl the contents; **do not shake.** Drug is stored in the refrigerator, protected from light, and must be warmed by standing at room temperature for at least 20 min or warmed in the hand for at least 8 min. Artificial warming methods should **NOT** be used.

SURFACTANT, PULMONARY/CALFACTANT
Infasurf
Bovine lung surfactant

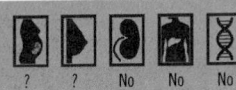

? ? No No No

Intratracheal suspension: 35 mg/mL phospholipids (3, 6 mL); contains 26 mg phosphatidylcholine, 0.7 mg protein, and 0.26 mg surfactant protein B per 1 mL

Prophylactic therapy: 3 mL/kg/dose intratracheally as soon as possible; up to a total of three doses may be given Q12 hr

Rescue therapy (treatment; see remarks): 3 mL/kg/dose intratracheally immediately after the diagnosis of RDS. May repeat dose as needed Q12 hr to **max.** of 3 doses total

Method of administration for previously listed therapies (see remarks): Suction infant prior to administration. Manufacturer recommends administration through a side-port adapter into the endotracheal tube with two attendants (one to instill drug and another to monitor and position patient). Each dose is divided into two aliquots of 1.5 mL/kg each; administer 1.5 mL/kg in each of

Continued

SURFACTANT, PULMONARY/CALFACTANT *continued*

two different positions (infant positioned with either the right or left side dependent). Drug is administered while ventilation is continued over 20 to 30 breaths for each aliquot, with small bursts timed only during the inspiratory cycles. A pause followed by evaluation of respiratory status and repositioning should separate the two aliquots. The drug has also been administered by divided dose into four equal aliquots and administered with repositioning in the prone, supine, right, and left lateral positions.

Common adverse effects include cyanosis, airway obstruction, bradycardia, reflux of surfactant into the endotracheal (ET) tube, requirement for manual ventilation, and reintubation. Monitor O_2 saturation and lung compliance after each dose such that oxygen therapy and ventilator pressure are adjusted as necessary.

All doses administered intratracheally via a 5-French feeding catheter. If suspension settles during storage, gently swirl the contents; **do not shake.** Drug is stored in the refrigerator, protected from light, and does not need to be warmed before administration. Unopened vials that have been warmed to room temperature (once only) may be refrigerated within 24 hr and stored for future use.

For rescue therapy, repeat doses may be administered as early as 6 hr after the previous dose for a total of up to four doses if the infant is still intubated and requires at least 30% inspired oxygen to maintain a $PaO_2 \geq 80$ torr.

SURFACTANT, PULMONARY/PORACTANT ALFA
Curosurf
Porcine lung surfactant

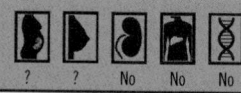

? ? No No No

Intratracheal suspension: 80 mg/mL (1.5, 3 mL): contains 76 mg phospholipids, 1 mg protein (0.45 mg surfactant protein B, and 0.59 mg surfactant protein C) per 1 mL drug

Rescue therapy (treatment): 2.5 mL/kg/dose (use birth weight) × 1 intratracheally, immediately following the diagnosis of RDS. May administer 1.25 mL/kg/dose Q12 hr × 2 doses as needed up to a **max. total dose** of 5 mL/kg

Method of administration (see remarks): Suction infant prior to administration. Each dose is divided into two aliquots, with each aliquot administered into one of the two main bronchi by positioning the infant with either the right or left side dependent. After the first aliquot is administered, remove the catheter from the ET tube and manually ventilate the infant with 100% oxygen at a rate of 40–60 breaths/min for 1 min. When the infant is stable, reposition the infant and administer the second dose with the same procedures. Then remove the catheter without flushing.

Currently approved by the US Food and Drug Administration (FDA) for the treatment (rescue therapy) of RDS. Transient episodes of bradycardia, decreased oxygen saturation, reflux of surfactant into the ET tube, and airway obstruction have occurred during dose administration. Monitor O_2 saturation and lung compliance after each dose and adjust oxygen therapy and ventilator pressure as necessary. Pulmonary hemorrhage has been reported.

All doses administered intratracheally via a 5-french feeding catheter. Suction infant prior to administration and 1 hr after surfactant instillation (unless signs of significant airway obstruction).

Drug is stored in the refrigerator and protected from light. Each vial of drug should be slowly warmed to room temperature and gently turned upside down for uniform suspension (**do not shake**) before administration. Unopened vials that have been warmed to room temperature (once only) may be refrigerated within 24 hr and stored for future use.

SYMDEKO

See Tezacaftor and Ivacaftor.

T

TACROLIMUS
Prograf, Astagraf XL, Envarsus XR, Protopic,
FK506, and generics
Immunosuppressant

    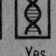

C   2   Yes   Yes   Yes

Caps (Prograf and generics): 0.5, 1, 5 mg
Extended release caps (Astagraf XL): 0.5, 1, 5 mg (Q24 hr dosing; see remarks)
Extended release tabs (Envarsus XR): 0.75, 1, 4 mg (Q24 hr dosing; see remarks)
Oral suspension: 0.5, 1 mg/mL
Injection (Prograf): 5 mg/mL (1 mL); contains alcohol and polyoxyl 60 hydrogenated castor oil
(cremophor)
Topical ointment (Protopic and generics): 0.03%, 0.1% (30, 60, 100 g)

SYSTEMIC USE:
**Infant, child, and adolescent (initial immediate release doses; titrate to therapeutic levels
and convert IV to PO as soon as possible; see remarks):**
  Liver transplantation:
    IV: 0.03–0.05 mg/kg/24 hr by continuous infusion
    PO: 0.15–0.2 mg/kg/24 hr ÷ Q12 hr
  Renal transplantation:
    IV: 0.06 mg/kg/hr by continuous infusion
    PO: 0.2–0.3 mg/kg/24 hr ÷ Q12 hr
      Astagraf XL (in combination with other immunosuppressants): 0.15–0.3 mg/kg/24 hr PO Q24
      hr; initial dose and post-reperfusion times vary with or without basiliximab induction
  Cardiac transplantation:
    IV: 0.01–0.03 mg/kg/24 hr by continuous infusion
    PO: 0.1–0.3 mg/kg/24 hr ÷ Q12 hr; use lower initial dose for those receiving cell depleting
    induction therapy
Adult (initial immediate release doses; titrate to therapeutic levels):
  IV:
    Liver or kidney transplantation: 0.03–0.05 mg/kg/24 hr by continuous infusion
    Cardiac transplantation: 0.01 mg/kg/24 hr by continuous infusion
  PO:
    Liver transplantation: 0.1–0.15 mg/kg/24 hr PO ÷ Q12 hr
    Kidney transplantation: 0.1–0.2 mg/kg/24 hr PO ÷ Q12 hr
    Cardiac transplantation: 0.075 mg/kg/24 hr PO ÷ Q12 hr
TOPICAL USE:
**Atopic dermatitis (discontinue treatment when symptoms resolve and reconsider diagnosis if no
improvement seen after 6 weeks; see remarks):**
  Child ≥2 to 15 yr old: Apply a thin layer of the 0.03% ointment to the affected skin areas BID and rub
  in gently and completely.
  Adolescent ≥16 yr and adult: Apply a thin layer of the 0.03% or 0.1% ointment to the affected skin
  areas BID and rub in gently and completely.

Avoid use in patients with prolonged cardiac QT intervals. IV dosage form **contraindicated** in
patients allergic to polyoxyl 60 hydrogenated castor oil (cremophor). Experience in pediatric
kidney transplantation is limited. Pediatric patients may require higher mg/kg doses than adults.
For BMT use (beginning 1 day before BMT), dose and therapeutic levels similar to those in liver
transplantation have been used.

Continued

TACROLIMUS *continued*

Major adverse events include tremor, headache, insomnia, diarrhea, constipation, hypertension, nausea, and renal dysfunction (increased risk with use of other nephrotoxic medications and with CYP 450 3A inhibitors). Hypokalemia, hypomagnesemia, hyperglycemia, confusion, depression, infections, lymphoma, liver enzyme elevation, optic neuropathy, and coagulation disorders may also occur. GI perforation, agranulocytosis, HUS, TTP, and hemolytic anemia have been reported.

Tacrolimus is a substrate of the CYP 450 3A4 drug metabolizing enzyme and P-gp transporter. A 1.5–2-fold higher initial standard dose up to a max. dose of 0.3 mg/kg/24 hr has been recommended for intermediate or extensive metabolizers for CYP 450 3A5. Calcium channel blockers, imidazole antifungals (ketoconazole, itraconazole, fluconazole, clotrimazole, posaconazole), macrolide antibiotics (erythromycin, clarithromycin, troleandomycin), cisapride, cimetidine, cyclosporine, danazol, herbal products containing schisandra sphenanthera extracts, methylprednisolone, grapefruit juice, Seville oranges, and severe diarrhea can increase tacrolimus serum levels. In contrast, carbamazepine, caspofungin, phenobarbital, phenytoin, rifampin, rifabutin, and sirolimus may decrease levels. Use with sirolimus may increase risk for hepatic artery thrombosis. **Avoid use** of live, attenuated vaccines. Use with other CYP 450 3A inhibitors and substrates has the potential to prolong the cardiac QT interval. Reduce dose in renal or hepatic insufficiency.

Monitor trough levels (just prior to a dose at steady state). Steady state is generally achieved after 2–5 days of continuous dosing. Interpretation will vary based on treatment protocol and assay methodology (whole blood ELISA vs. MEIA vs. HPLC). Whole blood trough concentrations of 5–20 ng/mL have been recommended in liver transplantation at 1–12 mo. Trough levels of 7–20 ng/mL (whole blood) for the first 3 mo and 5–15 ng/mL after 3 mo have been recommended in renal transplantation. African Americans may need to be titrated to higher dosages. Patients with liver function changes during direct-acting antiviral therapy related to hepatitis C may alter tacrolimus pharmacokinetics, therefore requiring enhanced monitoring.

Tacrolimus therapy generally should be initiated 6 hr or more after transplantation. PO is the preferred route of administration, and all PO dosage forms should be administered on an empty stomach (1 hr before and 2 hr after meals).

Astagraf XL (extended release capsule): Safety and efficacy have been established for de novo and stable (receiving immediate release dosage form) pediatric kidney transplant patients. A mg-per-mg conversion from immediate release dosage form to Astagraf XL has been recommended.

Envarsus XR (extended release tablet): Currently labeled for use in adult kidney transplant patients (de novo and stable on immediate release tacrolimus). When converting to Envarsus XR from immediate release dosage form, initiate at 80% of the established immediate release dosage form.

All extended release formulations are NOT interchangeable. IV infusions should be administered at concentrations between 0.004 and 0.02 mg/mL diluted with NS or D_5W.

TOPICAL USE: Not recommended for use in patients with skin conditions with a skin barrier defect with the potential for systemic absorption. **Do not use** in children <2 yr, immunocompromised patients, or with occlusive dressings (promotes systemic absorption). Approved as a second-line therapy for short-term and intermittent treatment of atopic dermatitis for patients who fail to respond, or do not tolerate, other approved therapies. Long-term safety is unknown. Skin burn sensation, pruritus, flu-like symptoms, allergic reaction, skin erythema, headache, and skin infection are the most common side effects. Application site edema has been reported. Although the risk is uncertain, the FDA has issued an alert about the potential cancer risk with the use of this product. See www.fda.gov/medwatch for the latest information.

TAZAROTENE
Arazlo, Fabior, Tazorac, and generics
Topical retinoid acid prodrug, keratolytic agent for acne or psoriasis

 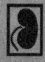   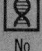

X	3	No	No	No

Topical cream:
   Tazorac and generics: 0.05%, 0.1% (30, 60 g); contains benzyl alcohol
Topical foam:
   Fabior and generics: 0.1% (50, 100 g)
Topical gel:
   Tazorac and generics: 0.05%, 0.1% (30, 100 g); contains benzyl alcohol
Topical lotion:
   Arazlo: 0.045% (45 g); contains EDTA and parabens

Acne:

   0.045% topical lotion (Tazorac):
     >9 yr and adult: Apply a thin layer of the lotion to affected areas once daily.
   0.01% topical cream, foam, or gel:
     ≥12 yr and adult: Apply a small amount of 0.1% strength dosage forms to affected areas QHS. Use thin film (2 mg/cm^2) for cream or gel dosage form and small amount for foam dosage form.
Psoriasis:
   ≥12 yr and adult: Apply a small amount of 0.05% gel (2 mg/cm^2) to affected areas QHS initially. If needed and tolerated, increase to 0.1% gel QHS. The cream dosage form may also be used the same way as the gel, but it is currently labeled for use in adults (≥18 yr).

Contraindicated in pregnancy. Pregnancy testing 2 wk prior to use and initiation of use during menstrual period have been recommended. **Avoid** use in abraded or eczematous skin or with other medications or cosmetics with drying effects, or medications that can cause photosensitivity.

Tazarotene is a retinoid prodrug that is converted to its active form, the cognate carboxylic acid of tazarotene (AGN 190299), by rapid deesterification in animals and humans.

Common side effects include erythema, dry skin, skin irritation/pain (including blistering and skin desquamation), pruritus, and worsening of psoriasis.

Avoid contact with mucous membranes. The foam dosage form is flammable; **avoid** fire, flame, or smoking during or immediately after use.

TERBINAFINE
Previously available as Lamisil, Lamisil AT, and generics
Antifungal

    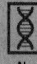

B	2	Yes	Yes	No

Tabs: 250 mg
Oral suspension: 25 mg/mL
Topical cream:
   Lamisil AT and generics [OTC]: 1% (12, 15, 30 g); contains benzyl alcohol
Topical spray:
   Lamisil AT [OTC]: 1% (15 mL); contains alcohol and propylene glycol

Tinea capitis:
   Child: 4–6 mg/kg/dose (**max. dose:** 250 mg) PO once daily, OR by the following once-daily dosage by weight category:
     10–20 kg: 62.5 mg
     20–40 kg: 125 mg

Continued

TERBINAFINE *continued*

>**40 kg:** 250 mg
Duration of therapy: *Trichophyton tonsurans:* 2—6 wk; *Microsprum canis:* 8—12 wk
Adult: 250 mg PO once daily × 4—6 wk
Onychomycosis:
Child and adolescent (limited data): PO once daily by weight category:
10—20 kg: 62.5 mg
20—40 kg: 125 mg
>**40 kg:** 250 mg
Adult: 250 mg PO once daily
Duration of therapy:
Fingernail infection: 6 wk
Toenail infection: 12 wk
Topical use for dermal mycosis:
≥**12 yr:**
Tinea pedis: Apply topically (cream or spray) interdigitally BID × 1 wk; if needed, apply the cream to the bottom or sides of the foot BID × 2 wk.
Tinea cruris/tinea corporis: Apply topically (cream or spray) to affected area once daily × 1 wk.
Pityriasis (tinea) versicolor: Apply spray to affected area once daily × 1 wk.

SYSTEMIC USE: Contraindicated in chronic or acute liver disease. Common side effects include headache, fever, cough, diarrhea, taste disorder, increased LFTs, GI disturbances, and rash. Severe dermatological reactions (e.g., SJS, TEN), hearing loss, neutropenia, thrombotic microangiopathy, and liver failure (some fatal) have been reported. Monitor AST/ALT at baseline and repeat with CBC if therapy is >6 wk. Signs and symptoms of liver disease may include persistent nausea, anorexia, fatigue, vomiting, right upper abdominal pain, or jaundice. Discontinue use immediately if biochemical or clinical evidence of liver injury develops.

Use with caution in renal impairment as terbinafine's clearance has been shown to decrease by ~50% in adults with CrCl ≤50 mL/min. Terbinafine inhibits CYP 450 2D6, thus increasing the effects/toxicity of 2D6 substrates such as amphetamines, risperidone, and fluoxetine.

Doses may be administered with or without food.

TOPICAL USE: Do not use on/in the eyes, mouth, nails, scalp, or vaginal areas. Local irritation, skin rash, xeroderma, pruritus, and contact dermatitis may occur. Apply to clean and dry affected area, and wash hands after each use. If using topical spray, hold spray 4—6 inches from the affected area during dose administration.

TERBUTALINE
Various generics; previously available as Brethine
β₂ adrenergic agonist

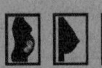   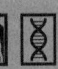

C   2   Yes   No   No

Tabs: 2.5, 5 mg
Oral suspension: 1 mg/mL
Injection: 1 mg/mL (1 mL)

Acute asthma exacerbation:
SC injection:
≤**12 yr:** 0.005—0.01 mg/kg/dose (**max. dose:** 0.4 mg/dose) Q15—20 min × 3; if needed, Q2—6 hr PRN
>**12 yr and adult:** 0.25 mg/dose Q20 min PRN × 3; **max. total dose:** 0.75 mg

TERBUTALINE *continued*

Continuous infusion, IV: 2—10 mCg/kg loading dose followed by infusion of 0.1—0.4 mCg/kg/min. May titrate in increments of 0.1—0.2 mCg/kg/min Q30 min depending on clinical response. Doses as high as 10 mCg/kg/min have been used. To prepare infusion: See p. iii.

Nebulization (use IV dosage form):
  <2 yr: 0.5 mg in 2.5 mL NS Q4—6 hr PRN
  2—9 yr: 1 mg in 2.5 mL NS Q4—6 hr PRN
  >9 yr: 1.5—2.5 mg in 2.5 mL NS Q4—6 hr PRN

Prevention and reversal of bronchospasms with asthma:
  Oral:
    ≤12 yr: Initial: 0.05 mg/kg/dose Q8 hr, increase as required. **Max. dose:** 0.15 mg/kg/dose Q8 hr or total of 5 mg/24 hr
    >12 yr and adult: 2.5—5 mg/dose PO Q6—8 hr
      Max. dose:
        12—15 yr: 7.5 mg/24 hr
        >15 yr: 15 mg/24 hr

Use of the IV and PO route should not be used for the prevention or prolonged treatment of preterm labor because of the potential for serious maternal cardiac events and even death. Nervousness, tremor, headache, nausea, tachycardia, arrhythmias, and palpitations may occur. Paradoxical bronchoconstriction may occur with excessive use; if it occurs, discontinue drug immediately. Injectable product may be used for nebulization. For acute asthma, nebulizations may be given more frequently than Q4—6 hr.

Monitor heart rate, blood pressure, respiratory rate, and serum potassium when using the continuous IV infusion route of administration. **Adjust dose in renal failure (see Chapter 31).**

TETRACYCLINE HCL
Various generics; previously available as
Sumycin
Antibiotic

D   2   Yes   Yes   No

Caps: 250, 500 mg
Oral suspension: 25 mg/mL

Do not use in children <8 yr.
Child ≥8 yr: 25—50 mg/kg/24 hr PO ÷ Q6 hr; **max. dose:** 3 g/24 hr
  Acne: 500 mg PO BID
Adult: 250—500 mg PO Q6 hr or 500 mg PO Q12 hr

Not recommended in patients <8 yr owing to tooth staining and decreased bone growth. Also **not recommended** for use in pregnancy because these side effects may occur in the fetus. The risk for these adverse effects is highest with long-term use. May cause nausea, GI upset, hepatotoxicity, stomatitis, rash, fever, and superinfection. Photosensitivity reaction may occur. **Avoid prolonged exposure to sunlight.**

Never use outdated tetracyclines because they may cause Fanconi-like syndrome. **Do not** give with dairy products or with any divalent cations (i.e., Fe^{2+}, Ca^{2+}, Mg^{2+}). Give 1 hr before or 2 hr after meals.

May decrease the effectiveness of oral contraceptives, increase serum digoxin levels, and increase effects of warfarin. Use with methoxyflurane increases risk for nephrotoxicity, and use with isotretinoin is associated with pseudotumor cerebri. **Adjust dose in renal failure (see Chapter 31).**
Short-term maternal use is not likely to cause harm to breastfeeding infants.

TEZACAFTOR AND IVACAFTOR
Symdeko
Cystic fibrosis transmembrane conductance regulator corrector and potentiator

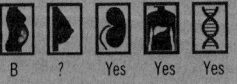

B   ?   Yes   Yes   Yes

Tabs (4-week supply in 4 weekly blister packs):
   Tezacaftor 50 mg and ivacaftor 75 mg (white tabs; 28 tabs) and ivacaftor 75 mg (light blue tabs; 28 tabs)
   Tezacaftor 100 mg and ivacaftor 150 mg (yellow tabs; 28 tabs) and ivacaftor 150 mg (light blue tabs; 28 tabs)

Child 6 to <12 yr:
   <30 kg: One tezacaftor 50 mg/75 mg ivacaftor PO QAM and one ivacaftor 75 mg PO every evening administered ∼12 hr apart
   ≥30 kg: One tezacaftor 100 mg/150 mg ivacaftor PO QAM and one ivacaftor 150 mg PO every evening administered ∼12 hr apart
Child ≥12 yr—adult: One tezacaftor 100 mg/150 mg ivacaftor PO QAM and one ivacaftor 150 mg PO every evening administered ∼12 hr apart
Dosage modification with hepatic impairment:

Child-Pugh Class	Morning Dose		Evening Dose
	Age 6 to <12 yr and <30 kg:	Age 6 to <12 yr and ≥30 kg, and ≥12 yr—adult:	All patients
Class A	No adjustment	No adjustment	No adjustment
Class B	One tablet of tezacaftor 50 mg/ivacaftor 75 mg PO QAM	One tablet of tezacaftor 100 mg/ivacaftor 150 mg PO QAM	No ivacaftor
Class C	One tablet of tezacaftor 50 mg/ivacaftor 75 mg PO QAM or less frequently	One tablet of tezacaftor 100 mg/ivacaftor 150 mg PO QAM or less frequently	No ivacaftor

Dosage modification with CYP 450 3A4 inhibitors:
   Moderate inhibitors (e.g., fluconazole, erythromycin): Do not administer any evening doses.
      Child 6 to <12 yr and <30 kg: Administer the following tablet PO on the following days only in the morning:

Tablet	Day 1	Day 2	Day 3	Day 4[a]
Tezacaftor 50 mg/ivacaftor 75 mg tab	One tablet		One tablet	
Ivacaftor 75 mg tab		One tablet		One tablet

[a]Continue dosing with tezacaftor 50 mg/ivacaftor 75 mg or ivacaftor 75 mg on alternate days.

      Child 6 to <12 yr and ≥30 kg, and ≥12 yr—adult: Administer the following tablet PO on the following days only in the morning:

Tablet	Day 1	Day 2	Day 3	Day 4[a]
Tezacaftor 100 mg/ivacaftor 150 mg tab	One tablet		One tablet	
Ivacaftor 150 mg tab		One tablet		One tablet

[a]Continue dosing with tezacaftor 100 mg/ivacaftor 150 mg or ivacaftor 150 mg on alternate days.

TEZACAFTOR AND IVACAFTOR *continued*

Strong inhibitors (e.g., ketoconazole, itraconazole, posaconazole, voriconazole, telithromycin, and clarithromycin): Do not administer any evening doses.

   Child 6 to <12 yr and <30 kg: One tezacaftor 50 mg/ivacaftor 75 mg PO in the morning on days 1 and 4, then continue with the same one tablet twice weekly (administered 3—4 days apart).

   Child 6 to <12 yr and ≥30 kg, and ≥12 yr—adult: One tezacaftor 100 mg/ivacaftor 150 mg PO in the morning on days 1 and 4, then continue with the same one tablet twice weekly (administered 3—4 days apart).

Works on CFTR trafficking defect by acting as a CFTR corrector (tezacaftor) and in combination with a CFTR potentiator (ivacaftor). Indicated for individuals with homozygous F508del CFTR mutation or who have at least one CFTR mutation that is responsive to this drug based on in vitro data and/or clinical evidence.

Common side effects include headache, nausea, sinus congestion, and dizziness. Increased liver enzymes and cataracts may occur; monitor baseline AST/ALT and ocular exam at baseline. Repeat AST/ALT every 3 months for the first year followed by annual assessments. Repeat ocular exams annually. May cause a false-positive urine drug screen for cannabinoids.

Use with caution with CrCl ≤30 mL/min and ESRD. Reduce dose with moderate/severe hepatic impairment or when initiating therapy while taking a CYP 450 3A4 inhibitor (see dosing section).

Tezacaftor and ivacaftor are substrates for CYP 450 3A4/3A5. Use with strong CYP 450 3A inducers (e.g., rifampin, rifabutin, carbamazepine, phenobarbital, phenytoin, St. John's wort) is not recommended. Tezacaftor and ivacaftor may increase the effects/toxicity of cyclosporine, digoxin, everolimus, sirolimus, tacrolimus, and warfarin. Always evaluate potential drug-drug interactions; see https://www.symdekohcp.com/drug-interactions. **Avoid** food or drink containing grapefruit or Seville oranges.

Administer all doses with high-fat foods to ensure absorption. If a dose (all dosage forms) is missed within 6 hr of a scheduled dose, administer a dose immediately. However, if the missed dose is >6 hr, skip that dose and resume therapy at the next scheduled dose. Never take a double dose for a missed dose.

THEOPHYLLINE
Theo-24, Elixophyllin, and generics
Bronchodilator, methylxanthine

| C | 2 | No | Yes | No |

Other dosage forms may exist.
Immediate release:
   Oral elixir/solution (Elixophyllin and generics): 80 mg/15 mL (473 mL); may contain up to 20% alcohol (alcohol-free preparations may be available)
Sustained/extended release (see remarks):
   Tabs:
      Q12 hr dosing (generics): 300, 450 mg
      Q24 hr dosing (generics): 400, 600 mg
   Caps (Q24 hr dosing: Theo-24 and generics): 100, 200, 300, 400 mg
   Sustained release forms should **not** be chewed or crushed. Capsules may be opened and contents may be sprinkled on food.

Dosing intervals are for immediate release preparations.
For sustained release preparations, divide daily dose >Q8—24 hr based on product.

Neonatal apnea:
   Loading dose: 5 mg/kg/dose PO × 1
   Maintenance: 3—6 mg/kg/24 hr PO ÷ Q6—8 hr

Continued

THEOPHYLLINE *continued*

Bronchospasm; PO:

Loading dose: 1 mg/kg/dose for each 2 mg/L desired increase in serum theophylline level

Maintenance, infant (<1 yr):

Preterm:

<24 days old (postnatal): 1 mg/kg/dose PO Q12 hr

≥24 days old (postnatal): 1.5 mg/kg/dose PO Q12 hr

Full-term up to 1 yr old: Total daily dose (mg) = [(0.2 × age in weeks) + 5] × (kg body weight)

≤6 mo: Divide daily dose Q8 hr

>6 mo: Divide daily dose Q6 hr

Maintenance, child >1 yr and adult without risk factors for altered clearance (see remarks):

<45 kg: Begin therapy at 12—14 mg/kg/24 hr ÷ Q4—6 hr up to **max. dose** of 300 mg/24 hr. If needed based on serum levels, gradually increase to 16—20 mg/kg/24 hr ÷ Q4—6 hr. **Max. dose:** 600 mg/24 hr

≥45 kg: Begin therapy with 300 mg/24 hr ÷ Q6—8 hr. If needed based on serum levels, gradually increase to 400—600 mg/24 hr ÷ Q6—8 hr.

Drug metabolism varies widely with age, drug formulation, and route of administration. Most common side effects and toxicities are nausea, vomiting, anorexia, abdominal pain, gastroesophageal reflux, nervousness, tachycardia, seizures, and arrhythmias.

Serum levels should be monitored. Therapeutic levels: bronchospasm: 10—20 mg/L; apnea: 7—13 mg/L. Half-life is age dependent: 30 hr (newborns); 6.9 hr (infants); 3.4 hr (children); 8.1 hr (adults). See Aminophylline for guidelines for serum level determinations. Liver impairment, cardiac failure, and sustained high fever may increase theophylline levels. Theophylline is a substrate for CYP 450 1A2. Levels are increased with allopurinol, alcohol, ciprofloxacin, cimetidine, clarithromycin, disulfiram, erythromycin, estrogen, isoniazid, propranolol, thiabendazole, and verapamil. Levels are decreased with carbamazepine, isoproterenol, phenobarbital, phenytoin, and rifampin. May cause increased skeletal muscle activity, agitation, and hyperactivity when used with doxapram, and increase quinine levels/toxicity.

Use ideal body weight in obese patients when calculating dosage because of poor distribution into body fat. Risk factors for increased clearance include: smoking, cystic fibrosis, hyperthyroidism, and high-protein diet. Factors for decreased clearance include CHF, correction of hyperthyroidism, fever, viral illness, sepsis, and high-carbohydrate diet.

Suggested dosage intervals for sustained release products (see following table):

THEOPHYLLINE SUSTAINED RELEASE PRODUCTS

Trade Name	Available Strengths	Dosage Interval
CAPSULES:		
Theo-24	100, 200, 300, 400 mg	Q24 hr
TABLETS:		
Theochron and generics	100, 200, 300, 450 mg	Q12 hr
Generics	400, 600 mg	Q24 hr

THIAMINE
Vitamin B$_1$, many generic products
Water-soluble vitamin

A/C   1   No   No   No

Tabs (OTC): 50, 100, 250 mg
Caps (OTC): 50, 100, 500 mg
Oral suspension: 25, 100 mg/mL

THIAMINE *continued*

Injection: 100 mg/mL (2 mL); may contain benzyl alcohol

For US RDA, see Chapter 21.

Beriberi (thiamine deficiency):

Child: 10—25 mg/dose IM/IV once daily (if critically ill) or 10—50 mg/dose PO once daily × 2 wk, followed by 5—10 mg/dose once daily × 1 mo

Adult: 10—20 mg/dose IM/IV TID (if critically ill) × 2 wk, followed by 5—30 mg/24 hr PO ÷ once daily or TID × 1 mo

Wernicke's encephalopathy syndrome:

Adult: 100 mg IV × 1, then 50—100 mg IM/IV once daily until patient resumes a normal diet. Initiate thiamine before starting glucose infusion.

Refeeding syndrome: see Chapter 11

Multivitamin preparations contain amounts meeting RDA requirements. Allergic reactions and anaphylaxis may occur, primarily with IV administration. Therapeutic range: 1.6—4 mg/dL. High-carbohydrate diets or IV dextrose solutions may increase thiamine requirements. Large doses may interfere with serum theophylline assay. Pregnancy category changes to "C" if used in doses above the RDA.

THIORIDAZINE
Various generics; previously available as Mellaril
Antipsychotic, phenothiazine derivative

 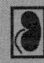

C   3   No   Yes   No

Tabs: 10, 25, 50, 100 mg

Refractory schizophrenia:

Child ≥6 yr—adolescent: Start with 0.5 mg/kg/24 hr PO ÷ BID—TID (**initial max.:** 50 mg/dose); dosage range: 0.5—3 mg/kg/24 hr PO ÷ BID—TID. **Max. dose:** 3 mg/kg/24 hr

Adult: Start with 150—300 mg/24 hr PO ÷ TID. Then gradually increase PRN to **max. dose** 800 mg/24 hr ÷ BID—QID.

Indicated for schizophrenia unresponsive to standard therapy. **Contraindicated** in severe CNS depression, brain damage, narrow-angle glaucoma, blood dyscrasias, and severe liver or cardiovascular disease. **DO NOT** co-administer with drugs that may inhibit the CYP 450 2D6 isoenzymes (e.g., SSRIs such as fluoxetine, fluvoxamine, paroxetine; and β-blockers such as propranolol and pindolol); drugs that may widen the QTc interval (e.g., disopyramide, procainamide, quinidine); and in patients with known reduced activity of CYP 450 2D6.

May cause drowsiness, extrapyramidal reactions, autonomic symptoms, ECG changes (QTc prolongation in a dose-dependent manner), arrhythmias, paradoxical reactions, and endocrine disturbances. Long-term use may cause tardive dyskinesia. Pigmentary retinopathy may occur with higher doses; a periodic eye exam is recommended. More autonomic symptoms and less extrapyramidal effects than chlorpromazine. Concurrent use with epinephrine can cause hypotension. Increased cardiac arrhythmias may occur with tricyclic antidepressants.

In an overdose situation, monitor ECG and avoid drugs that can widen QTc interval.

TIAGABINE
Gabitril and generics
Anticonvulsant

    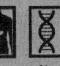

C   ?   No   Yes   No

Tabs: 2, 4, 12, 16 mg

Continued

TIAGABINE *continued*

Oral suspension: 1 mg/mL

Adjunctive therapy for refractory seizures (see remarks):
Child ≥2 yr (limited data from a safety and tolerability study in 52 children 2—17 yr, mean 9.3 + 4.1): Initial dose of 0.25 mg/kg/24 hr PO ÷ TID × 4 wk. Dosage was increased at 4-wk intervals to 0.5, 1, and 1.5 mg/kg/24 hr until an effective and well-tolerated dose was established. Criteria for dose increase required tolerance of the current dosage level and <50% reduction in seizures. Patients receiving enzyme-inducing antiepileptic drugs (AEDs) received a **max. daily dose** of 0.73 + 0.44 mg/kg/24 hr, and patients receiving non-enzyme-inducing AEDs received a **max.** of 0.61 + 0.32 mg/kg/24 hr.

Adjunctive therapy for partial seizures (dosage based on use with enzyme-inducing AEDs; see remarks). NOTE: Patients receiving non-enzyme-inducing AEDs had tiagabine blood levels about two times higher than patients receiving enzyme-inducing AEDs.
≥12 yr and adult: Start at 4 mg PO once daily × 7 days. If needed, increase dose to 8 mg/24 hr PO ÷ BID. Dosage may be increased further by 4—8 mg/24 hr at weekly intervals (daily doses may be divided BID—QID) until a clinical response is achieved or up to specified **max. dose.**
Max. dose:
12—18 yr: 32 mg/24 hr
Adult: 56 mg/24 hr

Use with caution in hepatic insufficiency (may need to reduce dose and/or increase dosing interval). Most common side effects include dizziness, somnolence, depression, confusion, and asthenia. Nervousness, tremor, nausea, abdominal pain, confusion, and difficulty in concentrating may also occur. Cognitive/neuropsychiatric symptoms resulting in nonconvulsive status epilepticus requiring subsequent dose reduction or drug discontinuation have been reported. Suicidal behavior or ideation, bullous dermatitis, and blurred vision have been reported. **Off-label use in patients WITHOUT epilepsy is discouraged** due to reports of seizures in these patients.

Tiagabine's clearance is increased by concurrent hepatic enzyme-inducing antiepileptic drugs (e.g., phenytoin, carbamazepine, and barbiturates), and St. John's wort. Lower doses or a slower titration for clinical response may be necessary for patients receiving non-enzyme-inducing drugs (e.g., valproate, gabapentin, and lamotrigine). **Avoid** abrupt discontinuation of drug.

TID dosing schedule may be preferred since BID schedule may not be well tolerated. Doses should be administered with food.

TIOTROPIUM
Spiriva HandiHaler, Spiriva Respimat
Anticholinergic agent, long-acting

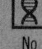

C   2   Yes   No   No

Aerosol inhaler:
Spiriva Respimat:
For asthma: 1.25 mCg/actuation (each cartridge weighs 4 g and provides either 28 or 60 actuations/inhaler); contains benzalkonium chloride and disodium EDTA
For COPD: 2.5 mCg/puff (each cartridge weighs 4 g and provides either 10, 28, or 60 actuations/inhaler); contains benzalkonium chloride and disodium EDTA
Inhalational capsules:
Spiriva HandiHaler: 18 mCg (boxes of 5s, 30s, or 90s with one HandiHaler device); contains milk protein

Asthma (maintenance therapy, see remarks):

TIOTROPIUM *continued*

Child ≥6 yr, adolescent, and adult:
  Spiriva Respimat: Inhale two 1.25 mCg actuations once daily; **max. dose:** 2.5 mCg/24 hr

Contraindicated in patients with ipratropium hypersensitivity reactions (e.g., angioedema, itching, or rash). Common side effects include headache, constipation, xerostomia, UTI, bronchitis, cough, pharyngitis, sinusitis, and URI. Bowel obstruction, angle-closure glaucoma, urinary retention, and bronchospasm have been reported. The pediatric adverse reaction profile is similar to adults.

Use as an add-on maintenance therapy for asthma along with inhaled corticosteroid. Maximum benefits may take up to 4–8 wk of continuous use. Doses >2.5 mCg/24 hr were not associated with greater efficacy in FEV_1 for adults with asthma.

Monitor for anticholinergic side effects in patients with moderate/severe renal impairment (eGFR <60 mL/min).

Administration of Spiriva Respimat 1.25 mCg × 2 delivered with the AeroChamber Plus Flow-Vu holding chamber with/without facemask by an in vitro study utilizing inspiratory flow rates for children 6–12 mo, 2–5 yr, and >5 yr has been shown to deliver a comparable adult dose on a mCg-per-body-weight basis. Despite a report of similar adverse reaction profile to adolescents and adults from a 12-wk placebo control trial (2.5 mCg/24 hr) in children 1–5 yr, the clinical efficacy and safety have not been fully established for children <6 years of age with asthma.

TOBRAMYCIN
Tobrex, TOBI, TOBI Podhaler, Bethkis, Kitabis Pak, and generics; previously available as Nebcin
Antibiotic, aminoglycoside

    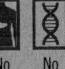

B/D   2   Yes   No   No

Injection: 10 mg/mL (2 mL), 40 mg/mL (2, 30, 50 mL); may contain phenol and bisulfites
Powder for injection: 1.2 g; preservative free
Ophthalmic ointment (Tobrex): 0.3% (3.5 g); contains 0.5% chlorobutanol
  In combination with dexamethasone (TobraDex): 0.3% tobramycin with 0.1% dexamethasone (3.5 g); contains 0.5% chlorobutanol
Ophthalmic solution (Tobrex and generics): 0.3% (5 mL)
  In combination with dexamethasone as an ophthalmic suspension (both products contain 0.01% benzalkonium chloride and EDTA):
    TobraDex and generics: 0.3% tobramycin with 0.1% dexamethasone (2.5, 5, 10 mL)
    TobraDex ST: 0.3% tobramycin with 0.05% dexamethasone (5 mL)
Nebulizer solution:
  Bethkis: 300 mg/4 mL (56s); preservative free
  TOBI, Kitabis Pak, and generics: 300 mg/5 mL (56s); preservative free
  170 mg/3.4 mL (mixed in 0.45% NS, preservative free, use with eFlow/Trio nebulizer)
Powder for inhalation:
  TOBI Podhaler: 28 mg capsules (224 capsules in 4 weekly packs with 2 Podhaler inhalation devices)

Initial empiric dosage; patient-specific dosage defined by therapeutic drug monitoring (see remarks)

Continued

TOBRAMYCIN *continued*

Neonate/infant, IM/IV (see following table):

Postconceptional age (wk)	Postnatal age (days)	Dose (mg/kg/dose)	Interval (hr)
≤29[a]	0–7	5	48
	8–28	4	36
	>28	4	24
30–34	0–7	4.5	36
	>7	4	24
≥35	ALL	4	24[b]

[a]Or significant asphyxia, PDA, indomethacin use, poor cardiac output, reduced renal function.
[b]Use Q36 hr interval for HIE patients receiving whole-body therapeutic cooling.

Child: 7.5 mg/kg/24 hr ÷ Q8 hr IV/IM
Cystic fibrosis (if available, use patient's previous therapeutic mg/kg dosage):
　　Conventional Q8 hr dosing: 7.5–10.5 mg/kg/24 hr ÷ Q8 hr IV
　　High-dose extended interval (once daily) dosing: 10–12 mg/kg/dose Q24 hr IV
Adult:
　　Conventional Q8 hr dosing: 3–6 mg/kg/24 hr ÷ Q8 hr IV/IM
　　High-dose extended interval: 4–7 mg/kg/dose Q24 hr IV/IM
Ophthalmic:
　Tobramycin:
　　Child and adult:
　　　Ophthalmic ointment: Apply 0.5-inch ribbon into conjunctival sac(s) BID–TID; for severe infections, apply Q3–4 hr initially, then reduce dose frequency.
　　　Ophthalmic drop: Instill 1–2 drops of solution to affected eye(s) Q4 hr; for severe infections, instill 2 drops Q30–60 min initially, then reduce dosing frequency.
　Tobramycin with dexamethasone:
　　≥2 yr and adult:
　　　Ophthalmic ointment: Apply 0.5-inch ribbon of ointment into conjunctival sac(s) TID–QID.
　　　Ophthalmic drop:
　　　　TobraDex: Instill 1–2 drop(s) of solution to affected eye(s) Q2 hr × 24–48 hr, then 1–2 drop(s) Q4–6 hr; increase dosing interval when signs and symptoms improve.
　　　　TobraDex ST: Instill 1 drop of solution to affected eye(s) Q2 hr × 24–48 hr, then 1 drop Q4–6 hr; increase dosing interval when signs and symptoms improve.
Inhalation:
　Cystic fibrosis prophylaxis therapy:
　　≥6 yr and adult:
　　　TOBI, Bethkis, Kitabis Pak, and generic nebs: 300 mg Q12 hr administered in repeated cycles of 28 days on drug followed by 28 days off drug
　　　Use with eFlow/Trio nebulizer: 170 mg Q12 hr administered in repeated cycles of 28 days on drug followed by 28 days off drug
　　　TOBI Podhaler: Inhale four 28-mg capsules (112 mg) Q12 hr administered in repeated cycles of 28 days on drug followed by 28 days off drug.

Use with caution in combination with neurotoxic, ototoxic, or nephrotoxic drugs; anesthetics or neuromuscular blocking agents; pre-existing renal, vestibular, or auditory impairment; and in patients with neuromuscular disorders. May cause ototoxicity, nephrotoxicity, and neuromuscular blockade. Serious allergic reactions, including anaphylaxis, and dermatologic reactions, including exfoliative dermatitis, toxic epidermal necrolysis, erythema multiforme, and Stevens-Johnson syndrome, have been reported rarely. **Ototoxic effects synergistic with furosemide.**

TOBRAMYCIN *continued*

Higher doses are recommended in patients with cystic fibrosis, neutropenia, or burns. **Adjust dose in renal failure (see Chapter 31).** Monitor peak and trough levels.

Therapeutic peak levels with conventional Q8 hr dosing:
  6—10 mg/L in general
  8—10 mg/L in pulmonary infections, neutropenia, osteomyelitis, and severe sepsis

Therapeutic trough levels with conventional Q8 hr dosing: <2 mg/L. Recommended serum sampling time at steady state: trough within 30 min prior to the third consecutive dose and peak 30—60 min after the administration of the third consecutive dose.

Therapeutic peak and trough goals for high-dose extended-interval dosing for cystic fibrosis:
  Peak: 20—40 mg/L; recommended serum sampling time at 30—60 min after the administration of the first dose
  Trough: <1 mg/L; recommended serum sampling time within 30 min before the second dose

Serum levels should be rechecked with changing renal function, poor clinical response, and at a minimum of once weekly for prolonged therapies.

To maximize bactericidal effects, an individualized peak concentration to target a peak/MIC ratio of 8—10:1 may be applied.

For initial dosing in obese patients, use an adjusted body weight (ABW). ABW = Ideal Body Weight + 0.4 (Total Body Weight — Ideal Body Weight)

INHALATIONAL USE: Transient voice alteration, bronchospasm, dyspnea, pharyngitis, and increased cough may occur. Transient tinnitus, decreased appetite, and hearing loss have been reported with nebulized dosage forms. Aphonia, discolored sputum, and malaise have been reported with the powder for inhalation. Use is not recommended with nephrotoxic, neurotoxic, or ototoxic medications, or when intravenous antibiotic therapy is prescribed. When used with other inhaled medications in cystic fibrosis, use the following order of administration: bronchodilator first, chest physiotherapy, other inhaled medications (if indicated), and tobramycin last. For TOBI Podhaler, inhale the entire contents of each capsule. To improve adherence with prophylactic inhalation therapy, initiate each 28-day inhalation cycle on the first day of an odd- or even-numbered month.

Pregnancy category is a "D" for injection and inhalation routes of administration and a "B" for the ophthalmic route.

TOLNAFTATE
Tinactin, many other brands and generics
Antifungal agent

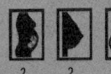   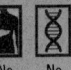

? ? No No No

Topical aerosol liquid [OTC]: 1% (150 g); may contain 29% vol/vol or 41% wt/wt alcohol
Aerosol powder [OTC]: 1% (133 g); contains 11% vol/vol alcohol and talc
Cream [OTC]: 1% (15, 30, 114 g)
Topical powder [OTC]: 1% (45 g)
Topical solution [OTC]: 1% (10, 15, 30 mL); may contain propylene glycol and/or parabens

Child (≥2 yr), adolescent, and adult:
  Topical for tinea pedis, tinea corporis, and tinea cruris: Apply 1—3 drops of solution, or small amount of liquid, cream, or powder to affected areas BID for 2—4 wk.

May cause mild irritation and sensitivity. Contact dermatitis has been reported. **Avoid** eye contact. **Do not use** for nail or scalp infections. Discontinue use if sensitization develops.
Pregnancy category not formally assigned by FDA.

TOPIRAMATE
Topamax, Topamax Sprinkle, Trokendi XR, Qudexy
XR, Eprontia, and generics
Anticonvulsant

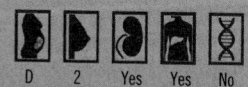

D   2   Yes   Yes   No

Caps, sprinkle:
   Topamax Sprinkle and generics: 15, 25 mg
Tabs:
   Topamax and generics: 25, 50, 100, 200 mg
Extended release caps, sprinkle (Q24 hr dosing; see remarks):
   Qudexy XR and generics: 25, 50, 100, 150, 200 mg
Extended release caps (Q24 hr dosing; see remarks):
   Trokendi XR: 25, 50, 100, 200 mg
Oral solution:
   Eprontia: 25 mg/mL (473 mL); contains parabens and polyethylene glycol
Oral suspension: 6, 14, 20 mg/mL ✍

Adjunctive therapy for partial onset seizures or Lennox-Gastaut syndrome (immediate release dosage forms):
   Child 2−16 yr: Start with 1−3 mg/kg/dose (**max. dose:** 25 mg/dose) PO QHS × 7 days, then increase by 1−3 mg/kg/24-hr increments at 1- to 2-wk intervals (divided daily dose BID) to response. Usual maintenance dose is 5−9 mg/kg/24 hr PO ÷ BID; **max. dose:** 400 mg/24 hr
   ≥17 yr and adult: Start with 25−50 mg PO QHS × 7 days, then increase by 25−50 mg/24 hr increments at 1-wk intervals until adequate response. Doses >50 mg should be divided BID. Usual maintenance dose: 100−200 mg BID. Doses above 1600 mg/24 hr have not been studied.

Adjunctive therapy for primary generalized tonic-clonic seizures (immediate release dosage forms):
   Child 2−16 yr: Use above initial dose and slower titration rate by reaching 6 mg/kg/24 hr by the end of 8 weeks.
   ≥17 yr and adult: Use above initial dose and slower titration rate by reaching 200 mg BID by the end of 8 weeks; **max. dose:** 1600 mg/24 hr

Monotherapy for partial onset seizures or primary generalized tonic-clonic seizures (immediate release dosage forms):
   Child 2 to <10 yr: Start with 25 mg PO QHS × 7 days; if needed and tolerated, may increase dose to 25 mg PO BID. May further increase by 25−50 mg/24 hr at weekly intervals over 5−7 wk up to the lower end of the following daily target maintenance dosing range (if needed and tolerated, increase to higher end of dosing range by increasing by 25−50 mg/24 hr at weekly intervals):
     ≤11 kg: 150−250 mg/24 hr ÷ BID
     12−22 kg: 200−300 mg/24 hr ÷ BID
     23−31 kg: 200−350 mg/24 hr ÷ BID
     32−38 kg: 250−350 mg/24 hr ÷ BID
     >38 kg: 250−400 mg/24 hr ÷ BID
   Child ≥10 yr and adult: Start with 25 mg PO BID × 7 days, then increase by 50 mg/24 hr increments at 1-wk intervals up to a **max. dose** of 100 mg PO BID at wk 4. If needed, dose may be further increased at weekly intervals by 100 mg/24 hr up to a recommended **max. dose** of 200 mg PO BID.

Migraine prophylaxis:
   Child 6 to <12 yr and ≥20 kg (limited data): Start with 15 mg PO once daily × 7 days, then increase to 25 mg PO BID × 7 days, then gradually increase dose to effect up to a target dose of 2−3 mg/kg/24 hr ÷ BID (**max. dose:** 200 mg/24 hr).
   Child ≥12 yr and adult: Titrate dosage to 50 mg PO BID with the following schedule:

TOPIRAMATE *continued*

	Morning PO Dose	Evening PO Dose
Week 1	None	25 mg
Week 2	25 mg	25 mg
Week 3	25 mg	50 mg
Week 4 and beyond	50 mg	50 mg

Use clinical outcome to guide dose and titration. Longer intervals between dose adjustments can be used.

Use with caution in renal and hepatic dysfunction (decreased clearance) and sulfa hypersensitivity. **Reduce dose by 50% when creatinine clearance is <70 mL/min.** Common side effects (incidence lower in children) include ataxia, cognitive dysfunction, dizziness, nystagmus, paresthesia, sedation, visual disturbances, nausea, dyspepsia, and kidney stones (higher urinary calcium/citrate ratio; incidence higher in children). Secondary angle closure glaucoma characterized by ocular pain, acute myopia, and increased intraocular pressure has been reported and may lead to blindness if left untreated. Patients should be instructed to seek immediate medical attention if they experience blurred vision or periorbital pain. Oligohidrosis and hyperthermia have been reported primarily in children and should be monitored, especially during hot weather and with use of drugs that predispose patients to heat-related disorders (e.g., carbonic anhydrase inhibitors and anticholinergics). Low serum bicarbonate levels, negative effects on growth (height and weight) in children, increased serum creatinine and glucose in children, and decreased bone mineral density have been reported in clinical trials. Hyperchloremic, non-anion gap metabolic acidosis, hyperammonemia (with or without encephalopathy), suicidal behavior or ideation, serious skin reactions (e.g., SJS and TEN), and false-positive sweat chloride test for cystic fibrosis have been reported.

Drug is metabolized by and inhibits the CYP 450 2C19 isoenzyme. Phenytoin, valproic acid, and carbamazepine may decrease topiramate levels. Topiramate may decrease valproic acid, digoxin, warfarin, and ethinyl estradiol (to decrease oral contraceptive efficacy) but may increase phenytoin levels/effects. Alcohol and CNS depressants may increase CNS side effects. Carbonic anhydrase inhibitors (e.g., acetazolamide) may increase risk of metabolic acidosis, nephrolithiasis, or paresthesia. Use with valproic acid may result in the development of hyperammonemia.

Safety and efficacy in migraine prophylaxis in pediatrics have not been established; an increase in serum creatinine has been reported in a clinical trial.

Qudexy XR and Trokendi XR are not bioequivalent and should not be interchanged. Doses may be administered with or without food. Capsule may be opened and sprinkled on small amount of food (e.g., 1 teaspoonful of applesauce) and swallowed whole (do not chew). Maintain adequate hydration to prevent kidney stone formation. If discontinuing therapy, gradually taper dosage.

TRAZODONE
Generics; previously available as Desyrel
*Antidepressant, serotonin reuptake inhibitor/
antagonist, triazolopyridine-derivative*

| C | 2 | Yes | Yes | No |

Tabs: 50, 100, 150, 300 mg
Oral suspension: 10 mg/mL

Insomnia with comorbid psychiatric disorders (limited data):
18 mo to <3 yr: Start at 1—2 mg/kg/dose (**max. dose:** 25 mg) PO QHS. If needed, increase by 12.5—25 mg Q2 wk up to a **max.** of 100 mg/24 hr.

Continued

TRAZODONE *continued*

3—5 yr: Start at 1—2 mg/kg/dose (**max. dose:** 50 mg) PO QHS; if needed, increase by 12.5—25 mg Q2 wk up to a **max.** of 150 mg/24 hr.

5 yr—adolescent: 25—50 mg PO QHS; if needed, increase by 12.5—25 mg Q2 wk up to a **max.** of 200 mg/24 hr. Daily dose may be divided BID—TID when used for palliative care.

Use with caution in pre-existing cardiac disease, initial recovery phase of MI, in patients receiving antihypertensive medications, renal and hepatic impairment (has not been evaluated), and electroconvulsive therapy. Common side effects include dizziness, drowsiness, dry mouth, and diarrhea. May cause angle-closure glaucoma in patients with anatomically narrow angles who do not have an iridectomy. Seizures, tardive dyskinesia, EPS, arrhythmias, priapism, blurred vision, neuromuscular weakness, anemia, orthostatic hypotension, and rash have been reported. Monitor for clinical worsening of depression and suicidal ideation/behavior following the initiation of therapy or after dose changes.

Trazodone is a CYP 450 3A4 isoenzyme substrate (may interact with inhibitors and inducers) and may increase digoxin levels and increase CNS effects of alcohol, barbiturates, and other CNS depressants. **Max.** antidepressant effect is seen at 2—6 wk.

TREPROSTINIL
Remodulin, Tyvaso, Tyvaso DPI, Orenitram, and generics
Prostaglandin I2 analogue, vasodilator

  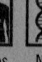 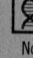

C   ?   Yes   Yes   No

Injection:
Remodulin and generics: 1 mg/mL (20 mL), 2.5 mg/mL (20 mL), 5 mg/mL (20 mL), 10 mg/mL (20 mL); contains metacresol

Inhalation solution:
Tyvaso: 0.6 mg/mL (2.9 mL; 4s and 28s); use with Tyvaso inhalation system

Powder for inhalation:
Tyvaso DPI: 16, 32, 48, 64 mCg (16 cartridges with 2 inhaler devices, 112 cartridges with 5 inhaler devices)

Extended release tab:
Orenitram: 0.125, 0.25, 1, 2.5, 5 mg

Pulmonary arterial hypertension (PAH):
IV/SC infusion:

Child (limited data): Initial dose of 2 nanogram/kg/min has been recommended with careful titration. Stable doses have been reported at 50—80 nanogram/kg/min with an unknown maximum dosage. Dosages as high as 350 and 170 nanogram/kg/min have been reported with the SC and IV routes, respectively.

Adult: Start at 1.25 nanogram/kg/min. If not tolerated, reduce to 0.625 nanogram/kg/min. If needed, increase dose at increments of 1.25 nanogram/kg/min per wk for the first 4 wk followed by 2.5 nanogram/kg/min per wk thereafter. Usual target dose: 40—80 nanogram/kg/min

Inhalation:

Child (limited data): 1—9 (6—54 mCg) patient-activated breaths Q6 hr. A retrospective report of 29 children with PAH receiving background therapy initially received 3 breaths (18 mCg) via oral inhalation QID and titrated doses weekly as tolerated to a **maximum** of 9 breaths (54 mCg) QID for ≥6 wk. Nineteen of 29 children had WHO functional class improvement (significant improvements in exercise tolerance and peak oxygen consumption). Four children had to discontinue therapy for reasons of O_2 desaturation (1), progression of PAH (1), and chest tightness with bronchospasms (2).

TREPROSTINIL *continued*

Adult: Start at 3 breaths (18 mCg) via oral inhalation Q4 hr four times a day during waking hours. Reduce dose to 1 or 2 breaths if not tolerated and subsequently increase to 3 breaths. If tolerated, increase dose by 3 additional inhalations at ~1–2 wk intervals to the target and **maximum** maintenance dose of 9 breaths (54 mCg) QID.

Use with caution in liver or renal impairment by titrating doses slowly. **Avoid use** with the oral dosage form in Child-Pugh class B and C. Treprostinil is primarily metabolized by the liver via CYP 450 2C8, and its metabolites are excreted primarily via the urinary route. Inhibitors (e.g., gemfibrozil) and inducers (e.g., rifampin) may increase and decrease treprostinil effects, respectively.

Flushing, muscle pain (especially with SC route), headaches, and diarrhea are common side effects with injectable routes. Central line Gram-negative catheter infections have been reported with the IV route. Recommendations for reducing this risk include using watertight seals in the drug delivery system and closed-hub systems, replacing the diluent with the diluent used for epoprostenol, and using the SC route. Thrombocytopenia has been reported with SC administration. Worsening of reactive airway symptoms, bronchospasm, cough, dizziness, muscle, bone or jaw pain, headache, syncope, and flushing may occur with the inhaled route. Headache, diarrhea, nausea, and flushing are common side effects with the oral dosage form in clinical trials.

Treprostinil has a longer $T_{1/2}$ than epoprostenol with better room temperature stability (depending on specific diluent used).

Do not abruptly withdraw therapy, and have a backup plan for interruptions with IV/SC continuous therapies (e.g., backup pumps and medications).

TRETINOIN—TOPICAL PREPARATIONS
Retin-A, Retin-A Micro, Altreno, Atralin, Avita,
Renova, Refissa, and many others
In combination with clindamycin: Veltin, Ziana,
and generics
In combination with benzoyl peroxide: Twyneo
Retinoic acid derivative, topical acne product

  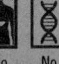

C   2   No   No   No

Cream (all strengths may contain parabens, benzyl alcohol, and edetate disodium):
  0.02% (20, 40, 60 g): Renova
  0.025% (20, 45 g): Avita, Retin-A, and generics
  0.05% (20, 40, 45 g): Refissa and generics
  0.1% (20, 45 g): Generics
Topical gel (all strengths may contain 90% alcohol, benzyl alcohol, propylene glycol, and trolamine):
  0.01% (15, 45 g): Retin-A and generics
  0.025% (15, 20, 45 g): Avita and generics
  0.04% (20, 45, 50 g): Retin-A Micro and generics
  0.05% (45 g): Atralin and generics
  0.06% and 0.08% (50 g): Retin-A Micro
  0.1% (20, 45, 50 g): Retin-A Micro and generics
Lotion (Altreno):
  0.05% (20, 45 g), contains benzyl alcohol, parabens, and trolamine
In combination with clindamycin:
  Topical gel (Veltin, Ziana, and generics): 0.025% tretinoin and 1.2% clindamycin (30, 60 g); may contain parabens, tromethamine, and propylene glycol

Continued

TRETINOIN—TOPICAL PREPARATIONS *continued*

In combination with benzoyl peroxide:
Topical cream (Twyneo): 0.1% tretinoin and 3% benzoyl peroxide (50 g)

Topical for acne:
Child ≥12 yr and adult (may be used as young as 8 yr as reported in the literature and specific product labeling; see remarks): Gently wash face with a mild soap, pat the skin dry, and wait 20 to 30 min before use. Initiate therapy with lower strengths (0.02% or 0.025% cream, or 0.01% gel) and apply a small pea-size amount to the affected areas of the face QHS or on alternate days. See remarks.

In combination with clindamycin:
Child ≥12 yr and adult: Gently wash face with a mild soap, pat the skin dry, and wait 20 to 30 min before use. Apply a pea-size amount to entire face QHS.

In combination with benzoyl peroxide:
Child ≥9 yr and adult: Apply a thin layer to affected areas once daily on clean and dry skin.

Contraindicated in sunburns. **Avoid** excessive sun exposure. If stinging or irritation occurs, decrease frequency of administration to every other day. **Avoid** contact with eyes, ears, nostrils, mouth, or open wounds. Local adverse effects include irritation, erythema, excessive dryness, blistering, crusting, hyperpigmentation or hypopigmentation, and acne flare-ups. Concomitant use of other topical acne products may lead to significant skin irritation. Onset of therapeutic benefits may be experienced within 2–3 wk with optimal effects in 6 wk. The gel dosage form is flammable and should not be exposed to heat or temperatures >120°F.

Lower minimum age (<12 yr) for use by specific product labeling:
Atralin gel: ≥10 yr
Altreno lotion: ≥9 yr

Retin-A Micro 0.04% topical gel has been used in children ≥8 yr as reported in the literature.

In combination with clindamycin (additional remarks from above): Contraindicated in regional enteritis, ulcerative colitis, or history of antibiotic-associated colitis. Prolonged use may result in fungal and bacterial superinfection, including *C. difficile*—associated diarrhea. Common side effects include burning sensation, desquamation, erythema, and xeroderma. See Clindamycin (topical use) for additional information.

In combination with benzoyl peroxide (additional remarks from above): Contraindicated with a history of hypersensitivity reactions to either components. Common side effects include pain at application site, application-site scaling, erythema, dry skin, pruritus, and irritation. See Benzoyl Peroxide for additional information.

TRIAMCINOLONE
Nasal preparations: Nasacort Allergy 24HR, Nasal Allergy 24 Hour, and generics
Topical preparations: Triderm, Kenalog, Oralone, Trianex, Tritocin, and generics
Injection preparations: Kenalog-10, Kenalog-40, Kenalog-80, generics, and others in kits
Corticosteroid

C/D   2   Yes   Yes   No

Nasal spray:
Nasacort Allergy 24HR, Nasal Allergy 24 Hour, and generics [OTC]: 55 mCg/actuation (60 actuations per 10.8 mL, 120 actuations per 16.9 mL); contains benzalkonium chloride, polysorbate 80, and EDTA

TRIAMCINOLONE *continued*

Cream:
   Triderm and generics: 0.1% (15, 28.4, 30, 80, 454 g); contains propylene glycol
   Generics: 0.025% (15, 80, 454 g), 0.5% (15 g)
Ointment:
   Generics: 0.025%, 0.1% (15, 80, 454 g), 0.5% (15 g)
   Trianex, Tritocin, and generics: 0.05% (110, 430 g)
Lotion: 0.025%, 0.1% (60 mL)
Topical aerosol:
   Kenalog and generics: 0.2 mg/2 second spray; each g of spray contains 0.147 mg triamcinolone acetate (63, 100 g); contains 10.3% alcohol
Dental paste:
   Oralone and generics: 0.1% (5 g)
See Chapter 10 for potency rankings and sizes of topical preparations.
Injection as acetonide: 10 mg/mL (Kenalog-10 and generics) (5 mL), 40 mg/mL (Kenalog-40 and generics) (1, 5, 10 mL), 80 mg/mL (Kenalog-80) (1, 5 mL); all strengths contains benzyl alcohol and polysorbate 80
   Kits (all contain benzyl alcohol and polysorbate 80):
      P-Care K40, Pod-Care 100K: 40 mg/mL (1 × 1 mL)
      P-Care K80, Pro-C-Dure 5: 40 mg/mL (2 × 1 mL)
      Pro-C-Dure 6: 40 mg/mL (3 × 1 mL)

Intranasal (titrate to lowest effective dose after symptoms are controlled; discontinue use if no relief of symptoms occurs after 3 wk of use):
   Child 2—5 yr: 1 spray in each nostril once daily (110 mCg/24 hr; starting and **max. dose**)
   Child 6—11 yr: Start with 1 spray in each nostril once daily (110 mCg/24 hr). If no benefit in 1 wk, dose may be increased to the **max. dose** of 2 sprays in each nostril once daily (220 mCg/24 hr). Decrease dose back to 1 spray each nostril when symptoms are controlled.
   ≥12 yr and adult: 2 sprays in each nostril once daily (220 mCg/24 hr; starting and **max. dose**). Decrease dose to 1 spray each nostril when symptoms are controlled.
Topical cream or ointment:
   Infant, child, and adult: Apply a thin film to affected areas BID—TID for topical concentrations of 0.1% or 0.5% and BID—QID for 0.025% or 0.05%.
Topical spray or lotion:
   Infant, child, and adult: Spray or apply to affected area TID—QID.
SYSTEMIC USE (see remarks):
   Anti-inflammatory and allergic condition:
      Child and adolescent (use 40 or 80 mg/mL strength, deep IM into gluteal muscle): 0.11—1.6 mg/kg/24 hr IM ÷ TID—QID
   Intralesional for dermatosis:
      ≥12 yr and adult (use 10 mg/mL strength): Inject up to 1 mg/site × 1 and may be repeated × 1 or more times weekly. May give separate doses in sites ≥1 cm apart, **not to exceed** 30 mg.

NASAL USE: Rare reports of bone mineral density loss and osteoporosis have been reported with prolonged use of inhaled dosage form. Nasal preparations may cause epistaxis, cough, fever, nausea, throat irritation, dyspepsia, and fungal infections (rarely). Shake intranasal dosage forms before each use.

TOPICAL USE: Topical preparations may cause dermal atrophy, telangiectasias, and hypopigmentation. HPA axis suppression, Cushing syndrome, and intracranial hypertension have been reported in children with topical use. Topical steroids should be used with caution on the face and in intertriginous areas. See Chapter 8. **Avoid** spraying the eye or inhaling the topical aerosol dosage form. Aerosol dosage form is flammable.

Continued

TRIAMCINOLONE *continued*

INJECTABLE USE: Anaphylaxis has been reported with use of the injectable dosage form. Dosage adjustment for hepatic failure with systemic use may be necessary. Triamcinolone is a substrate of the CYP 450 3A4 enzyme; inhibitors of this enzyme may increase risk for side effects. **Use with caution** in thyroid dysfunction, respiratory TB, ocular herpes simplex, peptic ulcer disease, osteoporosis, hypertension, CHF, myasthenia gravis, ulcerative colitis, and renal dysfunction. With systemic use, pregnancy category changes to "D" if used in the first trimester. **Avoid** IV administration with injectable dosage forms. Injectable forms contain benzyl alcohol.

TRIAMTERENE
Dyrenium and generics
Diuretic, potassium sparing

   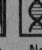

C/D   ?   Yes   Yes   No

Caps: 50, 100 mg

Hypertension:
  Child: 1—2 mg/kg/24 hr PO ÷ BID. May increase up to a **max.** of 3—4 mg/kg/24 hr up to 300 mg/24 hr
  Adult: 50—100 mg/24 hr ÷ once daily—BID PO; **max. dose:** 300 mg/24 hr

Do not use if GFR <10 mL/hr or in severe hepatic disease. **Adjust dose in renal impairment (see Chapter 31)** and cirrhosis. Monitor serum electrolytes. May cause hyperkalemia, hyponatremia, hypomagnesemia, and metabolic acidosis. Interstitial nephritis, thrombocytopenia, and anaphylaxis have been reported.

Concurrent use of ACE inhibitors may increase serum potassium. **Use with caution** when administering medications with high potassium load (e.g., some penicillins) and in patients with hepatic impairment or on high-potassium diets. Cimetidine may increase effects. This drug is also available as a combination product with hydrochlorothiazide; erythema multiforme and toxic epidermal necrolysis have been reported with this combination product. Administer doses with food to minimize GI upset. Pregnancy category changes to "D" if used in pregnancy-induced hypertension.

TRIFLURIDINE
Generics; previously available as Viroptic
Antiviral, ophthalmic

    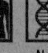

C   ?   No   No   No

Ophthalmic solution: 1% (7.5 mL); contains thimerosal

Herpes keratoconjunctivitis:
  ≥6 yr, adolescent, and adult: Instill 1 drop into affected eye(s) Q2 hr while awake up to a **maximum** of 9 drops/24 hr. Reduce dose when there is re-epithelialization of the corneal ulcer to 1 drop Q4 hr (**minimum** 5 drops/24 hr) × 7 days. If improvement does not occur in 7—14 days, consider alternative therapy. **DO NOT EXCEED** 21 days of treatment.

Burning sensation in eyes and palpebral edema are common side effects. Rare cross sensitivity with idoxuridine, increased intraocular pressure, keratoconjunctivitis, and ocular hyperemia have been reported.

Avoid touching the applicator tip to eye, fingers, or other surfaces, and do not wear contact lenses during treatment of ocular infections. Apply pressure to the lacrimal sac during and for 1—2 min after dose administration to reduce risk of systemic absorption.

TRIFLURIDINE *continued*

Store medication in the refrigerator (2—8°C). Storage at room temperature will result in a decrease in pH to cause stinging and ocular discomfort when in use.

TRIKAFTA

See Elexacaftor/Tezacaftor/Ivacaftor.

TRIMETHOBENZAMIDE HCL
Tigan and generics
Antiemetic

    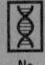

?	3	Yes	Yes	No

Caps: 300 mg
Injection (Tigan): 100 mg/mL (2 mL)

Nausea/Vomiting:
  Child (PO): 15—20 mg/kg/24 hr ÷ TID—QID
    Alternative dosing:
      <13.6 kg: 100 mg TID—QID
      13.6—40 kg: 100—200 mg/dose TID—QID
      >40 kg: 300 mg/dose TID—QID
  Adult:
    PO: 300 mg/dose TID—QID
    IM: 200 mg/dose TID—QID

Do not use in premature or newborn infants. **Avoid** use in patients with hepatotoxicity, acute vomiting, medications with CNS depressant effects, or allergic reaction. CNS disturbances are common in children (extrapyramidal symptoms, drowsiness, confusion, dizziness). Hypotension, especially with IM use, may occur. **IM not recommended in children.** Consider reducing dosage in the presence of renal impairment since a significant amount of drug is excreted and eliminated by the kidney.

TRIMETHOPRIM AND SULFAMETHOXAZOLE

See Sulfamethoxazole and Trimethoprim.

U

URSODIOL
Urso 250, Urso Forte, Reltone, and generics;
previously available as Actigall
Gallstone solubilizing agent, cholelitholytic agent

    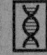

B	1	No	Yes	No

Oral suspension: 20, 25, 50, 60 mg/mL
Caps:
  Generics: 200, 300, 400 mg
  Reltone: 200, 400 mg

Continued

URSODIOL *continued*

Tabs:
    Urso 250 and generics: 250 mg
    Urso Forte and generics: 500 mg

Biliary atresia:
    Infant and child (limited data): 10—20 mg/kg/24 hr ÷ BID—TID PO; higher doses of
        20—36 mg/kg/24 hr have been reported in neonates and infants receiving the Kasai
        procedure
Pruritus from cholestasis:
    Infant, child, and adolescent (limited data): 15—30 mg/kg/24 hr ÷ once daily—BID PO
TPN-induced cholestasis:
    Infant and child (limited data): 10—30 mg/kg/24 hr ÷ TID PO
Cystic fibrosis (to improve fatty acid metabolism in liver disease; limited data):
    Child: 15—30 mg/kg/24 hr ÷ BID—TID PO
Gallstone dissolution:
    Adult: 8—10 mg/kg/24 hr ÷ BID—TID PO

Contraindicated in calcified cholesterol stones, radiopaque stones, bile pigment stones,
or stones >20 mm in diameter. **Use with caution** in patients with nonvisualizing
gallbladder and chronic liver disease. May cause GI disturbance, rash, arthralgias, anxiety,
headache, and elevated liver enzymes (elevated ALT, AST, alkaline phosphatase, bilirubin, GGT).
Monitor LFTs every month for the first 3 months after initiating therapy and every 6 months
thereafter. Thrombocytopenia has been reported in clinical trials.

Aluminum-containing antacids, cholestyramine, and oral contraceptives decrease ursodiol
effectiveness. Dissolution of stones may take several months. Stone recurrence occurs in 30% to
50% of patients within 5 yr.

V

VALACYCLOVIR
Valtrex and generics
Antiviral agent

        B   1   Yes   Yes   No

Tabs/caplets: 500, 1000 mg
Oral suspension: 50 mg/mL

Child: Recommended dosages based on steady-state pharmacokinetic data in
immunocompromised children. Efficacy data are incomplete.
    To mimic an IV acyclovir regimen of 250 mg/m²/dose or 10 mg/kg/dose TID:
        30 mg/kg/dose PO TID OR alternatively by weight:
            4—12 kg: 250 mg PO TID
            13—21 kg: 500 mg PO TID
            22—29 kg: 750 mg PO TID
            ≥30 kg: 1000 mg PO TID
    To mimic a PO acyclovir regimen of 20 mg/kg/dose 4 or 5 times a day:
        20 mg/kg/dose PO TID OR alternatively by weight:
            6—19 kg: 250 mg PO TID
            20—31 kg: 500 mg PO TID
            ≥32 kg: 750 mg PO TID

VALACYCLOVIR *continued*

Varicella zoster (chickenpox; immunocompetent patient; initiate therapy at earliest signs or symptoms, within 24 hr of rash onset):
  Infant ≥3 mo, child, and adolescent: 20 mg/kg/dose PO TID × 5 days; **max. dose:** 1 g/dose TID
HSV genital herpes (immunocompetent):
  Child ≥3 mo—11 yr (limited data):
    Initial episode: 20 mg/kg/dose PO Q12 hr (**max. dose:** 1000 mg/dose) × 7—10 days or longer if lesions are not completely healed
    Recurrent episodes: 20 mg/kg/dose PO Q12 hr (**max. dose:** 1000 mg/dose) × 5—10 days; most effective when therapy is initiated within 1 day of lesion appearance
    Suppressive therapy: 20 mg/kg/dose PO Q24 hr (**max. dose:** 1000 mg/dose)
  Adolescent and adult:
    Initial episode: 1 g/dose PO BID × 10 days or longer if lesions are not completely healed
    Recurrent episodes: 500 mg/dose PO BID × 3 days or 1000 mg PO once daily × 5 days
    Suppressive therapy:
      Immunocompetent patient: 500—1000 mg/dose PO once daily × 1 year, then reassess for recurrences. Patients with <9 recurrences per yr may be dosed at 500 mg/dose PO once daily × 1 yr.
Herpes zoster (shingles, immunocompetent; initiate therapy within 48—72 hr of onset of rash; see remarks):
  Child ≥2 yr and adolescent: 20 mg/kg/dose PO Q8 hr; **max. dose:** 1000 mg/dose for a minimum of 7—10 days and until lesions have crusted over
  Adult (immunocompetent): 1 g/dose PO Q8 hr for a minimum of 7—10 days and until lesions have crusted over
Herpes labialis (cold sores; initiated at earliest symptoms):
  ≥12 yr and adult:
    Immunocompetent: 2 g/dose PO Q12 hr × 2 doses (1 day)
    HIV positive: 1 g/dose PO Q12 hr × 5—10 days. For chronic suppressive therapy, 500 mg PO Q12 hr

This pro-drug is metabolized to acyclovir and L-valine with better oral absorption than acyclovir. **Use with caution in hepatic or renal insufficiency (adjust dose; see Chapter 31).** Thrombotic thrombocytopenic purpura/hemolytic uremic syndrome (TTP/HUS) has been reported in patients with advanced HIV infection and in bone marrow and renal transplant recipients. Probenecid or cimetidine can reduce the rate of conversion to acyclovir. Headache, nausea, and abdominal pain are common adverse events in adults. Headache is common in children. See Acyclovir for additional drug interactions and adverse effects.

For initial episodes of genital herpes, therapy is most effective when initiated within 48 hr of symptom onset. Therapy should be initiated immediately after the onset of symptoms in recurrent episodes (no efficacy data when initiating therapy >24 hr after onset of symptoms). Data are not available for use as suppressive therapy for periods >1 yr.

Valacyclovir **CANNOT** be substituted for acyclovir on a one-to-one basis. Doses may be administered with or without food.

VALGANCICLOVIR
Valcyte and generics
Antiviral agent

C 3 Yes Yes No

Tabs: 450 mg
Oral solution: 50 mg/mL (88 mL); contains saccharin and sodium benzoate
Oral suspension: 60 mg/mL

Continued

VALGANCICLOVIR *continued*

Neonate and infant:

Symptomatic congenital CMV (from pharmacokinetic [PK] data in 8 infants 4—90 days old [mean: 20 days] and 24 neonates 8—34 days old): 16 mg/kg/dose PO Q12 hr produced similar levels to IV ganciclovir 6 mg/kg/dose BID. A comparison of 6 weeks vs. 6 months of therapy in 96 neonates (>32 wk gestation and ≥1.8 kg) showed modest improvement in long-term hearing and developmental outcomes at 1—2 yr of age with the longer duration of therapy of 6 months.

Child (1 mo—16 yr):

CMV treatment for mild/moderate infection for solid organ transplant recipients (see remarks): Q12 hr PO dosage calculated with the following equation:

mg dose (**max. dose:** 900 mg) = 7 × BSA × CrCl. BSA is determined by the Mosteller equation and CrCl is determined by a modified Schwartz equation (**max. value:** 150 mL/min/1.73m²).

Mosteller BSA (m²) equation: square root of [(height [cm] × weight [kg]) ÷ 3600]

Modified Schwartz (mL/min/1.73 m²) equation (max. value: 150 mL/min/1.73 m²): k × height (cm) ÷ serum creatinine (mg/dL); where k = 0.33 if patient is <1 yr old with low birth weight for gestational age; k = 0.45 if patient is <1 yr old with birth weight appropriate for gestational age or if patient is 1 to <2 yr old; k = 0.55 if males 2 to <13 yr old and females aged 2 to <16 yr old; or k = 0.7 if male 13—16 yr old

Duration of therapy for treatment regimen: Minimum of 2 weeks until symptoms resolve, and until 1 or 2 consecutive weekly CMV viral loads are undetectable or below a test-specific threshold level

CMV prophylaxis in kidney (4 mo—16 yr), heart (1 mo—16 yr), or liver (4 mo—16 yr) transplantation (see remarks): Q24 hr PO dosage initiated within 10 days of transplantation is calculated with the following equation:

Daily mg dose (max. dose: 900 mg) = 7 × BSA × CrCl. BSA is determined by the Mosteller equation and CrCl is determined by a modified Schwartz equation (**max. value:** 150 mL/min/1.73 m²).

Mosteller BSA (m2) equation: square root of [(height [cm] × weight [kg]) ÷ 3600]

Modified Schwartz (mL/min/1.73 m²) equation (max. value: 150 mL/min/1.73 m²): k × height (cm) ÷ serum creatinine (mg/dL); where k = 0.33 if patient is <1 yr old with low birth weight for gestational age; k = 0.45 if patient is <1 yr old with birth weight appropriate for gestational age or if patient is 1 to <2 yr old; k = 0.55 if males 2 to <13 yr old and females aged 2 to <16 yr old; or k = 0.7 for males 13—16 yr old

Duration of therapy for prophylaxis:

Kidney transplantation (≥4 mo to 16 yr): 200 days

Heart transplantation (≥1 mo to 16 yr): 100 days

Liver transplantation (≥4 mo to 16 yr): 100—200 days; limited data

Adolescent (>16 yr) and adult:

CMV retinitis:

Induction therapy: 900 mg PO BID × 14—21 days with food

Maintenance therapy: 900 mg PO once daily with food for a minimum of 3—6 mo

CMV treatment of mild/moderate infection in solid organ transplant recipients: 900 mg PO BID for a minimum of 2 wk until symptoms resolve and until 1 or 2 consecutive weekly CMV viral load is undetectable or below a test-specific threshold level

CMV prophylaxis in heart, kidney, and kidney-pancreas transplantation: 900 mg PO once daily starting within 10 days of transplantation until 100 days post heart or kidney-pancreas transplantation; or until 200 days post kidney transplantation

This pro-drug is metabolized to ganciclovir with better oral absorption than ganciclovir. **Contraindicated** with hypersensitivity to valganciclovir/ganciclovir; ANC <500 mm³; platelets <25,000 mm³; hemoglobin <8 g/dL; and patients on hemodialysis. **Use with caution in renal insufficiency (adjust dose; see Chapter 31)**, preexisting bone marrow suppression, or receiving

VALGANCICLOVIR *continued*

myelosuppressive drugs or irradiation. Has not been evaluated in hepatic impairment. May cause headache, insomnia, peripheral neuropathy, diarrhea, vomiting, neutropenia, anemia, and thrombocytopenia. Neutropenia incidence is greater at day 200 vs. day 100 in pediatric kidney transplant patients.

Use effective contraception during and for at least 90 days after therapy; may impair fertility in men and women. See Ganciclovir for drug interactions and additional adverse effects.

Monitor CBC with differential, platelets, and serum creatinine at baseline and periodically during therapy. Consider changes in serum creatinine and body changes to height and body weight for prophylaxis dosing.

Valganciclovir **CANNOT** be substituted for ganciclovir on a one-to-one basis. All doses are administered with food. **Avoid** direct skin or mucous membrane contact with broken or crushed tablets.

VALPROIC ACID/VALPROATE SODIUM
Generics; previously available as Depakene (PO)
and Depacon (IV)
Depakote: See Divalproex Sodium
Anticonvulsant

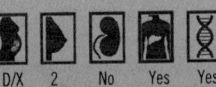

D/X   2   No   Yes   Yes

VALPROIC ACID:
Caps: 250 mg
Oral solution: 250 mg/5 mL (473 mL); may contain parabens
VALPROATE SODIUM:
Injection: 100 mg/mL (5 mL); contains EDTA

Dosages based on valproic acid or valproate sodium. See remarks regarding use of extended release dosage forms such as Depakote ER.

Seizures (PO):
 Initial: 10—15 mg/kg/24 hr ÷ once daily—TID
 Increment: 5—10 mg/kg/24 hr at weekly intervals to **max. dose** of 60 mg/kg/24 hr
 Maintenance: 30—60 mg/kg/24 hr ÷ BID—TID. Due to drug interactions, higher doses (up to 100 mg/kg/24 hr ÷ TID—QID) may be required in children on other anticonvulsants. If using divalproex sodium (Depakote or Depakote Sprinkle), divide daily dose BID.

Intravenous route (use only when PO is not possible):
 Use same PO daily dose ÷ Q6 hr. Convert back to PO as soon as possible.

Rectal route (use syrup diluted 1:1 with water, given PR as a retention enema; limited data):
 Load: 20 mg/kg/dose
 Maintenance: 10—15 mg/kg/dose Q8 hr

Migraine prophylaxis:
 Child (limited data): Start at 10—15 mg/kg/24 hr PO ÷ BID (**max. initial dose:** 250 mg/dose). If needed, increase dose over 4—6 wk to 40—45 mg/kg/24 hr PO ÷ BID up to a **maximum** of 1000 mg/24 hr. Alternative dosing for adolescent ≥17 yr is 250 mg PO BID initially titrated up to a **maximum** of 1000 mg/24 hr.
 Adult: Start with 500 mg/24 hr ÷ PO BID. Dose may be gradually increased to a **max.** of 1000 mg/24 hr ÷ PO BID. If using divalproex sodium extended release tablets, administer daily dose once daily.

Contraindicated in hepatic disease, pregnancy (for migraine indication), urea cycle disorders (e.g., OTC deficiency), mitochondrial disorders with mutations in DNA polymerase γ (e.g., Alpers-Huttenlocher syndrome), and children <2 yr suspected of the aforementioned

Continued

VALPROIC ACID/VALPROATE SODIUM *continued*

mitochondrial disorder. May cause GI, liver, blood, and CNS toxicity; weight gain; transient alopecia; pancreatitis (potentially life-threatening); nausea; sedation; vomiting; headache; thrombocytopenia (dose-related); platelet dysfunction; rash (especially with lamotrigine); and hyperammonemia. Hepatic failure has occurred especially in children <2 yr (especially those receiving multiple anticonvulsants, with congenital metabolic disorders, with severe seizure disorders with mental retardation, and with organic brain disease). Idiosyncratic life-threatening pancreatitis has been reported in children and adults. Hyperammonemic encephalopathy has been reported in patients with urea cycle disorders. Suicidal behavior or ideation, male infertility, elevated testosterone, decreased bone mineral density, DRESS, encephalopathy without elevated ammonia levels, hair texture/color changes, and nail/nail bed disorders have been reported.

Valproic acid is a substrate for CYP 450 2C19 isoenzyme and an inhibitor of CYP 450 2C9, 2D6, and 3A3/4 (weak). It increases amitriptyline/nortriptyline, rufinamide, phenytoin, propofol, diazepam, and phenobarbital levels. Concomitant estrogen-containing contraceptives, phenytoin, phenobarbital, topiramate, meropenem, cholestyramine, and carbamazepine may decrease valproic acid levels. Amitriptyline or nortriptyline may increase valproic acid levels. May interfere with urine ketone and thyroid tests.

Do not give syrup with carbonated beverages. Use of IV route has not been evaluated for >14 days of continuous use. Infuse IV over 1 hr up to a **max. rate** of 20 mg/min. Depakote and Depakote ER are **NOT** bioequivalent; see package insert for dose conversion. Depakote ER is intended for once daily administration and may require higher daily doses when converting from other dosage forms.

Therapeutic levels: 50–100 mg/L. Recommendations for serum sampling at steady state: Obtain trough level within 30 min prior to the next scheduled dose after 2–3 days of continuous dosing. Levels of 50–60 mg/L and as high as 85 mg/L have been recommended for bipolar disorders. Monitor CBC and LFTs prior to and during therapy.

Valproic acid and divalproex should not be used in pregnant women. Increased risk of neural tube defects, decreased child IQ scores, craniofacial defects, and cardiovascular malformations have been reported in babies exposed to valproic acid and divalproex sodium.

Pregnancy category is "X" when used for migraine prophylaxis and is "D" for all other indications.

VALSARTAN
Diovan and generics
Angiotensin II receptor blocker, antihypertensive agent

D   3   Yes   Yes   No

Tabs: 40, 80, 160, 320 mg
Oral solution: 4 mg/mL (120, 473 mL); may contain parabens and propylene glycol
Oral suspension: 4 mg/mL

Hypertension (see remarks):

Infant ≥6 mo and ≥6 kg (limited data): Start at 1 mg/kg/dose PO once daily; if needed, increase dose every 2 weeks up to a **maximum** of 4 mg/kg/24 hr. Usual range: 0.25–4 mg/kg/dose once daily

Child 1–16 yr: Start at 1 or 2 mg/kg/dose PO once daily (**max. dose:** 40 mg/24 hr). Usual dosage range: 1–4 mg/kg/dose once daily; **max. dose:** 4 mg/kg/24 hr up to 160 mg/24 hr

Alternative dosage for child 1–5 yr (≥8 kg; limited data): A reported range of 0.4–3.4 mg/kg/dose PO once daily with the following **maximum doses:**

<18 kg: 40 mg/24 hr
≥18 kg: 80 mg/24 hr

VALSARTAN *continued*

Adolescent ≥17 yr and adult (non-volume-depleted status): Start 80 or 160 mg PO once daily; usual dose range is 80—320 mg once daily. **Max. dose:** 320 mg/24 hr

Contraindicated with aliskiren use in patients with diabetes. Discontinue use immediately when pregnancy is detected. **Use with caution** in renal (CrCl <30 mL/min) and liver insufficiency, heart failure, post-myocardial infarction, renal artery stenosis, renal function changes, and volume depletion.

Hypotension, dizziness, headache, cough, and increases in BUN and sCr are common side effects. Hyperkalemia (most commonly reported in children <6 yr with underlying renal disease in clinical trials; also consider salt substitutes, foods, and medications which may increase potassium levels), bullous dermatitis, angioedema, acute renal failure, and dysgeusia have been reported. May increase lithium levels resulting in toxicity for those receiving concurrent lithium therapy; monitor lithium levels closely.

Onset of initial antihypertensive effects is 2 hr with maximum effects after 2—4 wk of chronic use. Patients may require higher doses of oral tablet dosage form than with the oral suspension due to increased bioavailability with the oral suspension.

VANCOMYCIN
Vancocin, Firvanq, and generics
Antibiotic, glycopeptide

  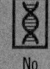

C/B   1   Yes   No   No

Injection: 0.5, 0.75, 1, 1.5, 5, 10 g
Premixed injection:
  In D_5W or NS: 500 mg/100 mL, 750 mg/150 mL, 1000 mg/200 mL
  In NS: 1250 mg/300 mL, 1500 mg/300 mL
Caps (Vancocin and generics): 125, 250 mg
Oral solution: 25 mg/mL
  Firvanq and generics: 25 mg/mL (80, 150, 300 mL); may contain sodium benzoate
  Firvanq: 50 mg/mL (150, 210, 300 mL); may contain sodium benzoate

Initial empiric dosage; patient-specific dosage defined by therapeutic drug monitoring (see remarks)
Neonate, IV (see following table for dosage interval):
  Bacteremia: 10 mg/kg/dose
  Meningitis, pneumonia: 15 mg/kg/dose

Postmenstrual Age (Weeks)[a]	Postnatal Age (Days)	Dosage Interval (hr)
≤29	0—14	18
	>14	12
30—36	0—14	12
	>14	8
37—44	0—7	12
	>7	8
≥45	All	6

[a]Postmenstrual age = gestational age + postnatal age.

Continued

VANCOMYCIN *continued*

Infant, child, adolescent, and adult, IV:

Age	General Dosage	CNS Infections, Endocarditis, Osteomyelitis, Pneumonia, and Septic Arthritis
1 mo—12 yr	15 mg/kg/dose Q6 hr	20 mg/kg/dose Q6 hr
Adolescent (>12 to <18 yr)[a]	15 mg/kg/dose Q6—8 hr	20 mg/kg/dose Q6—8 hr
Adult (≥18 yr)	15 mg/kg/dose Q8—12 hr	20 mg/kg/dose (max. 2 g) Q8—12 hr

[a]Use Q8 hr dosing interval for older adolescent.

Clostridium difficile colitis (**PR route of administration may be preferable for complete ileus**):
　　Child: 40—50 mg/kg/24 hr ÷ Q6 hr PO × 7—10 days
　　　　Max dose: 500 mg/24 hr; higher maximum of 2 g/24 hr have also been used for severe/fulminant disease
　　Adult: 125 mg/dose PO Q6 hr × 7—10 days; dosages as high as 2 g/24 hr ÷ Q6—8 hr have also been used for severe/fulminant disease
Endocarditis prophylaxis for GU or GI (excluding esophageal) procedures (complete all antibiotic dose infusion[s] within 30 min of starting procedure):
　　Moderate-risk patients allergic to ampicillin or amoxicillin:
　　　　Child: 20 mg/kg/dose (**max.** 1 g/dose) IV over 1—2 hr × 1
　　　　Adult: 1 g/dose IV over 1—2 hr × 1
　　High-risk patients allergic to ampicillin or amoxicillin:
　　　　Child and adult: Same vancomycin IV dose as moderate-risk patients plus gentamicin 1.5 mg/kg/dose (**max. dose:** 120 mg/dose) IV/IM ×1

Ototoxicity and nephrotoxicity may occur and may be exacerbated with concurrent aminoglycoside use. Greater nephrotoxicity risk has been associated with higher therapeutic serum trough concentrations (≥15 mg/mL), concurrent piperacillin/tazobactam therapy, and receiving furosemide in the intensive care unit. **Adjust dose in renal failure (see Chapter 31).** Use total body weight for obese patients when calculating dosages. Low concentrations of the drug may appear in CSF with inflamed meninges. Nausea, vomiting, and drug-induced erythroderma are common with IV use. Vancomycin infusion reaction is associated with rapid IV infusion. Infuse over 60 min (may infuse over 120 min if 60-min infusion is not tolerated). **NOTE:** Diphenhydramine is used to reverse the infusion reaction. Allergic reactions (including drug rash with eosinophilia and systemic symptoms [DRESS]), neutropenia, and immune-mediated thrombocytopenia have been reported. Serious skin reactions (e.g., SJS, TEN) have been reported in association with use of both IV and oral routes of administration.

Although current extrapolated adult guidelines suggest measuring only trough levels, an additional post-distributional level may be useful in characterizing enhanced/altered drug clearance for quicker dosage modification to attain target levels; this may be useful for infants with known faster clearance and patients in renal compromise. Consult a pharmacist.

The following therapeutic trough level recommendations are based on the assumption that the pathogen's vancomycin MIC is ≤1 mg/L.

Indication	Goal Trough Level
Uncomplicated skin and soft tissue infection, uncomplicated bacteremia, febrile neutropenia, sepsis	10—14 mg/L
CNS infections, endocarditis, pneumonia, osteomyelitis, septic arthritis	14—17 mg/L

VANCOMYCIN *continued*

Peak level measurement (20–50 mg/L) has also been recommended for patients with burns, clinically nonresponsiveness in 72 hr of therapy, persistent positive cultures, and CNS infections (≥30 mg/L).

Recommended serum sampling time at steady state: Trough within 30 min prior to the fourth consecutive dose and peak 60 min after the administration of the fourth consecutive dose. Infants with faster elimination (shorter $T_{1/2}$) may be sampled around the third consecutive dose.

Recent evidence strongly suggests moving away from serum trough vancomycin monitoring to a pharmacokinetic/pharmacodynamics (PK/PD) target of area under the curve (AUC) to MIC ratio. An $AUC_{(24)}$ of 400–600 mg*h/L is associated with clinical efficacy and reduced risk for AKI. Vancomycin therapeutic monitoring guidelines were revised in 2020 by the IDSA in collaboration with PIDS, SIDP, and ASHP. Consult with an ID specialist and pharmacist to see how this monitoring method is best operationalized at your institution.

ORAL USE for *C. difficile*: Vancomycin (PO) or metronidazole (PO) is currently the recommended first-line therapy for children, whereas vancomycin (PO) or fidaxomicin (PO) is recommended for adults. See *Clinical Infectious Diseases* 66(7):e1–e48 for the 2017 IDSA/SHEA Clinical Practice Guidelines. Common adverse effects with oral vancomycin capsules in adults include nausea, abdominal pain, and hypokalemia.

Pregnancy category "C" for the intravenous route and "B" for the oral route of administration.

VARICELLA-ZOSTER IMMUNE GLOBULIN (HUMAN)					
VariZig, VZIG					
Hyperimmune globulin, varicella-zoster	C	2	No	No	No

Injection: 125 Units (1.2 mL); contains 10% maltose, 0.03% polysorbate 80, and <40 mCg/mL IgA; preservative free. May contain low levels of anti-protein S antibodies

Infant, child, and adolescent: Dose should be given within 48 hr of varicella exposure and no later than 96 hr postexposure. IM administration:

  <2 kg: 62.5 Units
  2.1–10 kg: 125 Units
  10.1–20 kg: 250 Units
  20.1–30 kg: 375 Units
  30.1–40 kg: 500 Units
  >40 kg: 625 Units
  Max. dose: 625 Units/dose

If patient is high risk and re-exposed to varicella for more than 3 weeks after a prior dose, another full dose may be given.

Contraindicated in severe thrombocytopenia due to IM injection, immunoglobulin A deficiency (anaphylactic reactions may occur), and known immunity to varicella zoster virus. See Chapter 16 for indications. Local discomfort, redness, and swelling at the injection site and headache may occur.

Hyperviscosity of the blood may increase risk for thrombotic events. Interferes with immune response to live virus vaccines such as measles, mumps, and rubella; defer administration of live vaccines 6 mo or longer after VZIG dose. See latest AAP *Red Book* for additional information.

Avoid IM injection into the gluteal region due to risk for sciatic nerve damage and **do not exceed** age-specific **single max. IM injection** volume.

VASOPRESSIN
Vasostrict and generics, 8-Arginine Vasopressin;
previously available as Pitressin
Antidiuretic hormone analog

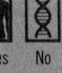

C 2 No Yes No

Injection:
   Vasostrict and generics: 20 Units/mL (aqueous) (1, 10 mL); may contain 0.5% chlorobutanol
Premixed injection in D₅W:
   Vasostrict: 0.2, 0.4, 0.6 Units/mL (100 mL)

Diabetes insipidus: Titrate dose to effect (see remarks).
   SC/IM:
      Child: 2.5–10 Units BID–QID
      Adult: 5–10 Units BID–TID
   Continuous infusion (child and adult; limited data): Start at 0.5 milliunit/kg/hr (0.0005 Units/kg/hr).
      Increase dosage by 0.5 milliunit/kg/hr every 10 min PRN up to **max. dose** of 10 milliunit/kg/hr (0.01 Units/kg/hr).
GI hemorrhage (IV; NOTE: dosage metric is Units/kg/min for children and Units/min for adults):
   Child (limited data): Start at 0.002–0.005 Units/kg/min. Increase dose as needed to **max. dose** of 0.01 Units/kg/min.
   Adult: Start at 0.2–0.4 Units/min. Increase dose as needed to **max. dose** of 0.8 Units/min.
Cardiac arrest, ventricular fibrillation, and pulseless ventricular tachycardia (limited data):
   Child (use following 2 doses of epinephrine; limited data): 0.4 Units/kg IV × 1
Vasodilatory shock with hypotension (unresponsive to fluids and pressors; NOTE: dosage metric is Units/kg/min for children and Units/min for adults):
   Infant, child, adolescent (various reports; limited data): 0.00017–0.008 Units/kg/min via continuous IV infusion in combination with pressors
   Adult: 0.01–0.04 Units/min via continuous IV infusion in combination with pressors

Use with caution in seizures, migraine, asthma, and renal, cardiac, or vascular diseases.
   Side effects include tremor, sweating, vertigo, abdominal discomfort, nausea, vomiting,
   urticaria, anaphylaxis, hypertension, and bradycardia. May cause vasoconstriction, water
   intoxication, bronchoconstriction, and decreased cardiac index. Drug interactions: lithium,
   demeclocycline, heparin, and alcohol reduces activity; carbamazepine, tricyclic antidepressants,
   fludrocortisone, and chlorpropamide increases activity. Hemodynamic monitoring is recommended
   when used with catecholamines, indomethacin, ganglionic blocking agents, and medications that
   may cause SIADH (e.g., SSRIs, TCAs, carbamazepine, and oxcarbazepine).
Do not abruptly discontinue IV infusion (taper dose). Patients with variceal hemorrhage and hepatic
   insufficiency may respond to lower dosages. Monitor fluid intake and output, urine specific gravity,
   urine and serum osmolality, plasma osmolality, and sodium.

VECURONIUM BROMIDE
Various generics; previously available as
Norcuron
Nondepolarizing neuromuscular blocking agent

C ? Yes Yes No

Injection: 10, 20 mg; contains mannitol

Neonate:
   Initial: 0.1 mg/kg/dose IV
   Maintenance: 0.03–0.15 mg/kg/dose IV Q1–2 hr PRN

VECURONIUM BROMIDE *continued*

Infants (>7 wk to 1 yr) (see remarks):
> **Initial:** 0.08—0.1 mg/kg/dose IV; reduce dose to 0.04—0.06 mg/kg/dose IV if used in combination with succinylcholine
> **Maintenance:** 0.05—0.1 mg/kg/dose IV Q1 hr PRN; may administer via continuous infusion at 0.06—0.09 mg/kg/hr IV

>1 yr—adult (see remarks):
> **Initial:** 0.08—0.1 mg/kg/dose IV; reduce dose to 0.04—0.06 mg/kg/dose IV if used in combination with succinylcholine
> **Maintenance:** 0.05—0.1 mg/kg/dose IV Q1 hr PRN; may administer via continuous infusion at 0.09—0.15 mg/kg/hr IV

Use with caution in patients with renal or hepatic impairment, and neuromuscular disease. Dose reduction may be necessary in hepatic insufficiency. Infants (7 wk to 1 yr) are more sensitive to the drug and may have a longer recovery time. Children (1—10 yr) may require higher doses and more frequent supplementation than adults. Enflurane, isoflurane, aminoglycosides, β-blockers, calcium channel blockers, clindamycin, furosemide, magnesium salts, quinidine, procainamide, and cyclosporine may increase the potency and duration of neuromuscular blockade. Calcium, caffeine, carbamazepine, phenytoin, steroids (chronic use), acetylcholinesterases, and azathioprine may decrease effects. May cause arrhythmias, rash, and bronchospasm. Severe anaphylactic reactions have been reported.

Neostigmine, pyridostigmine, or edrophonium is an antidote. Onset of action within 1—3 min. Duration is 30—40 min. **See Chapter 1 for rapid sequence intubation.**

VERAPAMIL
Calan SR, Verelan, Verelan PM, and generics;
previously available as Calan
Calcium channel blocker

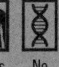

C   2   Yes   Yes   No

Tabs: 40, 80, 120 mg
Extended/sustained release tabs (Calan SR and generics): 120, 180, 240 mg
Extended/sustained release caps (for Q24 hr dosing):
> **Verelan:** 120, 180, 240, 360 mg
> **Verelan PM:** 100, 200, 240, 300, 360 mg
> **Generics:** 100, 120, 180, 200, 240, 300, 360 mg

Injection: 2.5 mg/mL (2, 4 mL)
Oral suspension: 50 mg/mL

IV for dysrhythmias: Give over 2—3 min. May repeat once after 30 min.
> **1—16 yr, for PSVT:** 0.1—0.3 mg/kg/dose IV × 1 may repeat dose in 30 min; **max. dose:** 5 mg first dose, 10 mg second dose
> **Adult, for SVT:** 5—10 mg (0.075—0.15 mg/kg) IV × 1 may administer second dose of 10 mg (0.15 mg/kg) 15—30 min later

Hypertension (PO):
> **Adult:**
>> **Immediate release dosage forms:** 120—360 mg/24 hr PO ÷ TID
>> **Sustained release dosage forms:** 200—480 mg/24 hr PO once daily. **Max. dose:** 480 mg/24 hr (400 mg/24 hr for Verelan PM)

No longer recommended as an antihypertensive agent for children. **Contraindications** include hypersensitivity, cardiogenic shock, severe CHF, sick sinus syndrome, or AV block. **Use with caution** in hepatic and renal **(reduce dose in renal insufficiency; see Chapter 31)** impairment.

Continued

VERAPAMIL *continued*

Owing to negative inotropic effects, verapamil should not be used to treat SVT in an emergency setting for infants. **Avoid IV use** in neonates and young infants due to apnea, bradycardia, and hypotension. May cause constipation, headache, dizziness, edema, and hypotension. EPS has been reported.

Monitor ECG. **Have calcium and isoproterenol available to reverse myocardial depression.** May decrease neuromuscular transmission in patients with Duchenne muscular dystrophy, and worsen myasthenia gravis.

Drug is a substrate of CYP 450 1A2 and 3A3/4, and an inhibitor of CYP 3A4 and P-gp transporter. Barbiturates, sulfinpyrazone, phenytoin, vitamin D, and rifampin may decrease serum levels/effects of verapamil; erythromycin, quinidine, and grapefruit juice may increase serum levels/effects. Verapamil may increase effects/toxicity of β-blockers (severe myocardial depression), carbamazepine, cyclosporine, sirolimus, everolimus, digoxin, ethanol, fentanyl, lithium, nondepolarizing muscle relaxants, prazosin, and tizanidine. Use with telithromycin has resulted in hypotension, bradyarrhythmias, and lactic acidosis. Bradycardia has been reported with concurrent use of clonidine, and increased bleeding times have been reported with use with aspirin. **Do not** crush or chew extended release dosage forms.

VIGABATRIN
Sabril, Vigadrone, and generics
Anticonvulsant

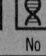

| C | 2 | Yes | Yes | No |

Tabs (Sabril and generics): 500 mg
Powder for oral solution (Sabril, Vigadrone, and generics): 500 mg per packet to be dissolved in 10 mL water (50s)

Infantile spams (1 mo—2 yr; see remarks for discontinuation of therapy): Start at 50 mg/kg/24 hr ÷ BID PO; if needed and tolerated, may titrate dosage upward by 25—50 mg/kg/24 hr increments Q3 days up to a **maximum** of 150 mg/kg/24 hr ÷ BID. Gradually withdraw therapy if no clinical benefit is seen in 2—4 wk.

Adjunctive therapy for refractory complex partial seizures (gradually withdraw therapy if no clinical benefit is seen in 3 mo; see remarks for discontinuation of therapy):
Child ≥2 yr and ≥10 kg, and adolescent ≤16 yr and ≤60 kg: If needed and tolerated, increase starting dose at weekly intervals to the recommended maintenance dose.

Weight (kg)	Starting Daily Dose (mg/24 hr ÷ BID)	Recommended Daily Maintenance Dose (mg/24 hr ÷ BID)
10—15	350	1050
>15—20	450	1300
>20—25	500	1500
>25—60	500	2000

Adolescent (≥17 yr) and adult (see remarks for discontinuation of therapy): Start at 500 mg BID PO; if needed and tolerated, increase daily dose by 500-mg increments at 7-day intervals. Usual recommended dose: 1500 mg BID; **max. dose: 6000 mg/24 hr.** Doses >3 g/24 hr have not been shown to provide additional benefit and are associated with more side effects.

Use with caution in renal impairment **(reduce dose; see Chapter 31)** and other CNS depressants (enhanced effects). Can cause progressive and permanent vision loss (risk increases with dose and duration); periodic vision testing is required. Common side effects in children and adults include rash, weight gain, GI disturbances, arthralgia, visual disturbances,

VIGABATRIN *continued*

vertigo, sedation, headache, confusion, and URIs. Liver failure, anemia, psychotic disorder, angioedema, Stevens-Johnson syndrome, TEN, alopecia, and suicidal ideation have been reported. Abnormal MRI signal changes (T2 signal and restricted diffusion in a symmetric pattern) and intramyelinic edema (in postmortem exams) have been reported in infants treated for infantile spasms.

Ketorolac, naproxen, and mefloquine may decrease the effect of vigabatrin. Vigabatrin may decrease the effects/levels of phenytoin but increase the levels/toxicity of carbamazepine.

Use in adjunctive therapy for refractory complex partial seizure has labeled indication for ≥10-yr-old patients when potential benefits outweigh the risk of vision loss.

DO NOT rapidly withdraw therapy. Dosage needs to be tapered when discontinuing therapy to minimize increased seizure frequency. The following tapering guidelines have been recommended:

Infant: Decrease by 25–50 mg/kg every 3–4 days.

Child: Decrease dose by $\frac{1}{3}$ every 7 days for 3 weeks.

Adult: Decrease by 1 g/24 hr every 7 days.

Doses may be administered with or without food. Access to this medication is restricted to prescribers and pharmacies registered under a special restricted distribution program (SABRIL REMS Program) in the United States. Call 888-457-4273 or see www.SabrilREMS.com for more information.

VITAMIN A Aquasol A and many generics *Vitamin, fat soluble*	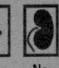 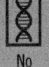

A/X 2 No No No

Caps [OTC]: 7500, 8000, 10,000, 25,000 IU
Tabs [OTC]: 10,000, 15,000 IU
Oral drops [OTC]: 750 mCg/0.3 mL (2500 IU/0.3 mL) (30 mL)
Sublingual tabs [OTC]: 5000 IU
Injection for IM use (Aquasol A): 50,000 IU/mL (2 mL); contains polysorbate 80 and chlorobutanol
Conversion: 10,000 IU is equivalent to 3000 mCg vitamin A.

US RDA: See Chapter 21.

Supplementation in measles (a third dose may be administered 2–4 wk after the second dose if patient has ocular signs of vitamin A deficiency or is severely malnourished; see remarks):
   <6 mo: 50,000 IU/dose once daily PO × 2 days
   Infant 6 mo to <1 yr: 100,000 IU/dose once daily PO × 2 days
   Child 1–5 yr: 200,000 IU/dose once daily PO × 2 days

Malabsorption syndrome prophylaxis:
   Child >8 yr and adult: 10,000–50,000 IU/dose once daily PO of water miscible product

Cystic fibrosis (usually dosed in cystic fibrosis specific multivitamins, but those with liver disease may require higher doses; monitor serum concentrations):
   Infant: 1500 IU/dose once daily PO
   Child 1–3 yr: 5000 IU/dose once daily PO
   Child 4–8 yr: 5000–10,000 IU/dose once daily PO
   Child ≥9 yr and adolescent: 10,000 IU/dose once daily PO

High doses above the US RDA are teratogenic (category X). The use of vitamin A in measles is recommended in children 6 mo–2 yr of age who are either hospitalized or who have any of the following risk factors: immunodeficiency, ophthalmologic evidence of vitamin A deficiency, impaired GI absorption, moderate to severe malnutrition, and recent immigration from areas with high measles mortality. May cause GI disturbance, rash, headache, increased ICP (pseudotumor cerebri), papilledema, and irritability. Large doses may increase the effects of warfarin. Mineral oil, cholestyramine, and neomycin will reduce vitamin A absorption. **Do not** assess vitamin A levels during an acute inflammatory condition as falsely low levels have been reported.

VITAMIN B₁

See Thiamine.

VITAMIN B₂

See Riboflavin.

VITAMIN B₃

See Niacin.

VITAMIN B₆

See Pyridoxine.

VITAMIN B₁₂

See Cyanocobalamin.

VITAMIN C

See Ascorbic Acid.

VITAMIN D₂

See Ergocalciferol.

VITAMIN D₃

See Cholecalciferol.

VITAMIN E/α-TOCOPHEROL
Aqueous Vitamin E, Nutr-E-Sol, and many others
including generics
Vitamin, fat soluble

A/C   2   No   No   No

Tabs [OTC]: 100, 200, 400 IU
Caps [OTC]: 100, 200, 400, 1000 IU
Oral solution (Aqueous Vitamin E and generics [OTC]): 50 IU/mL (12, 30 mL); may contain propylene glycol, polysorbate 80, and saccharin
Oral liquid (Nutr-E-sol) [OTC]: 400 IU/15 mL (473 mL)
Conversion: 400 IU is equivalent to 180 mg of vitamin E

US RDA: See Chapter 21.

VITAMIN E/α-TOCOPHEROL *continued*

Vitamin E deficiency and liver disease, PO: Monitor levels closely and use water miscible form (especially with malabsorption).
Neonate: 25—50 IU/kg/24 hr
Infant, child, and adolescent: 10—50 IU/kg/24 hr
Cystic fibrosis supplementation (use water miscible form; usually dosed in cystic fibrosis specific multivitamins): 5—10 IU/kg/24 hr PO once daily; **max. dose:** 400 IU/24 hr

Adverse reactions include GI distress, rash, headache, gonadal dysfunction, decreased serum thyroxine and triiodothyronine, and blurred vision. Necrotizing enterocolitis has been associated with large doses (>200 units/24 hr) of a hyperosmolar product administered to low birth weight infants. May increase hypoprothrombinemic response of oral anticoagulants (e.g., warfarin), especially in doses >400 IU/24 hr.

In malabsorption, water miscible preparations are better absorbed. Therapeutic levels: 6—14 mg/L. Pregnancy category changes to "C" if used in doses above the US RDA.

VITAMIN K

See Phytonadione.

VORICONAZOLE
Vfend and generics
Antifungal, triazole

D   3   Yes   Yes   Yes

Tabs: 50, 200 mg; contains povidone
Oral suspension: 40 mg/mL (75 mL); may contain sodium benzoate
Injection: 200 mg; contains 3200 mg sulfobutyl ether β-cyclodextrin (SBECD) (see remarks)

Empiric doses; consider drug interactions and pharmacogenomic based recommendations (see remarks). Between-patient and inter-occasion pharmacokinetic variability is high. *Monitor trough level and adjust dose accordingly.*

Infant and child <2 yr (limited data): Start with 9 mg/kg/dose IV/PO Q12 hr; monitor levels and adjust dose. Median dose of 31.5 mg/kg/24 hr ÷ 12 hr (range: 12—71 mg/kg/24 hr) has been reported to achieve target trough levels.

Child 2—≤12 yr and 12—14 yr weighing <50 kg:
  Invasive aspergillosis, candidemia (nonneutropenic), other deep tissue *Candida* infections, or other rare molds (e.g., *Scedosporium* and *Fusarium*):
    Loading dose: 9 mg/kg/dose IV Q12 hr × 2 followed by maintenance dose
    Maintenance dose: 8 mg/kg/dose IV Q12 hr and convert to the oral suspension dosage form after significant clinical improvement at a dose of 9 mg/kg/dose PO Q12 hr (**max. dose:** 350 mg Q12 hr). The oral suspension dosage form was used in clinical trials, and the bioequivalence of this dosage form and tablets has not been evaluated in children. Dosage increments and decrements of 1 mg/kg (or 50 mg) steps have been recommended for those with inadequate response and who are unable to tolerate their dosage level, respectively.
  Esophageal candidiasis:
    Treatment:
      IV: 4 mg/kg/dose Q12 hr
      PO: 9 mg/kg/dose Q12 hr; **max. dose:** 350 mg Q12 hr
  Prophylaxis for candidiasis in high-risk AML, ALL, and allogeneic HSCT patients (limited data):
    IV: 9 mg/kg/dose Q12 hr × 2 doses followed by 8 mg/kg/dose Q12 hr
    PO (oral suspension): 9 mg/kg/dose Q12 hr; **max. dose:** 350 mg/dose

Continued

VORICONAZOLE *continued*

Child 12—<15 yr weighing ≥50 kg, >15 yr (any weight), and adult:
  Invasive aspergillosis, candidemia (nonneutropenic), fusariosis, scedosporiosis, or other serious fungal infections:
  Loading dose: 6 mg/kg/dose IV Q12 hr × 2 doses followed by maintenance dose
  Maintenance dose:
    Candidemia (nonneutropenic): 3—4 mg/kg/dose IV Q12 hr
    Invasive aspergillosis, fusariosis, scedosporiosis, or other serious fungal infections: 4 mg/kg/dose IV Q12 hr; if patient unable to tolerate, reduce dose to 3 mg/kg/dose IV Q12 hr
  PO maintenance dose: Initial dose may be increased to the maximum dose when response is inadequate; if dose is not tolerated, reduce dose by 50 mg decrements, until tolerated, with minimum of the initial recommended dose.
    <40 kg: 100 mg Q12 hr
    ≥40 kg: 200 mg Q12 hr
  Esophageal candidiasis (secondary therapy; treat for a minimum of 14 days and until 7 days after resolution of symptoms): Initial dose may be increased to the maximum dose when response is inadequate by 50 mg increments for patients <40 kg and by 100 mg increments for ≥40 kg. If a titrated dose is not tolerated, reduce dose by 50 mg decrements until tolerated with the minimum of the initial recommended dose.
    <40 kg: 100 mg Q12 hr
    ≥40 kg: 200 mg Q12 hr

Contraindicated with concomitant administration with rifampin, carbamazepine, long-acting barbiturates, ritonavir, efavirenz, rifabutin, ergot alkaloids, or St. John's wort (decreases voriconazole levels); and with terfenadine, astemizole, cisapride, pimozide, naloxegol, tolvaptan, quinidine, or sirolimus (voriconazole increases levels of these drugs to increase side effects). **Use with caution** in proarrhythmic conditions (e.g., congenital/acquired QTc prolongation, cardiomyopathy, and sinus bradycardia), severe hepatic disease, and galactose intolerance. Concurrent use with CYP 450 3A4 substrates that can lead to prolonged QTc interval (e.g., cisapride, ivabradine, pimozide, and quinidine) is **contraindicated**.

Drug is a substrate and inhibitor for CYP 450 2C9, 2C19 (major substrate), and 3A4 isoenzymes. Always check for interactions for risk of potential toxicities and use recommendation when used with other medications that have similar CYP 450 substrate characteristics. Specific CYP 2C19 phenotype and use recommendation for children and adults are as follows:

CYP 450 2C19 Phenotype	Pediatric Use Recommendation	Adult Use Recommendation
Ultrarapid metabolizer	Use alternative medication[a]	Use alternative medication[a]
Rapid metabolizer	Initiate with standard dosing with TDM[b]	Use alternative medication[a]
Intermediate metabolizer	Initiate with standard dosing with TDM[b]	Initiate with standard dosing with TDM[b]
Poor metabolizer	Use alternative medication[a]; if voriconazole must be used, use a lower dose with TDM[b]	Use alternative medication[a]; if voriconazole must be used, use a lower dose with TDM[b]

[a]Alternative medication should not be dependent on CYP 2C19 metabolism and may include agents such as isavuconazole, liposomal amphotericin B, and posaconazole.
[b]TDM = therapeutic drug monitoring

VORICONAZOLE *continued*

Currently approved for use in invasive aspergillosis; candidemia, and disseminated candidiasis in skin, abdomen, kidney, bladder wall, and wounds; candidal esophagitis; and serious infections caused by *Fusarium* species and *Scedosporium apiospermum* in children ≥2 yr of age.

Common side effects include GI disturbances, fever, headache, hepatic abnormalities, photosensitivity (higher incidence in children; **avoid** direct sunlight and use protective measures), rash (6%), and visual disturbances (30%). Use with drugs associated with UV reactivation (e.g., methotrexate) increases risk for photosensitivity. Discontinue therapy with a dermatological follow up for those who develop photosensitivity reactions as squamous cell carcinoma and melanoma have been reported in those who experience this adverse reaction, especially with long-term use. Serious but rare side effects include anaphylaxis, liver or renal failure, and Stevens-Johnson syndrome. DRESS has been reported. Pancreatitis has been reported in children. Monitoring serum transaminase and bilirubin levels weekly for the first month of therapy followed by reduced frequency has been recommended. Higher frequency of LFT elevations has been reported with children.

Correct potassium, magnesium, and calcium levels before and during voriconazole therapy. **Adjust dose in hepatic impairment** by decreasing only the maintenance dose by 50% for patients with a Child-Pugh class A or B. **Do not use** IV dosage form for patients with GFR <50 mL/min because of accumulation of the cyclodextrin excipient; switch to oral therapy if possible. Patients receiving concurrent phenytoin should increase their voriconazole maintenance doses (IV: 5 mg/kg/dose Q12 hr; PO: double the usual dose).

Inter-occasion pharmacokinetic variability is high, thus requiring serum level monitoring. Therapeutic levels: trough: 1—5.5 mg/L. Levels <1 mg/L have resulted in treatment failures and levels >5.5 mg/L have resulted in neurotoxicity such as encephalopathy. Recommended serum sampling time: obtain trough within 30 min prior to a dose. Steady state is typically achieved after 5—7 days of initiating therapy.

Oral bioequivalence of the oral suspension and tablet has not been evaluated in children. Administer IV over 1—2 hr with a **max. rate** of 3 mg/kg/hr at a concentration ≤5 mg/mL. Administer oral doses 1 hr before and after meals.

W

WARFARIN
Jantoven and generics; previously available as Coumadin
Anticoagulant

| D/X | 1 | Yes | Yes | Yes |

Tabs: 1, 2, 2.5, 3, 4, 5, 6, 7.5, 10 mg

Infant and child (see remarks): To achieve an INR between 2 and 3.5 directed by specific indication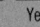

Loading dose on day 1:

Baseline INR ≤1.3: 0.2 mg/kg/dose PO; **max. dose:** 7.5 mg/dose

Liver dysfunction, baseline INR >1.3, cardiopulmonary bypass within previous 10 days, NPO status/poor nutrition, receiving broad spectrum antibiotics, receiving medications that significantly inhibit CYP 450 2C9, or slow metabolizers of warfarin (see remarks): 0.05—0.1 mg/kg/dose PO; **max. dose:** 5 mg/dose

Immediate postoperative period after a Fontan procedure: 0.05 mg/kg/dose PO; **max. dose:** 2.5 mg/dose

Loading dose on days 2—4:

Continued

WARFARIN *continued*

Day 2		Days 3 & 4	
INR Level	**Dose Adjustment**	**INR Level**	**Dose Adjustment**
1.1—1.3	Repeat day 1 loading dose	1.1—1.4	Increase previous dose by 20%—50%
1.4—1.9	Decrease day 1 loading dose by 50%	1.5—1.9	Continue current dose
≥2	Hold dose for 24 hr, then give 50% of day 1 loading dose on day 3	2—3	Use 25%—50% of day 1 loading dose
		3.1—3.5	Use 25% of day 1 loading dose
		>3.5	Hold dose until INR <3.5, then restart at ≤25% of day 1 loading dose

Maintenance dose (therapy day ≥5):

Goal INR 2—3		Goal INR 2.5—3.5	
INR	**Dose Adjustment**	**INR**	**Dose Adjustment**
1.1—1.4	Increase previous dose by 20%	1.1—1.9	Increase previous dose by 20%
1.5—1.9	Increase previous dose by 10%	2—2.4	Increase previous dose by 10%
2—3	No change	2.5—3.5	No change
3.1—3.5	Decrease previous dose by 10%	3.6—4	Decrease previous dose by 50% for one dose, then restart at a dose (prior to 50% dose decrease) decreased by 20% the next day
>3.5	Hold dose until INR <3.5, then restart at 20% less than the last dose	>4	Hold dose for 1 day, then restart at a dose decreased by 20% of the last dose

Usual maintenance dose for INR goal of 2—3 (see remarks): ~0.1 mg/kg/24 hr PO once daily; range: 0.05—0.34 mg/kg/24 hr. Reported average dosages include the following:

Infant <1 yr: 0.33 mg/kg/24 hr PO once daily

Adolescent 11—18 yr: 0.09 mg/kg/24 hr PO once daily

Adult (see remarks): 2.5—10 mg PO once daily × 2—3 days. Adjust dose to achieve the desired INR or PT. Maintenance dose range: 2—10 mg/24 hr PO once daily

Contraindicated in severe liver or kidney disease, uncontrolled bleeding, GI ulcers, and malignant hypertension. Acts on vitamin K—dependent coagulation factors II, VII, IX, and X. Side effects include fever, skin lesions, skin necrosis (especially in protein C deficiency), anorexia, nausea, vomiting, diarrhea, hemorrhage, and hemoptysis.

Warfarin is a substrate for CYP 450 1A2, 2C8, 2C9, 2C18, 2C19, and 3A3/4. Amiodarone, azole antifungals (e.g., fluconazole, voriconazole), broad spectrum antibiotics (e.g., cefepime, meropenem, piperacillin/tazobactam), chloramphenicol, chloral hydrate, cimetidine, corticosteroids, delavirdine, fluoroquinolones (e.g., ciprofloxacin, levofloxacin), fluoxetine, metronidazole, indomethacin, large doses of vitamins A or E, nonsteroidal anti-inflammatory agents, omeprazole, oxandrolone, quinidine, salicylates, SSRIs (e.g., fluoxetine, paroxetine, sertraline), sulfonamides, and zafirlukast may increase warfarin's effect. Ascorbic acid, barbiturates, carbamazepine, cholestyramine, dicloxacillin, griseofulvin, oral contraceptives, nafcillin, ribavirin, rifampin, spironolactone, sucralfate, and vitamin K (including foods with high content) may decrease warfarin's effect.

WARFARIN *continued*

Younger children generally require higher doses to achieve desired effect. Children receiving Fontan cardiac surgery may require smaller doses than children with either congenital heart disease (without Fontan) or no congenital heart disease. (See *Chest* 2004;126:645–687S and *Blood* 1999;94 [9]:3007–3014 for additional information.)

Lower doses should be considered for patients with pharmacogenetic variations in CYP 2C9 (e.g., *2 and *3 alleles) and VKORC1 (e.g., 1639G>A allele) enzymes, especially in European ancestry. Elderly and/or debilitated patients, and patients with a potential to exhibit greater than expected PT/INR response to warfarin should also consider using lower doses.

Z

ZIDOVUDINE
Retrovir, AZT, and generics
Antiviral agent, nucleoside analogue reverse transcriptase inhibitor

C   2   Yes   Yes   No

Caps: 100 mg
Tabs: 300 mg
Oral syrup: 50 mg/5 mL (240 mL); contains 0.2% sodium benzoate
Injection: 10 mg/mL (20 mL); preservative-free solution (vial stoppers may contain latex)
In combination with lamivudine (3TC) as Combivir and generics:
   Tabs: 300 mg zidovudine + 150 mg lamivudine
In combination with abacavir and lamivudine (3TC) as Trizivir and generics:
   Tabs: 300 mg zidovudine + 300 mg abacavir + 150 mg lamivudine

HIV: See https://clinicalinfo.hiv.gov/en/guidelines
Prevention of HIV vertical transmission (low- and high-risk cases) and presumptive treatment:
   14–34 weeks of pregnancy (maternal dosing):
      Until labor (see perinatal guidelines for currently recommended combination antiretroviral therapies, which may or may not include zidovudine): 600 mg/24 hr PO ÷ BID–TID
   During labor (maternal dosing; dosage based on maternal total body weight): 2 mg/kg/dose IV over 1 hour followed by 1 mg/kg/hr IV infusion for 2 hours. For scheduled cesarean delivery, initiate this regimen 3 hr prior to surgery.
   Neonate and infant (initiate therapy within 6–12 hr of birth):

Gestational Age (wk)	Oral (PO) Dosage	Intravenous (IV) Dosage[a]
<30	**Birth to 4 wk of age:** 2 mg/kg/dose Q12 hr **4 to 8–10 wk of age:** 3 mg/kg/dose Q12 hr **>8–10 wk of age[b]:** 12 mg/kg/dose Q12 hr	**Birth to 4 wk of age:** 1.5 mg/kg/dose Q12 hr **4 to 8–10 wk of age:** 2.25 mg/kg/dose Q12 hr **>8–10 wk of age[b]:** 9 mg/kg/dose Q12 hr

Continued

ZIDOVUDINE *continued*

Gestational Age (wk)	Oral (PO) Dosage	Intravenous (IV) Dosage[a]
30—34		
	Birth to 2 wk of age: 2 mg/kg/dose Q12 hr	**Birth to 2 wk of age:** 1.5 mg/kg/dose Q12 hr
	2 to 6—8 wk of age: 3 mg/kg/dose Q12 hr	**2 to 6—8 wk of age:** 2.25 mg/kg/dose Q12 hr
	>6—8 wk of age[b]**:** 12 mg/kg/dose Q12 hr	**>6—8 wk of age**[b]**:** 9 mg/kg/dose Q12 hr
≥35		
	Birth to 4 wk of age: 4 mg/kg/dose Q12 hr	**Birth to 4 wk of age:** 3 mg/kg/dose Q12 hr
	>4 wk of age[b]**:** 12 mg/kg/dose Q12 hr	**>4 wk of age**[b]**:** 9 mg/kg/dose Q12 hr

[a]Convert to PO route when possible.
[b]Make this dose increase only for infants with confirmed HIV infection.

HIV postexposure prophylaxis (all therapies to begin within 2 hr of exposure if possible for a total of 28 days): See https://clinicalinfo.hiv.gov/en/guidelines for the most recent preferred and alternative regimens. Zidovudine is dosed using HIV treatment doses and used in combination with lamivudine and additional antiretroviral agent(s).

See https://clinicalinfo.hiv.gov/en/guidelines for additional remarks.

Use with caution in patients with impaired renal or hepatic function. Dosage reduction is recommended in severe renal impairment and may be necessary in hepatic dysfunction. Drug penetrates well into the CNS. Most common side effects include: anemia, granulocytopenia, nausea, and headache (dosage reduction, erythropoietin, filgrastim/GCSF, or discontinuance may be required depending on event). Seizures, confusion, rash, myositis, myopathy (use >1 yr), hepatitis, and elevated liver enzymes have been reported. Macrocytosis is noted after 4 wk of therapy and can be used as an indicator of compliance. Lactic acidosis and severe hepatomegaly with steatosis, including fatal cases, have been reported. Neutropenia and severe anemia have been reported in advanced HIV disease. Use of injectable dosage form may cause allergic reactions in latex-sensitive individuals.

Do not use in combination with stavudine because of poor antiretroviral effect. Effects of interacting drugs include: increased toxicity (acyclovir, trimethoprim-sulfamethoxazole); increased hematological toxicity (ganciclovir, interferon-alpha, marrow suppressive drugs); and granulocytopenia (drugs that affect glucuronidation). Methadone, atovaquone, cimetidine, valproic acid, probenecid, and fluconazole may increase levels of zidovudine, whereas rifampin, rifabutin, and clarithromycin may decrease levels.

Do not administer IM. IV form is incompatible with blood product infusions and should be infused over 1 hr (intermittent IV dosing). Despite manufacturer recommendations of administering oral doses 30 min prior to or 1 hr after meals, doses may be administered with food.

ZINC SALTS, SYSTEMIC
Galzin, Orazinc, and generics
Trace mineral

A/C   2   Yes   No   No

Sulfate salt (23% elemental Zn):
   Tabs as sulfate (Orazinc and generics) [OTC]: 66, 110, 220 mg

ZINC SALTS, SYSTEMIC *continued*

Caps as sulfate (Orazinc and generics) [OTC]: 220 mg
Liquid as sulfate: 10 mg elemental Zn/mL
Injection as sulfate; preparations may be preservative free:
  1 mg elemental Zn/mL (10 mL)
  3 mg elemental Zn/mL (10 mL)
  5 mg elemental Zn/mL (5 mL)
Acetate salt (30% elemental Zn):
  Caps as acetate (Galzin): 25, 50 mg elemental per capsule
  Liquid as acetate: 5 mg elemental Zn/mL, 10 mg elemental Zn/mL
Chloride salt (48% elemental Zn):
  Injection as chloride: 1 mg elemental Zn/mL (10 mL)

Zinc deficiency (see remarks):
  Infant and child: 0.5—2 mg elemental Zn/kg/24 hr PO ÷ once daily—TID
  Adult: 25—50 mg elemental Zn/dose (100—220 mg Zn sulfate/dose) PO TID
Wilson disease:
  Child ≥5—<10 yr: 75 mg elemental Zn /24 hr PO ÷ TID
  Child ≥10 yr and adolescent: 75—150 mg elemental Zn /24 hr PO ÷ TID
US RDA: See Chapter 21.
For supplementation in parenteral nutrition, see Chapter 21.

Nausea, vomiting, GI disturbances, leukopenia, and diaphoresis may occur. Gastric ulcers, hypotension, and tachycardia may occur at high doses. Patients with excessive losses (burns) or impaired absorption require higher doses. Therapeutic levels: 70—130 mCg/dL.

Parenteral products may contain aluminum; **use with caution** in renal impairment. May decrease the absorption of penicillamine, tetracycline, and fluoroquinolones (e.g., ciprofloxacin). Drugs that increase gastric pH (e.g., H_2 antagonists and proton pump inhibitors) can reduce the absorption of zinc. Excessive zinc administration can cause copper deficiency.

Approximately 20%—30% of oral dose is absorbed. Oral doses may be administered with food if GI upset occurs. Pregnancy category is "A" for zinc acetate and "C" for all other salt forms.

ZOLMITRIPTAN
Zomig and generics previously available as
Zomig ZMT
Antimigraine agent, selective serotonin agonist

   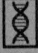

| C | 3 | Yes | Yes | No |

Tabs:
  Zomig and generics: 2.5 mg (scored), 5 mg
Oral disintegrating tabs (ODT):
  Generics: 2.5, 5 mg; contains aspartame
Nasal spray:
  Zomig and generics: 2.5 mg single unit nasal spray (6s), 5 mg single unit nasal spray (1s, 6s)

Treatment of acute migraines with or without aura:
  Nasal (safety of an average of >4 headaches in a 30-day period has not been established; see remarks):
    ≥12 yr and adult: Start with 2.5 mg inhaled into a single nostril × 1. If needed in 2 hr, a second dose may be administered. Dose may be increased to a **maximum** single dose of 5 mg if needed.
    Max. daily dose: 10 mg/24 hr

Continued

ZOLMITRIPTAN *continued*

>   **Patients receiving concurrent cimetidine:** Limit maximum doses to 2.5 mg as the **max. single dose** and **do not exceed** 5 mg in any 24 hr period.

Oral (use not recommended in children; safety and efficacy in children have not been established with the oral route. One randomized placebo-controlled trial in 696 adolescents 12−17 yr old did not establish efficacy and had similar adverse events as seen in adult trials):

>   **Adult (safety of an average of >3 headaches in a 30-day period has not been established; see remarks):**
>
>   **PO tabs:** Start with 1.25 or 2.5 mg PO × 1. If needed in 2 hr, a second dose may be administered. Dose may be increased to a **maximum** single dose of 5 mg if needed. **Max. daily dose:** 10 mg/24 hr
>
>   **ODT tabs:** Use the same dosage recommendation for PO tabs but with a 2.5 mg initial dose.
>
>   **Patients receiving concurrent cimetidine:** Limit **maximum** doses to 2.5 mg as the **max. single dose** and **do not exceed** 5 mg in any 24 hr period for both PO and ODT tabs.

Contraindicated in ischemic bowel disease; ischemic coronary artery disease; uncontrolled hypertension; peripheral vascular disease; history of stroke or TIA, arrhythmias, hemiplegic, or basilar migraine; significant cardiovascular disease; and coronary artery vasospasm.

Do not administer with any ergot-containing medications, any other 5-HT1 agonist (e.g., triptans), methylene blue, or within 2 wk of discontinuing an MAO inhibitor or linezolid. Cimetidine may increase the zolmitriptan levels; see dosage section for reduced maximum dosage. Patients with multiple cardiovascular risk factors and negative cardiovascular evaluation should have their first dose administered in a medically supervised facility.

Use **not** recommended in moderate/severe hepatic impairment. Severe renal impairment (CrCl 5−25 mL/min) reduces zolmitriptan clearance by 25%.

Common adverse reactions for all dosage forms unless otherwise indicated include nausea, taste alteration (nasal route), xerostomia, dizziness, hyperesthesia (nasal route), paresthesia, somnolence, sensation of hot and cold, throat pain, and asthenia (oral route). Hypertension, coronary artery spasm, MI, cerebral hemorrhage, and headaches have been reported.

For intranasal use, blow nose gently prior to dosing. Block opposite nostril while administering dose by breathing in gently.

When using the ODT, place the whole tablet on the tongue, allow the tablet to dissolve, and swallow with saliva. Administration with liquids is optional. **Do not** break the ODT tablet.

ZONISAMIDE
Zonegran, Zonisade, and generics
Anticonvulsant

C   3   Yes   Yes   No

Caps:
>   **Zonegran:** 25, 100 mg
>   **Generics:** 25, 50, 100 mg

Oral suspension:
>   **Zonisade:** 20 mg/mL (150 mL); contains sodium benzoate

Oral syrup: 10 mg/mL

Infant, child, and adolescent <16 yr:
>   **Adjunctive therapy for partial seizures (limited data):**
>
>   **<5 yr:** Start with 1−2 mg/kg/24 hr PO ÷ BID. Increase dosage by 0.5−1 mg/kg/24 hr Q2 wk to the usual dosage range of 5−8 mg/kg/24 hr PO ÷ BID.

ZONISAMIDE *continued*

5—<16 yr: Start with 0.5—1 mg/kg/24 hr PO ÷ once daily—BID. Increase dosage by 0.5—1 mg/kg/ 24 hr ÷ BID Q2 wk to the usual dosage range of 5—8 mg/kg/24 hr PO ÷ once daily—BID. Suggested maximum dose: 12 mg/kg/24 hr or 500 mg/24 hr; whichever is less

Infantile spasms (regimen that was effective in a small study from Japan; additional studies needed): Start with 2—4 mg/kg/24 hr PO ÷ BID. Then increase by 2—5 mg/kg/24 hr every 2—4 days until seizures disappear, up to a **maximum** of 20 mg/kg/24 hr.

Adolescent ≥16 yr—adult:

Adjunctive therapy for partial seizures: 100 mg PO once daily × 2 wk. Dose may be increased to 200 mg PO once daily × 2 wk. Additional dosage increments of 100 mg/24 hr can be made at 2-wk intervals to allow attainment of steady-state levels. Effective doses have ranged from 100—600 mg/24 hr ÷ once daily—BID (BID dosing may provide better efficacy). No additional benefit has been shown for doses >400 mg/24 hr.

Because zonisamide is a sulfonamide, it is **contraindicated** in patients allergic to sulfonamides (may result in Stevens-Johnson syndrome or TEN). Common side effects of drowsiness (especially at higher doses), ataxia, anorexia, gastrointestinal discomfort, headache, rash, and pruritus usually occur early in therapy and can be minimized with slow dose titration. Children are at increased risk for hyperthermia and oligohydrosis, especially in warm or hot weather. Suicidal behavior or ideation, acute pancreatitis, urolithiasis, metabolic acidosis (more frequent and severe in younger patients), DRESS/multiorgan hypersensitivity, rhabdomyolysis, metabolic acidosis, hyperammonemia/encephalopathy, acute myopia, glaucoma, and elevated creatinine phosphokinase have been reported.

Although not fully delineated, therapeutic serum levels of 20—30 mg/L have been suggested as higher rates of adverse reactions have been seen at levels >30 mg/L.

Zonisamide is a CYP 450 3A4 substrate. Phenytoin, carbamazepine, and phenobarbital can decrease levels of zonisamide.

Use with caution in renal or hepatic impairment; slower dose titration and more frequent monitoring is recommended. **Do not use** if GFR is <50 mL/min. **Avoid** abrupt discontinuation or radical dose reductions. Swallow capsules whole and **do not** crush or chew.

Chapter 31

Drugs in Kidney Failure

Elizabeth A.S. Goswami, PharmD and Katherine Hapgood, PharmD

See additional content online.

I. DOSE ADJUSTMENT METHODS

A. Maintenance Dose

In patients with kidney insufficiency, the dose may be adjusted using the following methods:

1. Lengthen intervals between individual doses, keeping normal dose.
2. Reduce number of individual doses, keeping interval between doses normal. For this method, percentage of usual dose is shown. For some medications and indications, specific dosing is provided.
3. A combination of the above

NOTE: Dose adjustments in these tables do not apply to patients in the neonatal period. For neonatal renal dosing, please consult a neonatal dosage reference (see Chapter 18). Dose modifications given are only approximations and may not be appropriate for all patients or indications. Recommendations for dose adjustments with reduced glomerular filtration rate (GFR) are often based on chronic kidney disease populations; it may not be appropriate to extrapolate these adjustments to acute kidney injury. **Each patient must be monitored closely for signs of drug toxicity, and serum levels must be measured when available; drug doses and intervals should be adjusted accordingly.** When in doubt, always consult a pharmacist and/or nephrologist who has expertise in renal dosing.

B. Dialysis

General recommendations are provided when available. However, factors such as patient age, indication for use, residual native kidney function, specific peritoneal dialysis (PD) or intermittent hemodialysis (IHD) prescription, and so on, will affect the medication dosing needs of each individual patient. Doses for IHD generally assume standard, thrice-weekly dialysis sessions with limited residual native kidney function. **Consult with a nephrologist or pharmacist who is familiar with medication dosing in dialysis before prescribing medications for a dialysis patient.**

C. Glomerular Filtration Rate Estimation

Estimated GFR (eGFR) in children may be calculated using the bedside CKiD equation[1]: $0.413 \times$ height (cm) / serum creatinine. Changes in serum creatinine lag changes in kidney function, and estimations may be inaccurate if serum creatinine is not at steady state. Additionally, in patients with reduced muscle mass or malnutrition, this equation may overestimate GFR. Other information such as trend in serum creatinine or presence of oliguria (<0.5 mL/kg/hr urine × 6 hr) or anuria may help interpret the appropriateness of the calculated eGFR. When in doubt, consult a nephrologist to help determine an accurate eGFR range for medication dosing.

II. ANTIMICROBIALS REQUIRING ADJUSTMENT IN KIDNEY FAILURE

(Table 31.1)

TABLE 31.1

ANTIMICROBIALS REQUIRING ADJUSTMENT IN KIDNEY FAILURE

		Adjustments Kidney Failure	
Medication	**eGFR (mL/min/1.73 m²)**	**Percentage of Usual Dose**	**Interval**
Acyclovir (IV)[2]	25–50	100%	Q12 hr
	10–25	100%	Q24 hr
	<10/IHD[a]/PD	50%	Q24 hr
Amantadine[b,3]	30–50	50%	Q24 hr
NOTE: On day 1, give normal dose, then decrease subsequent doses based on renal function.	15–29	50%	Q48 hr
	<15/IHD/PD	100%	Q7 days
Amikacin[4]	<60/IHD/PD	Administer a standard, one-time dose. Determine the appropriate interval for redosing based on serum concentrations. For IHD, redose based on concentrations. Optimal pharmacokinetic targets may be difficult to reach in patients with impaired kidney function; consider alternative agents.	
Amoxicillin[5,6]	10–29	50%–100%	Q12 hr
NOTE: Do not administer 875 mg immediate-release tablets with eGFR <30 mL/min/1.73 m².	<10/IHD[a]/PD	50%–100%	Q24 hr
Amoxicillin/clavulanate[5-7]	10–29	50%–100%	Q12 hr
NOTE: Do not administer 875 mg immediate-release or 1000 mg XR extended-release tablet with eGFR <30 mL/min/1.73 m².	<10/IHD[a]/PD	50%–100%	Q24 hr
Amphotericin B	No guidelines established.		
Ampicillin (IV)[5]	10–29	100%	Q8 hr
	<10/IHD[a]/PD	100%	Q12 hr
Ampicillin/sulbactam[8]	15–29	100%	Q12 hr
	<15/IHD[c]/PD	100%	Q24 hr
Aztreonam[b,5,9]	10–30	50%–66%	Q6–8 hr
NOTE: Administer full dose for initial dose, then adjust subsequent doses for kidney function.	<10/IHD/PD	25%–33%	Q6–8 hr
	IHD: Administer 12% of the full dose as an additional supplemental dose after dialysis in severe infections.		

Continued

TABLE 31.1

ANTIMICROBIALS REQUIRING ADJUSTMENT IN KIDNEY FAILURE—CONT'D

	Adjustments Kidney Failure		
Medication	eGFR (mL/min/1.73 m^2)	Percentage of Usual Dose	Interval
Cefaclor[5]	<10/IHD^c/PD	50%	Q8–12 hr
Cefadroxil[5]	10–29/IHD^a	100%	Q24 hr
	<10/PD	100%	Q36 hr
Cefazolin[5,10]	11–34	50%	Q12 hr
NOTE: Administer full dose for initial	≤10	50%	Q24 hr
dose, then adjust subsequent doses for kidney function.	IHD^a/PD	25 mg/kg	Q24 hr
Cefdinir[11]	<30	7 mg/kg (max 300 mg)	Q24 hr
	IHD^c/PD	7 mg/kg (max 300 mg)	Q48 hr
Cefepime[12]	30–60	100%	Q12 hr
NOTE: Administer full dose for initial	10–29	100%	Q24 hr
dose, then adjust subsequent doses for kidney function.	<10/PD/IHD^a	50%	Q24 hr
cefiderocol	>120	100%	Q6h
	30–59	75%	Q8h
	15–29	50%	Q8h
	<15/HDa/PD	38%	Q12h
Cefixime[b,14]	21–60/IHD	75%	Q12–24 hr
	<20/PD	50%	Q12–24 hr
Cefotaxime[5]	30–50	100%	Q8–12 hr
	10–29	100%	Q12 hr
	<10/IHD^a/PD	100%	Q24 hr
Cefotetan[5,15]	10–30	50%	Q12 hr
	<10/IHD^a/PD	50%	Q24 hr
Cefoxitin[16]	30–50	100%	Q8 hr
	10–30	100%	Q12 hr
	<10/IHD^c/PD	100%	Q24 hr
Cefpodoxime[17]	<30	100%	Q24 hr
	IHD	Administer thrice weekly after dialysis sessions.	
Cefprozil[18]	<30/IHD^a/PD	50%	Q12–24 hr
Ceftaroline[19]	31–50	66%	Q8–12 hr
	15–30	50%	Q8–12 hr
	<15/IHD^a/PD	33%	Q8–12 hr
Ceftazidime[5,20]	31–50	100%	Q12 hr
NOTE: Administer full dose for initial	10–30	100%	Q24 hr
dose, then adjust subsequent doses for kidney function.[4]	<10/IHD^a/PD	50%	Q24 hr

Ceftozolane/tazobactam[21]	30–50	50%	
NOTE: the manufacturer recommends against the use in pediatric patients with eGFR below 50 mL/min/1.73 m2. Doses based on adult recommendations.	15–29	25%	
	<15/HD	50–75% THEN	
		10–15%	
Cefuroxime (IV)[22]	10–20	100%	Q12 hr
	<10/IHD[c]/PD	100%	Q24 hr
Cephalexin[5]	30–50	100%	Q8 hr
	10–29	100%	Q12 hr
	<10/IHD[a]/PD	100%	Q24 hr
Ciprofloxacin[5]	10–29	100%	Q18 hr
	<10/IHD[a]/PD	100%	Q24 hr
Clarithromycin[23]	<30/IHD[a]/PD	50%	Q12 hr
Ertapenem[b,24]	≤30/IHD/PD	50%	Q12–24 hr
	IHD: If administered within 6 hr before dialysis, administer 30% of the normal daily dose as a supplemental dose after dialysis.		
Erythromycin[5,25-26]	Prophylaxis: no adjustment required Treatment: <10/IHD/PD: Hearing loss has been seen with normal doses in renal insufficiency, particularly in the elderly. Some recommend 50%–75% Q6–12 hr for treatment. Dose reduction may result in failure to achieve pharmacodynamic targets. Consider alternate therapy when possible. Weigh risks/benefits and individualize dose if required to treat serious infections.		
Ethambutol[b,27]	<30, IHD[a]	100%	3 times weekly
	PD		Data are not available. Begin with IHD dosing. Monitor closely and consider therapeutic drug monitoring.
Famciclovir[b,28]	Dose adjustments recommended for adult patients vary by indication. See package insert.		
Fluconazole[5,4,6]	10–50	50%	Q24 hr
NOTE: No adjustment required for single-dose regimen. Administer 100% of initial loading dose.	<10/PD	50%	Q48 hr
	IHD	100%	After each dialysis session
Flucytosine[29-30]	21–40	100%	Q12 hr
NOTE: If available, therapeutic drug monitoring should be used to guide optimal dosing. Use extreme caution in children with kidney impairment.	10–20	100%	Q24 hr
	<10	100%	Q48 hr
	IHD	100%	After each dialysis session
Foscarnet[31]	Dose adjustments vary by indication. See package insert for adjustments for induction and maintenance.		
Ganciclovir[32]	INDUCTION IV		
	50–69	2.5 mg/kg	Q12 hr
	25–49	2.5 mg/kg	Q24 hr
	10–24	1.25 mg/kg	Q24 hr
	<10/PD/IHD[a]	1.25 mg/kg	Thrice weekly

31

Continued

TABLE 31.1

ANTIMICROBIALS REQUIRING ADJUSTMENT IN KIDNEY FAILURE—CONT'D

	Adjustments Kidney Failure		
Medication	**eGFR (mL/min/1.73 m^2)**	**Percentage of Usual Dose**	**Interval**
	MAINTENANCE IV		
	50–69	2.5 mg/kg	Q24 hr
	25–49	1.25 mg/kg	Q24 hr
	10–24	0.625 mg/kg	Q24 hr
	<10/PD/IHD[a]	0.625 mg/kg	Thrice weekly
Gentamicin[4]	<50/IHD/PD	Administer standard initial dose. Determine appropriate interval for redosing based on serum concentrations. Optimal pharmacokinetic targets may be difficult to reach in patients with impaired kidney function. Consider alternative agents.	
Imipenem/cilastatin[b,33] NOTE: Patients with eGFR ≤15 should not receive imipenem/cilastatin unless dialysis will be initiated within 48 hr. Seizure risk increased with decreased kidney function.	60-89	75–80%	Q6–8 hr
	30–59	50–60%	Q6 hr
	10–29	40–50%	Q6–12 hr
	<10/IHD[a]	50%	Q24 hr
Isoniazid[6]	IHD[a]	100%	Q24 hr
Lamivudine[b,34] NOTE: Administer full dose for initial dose, then adjust subsequent doses for kidney function. If eGFR <5 or IHD, administer 33% of full dose as initial dose.	30–50	100%	Q24 hr
	15–29	66%	Q24 hr
	5–14	33%	Q24 hr
	<5/IHD[a]/PD	17%	Q24 hr
Levofloxacin[5,35] NOTE: Administer full dose for initial dose, then adjust subsequent doses for kidney function.	Q12 hr dosing		
	10–29	100%	Q24 hr
	<10/IHD/PD	100%	Q48 hr
	Q24 hr dosing		
	10–29	100%	Q48h
	<10/IHD/PD	67%	Q48 hr
Meropenem[b,36–37] Note: For GFR <30, maximum dose is 1000 mg	30–50	100%	Q12 hr
	10–29	50%	Q12 hr
	<10/PD	50%	Q24 hr
	IHD[a]	25 mg/kg	Q24 hr
Metronidazole[5,38]	<10/IHD[c]/PD	Renally eliminated metabolites may accumulate and lead to adverse events. Monitor patient. Though no dose adjustment is recommended by the manufacturer, some recommend a dose of 4 mg/kg at standard intervals. We prefer standard dosing with careful monitoring.	

Oseltamivir[b,39]	INFLUENZA TREATMENT		
	31–60	50%	Q12 hr
	11–30	50%	Q24 hr
	IHD	50%	Once, then after each dialysis session
	PD	50%	Once
	INFLUENZA PROPHYLAXIS		
	31–60	50%	Q24 hr
	10–30	50%	Q48 hr
	IHD	50%	Once, then after every-other dialysis session
	PD	50%	Weekly for duration of prophylaxis
Penicillin G—aqueous (K+, Na+) (IV)[5] NOTE: Administer full dose for initial dose, then adjust subsequent doses for kidney function.	10–50 <10/IHD[a]/PD	75% 50%	Q4–6 hr Q4–6 hr
Penicillin V K+ (PO)[40] NOTE: No dose adjustment required for twice-daily prophylaxis dosing. The manufacturer makes no recommendations for renal dose adjustments. Extending the interval has been suggested.	<10/IHD[a]/PD	100%	Q8 hr
Pentamidine[5] NOTE: Adjustment is not required for monthly prophylaxis.	10–30 <10/IHD[a]/PD	100% 100%	Q36 hr Q48 hr
Piperacillin/tazobactam[41]	20–40 <20 IHD[a]/PD	70% 50% 50%	Q6 hr Q6 hr Q8 hr
Posaconazole[42]	<50	Consider risks and benefits of use of the IV product as solubilizing agent may accumulate. Monitor SCr and consider changing to PO if signs of toxicity. With PO products, exposure may vary, and breakthrough infections may occur.	
Rifabutin[43]	<30	50%–100%	Q24 hr
Streptomycin sulfate[b,5,44] NOTE: Determine appropriate interval for redosing based on serum concentration when available. Patients with impaired kidney function are at risk for severe neurotoxicities, and a single dose may result in high levels for several days.	10–50 <10 IHD/PD	100% 100% 100%	Q24–72 hr Q72–96 hr Administer 2–3 times weekly after dialysis.

Continued

TABLE 31.1

ANTIMICROBIALS REQUIRING ADJUSTMENT IN KIDNEY FAILURE—CONT'D

Medication	eGFR (mL/min/1.73 m²)	Adjustments Kidney Failure	
		Percentage of Usual Dose	Interval
Sulfamethoxazole/trimethoprim[45] NOTE: No adjustment recommended for 2–3 times weekly prophylaxis dosing. The manufacturer recommends against use with GFR <15.	<30/IHD[a]/PD	50%	Q8–12 hr
Tetracycline[b,5]	10–50	100%	Q12–24 hr
	<10	100%	Q24 hr
Tobramycin[4]	<60	Administer standard initial dose. Determine appropriate interval for redosing based on serum concentrations. Optimal pharmacokinetic targets may be difficult to reach in patients with impaired kidney function. Consider alternative agents.	
Valacyclovir[b,46–47] NOTE: For IHD for all indications, dose for eGFR <10 and administer dose after dialysis. For PD for all indications, administer 500 mg Q48 hr.	HERPES ZOSTER (ADULTS)		
	30–49	100%	Q12 hr
	10–29	100%	Q24 hr
	<10/IHD[a]	50%	Q24 hr
	GENITAL HERPES (ADOLESCENTS/ADULTS): INITIAL EPISODE		
	10–29	100%	Q24 hr
	<10	50%	Q24 hr
	GENITAL HERPES (ADOLESCENTS/ADULTS): RECURRENT EPISODE		
	<30	100%	Q24 hr
	GENITAL HERPES (ADOLESCENTS/ADULTS): SUPPRESSIVE		
	<30	500 mg OR	Q24 hr (for usual dose of 1 g Q24 hr)
		500 mg	Q48 hr (for usual dose of 500 mg Q24 hr)
	HERPES LABIALIS (ADOLESCENTS/ADULTS)		
	30–49	50%	Q12 hr ×2 doses
	10–29	25%	Q12 hr ×2 doses
	<10	25%	Single dose
Valganciclovir[6,48–49] NOTE: For dosing in children, a maximum eGFR value of 150 mL/min/1.73 m2 should be used to calculate the dose. Calculate eGFR = k × height (cm) /	CHILDREN		
	Normal dosing accounts for kidney function: Once daily dose (mg) = 7× body surface area × creatinine clearance.		
	ADULTS—INDUCTION		
	40–59	450 mg	Q12 hr

	25–39	450 mg	Q24 hr
creatinine. Consider use of k = 0.413 when enzymatic creatinine assays are used. Original labeling includes the following when SCr calculated via Jaffe method: k = 0.33 in infants aged <1 year, with low birth weight for gestational age, 0.45 in infants aged <1 year, with birth weight appropriate for gestational age, 0.45 in children aged 1 to <2 years, 0.55 in boys aged 2 to <13 years and girls aged 2 to <16 years, and 0.7 in boys aged 13–16 years.	10–24	450 mg	Q48 hr
	<10/IHD[a] (limited data; consider ganciclovir)	200 mg	Thrice weekly
	ADULTS–MAINTENANCE		
	40–59	450 mg	Q24 hr
	25–39	450 mg	Q48 hr
	10–24	450 mg	Twice weekly
	<10/IHD[a] (limited data; consider ganciclovir)	100 mg	Thrice weekly
Vancomycin[4]	<50		Administer standard initial dose. Determine appropriate interval for redosing based on serum concentrations.
	IHD/PD		Administer standard initial dose. Obtain serum concentration after dialysis to determine need to redose. Obtain levels 4–6 hr after dialysis to allow for redistribution from peripheral compartment. If patient is unstable, may obtain sooner with knowledge that concentration may be lower than steady state.

[a]For IHD administer after dialysis on dialysis days.
[b]In adults; guidelines not established in children.
[c]Administer a supplemental dose after dialysis.
eGFR, Estimated glomerular filtration rate; *HIV*, human immunodeficiency virus; *hr*, hour; *IHD*, intermittent hemodialysis; *IM*, intramuscular; *IV*, intravenous; *K+*, potassium; *Na+*, sodium; *PD*, peritoneal dialysis; *PO*, oral; *Q*, every.

III. NON-ANTIMICROBIALS REQUIRING ADJUSTMENT IN KIDNEY FAILURE

(Table 31.2)

TABLE 31.2

NON-ANTIMICROBIALS REQUIRING ADJUSTMENT IN KIDNEY FAILURE

	Adjustments in Kidney Failure		
Medication	**eGFR**	**Percentage of Usual Dose**	**Interval**
Acetaminophen[5]	10–50	100%	Q6 hr
	<10/IHD/PD	100%	Q8 hr
Acetazolamide[5]	10–50	100%	Q12 hr
	<10/IHD/PD	Avoid use.	

Continued

TABLE 31.2

NON-ANTIMICROBIALS REQUIRING ADJUSTMENT IN KIDNEY FAILURE—CONT'D

	Adjustments in Kidney Failure		
Medication	**eGFR**	**Percentage of Usual Dose**	**Interval**
Allopurinol[5]	10–50	50%	Q6–24 hr
	<10/IHD/PD	30%	Q6–24 hr
Aminocaproic acid[b,50–51] Use with caution in patients with renal dysfunction. Can cause renal failure.	<60/Oliguria/ ESRD	12%–25%	Q4–6 hr, continuous
	IHD	No reduction needed	
Aspirin[5]	10–50	100%	Q4–24 hr
	IHD[a]	100%	Q24 hr
	<10/PD	Avoid use for analgesia and anti-inflammatory indications.	
Atenolol[5]	30–50	1 mg/kg up to 50 mg	Q24 hr
	10–29	1 mg/kg up to 50 mg	Q48 hr
	<10/IHD[a]/PD	1 mg/kg up to 25 mg	Q48 hr
Azathioprine[5,52]	10–50	75%	Q24 hr
	<10/IHD[a]/PD	50%	Q24 hr
Bismuth subsalicylate[b,52]	<50/IHD/PD	Avoid use in patients with renal failure.	
Bosentan[53]	Dose adjustment not required. Significant clearance by dialysis is not expected.		
Calcium supplements	<25	May require dosage adjustment depending on calcium level.	
Captopril[4,52]	10–50	75%	Q6–8 hr
	<10/IHD[a]/PD	50%	Q6–8 hr
Carbamazepine[5]	<10/IHD/PD	75%	Q8–12 hr
Cetirizine[5,6,52]	10-29/IHD/PD	50%	Q24 hr
	≤10	Use not recommended. Some consider 50% Q24 hr in this population.	
Chloroquine[5,6] NOTE: Dose adjustment recommended for long-term use.	<10/IHD/PD	50%	Depends on indication
Chlorothiazide[52,54]	<30	May be ineffective	
	<10	Use not recommended	
Clobazam[55]	<30	Use with caution; has not been studied	
Dabigatran[56]	<50	Avoid use.	
Desloratadine[b,57]	<50	100%	Q48 hr
Digoxin[5]	DIGITALIZING DOSE		
	ESRD	50%	NA
	MAINTENANCE DOSE		
	30–50	75%	Q12–24 hr

	10–29	50%	Q12–24 hr
		OR 100%	Q36 hr
	<10/IHD/PD	25%	Q12–24 hr
		OR 100%	Q48 hr
Disopyramide[b,58]	30–40	100%	Q8 hr
NOTE: Avoid continuous release product with eGFR <40.	15–30	100%	Q12 hr
	<15	100%	Q24 hr
EDTA calcium disodium[b,59]	IV: ADULT SERUM CREATININE-BASED DOSING		
NOTE: Do not administer in patients with anuria or severe oliguria.	≤2 mg/dL	1 g/m²	Q24 hr ×5 days
	2–3 mg/dL	500 mg/m²	Q24 hr ×5 days
	3–4 mg/dL	500 mg/m²	Q48 hr ×3 doses
	>4 mg/dL	500 mg/m²	Once weekly
Enalapril/Enalaprilat[5,52,60]	10–50	75%	Q12–24 hr
NOTE: Manufacturer does not recommend in pediatric patients GFR <30 mL/min/1.73 m².	<10/IHD[a]/PD	50%	Q12–24 hr
Enoxaparin[b,6,52]	<30	100%	Q24 hr
	IHD/PD	Serious bleeding complications may occur. Avoid use. If used, reduce dose and monitor anti-Xa activity.	
Epoprostenol[61]	Manufacturer does not recommend renal dose reduction. Titrate to clinical effect.		
Famotidine[5,62]	30–50	100%	Q24 hr
	10–29	50%	Q24 hr
	<10/IHD/PD	25%	Q24 hr
Felbamate[b,5,52,63]	<50/IHD[a]	50%	Q6–8 hr
Fentanyl[5,52,64–68]	INJECTION		
	<50	Manufacturer does not recommend dose reduction. Titrate to clinical effect.	
	PATCH		
	Limit use to non-opioid-naïve adult patients. Titrate after 72 hr from initial transdermal exposure.		
	Mild–moderate impairment[b]	12.5–25 mcg patch	Q72 hr
	Severe impairment	Not recommended by manufacturer	
Fexofenadine[5,52]	<50/IHD/PD	100%	Q24 hr
Flecainide[b,69]	<35	50%	Q12 hr
Furosemide	Avoid use in oliguria.		
Gabapentin[5,70]	30–59	75%	Q12 hr
	15–29	75%	Q24 hr
	<15/IHD[c]/PD	75%	Q48 hr
Hydralazine[d,5,6]	10–50	100%	Q8 hr
	<10/IHD/PD	100%	Q12–24 hr
Iloprost[b,71]	IHD/PD	Dose adjustment not required. Use with caution; has not been studied.	
Insulin (regular)[e,5,52]	10–50	75%	No change
	<10/IHD/PD	50%	No change
Ivacaftor[72]	<30	Use with caution, not studied.	

31

Continued

TABLE 31.2

NON-ANTIMICROBIALS REQUIRING ADJUSTMENT IN KIDNEY FAILURE—CONT'D

		Adjustments in Kidney Failure	
Medication	**eGFR**	**Percentage of Usual Dose**	**Interval**
Lacosamide[b,73]	<30	75% Maximum adult dose: 300 mg/24-hr period	Q12 hr
	IHD	Administer 50% dose supplementation after 4-hr dialysis session.	
Levetiracetam[5,74,75]	CHILDREN		
	<50	50%	Q12 hr
	IHD[f]/PD	50%	Q24 hr
	ADULTS – IMMEDIATE RELEASE		
	50–80	500–1000 mg	Q12 hr
	30–50	250–750 mg	Q12 hr
	<30	250–500 mg	Q12 hr
	IHD[f]/PD	500–1000 mg	Q24 hr
	ADULTS – EXTENDED RELEASE		
	50–80	1000–2000 mg	Q24 hr
	30–50	500–1500 mg	Q24 hr
	<30	500–1000	Q24 hr
	IHD[f]/PD	Use of immediate release product recommended	
Lisinopril[b,76]	10–50	50%	Q24 hr
	<10/IHD[a]/PD	25%	Q24 hr
Lithium[5,52,77–78] NOTE: Monitor serum concentrations. Lithium concentrations rebound after dialysis.	10–50	50%–75%	Q8–12 hr
	<10	25%–50%	Q8–12 hr
	IHD[a]/PD	25%–50%	Q8–12 hr
Loratadine[5]	<10/IHD/PD	100%	Q24–48 hr
Lumacaftor + Ivacaftor[79]	<30	Use with caution.	
Meperidine[5,6,52,80] NOTE: Accumulation of normeperidine can lead to tremors and seizures. Limit duration to ≤48 hr in all patients. Avoid use in patients with kidney dysfunction.	10–50	75%	Avoid use, especially repeat administrations.
	<10	50%	Avoid use, especially repeat administrations.
	IHD/PD	Avoid use.	
Methadone[5,52]	<10/IHD/PD	50%–75%	Q8–12 hr
Metoclopramide[5]	30–50	75%	No change
	10–30	50%	No change
	<10/IHD/PD	25%	No change

Drug			
Midazolam[5,81]	<10	50%	No change
NOTE: Metabolite α-hydroxymidazolam can accumulate in kidney failure, leading to prolonged sedation after midazolam is discontinued.			
Milrinone[82–83]	50		0.43 mCg/kg/min
NOTE: Initial doses suggested by	40		0.38 mCg/kg/min
manufacturer. Interpatient	30		0.33 mCg/kg/min
variability is common.	20		0.28 mCg/kg/min
Individualized doses and titration	10		0.23 mCg/kg/min
to hemodynamic and clinical response may be necessary.	5		0.2 mCg/kg/min
Morphine[5,66–68,84]	10–50	75%	No change
NOTE: Consider other agents in	<10/IHD/PD	50%	No change
patients with moderate to severe renal dysfunction or who receive dialysis. Glucuronide metabolites may accumulate, increasing risk of respiratory depression and sedation.			
Neostigmine[b,5,52]	10–50	50%	No change
	<10	25%	No change
Oxcarbazepine[b,85–86]	IMMEDIATE-RELEASE		
	<30	Initial dose: 50%. Titrate slowly.	Q12 hr
	EXTENDED-RELEASE		
	<30	Initial adult dose: 300 mg	Q24 hr
Pancuronium bromide[5,52,87]	10–50	50%	No change
	<10/IHD/PD	Avoid use. Prolonged neuromuscular blockade may result; half-life is doubled in renal failure.	
Phenazopyridine[52]	50–80	100%	Q8–16 hr
	<50	Contraindicated. Risk of nephrotoxicity, methemoglobinemia, and hemolytic anemia	
Phenobarbital[5,52,88]	<10/IHD[f]/PD	100%	Q12–24 hr
NOTE: Therapeutic drug monitoring encouraged. Titrate to level and therapeutic effect.			
Primidone[5]	10–50	100%	Q12–24 hr
NOTE: Due to complex metabolism, it	<10/IHD[a]	100%	Q24 hr
is preferred to use other options when available for patients with kidney failure.			
Quinidine[5,52]	<10/IHD[a]/PD	75%	Q6–12 hr
Sodium phenylacetate and sodium benzoate[89]	<50	Use with caution and close monitoring.	
Spironolactone[5,52]	30–50	100%	Q24 hr
	<30	Avoid use due to risk of hyperkalemia.	

Continued

31

TABLE 31.2

NON-ANTIMICROBIALS REQUIRING ADJUSTMENT IN KIDNEY FAILURE—CONT'D

	Adjustments in Kidney Failure		
		Percentage of Usual	
Medication	eGFR	Dose	Interval
Terbutaline[52,90–91]	<50	Renally eliminated; use with caution. No specific dose adjustment available	
Tezacaftor + Ivacaftor[92]	<30	Use with caution.	
Treprostinil[93–94]	Manufacturer does not recommend dose reduction. Use with caution and titrate slowly as increased exposure is expected.		
Triamterene[5,52]	<50/IHD/PD	Do not use due to risk of hyperkalemia.	
Verapamil[95–96]	<10	Dose reduction may be needed; use caution. Monitor blood pressure, ECG for PR prolongation, and other signs of overdose.	
Vigabatrin[97]	50–80	75%	Q12 hr
	30–50	50%	Q12 hr
	10–30	25%	Q12 hr

[a]For IHD administer after dialysis on dialysis days.
[b]In adults; guidelines not established in children.
[c]Administer supplemental dose after every 4 hours of dialysis, based on daily dose as follows (daily dose/recommended supplemental dose): 100 mg/125 mg; 125 mg/150 mg; 150 mg/200 mg; 200 mg/250 mg; 300 mg/350 mg.
[d]Dose interval varies for rapid and slow acetylators with normal and impaired renal function.
[e]Renal failure may cause hyposensitivity or hypersensitivity to insulin. Empiric dosing recommendations may not be appropriate for all patients; adjust to clinical response and blood glucose.
[f]Administer a supplemental dose after dialysis.
D, Dose reduction; *ECG*, electrocardiogram; *EDTA*, ethylenediaminetetraacetic acid; *eGFR*, estimated glomerular filtration rate; *ESRD*, end-stage renal disease; *GI*, gastrointestinal; *I*, interval extension; *IHD*, intermittent hemodialysis; *IM*, intramuscular; *IV*, intravenous; *MHD*, 10-monohydroxy metabolite; *NA*, not applicable; *PD*, peritoneal dialysis; *PO*, oral; *Q*, every; *SubQ*, subcutaneous; $t_{1/2}$, half-life.

REFERENCES

A complete list of references can be found online.

Index

Note: Page numbers followed by "f" indicate figures "t" indicate tables and "b" indicate boxes.

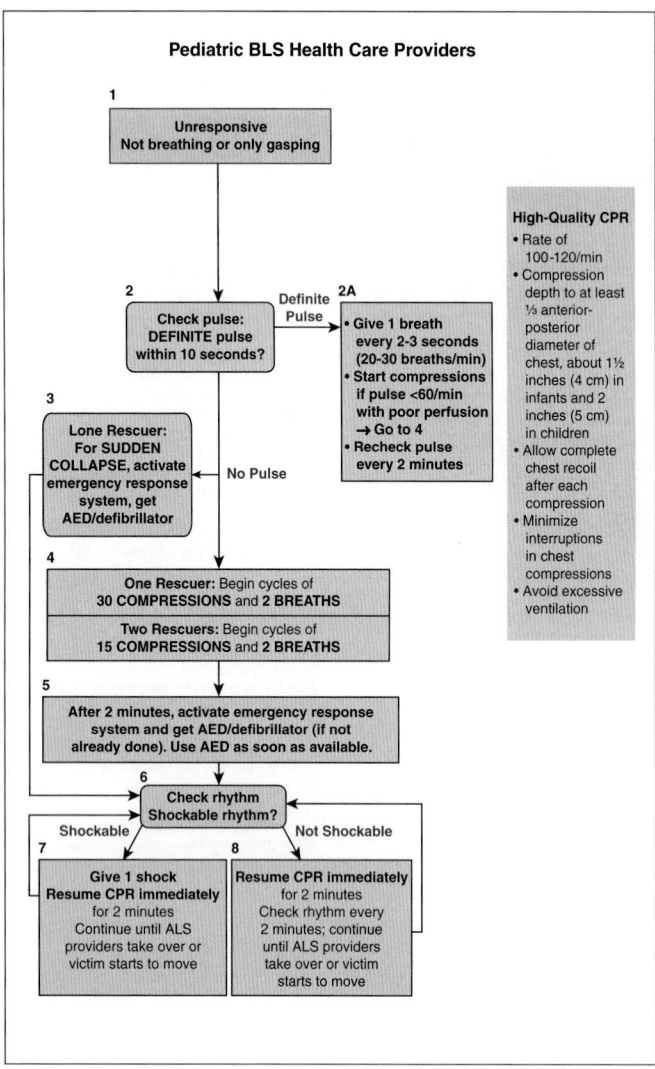

Pediatric BLS health care providers algorithm. (From Topjian AA, Raymond TT, Atkins D, et al. Part 4: Pediatric basic and advanced life support: 2020 American Heart Association Guidelines for Cardiopulmonary Resuscitation and Emergency Cardiovascular Care. *Circulation*. 2020;142[16_suppl_2]:S469–S523. http://dx.doi.org/10.1161/CIR.0000000000000901)

"Special thanks to Caitlin O'Brien MD, MPH for her expert guidance with the pediatric resuscitation algorithms."

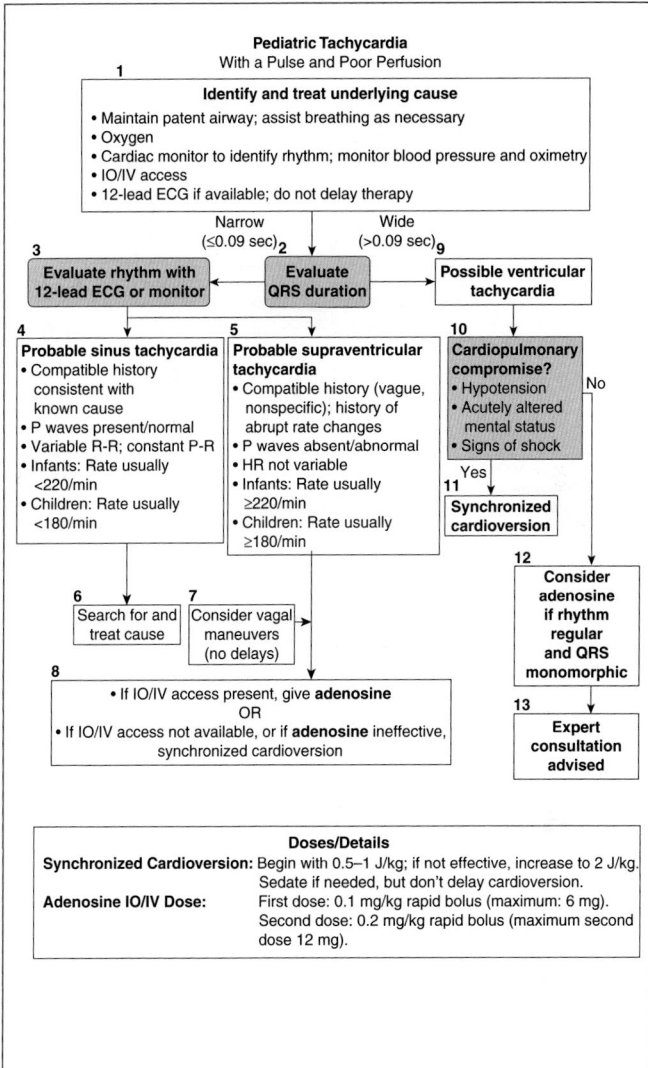

Pediatric tachycardia algorithm. (From Topjian AA, Raymond TT, Atkins D, et al. Part 4: Pediatric basic and advanced life support: 2020 American Heart Association Guidelines for Cardiopulmonary Resuscitation and Emergency Cardiovascular Care. *Circulation*. 2020;142[16_suppl_2]:S469–S523. http://dx.doi.org/10.1161/CIR.0000000000000901)

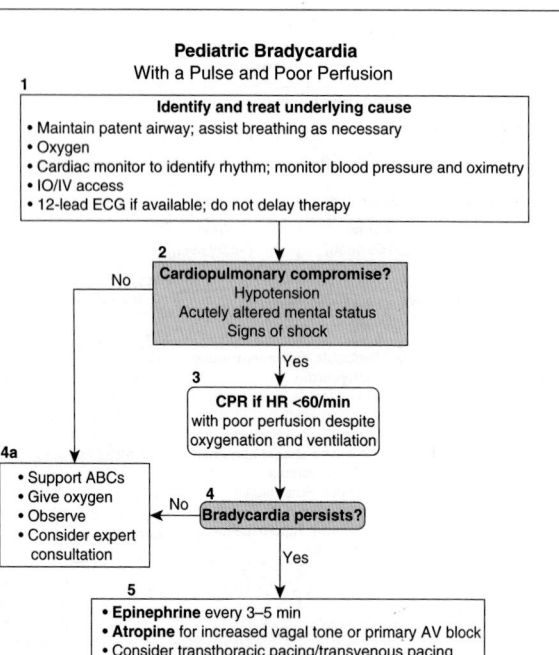

Pediatric Bradycardia
With a Pulse and Poor Perfusion

1
Identify and treat underlying cause
- Maintain patent airway; assist breathing as necessary
- Oxygen
- Cardiac monitor to identify rhythm; monitor blood pressure and oximetry
- IO/IV access
- 12-lead ECG if available; do not delay therapy

2
Cardiopulmonary compromise?
Hypotension
Acutely altered mental status
Signs of shock

No → / Yes ↓

3
CPR if HR <60/min
with poor perfusion despite
oxygenation and ventilation

4a
- Support ABCs
- Give oxygen
- Observe
- Consider expert consultation

No ← **4** **Bradycardia persists?**

Yes ↓

5
- **Epinephrine** every 3–5 min
- **Atropine** for increased vagal tone or primary AV block
- Consider transthoracic pacing/transvenous pacing
- Treat underlying causes

6
If pulseless arrest develops, go to Cardiac Arrest algorithm

Doses/Details
Epinephrine IO/IV Dose: 0.01 mg/kg (0.1 mg/mL concentration). Max dose: 1 mg (10 mL). Repeat every 3–5 minutes. If IO/IV access not available but endotracheal (ET) tube in place, may give ET dose: 0.1 mg/kg (1 mg/mL concentration, max 2.5 mg).
Atropine IO/IV Dose: 0.02 mg/kg. May repeat once after 5 min. Minimum dose 0.1 mg and maximum single dose 0.5 mg.

Pediatric bradycardia algorithm. (From Topjian AA, Raymond TT, Atkins D, et al. Part 4: Pediatric basic and advanced life support: 2020 American Heart Association Guidelines for Cardiopulmonary Resuscitation and Emergency Cardiovascular Care. *Circulation.* 2020;142[16_suppl_2]:S469-S523. http://dx.doi.org/10.1161/CIR.0000000000000901)